Cancer Nursing:
Care in Context

Also of Interest:

Evidence-Based Palliative Care
HH Abu-Saad
978-0-6320-5818-1

Cancer Care for Adolescents and Young Adults
Edited by Daniel Kelly and Faith Gibson
978-1-4051-3094-3

Cancer in Children and Young People
(John Wiley and Sons)
Faith Gibson and Louise Soames
978-0-4700-5867-1

An Introduction to Cancer Care
(John Wiley and Sons)
Tracey McCready
978-1-8615-6460-3

Cancer Nursing: Care in Context

Second Edition

Edited by

Jessica Corner

Director for Improving Cancer Services
Macmillan Cancer Support
and
Professor of Cancer and Palliative Care
School of Nursing and Midwifery
University of Southampton
Southampton
UK

and

Christopher Bailey

Senior Research Fellow
School of Nursing and Midwifery
University of Southampton
Southampton
UK

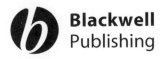

Blackwell
Publishing

Blackwell Publishing editorial offices:
Blackwell Publishing Ltd, 9600 Garsington Road, Oxford OX4 2DQ, UK
Tel: +44 (0)1865 776868
Blackwell Publishing Inc., 350 Main Street, Malden, MA 02148-5020, USA
Tel: +1 781 388 8250
Blackwell Publishing Asia Pty Ltd, 550 Swanston Street, Carlton, Victoria 3053, Australia
Tel: +61 (0)3 8359 1011

First published 2008 by Blackwell Publishing Ltd

ISBN-13: 978-1-4051-2253-5

Library of Congress Cataloging-in-Publication Data

Cancer nursing : care in context / edited by Jessica Corner and Christopher Bailey. – 2nd ed.
p. ; cm.
Includes bibliographical references and index.
ISBN-13: 978-1-4051-2253-5 (pbk. : alk. paper)
ISBN-10: 1-4051-2253-6 (pbk. : alk. paper)   1. Cancer–Nursing.   I. Corner, Jessica.   II. Bailey, Christopher.
[DNLM: 1. Oncologic Nursing–methods.   2. Neoplasms–nursing. WY 156 C2194 2008]
RC266.C355 2008
616.99′40231–dc22
2007025830

A catalogue record for this title is available from the British Library

Set in 11/12pt Adobe Garamond by SNP Best-set Typesetter Ltd., Hong Kong
Printed and bound in Singapore by C.O.S. Printers Pte Ltd

The publisher's policy is to use permanent paper from mills that operate a sustainable forestry policy, and which has been manufactured from pulp processed using acid-free and elementary chlorine-free practices. Furthermore, the publisher ensures that the text paper and cover board used have met acceptable environmental accreditation standards.

For further information on Blackwell Publishing, visit our website:
www.blackwellpublishing.com

Contents

Part 4: The Management of Cancer-related Problems   445

Part 5: Needs and Priorities in Cancer Care   573

Contributors

Audrey Ardern-Jones
Senior Clinical Nurse Specialist in Cancer
Genetics
Genetics Department
The Royal Marsden NHS Foundation Trust
Sutton, Surrey

Christopher Bailey
Senior Research Fellow
School of Nursing and Midwifery
University of Southampton
Southampton

Lynne Colbourne
Advanced Nurse Practitioner
Gloucestershire Hospitals NHS Foundation Trust
Cheltenham General Hospital
Cheltenham, Gloucestershire

Jessica Corner
Director for Improving Cancer Services
Macmillan Cancer Support
and
Professor of Cancer and Palliative Care
School of Nursing and Midwifery
University of Southampton
Southampton

Alan Cribb
Professor of Bioethics and Education
Centre for Public Policy Research
King's College London
London

Elizabeth Davies
Senior Lecturer in Cancer Registration
King's College London
London

Rebecca Doherty
Genetic Counsellor
The Royal Marsden NHS Foundation Trust
Sutton, Surrey

Lisa Dougherty
Clinical Nurse Specialist
Royal Marsden Hospital
London

Ruth Dunleavey
Clinical Nurse Specialist
St Vincent's Hospital
New South Wales
Sydney, Australia

Rosalind Eeles
Reader in Clinical Cancer Genetics, Honorary
Consultant in Cancer Genetics and Clinical
Oncology Team Leader, Translational Cancer
Genetics Team
Institute of Cancer Research
and
Head of Cancer Genetics Unit
Royal Marsden NHS Foundation Trust
Sutton, Surrey

Sara Faithfull
Director of Studies: Doctorate of Clinical Practice
Division of Health and Social Care
Faculty of Health and Medical Sciences
University of Surrey
Guildford, Surrey

Deborah Fenlon
Senior Research Fellow
School of Nursing and Midwifery
University of Southampton
Southampton

Claire Foster
Reader and Head of Macmillan Research Unit
Macmillan Research Unit
University of Southampton
Southampton

Yasmin Gunaratnam
Senior Research Fellow
University of Central Lancashire
Preston, Lancashire

Caroline Hoffman
Clinical Director and Research Co-ordinator
Breast Cancer Haven
London

Jane Hopkinson
Macmillan Senior Research Fellow
Macmillan Research Unit
University of Southampton
Southampton

Meinir Krishnasamy
Clinician-Researcher, Nursing
Supportive Care Research Group
The Peter MacCallum Cancer Centre
Melbourne
Victoria, Australia

Anne Lanceley
Clinical Research Fellow
UCL EGA Institute for Women's Health
Gynaecological Cancer Research Centre
University College London
London

Vivian Mak
Information Analyst
King's College London
London

Alastair Munro
Professor of Radiation Oncology
Department of Surgery and Molecular
Oncology
Ninewells Hospital and Medical School
Dundee, Scotland

Stephen O'Connor
Senior Lecturer in Cancer and Palliative
Care
School of Continuing and Advanced
Practice
Faculty of Society and Health
Buckinghamshire New University
Buckinghamshire

Sheila Payne
Help the Hospices Chair in Hospice Studies
University of Lancaster
Lancaster

Hilary Plant
Visiting Research Fellow
Florence Nightingale School of Nursing and
Midwifery
London

Annabel Pollard
Director, Clinical Psychology Services
The Peter MacCallum Cancer Centre
Melbourne
Victoria, Australia

Nancy Preston
Independent Researcher
Preston, Lancashire

Fay Scullion
Senior Macmillan Development Manager
Macmillan Cancer Support
York

Sarah Thomas
Clinical Nurse Specialist in Cancer Genetics
Genetics Department
The Royal Marsden NHS Foundation
Trust
Sutton, Surrey

Jenny Thompson
Freelance Lecturer and Writer
Moorbank Farmhouse
Crowhurst, Sussex

Jenny Walton
Macmillan Cancer Voices Trainer
Patient Representative
Humber and Yorkshire Coast
Cancer Network

Mary Wells
Lecturer and Clinical Research Fellow in
Cancer Nursing
School of Nursing and Midwifery
University of Dundee
Dundee, Scotland

Isabel White
Cancer Research UK Nursing Research
Training Fellow
European Institute of Health and Medical
Sciences (EIHMS)
University of Surrey
Guildford, Surrey

Anne Williams
Cancer Nursing Research Fellow/Specialist
Lymphoedema Nurse
Napier University/NHS Lothian
Edinburgh, Scotland

David Wright
Macmillan Senior Research Fellow
Macmillan Research Unit
University of Southampton
Southampton

Foreword

Major advances have been made on cancer over the past 30 years, with important developments in basic science, diagnostics, treatment, care of individuals affected by cancer and in organisation of cancer services. When I qualified as a doctor in 1977 CT scanning was in its infancy and neither MRI nor PET scanning were on the horizon; early scientific work to understand cell signalling pathways was underway, but the introduction of therapies targeted against these pathways was still a dream; the diagnosis of cancer was often not discussed with the patient and multidisciplinary team working was the exception not the rule.

Amongst the most important developments during my working life have been those related to cancer nursing. Nurse specialist roles have evolved for palliative care, chemotherapy, breast cancer and more recently for other cancers. Nurse consultant and nurse practitioner roles have been introduced in areas such as endoscopy and breast assessment. Nurses are now recognised as integral members of every multidisciplinary cancer team. The increasing complexity of cancer management has led to developments of the roles of nurses working on hospital wards, in outpatient settings and in the community.

However, there is still much to be done to achieve our goal of delivering optional care. We know that there are still many deficiencies in the care we provide in this country. The needs of those affected by cancer for information, good face-to-face communication and well coordinated care are still not always recognised or met. Patients may need support throughout their care pathway, but we know they can sometimes feel abandoned after the completion of primary treatment.

In order to deliver optimal care cancer nurses need access to information and education for themselves about all aspects of cancer, but especially about the multiplicity of roles that a cancer nurse may currently fulfil. These roles include assessment of an individual's needs, communication, coordination of care, education of patients and families, delivery of treatment and provision of comfort.

This second edition of *Cancer Nursing: Care in Context* provides an invaluable resource for aspiring and existing cancer nurses and for those who work alongside them in the delivery of multidisciplinary care. Jessica Corner and Chris Bailey have brought together a powerful team with availability to write eloquently and passionately about their areas of expertise. The authors have drawn on their direct experience to make this a most informative and readable text book.

Professor Mike Richards
National Cancer Director

Preface

This book is something of a departure from the standard textbook. Most are a source of knowledge about a particular disease, treatments, and health care practices. The function of a textbook is to compile in a single volume the 'state of the art' and the latest research evidence; to create a source of reference for knowledge, offering a kind of 'truth' in relation to what is known about, and what might constitute best practice in a given area. There are many such texts on cancer, cancer treatment, and cancer nursing on library and bookshop shelves. This book is not intended to replace these excellent texts; rather, the intention is to offer a different perspective.

An attempt is made here to reveal cancer as an experience that is socially and culturally determined in unique and powerful ways. It is acknowledged that there are many discourses or knowledge systems that surround cancer; indeed, several contrasting discourses may be found within the pages of this book. At times these are made manifest by the author; elsewhere the text is less self-conscious in this respect and adheres to a particular tradition or language. In general, however, it is acknowledged that cancer discourses dictate society's, individual, and collective responses to the disease and to the people who have it, and it is these that in turn shape our understanding of cancer.

To work effectively with cancer, nurses need to understand their reactions to the disease, and the reactions of others. Nurses need to move between biomedical and lay understanding of cancer and how it is treated, and to be aware of the failings of professional carers and health care in supporting people who have cancer. Complex dynamics within society, and within professional and organisational contexts, determine how cancer is managed and understood. Knowing that such processes are at large, and how these may affect one's own response to someone who is ill, or how treatment and care for a particular condition is constructed, is, we believe, the basis for caring. This book therefore offers a critical exploration of the forces that shape the delivery of cancer care, and this is given priority over the need to assimilate biomedical knowledge about cancer and its treatment. Access to the latter is offered throughout the book, and is set alongside a critical exploration of cancer care, personal accounts by people who have cancer, and reviews of research into care and treatment.

The stance taken is that change needs to happen so that the many and complex needs of people with cancer and their families are met more completely than at present; nurses have much to offer here, and may themselves be powerful agents of change. Perhaps this book takes a small step towards empowering nurses to develop alternatives for people with cancer, offering choices over how cancer is understood, and promoting the role of nursing in managing the day-to-day experience of cancer and its treatment.

Contributions to the book are from different perspectives and there is no claim that they speak with a single voice; it is a collection of differing but convergent viewpoints. A number of recurring themes draws the accounts together. The text as a whole takes a critical standpoint; all is not right with how cancer care is currently managed, therefore questions are raised about existing practice and whether this serves the interests of those who require care. Through the themes selected, discussion takes one beyond established orthodoxy, though the perspective of caring and the contribution of nursing are central.

At the outset, it was decided that this book should help nurses to access experiences of what it is like to have cancer, to receive treatment for cancer, or to care for someone who has cancer, since these are life changing and life defining. Unless one is able to think about what it must be like to experience cancer, it is not possible to understand what is needed. This has been achieved through the use of personal accounts derived from a variety of sources. Through the accounts the book adheres to a belief that in caring it is essential that nurses draw on the personal narratives, or stories, of people who are sick. In using personal accounts the book offers the reader knowledge through experience, albeit somewhat vicariously. The personal accounts, and indeed parts of the text itself, could be used as a focus for discussion or guided reflection; this is, we believe, the foundation for developing and changing practice. The book does not represent a single or final version of knowledge in cancer care; throughout, core texts, seminal works, and research studies are introduced so that readers can access and read these for themselves. The book therefore could be seen as a springboard from which the reader may begin his or her own journey of caring and scholarship in this intensely challenging area of health care.

For this second edition of the textbook we have retained many of the chapters from the first edition and updated them. We have also reflected the stronger voice and involvement of people with cancer as users of cancer services, and the opportunities that now exist for partnership working with professionals in shaping cancer services, research, and practice. Also, since publishing the first edition data have become available evidencing that longer survival is being achieved for key disease sites. The needs of increasing numbers of people who will live with cancer as part of their lives are addressed as are strategies needed to manage the effects of cancer beyond the treatment phase of illness.

The book has been organised into five parts. In the first, entitled Cancer, Care, and Society, cancer is set in context and the notion of cancer discourses and the responses of society, health care, and health carers are introduced and explained, as are some suggestions for escaping the defensive dynamics engendered by these. This discussion is set alongside the science of cancer epidemiology and a discussion about developments in cancer management. Part 2 deals with the experience of cancer from the perspectives of the person who is ill, family members, and health professionals. This is developed in Part 3, which offers detailed insight into the experience of cancer treatment, and the role of nurses in administering treatment and helping people with cancer to manage the effects of treatment. Part 4 explores the nursing management of problems related to cancer, redefining the more biomedically driven term 'symptom' as 'problem', and placing nursing in a central position in helping people to manage problems. Finally, Part 5 identifies and reviews a number of needs and priorities in cancer care, including perspectives on the needs of particular groups such as children and adolescents, the elderly, and working with ethnicity and difference. The themes of living with cancer long term, self-management and self-care, palliative care, and research in cancer care are also addressed.

Jessica Corner
Christopher Bailey

Part 1

Cancer, Care, and Society

CHAPTER ONE

What is cancer?

Jessica Corner

'Cancer' is the term used to denote a group of diseases sharing common characteristics, represented by each site of the body from which these arise. Many are quite different in nature, rate of progression, sequelae, treatment and outcome. While important progress has been made in the management of cancer, and palliation of symptoms and survival rates for cancer are improving for a number of cancer sites, cancer remains the cause of a quarter of all deaths in Europe.[1] Worldwide, 12% of people die from cancer, more than twice the number who die from AIDS, and in resource-rich countries one in four people die of the disease.[2] The effects of the disease process, the protracted nature of treatment, and the psychological impact of cancer mean that the implications for the individual reach beyond many other acute and chronic conditions. As Donovan and Girton highlight:[3]

> The magnitude of the problem of cancer in our society is only partially reflected by statistics on mortality and morbidity. These figures do not tell of the panic inherent in the mere thought of cancer, the role changes and conflicts that may arise when cancer is treated, or the dozens of other problems encountered by the person who faces a diagnosis of cancer. Since cancer is frequently a chronic disease with periods of acute intensive illness interspersed with the constant threat of death, the patient with a diagnosis of cancer must face the problems of each of these kinds of illnesses.

In being used to describe disease, cancer serves only as an umbrella term to draw together a large group of diseases (more than 100) with certain characteristics, rather in the way the term 'arthritis' is used. The difficulty with the term 'cancer' is that it is loaded with meanings for people, and these are inevitably negative. Understanding 'what cancer is' is therefore complex. One way of understanding cancer is to explore how it is manifested within the population. The science of disease within populations – epidemiology – is discussed by Elizabeth Davies and Vivian Mak later in this section. Cancer is a common condition: one in three people will develop cancer at some point in their lives. More than 270 000 people in the UK develop cancer each year. Although cancer can develop at any age, most people with cancer are over 65 years old.[1] At least 7.5 million new cancers are diagnosed each year in the world; cancer thus represents a huge burden of disease.[1] In the UK, four cancers account for over half of all cases: these are lung, breast, colorectal and prostate cancers. Figure 1.1 shows the 20 most common cancers in men and women in the UK, and Figure 1.2 shows a comparison between common cancers for developed and developing countries of the world, since these are different and reflect environmental factors contributing to cancer. Liver cancer is common in developing countries, where it is related to hepatitis B virus and food contaminated with aphlatoxin. In contrast, breast cancer is most common in developed countries.[2]

Figure 1.3 shows the most common cancers in men and women. These are somewhat different,

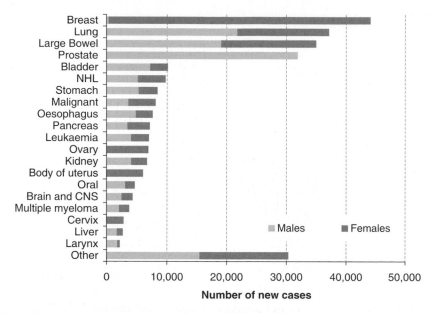

Figure 1.1   The 20 most commonly diagnosed cancers (excluding non-melanoma skin cancer) in the UK, 2003. NHL, non-Hodgkin's lymphoma; CNS central nervous system. Reproduced with permission from Cancer Research UK (2004). *Cancerstats Monograph.* London: Cancer Research UK.[1]

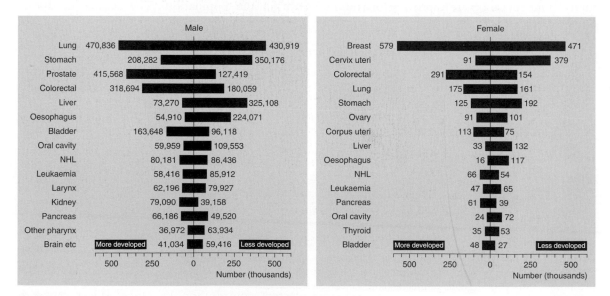

Figure 1.2   Comparison of the most common cancers in more and less developed countries in 2000. NHL, non-Hodgkin's lymphoma. Reproduced with permission from Stewart B. and Leihues P. (eds.) (2003). *World Cancer Report.* Lyons: International Agency for Research on Cancer.[2]

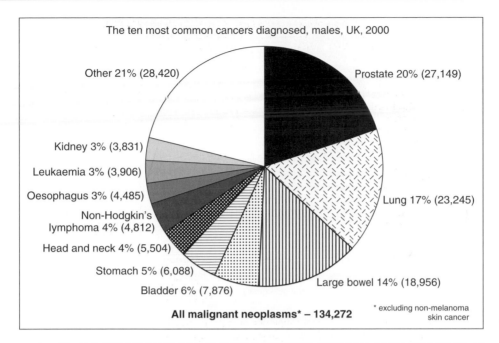

The ten most common cancers diagnosed, males, UK, 2000

Other 21% (28,420)

Prostate 20% (27,149)

Lung 17% (23,245)

Kidney 3% (3,831)

Leukaemia 3% (3,906)

Oesophagus 3% (4,485)

Non-Hodgkin's lymphoma 4% (4,812)

Head and neck 4% (5,504)

Stomach 5% (6,088)

Large bowel 14% (18,956)

Bladder 6% (7,876)

All malignant neoplasms* – 134,272

* excluding non-melanoma skin cancer

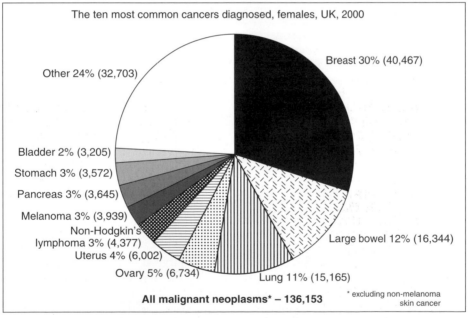

The ten most common cancers diagnosed, females, UK, 2000

Other 24% (32,703)

Breast 30% (40,467)

Bladder 2% (3,205)

Stomach 3% (3,572)

Pancreas 3% (3,645)

Melanoma 3% (3,939)

Non-Hodgkin's lymphoma 3% (4,377)

Uterus 4% (6,002)

Ovary 5% (6,734)

Large bowel 12% (16,344)

Lung 11% (15,165)

All malignant neoplasms* – 136,153

* excluding non-melanoma skin cancer

Figure 1.3 The most common cancers in men and women. Reproduced with permission from Cancer Research UK (2004). *Cancerstats Monograph*. London: Cancer Research UK.[1]

with lung cancer the most common for men, and breast cancer for women. Figure 1.4 shows the relative percentage of people who survive 5 years after diagnosis; this is an indicator of the chance of being cured of any particular cancer. Some cancers, such as skin cancer, if melanoma is excluded, have a very high chance of cure, whereas others, such as cancer of the lung and pancreas, have very low 5-year survival rates. The stage of the disease at diagnosis is an important

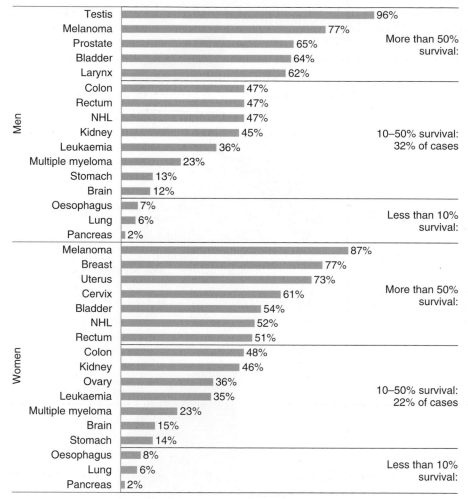

Figure 1.4 The relative percentage of people who survive 5 years after diagnosis. Reproduced with permission from Cancer Research UK (2004). *Cancerstats Monograph*. London: Cancer Research UK.[1]

determinant of survival. Survival for cancers detected and treated early is invariably better.[1] In the UK in 2002 there were 151 000 cancer deaths: lung cancer accounted for 22% of these and is the most common cause of cancer death; breast cancer accounted for 8% and is the leading cause of cancer death in women. In developed countries cancer is the cause of one in four deaths.[2] The lifetime risk of developing cancer of different sites is shown in Table 1.1. Survival from cancer is also related to socio-economic status, with people who are from more deprived socio-economic circumstances having both higher cancer incidences and

poorer survival chances, reflecting both exposure to risk factors, behaviour and access to health care.[4]

Interestingly, cancer is unusual among diseases, in that in professional discussion in oncology, 'survival' is used as a benchmark for measuring outcome and the effectiveness of treatment. Outcomes are discussed in terms of an individual's chances of survival, measured formally as relative 5-year survival rates. Treatment choices are made on the basis of assessment of an individual's survival chance offset against attendant levels of toxicity for any given course of treatment.

Table 1.1 Estimates of the percentage out of a cohort who developed cancer by the age of 65 years, and over a lifetime, England and Wales, 1997. Reproduced with permission from Cancer Research UK (2004). *Cancerstats Monograph*. London: Cancer Research UK.[1]

	Males			Females		
	% of cohort who develop cancer:		**Lifetime risk**	**% of cohort who develop cancer:**		**Lifetime risk**
	by age 65	**over lifetime**		**by age 65**	**over lifetime**	
Bladder	0.7	3.3	1 in 30	0.2	1.3	1 in 79
Brain and CNS	0.4	0.7	1 in 147	0.3	0.5	1 in 207
Breast	–	–	–	5.6	10.9	1 in 9
Cervix	–	–	–	0.6	0.9	1 in 116
Kidney	0.4	1.1	1 in 89	0.2	0.6	1 in 162
Large bowel	1.4	5.7	1 in 18	1.1	4.9	1 in 20
Leukaemia	0.4	1.0	1 in 95	0.3	0.8	1 in 127
Lung	1.7	8.0	1 in 13	1.0	4.3	1 in 23
Melanoma	0.4	0.7	1 in 147	0.5	0.9	1 in 117
Multiple myeloma	0.1	0.6	1 in 177	0.1	0.5	1 in 204
Non-Hodgkin lymphoma	0.6	1.4	1 in 69	0.4	1.2	1 in 83
Oesophagus	0.4	1.3	1 in 75	0.2	1.1	1 in 95
Ovary	–	–	–	0.9	2.1	1 in 48
Pancreas	0.3	1.0	1 in 96	0.2	1.1	1 in 95
Prostate	0.9	7.3	1 in 14	–	–	–
Stomach	0.5	2.3	1 in 44	0.2	1.2	1 in 86
Uterus	–	–	–	0.6	1.4	1 in 73

The possibility of death is immediate, and avoiding this as a goal predominates, reinforcing and responding to social and cultural images of cancer.

Biological understanding of cancer has become much more detailed in recent years, owing to discoveries in molecular biology and genetics. These discoveries in turn suggest new avenues by which treatment may be targeted at specific points in the natural history of cells in which cancer may originate. Weinberg eloquently describes the defining features of cancer at a cellular level:[5]

> Almost every tissue in the body can spawn malignancies; some even yield several types. What is more each cancer has unique features . . . the basic processes that produce these diverse tumours appear to be quite similar . . . 30 trillion cells of the normal, healthy body live in a complex, interdependent condominium, regulating one another's proliferation. Indeed, normal cells reproduce only when instructed to do so by other cells in their vicinity. Such unceasing collaboration ensures that each tissue maintains a size and architecture appropriate to the body's needs.
>
> Cancer cells, in stark contrast, violate this scheme; they become deaf to the usual controls on proliferation and follow their own internal agenda for reproduction. They also possess an even more insidious property – the ability to migrate from the site where they began, invading nearby tissues and forming masses at distant sites in the body. Tumours composed of such malignant cells become more aggressive over time, and they become lethal when they disrupt the tissues and organs needed for the survival of the body as a whole [p.3].

This description immediately transports us into a world deep inside the body, to a kind of internal city of citizen cells. Cancer is the sinister anarchistic force that threatens this internal society, and signals its ultimate demise; pictured in this way, fear of cancer and feeling the need to fight cancer seem natural responses.

A closer look at this deep internal world reveals a far less sinister sequence of mechanical or system failures, which, when they occur together, lead to the formation of a cancer. The aim of cancer science is to understand fully these mechanisms and eventually to find ways of correcting the mechanical failure, or to counteract the deleterious effects of it. The steps in the biological development of cancer outlined by Weinberg are shown in Figure 1.5.[5]

There is a number of mechanisms that either alone or in combination causes abnormalities in cell growth and multiplication. For a cancer to develop, it probably requires several to occur together.

Hanahan and Weinberg state that tumorigenesis is a multistep process whereby human cells are progressively transformed into highly malignant derivatives.[6] They suggest that 'tumour development proceeds via a process analagous to Darwinian evolution, in which a succession of genetic changes, each conferring one or another type of growth advantage, leads to the progressive conversion of normal cells into cancer cells' (p.57). They characterise these genetic changes as six alterations in cell physiology that collectively dictate maligant growth as follows:

1. *the development of self-sufficiency in growth signals* – in normal cells stimulatory signals that bind receptors on the cell membrane trigger the cell to move from a quiescent state into an active proliferative state in order for cell division to take place. Normal cells cannot multiply without such external stimulator signals. Tumour cells, on the other hand, generate their own internal growth signals and therefore are much less dependent on stimulation from the normal tissue environment; they acquire 'growth signal autonomy'

2. *acquired insensitiviy to antigrowth signals* – in normal tissue multiple antiproliferative signals operate to maintain cellular quiesence and tissue homeostasis. In cancer cells genetic changes render cells insensitive to antigrowth factors. Alterations, or mutations, in genes within human cells contribute to abnormalities in cell growth. The mutations occur through errors in the replication of deoxyribonucleic acid (DNA) during cell division and may occur after exposure to a carcinogen. Mutations that activate the normal functions of the cell are called proto-oncogenes.[7] Tumour suppressor genes inactivate cell proliferation and if they fail to do this, cell growth may continue when it is no longer needed

3. *evading apoptosis* – the ability of tumour cell populations to expand in number is determined not only by the rate of cell proliferation but also by the rate of cell attrition. Acquired resistance towards programmed cell death or apoptosis is a hallmark of most types of cancer. The cell cycle is the name given to the process of cell division and is likened to a kind of clock that is set to a particular speed and rhythm.[5] The cell cycle proceeds in a series of phases; this results in the cell's DNA being replicated and the cell, and its DNA, dividing and becoming two daughter cells. Initially, the cell increases in size and prepares to copy its DNA ready for cell division. Then the chromosomes are replicated and the cell prepares to divide. Finally mitosis, or cell division, occurs. The cell then rests until it prepares to divide again. This cycle is controlled within the cell by cyclins and cyclin-dependent kinases or enzymes.[7] Normally mechanisms of control prevent cells within the body continuing to divide and proliferate unless this is required. Tumour suppressor proteins within the cell can either block the activity of these cell cyclins, and therefore cause the cell cycle, and cell division, to pause; or, if excessive amounts of cyclins are produced by the cell, then cell division may proceed unchecked.[8] Further cellular mechanisms exist to prevent uncontrolled cell division, for example, a process known as apoptosis. This is a mechanism whereby an abnormality in the cell's DNA is recognised within the cell and its own death is brought about as a consequence. The p53 protein is involved in apoptosis; disruptions in the gene involved in the production of p53 may mean that abnormal cells can avoid apoptosis. Cancer cells may also produce proteins that prevent apoptosis. If apoptosis is avoided then an abnormal cell will continue to divide and replicate itself, perhaps indefinitely[5]

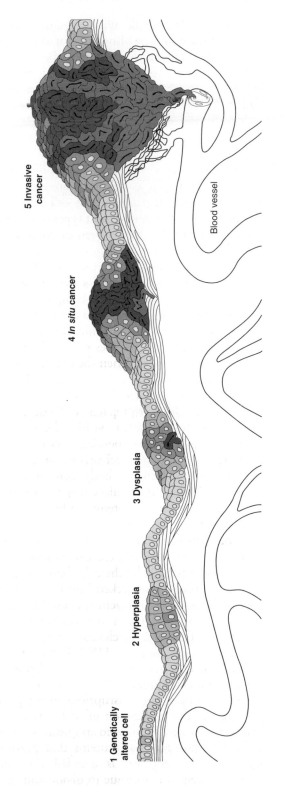

1 Genetically altered cell

2 Hyperplasia

3 Dysplasia

4 In situ cancer

5 Invasive cancer

Blood vessel

1 Tumour development begins when some cell ( ) within a normal population ( ) sustains a genetic mutation that increases its propensity to proliferate when it would normally rest.

2 The altered cell and its descendants continue to look normal, but they reproduce too much – a condition termed hyperplasia. After years, one in a million of these cells ( ) suffers another mutation that further loosens control on cell growth.

3 In addition to proliferating excessively, the offspring of this cell appear abnormal in shape and in orientation; the tissue is now said to exhibit dysplasia. Once again, after a time, a rare mutation that alters cell behaviour occurs ( ).

4 The affected cells become still more abnormal in growth and appearance. If the tumour has not yet broken through any boundaries between tissues, it is called *in situ* cancer. This tumour may remain contained indefinitely; however, some cells may eventually acquire additional mutations ( ).

5 If the genetic changes allow the tumour to begin invading underlying tissue and to shed cells into the blood or lymph, the mass is considered to have become malignant. The renegade cells are likely to establish new tumours (metastases) throughout the body; these may become lethal by disrupting a vital organ.

Figure 1.5 Tumour development occurs in stages. The creation of malignant tumour in epithelial tissues is depicted schematically. Epithelial cancers (carcinomas) are the most common malignancies. The mass seen here emerges as a result of mutations in four genes, but the number of genes involved can vary. Reproduced with permission from Weinberg R.A. (1996). How cancer arises. *Scientific American* **275**, 62–70.[5]

4. *limitless replication potential* – acquired disruption in cell-to-cell signalling to control cell proliferation does not on its own ensure tumour growth. Cells carry an intrinsic programme that limits their multiplication. A mechanism exists within the body to regulate and monitor the number of times any single cell can replicate itself. Normally this occurs 50 to 60 times before a cell becomes senescent and eventually dies.[5] This is dictated by the length of telomeres or sections at the ends of chromosomes; these become slightly shortened each time a cell multiplies, and once below a critical length the cell stops dividing. In cancer cells, an enzyme, telomerase, is produced, which replaces the effect of the telomeres becoming shortened. This enzyme promotes excessive growth and cell multiplication; again, this may be part of the process by which a tumour forms

5. *sustained angiogenesis* – in order to continue growth and proliferation, cells need to be in close proximity to a capillary blood vessel, therefore malignant lesions, if they are to survive, need to develop the potential to encourage blood vessel growth or angiogenesis. Hanahan and Weinberg suggest that this occurs in a series of steps with angiogenesis being activated in midstage lesions before a full tumour develops.[6] The appearance of angiogenic capability is the result of subtle changes in the balance of angiogensis inducers and inhibitors, commonly through alterations in gene transcriptions causing alterations in the complex homeostatic regulation of normal tissues

6. *tissue invasion and metastases* – in most types of cancer, the primary tumour eventually develops 'pioneer cells' that invade adjacent tissues or travel to distant sites, where they may develop into new cell colonies. Invasion and metastases are very complex processes that are incompletely understood. Proteins involved in the tethering of cells to their surrounding tissue are altered in cells possessing invasive or metastatic capabilities.

If these various mechanisms involved in cell growth and multiplication are disrupted, or where normal control mechanisms alter or fail, abnormal tissue growth will result. Thus, according to Weinberg, cancer occurs directly as a result of 'runaway cell proliferation'.[5] He concludes:

> Still, despite so much insight into cause, new therapies have so far remained elusive. One reason is that tumour cells differ only minimally from healthy ones; a minute fraction of the tens of thousands of genes in a cell suffers damage during malignant transformation. Thus, normal friend and malignant foe are woven of similar cloth, and any fire directed against the enemy may do as much damage to normal tissue as to the intended target [p.14].

Weinberg returns to using metaphor to explain cancer. This time the intercellular world is not likened to reproduction or architecture, but to 'war', to be waged against runaway cells in an attempt to control cancer. Science and scientists make use of such metaphors and other techniques more familiar in literature, as devices to help reveal and articulate scientific facts. In doing this spaces are created in which such facts can become material or real when they are not in themselves visible; for example, as in the complex activities within the cell already described.[9] What is important is to understand how these metaphors may also become part of a wider social or cultural understanding of cancer, and themselves create 'what cancer is'.[10,11] There is an important cyclical process here. Cancer, the 'killer disease', becomes understood as a monstrous aberration of anarchistic runaway cell 'beings', an antisocial process working against the collective organism with grave or even fatal results. This is a powerful image, real to some extent because cancer is common and many people die from it (although, in developed countries, not as many as die from cardiovascular disease, which does not seem to engender such negative images). The 'runaway, anarchistic monster' is also a powerful and difficult image for people who have the disease to experience within themselves, when cancer is visible, in the main, only through physical, embodied sensations such as pain or fatigue. Perhaps, given this, scientists should be more careful with the metaphoric and narrative devices they use to explain complex, 'invisible' facts.

Cancer is part of our culture, understood as a dreaded disease, feared perhaps more than any other disease, associated with inevitable death, and a death that is painful and unpleasant. Stories of people with cancer, especially celebrities who have cancer, frequently appear in newspapers and magazines. Jackie Stacey has explored how popular cultural narratives are used to tell people's stories of having cancer.[10] These, like fictional tales, or screenplays, follow a path through time, usually involving a heroic figure who struggles to overcome difficulties in the name of truth, justice, or love. The stories, like those in films or books, often involve tales of monsters and heroic recoveries. While the stories are real, in that they are about real people and cancer, in the way that they are told they are constructed to fit this familiar fictional form. She says:[10]

> Cancer never really invades the body as such, but rather reproduces itself from within. Malignant growths secretly proliferate. Like the monster of screen horror, it threatens bodily order and takes over its regulating systems. Horror films often tell tales of the conquering of monsters. Invaders from outside . . . threaten the order of human society and must be exterminated in the name of civilisation. More often than not, the monstrous threat invades the body. Occupied by an alien force or physical presence, the innocent human victims lose control of the body and its functions. Be it vampires, ghouls or monsters from outer space, the horror narrative explores the boundaries between human and non-human, between life and death and between self and other. Its resolution requires the expulsion of the alien from the physical and social body it threatens, and the reestablishment of human order and stability. The heroes (the good scientists, the decent citizens, the protective fathers – and very occasionally the Sigourney Weavers) fight the monster to its death and return the rule of law to its rightful supremacy. Stories of surviving cancer fit easily into these patterns of journey from chaos to control. They combine the masculine heroics of such adventure narratives with the feminine suffering and sacrifice of melodramas [p.10].

These stories use language laced with metaphor; people with cancer 'battle' for their survival, and cancer treatment is represented as a military campaign; the oncologist is at war against a killer disease, and cancer treatments are his ammunition. It seems that society as a whole is at war with cancer. As Susan DiGiacomo states:

In a society that has declared 'war on cancer' the cancer patient is a victim, held hostage by a disease that has invaded his body, which becomes the battle field on which the war is fought. The dissimilar meanings of corruption and battle combine to promote medical paternalism and authoritarianism. No effort is spared to defeat so evil an enemy, and no general needs to explain his orders.[11]

The metaphors surrounding cancer also reflect changing attitudes within society towards death.[12] Today, as a result of longevity, it is possible for death not to be experienced within a family for a generation. Death has become something that is not part of our daily lives; unlike in premodern times, our relationship with death has increasingly become one of denial of its possibility, rather than an ever-present reality. In this situation, cancer has become a symbol of death itself. On every occasion it presents itself to us it forces cracks into man's armoury that represses fear of death. As De Beauvoir concludes in her account of her experience of her mother's death from cancer:[13]

> You do not die from being born, nor from having lived, nor from old age. You die from *something*. The knowledge that because of her age my mother's life must soon come to an end did not lessen the horrible surprise: she had sarcoma. Cancer, thrombosis, pneumonia: it is as violent and unforeseen as an engine stopping in the middle of the sky. My mother encouraged one to be optimistic when, crippled with arthritis and dying, she asserted the infinite value of each instant; but her vain tenaciousness also ripped and tore the reassuring curtain of everyday triviality. There is no such thing as a natural death: nothing that happens to man is ever natural, since his presence calls the world into question. All men must die: but for every man his death is an accident and, even if he knows and consents to it, an unjustifiable violation [p.92].

If cancer is understood as a disease through the use of metaphor, it is also in turn a powerful metaphor.[14] Cancer is a word that is ubiquitous; it is used to suggest many things, such as, all that is bad in society, or a pervasive fault in a machine, or a flaw in how an organisation is functioning. The cancer metaphor has developed a meaning within our culture that is both part and not part of cancer the disease; it develops a life of its own, and may or may not in the end reflect the disease in any direct way. The more established the meanings surrounding cancer become, the more these then shape people's expectations and fears of the disease; the process is insidious.

Cancer is all around us, quite literally because of the numbers of people who have cancer or who will be affected by cancer because someone they know has it. It is also all around us in the way in which it is part of our culture, and how we use what we believe about cancer to convey what we mean about other things; this in turn affects how we respond when we come across someone who has cancer. It is understanding this, and finding ways of responding to this complex interrelationship between disease and its various constructions for individuals, for professionals, and for health care, that is the foundation of caring.[15,16]

What is cancer? This is an unanswerable question: it is many things, it is what you make it, and it is what others make of it.

References

1. Cancer Research UK (2004). *Cancerstats Monograph.* London: Cancer Research UK.
2. Stewart B. and Leihues P. (eds.) (2003). *World Cancer Report.* Lyons: International Ageny for Research on Cancer.
3. Donovan M.I. and Girton S.E. (1984). *Cancer Care Nursing*, 2nd edition. Norwalk, CT: Appleton Century Crofts, p. 15.
4. Kogevinas M., Pearce N., Susser M. and Bofetta P. (eds.) (1997). *Social Inequalities and Cancer.* Lyons: International Agency for Research on Cancer.
5. Weinberg R.A. (1996). How cancer arises. *Scientific American* **275**, 62–70.
6. Hanahan D. and Weinberg R.A. (2000). The hallmarks of cancer. *Cell* **100**, 57–70.
7. Yarnold J.R. (1996). What are cancer genes and how do they upset cell behavior? In Yarnold J.R., Stratton M. and McMillan T.J. (eds.) *Molecular Biology for Oncologists*, 2nd edition. London: Chapman and Hall
8. Carr A.M. (1996). Cell cycle control and cancer. In Yarnold J.R., Stratton M. and McMillan T.J. (eds.) *Molecular Biology for Oncologists*, 2nd edition. London: Chapman and Hall.
9. Lenoir T. (1998). Inscription practices and the materialities of communication. In Lenoir T. (ed.) *Inscribing Science: Scientific Texts and the Materiality of Communication.* Stanford, CA: Stanford University Press.
10. Stacey J. (1997). *Teratologies: a Cultural Study of Cancer.* London: Routledge.
11. DiGiacomo S.M. (1987). Biomedicine as a cultural system: an anthropologist in the kingdom of the sick. In Baer H.A. (ed.) *Encounters with Biomedicine: Case Studies in Medical Anthropology.* New York: Gordon and Breach, p. 323.
12. Sontag S. (1977). *Illness as Metaphor.* London: Allen Lane.
13. De Beauvoir S. (1969). *A Very Easy Death.* London: Penguin, p. 92.
14. Reisfield G.M. and Wilson G.R. (2004). Use of metaphor in the discourses on cancer. *Journal of Clinical Oncology* **22**, 4024–4027.
15. Corner J. (1997). Nursing and the counter culture for cancer. *European Journal of Cancer Care* **6**, 174–181.
16. Hunsker Hawkins A. (1999). *Reconstructing Illness: Studies in Pathography*, 2nd edition. West Lafayette, Indiana: Purdue.

CHAPTER TWO

Knowledge and caring: a philosophical and personal perspective

Alan Cribb

Preamble

Most days after I got home from school I would sit on a stool by the kitchen work surface and talk to my mum. She would be making dinner for the family and I have particularly clear memories of her preparing vegetables – peeling and chopping them while I pinched bits. I was eager to report the details of my day and to give her the benefit of my opinion on all manner of things. I was very interested in science at the time, having been fired by the thought that everything is made of molecules! Not only did it not occur to me to help but I don't think it ever occurred to me to ask about her or her day (she would just have returned from work), or about whether she had anything on her mind. It was one-way traffic. She would listen quietly, sometimes asking questions, occasionally offering advice. I suppose if I know anything worth knowing about care I started to learn it at times like that – being cared for body and soul as a matter of routine, and scarcely appreciating it. So writing about caring seems a bit odd.

Knowledge is a different matter. Knowledge belongs in books. School was about knowledge and I carried some of it home in my physics and chemistry textbooks, shut away in my school bag. Many people think knowledge ought to be only written about in the third person, that it is something formal and impersonal. There are academic conventions to adhere to (Bloggs, 1997). If one is going to write about knowledge one had better be on one's best behaviour. Furthermore, one had better sound like an intellectual. Epistemological analysis demands a rigorous idiom (that sort of thing).

So there is the problem – how to write about these two different concerns together; how to do justice to my mum and the science textbooks. I have to admit at once that I cannot. I am in a textbook and I will have to be fairly 'textbookish', but from time to time I may also have to rebel.

PART ONE – PICTURES OF KNOWLEDGE

Two worlds

I want to start by reinforcing some of the contrasts in the preamble, by drawing a tidy distinction between two worlds – the scientific world (or more precisely the 'world as known by science') and the 'human world'. No doubt, like all such distinctions, it should not be drawn too tidily, and it may even collapse under close inspection; but there will be time for qualifications later. I want to argue that the reason for emphasising this contrast is because it plays a very important role in so much of modern life. It shapes so much of what we do and think.

Consider the furniture in your home. Items of furniture will have stories attached to them. Simple stories: 'This was a present from x'; 'This was a bargain from y'. Elaborate stories: 'Remember the first meal we had at this table, when I hardly knew you . . .'; 'This bed could tell a few tales . . .'. But suppose we are asked whether these stories are *really* about the furniture. Are they not only projections of our concerns, which we 'tag' onto them? Surely, it could be said, if we want to know about tables we should turn to science. Chemistry can help us to understand the material constitution of a table, and physics its ultimate constitution. The table is *really* some sort of configuration of energy. It appears to our common-sense eyes to be brown and solid, but in itself it is not even these things. Appearances are deceptive.

Of course, for virtually all domestic purposes we do not need to concern ourselves with the 'science of furniture' (although we might note in passing that the furniture industry employs people with expertise in material sciences, ergonomics, etc). We can manage very well with common sense or 'lay beliefs'. But at the back of our minds we know that, at least with regard to material things like furniture, common sense is second rate. Our lay judgements are unreliable and sometimes plain wrong. Most people could make sensible guesses about which materials are most hazardous in a fire, but most people would get some of it wrong. This is one of many ways to 'die of ignorance'. What applies to furniture is certainly true for microwave ovens and television sets, and all the paraphernalia of modern life. The lay realm is one of opinion, guesswork, and myth. It is part of the real world but it is also shaded from it by various degrees of scientific ignorance.

None of this would be of much consequence if it only applied to domestic furniture, but it is possible to see this as a mere instance of a general truth. The modern world is, according to many perspectives, one in which lay beliefs have been eroded, demoted, replaced, and transformed by scientific knowledge. Secularisation is perhaps the most significant example of this change. A cosmos that has a personal creator at its heart has been superseded by a Godless, 'cold' universe. Human beings do not have an exceptional place in the meaning and the mystery of the world; they have emerged 'ordinarily' out of the processes of evolution, and they are biological rather than theologi-

cal creations. Many other parallel and allied shifts have taken place. Weber calls this process, by which the 'magic' is taken out of the world by a modern, scientific, rationalistic spirit, 'disenchantment'. When we see lambs or daffodils they may speak to us of hope and renewal, of an underlying sense of purpose, of belonging. But we also know that they are just natural 'blind' phenomena, and in a sense meaningless ones, and that our metaphysical interpretations of them are misleading. (I am deliberately overstating this. Of course it is possible, indeed probably the norm, to entertain both 'scientific' and 'lay' beliefs at the same time, to live, as it were, in two worlds. I will come back to this shortly.)

Furthermore, what I am calling the human world is being displaced and colonised not only by the natural sciences, but also by the social or 'human sciences'. Every facet of our lives is subject to increasing quantities of sociological and psychological research. Here also, personal and common-sense opinion is set beside 'more expert' analyses. An individual struggling with an incident of crime, or divorce, or illness will make their own interpretations of events. But much of the social scientific research will be designed to transcend these interpretations, to identify the underlying explanations, the underlying reality. A wife may go to the doctor on behalf of her husband because 'he's too busy at work'. But a sociological eye will see that the couple are acting out gendered roles. Over time, as with the natural sciences, these social scientific lessons will become incorporated into a changed set of lay beliefs. Thus, for example, someone suffering from grief might anticipate that their experience may come in certain well-documented packages – in complex and contradictory feelings, in waves, in stages and so on.

It seems to me that most of us live in two worlds. The 'scientific world' has not expanded to fill every corner of our experience, and even in those areas where it is generally deemed to uncover the real nature of things many people do not regard it as sufficient. So, even in the most secularised and scientifically minded cultures, people still live in a relatively enchanted world. This may be experienced as a source of tension or 'dissonance' in individuals' lives. They may, for example, be aware of a gap between their relatively 'tough-minded' public persona in which they account for the behaviour of others in sociologically and psychologically informed ways (say as 'rational economic consumers'), and their 'tender-minded' private self (who takes romantic love seriously and sees their loved one as someone of unique and infinite worth) They may rely on the predictability of a scientific and technological infrastructure, while pursuing scientifically dubious or even antiscientific belief systems. We cannot but acknowledge the explanatory power and the usefulness of scientific ways of thinking, but we do not want to live in a cold world. Disinterested rational abstract inquiry helps us to gain mastery over our environment but in doing so it makes it less hospitable. How will we be better off if we gain control of the world but lose our soul and our home?

As I've already indicated, this contrast between the scientific and the human worlds is in many ways too simplistic, and it is tempting to overstate the dominance of a scientific perspective. I therefore want to make some remarks designed to qualify and challenge the impression I have given up to this point. But I will also insist that something like this crude picture is a crucially important ingredient of life in the modern world.

Commentary 2.1

> Reading through this chapter some time after it was drafted, I think I see what I am trying to do and say in it. It is very much a personal piece (maybe a self-indulgent one); I am not trying to say anything original but simply to sort out ideas about knowledge and caring, some of which have come from studying philosophy and some from my personal life. I want to take issue with the view that knowledge and caring are two entirely different things, the former being 'clever' and the latter 'natural'. I am starting by looking at some ideas of what real knowledge is. The aim is to prompt the reader into reflections on their own ideas about knowledge and caring, and the relationship between them.

Real knowledge (mark 1)

Here are some objections to the picture set out in the last section. First, why speak of 'science' when really I am drawing a contrast between expert

knowledge and lay beliefs? Surely most forms of knowledge are not scientific, and am I not stretching a point even by parcelling sociology and psychology in with the natural sciences? Second, the various sciences have not had such indisputable success. At best they offer one kind of explanation of one aspect of the world – they are not a substitute for theological, historical, or cultural accounts of the world. Third, many people – even in the 'most advanced' societies – would, as I have hinted, see science as something on the margins of their life, as something largely irrelevant to their central concerns. How can this be reconciled with the picture of the scientific world inexorably displacing and colonising the human world? All these objections have merit, and they help to add some confusion to what is, after all, a confusing scene.

The rationale for starting with the tidy distinction, and the crude picture, is that it reflects a powerful current (arguably *the* current) of modernisation – the idea that human progress comes from the growth and application of knowledge, and that above all *real* knowledge is scientific knowledge. This is one of the ruling ideas of modern societies. Constant attempts are made to dethrone it and to kill it off, but it is not easily dislodged.

The philosophical version of this ruling idea is called 'positivism'. There are many variants of philosophical positivism, and many internal and external controversies about them, but it is worth briefly sketching out some of the key components of what might be called classical, or naive, positivism.

- *Methodological monism* – a fancy name for the idea that there is only one kind of method suitable for the production of knowledge. The natural sciences are typically taken to be paradigms of knowledge. Many traditional belief systems (especially metaphysical theories about transcendent realities, but also 'thisworldly' ideological, moral, or aesthetic judgements) are seen to be without warrant, or even without meaning. In general, a sharp demarcation is made between real knowledge, which satisfies appropriate methodological rigours, and mere belief, superstition, and plain nonsense, which falls beyond the line.

- *The quest for generalisations and structures* – the most favoured method involves the discovery, formulation, and testing of law-like generalisations that describe particular cases or events as instances of some general phenomena. (For example: this bucket of water conducts electricity because substances with such and such properties conduct electricity; this economy is suffering from inflation because economies with such and such properties always do so.) So the generalising manoeuvre is accompanied by another one – the identification of the underlying combination of properties or 'structures' that help to explain the phenomena. We cannot understand the nature of water or economies, or anything at all for that matter, by looking at their surfaces. We need to understand their inner constitution, the reality beyond the surface appearance.

- *Prediction and control* – the value of law-like generalisations is that they put us in a better position to intervene in events with predictable results, i.e. they enable us to exercise greater control over events. The capacity for effective technologies (including both mechanical engineering and social engineering) is enhanced.

- *Reductionism* – the shift from surface appearances to underlying structures is sometimes called reductionism. Although this is principally about explaining things, it also suggests that something is 'taken away' by the explanatory move. All manner of things are rendered mere appearance, not fully real. There are many forms of reductionism, some of which are very radical and, if accepted, denude the world of all kinds of phenomena. 'Physicalism' is the thesis that everything can be explained by the laws of physics. This is the adult version of my juvenile enthusiasm about everything being made of molecules. If, as seems plausible, everything is made of matter or energy, why not try to explain everything (tea parties as well as tea cups) in purely physical terms? (Sociology also practises many types of reductionism, the most extreme being the predominantly antipositivist 'social construction of reality' thesis. Here it turns out that many seemingly substantial things do not really exist in their own right but only as a product of human languages and practices.)

Whether or not positivism has been successful as a philosophical position (and a huge amount of work has gone into arguing that it has not), it has certainly been extremely influential both in the academic sphere and in the wider community. In the academic sphere its influence is shown, for example, by the incorporation of scientific methodologies into a wide range of subject areas. Indeed, in many areas 'research' is more or less equated with scientific style research. Some of its immense impact on the wider culture is indicated in the previous section.

Before considering some of the main antipositivist arguments, I will say a little more about the wider cultural associations of the sharp demarcation between real 'expert' knowledge and mere 'lay' belief. I want to summarise a conception of real knowledge that has widespread currency, which I will call 'the encyclopaedic picture of knowledge'.

In this picture, knowledge is represented by an encyclopaedia. It is something solid, substantial – something in which we can have confidence. It is also something that can be written down, that can exist in an impersonal form and can be used as a common resource. Of course, more would have to be added to complete a full drawing of this picture, but the idea of an encyclopaedia will do for a thumbnail sketch.

A similar picture is evoked by the idea of a non-fiction library. Here knowledge is arranged by subject as well as alphabetically. Time and space are mapped through the history and geography of the world, period by period, region by region. The natural and physical aspects of the world are covered by biological and physical sciences. We can 'zoom in' to organs, cells, genes, and so on, or 'zoom out' to solar systems, galaxies, and beyond. Human culture is stored in all its religious, aesthetic, practical, and technological varieties. Some encyclopaedias are organised in a similar manner, and are, in effect, 'portable libraries'. We can imagine them as a record of all accumulated knowledge, organised into an interconnected and mutually supportive matrix.

If we operate with a picture like this, we may also picture learning as 'studying'. There we are at the beginning of a course; over the horizon the exams are looming, and the problem is how are we going to get all the knowledge in the books on our shelves into our heads in time. When we go into the library and the stacks of books multiply, it is natural to panic – our heads are so 'empty'!

But there is also something rather dead or inert about an encyclopaedia. We seem to be able to get along with life very well while it gathers dust. Many of the things we know, we learn without recourse to books, and furthermore there are many things we would be foolish to try and learn from books. (This is the sense in which caring doesn't belong in textbooks.) Libraries are all very well, but surely virtually everything that matters goes on outside libraries? Are we not right to regard someone who does not appear to realise this as rather foolish and callow?

Here I am only playing with impressions, and with vague outlines and contrasts. But I think there are important clues in these contrasts between the 'bookish' and the 'non-bookish' parts of life; clues that point in the direction of another picture of 'real knowledge', a picture that does not place our everyday, practical, and personal knowledge in the box labelled 'seconds', and that helps to restore the primacy of the human world.

Real knowledge (mark 2)

'And now for something completely different.' This was one of the catch phrases of the Monty Python team. It was used – cleverly – to provide continuity when there wasn't any, but it will do for me as well, because I intend to say something about humour.

Nearly everyone knows how to be funny, and some people are very good at it. There are few people who go around being self-consciously and deliberately funny (and this is very difficult to carry off successfully and without causing annoyance), but we can all try to see 'the funny side of things'. Smiles and laughter are a very large element of the compound that makes life tolerable. Although they can be used divisively, their natural tendency is to draw people together. They are part of the warmth and the enchantment of the world. Even if we come to the conclusion that the universe is meaningless, they help us to 'look on the bright side of life'.

But although we can perfectly properly say that someone knows how to be funny, or knows how to see the funny side of life, we would not expect to find this kind of knowledge in a book. In fact, we know it is exceedingly difficult to theorise about humour and that someone who does so might in any case (or as a result) be pretty humourless. Writing about humour is at best a small part of knowing about humour, and we are inclined to say that the real knowledge falls outside books. There are many sorts of things about which this is true. Perhaps the most obvious set is 'physical' skills such as swimming, typing, or driving a car. But there are other more general and more fundamental sorts of knowledge that fall into the same category, such as speaking English (or another natural language), or – equally important for our purposes – knowing how to conduct a conversation. Indeed, these relatively conspicuous examples are only the tip of the iceberg, or rather they are some of the prominent features of the human face obscured by the currency of 'encyclopaedic knowledge'.

These reflections serve as an introduction to a 'mark 2' picture of real knowledge, which I will call 'the personal resource picture'. In some ways (but not all) this can be seen as the opposite of the mark 1 picture. According to this conception, knowledge is personal, not impersonal. Real knowledge *cannot* be written down; rather it can only exist as part of the outlook, dispositions, and skills of people. (Of course some 'shadows' of it can be written down, just as something of the knowledge of someone who is an expert cook can be written into cookery books.) This sort of knowledge is not acquired by studying, but by doing, by living. Here experience and practice make all the difference, and being able to recite 'knowledge' counts for little or nothing.

Similar distinctions are sometimes made by differentiating between 'knowledge' and 'skills', or between 'theoretical knowledge' and 'practical knowledge'. But these other terms can be misleading if they suggest that the former type of knowledge is intellectual or mind-centred and the latter is essentially technical or physical (and body-centred). Stupid divisions have often been made between 'working with one's brain' and 'working with one's hands'. These divisions are conceptually stupid because human activities (with very few exceptions) are not delegated to parts of persons, and because an individual is a single unified 'embodied intelligence', not a strange combination of a thinking disembodied executive with an unthinking physical workforce. And, as I have indicated, this division is also closely bound up with peculiar social divisions, which link kinds of work with personal and social status. The personal resource picture of knowledge, therefore, is not meant to pick out only practical skills, except in the sense that all knowledge involves 'skills that have to be practised'. These include thinking skills and theoretical skills. Thus it is not only being a good piano player or being a good listener that involves personal knowledge, but also being a good historian or physicist. In all of these cases, the real embodied knowledge cannot be written down. (This is not to dismiss completely the kind of knowledge that can be written down. But note that this does not consist entirely of the sort of abstract impersonal truths that the encyclopaedic picture would suggest; rather, much of it represents 'personal voices' with whom we, as readers, are in conversation.)

Commentary 2.2

My main preoccupation here seems to be with the relationship between 'book knowledge' and 'personal knowledge'. Is one more basic than the other? Is one more important than the other? How do they fit together? Perhaps this is only a personal preoccupation – something I've got a 'hang up' about. But I suspect it is something of general relevance. Everyone has to do more and more exams and assessments. More and more academic books are being produced and read. Yet it is clear to most people that there is much more to learning and development than the learning that takes place 'on paper'. These days, is enough emphasis placed on 'the university of life'?

Knowledge mark 2 belongs squarely to the human world rather than 'the world as known by science'. Indeed, it helps us to see how the latter is not independent of the former but is supported and sustained by it. The naive positivist would picture 'the world as known by science' as the real world, the solid foundation underpinning the 'apparent' world of everyday human affairs. But it is equally possible to see our everyday experience – of furniture, and friends and so on – as primary, as providing the frame of reference that makes possible the various abstractions of science and expert knowledge, and as providing the only real context in which these abstractions can be applied and tested. This is the message of the most influential antipositivist philosophies of knowledge, such as the 'phenomenological' and 'hermeneutic' approaches. This is not the place to do justice to these approaches, but a short summary of their central tenets will serve to sum up much of the ground I have covered so far.

These approaches emphasise the distinctiveness and the priority of the human world, the world of our consciousness and language. If we had to do an inventory of the kinds of things there are, we ought to be struck by the immediacy and all-pervasiveness of some apparently non-physical things – namely, states of mind and meanings. (Some thinkers would argue that these are the only things whose existence we can be sure of!) Human history and culture are made up of meanings and stories, as are our individual lives, and all of these things can only be properly understood and known about by taking these meanings seriously, rather than dismissing them in favour of some spurious 'science'. In fact, the stories that weave our domestic furniture into our lives indicate a reality just as substantial as the stories that scientists tell about the material of which they are made.

This suggests a different relationship between expert and lay 'knower'. Instead of seeing the lay person as 'falling short' of knowledge, as essentially ignorant, these approaches see the processes of 'everyday knowing' as entirely continuous with, and the basis of, more specialised forms of knowledge. Many important forms of expertise are simply more practised, more disciplined, and hence more developed versions of so-called ordinary 'lay' practices. In these instances there are differences of degree rather than kind. The basic (and perhaps also the highest) form of expertise, which is open to all, is to know how to operate as a member of the human community, to be able to understand what others are saying, to have a sense of what matters, and to be able to contribute to one another's lives and well-being.

Parenthesis

I remember the shock when Dad rang to say Mum had got cancer the first time. It was a few minutes before I reacted. I sat down and kept looking in the direction of the television programme I had been watching. Outwardly the world was the same but it had been transformed. After a few minutes the first signs of this began to trickle through in waves of messy and contradictory feelings. Of course, I had no idea about the long years of upheaval ahead – the activity, the waiting, the uncertainty, the drama, and the routine that would dominate our lives, a flood that would sweep us and all our lives along, hurling the familiar aside, ripping up our bearings, and yet demanding sanity and steadiness. In that first few days it was relatively simple: there was concern for Mum and Dad, there was the imperative to be 'OK', there was hurt and fear to be kept at bay, and there was the urgent need to understand what was happening at the hospital; what the successive tests indicated, what the implications were, what was being done, what more could be done.

Those early hospital visits had two aspects. Here was the site of intervention, here were drips and dressings, here was technical expertise. Yet there was my mum, out of place, and with her spirit quietened. She was also determined to be OK, but with a burden she couldn't quite displace from her face. The face of health care and my mum's face locked together. With the foolishness of a young man, I wanted a quick technical fix; I was impatient for progress, I wanted to reassure everyone (not least myself) that everything would soon be alright. But, of course, even if a relatively quick fix had been possible it would not have met Mum's immediate needs. Her life was overturned, she was away from her home, surrounded by strangers and strangeness, the 'taken for granted' gone, and she was alone.

PART TWO – CARING KNOWLEDGE

What are the connections between knowledge and caring? There are many, and they depend, of course, on what we mean by 'caring'. I will sketch out two possible connections by way of an introduction to this half of the chapter.

First, *caring can be seen as an application of knowledge* – in order to care for someone (assuming a health service context for now), there are a great many things we need to know. Some of these things fall clearly into the category of scientific and technical knowledge. Diagnostic procedures, from pulse rates and temperatures to sophisticated imaging techniques, are one example. They enable us to look below the surface, to get beyond the individual's subjectivity. Someone may feel perfectly well, with no desire to be a patient, but a routine screening procedure or the investigation of some apparently trivial anomaly might uncover a 'problem', and a whole clinical journey begins. Despite proper concerns about the medicalisation of life, most of us, most of the time, are grateful for the instruments and techniques of clinical science. However, most of us, most of the time, are in some respects 'squeezed out' by clinical science. When we are unwell we are both the centre of attention and also 'on the margins' – hanging around in the waiting room of science. There are clearly other non-scientific sorts of things we need to know in order to care for someone. We may need to know a great deal about them (depending on how extensive our interactions with them are), e.g. how they feel, what their hopes, fears, memories, beliefs, opinions are; we may need to know about their home life, friends and relatives, work, leisure, cultural and religious life. In short, we need to get to know about them as a person, and the social and cultural network that shapes their identity.

But this takes us into a different realm, and a second sort of connection between knowledge and caring. Up to now the implication has been that knowledge is a mine of general and specific 'information' that we deploy when we care for someone, and that we need different sorts of knowledge because people are complex beings. This is to rely on an encyclopaedic picture of knowledge. But as we have already seen, this is an inadequate picture for many purposes. What is crucial is not knowing in the abstract, but embodied knowledge, or know-how. To care for someone, even if that someone is construed as an object of scientific knowledge, I have to be prepared to work *with* that person. To care for someone *as a person* I have, to some extent, to get *to know them,* and not just 'about them' in the abstract. Indeed, a substantial component of caring for someone is precisely paying attention to, and concerning oneself with, the person for whom one is caring. This is one of the respects in which caring can be seen as a form of knowledge, and not merely the application of knowledge. This may seem an odd way of talking but it serves to emphasise a number of things, which I will merely assert here.

Caring is not some warm, 'wishy-washy' feeling but an exacting and demanding set of skills, which exercises all of our faculties and judgement (including our 'emotional judgement'); it is a form of know-how that admits of degrees of expertise and is developed through practice and experience as well as reflection. To be 'a caring person' is not an alternative to being an intelligent person, it is necessarily an exercise of intelligence.

In what follows I hope to illustrate and defend these assertions, and also to indicate some of the challenges of caring as a form of expertise. In particular I want to look at: (a) the relation between technical and person-centred elements of caring; (b) the idea of 'emotional expertise'; and (c) the ways in which cultural and institutional contexts affect the possibilities of caring. These issues are closely interrelated but here I will separate them out as far as I can. But I will start with another and different distinction, which could be a source of confusion. Caring has both a practical and an affective side. We can use the label *'caring for'* to indicate the practical dimension of caring. If I care for someone then I look after them, give them food or medicines, tend to their needs, and make sure the environment is suitable for them, that they are comfortable or sufficiently stimulated, etc. I might also care for them by listening to them, by treating them with respect, by ensuring that they don't feel ignored, etc. We can use the label *'caring about'* to indicate the affective dimension of caring. If I care about someone then I have feelings of concern or regard towards them, and to some degree their welfare matters to me. If we care about someone, we are inclined to want to look after them, but the two do not necessarily coincide. At least up to a point we can care for someone without caring about them, and vice versa.

Technical and person-centred caring

In drawing a distinction between technical and person-centred facets of care, I am not referring to the practical/affective distinction discussed above; rather, I mean to draw attention to two interconnected elements of practical care, or 'caring for'. What I mean by technical care is all the care that derives from technical knowledge, or, more precisely, knowledge that treats the individual as an object to which generalisations apply. What I mean by person-centred care is care that depends upon regarding the individual as a unique subject, as a particular person with a distinct biography, outlook, and set of preferences. In the main, 'technical caring' and 'person-centred caring' are complementary.

Human beings can be seen quite properly as both part of the 'world as known by science', and part of the human world. They are made up of both matter and meaning. If we want to understand them, and care for them, we must take equally seriously those aspects of them that can be generalised about and those that cannot. It is not very easy to draw a definite line here, but some things are certainly appropriate objects for technical knowledge (e.g. blood, bones, and bodies generally), and some things certainly require a more person-centred approach (e.g. listening to someone's 'story'). Both these aspects of care are important. If we are interested in 'technical success', we are likely to focus on health 'outcomes'; if we are interested in 'success with persons', we might look at whether the person feels valued.

These two aspects of care are often complementary but there are also respects in which they can be in tension with one another. They are complementary because if we want to achieve good outcomes this itself can provide motivation to work closely with a patient and treat them with respect. Their compliance and/or their positive state of mind might contribute to the technical success we want. This gives us an instrumental and derivative reason to value people (although the real direction of derivation is the opposite – technical success is valuable because people are valuable). It is tempting to emphasise this complementariness, and indeed to go further and say that we should not even separate out these two elements of caring, that there is only good caring, which must integrate these elements. This may be true in practice but it is also necessary to be aware of the possible tensions between these elements.

A mind set, or a set of practices, which is geared to treating people as objects for technical intervention is not necessarily one well suited to responding to persons. Partly this relates to the costs of a 'conveyor belt' approach to human dignity and sensibilities, but it has widespread ramifications. Many of the routine, but important, issues in health care ethics spring out of these tensions. For example, a specific drug may be routinely prescribed and regarded as optimal for a specific condition, but should it be prescribed if the patient has a considered preference for something else and there are alternatives available? A father wishes to delay a critical operation on his daughter until after his partner flies in from overseas – how far should these wishes be respected? Whatever is for the best here, these alternatives may not even come to light unless the environment is relatively 'person-centred'.

Achieving the right balance between these two elements of care will serve as an example of why caring is an exacting business. Not only does it potentially call upon a wide range of knowledge but it depends upon integrating different sorts of considerations together. This means paying attention to both technical and personal factors, and gaining confidence and experience in making continuous practical and moral judgements. However, this example may give the impression that what I principally have in mind is some kind of cognitive or intellectual challenge – the difficulty of 'weighing together' different considerations. Although I am happy to see this as an intellectually exacting process, I also have in mind the fact that it is, at the same time, emotionally exacting, and that it is the need for 'emotional expertise' that marks out the real challenge, and the special intelligence, of caring.

Emotional expertise

I am using the expression 'emotional expertise' to refer to the know-how at the heart of caring. Some people will dislike the expression and the whole idea of emotional expertise. There is a common view that emotions are things that 'just happen' to us; that we 'suffer' them rather than 'do' them. This being the case, how does it make sense to talk of developing expertise with regard to them? In addition, does not talk of expertise imply that there are 'emotional experts', that some people are 'good at emotions' and other people 'bad at emotions', and is this not unnecessarily elitist and divisive? I have sympathy for these thoughts, and I have deliberately chosen the label 'emotional expertise' because it provokes them, but on balance I see these reactions as misguided. I think that in some respects: (a) we are responsible for emotions; and (b) it is possible to be more or less skilful and conscientious in the exercise of these responsibilities. What is more, this is not just my opinion but it is a view endorsed by a great deal of ancient and modern thought and scholarship. Of course, 'emotional expertise' is an umbrella term, and using it may obscure many complexities and controversies; there would no doubt be disagreement about its components and how they can be combined.

One tradition with bearing on this matter is discussion of 'the virtues', i.e. admirable and desirable qualities of character, such as courage or wisdom. Although 'virtues' may sound like an archaic term, we still operate with closely related ideas. For example, we write 'character references' for people, and in so doing we may talk of their honesty, loyalty, tenacity, fairness, balance, and so on. We admire friends or acquaintances for who they are and not just for what they achieve. If we are bringing up children we typically want them to be 'good' – to be people whom others respect for their integrity and dispositions. In all of these cases, we are concerned with 'the virtues'. In Western academic philosophy, the discussion of the virtues normally begins with reference to Aristotle's ethics but there has been a continuing thread of discussion on this theme, and virtue theory, including Aristotle's related work, has had a substantial revival during the past 20 years.

I cannot do justice to these academic debates here. But perhaps I can indicate a few important issues arising from them. First, we are inclined to hold people as *to some extent* responsible for their character (although, of course, many other factors outside an individual's control help to determine character). Both religious teachings and the huge self-improvement industry are testament to the belief that we can make a difference to the ways we think and act, to the kinds of people we are. Second, character is not just about how we reason at some abstract level, but it is also about how we feel about things, how we respond to things, and what our inclinations and desires are. If both of these claims are true then it follows that we are to some degree responsible for our emotional life, that it is possible to conceive of emotional development, perhaps even of emotional education or learning. This, in broad terms, is certainly what is entailed by much of the literature on the virtues.

Commentary 2.3

I suppose what I am getting at here is fairly straightforward: there are people we admire because they are good with others. They may possess talents and skills in this regard that we may not. Do we think that these qualities are just part of life's lottery, or do we, to some degree, feel that these 'role models' have earned our respect? I think the latter. Furthermore, if we want to aspire to some of these admirable qualities I think we need to try to become more clear about what these talents are and how they can be developed.

Perhaps I can make this seem more plausible by using an example. Imagine a young man who is very jealous about his girlfriend. If he sees her talking for any time to other people he feels anxious and resentful, and these feelings can easily collapse into despair or anger. We might say that he 'cannot help' feeling like that, perhaps even that these feelings are 'natural'. We might feel sorry for him (and his girlfriend!). It is unfair to say that he should just 'snap out of it'. But notice what a difference the facts make. Suppose his girlfriend has never given him any reason to be jealous; suppose we have it on the best authority that nothing in her actions or in her heart should give him cause to worry. We would surely draw this to his attention. We would ask him to re-appraise the situation, and over the course of time we would hope that he would come to see things differently and, as a result, to some degree to feel

differently. If we were speaking bluntly we might say, 'You've got to learn not to feel like that!'

Now this example works because so many emotions, including jealousy, are intimately related to our beliefs about the world. So if our beliefs are unreasonable (or irrational), then the emotions that relate to them will be, to use a neutral-sounding phrase, 'somehow inappropriate'. Of course you cannot just switch your beliefs or feelings on or off. It takes time and practice to change. Consider a visitor who is frightened by being close to a cancer patient, or a novice nurse who feels nervous and inadequate when performing routine procedures. In these cases too we might be sympathetic while, at the same time, hoping that they would learn not to have these feelings. Notice that this is about emotional change and not just about covering feelings up, which is also a necessary, but different, aspect of managing our emotions. In all the examples above we might expect the individuals to attempt to cover up their feelings as a short-term strategy; in other instances, it may be necessary to learn to 'put up a front' in the longer term. (Managing our own emotions involves a combination of change and 'acting' – here I am discussing the former rather than the latter, but I ought to at least make reference to the need for some 'acting', and of course the inherent problems of inauthenticity and self-alienation.)

Virtue theory is based on the insight that our understanding, feelings, and dispositions form compounds such that we cannot effectively develop these elements separately. Someone who is prudent (or honest, etc) sees the world in certain ways, feels in certain ways, and acts in certain ways; this is what is involved in having a virtue. Of course there is room for debate about which set of virtues we believe people in general should aspire to (and also about the virtues most fitting for certain roles or positions). Similarly, it is unclear exactly how far, and in what respects, our character is capable of being shaped by our learning and practice. However, it would seem foolish and irresponsible (and fly in the face of our experience) to dismiss completely the notion of character development, and with it the notion of emotional learning and growth.

This discussion of virtues has concentrated primarily on self-development and on managing our own emotions, but what has this got to do with caring for others? Perhaps it is obvious. The jealous boyfriend is not in a good position to care for his girlfriend. The visitor who is frightened of cancer is not well placed to care for the patient. The nurse who feels self-conscious and inadequate is going to be less helpful to her patients than she might be. We cannot really aspire to deal with other people's concerns and feelings unless we are dealing with our own. I will not stress this point again but I hope that it will be seen as the back-cloth to what follows.

As we have seen, a crucial aspect of caring for persons is to relate to them as persons and not as objects. There are other aspects of caring that do not depend quite so much on this. For example, we could say that a government cares – practically cares – for the population by introducing clean-air legislation (or other health-protection mechanisms). In the case of these interventions, people can be treated as biological creatures (although there will usually be accompanying processes of consultation and education as well). One way of bringing out the differences is to ask how far the technology in our hospitals and health centres could take over from human beings. There are, no doubt, areas where it makes little or no difference whether a machine or a human being does the caring, but there are others where it seems to make all the difference in the world. If we are in a room full only of technology, we are still alone. Here, again, is the double-aspect of persons – we are made of both matter and meaning, of both stuff and subjectivity. If we are to be 'treated' properly then both components need responding to, and our subjectivity can only be recognised and responded to by another's subjective awareness. Of course, if a human carer behaves exactly like a piece of technology, like a sophisticated robot going through procedures, then the fact that they are a person makes no difference. What is this special ingredient of caring of which human beings are capable? I will borrow the term 'emotional labour' to describe it.

A number of social scientists and feminist scholars has used this term to indicate a substantial and vital, but typically neglected, sphere of human activity and relationship, i.e. the hard work that goes into acknowledging and meeting one another's emotional needs. Most of this work is unpaid, but it goes on in every setting and context. It is largely and characteristically undertaken by women. It is often informal and invisible – it tends to take place 'behind the scenes', to be off the official agenda (some parts of health care, and pastoral care in education are, to varying degrees, exceptions). In a climate in which measurable public 'outputs' are valued, emotional labour is likely to be grossly undervalued, if not unnoticed. (This is itself a good enough reason to adopt the term.)

Different scholars will write about different facets of emotional labour, and will continue, no doubt, to use the term to mean rather different things. It is, I think, a strength of the term that it can be used to refer to a wide range of things. But here I am borrowing it simply to help capture some of what is entailed by the affective aspect of caring. To think of caring as 'hard work' suggests not only that it is strenuous but also that it is skilful. To talk of 'caring' may sound wishy-washy to many people; to talk of 'emotional labour' sounds – I think helpfully – as if you might be indicating a form of expertise, a demanding discipline. (However, there is the danger that we might start thinking of the affective aspect of caring as if it were some technical and highly esoteric skill, which would be most unfortunate.)

One way of indicating some of the expertise required to be an effective 'emotion worker' is to consider the range of relevant factors. Clearly, affective care has to be responsive to circumstances and to individuals. There is something farcical about thinking one could go around indiscriminately caring for people. Furthermore, it is downright intrusive and disrespectful to assume a licence to work upon other people's emotional well-being. Most of the time all we need to achieve is what might be called 'good manners', by being polite, and hopefully reasonably kind and sensitive to the people we meet. As part of this process we may notice that they appear upset, or anxious, or cross, and we may tailor our words and deeds to their manner to some degree, but it is not generally part of our brief to do more than that. Everything depends upon our relationship with them, and the circumstances under which we are meeting. Are they friends or strangers? Are we in a bus queue or in a self-help group?

The same applies within health care settings: just because we are in a professional role and are practically caring for someone, it does not follow that we should be paying any *special* attention to their specific emotional or psychological needs. Most importantly, they may not want that sort of attention; in addition, it may not be a fitting part of the task in hand. The 'emotional labour' required may be fairly circumscribed. Someone who is taking blood samples from a series of patients in a waiting room needs to be able to be as reassuring and as gentle as possible, while doing their job effectively and efficiently. It is also useful to be able to recognise, and to be patient with, individuals who are unusually frightened of that procedure. But it would be completely out of place for them to strike up a conversation about the patient's deeper worries. What is fitting will thus depend, amongst other things, upon (a) what the individual person needs and wants; (b) the nature of the professional role; (c) whether the relationship has a history and/or a future; and (d) the particular characteristics and personal styles of the two people involved.

Furthermore, 'emotional labour' rarely occurs on its own, and this makes even greater demands. Most of the time when we are caring for someone, we are doing something practical or technical. As a necessary part of these practical interventions, we will have regard to emotional matters. We may choose to comfort someone physically, or to listen to their point of view, or provide some occasional companionship, but in order to do these things well we often need to be fully engaged with the whole of their care. If we are listening to someone who is about to be discharged home and is concerned about how they are going to cope, it helps if we have some insight into what they are saying (and in turn this may involve a knowledge of their clinical condition, their medication, their attitudes, their family, home services, etc). This is not necessarily because we are in a better position to do something about their concerns (although we may be) but because we are better able to listen, better able to hear what they are saying and to understand it. Sometimes people just need attention and recognition, but often what they really

value is 'informed attention'. It is this compound of technical and emotional expertise that is so characteristic of health care and particularly of nursing.

Supporting care

Until now I have concentrated on the difference that individuals can make, but it is not all a question of individual responsibility. In many respects individuals can only do what circumstances allow, and we all require the support of each other and of the right policies and cultures. There are some deep philosophical and practical questions raised here, which I will pass over very quickly. First, it is very difficult to separate out individual and collective responsibility. The debate about criminality is a familiar one – how far, and when exactly, should we hold individuals responsible for a crime rather than seek explanations in the various pressures and contexts that help to shape them? It is broadly the same debate with virtues as with vices. In professional roles we should certainly expect that individual practitioners will be motivated not to fall below certain minimal standards of practice, but can the wider society expect them to be motivated to aspire to, and strive for, ideals of best practice? I would argue that the latter is an unrealistic expectation unless a good deal of thought and effort is put into creating supportive contexts for professional work. This takes us on to a second set of puzzles, i.e. what counts as a 'supportive context'.

Commentary 2.4

In this final section I am trying to correct a possible overemphasis in the previous discussion. What I have called personal knowledge is essential but it cannot stand on its own. It is no good simply saying that everyone should 'pull themselves up by their own boot straps', and miraculously develop the caring virtues. We need to think hard as a society (and institutionally) about how we can support each other's development. We need to understand more about personal knowledge and 'emotional expertise' in particular. I think it is partly about putting these discussions firmly at the top of the agenda along with other important topics such as budgets, etc.

I will not try to solve these puzzles in this chapter (nor could I!) but I will try to suggest some factors that need to be borne in mind. These questions about fashioning the context of professional work can draw upon a variety of forms of knowledge. There is a lot of relevant work in management studies, organisational theory, economics, social psychology, social policy, sociology, and so on, as well as practical expertise relating to leadership or team working, etc. But, as always, it is vital that those who are developing or applying these forms of knowledge are asking the 'right questions'. It seems to me that all too often those voices that are most influential in policy making neglect important questions. Efficiency and health gain are most important but we also need to ask 'How can institutions and cultures be developed in ways that underpin and that foster "caring expertise"?'. Health care is about health and care, and it is foolish to assume that these two are the same and that whatever delivers one will deliver the other. (Of course, some people may wish to develop the argument that at some level these two concepts converge in important ways – but that is a different matter.)

There are two related sets of reasons for this relative neglect of caring:

- a policy climate increasingly dominated by 'outputs', the language of audit and the use of performance indicators, which by their very nature are reductionist
- the ambiguities and complexities surrounding the notion of caring, which make it difficult to have a confident public debate about, let alone to accommodate this debate to, an 'output-orientated' policy climate.

Both of these sets of reasons are worth attending to and I will say a little more about the relationships between them shortly. But on this occasion I have concentrated more on this second set of reasons. I am conscious of the difficulties of treating caring with due seriousness. It is all too easy to retreat into sentimentality or wishful thinking, and to deal in vague generalisations. We are inclined to see it as a question of instinct or intuition, perhaps something it is counter-productive to theorise about (rather like humour). I think

there is a lot to be said for this attitude; there is a limit to how far we should, as individuals, be self-conscious and analytical about dispositions and skills that need to become 'second nature' if they are to be truly effective. But I believe we do need to be self-conscious about these questions as citizens, or as professional groups, and to ask how we, collectively, can create conditions under which this particular embodied form of knowledge can be acknowledged and nourished. One issue that can be used to illustrate this sort of question is the use of time. It is a crucial issue because underlying the output-orientated culture is the imperative to allocate public resources efficiently. The time of health professionals is, in every sense, the most valuable resource of health services and is itself necessarily rationed.

Anyone who has visited their general practitioner (GP) will understand how time creates certain caring possibilities. There is a limit to what can be done in a 5–10-minute consultation. A GP, especially if they are of a holistic persuasion, may well ask about your home or work circumstances – are you under stress, or do you have specific problems that are keeping you awake? They may also ask about your diet, exercise patterns, and so on, and they will have to consider whatever condition or concern brought you there in the first place. All of this is good practice and may well throw up important clues to improving your health. But the time pressures on the consultation will powerfully shape the structure and the 'feeling' of the interaction. The process will nearly always be informed by the move towards some 'intervention' on the part of the GP, whether it be encouragement, advice, treatment, or referral. Two things will rarely be possible: (a) the doctor simply listening to an extended account of this range of life-related problems, prompted by their questioning; and (b) a careful negotiation of a shared understanding of some of these factors. Yet both of these things can be, depending on the case at hand, vital foundations for certain forms of caring. This shortcoming is not necessarily a problem – the limitations on these particular consultations are widely understood and accepted. But if, under budgetary pressures, a predominantly instrumental style of interaction increasingly comes to be seen as the appropriate model of personal interaction across a range of settings, the potential for caring relationships in professional health services will be greatly diminished.

There are many other things we need to understand in more depth. For example, what sorts of professional support enable different practitioners to sustain person-centred caring over years? How can we effectively encourage practitioners to find their own style of 'emotional expertise' and to know when they are at the limits of their competence? How can we create settings with the right balance of generalist and specialist 'emotional expertise'? Above all, how can policy making give proportionate emphasis to both technical and person-centred facets of care, and to both 'health gain' and caring processes? The first step to a better understanding is to ensure that we give proper respect to, and consideration of, the whole range of forms of expertise that people possess. We should not take caring for granted; we should not assume that we understand it, we should not treat is as a fixed 'natural resource' that can be deployed in any set of circumstances. It is a precarious and priceless form of knowledge.

Postscript

I do not really want to say anything about my mum's death or dying. It still seems too private to talk about (especially in such a public place). And I certainly don't want to imply that there is some kind of wisdom, some kind of caring, that could 'make it right'. Suffering cannot be denied. But, of course, there are also good things and gratitude. All of those people who supported her, and us, through the upheavals of her last few years did something immensely precious. Friends, neighbours and colleagues spring to mind, but so do people who were once strangers, people who were 'just doing their job'. There were mistakes, misunderstandings, insensitivities, and general clumsiness mixed up in all of this, but what should we expect? Human beings are pretty imperfect creatures and caring is such a demanding business. Care has so many faces, and serves so many ends, and different compounds are needed from instance to instance.

I am grateful for the technical expertise, for the people who listened or provided companionship, for those who understood the practical routines, for the kind touches, for the opportunities for laughter and for many other things. It seems to me – and I admit I'm biased – that both my parents were exceptionally brave and good during these ordeals (although of course they 'failed' too sometimes), and they were lucky to have each other and their family around. There is a limit to what 'professional carers' can do, and there is a limit to what can be expected of them. Yet, at the same time, within these limits there is scope for an infinite amount of good.

At the thanksgiving service for my mum, as before and since, people celebrated her. They spoke about her gentle and sympathetic nature. In my opinion gentleness cannot be overrated, but I don't see these good qualities as entirely passive or as just 'natural', such that they cannot be learned or practised. It seems possible for us to be more or less alive to other people's needs. Our capacity for this may vary from time to time and according to many other factors. But some people seem to be very good at it. They are able to generate a powerful current of attention that places other people at the centre of things. This is how my mum's friends and (albeit in different ways) her patients and acquaintances knew her and remember her.

Acknowledgements and further reading

First, I would like to say thank you to my mum, Joan Ashton Cribb. Thanks are also due to a few close friends and colleagues who encouraged me to write this chapter and gave me helpful comments on it. There are other debts unacknowledged in the text; indeed, I do not claim any originality for what I have written. I have no doubt been influenced by many things, only some of which I could even bring to mind. One of the more conspicuous influences (to those with an interest in philosophy) is Gilbert Ryle's discussion of 'Knowing how and knowing that' and subsequent work on the same theme (Ryle G. (1945). *Proceedings of the Aristotelian Society* **XLVI**, 1–16;

Nyiri J.C. and Smith B. (1988). *Practical Knowledge: Outline of a Theory of Traditions and Skills.* London: Croom Helm.). There are plenty of references to work on 'caring' in other chapters but I have explicitly drawn on two traditions of related work – virtue theory and work on emotional labour in health care (see for example, Pence G. (1984). Recent work on the virtues, *American Philosophical Quarterly* **21**, 281–297; Smith P. (1992). *The Emotional Labour of Nursing.* Basingstoke: Macmillan Press, Basingstoke).

For those interested in thinking in greater depth about some of the issues raised in this chapter, I suggest a couple of possible starting points – Hollis M. (1994). *The Philosophy of Social Science, an Introduction.* Cambridge: Cambridge University Press; Oakley J. (1992). *Morality and the Emotions.* London: Routledge.

CHAPTER THREE

Cancer, care, and society

Christopher Bailey

Cancer probably affects most of us in some way, directly or indirectly. We may, professionally or informally, provide care for someone who has cancer. We may have or have had cancer ourselves. Someone we know has probably had cancer. We hear about it, read about it, and see images of it. Cancer and cancer treatments are sometimes written about in our newspapers in terms that evoke images of war, weaponry, and violent assault. The chief executive of a major cancer charity, for example, is quoted as saying that tamoxifen is 'an important addition to the armoury of therapies' available to treat women with breast cancer;[1] another drug is described as 'targeting' cell protein and 'suffocating' the tumour 'to death'.[2] An article from 2005 describes scientists as claiming to be developing a system to 'kill cancer cells with a single blast of ultrasound', and quotes a doctor as explaining that 'the ultrasound-activated bubbles target with single-cell precision so that the technique is like sniping at specific cancer cells'.[3] *The Sun* newspaper reported that the breast cancer drug Herceptin (Genentech, Inc) 'seeks out problem genes and locks onto them' using monoclonal antibodies like 'mini-rockets'.[4] Another article from *The Sun* speaks of the 'latest weapon in the war on cancer' as 'microscopic missiles which seek out and destroy tumour cells':

> The futuristic treatment . . . mirrors the nano-bots used by the Borg in *Star Trek: The Next Generation*.

> Tiny beads, called nanoparticles, bombard tumour cells with cancer killing drugs while leaving healthy ones unharmed . . . Depending on the type of tumour they're targeting, the particles will latch on to the outside of cancer cells and stop them working, or penetrate the cells and destroy them.
>
> *The Sun*, 3 November 2005[5]

The message behind this kind of language seems to be that cancer is such a formidable challenge that in order to confront it, we must draw upon the fighting spirit that sustains us, against the odds, in wartime, and upon our belief in the superiority of our technology and military power.

There is another kind of message about cancer and cancer treatment in the media that is softer and less confrontational. This is that some treatments offer to prevent or protect us from cancer. Embryo selection, for example, although controversial, is seen by some as a possible means of allowing women with a history of breast cancer to have healthy children. So for some people, this is 'good preventative medicine', for others, it is part of a distasteful 'quest for perfection'.[6] Some cancer experts speak of the potential of lifestyle changes to achieve long-term control of cancer and make cancer 'like diabetes':

> More than a third of cancer deaths worldwide have preventable causes that could be tackled by changing people's behaviour and their environment . . . The impact of smoking on several cancers is well known,

but alcohol use, unsafe sex, low fruit and vegetable intake, obesity, lack of exercise, contaminated injections and indoor smoke from fuels are also risks that could be reduced.

The Guardian, 18 November 2005[7]

Vaccination against cancer is described in terms that mirror the language applied to other forms of preventable disease:

Vaccination against cervical cancer could become as common in schools as jabs against meningitis are now, following the dramatic results of the latest clinical trials.

The Guardian, 8 October 2005[8]

Perhaps what cancer stories in the media demonstrate is that in some ways we are moving away from a position of highest alert against cancer as a deadly and imminent threat, to a position that reflects greater confidence in our ability to protect ourselves, metaphorically speaking, without always being on the offensive. This must surely be a less frantic frame of mind for us, as a society, to be in. In some cases, we can see the two positions side by side, and perhaps this is a more accurate representation of where we are collectively. The same article that speaks of the possibility of creating a vaccine to 'protect' against human papilloma virus, for example, also refers to the possibility of treating cancer by teaching the immune system 'to recognise the enemy within – and attack it before it causes potentially fatal disease'.[8]

'Cancer' is sometimes applied metaphorically to situations outside health care, to express horror at the threat to some cherished, and previously vigorous and healthy part of society:

Nigeria's Anglican Church says that the US branch of the church is a 'cancerous lump' that should be 'excised'. Nigerian bishops were responding to a proposal from the Archbishop of Canterbury Rowan Williams last week. He had suggested the introduction of a two-tier system of church membership to avoid complete disintegration over the issue of homosexuality . . . 'A cancerous lump in the body should be excised if it has defied every known cure', [the Nigerian bishops] say. 'To attempt to condition the whole body to accommodate it will lead to the avoidable death of the patient.'

BBC News, 4 July 2006[9]

In 1997 the Labour Party denounced the private finance initiative (PFI) as creeping privatisation. They asked senior doctors to sign a letter in which they described the internal market as a cancer eating away at the NHS . . . If the government does not heed the doctors' warnings, the cancer they correctly diagnosed eight years ago will destroy the NHS.

The Guardian, 27 June 2005[10]

Frank Field yesterday launched the latest salvo in his post-resignation fightback with an assault on spin doctors, whose activities he called a cancer at the heart of the Government . . . He said: 'Sadly, this whole episode shows the real need for that. In the long run, you cannot run a government like this. It's a cancer that will eat away at the heart of our very existence and undermine the way ministers behave'.

The Guardian, 4 August 1998[11]

This is another side of the war with cancer, where cancer is attacking the healthy social body, as opposed to the physical body. Here, cancer is a *moral* threat, something unremittingly *bad*. For those whose lives are affected by cancer, the implication can clearly be that there is something bad about their lives, their loved ones, or *them*.

Susan Sontag believed that cancer 'is a metaphor for what is most ferociously energetic, and these energies constitute the ultimate insult to the natural order' (p.72).[12] It is, she suggests, a metaphor for what is *not* good and *not* right, for forces opposed to the flourishing and harmonious side of our lives. In health care, the 'war against cancer' goes on; but the importance to us of the *idea* of health extends beyond formal health care systems. If parts of society 'have cancer' they too might need treatment to put them right: the 'cancerous lump' must be 'cut away'. Health and health care thus provide a model for maintaining order that applies not only to our physical selves, but also to ourselves as good citizens and to the good governance of our institutions. The importance we place on the 'war against cancer' reflects not only our desire to put our bodies right, but also our determination to keep ourselves and our communities in good working order.

Cancer is part of the everyday lives of thousands of people, yet it often seems anything but 'everyday'. Each day thousands of people learn, or realise, or suspect, or fear that they have cancer; they learn that their mother or father, or son or daughter, or wife or husband or partner, or friend, or neighbour or aunt, cousin, niece, or nephew has cancer. We don't even have to have cancer to be frightened of it. Here, a researcher working with people with cancer is talking about her fears:[13]

> When I started working with people with cancer (five years ago, and before engaging in my current work at this research unit) it was at the front-lines in more of a supportive role. For the first couple of months I had dreams that I had cancer and I would feel overwhelmed when I met roomfuls of people with cancer . . . the way that I think that most people think that cancer is the harbinger of death. It took me a couple of months to integrate the work and for the nightmares to stop [p.279].

Claudine Herzlich and Janine Pierret, French sociologists whose studies of illness are based on collections of personal experiences, refer to cancer as the 'most frightening illness of all'.[14] It is so frightening in fact that cancer is a word that sometimes cannot be spoken: a word that, if spoken, 'condemns the sufferer', as if by magic. In France, say Herzlich and Pierret, it is rarely publicly acknowledged that people have died of cancer; rather, they are said to have died after 'a long and painful illness'. They record conversations that reflect the 'quasi-magic image' or the 'phantasms' of contagion, which affect both people with cancer and those who are not ill themselves.

Despite modern pathology, which has transformed much of our understanding of illness, anxiety in our society still 'crystallises' around one 'scourge' of illness that is totally associated with death: cancer, according to Herzlich and Pierret, has become the 'very embodiment of physical suffering' for us.[14] It is the 'specific illness of our society', '*the* illness of our time', so dominant that it sometimes seems to be the '*only* illness' (p.55). Cancer, they say, is the modern equivalent of the 'age-old scourges', and like diseases in the past, it is 'fraught with phantasms of rot invading the body, and animals that gnaw and destroy it' (p.56).

They point to two 'conceptions' or themes in the aetiology of cancer, which illustrate how cancer has become the 'prototype' of modern illness:

> One of them sees it as an illness of the individual, the other as a disorder of our way of life and of society. In fact . . . *cancer is the illness of individuals in their relations with society.* It is indeed an illness of the individual, but this individual can only be conceived of in relation with society as a whole. At the same time cancer is also an illness produced by society, but one that manifests the flaws of the present-day individual [p.62].

Cancer is sometimes seen as a development of certain psychological characteristics, such as repressed or anaesthetised feelings, resignation in the face of life, lack of self-confidence, or an inability to express energy, particularly sexual energy, freely. Deborah Lupton, for example, has drawn attention to the link made between breast cancer and suppression of anger and trying to be 'nice'.[15] The contemporary image of the 'cancer personality' is, Sontag writes, a 'forlorn, self-hating, emotionally inert creature'.[12] Herzlich and Pierret do not agree, however, that this 'schema' reflects the majority of people's ideas of 'cancer as an individual disease'.[14] They emphasise instead that people see themselves as predisposed towards the disease (for example, because they have relatives with cancer), or as 'favourable terrain' for it. At the same time, people often believe that their environment determines their individual behaviour: the ideas of cancer as an individual illness and cancer as an illness produced by society (for example, by pollution) co-exist. Herzlich and Pierret conclude that cancer is experienced both as 'timeless scourge' and as part of the dangers of modern life:[14]

> 'Is cancer a part of myself, or does it come to me from the outside world?' the sick person wonders [p.65].

In the UK, Clive Seale has written extensively on the impact of cancer in the media.[16–20] Seale questions Susan Sontag's view that the language of cancer in both popular and scientific culture is purely militaristic. He proposes that the language we associate with stories of personal experiences of cancer often uses sporting rather than military imagery. Words such as 'fight', 'victory' and 'defence', he argues, can have non-military connotations even if they refer metaphorically to a military context.[16]

Seale's analysis of English language newspaper articles suggests that the language used in stories of personal experiences of cancer often refers both to sporting and military activity. Stories about people with cancer who have some sporting connection are also common. He argues that language with purely military connotations is probably more prevalent in reports of new cures and treatments than it is in accounts of personal experiences of cancer; but it is more appropriate, he says, to describe the language in personal accounts of people with cancer as 'struggle language':[16]

> in which sporting connotations are evoked through the use of military metaphors. This relies on an underlying conception of sport as standing for a life and death struggle. The military arena, on the other hand, is less in tune with contemporary sensibilities, where the celebration of naked violence is often repressed as an illicit pleasure [p.325].

Seale asks us to consider whether there is any real evidence to show, as Sontag and others have argued, that war metaphors have a harmful effect on people who have, or who are concerned about, cancer.[12,16] He suggests that struggle language may actually have an inspiring or supportive effect, and reminds us of those anthropologists:[16]

> who have argued for the therapeutic value of rehearsing illness narratives in a public context [p.326].

Essentially, the argument here is that finding an acceptable way of telling the story of our cancer helps us to live with the illness:[16]

> Sports stories allow cancer to be portrayed as a psychological and spiritual journey, with progression towards a satisfying resolution even where death lies at the end . . . [p.326].

Deborah Lupton, who has written on the representation of breast cancer in the popular press in Australia, makes a slightly different point.[15] In her analysis, the use of phrases that emphasise the positive impact of fighting qualities on cancer survival 'depict the stereotypical passive feminine role as threatening to health' (p.78). At the same time, because women who delay having children, for example to pursue a career, were identified as being at increased risk of developing breast cancer, this expression of female assertiveness was also made to seem dangerous. Women, Lupton suggests, were 'blamed' in press accounts 'regardless of which role they chose to take' (p.78):

> This discourse of victim blaming was central in press representations of breast cancer. In the face of this devastating and dread disease, the press sought to locate the responsibility upon individual women for changing their lifestyles in order to avoid developing breast cancer. The overwhelming message was that 'women should do something to protect themselves' . . . Women who failed to perform . . . recommended actions, press accounts implied, were irresponsible and neglectful of their own health [p.85].

Whether we experience cancer personally, as an individual who is given this diagnosis; or personally through a partner, friend, or relative; or personally, as someone whose responsibility it is to support and care for someone else who has cancer; whether we experience cancer indirectly, through the airwaves, on the screen, on the page, or on the billboard; however we experience it, we are almost always moved by it, and often we find ourselves feeling the need to respond, to shake off a mood, offer some form of help, or perhaps to avoid the subject altogether. It is difficult to see how we can avoid having some stance, some collection of thoughts and feelings, some mixture of the rational and irrational that is evoked by cancer.

My own feelings about cancer and about working with people with cancer have changed over time. When I started out as a student nurse I found cancer a difficult illness, and what sticks in my mind is a feeling that I didn't really know what it was, what kind of 'disease' or 'illness' it was. Caring for people recovering from abdominal surgery for cancer of the colon or rectum seemed to me, as a raw recruit to nursing, to be almost impossibly complicated. People's bodies, after surgery, seemed so radically altered, pieced together, that I was quite disorientated. I marvelled at the dexterity and matter-of-factness of more experienced nurses (who were, in reality, probably only recently or only just qualified).

Cancer was a mysterious disease, and treatment sometimes left people scarred or permanently altered, bowel rerouted to the abdominal wall and protruding discoloured into a large bag. Yet over time, with support from others, a sense of being orientated again, and of the wholeness of people, together with a consciousness of the effects of illness and surgery, returned, though it is probably true to say that a sense of the impact (or collision) of illness and treatment in cancer has remained with me. It is, overall, a feeling I welcome, because it is an incentive not to accept the status quo, a powerful message that we must always question whether accepted or 'normal' practice serves the interests of those who require health care.

Cancer, and sometimes treatment for cancer, can appear to elbow out the person at the centre who is experiencing it; it can be so intimidating, and cause such physical and mental upheavals. The treatment we provide for it is sometimes traumatic, and the feelings it evokes can weigh heavily on us. I wonder sometimes how those more experienced nurses worked with such composure. Was it the composure of confidence or understanding, or did it sometimes include a kind of detachment? Do we sometimes push our feelings about a disease like cancer to the back of our minds? How often have we said, or heard our colleagues say, that if you thought about it all the time, you couldn't do it, almost as if this was a necessary skill for the job? But, don't we all 'think about it' a lot as well? Thinking about it, about cancer, about how it affects people, how it affects us, about how, as a society, we respond to it, both in health care and more widely, in the media, across the dining table, may be vital to understanding. But thinking alone, about such a strange and difficult thing as cancer, may not take us far enough. Talking about it, with our colleagues, our family or friends, with the people we care for, may take us further if we can do it reciprocally and supportively. Indeed, dialogue may be one means of creating the mutual support and the opportunity to express ourselves that we need to be able to understand cancer, our feelings about it, and what we want to achieve professionally. Without this further mutual, exploratory dimension, how easy is it to review

and build upon the joys and sadnesses of the day's or the week's events?

Hochschild writes of our ability to reflectively assess when a feeling is inappropriate and to manage or to *work on* our feelings.[21] This 'emotion work' is different from emotion control or suppression, which, Hochschild suggests, imply an effort to stifle or prevent feeling. Emotion work means shaping as well as suppressing our feelings; it involves invoking desired feelings that are not initially present. Hochschild speaks of 'emotion–work systems', in which dialogue with others – friends, perhaps – assists the process of working on or shaping our feelings; and of being conscious of a moment of 'pinch' or discrepancy between what we feel and what we want to feel.[21] The purpose of working on our feelings is to eliminate this 'pinch'.

In nursing, some theorists have used similar ideas to describe reflective practice. Chris Johns, for example, has written a series of papers and books on the theme of enabling practitioners to learn through reflection on experience.[22–29] By reflecting on experience, Johns believes, we can begin to see the contradictions between the way we think, feel and act, and the values we aspire to in our practice. For him, reflective practice is a way of exploring new ways of acting to realise our values in reality.[29]

Reflection, says Johns:[24]

> offers practitioners a window to look inside themselves and know who they are as they strive towards understanding and realizing the meaning of desirable work in their everyday practices. The practitioner can expose, confront and understand the contradictions between the way she practices and what is desirable. It is the commitment to achieve desirable work that empowers the practitioner to take action to appropriately resolve these contradictions [p.1137].

To achieve this, Johns has developed and repeatedly refined a model of structured reflection. Practitioners are introduced to structured reflection through a 'constant process of analysing supervision dialogue', in the course of which they are given the opportunity to:[22]

> tell their stories of practice and . . . identify, confront and resolve the contradictions between what the

practitioners aim to achieve and actual practice . . . [p.230].

The practitioner is encouraged to reflect on his or her experience with a supervisor who helps to direct the process of exploration and is available during difficult or painful issues. Johns uses the example of supervision dialogue between himself and Caitlin, a team leader on a medical ward, to illustrate the practical applications of structured (or *guided*) reflection.[23] Supervisor and practitioner discuss the care provided for Ray, who has a meningioma. Ray's drug therapy has been discontinued, and as things stand he will soon die, though not at home, as a decision has been taken to keep him in hospital. The dialogue focuses on the question of why Ray has not been asked to participate in the process of reviewing his care, whereas his wife, Lucy, has. Johns, the supervisor, introduces some ideas about dying people and their need to communicate, which, he says, produce an 'a-ha' moment for Caitlin, an 'opening of shutters'. Caitlin takes the decision to be much more open with Ray about his care and treatment, and to engage more closely with his wife Lucy's feelings of unhappiness. Doing so enables Caitlin to facilitate the saying of goodbyes between Ray and Lucy. Johns comments:[23]

> Choosing to give herself to these people is a momentous leap of faith for Caitlin, a metaphoric cocktail of emotions that were difficult to manage and threatened to sweep her away. Perhaps it would be easier for her to remain detached and task-focused so she does not have to concern herself with these issues. Yet, she can no longer do this within her concern for this family and her beliefs about caring [p.37].

For Johns, 'remaining available' or 'true presence' is at the heart of caring: Caitlin's 'leap of faith' is her decision to become more fully open to Ray and Lucy's experience – to 'open the shutters'. Johns' account of his encounter with Tom, who has Parkinson's disease, shows something of what being 'available' can mean:[26]

> He loved his shave. His happiness was for me to take 'Murray Mints', his gift back for my attention, my respect and kindness. In seeking to connect with me, he needed to give something back. By accepting I could honour this need and he could honour himself.

We began to tune into a reciprocal relationship, where I could respond with an appropriate level of involvement with Tom. In this way I synchronized our rhythms of relating to each other at this moment. In tune with him, I was most available to him. I was conscious about how I paid him attention that responded to his feelings and needs, which had made him so happy that morning when he had been so miserable [p.20].

Being 'available', Johns believes, is a 'key therapeutic role' (p.22).[26] For Benner and Wrubel, 'involvement and caring may lead one to experience loss and pain, but they also make joy and fulfilment possible' (p.3).[30] And yet, as Johns acknowledges, there are forces that 'squash' or 'minimise' caring values.[24] The low status and lesser rewards of nursing relative to medical practice, for example, may have led nurses to adopt the values of the dominant group. Caring, it is feared, may have been reduced to a subculture, and it is for this reason that effective means of creating the conditions under which caring beliefs can be realised are urgently needed.[22] It is within the context of this 'minimisation of caring values' that Johns seeks to develop reflective practice, and to establish it as an engine for the regeneration of care.

Caitlin, we must remember, must be well supported to enable her to take the steps she does.[23] She has 'contracted' to meet her supervisor for one hour every three weeks; between meetings she keeps a reflective journal, in which she records her experiences and her responses, guided by a series of 'reflective cues'. Like Benner and Wrubel,[30] Johns believes it is a mistake to think that caring is the cause of 'burnout' and that we should therefore 'protect' ourselves from caring, as if it were a threat:[30]

> Rather, the loss of caring is the sickness, and the return of caring the recovery . . . Although disengagement may numb pain, one is also numbed to the resources and support of others in the situation. Recovery requires rest and respite, but it also requires the reintegration of concern and involvement [p.373].

Rather than seeing caring as the cause of stress, we should hold institutions and systems responsible if they fail to provide the means of developing and sustaining caring practices.[22] Johns explains:[23]

> However profound this process of becoming may seem, it is dependent on the supervisor being available to work with the practitioner. My key role was to balance high challenge with necessary support, so Caitlin did not feel threatened, which would inhibit learning. This was helped by establishing our therapeutic working relationship over several months. How I interpret and respond to Caitlin was a role model of 'being available' for her patients [p.38].

Johns supports and is 'available' for Caitlin through the process of guided reflection in the same way that she is becoming 'available' for people like Ray and Lucy, in a supportive and exploring therapeutic relationship.

It is over 40 years since Isabel Menzies published her famous paper on the organisation of the nursing workforce in a London teaching hospital.[31] Some, myself included, would argue that it still has the power to influence our understanding of the forces that shape the way that nurses work. Menzies believed that the nurses she studied were organised collectively (or socially) in a way that suggested they were trying to defend or protect themselves from anxiety.

Menzies, who was working for the Tavistock Institute of Human Relations in London, was asked for help by the hospital in a project to facilitate organisational change within its nursing service. Trained nurses were, she says, employed to a large extent in 'administrative, teaching, and supervisory roles', while the student nurses were 'in effect, the nursing staff of the hospital at the operational level with patients' (p.44).[31] She describes a situation in which the demand for care within the hospital was such that staffing needs took priority over training needs. The researchers from the Tavistock Institute set about exploring this situation by conducting a series of interviews with nurses, medical and 'lay' staff, and by carrying out observational studies in clinical areas. Over and over again the researchers encountered such high levels of tension, distress, and anxiety among staff that they found it hard to understand how individuals were able to tolerate it. In fact, Menzies reports, there was a great deal of evidence to suggest that nurses were not able to tolerate

such anxiety, and, 'in one form or another, withdrawal from duty was common' (p.45). Menzies explores the nature of the anxiety she believed she had identified in the nurses in this study from a psychoanalytic perspective; and more than 40 years on, her powerful account still thoroughly merits re-reading. Nurses, she says, are:

> . . . in constant contact with people who are physically ill or injured, often seriously. The recovery of patients is not certain and will not always be complete. Nursing patients who have incurable diseases is one of the nurse's most distressing tasks. Nurses are confronted with the threat and reality of suffering and death as few lay people are. Their work involves carrying out tasks which, by ordinary standards, are distasteful, disgusting and frightening. Intimate physical contact with patients arouses strong libidinal and erotic wishes and impulses that may be very difficult to control. The work situation arouses very strong and mixed feelings in the nurse: pity, compassion, and love; guilt and anxiety; hatred and resentment of the patients who arouse those strong feelings; envy of the care given to the patient [p.46].

Nurses, in particular, must:

> allow the projection into them of such feelings as depression and anxiety, fear of the patient and his illness, disgust at the illness and the necessary nursing tasks. Patients and relatives treat the staff in such a way as to ensure that the nurses experience these feelings instead of – or partly instead of – themselves . . . Thus, to the nurses' own deep and intense anxieties are psychically added those of the other people concerned [p.49].

The extraordinary context in which nursing takes place affects us in very powerful ways. The very nature of caring for seriously ill or dying people evokes feelings so strong that they may shape the pattern of work in ways of which we are only partly conscious. In other words, we may organise our care in the way we do to minimise the impact of the situation on us, restricting what we do rather than expanding and exploring the possibilities of care – what Johns might describe as 'squashing' caring values.[24]

Menzies argues that a social organisation such as the nursing service in a hospital develops a mode of functioning that is influenced by a number of interacting factors. These include the organisation's primary task, the technologies available for performing that task, and the needs of the members of the organisation, particularly their need for social and psychological satisfaction and for support in the task of dealing with anxiety. This need, Menzies believes, is especially important.[31] To an extent, indeed, the mode of functioning of a social organisation may be determined by the psychological needs of its members (p.50). The way we care for people with cancer could be shaped or determined, that is to say, by our experience of cancer and the feelings that flow from it. Anxiety, as well as positive, constructive feelings, are part of our experience of caring, and from time to time might lead us to pull in our horns on a personal level and circle the wagons on an organisational level, in an attempt to protect ourselves from harm. Chris Johns' guided reflection is, in effect, a way of helping us to manage the experience of caring for people constructively, a way of providing the support we need to avoid 'pulling in our horns', or 'putting up the shutters' in situations where issues and feelings seem just too intimidating.

Isabel Menzies[31] argues that when members of an organisation are struggling against anxiety, defence mechanisms develop and become part of the organisation. For example, if a nurse experiences anxiety as a result of the closeness and intensity of her relationship with people under her care, the nursing service:

> may attempt to protect her by splitting up her contact with patients. It is hardly too much to say that the nurse does not nurse patients. The total workload of the ward or department is broken down into lists of tasks, each of which is allocated to a particular nurse . . . This prevents her from coming effectively into contact with the totality of any one patient and his illness and offers some protection from the anxiety this arouses [p.51].

The feelings we experience in nursing, unmanaged and unsupported, may cause us to limit our contact with people, or to avoid certain difficult aspects of our relationships with the people we care for in our work. In a more recent language of caring, we are not 'fully present' or 'available'. Some recent research in nursing has suggested that the idea of being fully 'present' or 'available' in caring situations is an idealisation, even fantasy, of what caring can actually be, and that it might be more realistic for nurses to aim to be 'good enough'.[32] Other research in palliative care has pointed to the way in which the notion of a 'good death' may be interpreted, in practice, as a 'good enough' death, with the emphasis on routine medical practices and a prioritisation of physical aspects of symptom management.[33]

It is interesting to reflect on the extent to which the need to protect ourselves is still a factor in the way that nursing is organised today. How much of nursing is a 'social defence system' established to help us avoid certain difficult feelings? And how may nursing change if our need for such strong defences were reduced by more supportive structures, by 'conditions where caring becomes possible'?[23]

Menzies concludes that in the institution she studied:[31]

> The characteristic feature of the social defence system . . . is its orientation to helping the individual avoid the experience of anxiety, guilt, doubt, and uncertainty . . . the potential anxieties in the nursing situation are felt to be too deep and dangerous for full confrontation, and to threaten personal disruption . . . In fact, of course, the attempt to avoid such confrontation can never be completely successful [p.63].

In her opinion, 'true mastery' of the feelings evoked by nursing is most likely to be achieved by 'a deep working-through' of intense situations, a theme familiar to us today, though it may be couched in terms of caring 'visualised and realised through guided reflection'.[24]

Benner and Wrubel describe caring as the producer of *stress* and *coping with* the lived experience of illness.[30] They explain that this is because what we care about *matters* to us and therefore is a potential source of concern to us; at the same time, if we care about something it means something to us, and we therefore commit ourselves to it and involve ourselves in it. This lays the groundwork for coping. Nurses, they say, 'help patients to recover caring, to appropriate meaning, and to maintain or re-establish connection' (p.2).

'Making contact', or understanding the 'lived experience of illness' is at the centre of their account of nursing: it is this principle of openness to others that empowers nurses to grasp the 'daily consequences' of illness, to 'convey acceptance and understanding', and to work with 'thoroughness and attentiveness'(see Benner and Wrubel,[30] Chapter 1). Like Chris Johns, Benner and Wrubel see the ability to be present in the special sense of being accessible and connected as the foundation of nursing as a caring occupation. In their example of 'presencing', a clinical nurse specialist, Mary, describes an interaction with Dave, who has lung cancer:[30]

> He was yelling that he wanted everything packed up. I felt a panic among the staff . . . I went into his room and he yelled at me: 'Are you listening?' I said yes pretty calmly, and he began crying softly and talking. He knew I was listening [p.15].

Mary explains that it is because she is not 'walking out of the door as she walks in' that her relationship with Dave is right; we might say that this is a way of describing 'making contact', or 'being accessible'. Benner and Wrubel[30] explain that it is this 'presence' that makes all the caring, nursing processes that Dave needs from Mary possible. As Mary says:

> . . . during the following weeks we spent some intensive time going over what needed to be accomplished . . . We began concentrating on his issues: chemotherapy at home, volunteers coming into his house, pain management. It was great, because with support he made the most of his time [p.15].

In *Anguish*, the American sociologists Anselm Strauss and Barney Glaser describe the hospital care and treatment of one woman with breast cancer ('Mrs Abel').[34] They introduce for the first time the theory of 'dying trajectories', which can be used as a way of interpreting situations in which it is acknowledged that an individual is going to die. Because the length of time it takes for someone to die varies, as does the certainty with which we can say they will actually die at a specified time, there are a number of possible dying 'trajectories'. A trajectory, Strauss and Glaser explain, 'has shape: it can be graphed. It plunges straight down; it moves slowly downward; it vacillates slowly . . .' (p.12).[34] Dying trajectories

are, they emphasise, what is *perceived* to be the course of dying, and may depart from the *actual* course of dying. They suggest that dying trajectories are an important part of the life of health care institutions: some areas, intensive therapy units for example, are, they say, 'quick dying wards'; others, like the oncology unit, are 'lingering wards'. Crucially, the number of deaths characteristic of a particular ward or unit, and the speed with which deaths characteristically occur, are factors that play a part in shaping the way in which nurses and doctors organise their work.

Mrs Abel, like other people with advanced cancer, was seen as having a 'lingering dying trajectory', a long-term course of dying in hospital: death is acknowledged as certain, though the precise point in time at which it will occur is not known. So the shape of her trajectory was 'of long duration' and moved 'slowly but steadily downward' (p.1). Strauss and Glaser describe how on Mrs Abel's floor staff saw terminal care as 'work', and found the physiological and psychological care of Mrs Abel 'distasteful' (p.6). They preferred to concentrate on people who were getting better, or who were dying less difficult deaths. Dying patients, they say, could 'unwittingly compete with other patients for attention': Mrs Abel, for example, 'continuously wished to talk . . . no matter how pressed they were' (p.7).

Work on the floor had many important 'temporal features' (p.6). There were schedules for feeding patients, bathing, turning in bed, dispensing drugs, administering tests, close observation, and giving treatments. In fact, say Strauss and Glaser, 'the total organisation of activity . . . during the course of dying is profoundly affected by temporal considerations' (p.9).

The story of Mrs Abel ties together an interest in 'temporal features' with another aspect of the organisation of care. Some aspects of care are termed 'non-accountable', which means that nurses and doctors have 'considerable freedom' or 'latitude' in these areas, and do not feel obliged to report, or account for *how* tasks or procedures are carried out (p.10). Strauss and Glaser feel particularly strongly that 'social psychological aspects' of care (relationships, for example) fall into this category. Because psychosocial care is 'non-accountable', it is 'unnoticed'. As such (and this is what happened in Mrs Abel's case), psycho-social care can be allowed to 'disintegrate' (p.10). The *temporal* dimension is vital to any hospital situation because it is a fundamental tool in the organisation of care. We effectively shape the care we give through our use of time. So when the time we spent on something is 'non-accountable' the consequences can be profound. Because the time we spend on psychosocial care is not recorded or accounted for, say Strauss and Glaser, even if we spend less and less time on it, it is unlikely that it will be noticed or that anything will be done to halt the consequences. Unaccountable aspects of care can simply disintegrate without our noticing it.

There are several factors, according to Strauss and Glaser, that change the way in which care is shaped and organised. Diagnosis and prognosis, a person's illness status, nurses' *expectations* are, they feel, particularly important influences. Care is disrupted, becomes problematic, when expectations (for example, 'approximations' of patients' dying trajectories) are not fulfilled. Patients are 'expected to die on schedule' (p.16), and 'when progress turns out to be unusual, personnel may experience a disquieting feeling of having missed certain steps . . . miscalculations can play havoc with the organisation of work' (pp.17–18).[34]

The picture of nurses and doctors we get from *Anguish* is of a group of people whose peace of mind depends upon their ability to predict key events; the last thing we might expect is for one of them to make a 'leap of faith', like Caitlin in Chris Johns' account.[23] But the staff in *Anguish* are not so different from the nurses in Isabel Menzies' study, who sought refuge from the powerful emotions evoked by illness in detachment from their work and from each other. We all, like Caitlin, need a mentor to throw our most difficult feelings about nursing at, and a place to rehearse difficult, unfamiliar nursing 'moves'.

Mrs Abel, the central figure in Strauss and Glaser's account of medical and nursing care,[34] provides a powerful example of how the image of 'the patient' can be constructed. For the researchers Mrs Abel is 'a case', upon which theory is grounded. And while it would be unfair to say that she is treated as if she were part of a laboratory experiment, she is the object of inquiry or inves-tigation, not a participant. She is not invited in, or given a footing in what is essentially her story. Unlike the participants in Chris Johns' accounts, Mrs Abel is not seen as a primary source of knowledge about her situation: rather, it is the researchers who know, and who exercise powers of analysis and illumination. In a similar way, according to Strauss and Glaser, Mrs Abel is seen by her nurses and doctors as having a certain range of behaviour open to her, and her illness is seen as having certain parameters, a certain scope, within which to unfold. When her behaviour takes a different course, or her illness unfolds in seemingly inexplicable ways, sanctions are imposed in an attempt to re-establish the familiar pattern of life on the floor. Mrs Abel is ostracised, bullied, cajoled, and ultimately, it seems, operated on in an attempt to restore order. As long as she remains a particular kind of 'patient', her behaviour and her illness will receive (one imagines) dutiful medical and nursing care. If, like an unruly actor, she departs from her script, every effort is made to persuade her to return to it. It is as if illness and illness behaviour are subject to a kind of contract, agreed between the most powerful members of a group, which stipulates that it is okay to act in certain ways, but not in others. A cancer like Mrs Abel's isn't usually associated with the kind of pain she says she is experiencing, so crying and monopolising people's time in the way she does is not what she *should*, as a good patient, *do*. For the nurses and doctors on Mrs Abel's floor, there is something insubstantial or unconvincing about the pain she describes, and something outrageous, even offensive, about her behaviour, because her mode of experience does not follow the anticipated and legitimate path.

Of course, the idea that there is such a thing as a socially sanctioned *role* to be adopted when we are ill is not new.

In *The Social System*, the American sociologist Talcott Parsons gives his famous analysis of medical practice.[35] He sees health as a 'ubiquitous practical problem in all societies' but points out that the influence of 'the therapeutic process' extends beyond health to 'problems of deviance and social control' (p.429). Medical practice is theorised as playing a part in the maintenance of balance in the social system as a whole. When we are ill, Parsons argues, we are unable to perform our social roles effectively. But because illness is not something that just happens to us willy-nilly, but also something towards which our unconscious may for various reasons impel us, it is also a factor in the functioning of the social system in the sense that it is part of our (consciously or unconsciously) willed (or 'motivated') interactions. There is a dimension of motivation to illness, so that:

> it becomes not merely an 'external' danger to be 'warded off' but an integral part of the social equilibrium itself. Illness may be treated as one mode of response to social pressures, among other things, as one way of evading social pressures. But it may also . . . have some possible positive functional significance [p.431].

Parsons claims that illness is a departure from normal functioning both biologically and socially. Illness changes us biologically, but it also changes our sense of ourselves in relation to others.

According to this particular sociological interpretation, medical practice provides the social system with a means of coping with illness that is achieved through the adoption of a series of defined and established roles. The principal roles in question are the medical practitioner, and the 'sick person'. The medical practitioner's role is 'collectivity oriented', and above all requires a high level of technical competence. He or she is an 'applied scientist', setting aside personal likes and dislikes when making a judgement, striving for neutrality and objectivity (p.435).[35]

Parsons identifies four groups of expectations associated with the 'sick role' (pp.436–437):

1. the sick person is exempted from 'normal social role responsibilities'
2. the sick person is in need of care and cannot make him or herself better
3. there is an obligation to want to get well
4. there is an obligation to seek help from a competent (that is medical) practitioner.

Crucially, the medical practitioner is seen as exercising a power of 'legitimation'; that is to say, the medical practitioner determines whether the 'sick person' is legitimately sick enough to be given exemption from normal responsibilities. The sick role is seen as involving not just exemptions but privileges, and Parsons argues that this may motivate individuals to attain or to sustain the status of sick person.[35] From the point of view of the social system it is imperative that the sick person is 'motivated' to recover; as Parsons sees it control of the motivational balance, tipped in order to favour as efficient and brisk an exit from the sick role as possible, rests in the hands of the medical establishment. Perhaps, in Mrs Abel's case, we can see legitimation faltering and the sick person's exemption from responsibilities losing its effect. Because the power of legitimation is exercised one-sidedly, Mrs Abel cannot herself establish that her pain is real. She steadily loses both credibility and respect in the eyes of the majority of her carers. Parsons' interpretation of the role of medical practice in the social system acknowledges the controlling role of medical practitioners in the health care system; the 'sick role' is identified as abnormal or deviant, with the sick person potentially motivated to remain formally designated as sick. In effect, this interpretation of the sick role establishes inequality as a principle of health care and in so doing leaves medical practice and the general public on opposite sides of a conflict of interests.

Parsons' concept of the patient's role belongs to a branch of the sociology of health and illness known as functionalism. Functionalism, in contrast to some more contemporary perspectives, sees relationships in health care as having been achieved through consensus, and the stance of medical practitioners towards their patients as both benevolent and directive at the same time. Lupton points out that in the functionalist model the relationship between doctor and patient is characterised by a preponderance of power in the hands of the doctor, but is not seen as conflicted: rather, the imbalance of power is seen as a necessary addition to medical knowledge, allowing medicine to exercise its benevolent function (p.7).[36] She comments, citing Turner:[37]

> While Parsons' work was ground-breaking in elucidating the social dimension of the medical encounter, the functionalist perspective has been subject to criticism based on its neglect of the potential conflict inherent

in the medical encounter. Critics argue that the functionalist position typifies patients as compliant, passive and grateful, while doctors are represented as universally beneficent, competent and altruistic [p.7].[36]

In our encounters with medicine and health care we are expected to behave with self-discipline. In addition to attending to our health care needs (narrowly defined), medicine and health care are a training ground for good, orderly citizenship. The self-discipline we express as advocates of healthy behaviours has a broader significance in the maintenance of a 'healthy' society through co-operative productive endeavour and the acceptance of benevolent power inequalities. As Herzlich and Pierret have pointed out, medicine is not simply 'one institution among others' (p.190); rather, it is a model for all present-day social institutions and therefore has a profound effect on our experience of our place in society.[14] By the end of the 19th and the beginning of the 20th centuries, they argue, the medical practitioner had come to represent science and its power, and medicine had claimed the right to determine the rules that society should follow. In support of this argument, they point to examples of medical regulation of sexuality, early childhood, and the relationship between health, the environment, and social conditions. Today, they argue, we are 'firmly entrenched' in the age of medicine, and all practices involving the body 'assume meaning in relation to medicine' (p.193): seeking medical care has become the norm and getting well is an obligation. Our tendency towards 'total adherence to the positive value of medicine' and 'the need to submit to it with complete docility' (p.195), mean that:[14]

> the physician 'knows'; he alone is in a position to state an opinion that can be considered the truth about the condition of the sick. The latter feel separated from the knowledge of their bodies, but they believe that this knowledge is present in another person who, for that very reason, is authorized to speak and prescribe. The sick acknowledge themselves to be in the hands of others, objects of their knowledge and their action [p.196].

While Parsons interprets medical supervision in an entirely positive way, it has been argued that our current relations with health care discourage us from reacting to illness in an autonomous way: we have become dependent on specialised interventions and have lost confidence in our own 'recuperative powers' and 'biological adaptability' (p.197).[14] Herzlich and Pierret quote one interviewee to this effect:[14]

> 'One is being infantilized', said a 25-year-old young woman . . . 'In the relations with the nurses, you just feel completely infantilized. Above all, don't try to speak about your feelings, or about your desires, or anything like that . . . just swallow your medications like a good girl, smile a lot, and especially don't think that you know what's good for you better than the nurse. That is to say: she always knows everything, *you must blindly obey her and not say anything* . . . just be there like a good girl' [p.198].

It has become increasingly difficult, given the medical view, for us to attribute any positive values at all to sickness and death, though these experiences have in the past been given meaning by communal social events and practices.[14] The professional medical viewpoint tends to define problems in its own terms, and medical practice can be seen as having a vested interest in controlling the nature and extent of the services it makes available. Thus, in effect, the lay perspective is set to one side and the physician–patient relationship becomes, contrary to functionalist teaching, inherently conflicted:[14]

> as the specialization that defines the field of the physician's intervention becomes more and more narrow [it] increasingly ignores the total reality perceived by the patient' [p.200].

One important effect of sociological frameworks such as the social constructionism represented in writers like Herzlich and Pierret,[14] Deborah Lupton,[15,36] and Bryan Turner[37] (in contrast to the functionalism of Talcott Parsons[35]) is to 'problematise' the doctor–patient relationship; that is to say, a critical space is opened up, which enables lay and professional participants in health care, as well as commentators, to set new goals beyond established orthodoxies. Social constructionism sketches out a rationale for the inequality and loss of autonomy experienced by individuals involved in formal health care, but instead of endorsing it, interprets it as a rather one-sided exercise of vested interests. The autonomy (or 'agency') of the lay person, together with a re-evaluation of his or her whole experience, is brought into view and identified as a necessary dimension of relationships in health care. The legitimacy of an imbalance of power, even attached to a rhetoric of philanthropy, is brought into question.

Having said that, we should remember that Michel Foucault, the French cultural historian, recognised the medical dominance of doctor–patient encounters, but saw it as a voluntary and necessary arrangement:[36]

> When discussing power in the medical encounter, the functionalist and the Foucauldian perspectives . . . overlap to some degree. In understanding power relations as productive rather than coercive, Foucauldian theory restates the assertion of classic functionalism that medical dominance is *necessary* for practitioners to take control in the medical encounter to fulfil the expectations of both parties, rather than a source of oppression . . . In this view, detachment, reserve, responsibility for the patient's well-being and an authoritarian stance must be maintained by the doctor, and the notion of patients being 'empowered' to take control in the encounter makes little sense, for such a change in the relationship calls into question the reason why the very encounter exists [pp.112–113].

Beresford points out that the last 20–30 years have seen the emergence of new movements of welfare users, and that government has sought to incorporate and respond to these.[38] New Labour, he argues, has highlighted 'participation, partnership, and empowerment' in social policy, but in reality:

> welfare users have had minimal involvement in welfare reform despite the significance attached to such reform and the massive impact it is having [p.501].

It is, he says, still unclear how the shift in power to patients and service users is to be achieved:

> The voices of disabled people, mental health service users and people with learning difficulties and older people are still largely marginal in social policy. One of the key developments in social policy in recent years

has been the recognition and inclusion of difference and the challenging of social divisions. This hasn't happened for service users *as service users*. If social policy is . . . to reflect commitments to equality and inclusion, this has to change [p.507].

Fundamental questions remain to be answered if problems of bias associated with knowledge linked to services and policy are to be addressed. How, for example,[38]

> can social policy, which doesn't fully and equally include service users, resist accusations of institutionalised discrimination, bias and presenting a partial picture [p.509]?

Carolyn Featherstone writes of modern society as one in which the body is 'an object of obsession'.[39] In fact, the body is a 'project', a means through which we set out to achieve social or material ends. Cancer, though, disrupts the 'body-as-project' through its power to stigmatise and fragment the image we have of our bodies both physically and emotionally. Featherstone draws attention to the role of writers like Michel Foucault and the symbolic interactionist Erving Goffman in providing a critical perspective on the notion of disease in Western culture. Naturalistic theories, which suggest that relationships in society (those between, for example, men and women, or different classes) are founded on the different strengths and weaknesses of our bodies, legitimise inequality because they deem such differences to be part of a natural and unchanging order.[39] Social constructionism, in contrast, looks upon the meaning our bodies have for us as being determined by social structures and encounters with others. When our bodies are affected by disease in such a way that the flow of everyday encounters is interrupted, or if our bodies conflict with dominant social representations, the experience is traumatic and we feel stigmatised.[39]

Featherstone suggests that Michel Foucault's development of the idea of 'discourse' (statements emanating from authoritative social groups that have the power to constitute reality of a kind) gives us the means to understand how medical practice is able to shape our sense of our bodies:[39]

'Discourse' is a key concept in Foucault's writings . . . 'discourse' is concerned with expert statements of powerful groups, i.e. statements which are taken seriously by a community of experts . . . we are talking about a mental model of reality, as used by expert groups. It will include the language, concepts and criteria of evaluation which are seen as legitimate for discussion of, for example, medical issues . . . The power of the medical profession is located in its discourse or ideas. Much of our thought about our bodies, then, is constrained by medical ideas which change over time [pp.166–167].

Our experience of our bodies in illness is constrained by medical discourse, which, though it changes over time, affects us as if it were part of a permanent order of nature, difficult, if not impossible, to resist. Holding on to a sense of our bodies as 'us' in the midst of intense medical discussion and cancer therapy is often beyond our means. We may be overpowered without being fully conscious of the loss (see Spence).[40]

Some sociological viewpoints have tended to see Western medicine in terms of its influence on (or 'medicalisation' of) the body. Bryan Turner, for example, writes of medicine as a key institution in the regulation of bodies: the body is 'socially constructed', made real to us (or 'fabricated') through scientific discourses in medicine.[41] Our bodies are controlled not just in health care but more widely in society through the exercise of medical power, which encourages us to exercise discipline over ourselves. The body, in this view, is 'problematised', can no longer be taken simply as a biological entity, and is seen instead more as a text, something written or laid down by powerful forces such as science or medicine. The need for a regulated body, a body under control and well-disciplined, is seen as originating in the emergence of Western capitalism, which requires 'docile and productive' bodies. Medicine, it is argued, is directed at creating such bodies:[41]

the growing importance of preventive medicine and the use of the concept of 'life-style' to regulate employees in order to manage corporate insurance demands have meant that there is a major intervention of medical ideas and practice into everyday reality – through diet, exercise, anti-smoking norms, sexual regulation of appropriate (that is 'healthy') partners, the regulation of childbirth, and the hygienic treatment of death [p.18].

The social constructionist perspective emphasises that medical knowledge is, like lay knowledge, constructed by and dependent on a particular society. Such knowledge is relative, and can be 'renegotiated', or undergo structural change, which incorporates changes in the relations between those who share in it, as when the doctor–patient relationship undergoes fundamental change. In health care we often behave in a way that suggests that medical knowledge represents essential truths; but from the 'post-structuralist' social constructionist point of view, this is because our society gives doctors (and scientists) special power over truth (as it once gave the church such power). Our behaviour in relation to nursing knowledge suggests that this possesses fewer essential truths, as if nurses do not enjoy quite the same social power as doctors. Social constructionism is a way of exploring the relative nature of such socially powerful bodies of knowledge as medicine; a way of understanding the social and historical conditions that give them their truth value. Renegotiation and a repositioning of less powerful social groups in a way that is more fully in accordance with interests that have been obscured by a very dominant body of knowledge, can theoretically follow.

Turner believes that the scientific medical curriculum, with its emphasis on acute illness and 'heroic medicine', maintains the dominance of the natural sciences; and that psychological, sociological, economic, political, and environmental causes of illness are excluded from systematic study, despite changes in the character of disease and the needs of an increasingly dependent population.[41] He suggests that health care should commit itself to an 'interdisciplinarity' based on the idea of the 'whole person as the focus of health care':

Scientific medicine is limited because it is based on a narrow, specialised and technical view of the human body as a machine which responds in a determinate way to the therapies derived from clinical experience and basic research [p.139].

Williams reminds us that disability theory offers an alternative to the scientific medical perspective.[42] He draws our attention to those who have rejected models of disability that focus on physical structure and function, activity, and social disadvantage, in favour of an approach that views disability as a form of social oppression, and as less to do with the body itself, than with the 'prejudices and barriers which mitigate against full participation on equal terms' (p.47).

In her paper on being an anthropologist in the 'kingdom of the sick', Susan DiGiacomo describes her experience of medical practice when she is diagnosed with Hodgkin's disease.[43] Much of her account is concerned with the encounters she has with doctors supervising her treatment. She sets out to 'demystify' her disease and her treatment, both as a means of 'staying sane' and to 'restore some sense of control':

> Treatments of indefinite length and uncertain outcome invariably inspire fear and rage, and rob the cancer patient of much of his personal autonomy. In such circumstances knowledge is the only kind of power available [p.316].

Hospital staff, she says, disapproved of her curiosity; and the hospital culture defined 'categories and persons – doctors and their patients' and their relationship to each other. As a service user, DiGiacomo finds the dynamics of health care controlling, and disapproving of knowledge and power being placed in the hands of the individual, and she experiences this as detrimental to her care and well-being. As an anthropologist, she believes that orthodox Western medicine ('biomedicine') is a cultural system that creates, or attempts to create, the reality of those involved in it. Powerful forces, like language, authority, organisational rules, and valuing of certain types of knowledge (the 'discourse' of biomedicine) combine to form a cultural system that is experienced as normality, though counter-systems exist and may be the chosen systems of different individuals.

The way we use language to represent disease and our bodies can be said to reflect our beliefs about disease, held individually or as a group. Cassell found that the patients he interviewed saw disease as 'an intrusive object rather than as a part of themselves', much as modern medicine does.[44] It seems particularly appropriate to us to refer to malignant tumours as 'its' or independent entities, as the people in Cassell's study did; though, he says, it is possible to conceive of a language for tumours that treats them as part of us. Cassell argues that it is the diseases themselves (and not merely the tumours) that are seen as objects. He found that symptoms and organs involved in the disease were referred to in the same impersonal way. Though Cassell remains undecided about whether the mind's view of the body, reflected in language, is culturally determined, or whether this view is 'biologically inherent' (neatly reflecting the line separating social constructionist and naturalistic, sociobiological viewpoints), he inclines to the latter. While the effect of speaking of disease as an 'it' may be to place distance between the person and the disease, Cassell concludes that it may be of greater therapeutic value to use language to reduce that distance:[44]

> words in their concrete reality may be a bridge through which the person can bring into his ken and perhaps even influence, parts of the body which until then reside in a mysterious inner world seemingly inaccessible to consciousness, much less to conscious action [p.146].

As a cultural system, DiGiacomo argues, biomedicine can sometimes be 'renegotiated': if patients hold strong beliefs in a counter-cultural system, a different way of constructing health care, they may be able, through dialogue, to modify the way that health care is made available to them.[43] Biomedicine, though, is very powerful, and can point to the many benefits and advantages it confers: it is often difficult, as an individual, to impose oneself upon this system, and doing so may carry the risk of being judged disruptive. Susan DiGiacomo's account in effect chronicles her own efforts to 'renegotiate' the terms of the system of biomedicine that puts forward her regime of care and treatment.[43]

Mathieson and Stam describe a different, but perhaps related type of 'negotiation' in their discussion of 'cancer narratives':[45]

> In negotiating their way through regimens of treatment, changing bodies and disrupted lives, the telling of one's own story takes on a renewed urgency. In the end, they are more than just 'stories' but the vehicle

for making sense of, not just an illness, but a life [p.284].

Thus 'renegotiation' can be seen as taking place both externally, in interaction with a system or culture, and internally, as a process of reinterpreting or remaking identity in the face of momentous personal events. Chronic illness, to use the term introduced in Michael Bury's famous paper,[46] can be interpreted as a special kind of disruptive experience – a *biographical* disruption – which leads to a fundamental rethinking of a person's biography and self-concept.[47] Charmaz, too, conceptualises illness as a form of assault on the self, in which 'former self-images' crumble away 'without a simultaneous development of equally valued new ones' (p.168).[48] While there is evidence that not all chronic illness is experienced in this way,[47] both Bury's and Charmaz's work serves to illustrate the force of Mathieson and Stam's arguments about the role of telling and retelling one's own story, or 'self-narrative', in the reconstruction, or 'renegotiation' of identity under conditions of illness.[45]

Frankenberg suggests that the world of biomedicine and the world of the patient diverge chronologically, especially in chronic disease, where the physician's involvement is much shorter than the patient's:[49]

the knowledge and understanding over time of the sickness trajectory enjoyed by technicians, nurses, and especially patients and their relatives may well be much greater than that of their physicians. In general, the physician may know more than the patient about acute disease in practical as well as in theoretical terms. He or she may have seen many discrete patients over a period of years; the chronic patient on the other hand has had the opportunity to study one patient over many years and continuously. A collection of such patients organised into a specific patient group may have much to teach not only about illness and sickness but also about disease [p.19].

Frankenberg offers a distinction between 'disease' and 'illness', consistent with a social constructionist perspective. By 'disease', Frankenberg means disturbances in body functions and performance seen in biological terms; 'illness', on the other hand, is concerned with the perceptions

individual sufferers have of what medical practitioners identify as disease:

Disease depends on the existence of the social organisation of biologists and the medically trained, and illness on a socially constructed sense of self which certainly does not exist in the same form in all societies [p.17].

Our sense of the nature of disease and illness and our related behaviour is specific to the way that we have developed, individually and historically, within a society. Frankenberg, who is making room for a 'renegotiation' of some widely held cultural assumptions by pointing to the relative nature of phenomena such as disease and illness, takes issue with sociologists who approach 'death-andying' as if it were one word; this, he points out, implies that all but the final stages of life can be 'reasonably analysed without reference to its most universal and inevitable end, and shifts responsibility for 'deathandying' to specialists, such as hospice workers and social scientists. Instead, he uses the word 'lifedeath' to refer to the part of life in which death is 'part of the not yet conscious', and 'deathlife' for life that is accompanied by 'consciousness of its not too far distant end' (p.18).

Arthur Kleinman also sees a contrast between patients' experiences of illness and the medical focus on disease, though he believes it is possible, indeed therapeutic, for clinicians to help patients to 'order' their experience.[50] What illness means to people, he says, should be interpreted by patients, families and practitioners together. The medical system, though, tends to detach practitioners from the experience of illness.

The cultural shaping of the experience of illness is reflected in the characteristic way we perceive and monitor our bodies. We are very careful about what we allow into our bodies, what we try to exclude, and how we manage material expelled from our bodies. We have a particular sense within communities and societies of what it means to 'take care of ourselves', and of what it means to lead a healthy life. We have social rules to manage contagion, as the rules for dealing with coughing, sneezing, and washing show. There are areas where the difference between good and bad practices becomes blurred, as with the taking of drugs in sport: some sections of the sporting world are more prohibitive than others, with the result that our sense of how to regulate our bodies becomes touched by ambiguity. Keeping our bodies in order – not too spotty, not too fat – carries a sense of obligation to others: our fellows, our communities may accuse us of 'letting ourselves go' if we put on weight, and failure to follow social rules of good bodily order may offend or threaten others, as is the case with spitting, or scratching ourselves.

Kleinman's explanation of disease (as opposed to illness) is that it is created when illness is 'recast' by the practitioner 'in terms of theories of disorder' (p.5); disease is an 'it', not a 'me' of personal experience, created within a specific system of names and classifications.[50] From the point of view of biomedical culture, disease is defined as, and confined to, changes in biological structure or function, but from a 'biopsychosocial' perspective, Kleinman argues, disease represents an interaction between 'body, self, and society' (p.6). The strong cultural position of biomedicine in Western societies means that the mechanism of disease (the way it alters biological structure or function) often represents its meaning. Cancer, whose mechanism and treatment we do not yet completely understand, is therefore:[50]

> an unsettling reminder of the obdurate grain of unpredictability and uncertainty and injustice . . . in the human condition. Cancer forces us to confront our lack of control over our own or others' death. Cancer points up our failure to explain and master much in our world. Perhaps most fundamentally, cancer symbolizes our need to make moral sense of 'why me?' that scientific explanations cannot provide [p.20].

He proposes an alternative approach to therapy, in which medical care is 'reconceptualised' and relations between medical practitioner and patient are renegotiated. This approach involves 'an empathetic witnessing of the existential experience of suffering' and 'practical coping with the major psychosocial crises that constitute the menacing chronicity of that experience' (p.10);[50] it is offered as a counter-blast to the biomedical specialist who, Kleinman suggests, does not:[50]

> credit the patient's subjective account until it can be quantified and . . . rendered more 'objective' . . . Illness experience is not legitimated by the biomedical specialist, for whom it obscures the traces of morbid physiological change [p.17].

Frankenberg, for one, expresses reservations about whether Kleinman's 'reconceptualisation' of medical care is as fundamental as it might seem (it may, he says, be 'radical' rather than 'revolutionary').[49] He points out that drawing a distinction between disease and illness does not mean that concepts of disease are rejected. Frankenberg implies that Kleinman's 'empathetic witnessing' amounts to a proposal that:

> the physician must learn the patient's interpretation and the nature of the illness, and then in turn, as part of the cure, teach the patient as much about the disease as is possible and necessary for treatment to be both carried out and complied with [p.16].

Consequently, power and control in the therapeutic encounter is retained by medical practice, and the patient remains suppliant, petitioning for dispensations. Frankenberg sees hospital patients' time as routinised and inflexible, with 'almost total disruption' of 'the natural rhythms of bodily desires' like sleeping, eating, evacuating waste, and enjoying sexual experience.[49] Healing and illness, he says, take place within a 'time view' that is the patient's own, and which is infrequently shared by physicians and nurses; medicine, analysing and treating the disease, is practised in another time, distant from the patient. In hospital, the argument goes, patients lose control over their own time to medical and nursing staff, who maintain the power relations of public health care. Radical change is beginning to take place with the rise of the user movement, but for Frankenberg such change is less than fundamental so long as it does nothing to affect the most deeply rooted processes of health care practice. Revolutionary change can only take place when patients 'take charge of their own time'. For healing to be established as part of our culture, medicine must 'renegotiate' its relationship with service users and other health care workers on the basis of equal partnership, and relinquish its control over the time of others, which enhances its power, diminishes the autonomy of others, and puts distance between it and the experience of illness.[49]

Susan DiGiacomo, who writes of cancer treatment as 'as brutally primitive as any inflicted by the leeches and barber-surgeons of old' (p.318), found her identity 'assailed' by hospital and by having cancer.[43] Cancer, she says, quoting Erving Goffman,[51] is a stigma that reduces a 'whole and usual person' to a 'tainted, discounted one', and as such affects the way that relationships between patients and their doctors are structured. She agrees with Susan Sontag that cancer and cancer treatment are often referred to with military terminology,[12] and that metaphorically speaking, cancer implies 'social deviance, social injustice, and political corruption'; the individual with cancer is caught up in the implications of catastrophe and evil. Having lost control of her work and her body, DiGiacomo was determined to keep control of her identity, including 'anthropologist', her professional identity. Knowledge, asking questions, was a means of avoiding becoming a victim; but when she approached doctors as colleagues, rather than superiors, she found they were both surprised and disapproving, and that conflict occasionally ensued. She experienced the social power relations incorporated in the formal health care setting as detrimental to well-being (or as Frankenberg might say, contrary to healing).

DiGiacomo tells how an eminent oncologist supervising her care treated detailed information about Hodgkin's disease as too dangerous to pass on to her, and as potentially damaging to her sanity; her anaesthetist and surgeon refused her husband access to the recovery room on the basis of custom ('pseudo-hygienic and pseudo-practical nonsense'); the purpose of attending for treatment simulation was misrepresented; radiation 'burns' were renamed radiation 'reaction'; and hair loss that was more extensive than predicted was explained as the result of increased 'traction' caused by her long hair.

She provides a number of examples of what Frankenberg[49] sees as the medical control of patient's time:

> I was told peremptorily to appear the next day for my first treatment. I got angry. I lived more than two hours' drive from the hospital and needed advance notice in order to organise my new commuter life. I refused to come in until the following Monday, and the reaction was one of surprise and indignation. It did not matter that no time frame had been specified, I should simply do what I was told without argument, regardless of the dislocation and inconvenience it caused me.
>
> I prepared for my weekly visits with my radiologist as I would prepare for any interview I would do as a field anthropologist. I thought out my questions beforehand, and conducted the interview from notes. I had to talk fast, because after the first five or ten minutes, my doctor began edging toward the examining room door, an indication she felt she had spent enough time answering my questions and had other important things to do. These visits were clearly for her benefit, so she could gauge my progress, not for mine [p.323].[43]

Ultimately, Susan DiGiacomo comes to feel that she has been 'bullied into accepting more treatment . . . made to submit, to comply, through the strategic manipulation of information' (p.325): she sees the counter-process of overcoming confrontation and submission as possible through a 'negotiation' with clinical practice.[43]

Reviewing her experience of hospital care and treatment for cancer, she comments that her refusal to participate in roles ordinarily assigned by the health care system enabled her to redefine her relationship with her doctors, and made apparent the meanings or beliefs which give the system structure and shape. People with cancer, DiGiacomo feels, are particularly subject to a process of depersonalisation; in other words, they 'become their disease'. Personal contact with health-service users is, she says, 'highly routinised', and doctors share the belief that a person's knowledge that she has cancer 'renders her so emotionally unstable that she is unable to confront and live with any reminders of the severity of her condition' (p.337). Patients are assumed to be unable to understand explanations, so information is withheld. Angry patients are seen as hostile or resentful rather than as having a legitimate grievance; responsibility for conflict is seen as that of the patient and not the doctor. Consultations do not allow time for questions, because they are dominated by the physical examination: the end of the consultation is indicated by a shuffling of papers or an opening of the door, making a private discussion public and therefore ending it.

Writing some 20 years ago now, DiGiacomo's experiences may sound implausible. But the manner in which individual health service users are still circumvented by care that finds it easier to manage a *clinic* rather than engage with a *person* is well illustrated by Helen Allan's account of caring and non-caring in a fertility unit:[32]

> The ability to combine caring and non-caring was achieved through an activity I have described as 'nursing the clinic' where the clinic and the doctor became the focus of nursing rather than the patient . . . Suki and Evelyn 'nursed the clinic' as they welcomed the patients, showed them into the consulting rooms and responded to doctors' demands. But they did not 'nurse' Joanna. It was not possible to know whether Joanna felt she was being ignored and my interpretation of non-caring raises interesting questions about what ethical justification there can be for emotional distance in the face of evident distress such as crying [p.54].

Susan DiGiacomo concludes that encounters between doctors and people with cancer are structured as they are to keep the individual in a position of ignorance, leaving the doctor in a better position to secure the patient's co-operation with dangerous and unpleasant forms of treatment.[43] The doctor emerges 'omniscient and omnipotent', which has the effect of reducing the ambiguity surrounding the patient's prognosis following treatment. 'Declaring a war on cancer' justifies the most extreme of measures, diminishes the necessity for openness and proportionality, and obscures the rationale for genuine consensus called for in a 'negotiation model' for practice. Some sociological work may actually 'aid and abet' situations in which patients are kept in relative ignorance by ascribing difficulties in communication to patients' own psychological states. Beneath the successful, technological public image of biomedicine, DiGiacomo sees a reality of uncertainty, ambiguity, and contradiction. Treatment decisions that rely on medical control of information lead to distrust and fear, and end with a sense of betrayal when treatment does not produce the desired result.

Negotiation and resolution begin when DiGiacomo is informed promptly of a change in her medical condition, and progress further as her GP begins to act in the role of advocate. According to her GP she is more afraid of 'being out of control and not in a position to make an informed decision' (p.328) than she is of her cancer; her most urgent need is therefore to 'comprehend my disease and its treatment to the fullest possible extent' (p.328).[43] A meeting, lasting for an hour, is held for her with both oncologist and radiologist, with questions submitted in advance, and a transcript of answers provided. She is given a copy of the full research protocol for an investigation of experimental treatments for Hodgkin's disease before beginning chemotherapy.

She questions the necessity for 12 cycles of chemotherapy, pointing out that the standard 'salvage' regime for patients who have 'failed' radiotherapy is six cycles. Her oncologist tells her that there is no way of knowing whether six cycles is sufficient, but DiGiacomo continues to believe that 'overestimating the required dosages might be as serious as underestimating them'. At the beginning of treatment, she experiences severe facial pains, gastrointestinal problems, immunosuppression, and fever, though no infection can be identified. She discusses the possibility of chemotherapy being ineffective, and is given details of her chances of survival if this were the case; talking about death with her doctor seems to demonstrate the value of a 'negotiation model' for clinical practice, which she glosses as 'each of us seeing the other in three dimensions instead of two' (p.332).

As DiGiacomo renegotiates the terms of her health care, insisting both that she is given detailed information and that her experience of treatment and illness, and insight into the effects upon herself, are fully acknowledged, we see practice turned 180 degrees away from Mrs Abel's predicament. Whereas Mrs Abel remained stranded, without credence or credibility and was ultimately acted upon (literally operated upon) blindly, in ignorance of her needs and wishes, DiGiacomo fights hard to win recognition of herself and of the grounds for her well-being. In her later dealings with her oncologist, she seems to experience greater acknowledgement of her own 'time view', her own 'illness-time', her sense of living 'lifedeath' not 'deathlife' (see Frankenberg[49]). Collaboration on medical decisions becomes part of their meetings:[43]

> He came to respect my ability to observe and report sensitively and accurately . . . as I began to negotiate more aggressively (and more successfully) for lower doses. This was no fiction of participation; it was based on mutual understanding of chemotherapy as a necessarily and inherently indeterminate process [p.333].

Being a 'collaborator' rather than 'an object of treatment' provides Susan DiGiacomo with a sense of empowerment, which relieves depression and fear, though it also means that she has to share her oncologist's worries. She believes that her persistent fever is a symptom of the damage chemotherapy is doing to her body: she feels she is being 'destroyed in order to be saved'. Eventually, treatment is halted and she concludes that her own explanation of her condition, that her body is unable to tolerate chemotherapy, is more credible than her doctor's belief that she has suffered an undetectable infection. She implies that her doctor is forced to acknowledge the strength of her case, and thus in a sense a new position has been negotiated on what counts as credible knowledge about illness: the medical explanation (or discourse) is finely balanced in terms of credibility with the personal one.

A long and difficult struggle, in the course of which a model for negotiation in clinical practice is mapped out, ends with the final word on a clinical problem going to the patient. At the end of the struggle, in the course of which biomedical culture has in a local way accepted compromise, opened its borders, DiGiacomo's oncologist acknowledges her time view, where illness is not experienced as a number of courses of chemotherapy but as degenerating physical integrity and impending collapse. A degree of parity is achieved as the relevance and significance of the personal experience of illness is conceded.

DelVecchio Good and her colleagues believe that in America, oncologists have 'a cultural mandate to instil hope' in their therapeutic dialogues (or 'narratives') with patients.[52] Like DiGiacomo, they identify a layer of uncertainty in medical knowledge about the outcomes of cancer and treatment that must compete with the cul-

tural imperative to offer hope. Their experience suggests that oncologists respond with expressions of 'time without horizons or of highly foreshortened horizons' to:

> create an experience of immediacy . . . Time horizons, through therapeutic discourse and interaction, are distinctly foreshortened, and experience is consciously composed 'for the moment'. Endings, though palpably present for participants in clinical encounters, are unspecified . . . Instilling hope 'for the moment' becomes a legitimate and realistic task in the world of clinical oncology . . . [pp.856–857].

Creating hope by focusing on the present is a source of anxiety for patients who are looking for certainty and lack of ambiguity about the course of their illness; but patients, DelVecchio Good claims, often contribute to the process of generating commitment to treatment and hope for the future seen in their encounters with doctors. Hope, and compliance with medical regimens, are values deeply rooted in Western culture. To begin with, DelVecchio Good believes, consultations with oncologists are structured so as to avoid suggestions of crisis or 'threat to daily existence'.[52] A sort of 'housekeeping' takes place in which the organisational aspects of getting to treatment appointments are sorted out, and the effect is to keep things 'unremarkable'. At the same time, metaphors of slow and patient struggle may be introduced, like 'climbing a mountain' and 'one step at a time', to suggest a process of steady achievement, which continues even when a dying trajectory is clearly under way. The mountain-climbing metaphor implies a kind of protest; it is:[52]

> an image which suggests that the oncologist will pull the patient to safer, higher ground . . . a metaphor which taps into American concepts that through mobilizing personal will, the patient has resources to engage in the struggle for higher ground, for cure or remission [p.857].

When challenged to respond to concerns about prognosis, DelVecchio Good finds that clinicians employ 'narratives of immediacy', which:[52]

> drew patients back into the everyday realities of living and of therapeutic housekeeping, of treatment

schedules, of dealing with immediate side-effects, of assessing the current efficacy of the latest therapy . . . endings are rarely made explicit and progression is measured in calibrated bits, even though disclosure is considered to be the norm . . . [p.858].

Ultimately, when death or dying becomes an unavoidable reality, these 'narratives of immediacy and hope, struggle and progress' fragment and collapse. Unambiguous medical assessment of the stage or likely progress of an illness may, DelVecchio Good suggests, come out into the open more frequently at this point, when other narratives fragment.

Perhaps this is the inevitable consequence of what DelVecchio Good calls 'the dominant American narrative', the cancer care story, which seems to offer frankness yet employs subplots of hope and encouragement to a soldierly willingness to shoulder necessary hardships in the battle to survive.[52] The brave and hopeful soldier is not prepared for the potentially shattering end of the narrative. We find it helpful to put our faith in the brave persona we project as providers of health care or are offered as recipients; but we would perhaps like to be able to care for people with cancer so that we and they can be ourselves as much as possible *and* manage treatment, care, and future, without the need for such precarious roles.

Neither Mrs Abel nor the nurses and doctors on her floor were able to express or acknowledge concerns freely.[34] Mrs Abel was hemmed in by a vicious circle of unresolved difficulties; nursing and medical staff resisted to the last any modification of the clinical story of cancer as they understood it. Caitlin, in contrast, takes 'a leap of faith' and immerses herself as openly as she can in the needs of her patient, Ray, and his partner Lucy.[23] Susan DiGiacomo fights doggedly to be given a seat at the table, to renegotiate the terms of her dialogue with health care and to be given a say in tipping the balance of decisions, even when 'expert' opinion is against her.[43]

It is not just a matter of rebelling against the system or trendy theory: what Mrs Abel and her carers lack, and what Caitlin and Susan DiGiacomo are struggling to achieve is a way of being in the world that is open to experience (both our own and that of others) and discriminating about what has meaning or what matters. Patricia Benner's word for this is 'agency', which she interprets as openness to matters of significance.[53] Agency develops with experiential learning:

> . . . what is learned in practice by the practitioner is considered knowledge even though it contains puzzles and cannot always be fully located in the currently explicated science . . . the knowledge of the practitioner goes both before and after science because what occurs in the natural field of clinical experience is more variegated and complex than can be captured at any one time by scientific experiment. What is known sets up the questions and influences what is noticed, and the actual clinical experience alters, extends, or disconfirms what is known in the scientific discourse. Experience . . . requires openness to the new situation, but that openness is constituted by what has gone before; it is not naïve and undifferentiated [pp.14–15].

Benner is interested in the agency of nurses as health care providers, in their 'sense of responsibility for the patient's well-being', which becomes more sensitive to possibilities as the skill of the practitioner increases, and which is manifested in:

> negotiating and managing physician's responses to the patient situation . . . and . . . being responsive to and advocating for the patient and family concerns in ways that more closely match the actual concerns and needs [pp.26–27].[53]

'Agency' thus conceived is the domain both of the caring professions *and* the recipients of health care, but comes into view as a possibility only when the traditional balance of power in health care is conceived as contingent on cultural and social practices (and therefore relative) rather than as absolute and essential, a part of the natural order. How indispensable 'agency' is to caring, how much a part of well-being, in or out of health care, probably depends upon one's perspective, one's beliefs given all the historical, social, and cultural influences that bear upon them. For me, 'agency' and 'being available' are ideas that try very hard to give us a sense of the closeness, insightfulness, inventiveness, and commitment of caring. They share an intense focus upon the individual, the nurse, the mentor. Sometimes they might seem to involve an intensity of focus on the practitioner that somehow excludes wider considerations, including the voice of those on whose behalf care is provided. Structures in health care can be constructed to be more or less controlling of others, according to how much or how little control is seen as necessary to care or 'manage'.

Health care and illness take place in the larger, collective arena. We designate people as 'well', or 'sick', or 'patient' according to shared rules; we respond to people who are 'patients' according to the conventions and accepted practices of the roles we see as our own or the positions we take in the groups to which we belong. If 'agency' and 'being available' are about being committed to respond with discrimination to the experience of others, and are in some way central to the idea of caring, caring also encompasses the wider social or cultural arena where experiences of health and illness acquire their distinctive character, and health care organisations develop their formulas and structures, their distinctive ways of operating.

It is easy to see health care as a monolith, immovable and unshakeable, but if we shake up the bits and pieces of our sense of what health care is, new arrangements come into view, to be espoused or discarded in their turn.

References

1. NHS go-ahead for new breast cancer drugs. *The Guardian*, 23 May 2006.
2. Two-drug therapy may slow breast cancer advance. *The Guardian*, 23 March 2006.
3. Ultrasound could replace mainstream cancer treatments. *The Guardian*, 25 October 2005.
4. Here's how treatment hits target. *The Sun*, 25 May 2006.
5. A cure that boldly goes . . . *The Sun*, 3 November 2005.
6. Watchdog approves embryo selection to help prevent cancer. *The Guardian*, 11 May 2006.
7. Lifestyle changes could stop a third of cancers, says study. *The Guardian*, 18 November 2005.
8. Schools may offer cervical cancer vaccination to all girls. *The Guardian*, 8 October 2005.
9. Nigeria bishops scorn US 'cancer'. BBC News, 4 July 2006. http://news.bbc.co.uk/1/hi/world/africa/5144036.stm (accessed 24 July 2007).
10. Comment & Analysis: As doctors, we see the cancer that eats away at the NHS. *The Guardian*, 27 June 2005.
11. Field attack on 'cancer' of spin doctors. *The Guardian*, 4 August 1998.
12. Sontag S. (1977). *Illness as Metaphor*. New York: Farrar, Strauss & Giroux.
13. Gould J. and Nelson J. (2005). Researchers reflect from the cancer precipice. *Reflective Practice* **6**, 277–284.
14. Herzlich P. and Pierret J. (1987). *Illness and Self in Society*. Baltimore, MD: Johns Hopkins University Press.
15. Lupton D. (1994). Femininity, responsibility, and the technological imperative: discourses on breast cancer in the Australian Press. *International Journal of Health Services* **24**, 73–89.
16. Seale C. (2001). Sporting cancer: struggle language in news reports of people with cancer. *Sociology of Health and Illness* **23**, 308–329.
17. Seale C. (2001). Cancer in the news: religious themes in news stories about people with cancer. *Health* **5**, 425–440.
18. Seale C. (2002). Cancer heroics: a study of news reports with particular reference to gender. *Sociology* **36**, 107–126.
19. Seale C. (2003). Health and media: an overview. *Sociology of Health and Illness* **25**, 513–531.
20. Seale C. (2005). New directions for critical internet health studies: representing cancer experience on the web. *Sociology of Health and Illness* **27**, 515–540.
21. Hochschild A.R. (1979). Emotion work, feeling rules, and social structure. *American Journal of Sociology* **85**, 551–575.
22. Johns C. (1995). Framing learning through reflection within Carper's fundamental ways of knowing in nursing. *Journal of Advanced Nursing* **22**, 226–234.
23. Johns C. (1997). Caitlin's story – realizing caring within everyday practice through guided reflections. *International Journal for Human Caring* **1**, 33–39.
24. Johns C. (1996). Visualising and realizing caring in practice through guided reflection. *Journal of Advanced Nursing* **24**, 1135–1143.
25. Johns C. (1996). Understanding and managing interpersonal conflict as a therapeutic nursing activity. *International Journal of Nursing Practice* **2**, 194–200.
26. Johns C. (1998). Caring through a reflective lens: giving meaning to being a reflective practitioner. *Nursing Inquiry* **5**, 18–24.
27. Johns C. (1999). Reflection as empowerment? *Nursing Inquiry* **6**, 241–249.
28. Johns C. (2001). Reflective practice: revealing the [he]art of caring. *International Journal of Nursing Practice* **7**, 237–245.
29. Johns C. (2002). *Guided Reflection: Advancing Practice*. Oxford: Blackwell Science.

30. Benner P. and Wrubel J. (1989). *The Primacy of Caring: Stress and Coping in Health and Illness*. Menlo Park, CA: Addison-Wesley.

31. Menzies I. (1959). The functioning of social systems as a defence against anxiety. In *Containing Anxiety in Institutions: Selected Essays Volume 1*. London: Free Association Books.

32. Allan H. (2001). A 'good enough' nurse: supporting patients in a fertility unit. *Nursing Inquiry* **8**, 51–60.

33. McNamara B. (2004) Good enough death: autonomy and choice in Australian palliative care. *Social Science and Medicine* **58**, 929–938.

34. Strauss A.L. and Glaser B.G. (1970). *Anguish: a Case History of a Dying Trajectory*. London: Martin Robinson.

35. Parsons T. (1951). *The Social System*. London: Routledge and Kegan Paul.

36. Lupton D. (1994). *Medicine as Culture: Illness, Disease and the Body in Western Societies*. London: Sage Publications.

37. Turner B.S. (1988). *Medical Power and Social Knowledge*. London: Sage Publications.

38. Beresford P. (2001). Service users, social policy and welfare. *Critical Social Policy* **21**, 494–512.

39. Featherstone C. (1996). Views of the body, stigma and the cancer patient experience. In Parry A. (ed.) *Sociology: Insights in Health Care*. London: Arnold.

40. Spence J. (1986). *Putting Myself in the Picture: a Political, Personal and Photographic Autobiography*. London: Camden Press.

41. Turner B.S. (1992). *Regulating Bodies*. London: Routledge.

42. Williams S.J. (2000). Chronic illness as biographical disruption or biographical disruption as chronic illness? Reflections on a core concept. *Sociology of Health and Illness* **22**, 40–67.

43. DiGiacomo S.M. (1987). Biomedicine as a cultural system: an anthropologist in the kingdom of the sick. In Baer H.A. (ed.) *Encounters with Biomedicine*. New York: Gordon and Breach.

44. Cassell E.J. (1976). Disease as an 'it': concepts of disease revealed by patients' presentation of symptoms. *Social Science and Medicine* **10**, 143–146.

45. Mathieson C.M. and Stam H.J. (1995). Renegotiating identity: cancer narratives. *Sociology of Health and Illness* **17**, 283–306.

46. Bury M. (1982) Chronic illness as biographical disruption. *Sociology of Health and Illness* **4**, 167–182.

47. Lawton J. (2003). Lay experiences of health and illness: past research and future agendas. *Sociology of Health and Illness* **25**, 23–40.

48. Charmaz K. (1983). Loss of self: a fundamental form of suffering in the chronically ill. *Sociology of Health and Illness* **5**, 168–195.

49. Frankenberg R. (1988). 'Your time or mine?' An anthropological view of the tragic temporal contradictions of biomedical practice. *International Journal of Health Services* **18**, 11–34.

50. Kleinman A. (1988). *The Illness Narratives: Suffering, Healing, and the Human Condition*. New York: Basic Books.

51. Goffman E. (1963). *Stigma: Notes on the Management of Spoiled Identity*. Englewood Cliffs, NJ: Prentice-Hall.

52. DelVecchio Good M.-J., Munakata T., Kobayashi Y., Mattingly C. and Good B.J. (1994). Oncology and narrative time. *Social Science and Medicine* **38**, 855–862.

53. Benner P., Tanner C. and Chesla C. (1992). From beginner to expert: gaining a differentiated clinical world in critical care nursing. *Advances in Nursing Science* **14**, 13–28.

CHAPTER FOUR

Cancer epidemiology

Elizabeth Davies and Vivian Mak

Introduction

Epidemiology is usually defined as 'the study of the distribution and determinants of disease in human populations'. Although it employs methods drawn from a wide range of areas including survey work, randomised controlled trials, and industrial quality control techniques, a defining quality of epidemiology data is that it refers to populations or groups of people rather than to particular individuals. As a result the discipline makes use of the uneven distribution of disease within and between populations to identify and explore clues to the possible causes of disease. However, the observation that one group in a population is statistically more likely to develop a disease does not allow the identification of particular individuals in that group that will develop a disease. In the UK there is a strong tradition of collecting epidemiological data for research and surveillance of population health, and of using this evidence and international comparisons to develop public health policy. Health professionals working in the cancer field therefore need some knowledge of epidemiology to understand both the populations in which they work and the rationale for the development of health policy. Also, although epidemiological data cannot answer questions about an individual with any certainty, patients do often ask questions about their disease and its treatment which may be of an epidemiological nature, and such findings are often reported in the media. Health professionals need to be able to answer patients' questions or direct then to other sources of information. This chapter aims to present an applied perspective on epidemiology by focusing on questions people with cancer often ask (see Box 4.1), using where possible examples of national and regional data for some of the more common cancers. It also describes some core epidemiological concepts, some common types of study, and some of the seminal studies in cancer epidemiology and international comparative work. References and sources for further information are included so that the reader can then apply the principles to other less common cancers.

Descriptive cancer epidemiology

Descriptive epidemiology is the study of trends in the incidence of disease over time, within population subgroups and by geographical area. It also concerns the subsequent survival of patients after the diagnosis of disease. Each year over 10 million cases of cancer occur around the world and it causes six million deaths a year.

How common is cancer in the UK?

There are several ways of describing how common a disease is within a population but this first requires a definition of a case of the disease. Since the 1950s, cancer has been defined using

Table 4.1 Most common cancers in England and Wales, 2000

Rank	Site	Number of registrations	Proportion of all cancers (%)
Males			
1	Prostate	27149	20
2	Lung	23245	17
3	Colorectal	18956	14
Females			
1	Breast	40467	30
2	Colorectal	16344	12
3	Lung	15165	11

Box 4.1 Epidemiological questions that people commonly ask about cancer

Descriptive epidemiology
• How common is cancer in the UK?
• Has cancer been becoming more or less common?
• Are more people dying from cancer?
• How common is this cancer in people my age?

Aetiological epidemiology
• How do we find out about the causes of cancer?
• Was it something I was exposed to?

Prevention and screening
• Could I have done anything to prevent it?
• Why isn't there screening/earlier diagnosis for this cancer?

Clinical epidemiology
• What are my chances of cure with this treatment?
• Should I undergo this treatment?
• What does this new study mean for me?

Public health policy
• What is the government/cancer network/hospital/ primary care trust doing to improve the outlook for people with cancer?
• Is the UK doing as well as countries of similar economic status?
• How is information about cancer routinely collected and used in the UK and elsewhere?

the World Health Organisation International Classification of Diseases (ICD) based on topographical features (site) and behaviour of cancer (whether benign or malignant). These classifications have been successively revised and the tenth edition – ICD-10 – is now in use. Since 1976 a specific International Classification of Disease in Oncology has been available – ICD-O, which is now in its third edition.[1] This includes information on histology (morphology), which is usually available from the pathology report, as this has now been recognised as an important determinant of survival and indicator of treatment.

Data on the number of people diagnosed with cancer each year are collected by cancer registries from hospitals, primary care trusts and hospices in the UK, coded and then sent to the National Cancer Intelligence Centre at the Office for National Statistics where national figures are collated. These figures show that cancer is a relatively common disease – more than one in three people in the UK will develop it at some time in their life, and cancer causes one in four deaths.[2] For men the most common types are prostate, lung, and colorectal, and in women breast, colorectal and lung (see Table 4.1). Together these sites account for around one half of all cancer diagnoses each year.

Epidemiological terms to describe 'commonness' or the frequency of a disease in the population are generally called 'rates'. An important distinction is made between the terms 'incidence' and 'prevalence'. Incidence refers to the transition between health and disease and usually means the number of patients newly diagnosed in a population in any given time period. This is often presented as the crude incidence rate per 100000 people in a population per year. The follow-up period may, however, be longer and expressed as a cumulative incidence for this length of time. An incidence rate is calculated using person-time as the denominator:

$$\text{Incidence rate (persons)} = \frac{\text{Number of persons who become diseased during a defined period}}{\text{Total person-time at risk during the follow-up period}}$$

To be accurate, the number of people affected must include all those patients with disease, not simply those seen and treated in hospital. For example, some patients may never attend hospital, they may be diagnosed clinically, by biopsy and microscopic diagnosis, or attend hospital only briefly for a formal pathological diagnosis before receiving palliative care in the community. Finally cancer may be discovered only at post mortem. If only the cases seen and treated in hospitals are counted, it is very likely that the true incidence of a disease in a population will be underestimated. Similarly, accurate data on the size of the population are as important as those on the number of cases. The population of interest may be a nation, a region or an administrative area such as in the UK a cancer network, or a primary care trust. In the UK these population figures are available from the Office for National Statistics where they are updated regularly using data from the census. It is usual to want to compare the incidence rates between different areas, but the age structure of the population of areas may differ markedly between themselves and over time, making it difficult to draw a conclusion about this. For example, some countries in Europe have an older population than others and we may want to know whether, taking this into account, they still have a higher incidence of cancer. In this situation an 'age-standardised rate' is used. This is a summary index designed to simplify comparison of cancer rates between different populations with different age structures. This is achieved by adjusting the rates with reference to a standard population with a standard age structure. By convention either the 'World standard' or the 'European standard' population is used. These may also be applied to administrative areas within countries. The key point to appreciate is that these populations do not exist as 'real' populations, but are simply a standard reference.

Prevalence refers to the state of having a disease and is the number of patients diagnosed with cancer in any given period and alive at a given point in time. It is often used as a measure of disease burden, and of the likely need for continuing care (e.g. follow-up, rehabilitation or support), and is therefore of use in planning health services. Because it is difficult to estimate what proportion of patients are completely cured, prevalence is estimated simply as the number of cancer survivors. For example, estimates suggest that approaching 3 million people in the European Union were diagnosed in the previous 5 years and remain alive.[3] In the UK, people diagnosed with cancer in the last 10 years represent just over 1% of the population. Another way of describing the impact of a disease on a population is to describe the mortality or mortality rate within the population. This is the incidence of death from cancer in the population within a given time period.

Has cancer been becoming more or less common?

Around the world, cancer has been becoming more common. In the UK, data collected by the Office for National Statistics show that both the number of new cases and the age-standardised incidence of cancer has increased in England and Wales since the 1970s for both men and women. The incidence in younger adults (men aged less than 65 years and women aged less than 55 years) has remained fairly stable during this time, and much of the increase is among older adults. This is partly due to better reporting of cases during this period, and an ageing population leading to greater longevity and a higher proportion of elderly.[2] Figure 4.1 shows the age-standardised incidence rates for cancer in South East England between 1960 and 2003.

Cancer is, of course, not one disease but a mix of many different ones, and aggregating data about these diseases will mask important differences. One cancer that has been increasing due to both increased detection and increased longevity is prostate cancer, and this is now the most common cancer in men. Figure 4.2 shows trends in the incidence of prostate cancer in South East England.

Since 1985, the overall incidence of prostate cancer has increased from 44.1 to 81.6 per

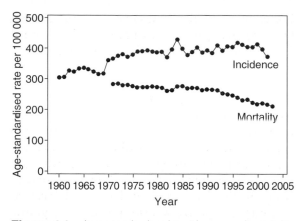

Figure 4.1 Age-standardised incidence and mortality rates for cancer in all sites in South East England 1960–2003.

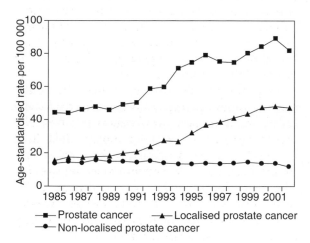

—■— Prostate cancer   —▲— Localised prostate cancer
—●— Non-localised prostate cancer

Figure 4.2 Trends in the age-standardised incidence rate for all prostate cancer in South East England 1985–2002.

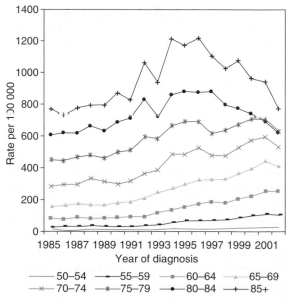

| 50–54 | 55–59 | 60–64 | 65–69 |
| 70–74 | 75–79 | 80–84 | 85+ |

Figure 4.3 Age-specific incidence rates of prostate cancer in South East England 1985–2002. Ages in years are shown in the key below.

100 000. The incidence of localised prostate cancer increased from 15.5 to 47.3 per 100 000, while the incidence of non-localised prostate cancer decreased slightly from 13.3 to 11.8 per 100 000. The rate of prostate cancer where there was no information about the extent of disease increased from 15.3 to 22.5 per 100 000. It is likely that the widespread use of a new diagnostic test prostate-specific antigen (PSA), particularly in the 1990s, explains the increase in localised prostate cancer.[4] In the European Union, prostate cancer is the fourth most commonly diagnosed cancer with around 157 000 new cases each year. Its incidence

has also been increasing in areas of Northern and Western Europe for the same reason.[3]

Are more people dying from cancer?

Data collected by the Office for National Statistics from the 1950s show that deaths from heart disease and infectious disease declined until the late 1990s. Similar data show that although the incidence of cancer has increased each year, the mortality, or rate of death, from cancer each year in the population has decreased during the same period. This has occurred for both men and women.[2] Figures for South East England also illustrate the same trend, and the decrease in mortality for males can be seen in the earlier Figure 4.1.

How common is this cancer in people my age?

Though some cancers such as testicular cancer occur in young adults, cancer is primarily a disease of older people. Again, the example of prostate cancer illustrates this well. The incidence rate within any particular age group can be easily calculated and this is called the age-specific incidence rate. Figure 4.3 shows these rates for prostate cancer from 1985 to 2002, and reveals that men aged over 85 years had the highest rate. These graphs allow the calculation of the annual percentage increase in incidence and show that men in their 50s and 60s had the highest annual increase. In most recent years of data the trends were distinctly different in different age groups. Rates declined in men aged over 80 years but increased in younger men.[4]

'Childhood cancer' is the term applied to cancer diagnosed in individuals before the age of 15 years and includes a wide range of diseases that differ from those affecting adults. In the UK leukaemias are the most common cancers affecting children (32%), followed by brain and spinal tumours (24%), and lympomas (10%).

Is cancer more common in people in the UK than elsewhere?

In general, cancer is a disease of people living in developed countries. This is partly because of the older age structure of the population in these countries, and partly because of exposure to risk factors for cancer associated with a more affluent lifestyle. A series of recent international collaborative studies has provided much more detailed information on how the incidence and survival differ for people living in the different European countries. Overall the most commonly diagnosed cancers in the European Union are bowel, breast, lung and prostate cancer. For men, however, the incidence of cancer in the UK appears lower than the overall European rate, ranking 19 out of 25. Hungary has the highest incidence rate largely due to the high rate of lung cancer, while Greece and Cyprus have the lowest. By contrast for women the cancer incidence rate is higher for the UK than the overall European rate, ranking seventh out of 25. Denmark has the highest incidence of cancer in women, while again Greece and Cyprus have the lowest rates.[3] Some cancers, for example cancers of the liver, cervix, or stomach, have a particularly high age-standardised rate in developing countries.

Aetiological epidemiology

Aetiology is the science of causes, and aetiological or analytic epidemiology is the study of risk factors for the occurrence of disease. To answer questions in this area, different kinds of studies are required from the descriptive trend studies already described – and in particular cohort or case–control studies.

How do we find out about the causes of cancer?

Although in everyday life we talk commonly and easily about one factor causing or producing a subsequent event, in epidemiology the term causality is used much more carefully, and usually with caveats. The reason is that it is unusual to find one-to-one relationships between any particular exposure and the onset of a disease. This is often due to the difficulty of measuring exposures or events that may have occurred a long time previously, and also because many common diseases including cancer are caused by many different factors – so called multifactorial causation. Different factors may have come into play at many different time points over a long latent period before the cancer develops and presents, creating a complex web of interacting causes. The causes closer to the event of cancer production are usually called proximal causes, and may themselves have their own determinants – commonly called distal causes. Epidemiology conceptualises cause in a probabilistic way as something (other things being equal) that increases the risk of a disease. Often many different factors and risks may be involved, and, to complicate matters further, some may decrease the risk of the disease.

Even with special analytical studies it is often very difficult to use epidemiological data to prove beyond doubt that a particular exposure is a definitive cause. This may need to be confirmed by an experiment – by either inducing cancer in animals or by intervening in a human population to prevent cancer. It is important to remember that even when factors are found that increase the risk of a disease at a population level, these are often very different from those that determine which individuals within the population develop the disease. The easily made assumption that relationships found at the population level will hold at an individual level is referred to as an ecological fallacy. It occurs because the ecological (population) effect fails to reflect the biological effect as it occurs at the individual level. Ecological bias occurs therefore when the measure of the association found at the group level is a distortion of any association occurring at individual level.

Epidemiological enquiry often begins by carefully describing an association observed between two factors, and then proceeds to deduce the extent to which causal inference is possible. If a difference in risk is discovered between two populations, then assessing the possibility of cause generally considers whether three factors may be operating – chance, bias and confounding.[5] These are described in turn.

Chance
Chance variation in the selection of a sample for any study can result in a false inference about the relevance of results to the whole population from which the sample was drawn. Tests of statistical significance have been designed to indicate how likely it is that a result in any sample arose by chance and is not in fact a real difference from the comparison group. The *P* value, which is given as a decimal, is the probability of obtaining (by play of chance) the observed distribution or a more extreme distribution, if no association truly exists. *P* values are influenced by both the size of the sample and the size or strength of the association. The larger the sample size, the higher the chance that the result is significant. Researchers usually set a probability value of less than 5% ($P < 0.05$) or 1% ($P < 0.01$) at which they call a finding 'statistically significant'.[6] This allows for the possibility that there is a one in 20 or one in 100 probability respectively that the difference could have arisen by chance. An increasingly used alternate measure is the confidence interval, which sets a range of values for the variable of study. The range is constructed so that it includes the range of values within which is it probable, given the sample size, that the true value falls. This specified probability is called the confidence level, and the end of the points of the confidence interval are called the confidence limits.[6] Associations between variables may be statistically significant but not causal, and it is also possible for a causal relationship to exist even if the association is not statistically significant. Small studies are often said to lack the power (size) to detect weak causal associations. Methods to increase the ability of an analysis to detect a given effect include increasing the sample size or pooling the results of several smaller studies together into a meta-analysis.

Bias
Bias can be defined as a systematic tendency for results to differ from the truth. The two most common sources of bias in epidemiological studies are selection bias and information bias. Selection bias occurs when the method of selecting study subjects into the groups being compared is not the same. This can also occur where participants differentially respond in one group or are recruited more commonly to one group rather than the other. Information bias occurs when the actual information collected from the two comparison groups is not the same. For example, participants in one group may inadvertently be asked questions or recall information in different ways from those in other groups. Alternatively, a researcher who is aware of or 'not blind' to the research hypothesis may consciously or otherwise seek out or observe more factors of causal interest in one group than another. Potential biases need to be thought through in the design of new studies, as it can be difficult to correct these at the analysis stage. In any study a judgement will finally need to be made about their likely presence and the strength of any effect on the results.

Confounding
Confounding refers to the tendency of factors of interest to cluster together so that the groups differ in the exposure of main interest but also on a number of other related factors. A confounding factor is one associated with, but not a consequence of, the exposure of interest, and with the proximal or distant cause of the disease under investigation. The effect of a confounding variable may be to exaggerate the degree of association between disease and exposure – a phenomenon called positive confounding – or to mask a true relationship – negative confounding. The effect of confounding can be diminished by good study design but, unlike the effects of bias, can be eliminated at analysis stage by using statistical techniques that control for the effect of potential confounders. Potential techniques include standardisation and multiple regression. However, it is only possible to control for confounding factors

that have been measured in any study. If confounding variables have not been measured, or measured imprecisely, then the effect cannot be controlled and residual confounding will remain in the results.

In assessing the likelihood that an association is causal, the possibility of chance, bias and confounding will need to be excluded. Sets of criteria for assessing causality have been developed to help with this. One such scheme is the Bradford Hill criteria set out in Box 4.2. Not all these criteria need apply in every case. Indeed in some instances a causal link may need to be assumed and prevention undertaken at a public-health level before the exact mechanism is understood.

Box 4.2   Bradford Hill criteria for assessing causality

1. *Strength*: does the relative risk differ greatly from unity or the correlation coefficient from zero? If so it is unlikely to be explained by bias and confounding.
2. *Independence*: does adjustment for known confounders markedly alter the association? If not residual confounding is unlikely.
3. *Specificity*: is the association specific to one combination of disease or exposure? This makes causality more likely but its absence does not exclude it (as some exposures may cause many different diseases).
4. *Consistency*: is the association found in different study populations and across different study designs? This provides evidence against bias, confounding and chance.
5. *Time sequence*: is the temporal sequence correct? This is essential to be able to argue against the possibility of reverse causality.
6. *Dose response*: is there a graded relationship between exposure and the risk of disease?
7. *Plausibility*: is the causal link biologically plausible? However, not all aetiological relationships can be explained in terms of current knowledge.
8. *Reversibility*: can the association be shown to be diminished by a preventative experiment?

Was it something I was exposed to?

The discussion so far shows how difficult it may be to answer this question. Nonetheless, a number of factors have been clearly linked to an increased occurrence of different cancers – cigarette smoke and lung cancer, asbestos and mesothelioma, radiation and haematological cancer, and sunlight exposure and skin cancer. A case–control study is a design commonly used by researchers wishing to identify risk factors for disease development. This kind of study compares the past history of exposure to the factor being investigated in a group of people who have a particular disease, with the exposure in the population at large. Those with the diseases are the 'cases' and those in the comparison group are 'controls'. Some of the first classic investigations of this kind were studies in the early 1950s investigating the link between smoking and lung cancer.[7] These researchers first studied the medical records of patients with and without lung cancer and compared their smoking history. A strong relationship, suggesting nine times the risk of lung cancer among smokers emerged, leading them to carry out a larger interview study questioning patients directly about their smoking history. Their next step was to conduct a longitudinal study to test their hypothesis prospectively.[8] For this they assembled a cohort study of 20 000 UK male doctors and followed them over time to investigate their health.[9] This allowed them to show that as well as smoking increasing the risk of lung cancer, the more individuals smoked and the longer they smoked the higher their risk of dying of lung cancer became. Smoking cessation was shown to reduce the risk.

Case–control and cohort studies have also shown that mesothelioma is linked to prior exposure to asbestos, mostly of men working to manufacture and use it in shipbuilding, and insulation. The link between radiation and leukaemia was established by observing risk in children exposed *in utero* to X-rays used for pelvimetry before childbirth. Studies after the explosion of atomic weapons in Japan at the end of the second world war found an increase in the rates of leukaemia very soon after. Rates were found to be 150 times greater for people who had been within 1 km of the blast.

Measures of disease risk

In situations where the researcher has information about outcome by following up a group of people exposed to a risk factor of interest and can compare this to the risk in another unexposed group, it is possible to make a calculation of the relative risk or the relative rate of a disease following that exposure. The relative rate is defined as the ratio of the incidence rate of the disease in the exposed group divided by the corresponding rate in the non-exposed group. A relative rate of 1.0 indicates that the incidence rates of disease in the exposed and non-exposed group are the same, and that there is therefore no association observed between the exposure and the disease in the data. A value greater than 1.0 indicates an increased risk among those exposed to the factor. On the other hand, a relative rate of less than 1.0 means that there is a decreased risk among the exposed. The value of the relative rate depends on the time period over which the rate is calculated, which must be specified. For example, in their 20-year follow-up study of British doctors Doll and Peto found that the annual mortality rate for lung cancer per 100 000 population was 140 among cigarette smokers and 10 for non-smokers, giving a relative risk of smoking of 14.[9]

In some situations the researcher does not have access to complete follow-up data from a whole cohort of individuals, and may need to rely on a case–control study as already discussed. An economical approach commonly used to study rare outcomes is to select research subjects on the basis of their disease status, and question them and a comparison group of selected controls about their prior exposure to the risk factor of interest. The researcher does not know the outcome for all the people exposed to the risk factor, so rather than calculating the relative rate as in a cohort study, the odds of the disease are calculated to give the odds ratio. This can give an unbiased estimate of the relative rate.

While the relative rate represents the likelihood of disease in exposed individuals relative to the unexposed, the population-attributable risk is a measure that provides information about the absolute effect of the exposure. Its value gives an indication of the number of cases among the exposed that can be attributed to the exposure and could therefore be avoided if exposure to the risk factor could be eliminated. It can therefore be used as a measure of the potential public-health impact of a particular exposure. For example, the population-attributable risk for smoking in lung cancer is 82%. In the absence of smoking this proportion of lung cancer cases could be avoided.

Prevention and screening

Could I have done anything to prevent it?

Primary prevention is the prevention of the disease by removing or avoiding the factors that are known to cause or promote its development. It is estimated that over one-half of all cancers could be avoided by removing exposure to cigarette smoke and by improving diet to include less fat and alcohol and more fruit, vegetables and fibre. Improved diet and exercise could also decrease obesity, which appears to be a risk factor for some cancers including breast, colorectal, oesophageal, endometrial and kidney cancer. Secondary prevention or screening is the prevention of disease after it has developed but before it becomes clinically manifest and begins causing problems for the patient. Tertiary prevention in the detection of disease at the earliest stage possible, when there is most chance of treating the disease and minimising its impact on either survival or quality of life.

Why isn't there screening/earlier diagnosis for my cancer?

Screening is an organised effort by a health care system to improve the outcome of a disease by reducing either the number of cases within the population or the severity of the disease in those who develop it. Screening is not the urgent referral of patients with clinical symptoms suggestive of disease, nor is it the application of tests to those in whom suggestive symptoms are discovered. Instead it is the consistent offer of a test to individuals without symptoms who are at a higher risk than other population groups of developing that disease. This screening test does not in itself diagnose the disease but simply indicates those who require further evaluation by more definitive tests. It is those diagnostic tests, not the screening test, that will determine if the disease is present. It is often assumed that screening must be a good thing because it is better to diagnose any disease and receive treatment for it earlier than later, but this is not always the case. A great deal depends on the natural history of the disease and the number of negative effects that the screening programme and early treatment may have. In the UK, national cancer screening programmes are in place for breast and cervical cancer. One for colorectal cancer is about to be implemented, another for prostate cancer is being considered. A careful evaluation of risks, benefits and costs is now mandatory before any screening test is introduced. One commonly used set of criteria for assessing a screening test is that developed by Wilson and Junger (see Box 4.3).

Box 4.3 Wilson and Junger criteria for accepting population screening

1. The condition sought should be an important health problem.
2. There should be accepted treatment for patients with recognised diseases.
3. Facilities for diagnosis and treatment should be available.
4. There should be a recognised latent or early symptomatic stage.
5. There should be a suitable test or examination.
6. The test should be acceptable to the population.
7. The natural history of the disease, including latent disease, should be adequately understood.
8. There should be an agreed policy on whom to treat.
9. The cost of case-finding (including diagnosis and treatment of patients diagnosed) should be economically balanced in relation to possible expenditure on medical care as a whole.
10. Case-finding should be a continuing process and not a one-off project.

The first criterion for introducing a screening test is that the disease is serious. While most cancers might appear to satisfy this criterion it must also be the case that treatment during the detectable preclinical phase must result in a better prognosis than treatment given after symptoms develop. While breast cancer and cervical cancer screening appear to fulfil this, screening for lung cancer does not detect early-stage disease that can make a sufficient difference to mortality. The prevalence of preclinical disease must also be high in the population to justify the development of the programme. The test must be inexpensive, easy to administer, valid, reliable, reproducible and cause minimal discomfort to individuals to whom it is offered.

The performance of any screening test is usually described in terms of its specificity and sensitivity and its ability to produce false-positive and false-negative results. Sensitivity is the chance that a screening test will be positive if the patient truly does have the disease. As a test becomes more sensitive, the proportion of patients who are incorrectly classified as false negative will decrease. Specificity, on the other hand, is the chance that a screening test is negative if the disease truly does not exist in an individual. A test that is highly specific will rarely be positive in an individual without the disease and will therefore produce a low proportion of patients with false-positive results. Ideally it would seem desirable for a screening test to be both highly sensitive and specific, but in reality after a certain point there is usually a trade-off between the two measures when an increase in one results in a decrease in the other.

Any screening procedure will induce anxiety both in patients undergoing the test and in those who test positive and require further investigations. Investigations and treatment may themselves result in risk. It is therefore important that the overall benefit gained by those individuals eventually diagnosed and treated far outweigh any negative effects on the screened population and on those diagnosed by screening and treated without receiving better outcomes.

The screening programme for breast cancer has been most thoroughly evaluated. Randomised controlled trials of mammography for women aged over 50 years show that the mortality has decreased in women offered screening compared with unscreened controls. The fact that the reduction has not been significant in all the trials has led to some controversy, but the consensus of all expert opinion is that if 70% of eligible women attend for screening there is a 25% reduction in breast cancer mortality. Seventy per cent attendance is the minimum standard for the UK screening programme, though in some areas of the country the uptake is much lower. The sensitivity of mammography for women aged over 50 years is around 80%, but it is far lower in younger women because their predominantly more-dense breasts make detection difficult. The specificity of mammography ranges from 82% to 97% and 6–8% of women recalled after their first-ever screen for further tests turn out to have cancer. The age range included in national screening was originally 50–64 years, but was increased to 70 years in 2004. Women attend special centres where two-view mammography is carried out by staff dedicated to screening. The programme is subject to rigorous quality assurance according to national standards.[3] Current issues for the screening service are to determine, in collaboration with cancer registries, the rates of cancers that present symptomatically between screening intervals. An issue emerging very recently from follow-up studies of the women in the early Scandinavian trials of breast screening is that of over-diagnosis. Although screening programmes lead to a reduction in the population mortality from breast cancer, they also lead to an increase in cancers that would otherwise not have presented or been treated.[10,11]

Clinical epidemiology

Clinical epidemiology is the application of the principles, methods and findings of epidemiology to the diagnosis, prognosis, appraisal of decisions about treatment, and evaluation of care. Its focus is not on the risk of disease in the general population, sometimes called 'public health epidemiology', but instead on the study of patients who have already developed the disease. Its aim is to determine the factors contributing to outcome of the disease (for example, rates of recovery, disability, or death) rather than to determine what caused the patient to develop it. There is some debate about the exact definition of clinical epidemiology, and the term is also sometimes used for studies that include any kind of clinical measurement. The principles of clinical epidemiology are also similar and overlap to some extent with those of the recently developed term 'evidence-based medicine' – the conscientious, explicit, and judicious use of current best evidence in making decisions about the care of individual patients.[12]

What are my chances of cure with this treatment?

This is one of the most obvious questions to ask, and although not all patients may directly seek such explicit information, it is certainly a question that health professionals will want to be able to answer for the patient groups they see. The difficulty of determining risk for an individual patient as opposed to risk for a group of patients applies, as described before in the section on risk (pp. 57–58). There are several ways of thinking about the survival of groups of patients, and a number of techniques can be applied to data collected about the death of patients at different points in time. The first requirement is that there is adequate follow-up information. The survival rate is the simplest expression of the survival – and corresponds to the proportion of survivors in any one group studied and followed for a particular period of time. It may also be called the cumulative survival rate, and logically this equals 1 minus the cumulative fatality rate. Survival is usually calculated for the period of 5 years after the diagnosis, though when considering diseases with a very poor prognosis, e.g. lung or brain cancer, 1- or 2-year survival rates may be used. On the other hand, where statistics have been routinely collected and held for longer periods it may be possible to calculate 10- or 20-year survival. In many cancers the 5-year survival rate is usually regarded as the rate of cure.

Another very common way of presenting survival information visually is by plotting a survival curve, often using the Kaplan–Meier method which accommodates the fact that not all patients will have been followed ultimately to death. This curve starts with 100% of the study population alive at time zero – usually the date of diagnosis – and shows the percentage of patients surviving at each successive point in time before the endpoint of the study. These curves provide information about the rate of decline in the number of patients remaining alive and the different points at which patients are lost. These curves are also often referred to as crude survival curves. They are so-termed not because of their inelegance, but because they do not take into account the deaths that would have occurred in the group of patients whether or not they had been diagnosed with

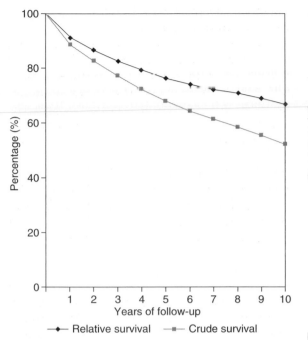

Figure 4.4 Period analysis of relative survival (1999–2003) for female breast cancer in South East England.

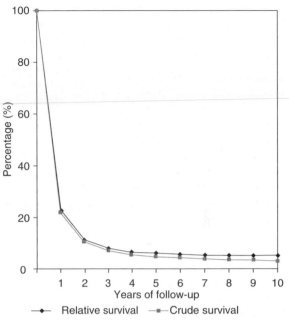

Figure 4.5 Period analysis of relative survival 1999–2003 for cancer of the lung in males in South East England.

cancer. In any group of similar-aged individuals, a number of people would have died from other causes. Information on other deaths is contained in a current 'life table', which summarises the combined mortality experience by age of a population in a particular period of time. From this can be calculated the survival of the diagnosed patient cohort relative to the general population. One way of understanding the relative survival is to see the general population survival – the background survival that might be expected – as running along at 100%, and to judge the drop in survival from that point to the relative survival curve for the group of interest as that attributable to having the particular diagnosis of cancer rather than to age. Figure 4.4 shows how the relative survival rate for women with breast cancer is higher than the crude survival. The difference between crude and relative survival is less pronounced for lung cancer as shown in Figure 4.5.

A method of providing even more specific information is to estimate the contribution to the risk of mortality for particular groups of patients; this may include age groups, stages of disease at

diagnosis, or those presenting with particular disabilities or co-morbid conditions. The proportional hazards model or Cox model estimates the risk that a patient in any of these groups will experience the hazard (usually death) in a given period of time.

As well as the nature of the survival analysis, it is important to be clear which population of patients it represents. Population-based analyses will include all patients known to have received the diagnosis in the entire resident population during the time period. This should be distinguished from a sample of patients diagnosed and treated in either primary or secondary care. Many selection factors operate to affect which patients are detected in primary care and which of these are referred on to secondary care and eventually receive treatment. Experience of seeing only patients treated in secondary care can give a distorted picture of the prognosis for a particular patient group. In addition, data from clinical trials may exclude older patients and those with co-morbidity. For example, clinical trials of one haematological cancer, myeloma, had historically included only patients aged under 65 years. Analysis of population data collected by the Thames Cancer Registry showed a high proportion of patients aged over 70 years, and led to the redesign of trials to determine the best treatment for this group (Steve Schey, personal communication).

Another increasingly topical issue is whether survival can be compared between different small areas of residence and even different hospitals. Because fewer patients die from their disease than are diagnosed, survival analyses require larger numbers than incidence analyses. For that reason comparison between larger populations is more robust than that between smaller areas. Indeed it has been argued that the average population of size of 100 000 in a UK primary care trust is too small a unit of analysis to determine meaningful differences between trusts on a year-on-year basis. Even comparisons of larger populations covered by cancer networks may reveal differences that are due to population characteristics, such as age structure, general health, and co-morbid conditions, as well as differences in treatment policy. On the other hand, performance tables of outcome are increasingly being used by the NHS. In cardiothoracic surgery, for example, post-operative mortality is now publicly available by named surgeon. Although most clinicians wish to know how their own hospital performs and how their patients survive, there are many concerns about the potential that over-simplistic or incorrect analyses have to damage public and patient confidence in individual hospitals. The chief methodological concern about published analyses is the degree to which referral patterns and case mix (prognostic factors) are, or can be, taken into account in assessing outcome. Co-morbidity is a major consideration in the clinical decision to refer and treat patients. It seems very likely that many specialist cancer centres treat patient populations that are skewed in two directions – towards those with the very best prognoses and towards those with complex problems that may have the worse prognoses. The problem is of whether like is being compared with like, as well as whether data can be obtained on all the possible factors of relevance. Whether and when it will be sensible to undertake these analyses will be a challenge for the cancer community as more data on individual patients are collected, and there is increasing pressure for more information to be made available.

Should I undergo this treatment?
The gold standard for the evaluation of cancer treatment is the randomised controlled trial. This is a planned test of a new treatment which compares the outcome in terms of symptom relief, quality of life, and survival for patients that receive and do not receive it. The key strength of this kind of trial is that, with their consent, patients are randomised to receive either the new treatment or the comparison treatment. This randomisation means that patients with different prognostic factors (that might affect the outcome after treatment) are likely to be distributed evenly between the two groups. This makes it much more likely that any difference observed is the result of the treatment being tested and not other factors. Trials require careful design and monitoring to ensure that they are ethical, feasible, acceptable for patients, measure the relevant range of outcomes, are large enough to detect a significant difference, and are stopped at the right time (i.e. if adverse effects emerge or the answer to the study question becomes clear beyond doubt).

Cohort studies of patients with a particular diagnosis can also provide relevant information for patients. They can, for example, tell them about their chances of return to work, the time they might expect to spend free from disability, or symptoms they may experience. However, the degree to which findings from cohort studies can be generalised will always depend on the breadth of the initial selection of patients and the adequacy of their follow-up. Because selection may be operating in determining which patients are included into cohort studies, and because there is no comparison group, cohort studies are not the best way to answer questions about the effectiveness of treatment. Again, predicting the outcome for the average patient does not easily translate into a prediction for any particular individual patient.

What does this new study mean for me?
The media often report the results of new treatment trials uncritically and somewhat overoptimistically in a way that may lead patients to expect

new treatments to be immediately available. Equally, the results of epidemiological studies may be reported as showing a relative increased risk of cancer occurrence in relation to a factor that is significant but represents a very small absolute increase in risk for any individual. Being asked to comment on a recently published study can therefore place health professionals in a difficult position. A good start is to explain a few important principles such as the need to consider the population studied or the groups of patients included, the likely generalisability of findings, and the need to confirm findings before practice is changed. However, for more detailed questions it is probably best to direct patients to more authoritative sources of information, such as fact sheets produced by major charities, and to provide reassurance that robust processes exist in the UK to ensure that new available evidence is discussed, debated and put into practice as soon as possible.

Public health policy

Although many researchers work with the hope that their findings will lead to improved public health policy or cancer services, attention to the quality of research evidence and ensuring its publication is rarely sufficient on its own to cause this. Innovators may use new knowledge to change their practice, and by their actions influence others, and in this way a new practice may diffuse throughout a health care system. However, this is usually a slow and patchy process. Creating a faster and more consistent change across an entire health care system requires a much more deliberate and organised effort. Getting evidence into practice requires a number of different events to occur. Evidence needs to be brought together, independently compared and considered, and a decision made about costs and benefits of putting it into practice. Political action needs to make that change a priority, release the resources to make change happen, decide what the mechanisms will be, over what timescale the change will occur, and how this will be monitored. Over the past 10 years there has been a consistent effort to do just this for cancer prevention and care in the UK.

What is this government/hospital/ primary care trust/cancer network doing to improve things?

The NHS Cancer Plan was published in 2000, and set out a range of specific objectives and targets linking prevention, diagnosis, treatment, care, and research for the first time.[13] It followed the 1999 *NHS Plan* – a 1-year plan to modernise the NHS by providing more staff and equipment to make services more effective and responsive to patient needs. It was also a practical implementation plan for the earlier *Calman–Hine Report* of 1995 that had set out the need for more consistent and specialised cancer services across the country.[14] *The NHS Cancer Plan* took forward the government's earlier 1997 public health agenda to cut the death rate in people aged under 75 years by at least one-fifth and to reduce adult smoking rates from 28% to 24% by 2010. In addition it set out to narrow the gap in cancer mortality and survival between the individuals living in most- and least-affluent areas, aimed to reduce smoking rates among manual groups from 32% in 1998 to 26% by 2010, and to set local targets for the areas with the highest rates. This was judged important because both the overall incidence and mortality rates of cancer are highest in areas of social deprivation. Although mortality is declining in the UK in all social groups, the absolute difference between affluent and deprived areas remains the same, or may even increase as those living in more affluent areas take up screening, stop smoking and change their diet earlier than those living in deprived areas. To reduce the gap, public health action may need to focus on people living in more deprived areas, and in 2004 an inequality target was set to reduce the cancer mortality gap between the richest fifth and the poorest fifth of primary care trusts by at least 6%. It is intended that this will be met by encouraging people to give up smoking, to present earlier to their general practitioners with symptoms, and to attend more regularly for screening, by extending the screening programme to 65–70-year-old women and ensuring the use of referral guidelines and better access to diagnostic tests for general practitioners.[14]

Smoking has proved a controversial public health issue to tackle but there has been gradual policy progress including a ban on advertising, stronger health warnings on cigarettes, anti-smoking campaigns, and more services to help people give up smoking. Most recently a ban on smoking in public places was introduced after much discussion, evidence of the success of such policies in parts of the US, and a free vote in the House of Commons. An initial proposal for a partial ban, exempting pubs that did not serve food was generally felt to disadvantage those living and working in pubs in more-deprived areas, which are more likely not to serve food.

In terms of other public health measures the previous *NHS Plan* had already focused on the role of diet, developing the five-a day programme encouraging people to eat more fruit and vegetables, and had developed a scheme to give free fruit to 4–6 year olds at school. *The NHS Cancer Plan* extended the breast cancer screening programme to include all women aged 65–70 years, and made it available to women over the age of 70 years on request. The cervical cancer screening programme was upgraded, pilots for implementation of colorectal cancer put in place, and more information provided for men about PSA testing to enable them to consider the costs of benefits of the test before making their choice.[13]

To deliver better cancer services, *The NHS Cancer Plan* sought to strengthen the ability of cancer networks to co-ordinate care and implement policies for better care. A major focus has been to decrease delay in diagnosis and treatment by setting targets for the time people waited after urgent referral or diagnosis to begin their treatment – the ultimate gaol being that no one should wait more than one month from urgent referral. Extra funding for scanners for diagnosis, treatment machines for radiotherapy, and the management of system change was also made available.[14]

Another policy focus has been the development of clear standards for care based on best available evidence. Following the *Calman–Hine Report* of 1995,[15] this was carried by the Improving Outcomes Guidance of the Clinical Outcomes Group of the Department of Health. Since 2000 the National Institute for Clinical Excellence (NICE) has developed and revised subsequent guidance. For cancer the guidance takes the form of a review of the evidence for effective care

carried out by an independent academic group, and a set of recommendations developed by a multidisciplinary expert group informed by wide stakeholder consultation. Such sets of guidance have now been produced for the most common cancers, and those for less common ones will be published soon after. Cancer networks are charged with developing local plans to implement these recommendations.

Is the UK doing as well as countries of similar economic status?

A major stimulus for these UK policy initiatives was the finding from European cancer registries study on cancer patients' survival and care (EUROCARE) studies that survival for patients with many of the major cancers in the UK lagged behind that for patients in the rest of Europe. It has been unclear exactly what the reason for this difference is but it is unlikely that it represents a chance finding. Whether it is a difference in stage at presentation, a difference in treatment given, or difference in the way the data are collected is unclear.[16] The assumption underlying policy initiatives so far has been that it may represent the presentation of patients at a later stage of the disease and a need for more consistent and organised treatment. The findings of the EUROCARE collaboration have also led to significant changes in cancer policy for different cancers in Denmark, Norway and Italy.[16]

How is information about cancer routinely collected and used in the UK?

As already mentioned, the Office for National Statistics collates data collected by the nine cancer registries in England and Wales and publishes annual statistics on cancer incidence and mortality. Annual data on incidence and mortality, and analyses of survival trends are also published for Scotland and Northern Ireland. The basis of these figures is data collected by cancer registries from the medical records and pathology records in hospitals, other electronic sources of data from hospitals, hospices, private hospitals, cancer screening programmes, other cancer registries, primary care, nursing homes, and death certificates. The registration dataset includes basic demographic information on age, sex, ethnicity, place of residence, information about the cancer including its site, its morphology and stage, and data on the first hospital the patient attended, where they received their first surgery, radiotherapy, hormonal, and chemotherapy treatment. This data is collected and coded by trained data officers and quality assured as it is entered to the cancer registry database. Registries follow up patient records for the first 6 months after diagnosis but do not actively collect follow-up information after this time. They receive death certificates for residents in their area who die from cancer, from the Office for National Statistics via the NHS Register. Registries never contact patients directly to check information or gather additional information for research. All data are kept securely and only reported as aggregate figures in reports. Until now patients have not been asked to give consent for their data to be collected and stored in the cancer registration dataset. Instead their consent has been implied and cancer registration is covered by section 60 of the Health and Social Care Act 2001 that exempts registries from having to seek consent from each individual on the basis that its purposes are in the interests of patients or the wider public. Currently, a leaflet explaining cancer registration is being piloted to ensure that patients do have information about the uses of these data, how their confidentiality is maintained, and how they may withdraw their details if they wish. The UK has the most comprehensive system of cancer registration in the world, and there has been some concern that if a large number of individuals chose to opt out of the process the quality of the data and their usefulness will be compromised. On the other hand, asking for explicit consent around the time of diagnosis could place an additional information burden on patients as they come to terms with the news of their diagnosis and are asked to make important decisions about treatment.

Much cancer research in the UK has made use of these aggregate cancer data with identifiable information removed. Identifiable data are currently only released back to organisations or individuals treating the patient, to the patient at their request, or to bona fide researchers who can justify the use of identifiable data, and have approval from a relevant research ethics committee and received a section 60 exemption.

Although the UK has the most comprehensive data on cancer in the world, it is increasingly recognised that more could be done to use these data effectively. Many of *The NHS Cancer Plan* targets require good information to monitor them. National plans for cancer intelligence aim to link cancer registration data to those contained in the hospital patient administration system and other datasets, and to obtain better information on ethnicity and staging of cancer.

More detailed information for patients on the epidemiology of individual cancers in the UK can be obtained from Cancer Research UK which produces a series of clear summary fact sheets for patients and professionals based on cancer registration data. Further information may be also obtained from the other organisations listed in Box 4.4.

Box 4.4   Sources of further information

- Cancer Research UK www.cancerresearchuk.org
- Cancerbackup www.cancerbackup.org.uk
- Macmillan Cancer Support www.macmillan.org.uk/Home.aspx
- National Cancer Screening programme www.cancer-screening.nhs.uk
- National Institute for Health and Clinical Excellence www.nice.nhs.uk
- UK Association of Cancer Registries www.ukacr.org
- Office for National Statistics www.statistics.gov.uk
- National Cancer Research Institute www.ncri.org.uk
- International Association of Cancer Registries www.iarc.com.fr

Most developed countries have been able to invest in the development of population-based registries collecting standard datasets and methods of analyses over many years. These may cover the whole nation or defined regions from which findings may be extrapolated to other areas. Countries from Africa, Central and South America, North America, Asia and Europe contribute to a compilation of cancer incidence across the world.[17] The International Association of Cancer Registries provides training and software support to individuals in countries aiming to develop their own registration system.

Acknowledgements
We thank Professor David Strachen for his clear teaching summaries of epidemiology to which we have referred in preparing this chapter, and to Professor Henrik Møller, Director of the Thames Cancer Registry for his comments on an earlier version of this chapter.

References

1. Fritz A., Percy C., Jack A. *et al.* (eds.) (2000). *World Health Organization. International Classification of Diseases for Oncology*, 3rd edition. Geneva: World Health Organisation.

2. Quinn M., Babb P., Brock A., Kirby L. and Jones J. Office for National Statistics. (2001). *Cancer Trends in England and Wales 1950–1999*. London: The Stationery Office.

3. Toms J.R. (2004). *CancerStats Monograph 2004*. London: Cancer Research UK.

4. Thames Cancer Registry. (2004). *Cancer in South East England 2002*. London: Thames Cancer Registry. www.tcr.org.uk (accessed 23 July 2007).

5. Hennekens C.H. and Buring J.E. (1987). *Epidemiology in Medicine*. Boston: Little Brown and Company.

6. Last J.M. (1998). *A Dictionary of Epidemiology*. New York: Oxford University Press.

7. Doll R. and Hill A.B. (1950). Smoking and carcinoma of the lung: preliminary report. *British Medical Journal* **2**, 739–748.

8. Doll R. and Hill A.B. (1971). A study of the aetiology of carcinoma of the lung. *British Medical Journal* **2**, 1271.

9. Doll R. and Peto R. (1976). Mortality in relation to smoking: 20 years observation on male British doctors. *British Medical Journal* **ii**, 1525–1536.

10. Zackrisson S., Andersson I., Janzon L., Manjer J. and Garne J.P. (2006). Rate of over-diagnosis of breast cancer 15 years after end of Malmö mammographic screening trial: follow-up study. *British Medical Journal* **332**, 609–692.

11. Moller H. and Davies E. (2006). Commentary: Over-diagnosis in breast cancer screening. *British Medical Journal* **332**, 691–692.

12. Sackett D., Richardson W.S., Rosenberg W. and Haynes R.B. (1997). *Evidence-based Medicine. How to Practice and Teach Evidence-based Medicine*. New York: Churchill Livingstone.

13. Department of Health. (2000). *The NHS Cancer Plan: A Plan for Investment, a Plan for Reform*. London: Department of Health.

14. Department of Health. (2004). *The NHS Cancer Plan and the New NHS: Providing a Patient-centred Service*. London: Department of Health.

15. Department of Health. (1995). *Calman–Hine Report. Expert Advisory Group on Cancer. A Policy Framework for Commissioning Cancer Services*. London: Department of Health.

16. Coleman M.P., Gatta G., Verdecchia A. *et al.* and the EUROCARE Working Group. (2003). EUROCARE-3 summary: cancer survival in Europe at the end of the 20th century. *Annals of Oncology* **14**, v128–149.

17. Parkin D.M., Whelan S.L., Ferlay J., Teppo L. and Thomas D.B. (eds.) (2002). *Cancer Incidence in Five Continents. Volume VIII*. Lyons: International Agency for Research on Cancer.

CHAPTER FIVE

Developments in the management of cancer

Alastair Munro

The title of this chapter is carefully chosen. It reflects the facts that not all developments are new and that there is more to cancer than treating it. Cancer does not exist in isolation, nor does its management. In terms of managing cancer we have to consider not just how we might try to control cancer, but also the context within which our efforts take place. The things we do are complex, and so is the context.

THE CONTEXT OF CANCER MANAGEMENT

Cancer affects individuals – but individuals exist in society and therefore any consideration of cancer that fails to place it within a social and economic context is inevitably incomplete. These issues are dealt with at length in other chapters in this book and are simply mentioned here as a reminder that developments in cancer will be affected by the times in which we live. Science and medicine are, after all, cultural activities.

Developments in the context of cancer management

In 1971 Richard Nixon famously declared war on cancer. Subsequently he lost the war, his reputation and the presidency. The main consequence of his declaration was to make the cure of cancer a high priority for medical research in the US and throughout the world. Society was encouraged to believe that cancer was a scourge that had to be, and could be, controlled. The application of science would solve the problem. Despite enormous investment over more than 30 years, the results of these efforts, from the point of view of society as a whole, have been modest. Given these modest achievements, we cannot assume that society will continue to fund cancer research at its current levels. Governments will demand value for money.

There is also the important question of, if resources are to be limited, what research questions should take priority. The Macmillan listening study showed that patients put a high priority on research into the impact cancer had on the lives of patients and their families.[1] This is in direct distinction to the emphasis on basic scientific research that has applied over the past decades. One consequence of this mismatch will be a continued increase in the number and importance of those charities (Macmillan Cancer Support, Marie Curie, Maggie's Centres) that attempt to support and inform patients and families affected by cancer. We should remember that even victories leave casualties and refugees in their wake.

Changing demographics

Cancer is a disease of ageing cells and, in the developed world, we are an ageing society. As people live longer, the prevalence of cancer rises and so, relative to other diseases, does cancer-related mortality. This leads to a series of gloomy prognostications concerning the 'epidemic' of cancer in the elderly. All of which ignores the simple fact that most of us accept that we have to die of something, and that not every 85 year old wants to cling desperately to life at any cost. We know surprisingly little about the attitudes of older people to the management of cancer: we tend to manage older patients as if they were simply slightly decrepit versions of their younger selves. All of us involved in managing patients with cancer need to have some knowledge of how to deal with the problems of older people facing cancer. The imperative to cure, felt by many oncologists, may be at odds with the values and hopes of many of their older patients. We will need to help older people explain themselves to us and, in return, we need to explain our interventions to them in terms that are neither dishonest nor intimidating. We need to design management policies that are both effective and acceptable to older patients.

The business of cancer

The relationship between medicine and society is changing. In order to attract publicity and resources medical researchers advertise their 'breakthroughs' in a way that, previously, would have been unthinkable. Drug companies use newspapers and television for product placement: even mediocre remedies are hailed as 'important advances'. The public is whipped up into a frenzy of expectation, only to be disappointed when the so-called breakthrough fails to have any demonstrable impact on what happens to their nearest and dearest. If, despite the positive messages from every news bulletin, they are told that they, or their friend or relative, will die from cancer, it is only natural that people will look around for someone to blame: sometimes themselves; sometimes multinational corporations; sometimes the health care system; sometimes individual practitioners. This, in turn, leads to defensive behaviour by those who consider themselves vulnerable to blame. Foods are suddenly removed from supermarket shelves because some minor additive has caused cancer in rats; family doctors send patients with minor symptoms to surgeons for investiga-

tions ('just in case') to exclude cancer. Clinical guidelines are used in a spirit of corporate protection rather than as a means of ensuring that each individual is offered the management that is most appropriate for them. Overall, there is a paradoxical paralysis: paradoxical, because action is commoner than reflection; paralysis, because thought is dominated by fear. These trends will develop and strengthen over the next decade. Cancer management will operate within a business model. Governance, economics, protocols, and risk assessments will dominate practice. Disasters will be less likely, but the opportunity cost could be a depersonalisation of care at every level, and from every perspective.

The belief that money conquers all

The market of spurious claims has another consequence. The notion arises that money is the solution to every problem. International comparisons are particularly invidious in this respect. The results of cancer treatment may appear to be better in the US, but this is not necessarily a result of greater expenditure or competence but may simply reflect the fact that we simply do not know very much about how cancer affects the millions of Americans with limited access to health care.

People come to believe that simply by paying money (for that wonder diet, for 'going private', for the new drug available for purchase on the internet, for a whole-body scan) every problem can be solved. A belief put most succinctly, in the context of AIDS, by the American writer Harold Brodkey: 'I want Clinton to save my life'. As if money and power were all that mattered.

With greater regulation of clinical practice, with costs for cancer management rising, with the widening of the socioeconomic chasm between those who have in abundance and those from whom what little they had has been taken, the number of individuals seeking cures on the open market will increase. For every person willing to pay, there is always someone eager to be paid.

The need for an evidence base

The increased regulation of cancer services is not just about containing costs, it is also about raising standards. The need to demonstrate objectively that any given intervention works is an essential part of this process. There should be evidence to support the use of an intervention: habit and custom are not enough, precedent is no guarantee of effectiveness.[2,3] The evidence-based approach applies just as much to nursing, and to oncology, as it does to any other branch of clinical activity.[4–7] Systematic reviews of the available data from randomised trials, for example those published in the Cochrane Library,[8,9] are a useful source of evidence upon which to base clinical practice.

Developments in global aspects of cancer management

Cancer in the developing world

Cancer is a global problem: 11 million people are diagnosed with cancer each year, the figure is expected to rise to 16 million by 2020.[10] All human societies are affected by cancer, there are, however, major international differences in the incidence of various forms of cancer and in the resources available to deal with them. More than 50% of the 7 million deaths from cancer each year are in the developing world,[11] countries in which resources for diagnosis and treatment are scarce. It costs £21 000 per annum to treat a patient with herceptin for advanced breast cancer; the annual per capita budget for health care in Uganda in 2001 was £10.[12] Even superficially similar tumours have very different presentations and management; oesophageal cancer in Johannesburg is a very different disease from oesophageal cancer in Birmingham. The World Health Organisation is currently preparing a strategy for cancer control which is based on advice, reports, and consultation rather than action. Unless and until the economies of the developing world are able to spend more on the health care of their citizens, cancer care for the majority of the world's inhabitants will be a theoretical possibility rather than a reality. In the meantime, harsh decisions have to made: morphine, rather than palliative radiotherapy, is the way to manage cancer-related pain in the developing world.

In the meantime, at least we have a reasonable statistical picture of what is happening, thanks to the Globocan initiative, sponsored by the World Health Organisation and run from the International Agency for Research on Cancer (IARC www.iarc.fr/). We can track the epidemic of HIV-related malignancies, we can look at epidemiological patterns of disease in space and time, and use the information to target scarce resources appropriately and to refine our knowledge of the interplay between inheritance and environment and how this might modify the susceptibility of a population to specific types of cancer.

The Breast Health Global Initiative (BHGI) has developed guidelines for the management of breast cancer in countries where resources for health care are scarce.[13] Such approaches will not bring the care offered to a villager in sub-Saharan Africa up to the level of that provided to a suburban Swede, but will help ensure that the money spent on the management of breast cancer in the developing world is spent effectively. This is important since, as citizens of the developing world adopt more Western lifestyles, the incidence of breast cancer increases,[14] and, unless there are effective programmes in place to deal with this increase, there will be a disproportionate increase in mortality from breast cancer in the developing world.

International differences

One of the main stimuli to the reorganisation of cancer services in the UK was the apparent demonstration that, in terms of international league tables of cancer survival, Britain was behind many other European countries (see Figure 5.1).

The primary source for this suspicion was the European Cancer Registries study on cancer patients' survival and care (EUROCARE study).[16–18] Unfortunately, although widely quoted, this study has several flaws. League tables inevitably oversimplify. Paradoxically, health care that is in overall terms better, may produce outcomes that are artefactually worse than those claimed by less-comprehensive systems of cancer care. In the UK in general, and in Scotland in particular, we have excellent data on cancer incidence and outcome for the entire population. We know who gets cancer, when they get it and what happens to them. In contrast, we know remarkably little about the management of cancer amongst the 45 million citizens of the US who do not have health insurance. If it takes money to

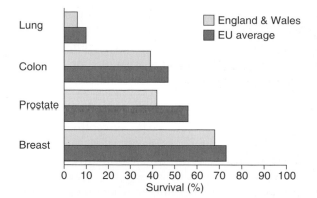

Figure 5.1 Cancer survival in the early 1990s: England and Wales lag behind Europe. Reproduced from *The NHS Cancer Plan*.[15] The graph suggests that, compared with the EU average, patients with cancer of the colon in England and Wales have a 5-year survival rate that is 10% less than the EU average. Data are not age standardised and the EU average may be overestimated and the British figures underestimated.

make a diagnosis then the poor are less likely to be diagnosed. If poorer people are never diagnosed then national statistics will, in comparison with a nation in which every patient with cancer is recorded, reflect the experience of a more affluent population. Since, for a variety of common-sense reasons,[19] well-off people with cancer are more likely to survive than poorer people with cancer, the result will be that the figures for cancer survival will be worse from the country with universal registration of incidence and outcome. The best results for cancer treatment will come from countries where all new patients are registered, where patients with poorer prognosis are lost to follow-up, and where all patients who are not known to have died from cancer are assumed to be cured. This is how some Swiss cancer statistics may have been derived and, unsurprisingly, Switzerland has amongst the best cancer survival statistics in Europe.

The Organisation for Economic Co-operation and Development (OECD) has recently published a careful and detailed comparative analysis of the quality of health care in the developed world (see Figure 5.2). They used 13 key indicators of quality, five of which are directly related to cancer management.[20] The OECD data, in contrast to the data shown in Figure 5.1, suggest that, in comparison with other developed countries, survival for patients with colorectal cancer is not significantly worse in the UK.

Rates of screening for breast cancer and cancer of the cervix are higher in the UK than they are in France or Italy, survival from breast cancer and cancer of the cervix is higher in the UK than it is in France or Germany. There is nothing in the OECD report to suggest that, when it comes to cancer management, and compared to other countries in the developed world, citizens of the UK are at any particular disadvantage. This is, of course, a highly political issue.

Developments in the economic aspects of cancer care

New interventions for all – affordable reality or the fantasy of the profligate?
The management of cancer is becoming increasingly expensive. New technologies for imaging or screening such as magnetic resonance imaging (MRI) and positron emission tomography (PET) scanning rarely substitute for the old, they are usually supplementary. The introduction, in the UK, of the National Institute for Health and Clinical Excellence (NICE) has, perhaps inadvertently, given us an insight into what one government in the developed world believes is a price worth paying for new technology in the management of cancer. The answer is simple: an intervention will be considered for funding if it costs less than about £30 000 per quality-adjusted life year (QALY) gained as a result of its introduction. This is, however, only part of the answer to the question 'What are we, as a society, prepared to pay for developments in cancer care?'. The issue of the multiplier has also to be addressed. A new drug used to treat a rare tumour might cost £22 000 per QALY and £15 000 per patient treated. If there were only 150 patients with that rare tumour in the UK each year, then the total bill would be £2.25 million per annum. If, however, the drug, again at a rate of £22 000 per QALY, was to be used in 35% of patients with lung cancer each year in the UK, then the total annual cost would work out at $0.35 \times 37450 \times 15000 =$

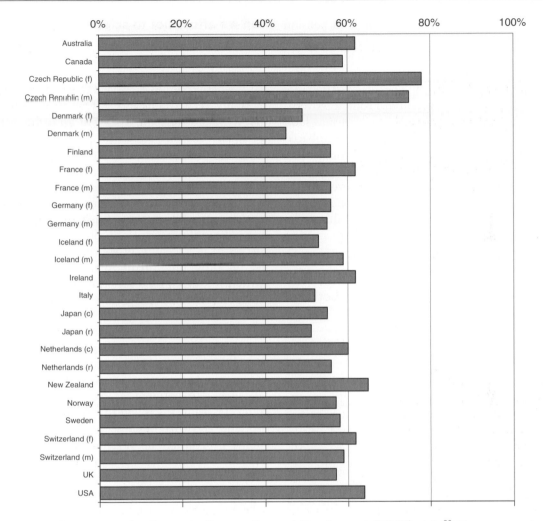

Figure 5.2 Organisation for Economic Co-operation and Development (OECD) data.[20] Five-year survival for colorectal cancer (2006) in the developed world. (m), men; (f), women; (c), colon; (r), rectum.

£19.7 million. Set against a total budget for cancer drugs in the UK of less than £200 million, this one intervention could cost 10% of the available budget and would, in overall economic terms, be unaffordable.

It is not easy to see a way forward that is both equitable and effective. Rather than give expensive interventions to all patients with a common tumour, it makes both clinical and economic sense to try to identify, before treatment, those patients who are going to respond and those who will not. The drug would then be given only to those likely to benefit, thus reducing the multiplier. The use of trastuzumab for breast cancer is an example of this approach.

Can we afford to allow people to give up smoking?

The economics of tobacco use are complex, the health consequences are straightforward: around 60% of lifelong smokers will die from smoking-related diseases. In one sense, smokers are a bargain. They smoke, pay taxes, retire, and promptly die. There may be some costs associated with their final illness but these are offset by savings in pension payments and the fact that they do not survive long enough to develop age-related illnesses. As initiatives to persuade people not to smoke gradually have an impact, there will be a delayed decrease in smoking-related mortality. From a government's point of view the problem is this: as soon as people stop smoking the revenue from tobacco taxation falls, however any savings in the costs of medical care will take several decades to percolate through. There is immediate loss of revenue, but any savings are deferred and, as mentioned above, the costs of providing pensions may, ultimately, be greater than the costs associated with treating smoking-related illness. (see Box 5.1).

Box 5.1   The economic relationship between smoking and health care in the UK

Cost to the UK health system of managing smoking-related illness:
£1.5 billion per annum

Cost to the UK economy of lives lost from smoking:
£80 billion per annum[a]

Tax revenues raised from duty on tobacco:
£8 billion per annum

Proportion of tax revenue raised from taxes on tobacco in the UK:
3.3%

Cost to UK exchequer of tobacco smuggling:
£2.5 billion per annum

NHS annual budget:
£70 billion

[a]the figure of £80 billion is based on a value of around £700 000 for a human life. Even if we valued life at 10% of this, smoking-related deaths would cost the UK £8 billion per year in lost lives.

The clear message is: we can afford to persuade people to stop smoking, we should try to persuade people to stop smoking, and any short-term losses will be offset by long-term savings. Even if the economic arguments were unconvincing, there would still be a moral imperative. Smoking causes misery and hardship to millions and it is morally dubious to do anything that encourages the habit.[21]

Can we afford not to screen for cancer?
Principles of screening

Screening programmes, in which asymptomatic individuals from the general population are tested to see whether or not they have cancer, may reduce mortality related to cancer. The assumption is, that by diagnosing the disease at an earlier stage, treatment is more likely to be successful. The choice of outcome measure for a screening programme is important. It is not 'fewer patients with advanced disease' or 'more patients suitable for treatment' or 'patients diagnosed by screening lived longer'. All of these measures are subject to bias. The only relevant criterion for judging the success of a screening programme is whether or not the programme reduced mortality from that particular cancer in the population as a whole. The evidence in favour of screening for cancer of the cervix is compelling. The evidence in favour of screening for breast cancer is somewhat less compelling. The evidence suggests that screening for colorectal cancer using faecal occult blood tests may significantly decrease mortality from colorectal cancer.[22] A national screening programme for colorectal cancer has already been launched in Scotland and there are also plans to introduce a similar programme in England and Wales.[23]

One of the problems with screening for cancer is that you may detect disease at a stage for which, if left untreated, there is no experience of its behaviour. DCIS (ductal carcinoma *in situ*) is now recognised as a pathological entity, largely as a result of mammographic screening for breast cancer. Although this condition is managed as if it were inevitably premalignant, there is no absolute proof that it is. There is an argument that breast screening leads to over-treatment of many women and that this over-treatment may compromise the effectiveness of mammographically based breast screening as a means of reducing mortality from breast cancer.[24–26] Similar controversy surrounds screening for prostate cancer using prostate-specific antigen (PSA). Are all the cancers detected by PSA screening clinically relevant? Which is worse, the threat and disruption caused by the so-called cancer, or that caused by the (perhaps unnecessary) treatment given to men with screen-detected tumours? The position is even more complicated when it comes to screening for lung cancer. Early tumours can be diagnosed when high-risk populations are screened using low-dose chest computerised tomography (CT). The problem is that many benign lung lesions are also detected. Although CT-based screening for lung cancer may, ultimately, become a sufficiently reliable screening test to be used for population-based screening, the currently available evidence suggests that it should not be used outwith a properly designed clinical trial.[27]

The issue of quality control is crucial to the conduct of a screening programme. If the screening test is not applied in a consistent and reproducible way, then the results may be misleading – causing problems with both false-positive and false-negative results. This is one of the more important arguments against *ad hoc* screening. Nevertheless, it is likely that demand for *ad hoc* screening will be driven by consumers: 'I want a cancer test'. The nuances of predictive value and the sometimes limited ability of tests to exclude particular diagnoses may be lost in the stampede to be tested.

The economics of screening for cancer

There are two main problems with the economics of cancer screening: the fallibility of screening tests and the problem of the multiplier. Screening tests are not 100% accurate, there are false-negative results (cancers missed) and false-positive results (the presence of cancer is erroneously suspected in someone who is entirely well). If a screening test is negative then a patient who actually has cancer may be falsely reassured by their test result and ignore early symptoms of the disease. In someone who is completely well, but whose screening test is falsely positive, we are in the very difficult position of having to prove the negative. This may involve invasive and potentially dangerous procedures, quite apart from the needless worry associated with actually being well but being told that cancer is suspected. The problem of the multiplier simply has to do with the fact that if we are screening a whole population then even a test that is inexpensive (say £5 per test) becomes a major expenditure when applied to 10 million people (a capital investment of £50 million for the test alone). If the false-positive rate is 0.1% then, on a population of 10 million tested, this translates to

10 000 healthy people who are exposed to the inconvenience, expense and psychological trauma associated with having to prove that they don't actually have cancer.

Screening for cancer may increase its incidence. Some screen-detected conditions, such as *in situ* changes in the breast or cervix, may be self-limiting – never destined to develop into invasive life-threatening illness. However, once they are detected by a screening programme they become illnesses that require treatment. Unsurprisingly, this treatment is usually highly effective. Whether, overall, we improve the health of the population by this type of approach is a controversial issue and lies at the root of much of the debate concerning the effectiveness of using mammography to screen for breast cancer.[24–26]

There are potential solutions. One is to use the power of molecular biology to improve the accuracy and precision of screening tests; another is to use combinations of simple tests for screening, rather than to rely on a single fallible test. We would use the power of computers and artificial intelligence techniques to work out that combination of test results that most accurately predicts the presence (or absence) of cancer. Another way to improve the effectiveness of screening is to target the screening test to those most at risk. This effectively raises the prevalence of cancer in the screened group and will, thereby, for any given level of test performance, improve the predictive value of a test. If you were using endoscopy to screen for oesophageal cancer in Sweden, and using a criterion of a body mass index (BMI) of $25\,kg/m^2$, you would have to perform 2200 endoscopies to detect one cancer in a population of obese men with reflux symptoms. If you raised the criterion for obesity to a BMI of $30\,kg/m^2$, then you would only have to perform 600 endoscopies to detect one cancer.[28]

Developments in the organisation of cancer care

The centralisation paradox and the rise of the multidisciplinary team

The centralisation paradox is straightforward: everybody wants to be treated as near as possible to their home; everybody wants to be treated by experts. The problem is obvious: since you cannot have an expert in every street, how do you ensure that patients receive the best possible care without having to travel excessive distances for treatment? The Calman–Hine report addressed this issue in the UK and came up with a series of recommendations: cancer specialists should concentrate on managing only two or three types of cancer (site specialisation); there should be cancer centres offering all specialist cancer services, and each cancer centre should be linked to one or more cancer units which would provide some, but not all, cancer services; there should be close links and co-operation between primary care and hospital-based services.[29] *The National Cancer Plan* further developed these recommendations and required that each patient with cancer should be discussed by a multidisciplinary team (MDT) with specific expertise and interest in that particular type of cancer.[15,30]

Cancer care in the UK is, nowadays, managed largely according to the principles set out in the Calman–Hine report.[29] There are over 30 cancer networks and the average population served by each network is 1.5 million. The original Calman–Hine proposal was that all radiotherapy services should be concentrated in the cancer centres. This has proved unpopular with both patients and staff,[31] and we have now moved to a model of devolved radiotherapy services.[32] Attendance at MDTs is now built into the job plans of pathologists, radiologists, surgeons, oncologists, and clinical nurse specialists. There is interesting prescriptive guidance on the requirements for multidisciplinary teams,[33] but very little evidence upon which to base the efficient and effective conduct of such teams. There is some evidence that the introduction of a MDT may influence survival. In Glasgow, the median survival for patients with inoperable non-small-cell lung cancer increased from 3.2 months to 6.6 months following the introduction of the MDT. The improvement appeared mainly to be due to a higher proportion of patients being treated with chemotherapy.[34] Our own, unpublished, data from Tayside shows that, for patients with node-positive colorectal cancer, the 3-year survival increased from 37.5% to 51% following the formation of the MDT.

Blurring professional boundaries

Increased demand for cancer services has provoked some rethinking of professional boundaries. Nurses and pharmacists now prescribe chemotherapy and run clinics, radiographers prescribe and plan radiotherapy.[35] Many of the roles traditionally taken by doctors have been taken on by others. This trend will, no doubt, continue, driven both by economics and the desire of non-medical professionals to make the best use of their education and talents. New approaches to training will be required. We will move beyond the competency-based approach that underpins much current practice, and move towards more generic skills: the ability to adapt personal roles to changing circumstances; the ability to function in a team; the ability to acquire new skills rapidly; the ability to view a substantive post as an opportunity for further learning, rather than as a career destination. This inevitably leads to a devaluation of what we might call 'craft skills': the ability, gained through learning and experience over many years, to perform a particular set of tasks appropriately and competently.[36]

Education is the key to many of the achievable developments in cancer management. Multiprofessional education for undergraduates is one method whereby mutual respect between professions may be fostered,[37] but not all professionals will have had the benefit of this approach to training. Electronic learning using web-based virtual lectures, tutorials and online assessments will further blur the boundaries between professions and will circumvent some of the difficulties that have arisen during previous attempts at multiprofessional education.[38,39]

Information technology

Computers are a ubiquitous presence in hospitals. There are clinical databases, prescribing databases, radiotherapy systems, laboratory systems and electronic imaging storage and retrieval systems. Few of these systems communicate with each other and only a small proportion of the vast amount of stored data is ever interrogated intelligently. A Martian looking at a modern hospital would see doctors and nurses as the servants, messengers carrying information between the masters, the computers. This will not continue. As technology becomes portable, and as wireless networks become feasible, we ought to be able to use computing equipment properly – at the bedside or in the clinic and in real time. Patients may also use computers and mobile technology (such as mobile phones) to communicate with those caring for them. Email and text messaging offer a powerful means for communication between patients and the clinical teams. Computer-assisted assessment of toxicity offers a means whereby patients can indicate what their real concerns are. It is important that older people are not left out of this process of electronic liberation: acceptability of computer systems to older patients must be part of the design specification.[40–42]

There is a vast amount of information about cancer and its management on the internet. Typing 'cancer' into Google produces 460 million hits; 'cancer treatment' 13.2 million hits; 'cancer research' 51.3 million hits. Some of this information is useful and true, much of it is disguised advertising, most of the rest is just plain crazy. The problem for people affected by cancer who wish to use the internet as a source of information is that they have no idea how to sort the true from the false, the advertising from dispassionate appraisal, the sane from the loopy. In the future, helping patients to navigate the labyrinth that is the internet will be an important part of cancer management. Most patients with cancer actively seek information about their disease and its management. We need to ensure that the information they find is both personally relevant and accurate.

Action at a distance

Telemedicine has been defined as 'the use of electronic information and communications technologies to provide and support healthcare when distance separates the participants'.[43] With improvements in IT in general, and with video links in particular, it will be increasingly possible to conduct clinical activities (consultations; review of clinical findings, and multidisciplinary team meetings) at a distance. Instead of a patient having to travel to a distant hospital for an expert opinion, it could simply be a matter of attending the local health centre and participating in a video-linked consultation with the hospital-based specialist.

The use of webcams and the internet would even extend this possibility to the patients' own homes. A community nurse could conduct part of their daily rounds by a series of scheduled web meetings with those patients who might not need physical care, but for whom the opportunity to discuss problems and receive advice is a crucial part of their care.

Care in the community

Hospital care is expensive. Not all sick patients with cancer need to be in hospital. Their needs may be equally, or perhaps better, met elsewhere. Care in the community represents a rare opportunity for financial pressures and societal pressures to act in the same direction: patients want to be as close to home as possible; specialist units want to accommodate only those patients for whom specialist care is necessary. However, if the hospital budget is completely independent of the budget for care in the community then the opportunity for logical process will be lost. If the number of patients cared for in the community is to increase, then additional funds will be required. Logic would dictate that these increased funds should come from the savings, in terms of efficiency, that the hospital is able to make through being able to discharge patients to the community. If the budgets are separate then funds will not move in the logical direction. The hospital's savings will be used to fund new treatments and initiatives within the hospital, the community will be left trying to do more work on the same budget. The community services will be over-stretched and fail, patients in the community will drift back to hospitals that have already given away the resources that would previously have been used for the care of those patients: everyone will suffer. Care in the community is an attractive concept, but only if there is a sensible integrated approach to the allocation of resources.

Developments in the intellectual aspects of cancer care

Thoughts about the origins of cancer

The classical view of the origins of cancer as a disease of cells can be traced back to Virchow in the mid-19th century and his famous statement 'I formulate the doctrine of pathological generation, and of neoplasia in the cellular pathological sense, in simple terms: *omnis cellula a cellula*'.[44] In other words, cancer begins when a cell goes wrong and gives rise to a lineage of cells that are, in behavioural terms, cancerous. The development of molecular biology in the mid-20th century, and in particular the elucidation of the structure of DNA and the genetic code in the 1950s, led to the belief that cancer might be explained in biochemical terms. The DNA in the nucleus of the cell governs cellular behaviour, cancer cells misbehave, therefore there must be something wrong with their DNA. In simple terms, there are two types of misbehaviour: gain of an abnormal function, which occurs when the cell acquires a gene ('oncogene') that confers some malignant properties; and loss of a normal function, when the cell loses a gene ('tumour suppressor gene') that would normally protect it against malignant transformation. The key issue here is that it is the loss of control of proliferation that is fundamental to the development of cancer. Cancer cells do not necessarily divide more rapidly than normal cells. It is just that the normal cells know when to stop dividing, and the cancer cells do not.

Recent research suggests that cancer may not arise from a single cell ('clonogen') that gives rise to the whole population of cancer cells. There may be multiple abnormal cells, arising at about the same time, all of which contribute to the development and growth of the tumour. This view emerges from a better appreciation that the origins of cancer lie in the interactions between cells and their environment. Very few cancers have purely genetic origins. Just as human development is the result of the interplay between nature and nurture, so cancer is a disease that represents the result of a changing environment acting upon more- or less-susceptible populations of cells.

Damage to the genetic material of a cell is called a mutation. Mutation is therefore inextricably intertwined with the origins of cancer. Every time a cell divides it provides an opportunity for mutation to occur. Human beings continuously renew themselves, a process that requires cell division. We each make, and dispose of, about 100 litres of slurpy stuff (gut cells, blood cells, lung cells, skin cells) each year. It takes about 2 500 000 000 000 000 cell divisions to produce a 50-year-old human being. In addition, our own bodies, as a result of our normal metabolic processes, expose us continuously to chemicals that cause mutations. Without even considering the effect of the environment (toxins, radiation), human beings generate 10 000 spontaneous mutations each day.[45,46] Against this background, cancer appears to be surprisingly uncommon.

The omic revolution

One current trend in cancer cell biology is to use the suffixes 'ome' and 'omic' to define areas of research activity. This is a manifestation of the 'omic revolution'.[47] Thus we have: genomics, the study of the total genetic material of a living entity; phenomics, the study of the complete set of phenotypes; proteomics, the study of the complete set of proteins in cells and fluids; the transcriptosome, that portion of the genome that is actively transcribed; metabolome, that portion of the transcribed genome that is metabolically active; 'omic space', a mathematical construct that defines the geometrical space within which all the other omics operate; and so on through epigenomics and ligandomics. The key issue here is not the coining of new words for old concepts but to emphasise that the omic approach involves looking at entities in their entirety. We are learning to appreciate, as Pope[a] did centuries ago, that simply trying to pass complex systems into manageable entities is, ultimately, an impoverished approach to the riches of biology. We need to look at the system as a whole, not just at its components. Just as the holistic approach is increasingly important in clinical medicine, so the systems approach is increasingly dominant in biological research. We are now a long way from the search for the mythical genes that 'cause' cancer or schizophrenia. The modern question is: 'what constellation of factors (genetic, epigenetic and environmental) combine in what ways to produce the particular biological phenomenon in which we are interested?'.

---

[a]'Like following life through creatures you dissect, You lose it in the moment you detect.' Alexander Pope (1688–1744) *Moral Essays*. Epistle i. Line 20.

Cell killing

The question 'when is a cell dead?' is deceptively complicated. The classical definition of a dead cancer cell is one that has lost its reproductive integrity, that is a cell which is incapable of division and is, in reproductive terms, doomed. The cell may appear morphologically normal; only when called upon to divide is its 'death' evident. Death by apoptosis or necrosis is a far less subtle process. The cell is dead in every sense of the word. In apoptosis the cell self-destructs in a programmed way, neatly breaking up into a set of packages that are disposed of in an orderly fashion. Necrosis is a more chaotic process. The cell is destroyed and there is a conspicuous inflammatory response with the unpackaged random fragments of cellular material being disposed of by phagocytosis.

Symbiosis versus eradication

Twenty years ago the governing concept of cancer treatment was the need to destroy every last cancer cell. Cure was the aim and, on the supposition that it only took one malignant cell remaining for the tumour to recur, all the cells of the tumour had to be destroyed. Increasingly we are becoming aware of the limitations of this approach. First, it is difficult on theoretical grounds to work out how even an extremely effective cytotoxic treatment might eradicate every last malignant cell. Fixed doses of cytotoxic agents kill a constant proportion of cancer cells, not a constant number. Starting with a tumour containing 10 000 000 000 cells, the first course of treatment may kill 9 000 000 000 cells, the sixth course will kill only 9000 cells and there will still be 1000 cancer cells remaining. Impressive quantities of cell killing do not necessarily translate into tumour cure. The failure of high-dose therapies may be an illustration of the limitations of this view of 'curative' cancer treatment.[48] Second, this view is based on the idea that a cancer starts at one time, and at one place, when a single cell acquires that set of abilities we define as malignant transformation. Everything that subsequently happens is the result of expansion of the original clone. This is by no means certain. Cells may undergo malignant transformations at different places and at different times. Cancer may be a multifocal disease, the concept of 'field change' has been around for a long time.[49] Given what we are learning about normal stem cells, we cannot even assume that metastases arise only when cells physically travel from a primary tumour to a site of implantation and secondary growth. The presence of cancer within the body may change the internal environment so that uncommitted stem cells, in the marrow for example, transform into malignant cells with the morphological features of breast cancer, even though neither they, nor their ancestors, have ever been anywhere near the breast.

We are now starting to draw finer distinctions: between cells that have some of the features of malignancy (such as ability to invade) but are not necessarily fully clonogenic, and those cells that, by themselves, are capable of reconstituting the tumour − tumour stem cells. It is possible that only a small proportion of malignant cells within a tumour have the quality of 'stemness'. These are, when it comes to cure, the crucial cells. Eradicate them and the tumour never returns; fail to eradicate them and, eventually, the tumour will recur. The key issue then becomes time: if the tumour never has sufficient time to regrow within an individual's natural lifespan then, in a pragmatic sense, this is tantamount to cure. This leads to a consideration of the concept of symbiosis, a set of circumstances in which the disease and its host co-exist peacefully (see Figure 5.3).

Cancer cells are present, but they are not causing symptoms nor are they compromising survival. Realistically, this may have been what so-called 'curative' therapies have been achieving. Rather than maintain the fiction that cancer is, in the classical sense, curable, we should perhaps turn our thoughts as to how best to achieve a reasonable symbiosis. A human being contains 100 000 000 000 000 (10^{14}) cells. A cancer 1 cm in diameter contains 1 000 000 000 (10^9) cells. By the time the number of cancer cells has been reduced to between 1 million (10^6) and 10 million (10^7), or thereabouts, the cancer is unlikely to produce symptoms or significant functional disturbance. This is a long way from 'cure'. However, if, for the duration of a patient's natural lifetime, we could keep the number of cancer cells below 10 million or so, we would have achieved, in the symbiotic sense, therapeutic success. Future

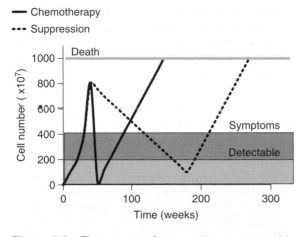

Figure 5.3 The concept of suppressive as opposed to eradicative therapy – and why it might sometimes be the better therapeutic strategy. At a size of 200×10^7 the tumour is detectable (for example by a rise in a serum marker), at a size of 400×10^7 it is symptomatic, at a size of 1000×10^7 it is fatal. Chemotherapy produces rapid, but transitory, response and survival time is short. With suppressive therapy, the response is slower but of longer duration. Both overall survival time, and time without significant symptoms is prolonged by the suppressive approach.

therapeutic strategies, particularly those based on biological approaches, will combine cell killing with the suppression of tumour cells. We will give up our attempts to hunt down every last potential clonogen.

Developments in the personal and familial aspects of cancer management

Individual beliefs and the flight from rationality

Clinicians involved in the care of patients with cancer are gradually learning to accept that patients' own beliefs are important. We are moving from 'complementary therapies have no scientific basis and you must not have them' through 'if you believe that a complementary therapy will help you, then it will probably do no harm and you might as well have it' towards 'how best might we incorporate complementary therapies into a man-

agement plan for this patient?'. In other words, we are moving from dismissal, through passive acceptance, and towards integration.

We still face the fundamental dilemma: the clash of systems of belief. Clinicians are supposed to be scientific, and science is supposed to be rational. If there is no plausible mechanism whereby a treatment might exert its effect then that therapy is likely to be dismissed. But absence of evidence is not evidence of absence. Chinese herbs can alleviate both subjective and objective toxicity related to chemotherapy for colorectal cancer.[50] The effect is there, we have no idea why it is there, but that does not mean that there is no biological mechanism for the effect: simply that we do not know what that mechanism is.

If orthodox medicine could provide all the answers then there would be little need for complementary therapies. Orthodox practitioners sometimes appear to forget that, following an endless series of unfulfilled promises, there may be some public disillusion. Everyone has seen or read that week's story about the latest breakthrough. Everyone is aware of the less newsworthy reality, they have watched relatives and friends die from the disease, despite the best efforts of orthodox practitioners. If we promised less, and delivered more, there would, perhaps, be less of a demand for alternative medicine. There are also other factors that may drive patients to seek alternative therapies. If we fail to explain ourselves properly, if we are arrogant and dismissive, if we pretend to have answers we do not have, then we can scarcely be surprised when our 'rational' advice is ignored.

Users of complementary and alternative medicines (CAM) tend to be younger, better off and female. Older people are less likely to use CAM. Patients with cancer, perhaps surprisingly, seem no more likely than the general population to use CAM. It will be interesting to see whether, as they grow older, younger people bring their enthusiasm for CAM into their later years or whether, as they age, they lose interest and simply accept what orthodox therapy has to offer.

If, as providers of health care, we are to acknowledge patients' rights to make their own choices then we will need to learn how best to incorporate CAM into orthodox therapies. We should not be forcing CAM upon reluctant or sceptical patients, but nor should we be denying it to those patients who believe it will help them. Leaving aside the vexed questions of evidence and belief, as clinicians we need to know three main things about any complementary or alternative therapy: is the complementary treatment toxic in its own right; is there any interaction between the complementary therapy and the conventional therapy that might increase the toxicity of either; is there any interaction between the complementary therapy and conventional therapy that might affect the efficacy of either? The evidence so far available suggests that acupuncture, aromatherapy, reflexology and spiritual healing are unlikely to cause direct harm.[51] Coffee enemas, some herbal medicinal products, osteopathy, and ozone therapy may occasionally cause serious complications and should not be used without careful consideration.

Social isolation and the decline of the family

The fabric of society is changing. Families are smaller and geographically more diffuse. The proportion of elderly people in the population is increasing. People are living longer after retirement. All of these factors will have effects upon patients with cancer and the support available to them. First, there is the simple financial question. As progressively fewer active workers have to support increasing numbers of retired people, will we have the financial resources to provide pensions and health care for the elderly? This is the tabloids' 'pensions time-bomb'. Then there are the questions about those things that are beyond price: if there are no children around, then who will provide emotional and practical support for elderly people with cancer? Things seem, at first consideration, grim. However, society shifts in a variety of ways and the rises in the rates of divorce and family breakdown may, in fact, enrich rather than impoverish the familial resources available to older people with cancer.

Other trends, such as the move towards retirement communities, may also be helpful: older people giving each other that support that their families are unable to provide. However things turn out in the next few decades, we can be certain that the social networks that support patients with cancer will be somewhat different from those that are currently in place. We will need to be able to adapt our management strategies to these changing social circumstances.

Support during and after treatment

The concept of supportive care for patients with cancer is a surprisingly recent development. There is a vast amount of information on supportive care for patients with cancer: 1.73 million hits on Google for 'supportive care' and cancer; 91 books on supportive care and cancer available online through Amazon (27 April 2006). Since the first publication in 1964,[52] there has been an exponential increase in the number of publications retrieved from Medline using the search criterion 'supportive care AND cancer' (see Figure 5.4). Many of these developments in the supportive care of patients with cancer are outlined elsewhere in this volume and in specific textbooks.[53,54] The importance of supportive care in cancer will continue to increase. As patients become more knowledgeable they will, quite rightly, demand more support. As cancer treatment becomes more complex, particularly with the integration of new therapies into the traditional triad of surgery, drugs and radiation, then the need to provide relief for treatment-related symptoms will increase. We already know that combining chemotherapy

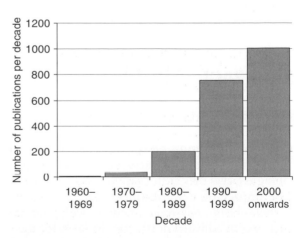

Figure 5.4 Publications identified by criterion 'supportive care AND cancer': Medline, by decade 1964 to 2006.

and radiation increases both tumour control and acute toxicity. As additional agents, such as inhibitors of signal transduction, are added in order further to improve tumour control, it is almost inevitable that patients will experience yet greater toxicity. We will need to derive regimens to mitigate these toxicities and enable patients to reap the benefits of these new approaches to treatment.

A patient's experience of cancer does not end when active treatment finishes. When treatment has been unsuccessful then they will need palliative care and support and, as mentioned previously, it is vital that this change may not be, from the patient's point of view, too abrupt. Even when treatment is successful, patients need support. There is good evidence that patients are psychologically at their most vulnerable at the end of a course of curative treatment.[55–59] Anxieties increase just at the time hospital visits become less frequent. This can be regarded as a withdrawal of support and interest and, again, is a transition that needs to be handled carefully. The concept of 'survivorship' explicitly acknowledges that patients who have been successfully treated for cancer have been through an experience that has changed their lives.[60,61] They, and their families, may have specific needs: for information, advice, and both physical and psychological support.[62–66] The problems don't end when treatment finishes. Increasing interest in the needs of cancer 'survivors' is evidenced by the growing number of publications addressing the support needs of people with cancer (see Figure 5.4).

THE PRACTICE OF ONCOLOGY

Developments in prevention

Changes in human behaviour

Worldwide, mortality rates for cancer are not falling as fast as they are for cardiovascular disease.[67] The impact of new treatments for cancer has, overall, been relatively modest with annual decreases in adjusted death rates of 1.5% for men and less than 1% for women in the developed world. Against this background, and considering the logistic and economic barriers to the delivery

of effective cancer therapy to the citizens of the developing world, it is clear that the most effective way to decrease the global burden of cancer would be through interventions that decrease the risks of the disease developing in the first place. Doll and Peto estimated that, in the US, over 80% of cancers were determined by environment or behaviour.[68] The Comparative Risk Assessment Collaborating Group (Cancer) identified nine risk factors for cancer that were related to environment or behaviour (see Box 5.2) and calculated their effects on the global burden of cancer.[69] They estimate that 37% of the 7 million deaths from cancer each year are caused by potentially remediable conditions: nearly 2.5 million people die each year from cancers that could have been prevented.[70]

Box 5.2 Nine main causes of preventable cancer worldwide

- Obesity – high body mass index
- Inadequate intake of fruit and vegetables
- Lack of physical exercise
- Smoking
- Excessive alcohol intake
- Unprotected sex with infected partner
- Environmental particulate pollution
- Household use of solid fuel
- Contaminated injections (hepatitis B and C).

Genetics applied to cancer prevention

Most cancers arise as a result of the interplay between genetic and environmental factors. We can do little about the genes we inherit but we can use our knowledge of an individual's genetic background to minimise their risk of developing cancer. There are several well-defined syndromes associated with an inherited susceptibility to cancer and these, together with possible means for lowering the associated risks of cancer, are outlined in Table 5.1.

Dominant inheritance implies that, on average, 50% of the offspring of an affected individual will inherit the increased susceptibility to cancer – it is the susceptibility that is inherited, not the cancer. Recessive inheritance implies that two-thirds of the normal siblings of an affected individual would be expected to be carriers of the condition: all

Table 5.1 Summary of the main dominantly inherited syndromes associated with increased susceptibility to cancer

Syndrome	Gene(s) implicated	Associated tumours and abnormalities	Strategies for prevention/ early diagnosis
Familial adenomatous polyposis (FAP)/ Gardner syndrome	APC	Colorectal cancer under the age of 25 years; papillary carcinoma of the thyroid; cancer of the ampulla of Vater; hepatoblastomas; primary brain tumours (Turcot syndrome); osteomas of the jaw; congenital hypertrophy of the retinal pigment epithelium (CHRPE)	Prophylactic panproctocolectomy
Hereditary non-polyposis colorectal cancer (HNPCC)	DNA mismatch repair genes (*MLH1; MSH2; MSH6*)	Colorectal cancer (typically in 40s and 50s)	Non-steroidal anti-inflammatory drugs; surveillance colonoscopy
HNPCC1	*MSH2*		
HNPCC2	*MLH1*	Endometrium, stomach, hepatobiliary (Lynch syndrome 1)	
HNPCC3	*PMS1*		
Peutz–Jeghers syndrome	*STK11*	Bowel cancer; breast cancer; freckles round the mouth	Surveillance colonoscopy; mammography
Multiple endocrine neoplasia (MEN)			
MEN type 1	Menin	Parathyroid tumours; islet cell tumours; pituitary tumours	Awareness of associations and paying attention to relevant symptoms
MEN type 2A	*RET*	Medullary carcinoma of the thyroid; phaeochromocytoma; parathyroid tumours	Regular screening of blood pressure, serum calcitonin and urinary catecholamines; prophylactic thyroidectomy
MEN type 2B	*RET*	Medullary carcinoma of the thyroid; phaeochromocytoma; mucosal neuromas; ganglioneuromas of the gut	Regular screening of blood pressure, serum calcitonin and urinary catecholamines; prophylactic thyroidectomy;
Li-Fraumeni	*P53*	Sarcomas; leukaemia; osteosarcomas; brain tumours; adrenocortical carcinomas	Very difficult, since pattern of tumours is so heterogeneous and varies from patient to patient
Familial breast cancer	*BRCA1; BRCA2*	Breast cancer; ovarian cancer; papillary serous carcinoma of the peritoneum; prostate cancer	Screening mammography; pelvic ultrasound; PSA (in males); prophylactic mastectomy; prophylactic oophorectomy
Familial cutaneous malignant melanoma	*CDNK2A; CDK4*	Cutaneous malignant melanoma	Avoid exposure to sunlight, careful surveillance
Basal cell naevus syndrome	*PTCH*	Basal cell carcinomas; medulloblastoma; bifid ribs	Careful surveillance, awareness of diagnosis (look for bifid ribs on X-ray)

Table 5.1 Continued

Syndrome	Gene(s) implicated	Associated tumours and abnormalities	Strategies for prevention/ early diagnosis
Von Hippel–Lindau	*VHL*	Renal cancer; phaeochromocytoma; haemangiomas of the cerebellum and retina	Urinary catecholamines
Neurofibromatosis			A difficult problem; maintain a high index of suspicion concerning any rapid changes in growth or character of any nodule
Type 1	*NF1*	Astrocytomas; primitive neuroectodermal tumours; optic gliomas; multiple neurofibromas	
Type 2	*NF2*	Acoustic neuromas; spinal tumours; meningiomas; multiple neurofibromas	

the offspring of an affected individual will be carriers. There are also several recessively inherited syndromes associated with inherited susceptibility to cancer. These include ataxia-telangiectasia, Bloom's syndrome and xeroderma pigmentosum.

The whole area of genetic prediction and prevention is fraught with moral and ethical difficulties.[70,71] How much do we want to know, what can we do to change our destiny, should we allow ourselves to have children, how much should we be told, when should we be told, who should do the telling? How do you discuss prophylactic mastectomy and oophorectomy with a young woman who is hoping to get married and have children? There is no guarantee that she will get breast cancer, just because she has a *BRCA* mutation. But she has already watched an aunt and a sister die from the disease.

The use of SNPs (single nucleotide polymorphisms) is about to make the whole business even more complicated. A SNP arises when one base in a DNA molecule is, with reasonable frequency, replaced by another. SNPs occur throughout the human genome, at a rate of one per several hundred bases, and can be thought of as identifiable markers along the length of the DNA. It has recently become possible to analyse many different SNPs rapidly and simultaneously,[72] and to associate the pattern of the SNPs with clinical outcomes and cancer risk.[73] Data on SNPs is widely available in public-access databases. The ease of this technology is both attractive and terrifying. Attractive, because it gives us a means of rapidly identifying associations between inheritance and disease; terrifying because it points to a future in which our individual SNP pattern might be used to dictate what we are allowed to do with our lives. If my SNP pattern identifies me as vulnerable to radiation-induced cellular damage then I should not be allowed to work in a nuclear power station. Conversely, if your SNP pattern indicates that you can easily metabolise the carcinogens present in tobacco then we might tell you that it is safe for you to smoke cigarettes.

Cancer vaccines

Vaccines have two potential roles in the management of cancer: prevention and treatment. The use of vaccines in the treatment of cancer is considered later on in this chapter.

Vaccines in cancer prevention

The main role of vaccines in modern medicine is in the prevention of infectious disease. Those cancers that are related to infection are therefore the main candidates for prevention using vaccines. Unfortunately, very few cancers are linked, either directly or indirectly, to infection. HIV infection is related to an increased incidence of malignancy (Kaposi's sarcoma; lymphomas; anal cancer; germ cell tumours; squamous carcinoma of the conjunctiva; cervical cancer) but there is, as yet, no effective vaccine against HIV. The development of effective anti-retroviral therapy has, however, lowered the incidence of malignant disease in patients who are HIV positive.[74,75] The problem of HIV-related malignancy is a major threat to the developing world. Given the unaffordability of anti-retroviral drugs in the developing world, a vaccine-based strategy is our best long-term prospect for dealing with the threat.

Cancer of the cervix is a tumour that is related to viral infection. The main culprit is the human papilloma virus (HPV) types 16, 18, 6, and 11. Effective vaccines against HPV are now available,[76] and offer the prospect of successfully controlling cervical cancer. The combination of vaccination and screening could, in theory at least, eradicate the disease.

Over 95% of cases of squamous cancer of the cervix are associated with HPV infection. The infection is usually acquired through sexual intercourse: if the infection could be prevented, then so could the cancer. The main approach to preventing HPV infection has been through vaccination. Two main commercial vaccines are currently being tested in large-scale clinical trials: a vaccine against HPV types 16 and 18;[76] a vaccine against HPV types 6, 11, 16 and 18.[77] Both have achieved proof of principle: there is evidence that vaccination prevents infection. The next stage of proof will be to show that preventing HIV infection prevents cancer of the cervix; the final proof will be to show that vaccination lowers mortality from cervical cancer in an immunised population.

In order to have their maximum effect these vaccines have to be given before first exposure to HPV, that is before a girl's first sexual intercourse. This poses ethical dilemmas. Some girls commence intercourse very young (at age 10 or 11 years), others do not. A population-based approach would, nevertheless, involve vaccinating all girls before their teenage years. This raises issues of informed consent – whose consent matters here, the child's or the parents'? Some have suggested that proof of HPV vaccination should be made a requirement for entry into secondary school. This may make sense from a public health perspective, but has an unpleasant element of coercion.[78]

Primary liver cancer is a major problem in the developing world. Although rare in the developed world, hepatocellular cancer is the fifth most common tumour worldwide. There is a clear association between infection with the hepatitis viruses B and C and primary liver cancer. The incidence of hepatocellular carcinoma in hepatitis B-positive patients with cirrhosis is 12%, the relative risk in carriers of hepatitis B compared with non-carriers is over 200.[79] Immunisation against hepatitis B is an effective method for controlling hepatocellular cancer related to infection with that virus.[80] Hepatitis C infection, by causing chronic liver disease, may also be associated with an increased risk of hepatocellular cancer. The recent rise in the incidence of primary liver cancers observed both in the West and in Japan may be related to increasing rates of infection with hepatitis C. There is, as yet, no vaccine against the hepatitis C virus and, consequently, hepatitis C may become an increasingly important cause of primary liver cancer throughout the world.[81]

Developments in diagnosis and staging

Molecular diagnosis

The diagnosis of cancer has traditionally depended upon a pathologist viewing a malignant cell under a microscope. This approach is, inevitably, invasive. To see the cell requires tissue, and to obtain tissue a biopsy is needed. As we move into an era of 'omic medicine' the potential exists for making the diagnosis of cancer by looking for molecular signatures in the components of peripheral blood. In proteomics we would look at the characteristic pattern of proteins associated with malignancy. We can also attempt to identify circulating malignant cells. In leukaemia this is an obvious and well-tested technology but the approach may now be extended to solid tumours. The technique of polymerase chain reaction (PCR), and elaborations thereupon, can be used to amplify small amounts of genetic material. Using this technology, it is possible to obtain detailed genetic information from the small number of tumour cells that can be found in the peripheral blood of patients with cancer. Current techniques are too unreliable for routine use but, as we develop this approach, it is possible to envisage non-invasive approaches to cancer that will yield useful diagnostic and prognostic information.[81–83] Cells other than tumour cells may also be important in this context: circulating endothelial cells may originate from the abnormal blood vessels formed by a growing tumours, and their detection may point to the presence of malignancy.[84]

Personalised medicine

It is hard to imagine clinical medicine as being ever, at any time, anything other than personalised. 'Personalised medicine' involves the use of genomic technologies to predict individuals' responses, in terms of both benefits and harms, to specific drugs.[85] By knowing what to expect, we will be able to put therapy for each individual on a rational basis. We would avoid giving drugs that, at the level of the individual person, would either not work or be so toxic as to negate any potential benefit. It is no coincidence that one of the earliest uses of the term 'personalised medicine' was in the *Wall Street Journal*.[86] There is money to made in this approach: if you can charge both for the predictive test, and for the drug treatment based on the results of that test, then, compared with simply charging for the drug, you have doubled your opportunity for profit. The idea that specific genetic sequences, which act as markers for particular susceptibilities, might be patented for use in commercial tests is somewhat against the spirit of science as co-operative enterprise. It may also hamper attempts to improve health care in the developing world.[87,88] It will be interesting to see whether the 21st century concept of 'personalised medicine' is able to deliver as much as it currently seems to promise.

Imaging

Developments in diagnostic imaging have had an enormous impact on the management of cancer over the past 25 years. Cross-sectional imaging with CT scanning and MRI have enabled us to map out the extent of disease in ways that could only have been dreamt of in the 1950s. We can determine whether clinically occult metastases have occurred (to lungs, to liver), and we can link the data from imaging the primary tumour directly to the equipment used for planning treatment with radiotherapy. One lesson we have learnt already: new imaging techniques are more likely to supplement, than to supplant, older techniques. MRI has not replaced CT scanning in staging

patients with cancer. There has also been considerable technological development within each of the classic imaging modalities (CT, MRI, ultrasound, nuclear medicine). A CT scan performed in 2006 is very different from one performed in 1995. The resolution of detail is greater, the scan takes far less time to perform, and the radiation dose to the patient is higher. The greater resolution is not always an advantage. It is likely to raise the incidence of false-positive scans and increase uncertainty for clinicians and anxiety for patients. What is the significance of a 5 mm opacity in the lung of a patient who had an operation for a node-negative cancer of the colon 4 years ago? How do you prove it is not a small metastasis? Could it be an innocent granuloma related to the patients' previous occupation as a worker in a jute mill? What should you tell the patient?

Similarly, ultrasound has moved a long way from the fuzzy fetal images of the 1970s: we now have colour Doppler (to show blood flow, or lack of it) and various endoluminal techniques that allow imaging from within hollow organs such as the oesophagus, rectum, ureter or aorta. Intra-operative ultrasound allows the surgeon to assess the state of the liver during surgery and can be very useful in discriminating between benign cysts and metastases within the substance of the liver. Open-coil MRI enables surgeon and radiologists to perform biopsies using magnetic resonance images, just as fluoroscopy, CT and ultrasound facilitate image-guided biopsy.

Optical coherence tomography (OCT) is a recently developed technique that may allow us to look at histology without the need for a biopsy. Using an OCT probe introduced with an endoscope it is possible to take high-resolution images of the oesophageal wall and, by visualising the architectural arrangement of the cells in the oesophageal wall, discriminate benign dysplasia from early cancer.[89]

Functional imaging

Traditional imaging procedures (CT, MRI, ultrasound) tell us a lot about anatomy, but very little about function. Positron emission tomography (PET) scanning offers the ability to image both structure and function simultaneously. PET scanning can be used to image metabolism in tumours (using 14-fluorodeoxyglucose, FDG); oxygen uptake in tumours and normal tissues (using 15-O_2), and it can also, using drugs labelled with isotopes, show drug distribution and metabolism. PET images are, compared to high-resolution CT images, fuzzy. This has led to the development of PET-CT techniques in which images taken by the two different techniques are registered with each other and fused.[90] This, in theory, gives us the spatial resolution of CT and the functional information of PET. On of the main uses of this approach in oncology has been in the investigation of mediastinal nodes in patients with lung cancer for whom surgery is being considered. PET-CT can be used to discriminate enlarged, but normal, nodes from nodes that are enlarged because they contain metastases.[91]

Interventional radiology

Interventional radiologists provide a repertoire of minimally invasive techniques that are extremely useful in the management of patients with cancer. Image-guided biopsies or cytological aspirates can enable the initial diagnosis, or that of recurrent disease, to be made without the need for major surgery. Examples would include percutaneous fine-needle aspirates of peripheral lung nodules, and ultrasound-guided biopsy of liver lesions in patients suspected of having colorectal cancer.

A stent is a rigid tube that can be used to relieve obstruction. Obstructing cancers of the gullet can be treated palliatively by self-expanding metal stents introduced via endoscope or by being passed over a guide wire.[92,93] A similar approach can be used for the relief of superior vena caval obstruction,[94] biliary obstruction,[95] and bronchial obstruction.[96] Plastic stents can be inserted from above or below into the ureter as a means of rapidly dealing with renal failure caused by obstruction of the renal tracts.

Trans-catheter embolisation is an interventional technique that directly targets the tumour vasculature. A catheter is introduced into vessels feeding the tumour and then material (alcohol, sponge, metal coils) that provokes clotting is squirted into the tumour. In effect, this produces infarction of the tumour. The approach can be used for palliative or pre-operative treatment for renal cancer,[97] or, combined with local infusion

of chemotherapy, for liver tumours.[98] Direct interference with the blood supply to a tumour is not a new concept. Shortly after his original description of the circulation of the blood (in 1639), William Harvey, in an attempt to treat a testicular tumour, ligated the testicular artery of a patient.[99]

Developments in cancer treatment

New targets and new approaches

As our knowledge of the basic mechanisms involved in malignant transformation has grown, then so has the sophistication of our attempts to manage the disease. Twenty-five years ago most cancer treatments were aimed at selectively killing cells that were actively dividing. The prime therapeutic target was DNA; if we could damage the DNA of replicating cells then we would prevent them dividing and, so the theory went, eradicate every last tumour cell. As mentioned previously, this picture is both incomplete and imperfect. It is the lack of control over cell division, rather than its rate, that is the key feature of the malignant process. Our attempts have therefore moved from a philosophy of 'let's kill them all' towards a more reasoned approach: 'what has made this particular group of cells misbehave, at this particular place and this particular time, and how might we best encourage them to revert to a more normal type of behaviour?'. In the current jargon, we start with 'target identification', finding out which gene (or gene product) has gone wrong. We then try to identify or design a drug that will restore normal function ('lead identification'). Once we have a potential therapeutic compound then we can look at close chemical relatives or directly tweak its molecular structure in order to identify that chemical that best restores normal activity ('lead optimisation'). Having found the best candidate we would then move into preclinical testing and then into clinical trials. This process is both very expensive and extremely time consuming. The clinical phase of development alone takes on average more than 6 years, and the whole process of bringing a drug to market may cost as much as $800 million.[100] Only a small proportion of candidate compounds ever make it to market and, as a result, those that do are very expensive indeed. Various measures are being introduced to try and speed up the process. The regulatory authorities, learning from the experience gained with HIV-AIDS, are providing fast-track procedures so that effective new treatments are not subjected to excessive bureaucratic delay. The drug companies themselves are also appreciating that contracting out the clinical testing, particularly to countries outwith Western Europe and the US, will improve accrual rates to trials: faster results at lower costs.[101] This all has implications for the future of academic oncology: testing drugs on behalf of companies has, up until now, been a fairly lucrative option for universities in the UK and US. Now that contract organisations are undercutting prices and producing more rapid results, this source of revenue is likely to diminish. The extent to which the cancer research agenda has been set by commercial interests is, in any event, a matter of some concern.[102]

The story of the development and marketing of the drug imatinib, used for the treatment of chronic myeloid leukaemia (CML) and gastro-intestinal stromal tumours (GIST) provides a useful illustration of the concepts and practicalities involved.

Signal transduction is that series of processes whereby events outwith a cell can influence events within the cell. A message from outside the cell is transmitted to the nucleus and, as a consequence, influences the behaviour of that cell (see Figure 5.5).

A crude mechanical description of the initial step in this process, involving the receptor tyrosine kinase, would go as follows. A messenger molecule (ligand) outwith the cell binds to the part of the tyrosine kinase that sticks out onto the

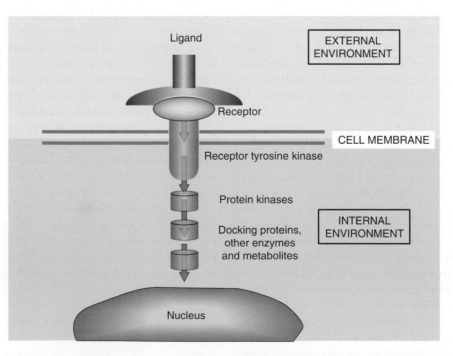

Figure 5.5 A schematic diagram of signal transduction. This is the process whereby information from outwith the cell influences events at the nucleus. Signal transduction pathways offer normal cells the ability to respond flexibly to changing external circumstances. In some cancer cells, signal transduction pathways are active, independently of outside events: it is as if a switch jammed in the 'on' postion. A molecule (ligand) binds to the receptor on the cell's surface. This triggers a cascade of messages, mediated by a series of enzymatic reactions, that eventually reach the nucleus. The enzymes, such as receptor tyrosine kinase and the protein kinases, involved in the transmission of these messages are potential targets for new anti-cancer drugs.

surface of the cell. This stimulates the tyrosine kinase to join to another tyrosine kinase molecule ('dimerisation'), as a result of which a phosphate molecule binds to the twinned molecules ('auto-phosphorylation'). The presence of this phosphate molecule causes the part of the tyrosine kinase molecule that is within the cell to become an active enzyme, which is able to transfer a phosphate molecule from the energy donor ATP to a target protein ('kinase activity'). The target protein gains energy and then is able, in turn, to use this energy to influence other events within the cell ('downstream signalling'). A vital feature of this process is that the activated tyrosine kinase forms a pocket within which the ATP can locate, and it is this physical act of location that allows the ATP to transfer energy to the target protein. Once the energy is transferred, the ATP changes shape and drifts out of the pocket, leaving it free for another ATP molecule and another transfer of energy. If the pocket is occupied by a molecule that fits it, just as ATP does, but does not give up energy and does not change shape, then the pocket is permanently occupied by an inert agent. Energy is not transferred, there is no signal, no matter what happens to the receptor on the cell surface, and no information will be passed on towards the nucleus.

The development of imatinib as an effective treatment for CML and GIST has been used to exemplify how we might develop targeted therapies.[103] The problem is that, like many so-called examples, it may represent an experience that is untypical. In CML and GIST, the majority of patients have abnormalities affecting the tyrosine kinase that is imatinib's target. However, for example in lung cancer, only about 10% of patients have mutations in the EGFR-related tyrosine kinase that is the target for the specific inhibitor gefitinib. When gefitinib was introduced as a new agent for treating lung cancer the assumption was that it would inhibit EGFR-related tyrosine kinase in all patients: it did not. Objective response rates were less than 20%.[104–106] EGFR expression did not predict response, but mutations in the EGFR-related tyrosine kinase did. These mutations had straightforward clinical correlates: responses were more likely in females, in patients with adenocarcinoma, in Japanese

patients, and in non-smokers.[107] So, as we consider the future of targeted therapies, we are left with the question which is the more reliable guide: imatinib or gefitinib; success for almost all patients or effective therapy for a small, but potentially identifiable, minority? Figures 5.6 and 5.7 illustrate the variability of response of gastrointestinal (GIST) tumours to imatinib. Figure 5.6 shows success; Figure 5.7 shows failure.

Gene therapy for cancer

If cancer is a disease of genes, then therapy aimed directly at correcting the genetic abnormality would appear to be an entirely logical therapeutic strategy. The logic may be impeccable but the clinical results have been largely disappointing. The promise that was offered when the first cancer-specific genes were identified has not been fulfilled. There are a number of reasons for this. The main obstacles to the clinical success of gene therapy are: delivery of the therapeutic gene to the target; persuading the target cells to incorporate the novel gene construct; and ensuring that the incorporated construct is safe and effective. Viruses provide an obvious means of transporting and inserting genes into the host genome, this is, after all, what they normally do. Unfortunately the use of live viruses is hazardous and there have been unexpected deaths in studies of gene therapy in humans.[108] As a result of this, and also because of concerns about rogue genes running amok in the human gene pool, there are now strict regulations governing this type of research. This imposes a further barrier to the rapid deployment of gene therapy for cancer. It is unlikely that the technical problems associated with gene therapy will be solved rapidly, and most of the techniques currently under trial may be too cumbersome for routine clinical use. RNA interference is a promising tool for gene therapy: it involves the use of small peptides to silence abnormal genes. The problem is, as ever, finding suitable vectors to convey the silencing peptides to the therapeutic target.[109]

Given the slow rate of progress so far, and the regulatory framework within which any advances must be made, it is unlikely that gene therapy will, within the next decade, have any major impact upon the management of cancer.

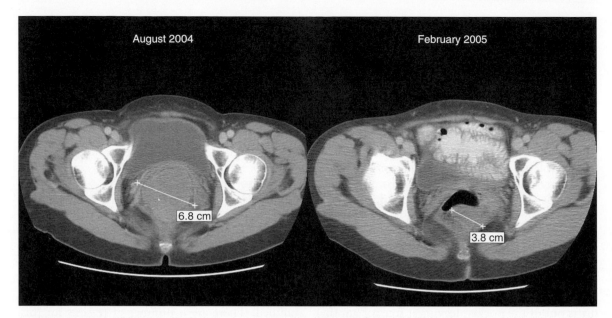

Figure 5.6   Gastrointestinal stromal tumours (GIST) of the rectum image on the left, pre-treatment showing extensive displacement of the bladder by a 6.8-cm-diameter tumour. On the right, after 6 months treatment with imatinib mesylate, the tumour has shrunk to a diameter of 3.8 cm. The patient remains well following surgical resection of the tumour in March 2005.

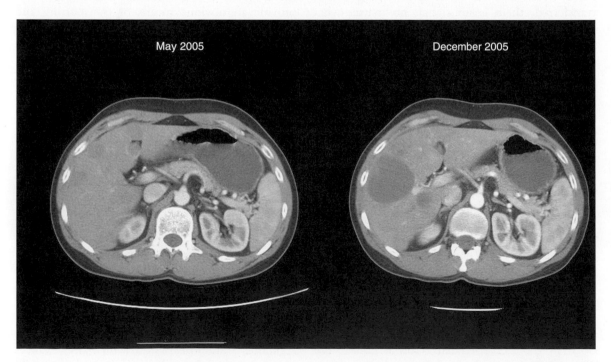

Figure 5.7   Primary resistance to imatinib mesylate in a patient with gastrointestinal stromal tumour (GIST) metastatic to the liver. There is clear progression of the liver lesion, despite treatment with imatinib mesylate, between May and December 2005.

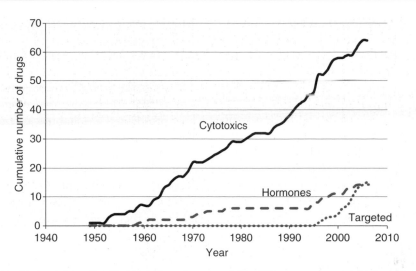

Figure 5.8 Data obtained from the Federal Drug Agency of the US on new approvals for cancer drugs 1949–2006. The plots are cumulative and show a rate at which new drugs are approved for treating cancer. The black line shows the curve for classically cytotoxic drugs; the dashed line shows the curve for hormonal therapies; the dotted line shows the curve for targeted therapies (drugs aimed at signal transduction pathways). There is no sense that targeted therapies are being approved at a faster rate than classically cytotoxic agents.

New drugs for old targets

Although the modern approach to target identification and the development of new therapeutic agents offers considerable promise we will, for the foreseeable future, still rely on cell killing as at least a part of our approach to treating cancer. We will still be trying to damage DNA, even though we increasingly appreciate that, by so doing we may be causing long-term harm. It is one of the great ironies of cancer treatment with either radiation or classically cytotoxic drugs that we can, with our therapies, cause the very disease that we are trying to cure. Secondary, treatment-induced, malignancies are becoming an increasingly important cause of death in those who have been successfully treated for cancer: 16% of all new cases of cancer in the US occur in that 3.5% of the population who are long-term survivors after being treated for cancer.[110]

Although little can be done about the genetic damage caused by agents designed to damage genetic material, it is possible to devise drugs that have less overall toxicity. Carboplatin is a derivative of cis-platinum that causes less damage to the kidneys than the parent compound (but does cause more damage to the bone marrow, particularly megakaryocytes). The idea of designing less toxic versions of active compounds is not a new one: cyclophosphamide is really just a less poisonous way of giving mustine.

Despite the move towards targeted therapies for cancer, there has been no recent decrease in the rate at which new, classically cytotoxic, drugs have come on to the market. Over the last decade, the rate of new Food and Drug Administration (FDA) approvals for drugs used in treating cancer has been the same for both types of drug (see Figure 5.8). The newly introduced, classically cytotoxic, drugs include: oxaliplatin – a cis-platinum derivative with activity against colorectal cancer; pemetrexed – an anti-folate with activity against mesothelioma; and clofarabine – a purine nucleoside analogue used in the treatment of leukaemia.

Old drugs in new clothes

The side-effects of drugs used in the treatment of cancer may sometimes depend upon the way the drug is formulated. Liposomes are small globules of lipid that can be used to encapsulate drugs. The liposomal preparations may be less toxic than the naked drug and the properties of the liposome itself may improve delivery of the active drug to the tumour. Liposomal preparations used in oncology include liposomal doxorubicin (Doxil), which is used in the treatment of ovarian cancer and HIV-related Kaposi's sarcoma. The liposome may be preferentially trapped within the abnormal vasculature of tumours and thus deliver high concentrations of the doxorubicin directly to the tumour. The main advantage is, however, that liposomal doxorubicin is far less toxic than doxorubicin itself. Hair loss is much less frequent, and lower cardiac toxicity means that the total cumulative dose of liposomal doxorubicin can be higher than the $500\,mg/m^2$ cap that limits the use of doxorubicin over the longer term. Other liposomal drugs used in oncology include: liposomal amphotericin, for the treatment of severe fungal infections; and liposomal daunorubicin for HIV-related Kaposi's sarcoma.

Polyethylene glycol (PEG) can also be used to modify the distribution and behaviour of drugs used in the treatment of cancer. This process, 'PEGylation' can prolong the duration of biological action of the drug, and has been useful in producing sustained-release preparations.

Many drugs that are of potential use in the treatment of cancer are poorly soluble in water. Since human beings are 50–60% water, this is a major limitation. Paclitaxel is particularly insoluble in water and so the standard preparation for intravenous use has had comparatively large quantities of ethanol and Cremophor EL (polyethoxylated castor oil) added to it as a vehicle to maintain solubility. Cremophor EL can cause allergic-type reactions and many of the hypersensitivity reactions associated with paclitaxel arise, not because of the drug itself, but because of the additional chemicals required to ensure solubility and stability. A variety of approaches have been taken to deal with this problem: filtration techniques; emulsions; liposomes. Only one approach has, so far, been approved by the FDA. This involves the use of nanoparticles bound to albumin (ABI-007, Abraxane). Preliminary testing suggests that this formulation of paclitaxel may be both safer and more effective.

Another development is to find ways of making cancer treatment more convenient. 5-fluorouracil (5-FU) has been used in cancer treatment for more than 30 years but it is somewhat cumbersome to administer effectively. It has a 10-minute half-life after intravenous injection and, when given by mouth, is not reliably absorbed. Giving folinic acid may prolong the effective period of action of 5-FU; giving the drug by continuous intravenous infusion is an obvious, but unwieldy, way to deal with its pharmacological limitations. The pro-drug capecitabine offers a convenient means of giving 5-FU orally and effectively mimics the pharmacology of continuously infused 5-FU. Capecitabine is first converted to 5'-DFCR by liver carboxylesterase the 5'-DFCR is converted to 5'-DFUR in the liver and tumour, and the 5'-DFUR is then converted to 5-FU by the enzyme thymidine phosphorylase which is preferentially expressed in tumour tissues.[111]

Vaccine therapy (immunotherapy) for cancer

Tumours are derived from our own normal cells and, unlike a kidney transplanted from a stranger, do not stimulate a strong immune response. Nevertheless there are identifiable, but subtle, differences between the antigens expressed by tumours and those expressed by the host tissues. These differences form the basis of the concept of 'tumour-associated antigens': antigens that uniquely identify malignant cells. The hunt for, and attacks based upon, these antigens is the basis for the immunotherapy of cancer.

Despite an attractive rationale, the clinical results have failed to meet expectations. There are several reasons for this: the antigenic differences between tumours and normal tissues are slight and, therefore, selective targeting is difficult; even when immune responses are evoked, they tend to be weak and have little impact upon clinical outcome; the immune system is far more subtle and complex than was originally appreciated – we enter the territory of unforeseen consequences.

Developments in decreasing the toxicity of treatment

Many cancers are now curable, but the costs, in terms of side-effects related to treatment, may be considerable. There are several ways in which toxicity can be mitigated without compromising cure. One is to develop new therapies that maintain effectiveness but with fewer adverse effects; examples include carboplatin (rather than cis-platinum); conformal radiotherapy (rather than treating with open fields).[112] The use of molecular profiling and pharmacogenomics may enable clinicians to identify individuals at particular risk of developing treatment complications after specific treatments. We would then be able either to avoid using the treatment in those particular patients or, if there were no effective alternative, to use modified doses and schedules. Examples of this approach already exist. Patients with Gilbert's syndrome (unconjugated hyperbilirubinaemia) are at particular risk of irinotecan-induced diarrhoea, and should not be treated with standard doses of the drug.[113]

In some circumstances we may have to accept that the treatment itself is bound to have adverse consequences and then to devise specific interventions that lessen the impact of treatment-related toxicity. Colony-stimulating factors (CSFs) can be used to lessen the myelosuppressive effects of chemotherapy. CSFs are involved in the control of normal haemopoiesis, they stimulate stem cells to divide and differentiate into mature functional cells. Filgrastim, pegfilgrastim, and sargramostim may all be used to prevent neutropenia (and, by extension, the risk of serious infection) in patients undergoing chemotherapy; epoietin and darbepoietin may be used to decrease the severity of anaemia, and have been advocated as alternatives to transfusion as a means of dealing with anaemia and fatigue arising from cancer and its treatment. Somewhat surprisingly, there is some evidence that decoctions of Chinese medicinal herbs may reduce the incidence of both neutropenia and of nausea in patients being treated with chemotherapy for colorectal cancer.[50]

Amifostine has been widely promoted as a clinically useful radioprotector, that is as a drug that may selectively protect normal tissues against the adverse effects of radiation. Despite decades of use, we still really do not know whether or not it has a role in clinical practice.[114,115] It may offer some protection against dry mouth in patients treated with radiotherapy for head and neck cancer and a recent meta-analysis suggests that it also protects against mucositis, radiation pneumonitis, and diarrhoea. This review also finds no evidence that amifostine protects tumours.[116] A detailed review of the evidence in 2002 concluded that the only clear indication for amifostine was in the prevention of radiation-induced xerostomia.[117] Publication bias and commercial sponsorship are major threats to the integrity of the literature on this topic: the literature search for the metaanalysis identified 33 potentially eligible trials, 10 of which had to be excluded on the grounds that they were duplicate publications.[116]

Anti-emetics are important in preventing and treating nausea and vomiting related to treatment for cancer. The vomiting associated with chemotherapy has three main phases: anticipatory, associated with apprehension and anxiety before any chemotherapy is actually given; acute, occurring within 48 hours of treatment; delayed, occurring several days after treatment. The development, during the 1980s, of the selective antagonists of the 5-hydroxytryptamine (5-HT$_3$) receptor was a major advance. Drugs such as ondansetron, granisetron and tropisetron have had a major impact upon our ability to deliver acceptable treatment, particularly with highly emetogenic drugs such as cis-platinum. Palonosetron is a recently developed 5-HT$_3$ receptor antagonist that has both high binding affinity and long plasma half-life. It may, therefore, have some therapeutic advantages over existing drugs. The results from two recent metaanalyses confirm that the combination of 5-HT$_3$ antagonist and dexamethasone is more effective than either alone, and that the addition of dexamethasone to a 5-HT$_3$ antagonist does not increase the incidence of adverse events.[118,119]

The neurokinin (NK) receptors are also important potential targets for anti-emetic drugs. Substance P is a tachykinin that is produced in the brainstem and which, by binding to the NK-1 receptor, can produce vomiting. Aprepitant specifically blocks the NK-1 receptor and, in combination with a 5-HT$_3$ antagonist and dexamethasone, may relieve vomiting in patients who have not had their vomiting adequately controlled by the standard therapy alone.[120,121]

Mucositis, which can be a side-effect both of drugs and of radiotherapy to the head and neck, can be an important cause of distress to patients being treated for cancer. It causes pain and difficulties with nutrition. Until recently, little could be done to alleviate the problem, although many attempts have been made. A Cochrane review has identified 71 evaluable randomised trials using a wide variety of interventions to prevent or treat mucositis: aciclovir, allopurinol mouthrinse, aloe vera, amifostine, antibiotic pastille or paste, benzydamine, beta carotene, calcium phosphate, camomile, chlorhexidine, clarithromycin, folinic acid, glutamine, GM-CSF, honey, hydrolytic enzymes, ice chips, iseganan, keratinocyte GF, misonidazole, oral care, pentoxifylline, povidone, prednisone, propantheline, prostaglandin, sucralfate, traumeel, and zinc sulphate.[122] Ice chips, antibiotic pastes and pastilles, amifostine, and hydrolytic enzymes were all of some benefit in reducing the severity of mucositis. More recently, growth factors have been used in attempts to maintain the integrity of the oral mucosa during chemotherapy. GM-CSF mouthwash is relatively ineffective, but palifermin (a recombinant humanised form of keratinocyte growth factor) shows promise as a mucosal protectant.[123]

Although diarrhoea and mucositis are often related toxicities – reflecting treatment-induced damage to the alimentary tract – diarrhoea can, in its own right, be a major problem after cancer treatment. There are two main categories of treatment-related diarrhoea: the acute and early; the late and chronic. There is no clear-cut relationship between the two syndromes: diarrhoea occurring acutely during treatment does not necessarily predict later problems with chronic diarrhoea.

The topoisomerase-1 inhibitor irinotecan is a potent cause of acute diarrhoea. This can, through dehydration, electrolyte imbalance, and secondary infection, become life-threatening.[124] The mechanism is believed to be mediated by gut bacteria which are able to reactivate an inactive metabolite of irinotecan. Other drugs, and radiotherapy, can cause diarrhoea by directly interfering with the ability of the gut lining to renew itself. Since irinotecan-induced diarrhoea arises through a specific mechanism it requires specific measures. Small-scale clinical studies have investigated the use of: Chinese herbal remedies; non absorbable antibiotics; activated charcoal; and glutamine. There is no clear evidence that any of these interventions are effective.[121] In the absence of an effective prophylactic regimen, the best management

policy for irinotecan-induced diarrhoea is prompt diagnosis and supportive care with intravenous fluids, loperamide, and, if necessary, antibiotics. Patients and their carers need to be aware of the problem and encouraged to seek medical advice if they develop diarrhoea after treatment. One potential pitfall is that the diarrhoea occurs in two phases: at and around the time of injection, and a delayed-onset phase several days later. The apparent lessening of symptoms after the first phase may give rise to a false sense of security.

The late effects of cancer treatment in general, and radiotherapy in particular, upon the bowel are becoming increasingly important. With the apparent rise in incidence of prostate cancer and with greater use of radiotherapy for rectal cancer, the number of patients surviving after pelvic irradiation is increasing. Many of these patients have significant, and occasionally debilitating, toxicity. These problems cannot simply be ignored, or regarded as the inevitable and unavoidable consequences of curative treatment. They can have a major impact on quality of life and should be investigated and treated properly. There are three main clinical syndromes: proctitis; anorectal dysfunction; small bowel diarrhoea. These syndromes may occur in conjunction with each other and this may lead to confusion. By taking the time to listen to patients' accounts of their symptoms it is, however, usually possible to work out what is going on.

The main symptoms of proctitis are rectal bleeding, mucus discharge from the rectum, irritation and pain. The hallmarks of proctitis are inflammation of the rectal wall, together with radiation-induced damage to the blood vessels (telangiectasia). The syndrome can be diagnosed on the basis of clinical history and proctoscopy. It usually occurs in patients who have a history of radical radiotherapy for prostate cancer and, in such patients, the radiation changes are often confined to the anterior wall of the rectum.

Anorectal dysfunction can occur after radiotherapy alone but, more often is found in patients who have been treated with both surgery and radiotherapy. The classical symptoms are of rectal discomfort, mucoid rectal discharge, faecal seepage, and difficulties with defecation. These difficulties are often manifest as a feeling of incomplete emptying so that, no sooner does a patient think that they have finished emptying their bowels than they have to start all over again ('prompt return to stool'). These sensations may recur frequently throughout the day and night, and so, with repeated and futile trips to the toilet, patients become exhausted and miserable. They attend clinic wearing a soiled pad and, when asked about their activities, are often housebound by virtue of embarrassment and fatigue. The pathophysiology of this problem is complex and probably involves a combination of decreased size of the rectal reservoir, decreased neuromuscular co-ordination, and deranged rectal sensation. The investigation of the syndrome is not straightforward: most of the useful information comes from the clinical history but specialised investigations, such as assessing rectal responses to pressure changes (manometry), may be helpful. Management is difficult. Promoting stool bulk may sometimes help, but can make things worse. If neuropathic pain is a dominating symptom then gabapentin, or a similar drug, may be helpful. Sometimes conversion to a permanent stoma offers the best quality of life. This option is often not considered by clinicians, since it implies therapeutic failure. However, for some patients with anorectal dysfunction, life is so unpleasant that a permanent stoma may seem a small price to pay for relief.

Diarrhoea, when it occurs as a late effect of treatment for cancer, can have a variety of causes. 'Radiation enteropathy' is not a simple diagnosis. Rather it represents a constellation of derangements of bowel structure and function that are related to previous radiotherapy. As such, it has a variety of causes and mechanisms. Since there is no one intervention that will adequately treat all causes, it is usually necessary to investigate patients who have chronic severe diarrhoea following treatment (see Table 5.2).

The reason that I have dealt with this issue at such length is because, in the UK at least, the problem is under-recognised, under-reported and under-treated. There are also other groups of patients with significant problems caused by treatment-related damage to normal tissues: infertility;[125–127] cardiac damage;[128–131] chronic fatigue and insomnia;[132,133] and cognitive impair-

ment.[134–138] These individuals may also be at a disadvantage because of a neglectful or nihilistic attitude to their problems. The principles that apply to the management of the adverse effects of cancer treatment upon the bowel apply at other sites. We need to recognise the clinical syndromes associated with treatment-related toxicity; formulate scoring systems, based on subjective and objective data, that allow the severity of the problems to be graded;[139] devise strategies for the appropriate investigation and assessment of patients with significant toxicity; and design, and prove the effectiveness of, interventions for each set of clinical problems. This process involves many individuals and specialties: patients; carers; nurses; family doctors; surgeons; oncologists; occupational therapists; dieticians; speech therapists; physiotherapists; specialist physicians (chest physicians, gastroenterologists, neurologists etc). There are very few MDTs dedicated to dealing with the problems that arise as a consequence of cancer treatment; most MDT's see their role as providing expertise at and around the time of diagnosis with little in the way of longer-term commitment. This is mainly because, in terms of their remit and their targets, this is all that is asked of them. However, what we cannot do at any level, whether individual or administrative, is simply ignore the misery and distress caused by the adverse consequences of cancer treatment.

New techniques in radiation oncology

Radiotherapy is a complex technological intervention and, as such, has been evolving over the past 110 years. The assumption is usually made that improved technology will lead to improved results. Although testable, this assumption is rarely tested. In part this reflects the difficulties of assessing complex clinical interventions, and in part it reflects an innate optimism: new is inevitably better. There is also an industrial agenda at work: just as a motor manufacturer wants to stimulate demand by adding new technologies (satellite navigation, cruise control, anti-lock brakes) to their vehicles, so the manufacturers of equipment

Table 5.2 Causes of diarrhoea after treatment for colorectal cancer

Cause	Investigation	Management
Rapid transit	Measure transit time	Loperamide; octreotide
Pancreatic insufficiency	Stool fat globules	Pancreatic enzyme supplements
	Faecal elastase and chymotrypsin	
	Serum or urinary isoamylase	
	NBT-PABA test	
	Pancreolauryl test	
	Secretin-pancreozymin test	
Stricture	Barium studies	Resection
	Colonoscopy	
Blind loop (bacterial overgrowth)	Glucose-hydrogen breath test	Metronidazole; probiotics
	Culture of duodenal aspirate	
Bile salt malabsorption	^{75}SeHCAT test	Cholestyramine
	Barium follow-through	
	^{99m}Tc-HPAO-labelled white blood cell scan	
Recurrent tumour	Colonoscopy	Appropriate treatment
	CT/MRI scan	
New primary	Colonoscopy	Appropriate treatment
	CT/MRI scan	
	Urinary 5-HIAA	
	Plasma VIP	
Disaccharide intolerance	Xylose absorption test	Modify diet (e.g. eliminate lactose); probiotics
Co-existent disease		
Thyrotoxicosis	Thyroid function	Carbimazole
Microscopic colitis	Colonoscopy and biopsy	Steroids
Drug therapy	Possible culprits	Trial of withdrawal
CMV infection	Colonoscopy and biopsy	Ganciclovir

NBT-PABA, *N*-benzoyl-L-tyrosyl-p-aminobenzoic acid; HCAT, ^{75}Se homotaurocholate; HPAO, technetium hexamethylpropylene-amine oxime; 5-HIAA, 5-hydroxyindole-acetic acid; VIP, vasoactive intestinal peptide; CMV, cytomegalovirus.

used for radiotherapy wish to convince us that we really need all the additional capabilities provided by this year's machine and that anything more than 2 years old is, effectively, obsolete. Some of the improvements are, like anti-lock brakes, genuinely useful features. Others, like leather seats, may only be of cosmetic interest. This is where rigorous evaluation should enter the process, but so rarely does. This is particularly true in the competitive US market where radiotherapy departments compete for custom and where it is important, for marketing purposes, to be seen to have the most up-to-date equipment. There is a real danger that the technology may drive a spurious 'need' rather than a genuine need driving the

development of necessary technology. Future developments in the technology of the delivery of radiation treatment will occur against this complex, confusing, and not always logical background.

Conformal radiotherapy

The principle of conformal therapy is not new, radiotherapists have always sought to shape the treated volume to conform to that of the tumour. The technology has however changed. Instead of cumbersome heavy blocks manually inserted into the path of the beam, we now have the ability to shape beams using devices built in to the head of the treatment machine: multi-leaf collimation. A series of finger-like processes project into the beam and their position can be adjusted, using integrated software, to produce complex shapes. The flexibility provided by this approach means that we can more accurately shape the volume that receives the highest dose of radiation, and so can more reliably spare adjacent normal tissues. Potentially, this may reduce adverse effects from any given dose of treatment or, conversely, permit the dose to be increased (with the possibility of a greater probability of controlling the tumour), while keeping the damage to normal tissues within acceptable limits.[112,140–142]

Intensity-modulated radiation therapy (IMRT)

In conformal radiotherapy each beam used to treat the tumour is of uniform intensity. If we consider the beam to be composed of little packets of energy ('photons'), then fluence is the technical term for the number of packets crossing a specified area in unit time. The beams used for straightforward conformal therapy have equal fluence across the profile of the beam. However, if we allow the intensity of the beam to vary across its profile, by considering the beam to be composed of a multitude of smaller beams each with its own fluence, then this gives us greater ability to sculpt and shape the dose to the target volume: a procedure that has been called dose-painting.[143] This is the essential concept behind IMRT – the intensity of the beam is altered (modulated) in order to provide more flexible geometry. IMRT is particularly valuable if we are trying to treat a concave treatment volume, for example when a tumour encases a vulnerable normal tissue such as the spinal cord. The techniques used for IMRT are complex both in principle and in practice,[144] but offer the real possibility of being able to deliver effective radiation doses to tumours previously considered to be untreatable, or the possibility of increasing tumour doses without increasing the risks of damage to normal tissues.

Image-guided radiotherapy

People move, even when they are lying still. Our lungs inflate and deflate, peristaltic waves ripple along our intestines, our bladders slowly fill, our hearts beat. In the old days of radiotherapy this did not matter very much. The volumes we treated

were, relative to the displacements caused by respiration or peristalsis, large. Nowadays, as we use conformal radiotherapy (XRT) and IMRT, the target volumes are smaller and even minor movements will be important – in order to treat the tumour you have to hit the target, and if the target moves beyond the beam the tumour will not be treated. As part of our planning procedures we can generate beam's-eye views: images of what the beam ought to be 'seeing' as it traverses the patient. If we store these images within the machine used to treat the patient we can use them to control whether or not the beam of radiation is switched on. Only when there is acceptable congruence between what the beam 'sees' and what it ought to be 'seeing' will the beam be switched on. If, as a result of movement, the target moves outwith the beam, it will switch itself off. This is the basic principle upon which image-guided therapy is based. Although the principle is simple, the procedures involved are complex – how good does the match have to be between reality and the image before the congruence is acceptable? How do you strike a compromise between perfection and feasibility?[145,146] If it takes an hour to treat one patient because of an insistence on absolute fidelity then this, in a busy department, is simply not a practical proposition.

Target definition

In order to hit a target, you first have to define it. In the past 30 years we have moved from a very basic approach to target definition, two plain X-ray pictures taken at right angles to each other, through 3D imaging using CT, to functional imaging using CT/PET fusion.[147] Now we treat not just shadows, but shadows with the metabolic properties of active cancer.

Fractionation – a continuing tale

When given with curative intent, radiotherapy is usually given as a series of treatments ('fractions') over a period of 3–7 weeks. The historical origins of this practice were physical, and to some extent economic, rather than biological but there are, nevertheless, good biological reasons for fractionating a course of radiotherapy.[148] In crude terms, fractionation enables us to do more damage to tumours and less damage to normal tissues. The problem is that we have, even after more than 100 years, surprisingly little information upon which to make rational choices concerning optimal fractionation regimens for specific tumour types.[149] This lack of basic information manifests itself as a wide variety of practice.[150] This lack of uniformity has implications that go well beyond the care of individual patients. If courses of radiotherapy are prolonged, for no reason other than custom, then this reduces overall capacity and may lead to increases in waiting times for treatment. Patients who wait longer for treatment may be less likely to be cured.[151] Since dose-per-fraction is a major influence on the late effects of radiation, simply decreasing the number of treatment sessions will not solve the problem of limited capacity. Over the next few years we should expect a series of clinical trials asking simple questions about optimal radiotherapeutic schedules: these trials may not directly improve cure rates but should enable us to make best use of our limited resources.

Combining therapies

Drugs and radiotherapy may act synergistically. The effect of both, when given together, may be greater than expected by simple addition: in terms of tumour control, it may be possible to add two and two to make five. This proposition always has to be considered in the light of the therapeutic ratio: it only makes good sense if there is synergy against the tumour and less synergistic effect upon the normal tissues. We have some evidence from head and neck cancer that synchronous chemotherapy and radiation is more effective than radiation alone,[152] but there is also some evidence that toxicity may also be increased and there is, as yet, no unequivocal evidence that the therapeutic ratio is improved. One interesting way forward is to combine targeted therapies with radiation and there is already one trial suggesting that adding cetuximab, which targets the epidermal growth factor receptor, to radiation is more effective than radiotherapy alone.[153]

Photodynamic therapy

Photodynamic therapy (PDT) is based on the principle that tumours will specifically take up chemicals ('photosensitisers') that, in response to illumination using visible light, will produce singlet oxygen molecules. Singlet oxygen is locally toxic and can produce cell death and obliterative vascular changes. These toxic effects are only found where there has been both uptake of the chemical and deposition of light. The selectivity of uptake with currently available photosensitisers is not particularly impressive: the tumour-to-normal tissue ratios are typically around 2 to 3. With current technology, the benefits from PDT at present are more to do with the localisation of light penetration, and subsequent sensitisation, than any selectivity of the photochemical for tumour cells.

The approach is only feasible for tumours that are accessible and relatively superficial. As technology develops, more tumours will be accessible using fibre optic sources, and higher light energy will enable the light to penetrate more deeply into tumours. Currently the limit of penetration is between 5 mm and 10 mm. A variety of photosensitisers are now available for clinical use.[154,155]

A similar approach ('photodynamic detection', PDD) can be used for delineating the extent of a tumour during surgery. If a brain tumour specifically takes up a photosensitiser then the neurosurgeon can assess its extent, during surgery, by simply applying light of the relevant wavelength to the area of interest. Where there is tumour, there is detectable fluorescence.

New techniques in surgery

Minimally invasive surgery

Surgery has traditionally used long incisions that permit direct inspection of the surgical field. The morbidity associated with surgery and the handling of sensitive tissues, such as the gut, can be considerable, and the typical hospital stay for a patient who needed abdominal surgery for cancer was 2–3 weeks. The same operation may now, using minimally invasive techniques, require only 3–5 days in hospital. The surgeon uses a laparoscope, inserted through a small ('keyhole') incision to view the tumour and adjacent organs. The surgical procedure is performed using specially designed instruments which can be introduced through other keyhole incisions. This type of surgery was previously confined to specialist centres but is now widely available and may, over the longer term, improve outcomes in cancer surgery.

Given these technological advances, the question now becomes — do we need the surgeon? Robotic techniques are being developed to improve the results of surgery for cancer.[156] At the moment the robotic devices supplement, rather than replace, the skills of the surgeon, but a future in which the surgeon is not the primary operator is at least conceivable.

Localised ablation

Extreme heat (radiofrequency ablation) or extreme cold (cryoablation) can be delivered to localised areas using probes that can be introduced laparoscopically. This permits the destruction of tumours, for example liver metastases, that cannot be removed surgically. Although unlikely to cure, these ablative procedures may prolong life in patients with unresectable metastatic disease.

Liver resection

Until fairly recently the idea that liver metastases could be resected with a view to curing patients was somewhat heretical. However, improvements in surgical technique mean that it is now commonplace to perform extensive surgery in an attempt to cure patients with liver metastases. The surgery is surprisingly well tolerated, and the questions we now must ask concern the role of chemotherapy as either a preparative regimen for patients about to have liver surgery or as post-operative adjuvant treatment in those patients whose liver disease has, apparently, been completely removed.

Improved reconstruction

Improvements in plastic and reconstructive surgery mean that large tissue defects can be replaced with tissue that is both functionally and cosmetically acceptable. This has meant that surgeons have been able to attempt more radical operations for patients with sarcomas or cancers of the head and neck. It has also meant that many women who have had mastectomy for breast cancer will now be routinely offered a reconstructive procedure.

Intra-operative radiotherapy, radiosurgery

The best way for a radiotherapist to visualise a tumour is to see it at open operation. A target that can be seen is a target that can be accurately irradiated, and so there is a compelling logic to the notion that radiotherapy might most appropriately be given at the time of surgical removal of a tumour. There are several obstacles to this logical approach. Most treatment machines are static and heavy so, either you have to move an anaesthetised patient with an open wound through the hospital to the radiotherapy department, or you must build a specialised operating theatre around a linear accelerator. Neither approach is really feasible for routine care. Another problem is biological: by giving treatment in a single session during the surgical procedure we sacrifice any benefits associated with fractionation. For established tumours this could be a limiting factor, but for microscopic residual disease left in the tumour bed this may be less of a problem.[157]

Recently a portable source of therapeutic X-rays has been developed that is no larger than a domestic electric drill. This means that it is now possible to deliver intra-operative radiotherapy without having to move the patient or having to build a specialised operating theatre. The technology is currently being evaluated in a randomised trial in the conservative treatment of breast cancer,[158] and may, in the future, have wider application.

The gamma knife uses a somewhat different approach and has been widely used in the treatment of tumours and other abnormalities within the central nervous system.[159,160] The gamma knife is essentially a focused array of cobalt beams that can be located using a stereotactic frame. The volume of interest is placed, using co-ordinates determined from diagnostic images, at the centre of the converging beams and so a high dose (12–20 Gy) can be delivered in a short overall time.

Developments in pain control and palliative care

A detailed discussion of this topic is well beyond the scope of this chapter and many of the issues are covered elsewhere in this book. The key developments in this area over recent years have been: better understanding of the molecular basis of individual variation in response to analgesics; better understanding of the pathophysiology of cancer-related pain; better delivery systems for analgesics (transdermal patches; and implanted pumps for spinal analgesia).

Summary and conclusions

On the basis of the developments discussed in this chapter it is possible to imagine two main directions of travel for the management of cancer in the future. We are in the middle of a dark wood facing a choice between two paths. Each path will take us to a distinct future: one future engendering cautious optimism; the other, considerable concern. We could call these futures A (the bleak outlook) and B (the more hopeful prospect).

Future A
The practice of oncology is left entirely to market forces. New drugs and new technologies are promoted on the basis of theoretical benefit, and the promise of increased income for their purveyors, and are never subjected to proper scrutiny. Clinicians and institutions adopt treatments because not to have them would lead to a loss of competitive edge. Compared to older, cheaper, interventions the new treatments may not be particularly effective and may cause more toxicity. The costs spiral out of control. Money is spent on drugs and technology and is not available for providing care. With the emphasis on the generation of income there is a decline in the importance and status of supportive care (unless it involves prescribing yet more expensive new drugs). Nurses are relegated to technical and custodial tasks; sometimes they are allowed to perform duties hitherto the preserve of physicians. This is mainly because they perform the tasks more competently and for less money. In an income-driven system there is no time to stop, to listen, or to console.

Only the rich can afford treatment and the principle of equal access for all is soon relinquished. Any improvements in outcome are small and can apply only to a small proportion of the population. A multiply-tiered system of care emerges, with a significant proportion of the population left without adequate care. Patients are empowered only in so far as their ability to pay and, with the belief that money can conquer all, those who can afford it are only too happy to comply with a system that offers them expensive new therapies.

Insurance companies establish the right to obtain access to genetic information on individuals seeking insurance. They use this information to set premiums based on individual genetic risks and some people may, on the basis of their SNP pattern, be denied any insurance at all or be charged exorbitant premiums. By eliminating their own risks, through the denial of service, the insurance companies are able to increase their profitability.

Public disillusion with the limited effectiveness and availability of expensive interventions combines with a decrease in respect for a profession seen to be motivated primarily by financial acquisitiveness, and causes a shift towards unproven complementary therapies. At least these treatments are usually cheaper than the conventional therapies, they are almost invariably less toxic and involve a degree of personal contact that, in the money-is-time world of orthodox practice, is often lacking. People who use complementary therapies may not live any longer, but at least they feel better.

There is little money to be made from the prevention of cancer, or from predictive and prognostic testing, and so these fields are left unexplored. The incidence of cancer rises along with the money to be made from it. A few do a little better, the majority fare substantially worse and, overall, the health and well-being of humankind suffers.

Future B
The practice of oncology is set firmly on a personal basis with each individual put at the centre of all processes and decisions. Ability to pay has no effect on the choices that are offered. The sharing of information (about choices, about therapies, about risks, about harms, about hopes, about concerns, about the extent to which knowledge is desired) is a crucial part of the therapeutic

process. There are no stock solutions. Each person affected by cancer has the opportunity and support to enable them to navigate their own path through the difficulties and problems that they encounter. Predictive and prognostic tests are a key part of the decision-making process. There is as much investment in this area as there is devising new treatments. As a result, the expense and misery caused by unnecessary and futile treatments is avoided. Patients who have been cured surgically are not given additional treatments 'just in case'. Patients are not given drugs to which their tumours will not respond, or to which their normal tissues are unduly sensitive. Targeted therapies become the rule, not the exception. Specific abnormalities associated with specific cancers are dealt with by specific treatments: no more blunderbuss.

Complementary therapies are not simply ignored or dismissed. They are investigated properly, and those that are of proven physical or psychological benefit are made freely available. Those that are harmful or ineffective are quietly forgotten.

Multidisciplinary teams take continuing interest in patients' management. They do not restrict their role to the initial phases of diagnosis and treatment but concern themselves with the long-term effects of management and facilitate the rehabilitation of patients following successful treatment.

The main emphasis in the management of cancer moves towards prevention. The tools of molecular biology are harnessed to explore key questions concerning the interactions between environment and inheritance. By understanding why a particular person developed a particular type of cancer at a particular time we take the first steps towards preventing similar individuals developing similar tumours in the future. We will adopt less patronising and more realistic approaches to advising the general public on how to adopt a more healthy approach to life. There will be less middle-class preaching and more actual engagement. By improving overall socio-economic standards, by reducing the size of the gap between the very rich and the very poor, and by improving education we will have dealt with many of the environmental factors that contribute to the incidence of cancer. Smoking will be banned in public places throughout the UK. People will give up smoking, not because they are forced to, but because they fail to see any point in continuing to smoke.

The incidence of cancer falls, those people who are unfortunate enough to develop the disease are treated with interventions of proven effectiveness and are actively involved in all decisions concerning their care. The overall burden of cancer is reduced and the health of the community improves.

Conclusion

These two futures are, of course, cartoons. The reality will lie somewhere between the two extremes. We do, however, as professionals working in health care, have some power to shape events. Many of the unpalatable aspects of Future A are already a reality. This has happened because we, and our colleagues, have reacted naively to developments. We should not be reacting to developments in cancer care. We should be shaping them, and shaping them for the betterment of all humankind.

References

1. Corner J., Wright D., Gunaratnum Y., McDonald J.W. and Foster C. (2007). The research priorities of patients attending UK cancer treatment centres: findings from a modified nominal group study. *British Journal of Cancer* **96**, 875–881.
2. Sackett D.L. (2002). Clinical epidemiology. What, who, and whither. *Journal of Clinical Epidemiology* **55**, 1161–1166.
3. Straus S.E. and McAlister F.A. (2000). Evidence-based medicine: a commentary on common criticisms. *Canadian Medical Association Journal* **163**, 837–841.
4. Bentzen S.M. (1998). Towards evidence based radiation oncology: improving the design, analysis, and reporting of clinical outcome studies in radiotherapy [comment]. *Radiotherapy and Oncology* **46**, 5–18.
5. McDonald L. (2001). Florence Nightingale and the early origins of evidence-based nursing. *Evidence Based Nursing* **4**, 68–69.
6. Overgaard J. and Bentzen S.M. (1998). Evidence based radiation oncology. *Radiotherapy and Oncology* **46**, 1–3.
7. Pape T.M. (2003). Evidence-based nursing practice: to infinity and beyond. *Journal of Continuing Education in Nursing* **34**, 154–161; quiz 89–90.

8. Munro A.J. (2001). Forum for applied cancer education and training. *European Journal of Cancer Care* **10**, 212–220.

9. The Cochrane Collaboration. www.cochrane.org/reviews/index.htm (accessed 13 September 2007).

10. World Health Organisation. (2006). *WHO Cancer Control Programme*. Geneva: World Health Organisation. www.who.int/cancer/en/ (accessed 24 July 2007).

11. World Health Organisation. (2005). *Global Programming Note: 2005–2007 Call for Resource Mobilisation and Engagement Opportunities*. Geneva: World Health Organisation.

12. World Health Organisation. (2006). *WHO Immunization Financing*. Geneva: World Health Organisation. www.who.int/immunization_financing/countries/uga/about/en/index.html (accessed 24 July 2007).

13. Anderson B.O., Shyyan R., Eniu A. *et al.* (2006). Breast cancer in limited-resource countries: an overview of the Breast Health Global Initiative 2005 guidelines. *Breast Journal* **12(suppl. 1)**, S3–15.

14. Parkin D.M. and Fernandez L.M. (2006). Use of statistics to assess the global burden of breast cancer. *Breast Journal* **12(suppl. 1)**, S70–80.

15. Department of Health. (2000). *The NHS Cancer Plan: a Plan for Investment, a Plan for Reform*. London: Department of Health.

16. Berrino F. (2003). The EUROCARE Study: strengths, limitations and perspectives of population-based, comparative survival studies. *Annals of Oncology* **14(suppl. 5)**, v9–13.

17. Berrino F., Sant M., Verdecchia A. *et al.* (1995). *Survival of Cancer Patients in Europe*. Lyons: International Agency for Research on Cancer.

18. Eurocare Working Group Resource Centre. (2003). *Eurocare: Survival of Cancer Patients in Europe*. www.eurocare.it/ (accessed 24 July 2007).

19. Munro A.J. (2005). Keynote comment: Deprivation and survival in patients with cancer: we know so much, but do so little. *The Lancet Oncology* **6**, 912–913.

20. Mattke S., Kelley E., Scherer P., Hurst J. and Gil Lapetra M.-L. (2006). *Health Care Quality Indicators Project – Initial Indicators Report*. Paris: Organisation for Economic Cooperation and Development.

21. Boyle P., Yasantha Ariyaratne M.A., Barrington R. *et al.* Tobacco: deadly in any form or disguise. *Lancet* **367**, 1710–1712.

22. Towler B., Irwig L., Glasziou P. *et al.* (1998). A systematic review of the effects of screening for colorectal cancer using the faecal occult blood test, hemoccult. *British Medical Journal* **317**, 559–565.

23. Atkin W.S. (2006) Impending or pending? The national bowel cancer screening programme. *British Medical Journal* **332**, 742–743.

24. Freedman D.A., Petitti D.B. and Robins J.M. (2004). On the efficacy of screening for breast cancer. *International Journal of Epidemiology* **33**, 43–55.

25. Olsen O. and Gotzsche P.C. (2001). Screening for breast cancer with mammography (Cochrane Review). *The Cochrane Library*, Issue 4. Oxford: Update Software.

26. Gotzsche P.C. (2004). On the benefits and harms of screening for breast cancer. *International Journal of Epidemiology* **33**, 56–64; discussion 9–73.

27. Strauss G.M., Dominioni L., Jett J.R. *et al.* (2005). Como international conference position statement: lung cancer screening for early diagnosis 5 years after the 1998 Varese conference. *Chest* **127**, 1146–1151.

28. Lagergren J. (2006). Controversies surrounding body mass, reflux, and risk of oesophageal adenocarcinoma. *The Lancet Oncology* **7**, 347–349.

29. Calman K. and Hine D. (1995). *A Policy Framework for Commissioning Cancer Services*. London: Department of Health.

30. Hall P. and Weaver L. (2001). Interdisciplinary education and teamwork: a long and winding road. *Medical Education* **35**, 867–875.

31. Allirajah D., Herbst K. and Morgan L. (2006). Free at the point of delivery? Exposing the hidden cost of hospital travel and parking for cancer patients. London: Macmillan Cancer Relief.

32. Board of the Faculty of Clinical Oncology. (2004). *Guidance on the Development and Management of Devolved Radiotherapy Services*. London: Royal College of Radiologists.

33. Department of Health. (2004). *Manual for Cancer Services*. London: Department of Health.

34. Forrest L.M., McMillan D.C., McArdle C.S. and Dunlop D.J. (2005). An evaluation of the impact of a multidisciplinary team, in a single centre, on treatment and survival in patients with inoperable non-small-cell lung cancer. *British Journal of Cancer* **93**, 977–978.

35. Board of the Faculty of Clinical Oncology. (2002). *Breaking the Mould: Roles, Responsibilities and Skills Mix in Departments of Clinical Oncology*. London: The Royal College of Radiologists, The Society and The College of Radiographers, The Royal College of Nursing, The Institute of Physics and Engineering in Medicine.

36. Sennett R. (2006). *The Culture of the New Capitalism*. New Haven, CT: Yale University Press.

37. McNair R.P. (2005). The case for educating health care students in professionalism as the core content of interprofessional education. *Medical Education* **39**, 456–464.

38. Mitchell B.S., McCrorie P. and Sedgwick P. (2004). Student attitudes towards anatomy teaching and learning in a multiprofessional context. *Medical Education* **38**, 737–748.

39. Rudland J.R. and Mires G.J. (2005). Characteristics of doctors and nurses as perceived by students entering medical school: implications for shared teaching. *Medical Education* **39**, 448–455.

40. Curzon P., Wilson J. and Whitney G. (2005). Successful strategies of older people for finding information, *Interacting with Computers* **17**, 660–671.

41. Dickinson A., Newell A.F., Smith M.J. and Hill R. (2005). Introducing the internet to the over-60's: developing an email system for older novice computer users. *Interacting with Computers* **17**, 621–642.

42. Milne S.A.D., Carmichael A., Sloan D., Eisma E. and Gregor P. (2005). Are guidelines enough? An introduction to designing web sites accessible to older people. *IBM Systems Journal* **44**, 557–571.

43. Division of Health Care Services. (1996). *Telemedicine: A Guide to Assessing Telecommunications in Health Care Committee on Evaluating Clinical Applications of Telemedicine.* Washington, DC: Institute of Medicine.

44. Virchow R. (1855) Every cell from a cell. *Virchows Archiv* **VIII**, 3.

45. Ames B.N. and Gold L.S. (1990). Too many rodent carcinogens: mitogenesis increases mutagenesis. *Science* **249**, 970–971.

46. Fraga C.G., Shigenaga M.K., Park J.W., Degan P. and Ames B.N. (1990). Oxidative damage to DNA during aging: 8-hydroxy-2′-deoxyguanosine in rat organ DNA and urine. *Proceedings of the National Academy of Sciences of the USA* **87**, 4533–4537.

47. Evans G.A. (2000). Designer science and the 'omic' revolution. *Nature Biotechnology* **18**, 27.

48. Leonard R.C., Lind M., Twelves C. *et al.* (2004). Conventional adjuvant chemotherapy versus single-cycle, autograft-supported, high-dose, late-intensification chemotherapy in high-risk breast cancer patients: a randomized trial. *Journal of the National Cancer Institute* **96**,1076–1083.

49. Slaughter D.P., Southwick H.W. and Smejkal W. (1953). Field cancerization in oral stratified squamous epithelium; clinical implications of multicentric origin. *Cancer* **6**, 963–968.

50. Taixiang W., Munro A.J. and Guanjian L. (2005) Chinese medical herbs for chemotherapy side effects in colorectal cancer patients (Cochrane Review). *The Cochrane Library*, Issue 1. Oxford: Update Software.

51. Ernst E. (2001). A primer of complementary and alternative medicine commonly used by cancer patients. *Medical Journal of Australia* **174**, 88–92.

52. Barnes D.M., Davis A.J., Moran T., Portillo C.J. and Koenig B.A. (1998). Informed consent in a multicultural cancer patient population: implications for nursing practice. *Nursing Ethics* **5**, 412–423.

53. Siegelman M.H. (1964). Advances in the supportive care of children with acute leukemia. *Medical Record and Annals* **57**, 439–441.

54. Berger A.M., Portenoy R.K. and Weissman D.E. (2002). *Principles and Practice of Palliative Care and Supportive Oncology.* New York: Lippincott Williams and Wilkins.

55. Faithfull S. and Wells E.M. (2003). *Supportive Care in Radiotherapy.* Edinburgh: Churchill Livingstone.

56. Deshields T., Tibbs T., Fan M.Y. *et al.* (2005). Ending treatment: the course of emotional adjustment and quality of life among breast cancer survivors immediately following radiation therapy. *Supportive Care in Cancer* **13**, 1018–1026.

57. Hipkins J., Whitworth M., Tarrier N. and Jayson G. (2004). Social support, anxiety and depression after chemotherapy for ovarian cancer: a prospective study. *British Journal of Health Psychology* **9**, 569–581.

58. Munro A.J. and Potter S. (1996). A quantitative approach to the distress caused by symptoms in patients treated with radical radiotherapy. *British Journal of Cancer* **74**, 640–647.

59. Shepherd K.L. and Fisher S.E. (2004). Prospective evaluation of quality of life in patients with oral and oropharyngeal cancer: from diagnosis to three months posttreatment. *Oral Oncology* **40**, 751–757.

60. Stam H., Grootenhuis M.A., Brons P.P., Caron H.N. and Last BF. (2005). Health-related quality of life in children and emotional reactions of parents following completion of cancer treatment. *Pediatric Blood and Cancer* **47**, 312–319.

61. Chabner B.A. (2003). Cancer therapy and survivorship. *Cancer Epidemiology Biomarkers and Prevention* **12**, 269s.

62. National Cancer Institute. (2006). *Cancer Survivorship Research.* http://dccps.nci.nih.gov/ocs/ (accessed 24 July 2007).

63. Bradley C.J. (2005). The need for online information on the economic consequences of cancer diagnosis, treatment, and survivorship. *Journal of Medical Internet Research* **7**, e29. http://www.pubmedcentral.nih.gov/articlerender.fcgi?artid=1550665 (accessed 3 August 2007).

64. Demark-Wahnefried W., Aziz N.M., Rowland J.H. and Pinto B.M. (2005). Riding the crest of the teachable moment: promoting long-term health after the diagnosis of cancer. *Journal of Clinical Oncology* **23**, 5814–5830.

65. Robison L.L. (2004). Cancer survivorship: unique opportunities for research. *Cancer Epidemiology Biomarkers and Prevention* **13**, 1093.

66. Zebrack B.J. and Zeltzer L.K. (2003). Quality of life issues and cancer survivorship. *Current Problems in Cancer* **27**, 198–211.

67. World Health Organisation. (2002). *The World Health Report 2002 – Reducing Risks, Promoting Healthy Life.* Geneva: World Health Organisation.

68. Doll R. and Peto R. (1981). The causes of cancer: quantitative estimates of avoidable risks of cancer in the United States today. *Journal of the National Cancer Institute* **66**, 1191–1308.

69. Burke W. and Press N. (2006). Ethical obligations and counseling challenges in cancer genetics. *Journal of the National Comprehensive Cancer Network* **4**, 185–191.

70. Danaei G., Vander Hoorn S., Lopez A.D., Murray C.J. and Ezzati M. (2005). Causes of cancer in the world: comparative risk assessment of nine behavioural and environmental risk factors. *Lancet* **366**, 1784–1793.

71. Evans J.P., Skrzynia C. and Burke W. (2001). The complexities of predictive genetic testing. *British Medical Journal* **322**, 1052–1056.

72. Engle L.J., Simpson C.L. and Landers J.E. (2006). Using high-throughput SNP technologies to study cancer. *Oncogene* **25**, 1594–1601.

73. Hu Z., Huo X., Lu D. *et al.* (2005). Functional polymorphisms of matrix metalloproteinase-9 are associated with risk of occurrence and metastasis of lung cancer. *Clinical Cancer Research* **11**, 5433–5439.

74. Crum N.F., Riffenburgh R.H., Wegner S. *et al.* (2006). Comparisons of causes of death and mortality rates among HIV-infected persons: analysis of the pre-, early, and late HAART (highly active antiretroviral therapy) eras. *Journal of Acquired Immune Deficiency Syndrome* **41**, 194–200.

75. Levi F., Randimbison L., Te V.C., Franceschi S. and La Vecchia C. (2004). Kaposi's sarcoma in Vaud and Neuchatel, Switzerland, 1978–2002. *European Journal of Cancer* **40**, 1630–1633.

76. Harper D.M., Franco E.L., Wheeler C. *et al.* (2004). Efficacy of a bivalent L1 virus-like particle vaccine in prevention of infection with human papillomavirus types 16 and 18 in young women: a randomized controlled trial. *Lancet* **364**, 1757–1765.

77. Villa L.L., Costa R.L.R., Petta C.A. *et al.* (2005). Prophylactic quadrivalent human papillomavirus (types 6, 11, 16, and 18) L1 virus-like particle vaccine in young women: a randomised double-blind placebo controlled multicentre phase II efficacy trial. *The Lancet Oncology* **6**, 271–278.

78. Zimmerman R.K. (2006). Ethical analysis of HPV vaccine policy options. *Vaccine* **24**, 4812–4820.

79. Beasley R.P., Lin C.-C., Hwang L.-Y. and Chien C.-S. (1981). Hepatocellular carcinoma and hepatitis B virus: a prospective study of 22707 men in Taiwan. *Lancet* **318**, 1129–1133.

80. Chang M.H., Chen T.H., Hsu H.M. *et al.* (2005). Prevention of hepatocellular carcinoma by universal vaccination against hepatitis B virus: the effect and problems. *Clinical Cancer Research* **11**, 7953–7957.

81. Kao J.H. and Chen D.S. (2005). Changing disease burden of hepatocellular carcinoma in the Far East and Southeast Asia. *Liver International* **25**, 696–703.

82. Bessa X., Elizalde J.I., Boix L. *et al.* (2001). Lack of prognostic influence of circulating tumor cells in peripheral blood of patients with colorectal cancer. *Gastroenterology* **120**, 1084–1092.

83. Bustin S.A. and Mueller R. (2006). Real-time reverse transcription PCR and the detection of occult disease in colorectal cancer. *Molecular Aspects of Medicine* **27**, 192–223.

84. Vlems F.A., Ruers T.J.M., Punt C.J.A., Wobbes T. and van Muijen G.N.P. (2003). Relevance of disseminated tumour cells in blood and bone marrow of patients with solid epithelial tumours in perspective. *European Journal of Surgical Oncology* **29**, 289–302.

85. Smirnov D.A., Foulk B.W., Doyle G.V. *et al.* (2006). Global gene expression profiling of circulating endothelial cells in patients with metastatic carcinomas. *Cancer Research* **66**, 2918–2922.

86. Science Policy Section, Royal Society of London. (2005). *Personalised Medicines: Hopes and Realities.* London: The Royal Society of London.

87. Langreth B.R. and Waldholz M. (1999). New era of personalized medicine: targeting drugs for each unique genetic profile. *Oncologist* **4**, 426–427.

88. World Health Organisation. (2002). *Genomics and World Health: Report of the Advisory Committee on Health Research.* Geneva: World Health Organisation.

89. Evans J.A., Poneros J.M., Bouma B.E. *et al.* (2006). Optical coherence tomography to identify intramucosal carcinoma and highgrade dysplasia in Barrett's esophagus. *Clinical Gastroenterology and Hepatology* **4**, 38–43.

90. von Schulthess G.K., Steinert H.C. and Hany T.F. (2006). Integrated PET/CT: current applications and future directions. *Radiology* **238**, 405–422.

91. Goerres G.W., von Schulthess G.K. and Steinert H.C. (2004). Why most PET of lung and head-and-neck cancer will be PET/CT. *Journal of Nuclear Medicine* **45(suppl. 1)**, 66S–71S.

92. Saranovic D., Djuric-Stefanovic A., Ivanovic A., Masulovic D. and Pesko P. (2005). Fluoroscopically guided insertion of self-expandable metal esophageal stents for palliative treatment of patients with malig-

nant stenosis of esophagus and cardia: comparison of uncovered and covered stent types. *Diseases of the Esophagus* **18**, 230–238.

93. Wenger U., Johnsson E., Bergquist H. *et al.* (2005). Health economic evaluation of stent or endoluminal brachytherapy as a palliative strategy in patients with incurable cancer of the oesophagus or gastrooesophageal junction: results of a randomized clinical trial. *European Journal of Gastroenterology and Hepatology* **17**, 1369–1377.

94. Rowell N.P. and Gleeson F.V. (2002). Steroids, radiotherapy, chemotherapy and stents for superior vena caval obstruction in carcinoma of the bronchus: a systematic review. *Clinical Oncology* **14**, 338–351.

95. Maire F., Hammel P., Ponsot P. *et al.* (2006). Long-term outcome of biliary and duodenal stents in palliative treatment of patients with unresectable adenocarcinoma of the head of pancreas. *American Journal of Gastroenterology* **101**, 735–742.

96. Walser E.M. (2005). Stent placement for tracheobronchial disease. *European Journal of Radiology* **55**, 321–330.

97. Munro N.P., Woodhams S., Nawrocki J.D., Fletcher M.S. and Thomas P.J. (2003). The role of transarterial embolization in the treatment of renal cell carcinoma. *BJU International* **92**, 240–244.

98. Brown D.B., Pilgram T.K., Darcy M.D. *et al.* (2005). Hepatic arterial chemoembolization for hepatocellular carcinoma: comparison of survival rates with different embolic agents. *Journal of Vascular and Interventional Radiology* **16**, 1661–1666.

99. Rugendorff E.W. and Wilson T. (1997). The history of urology on postage stamps and cancellations. *Journal of Urology* **158**, 1335–1339.

100. DiMasi J.A., Hansen R.W. and Grabowski H.G. (2003). The price of innovation: new estimates of drug development costs. *Journal of Health Economics* **22**, 151–185.

101. Wadman M. (2006). The quiet rise of the clinical contractor. *Nature* **441**, 22–23.

102. Delaney B. (2006). Is society losing control of the medical research agenda? *British Medical Journal* **332**, 1063–1064.

103. Sawyers C. (2004). Targeted cancer therapy. *Nature* **432**, 294–297.

104. Fukuoka M., Yano S., Giaccone G. *et al.* (2003). Multi-institutional randomized phase II trial of gefitinib for previously treated patients with advanced non-small-cell lung cancer. *Journal of Clinical Oncology* **21**, 2237–2246.

105. Johnson D.H. and Arteaga C.L. (2003). Gefitinib in recurrent non-small-cell lung cancer: an IDEAL trial? *Journal of Clinical Oncology* **21**, 2227–2229.

106. Kris M.G., Natale R.B., Herbst R.S. *et al.* (2003). Efficacy of gefitinib, an inhibitor of the epidermal growth factor receptor tyrosine kinase, in symptomatic patients with non-small cell lung cancer: a randomized trial. *Journal of the American Medical Association* **290**, 2149–2158.

107. Dowell J.E. and Minna J.D. (2005). Chasing mutations in the epidermal growth factor in lung cancer. *New England Journal of Medicine* **352**, 830–832.

108. Verma I.M. and Weitzman M.D. (2005). Gene therapy: twenty-first century medicine. *Annual Review of Biochemistry* **74**, 711–738.

109. Pai S.I., Lin Y.Y., Macaes B. *et al.* (2006). Prospects of RNA interference therapy for cancer. *Gene Therapy* **13**, 464–477.

110. Travis L.B., Rabkin C.S., Brown L.M. *et al.* (2006). Cancer survivorship – genetic susceptibility and second primary cancers: research strategies and recommendations. *Journal of the National Cancer Institute* **98**, 15–25.

111. Di Costanzo F., Sdrobolini A. and Gasperoni S. Capecitabine, a new oral fluoropyrimidine for the treatment of colorectal cancer. *Critical Reviews in Oncology and Hematology* **35**, 101–108.

112. Dearnaley D.P., Khoo V.S., Norman A.R. *et al.* (1999). Comparison of radiation side-effects of conformal and conventional radiotherapy in prostate cancer: a randomised trial. *Lancet* **353**, 267–272.

113. Rouits E., Boisdron-Celle M., Dumont A. *et al.* Relevance of different UGT1A1 polymorphisms in irinotecan-induced toxicity: a molecular and clinical study of 75 patients. *Clinical Cancer Research* **10**, 5151–5159.

114. Brizel D. (2003). Does amifostine have a role in chemoradiation treatment? *The Lancet Oncology* **4**, 378–380.

115. Overgaard J. (2003). Does amifostine have a role in chemoradiation treatment? *The Lancet Oncology* **4**, 380–381.

116. Sasse A.D., Clark L.G., Sasse E.C. and Clark O.A. (2006). Amifostine reduces side effects and improves complete response rate during radiotherapy: results of a metaanalysis. *International Journal of Radiation Oncology Biology Physics* **64**, 784–791.

117. Schuchter L.M., Hensley M.L., Meropol N.J. and Winer E.P. (2002). 2002 update of recommendations for the use of chemotherapy and radiotherapy protectants: clinical practice guidelines of the American Society of Clinical Oncology. *Journal of Clinical Oncology* **20**, 2895–2903.

118. Kovac A.L. (2006). Meta-analysis of the use of rescue antiemetics following PONV prophylactic failure with 5-HT$_3$ antagonist/dexamethasone versus single-agent therapies. *Annals of Pharmacotherapy* **40**, 873–887.

119. Leslie J.B., Gan T.J. Meta-analysis of the safety of 5-HT$_3$ antagonists with dexamethasone or droperidol for prevention of PONV (May). *Annals of Pharmacotherapy* **40**, 856–872.

120. de Wit R., Herrstedt J., Rapoport B. *et al.* (2004). The oral NK1 antagonist, aprepitant, given with standard antiemetics provides protection against nausea and vomiting over multiple cycles of cisplatin based chemotherapy: a combined analysis of two randomised, placebo-controlled phase III clinical trials. *European Journal of Cancer* **40**, 403–410.

121. Sharma R., Tobin P. and Clarke S.J. (2005). Management of chemotherapy-induced nausea, vomiting, oral mucositis, and diarrhoea. *The Lancet Oncology* **6**, 93–102.

122. Worthington H., Clarkson J. and Eden O. (2006). Interventions for preventing oral mucositis for patients with cancer receiving treatment (Cochrane Review). *The Cochrane Library*, Issue 2. Oxford: Update Software.

123. Stiff P.J., Emmanouilides C., Bensinger W.I. *et al.* (2006). Palifermin reduces patient-reported mouth and throat soreness and improves patient functioning in the hematopoietic stem-cell transplantation setting. *Journal of Clinical Oncology* **24**, 5186–5193.

124. Rothenberg M.L., Meropol N.J., Poplin E.A., Van Cutsem E. and Wadler S. (2001). Mortality associated with irinotecan plus bolus fluorouracil/leucovorin: summary findings of an independent panel. *Journal of Clinical Oncology* **19**, 3801–3807.

125. Lee S.J., Schover L.R., Partridge A.H. *et al.* (2006). American Society of Clinical Oncology recommendations on fertility preservation in cancer patients. *Journal of Clinical Oncology* **24**, 2917–2931, errata 5790.

126. Knobf M.T. (2006). Reproductive and hormonal sequelae of chemotherapy in women. Premature menopause and impaired fertility can result, effects that are especially disturbing to young women. *American Journal of Nursing* **106(3 suppl.)**, 60–65.

127. Schover L.R. (2005) Sexuality and fertility after cancer. *Hematology* **1**, 523–527.

128. Lipshultz S.E., Rifai N., Dalton V.M. *et al.* (2004). The effect of dexrazoxane on myocardial injury in doxorubicin-treated children with acute lymphoblastic leukemia. *New England Journal of Medicine* **351**, 145–153.

129. Minotti G., Menna P., Salvatorelli E., Cairo G. and Gianni L. (2004). Anthracyclines: molecular advances and pharmacologic developments in antitumor activity and cardiotoxicity. *Pharmacological Reviews* **56**, 185–229.

130. Senkus-Konefka E. and Jassem J. (2006). Complications of breast-cancer radiotherapy. *Clinical Oncology* **18**, 229–235.

131. Wouters K.A., Kremer L.C., Miller T.L., Herman E.H. and Lipshultz S.E. (2005). Protecting against anthracycline-induced myocardial damage: a review of the most promising strategies. *British Journal of Haematology* **131**, 561–578.

132. Hjermstad M.J., Fossa S.D., Oldervoll L. *et al.* (2005). Fatigue in long-term Hodgkin's disease survivors: a follow-up study. *Journal of Clinical Oncology* **23**, 6587–6595.

133. Savard J., Simard S., Hervouet S. *et al.* (2005). Insomnia in men treated with radical prostatectomy for prostate cancer. *Psycho-oncology* **14**, 147–156.

134. Jansen C.E., Miaskowski C., Dodd M., Dowling G. and Kramer J. (2005). A metaanalysis of studies of the effects of cancer chemotherapy on various domains of cognitive function. *Cancer* **104**, 2222–2233.

135. Matsuda T., Takayama T., Tashiro M. *et al.* (2005). Mild cognitive impairment after adjuvant chemotherapy in breast cancer patients – evaluation of appropriate research design and methodology to measure symptoms. *Breast Cancer* **12**, 279–287.

136. Phillips K.A. and Bernhard J. (2003). Adjuvant breast cancer treatment and cognitive function: current knowledge and research directions. *Journal of the National Cancer Institute* **95**, 190–197.

137. Shahinian V.B., Kuo Y.F., Freeman J.L. and Goodwin J.S. (2006). Risk of the 'androgen deprivation syndrome' in men receiving androgen deprivation for prostate cancer. *Archives of Internal Medicine* **166**, 465–471.

138. Shilling V., Jenkins V., Fallowfield L. and Howell T. (2003). The effects of hormone therapy on cognition in breast cancer. *Journal of Steroid Biochemistry and Molecular Biology* **86**, 405–412.

139. National Cancer Institute Cancer Therapy Evaluation Program (NCI-CTEP). (2003). *Common Terminology Criteria for Adverse Events v3.0 (CTCAE)*. Washington, DC: National Cancer Institute.

140. Koper P.C., Stroom J.C., van Putten W.L. *et al.* (1999). Acute morbidity reduction using 3DCRT for prostate carcinoma: a randomized study. *International Journal of Radiation Oncology Biology Physics* **43**, 727–734.

141. van Tol-Geerdink J.J., Stalmeier P.F.M., Pasker-de Jong P.C.M. *et al.* (2006). Systematic review of the effect of radiation dose on tumor control and morbidity in the treatment of prostate cancer by 3DCRT. *International Journal of Radiation Oncology Biology Physics* **64**, 534–543.

142. Zietman A.L., DeSilvio M.L., Slater J.D. *et al.* (2005). Comparison of conventional-dose vs high-dose conformal radiation therapy in clinically localized adenocarcinoma of the prostate: a randomized controlled trial.

Journal of the American Medical Association **294**, 1233–1239.

143. Bentzen S.M. (2005). Theragnostic imaging for radiation oncology: dose-painting by numbers. *The Lancet Oncology* **6**, 112–117.

144. Webb S. (2005). Intensity-modulated radiation therapy (IMRT): a clinical reality for cancer treatment, 'any fool can understand this'. The 2004 Silvanus Thompson Memorial Lecture. *British Journal of Radiology* **78**, S64–72.

145. Jaffray D.A. (2005). Emergent technologies for 3-dimensional image-guided radiation delivery. *Seminars in Radiation and Oncology* **15**, 208–216.

146. Ling C.C., Yorke E. and Fuks Z. (2006). From IMRT to IGRT: frontierland or neverland? *Radiotherapy and Oncology* **78**, 119–122.

147. Jarritt P.H., Hounsell A.R., Carson K.J. *et al.* (2005). Use of combined PET/CT images for radiotherapy planning: initial experiences in lung cancer. *British Journal of Radiology* **28(suppl.)**, 33–40.

148. Withers H.R. (1992). Biological basis of radiation therapy for cancer. *Lancet* **339**, 156–159.

149. Board of the Faculty of Clinical Oncology. (2006). *Radiotherapy Dose-Fractionation*. London: Royal College of Radiologists.

150. Williams M.V., James N.D., Summers E.T., Barrett A. and Ash D.V. (2006). National survey of radiotherapy fractionation practice in 2003. *Clinical Oncology* **18**, 3–14.

151. Wyatt R.M., Beddoe A.H. and Dale R.G. (2003). The effects of delays in radiotherapy treatment on tumour control. *Physics in Medicine and Biology* **48**, 139–155.

152. Pignon J.P., Baujat B. and Bourhis J. (2005). Apport des meta-analyses sur données individuelles au traitement des cancers ORL. *Cancer/Radiotherapie* **9**, 31–36.

153. Bonner J.A., Harari P.M., Giralt J. *et al.* (2006). Radiotherapy plus cetuximab for squamous-cell carcinoma of the head and neck. *New England Journal of Medicine* **354**, 567–578.

154. Allison R.R., Bagnato V.S., Cuenca R., Downie G.H. and Sibata C.H. (2006). The future of photodynamic therapy in oncology. *Future Oncology* **2**, 53–71.

155. Patrice T., Olivier D. and Bourre L. (2006). PDT in clinics: indications, results, and markets. *Journal of Environmental Pathology, Toxicology and Oncology* **25**, 467–486.

156. Berlinger N.T. (2006). Robotic surgery – squeezing into tight places. *New England Journal of Medicine* **354**, 2099–2101.

157. Enderling H., Anderson A.R., Chaplain M.A., Munro A.J. and Vaidya J.S. (2006). Mathematical modelling of radiotherapy strategies for early breast cancer. *Journal of Theoretical Biology* **241**, 158–171.

158. USC Department of Surgery. Intra-operative radiotherapy. Advanced Technology for the Treatment of Breast Cancer. www.targittial.com.whatistrgttrial.htm (accessed 24 July 2007).

159. Andrews D.W., Scott C.B., Sperduto P.W. *et al.* (2004). Whole brain radiation therapy with or without stereotactic radiosurgery boost for patients with one to three brain metastases: Phase III results of the RTOG 9508 randomised trial. *Lancet* **363**, 1665–1672.

160. Bhatnagar A.K., Flickinger J.C., Kondziolka D. and Lunsford L.D. (2006). Stereotactic radiosurgery for four or more intracranial metastases. *International Journal of Radiation Oncology, Biology, Physics* **64**, 898–903.

Part 2

The Experience
of Cancer

Introduction

Benner and Wrubel make an important point when they note that nursing and other caring practices have become paradoxical in a highly technical culture that seeks technological breakthroughs for all problems of illness.[1] Taking the example of heart transplants as an important medical 'breakthrough', they remind us that:

> Few notice that the intensive medical and nursing follow-up – solving the day to day problems of living with a transplanted organ, treating sores in the mouth due to immunosuppression, coping with a new hormonal milieu, promptly recognising and responding to infection and rejection – were all caring 'breakthroughs' that led to the eventual success of heart transplantation. These essential day to day nursing-care issues had to be solved in order to make heart transplantation a viable therapy. Yet they are all overlooked in the scientific and popular media coverage of the transplant story [p.xv].

This book attempts to celebrate such caring practices in cancer care, while also providing insights into the areas where nurses need to direct their attention, and explore the demands and skills of caring practices, wherever they are found and whoever should practise them.

Much has been written about the experience of cancer; it is also the focus of an ever-increasing body of research. This section sets out to explore this experience, and to pursue themes that may receive less attention: families and carers, professionals as well as lay people, who experience the disease through others. The theme is to explore in some detail an insider perspective (at least to the extent that one can get near to this) on what it is like to have cancer, and the problems and demands it brings, as well as the strategies people use to cope. The aim is to assist nurses to develop insight into what is needed in providing care.

People with cancer do not experience their illness alone. The experience of those close to them is of critical importance, for two reasons: first, because we know relatively little about the impact of cancer on relatives and friends, or for that matter on health professionals, and yet they are the most important sources of support for people with the disease. They will be responsible in many instances for a large proportion of the care and support that may be needed between episodes of formal treatment or institutional care. Cancer utterly disrupts people's lives; likewise, it disrupts in equal measure the lives of those around them. Second, through their actions and reactions, those who are close to people with cancer, whether family members or friends, or health care professionals, determine the experience of cancer for the people who have the disease.

This section provides insights into these issues and also explores what goes wrong in care, and the possible reasons behind our occasional inability to care. Thoughtful ideas around how nursing and nurses might take on a greater therapeutic role in the emotional lives of people affected by cancer are offered. Mary Wells begins this section with a detailed overview of the impact cancer has on people who are diagnosed as having cancer. Hilary Plant draws on her research and the accounts of people experiencing the impact of a family member or friend having cancer, to elucidate the experience of cancer within the family. In the concluding chapters Anne Lanceley begins to develop theory about nursing as a therapeutic endeavour in cancer care, the dynamics of therapeutic relationships in this context, and strategies and skills needed by nurses. She also exposes the barriers that exist for nurses working therapeutically; not the least of these is the sheer emotional burden that this imposes.

Reference

1. Benner P. and Wrubel J. (1988). *The Primacy of Caring: Stress and Coping in Health and Illness.* Menlo Park, CA: Addison-Wesley.

CHAPTER SIX

The impact of cancer

Mary Wells

Navigating your way through cancer and its treatment is rather like being dropped in a strange city, without a map or compass. There are no landmarks that you recognise and no familiar features. This city has no signs, no one speaks your language and your requests for help are incomprehensible: they are unable to help you.[1]

A diagnosis of cancer is profoundly shocking not just for its immediate impact but because it represents, for most people, the loss of present familiarity and the loss of a sense of future. The words of a young woman with head and neck cancer (above) illustrate the overwhelming sense of being thrown into a completely different place and feeling completely lost. Although survival rates continue to increase, and advances in treatment and support offer considerable hope for improved quality of life, the impact of cancer still 'hits you like a punch in the stomach'.[2]

Cancer changes lives, but the way in which it does so is as variable as the disease itself. The word 'cancer' is an all-encompassing label for more than 100 different types of cancer, many of which have very different manifestations, courses and consequences. As Frank states:

There is no 'right thing to say to a cancer patient', because the 'cancer patient' as a generic entity does not exist. There are only persons who are different to start with, having different experiences according to the contingencies of their diseases.

The importance of recognising the person beneath the diagnosis cannot be over emphasised. It is impossible to generalise about the effects a cancer diagnosis, or its treatment and aftermath, may have on a person. The impact, for example, of mutilating surgery such as mastectomy for breast cancer, or the lingering concerns an individual with an early cancer of the larynx cured by radiotherapy may have, can vary considerably between individuals, and may not immediately reflect expectations by health carers. How the person defines themselves and what he or she does for a living also has a major influence. Consider, for example, the devastating impact that severe peripheral neuropathy as a result of vinca alkaloid chemotherapy might have on a professional violinist or furniture maker, as opposed to someone who does not use their hands to make a living. The apparent nature and stage of the cancer or the severity of treatment-related side effects is not always revealed by a person's emotional reaction or apparent adjustment to living with the disease.[3]

The emotional impact of cancer will depend on a variety of factors, such as the experiences leading up to the communication of a diagnosis of cancer, the individual's perception of cancer and its meaning, the disruption the disease and treatment causes to normal life, perceptions surrounding treatment and its effects, experiences of past traumatic events, and individual personality and coping styles.[4,5]

This chapter explores the ways in which cancer changes and influences the lives of those who are affected by the disease, and wherever possible, uses people's own words to describe the impact of living with cancer.

The context of cancer

The word cancer precipitates strong emotional reactions, including fear, despair, deep shock and sometimes secrecy. Historically, cancer has been associated with contagion, suffering, pain, and death.[6–8] For many these associations are deeply embedded and, despite evidence for both improved survival and better quality of life through advances in treatment and symptom control, there remains a common perception that a diagnosis of cancer means certain death.

Benner and Wrubel propose that in order to overcome the negativity that cancer engenders, there is a need for wholesale cultural redefinition of the disease, so that it is understood instead as a chronic or potentially curable disease.[9] Although cancer shares similarities with other chronic diseases, Tritter argues that the chronic illness label is not useful.[10] He suggests that cancer is different from other chronic illnesses in a number of ways, including its complexity and variety, its strong association with death and its high profile in the media. Little also questions the appropriateness of conceptualising cancer as a chronic illness.[11] He suggests that people who *survive* cancer cannot be said to be suffering from a chronic illness, but that 'the suffering caused by confrontation with one's own death, by the threat of recurrence, by disruption in close relationships, the physical disabilities brought about by treatment, and encounters with implicit and explicit discrimination, is real and present, and it may be chronic' (p.202). There is no doubt that the experience of having cancer causes ambiguity and disruption in many areas of life, and that this may never be completely resolved, even when a person is 'cured'.

Cancer rarely takes a linear or predictable course from diagnosis to treatment, cure or death. More often cancer and its treatment produce episodes of acute illness and treatment with periods of relative health and normality. However, there are a number of particularly difficult points in a person's experience of cancer, including waiting for diagnosis, receiving the diagnosis, going through treatment, and trying to get back to normal.[12] The cancer trajectory as shown in Figure 6.1 is an over-simplification of the journey experienced by people with cancer, as it implies a progression through a number of discrete stages. Although it is a useful framework for

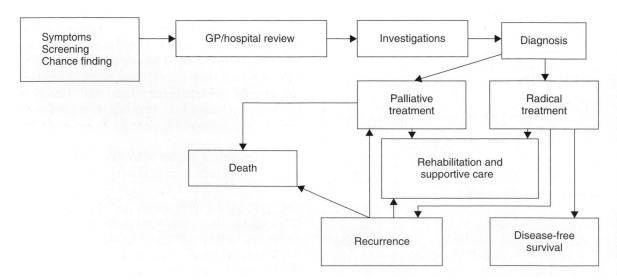

Figure 6.1 The cancer trajectory.

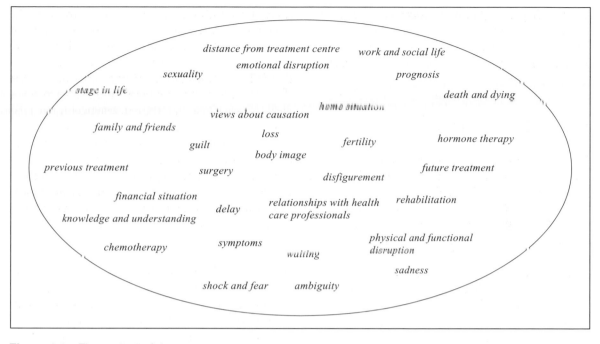

Figure 6.2   The context of the cancer experience.

considering the critical phases of the journey, it de-contextualises these important stages. At any stage, or indeed at every stage, the context in which the person experiences investigations, hospital appointments, treatment or supportive care is completely individual. Figure 6.2 illustrates just some of the many feelings, emotions, concerns and contextual influences that may have an impact on the individual's experience.

Diagnosis

Diagnosis is rarely the real beginning of the disease, as the cancer may have taken months or even years to develop before a diagnosis is actually triggered. However, it is the point at which cancer becomes a reality, and therefore represents an appropriate place to start.

The shock of receiving a cancer diagnosis can be overwhelming, and although most people express acute distress and fear at the news, many also experience profound feelings of disbelief or even outright denial. The accounts below illustrate some of these reactions. The first is an extract from an interview with a 71-year-old man diagnosed with carcinoma of the larynx.

> When he told me I'd got cancer – he bloody frightened me to death, he did. I went out, didn't I, went out cold . . . frightened me to death . . . I remember going down, sitting down and thinking that was it.[13]

Many people describe the feeling of almost being displaced from themselves, as if they are watching someone on stage or television that isn't really them. As this 48-year-old woman with carcinoma of the tongue explained, there is a sense of unreality about being told of a cancer diagnosis and it can be extremely difficult to take it all in.

> The first thing he more or less said was, 'I don't beat about the bush', he said 'what you've got, you've got a cancer,' and that's when it sort of hit me, because you're sort of mesmerised really, you sort of go into space, you think he can't be talking about me, he's probably wrong, he must be talking about someone else, but he said 'you have', he said 'you've got a cancer'. I think that was the worst time, because you come out of there thinking no, he's got it all wrong, he's got me muddled with somebody else.[13]

Communicating a diagnosis of cancer

Despite the immense shock of receiving a diagnosis of cancer, almost all patients remember how their diagnosis was communicated. A recent qualitative study explored patients' and families' experiences and wishes of being told about their cancer, and found that the *way* in which information is shared was as important as the content of the communication. Six attributes held by health professionals were identified as most important:[14]

- playing it straight (being honest and direct)
- making it clear (using language that can be understood)
- showing you care
- giving time
- pacing information (appreciating the importance of timing, understanding and readiness to receive information at different stages)
- staying the course (communicating a sense of being there for the person now and in the future, whether or not the cancer progresses).

When health care professionals did not demonstrate these attributes, patients were generally dissatisfied with the way in which information was disclosed. In terms of *what* they wanted to be told, patients showed that the two most important areas were information about prognosis and the provision of hopeful messages. Although patients wanted accurate information about what was likely to happen in the future, they also wanted to be able to maintain hope. Sometimes this involved 'living parallel realities' in which they acknowledged that the cancer was terminal but still hoped for a cure. Health professionals could maintain hope in a number of ways, including 'leaving the door open' for a more hopeful outcome, being honest about difficult subjects, presenting sensitive and timely information about palliative care, respecting patients' wishes to pursue alternative treatments, and being sensitive to changing information needs.

Communicating a diagnosis of cancer is difficult for health professionals as well as for the person who is receiving the news. Frequently the diagnosis of cancer is communicated in a busy outpatient clinic where time and space is limited. Patients often feel that they were too shocked or upset to know what to ask at the time, which adds to the distress and uncertainty felt between hospital appointments. Specialist nurses often play an important role during these periods, and it is important that they make it clear to patients that they are available to talk. Models of 'breaking bad news' provide a useful framework for discussing difficult emotional issues as well as imparting actual news. Box 6.1 outlines the S-P-I-K-E-S strategy, which emphasises the importance of attention to the setting, content and portrayal of information.[15]

Information

Providing information at all stages of the cancer trajectory is recognised as extremely important, and there has been a rapid increase in the amount and variety of information available to patients with cancer in recent years. The worldwide web has made it possible for most people to access high-quality information about cancer as well as inaccurate or biased information, which is often aimed at persuading vulnerable people to spend money on alternative or commercial products with no proven benefit. Clearly there are many huge advantages to the immediate availability of reliable information, such as that produced by Cancerbackup (www.cancerbackup.org.uk), but many patients are overwhelmed by the range and amount of information available, not knowing what to read and how to interpret it. The possibility of an 'inverse information law' also exists, whereby the people who most need information are least likely to have access to new technologies.[16] Additionally, studies show that the majority of patients still prefer to interact with health care professionals rather than use a computer or receive a booklet.[17]

A large UK survey of more than 2000 patients found that 87% preferred to be given as much information as possible, whether good or bad.[18] Other studies have revealed that certain groups of patients are more likely to be provided with information, including those with breast cancer,[17,19] and those who are more affluent.[20] These worrying findings suggest that the inverse information law applies across the board, and that people from

Box 6.1   Discussing difficult news or emotional issues: The S-P-I-K-E-S strategy

- *Setting (S)*:
  - privacy – create a sense of privacy and minimise disruptions as far as possible
  - involve significant others – appointing a 'spokesperson' may be helpful. Be aware of family situation and relationships
  - sit down – communicate a sense of partnership
  - look attentive and calm – maintain eye contact as much as possible but break off momentarily if the person is upset, so as to reduce intensity
  - listening mode – allow silence, do not interrupt, repeat important words, acknowledge what is said
  - availability – communicate any time restraints, reduce possible interruptions.
- *Perception (P)* – ask what the person thinks, feels and expects before you tell them. Check what they have been told and what they understand.
- *Invitation (I)* – ask what the person wants to know and when they want to know it.
- *Knowledge (K)* – provide some warning that you are going to talk about something difficult so that the person has a few more seconds to prepare. Avoid technical language and where possible use terms that the person themselves has used, providing information in small chunks. Be honest but do not destroy hope.
- *Empathy (E)*:
  - listen for and identify emotions being expressed, and if emotions are not being expressed, ask how the person feels about what has been said
  - identify the cause of the emotion(s)
  - show the person that you have made a connection between the cause (e.g. the diagnosis) and the emotion itself (e.g. profound shock)
  - validate the person's feelings by communicating to them that their emotions are understandable, normal and valid.
- *Strategy and summary (S)* – check intermittently that the person understands the information and that you are communicating about the same thing. At the end of the discussion summarise what has been said and ensure that a clear plan of action or future contact is communicated.

Adapted from Buckman (2005).[15]

deprived backgrounds who are more likely to have poor-prognosis cancers such as lung cancer may be systematically disadvantaged. However, it must be recognised that people differ enormously in their preferences for information, including the nature, timing and amount with which they feel comfortable. As Leydon and coworkers point out, people 'oscillate between the desire for information and the avoidance of new information' (p.912).[21] This qualitative study of 24 patients with varying diagnoses identified the themes of faith, hope and charity to explain patients' attitude to gaining and using information. Patients had *faith* in medical staff and often settled for the information they were given, feeling that asking for more might be frightening, confusing or frowned upon. Several patients felt that seeking further information could undermine their efforts to maintain *hope*, get on with life and be positive. Many were very aware of other people who were worse off or more deserving, and this often influ-

enced how much they sought information or approached busy staff whose time might be needed by others (*charity*).

Individual beliefs about cancer and its causation

It is normal to want to understand a disease or symptom that has such a profound impact on your life, and it can be deeply troubling if there is no explanation for it. Although some people find it helpful to be able to attribute their disease to a particular cause (e.g. mesothelioma and exposure to asbestos or lung cancer and smoking), such attributions can also foster bitterness, guilt, anger and regret. Where there is no obvious source of blame, many people still spend a great deal of time searching for meaning, motivated by a strong desire to make sense of the situation. This search may help the person to adapt and regain control, and it may occur at any stage. Taylor has devised a conceptual framework for the search for meaning, which includes four key components:[22]

- identifying causal explanations, which may change over time and differ according to cultural background
- selective incidence – asking questions such as 'Why did this happen to me and not someone else?'
- responsibility – considering who or what is to blame? If a person perceives that they can modify their behaviour or lifestyle to reduce their susceptibility to recurrence they may feel more in control than if they feel that inherent personality factors are to blame[23]
- significance of the experience – some individuals construe benefits from their cancer.

Individuals will respond in different ways to this search, showing resignation (passive acceptance), remonstration (lack of acceptance and discontent), or reconciliation (significance found and accepted).

A phenomenological view of adjustment and cancer emphasises the inextricable link between the meaning and context of the illness experience and the person's ability to cope with the disease.[9] The individual construction of meaning is to a large extent dependent on personal beliefs, characteristics, and events, past and present.[5,24]

The sociological and anthropological literature identifies that the meaning of illness is attributed as a result of socially determined cultural interpretations and networks, and that an individual's own interpretation and explanation for illness and its symptoms are highly significant to the 'legitimisation' of disease.[25–28] The acceptance of someone's 'popular' explanation is important, as it 'permits patients to satisfactorily integrate their illness in a context where the need for coherence in the face of a break with life is essential'.[29]

Assigning meaning to illness helps to reduce or even resolve suffering.[24] Nurses can greatly assist with the process of finding meaning, by letting an individual tell their own story surrounding their illness, and helping them place this in context, thus reinforcing and showing acceptance of their feelings and explanations. This 'illness narrative'

has been recognised as an important means by which understanding of the meaning of illness can be developed by an individual, and may be of enormous therapeutic value (see Care strategy 6.1).[25,30–32]

The situation in which the diagnosis occurs

An individual's reaction to a diagnosis of cancer is to some extent dependent on the way in which the disease presents itself and is first acknowledged. Significant factors include whether or not the person suspected they had cancer, expects to be told they have cancer, or experiences a delay in diagnosis.

The advent of 'one-stop' clinics for patients with common cancers such as breast cancer has streamlined the process of diagnosis and has significantly reduced waiting times for results and treatment. Although there are clearly many advantages to receiving a quick diagnosis, it can be particularly shocking for people who did not expect to be told they have cancer. Where cancer has been detected through a routine screening test with little prior counselling, there may have been no time to consider the possibility that anything serious is wrong. Patients have often described turning up for an outpatient appointment alone because they had no idea they would be given such devastating news.

Others who have suspected cancer for some time may be relieved to find out their diagnosis, since it ends some of the uncertainty. The example below illustrates this:

> He took a sample and after a week I had an appointment with him again, and then he told me it was malignant, that is was cancer. And to tell you the truth, I was very comfortable with it. He told me exactly how it was. And he told me how it was progressing and even if this is a disease that people don't like very much, I was very content to finally know what was wrong with me. Having been like this for a few years, I was always getting lower and lower. I was worse and worse all the time. I almost cheered up just to know what it was . . . You have been fighting some ghost that you don't know what it is, nothing. That was absolutely the worst thing about the whole thing.[35]

Care strategy 6.1   Facilitating narratives

Facilitating the process in which someone can 'tell their story' acknowledges who they are as a person, and values their interpretation of how their identity has been disrupted as a result of cancer. The construction of such a narrative enables the individual to make sense of what is happening, as well as to incorporate their illness into the context of their life in its wider sense. This can help enormously to 'normalise' their experience.

Time, space and privacy are essential. Being sensitive to metaphors, stories about apparently unrelated events in people's lives, jokes, and 'throw away' remarks is also very important. Some people will find it much easier to express difficult emotions through humour or a story about something they did before they were diagnosed, therefore it is vital that nurses listen carefully to such cues. Others will talk directly about 'how it all started' without needing encouragement. However, asking about the following aspects of the experience may assist the expression of a narrative or story:

- describing what happened around the time of the diagnosis, and their thoughts and feelings
- describing how things have changed since the diagnosis – friends, family, work, relationships, roles – for better and for worse
- what the treatment and its effects have been like
- what 'normal' life is like now
- how they feel they have changed since the diagnosis
- how they make sense of the cancer and whether they think there are any explanations
- what is most important in life now
- how they see the future
- what has been the most significant change in their life as a result of the diagnosis.

Clearly this is not a list of direct questions, but a series of potential areas of discussion. Some people may find it easier to express themselves using art, photographs or writing, and it may be possible to encourage them to tell their story using these mediums, even if they find it difficult to talk. Hearing other people's stories can also be beneficial. In a questionnaire study, Chelf et al. found that 85% of people who attended a storytelling workshop gained hope from hearing others' stories of living with cancer.[33]

Time to 'debrief' is important, as retelling many aspects of the narrative may provoke feelings and reactions that require support within the safety of the therapeutic relationship. As Atwood describes,[34] the story may only make sense afterwards, and there needs to be time to reflect on its meaning:

When you are in the middle of a story it isn't a story at all, but only a confusion; a dark roaring, a blindness, a wreckage of shattered glass and splintered wood; like a house in a whirlwind, or else a boat crushed by the icebergs or swept over the rapids, and all aboard powerless to stop it. It's only afterwards that it becomes anything like a story at all. When you are telling it, to yourself or to someone else [p.346].

Delays in diagnosis can have a significant impact on outcome, therefore it is not surprising that they often evoke feelings of anger, guilt and blame. The nature and length of the delay may colour an individual's reactions to the diagnosis and his or her ability to cope and adjust. Reasons for delay are often multifactorial and can include failure by a general practitioner or other health professional to recognise symptoms suggestive of cancer, difficulties in detecting the cancer using routine diagnostic procedures, and delays on the part of the patient. In recent years, considerable resource has been directed towards improvements in referral and diagnosis but we also need to understand more about the delays that are effectively caused by patients themselves due to fear, stigma, denial, guilt, and not taking symptoms seriously. A qualitative study of patients with lung cancer revealed that contrary to the widely held view that lung cancer is silent until far advanced, patients experienced symptoms for many months before their diagnosis but tended not to attribute these to serious illness.[36] It appeared that those who smoked felt undeserving of medical care and expected to be treated less promptly.

One of the problems in diagnosing cancer promptly and accurately is that cancer is essentially a disease of older people who already have concomitant disease, therefore symptoms may be masked or interpreted wrongly.[37] Lack of awareness of the likelihood of cancer, and delay in seeking help are common in older people. Edlund and Sneed studied the attitudes and reactions of 133 people of all ages, newly diagnosed with cancer, and found that people over the age of 70 years were significantly less positive about the outcome of their disease, believing that nothing could be done.[38] However, they were also significantly less psychologically distressed than other age groups. This may be because older people are more resigned to the idea of illness and death than younger people, or it may reflect the attitude of society and the health care system to the elderly; since they are no longer economically useful, older people may have a sense of time having run out.

For those who have delayed seeking help for signs of cancer, guilt and self-reproach may complicate acceptance of treatment, and psychological recovery.[39] Paradoxically, fear of criticism by doctors and health professionals may play a part in extending delay. Family members may also feel responsible for not acting sooner, or may be frustrated in being unable to convince someone to visit their doctor.

For some, a conscious decision is taken not to seek treatment, and these people may delay their diagnosis until it becomes impossible to manage their symptoms, or until they need emergency care. Reasons for delaying diagnosis include family responsibilities such as being the main carer for someone else, and personal issues such as fear, embarrassment, stigma, and ignorance. Some people find it more and more difficult as time goes on to admit that something is wrong. It is not uncommon for an obvious cancer to be hidden from a partner for months or years, undressing in the dark and making other excuses for odour arising from the tumour. Fungating tumours in intimate places such as the breast, anus, vulva or penis, for example, may cause embarrassment, and therefore delay in seeking help for them. A mixture of guilt and relief may result when finally 'found out'.

As a professional carer it is sometimes hard to understand how someone could hide a cancer for so long, particularly when, in the case of a fungating wound, it is manifestly malodourous, weeping,

raw and often extensive. Feelings of self-disgust, fear of rejection, judgement and blame, or anticipating punishment may be commonly experienced.[40] A supportive and non-judgemental approach is important in caring for such individuals, as the expectation of further rejection can be very powerful.

Attributing personal responsibility onto illness can lead to feelings of guilt, self-blame, and shame.[41] Guilt and isolation can be felt because of a belief that cancer is a result of past wrongdoing or sinful behaviour, and cancer can be perceived as a 'punishment' and therefore deserved in some way. For example, lung cancer in someone who has smoked heavily can be accompanied by feelings of guilt and self-reproach; these may also be reinforced by unsympathetic health professionals. Guilt may also, however, be a means by which some individuals define themselves in order to preserve feelings of being in control. In this way guilt may permit protection from other more difficult emotions engendered by life-threatening illness.[42]

Sontag argues that recent psychological theories associating cancer with personality type may result in people feeling culpable for it.[8] In addition, media attention surrounding prevention through diet and self-examination has encouraged notions of blame and fault in those who develop the disease. This is exaggerated by a health care culture that promotes a non-judgemental attitude towards consumers of care, yet at the same time strongly emphasises individual responsibility for health and illness. Thus, the health care system can simultaneously relieve and reinstate guilt.

Individual personality and coping style

There has been considerable controversy about the extent to which an individual's personality and coping style actually affect their outcome, but it is widely acknowledged that different coping styles do exist and that individuals display a number of different reactions to their diagnosis. The expanding field of 'psycho-oncology' has provided a large number of different theories of adjustment and adaptation to cancer and its treatment. While it is impossible to generalise about an individual's reaction to cancer, these theories may be useful in the recognition of common reactions and the facilitation of emotional expression.

A number of the theories highlight stages that an individual may pass through in adjusting to the news of a diagnosis of cancer.[43,44] These include shock, numbness, and disbelief, lasting for days to weeks; acute distress, which may manifest itself as anger or anxiety, lasting for weeks to months; depression, or despair, and gradual acceptance, which may take several months or even years. While these theories are useful, they are also problematic in that they suggest that such emotional reactions are universally experienced and that progression through such stages of adjustment is serial and occurs in a forward direction, thus portraying an overly constrained notion of what is 'normal' and 'healthy' adjustment.

The work of Greer *et al.* has been extremely influential in our understanding of patients' adjustment to cancer.[45] These authors interviewed 69 women with breast cancer and identified five distinct adjustment styles:

- fighting spirit
- avoidance and denial
- fatalism
- anxious preoccupation
- helplessness and hopelessness.

A person who adopts a fighting spirit towards her cancer may perceive the threat of cancer as a challenge that she is determined to overcome, expressing this with the following kinds of response: 'I'm not giving up', 'This is not going to get me', 'I'm going to fight it'. Someone who avoids or denies their disease may have an equally strong response, ignoring the fact that it is anything to do with them. Those who feel fatalistic, helpless, hopeless or excessively anxious are less able to take control of the situation and may be more overwhelmed by the diagnosis.

How far health professionals should collude with or refute an attitude of denial is not straightforward. On balance it is considered unwise and possibly harmful to attempt forcefully to break through a patient's denial; however, to collude and encourage such denial might be equally harmful. Over-zealous health care professionals can insist on truth telling at times when a patient is not ready or able to deal with the impact of what they are being told. Careful and sensitive discussion in a safe, therapeutic relationship will often provide an opening for such dialogue, without removing the ability for the person to hold on to control of the situation.

Those who are fatalistic about their disease, and do not believe they have any control, may express this through passive acceptance: 'You can't do anything and if you can't do anything about it there's no point worrying about it, so you have to make the best of it . . . I think you might as well make the best of it, otherwise you give up and get worried about it, no point in doing that'.[13]

Comments such as 'You are the expert' or 'I'm in your hands' may frequently be said to doctors or nurses, by individuals who feel safer leaving any decisions to their professional carers. This passive attitude may make it difficult for the person to access help or believe in their ability to influence the course of events, but it may also protect against the sometimes overwhelming burden of having cancer. There are probably times in most people's illness when placing responsibility and trust in others is an essential part of maintaining psychological stability. As one man said, 'when you're not feeling well you don't feel very safe, you just want somebody to make it go away'.[13]

Anxious preoccupation is a term used to describe someone who finds it difficult to think of anything other than their illness and looks for constant reassurance. They may seek alternative medicine or excessive amounts of information, worrying that every symptom is a sign of recurrent disease: 'I don't know what is going on . . . am I OK or am I not . . . I go over and over it in my mind'.[13] These adjustment styles are not necessarily pathological or negative, although they might indicate anxiety or depression, which could warrant psychological intervention. Many people will alternate between a variety of reactions to their situation, while others remain positive and in control throughout their illness.

Someone who has 'given up' and is overwhelmed by the cancer and cannot see any way out may be said to have adopted a 'helpless/

hopeless' adjustment style. This particular response has been most strongly linked with a poor outlook. Greer *et al.* followed their sample of women with breast cancer over a 15-year period and found that the responses of fighting spirit and denial were positively associated with longer survival, and that the helpless/hopeless response was correlated with a poorer outcome.[45–47] Although the study provoked considerable interest in the relationship between cancer and the mind, the idea that a single coping style is possible to identify and that this is stable and durable over time is problematic. The original study also neglected the possible influence of other factors including prognostic indicators, support and subsequent life events. A larger and more recent cohort study, which did control for known prognostic factors, confirmed that a helpless/hopeless outlook still exerted a significantly detrimental effect on disease-free survival, although no sustained link between fighting spirit and improved survival was found.[48] Despite such individually convincing findings, a recent systematic review concluded that there is little overall evidence to support an association between coping style and survival from cancer.[49]

Petticrew *et al.* also suggest that the tendency to associate certain coping styles with improved survival has led to a pressure on patients to cope in a certain way, thus adding to their psychological burden.[49] Feelings of anger, anxiety, sadness and despondency are entirely appropriate responses to a life-threatening event, such as a diagnosis of cancer, and these emotions are unlikely to go away completely unless the threat of the disease is also removed. However, when these feelings persist and are overwhelming they can become damaging. It is estimated that about one-third of people with cancer suffer from clinically significant anxiety and depression.[50]

Adjustment to cancer

Brennan argues that coping theories do not go far enough in explaining the way in which a person adapts over time to having cancer.[51] How well an individual adjusts to a life-threatening illness such as cancer is thought to depend largely on the way in which they appraise the 'catastrophic threat'

imposed by the diagnosis. How the person perceives the magnitude and consequences of the threat, and how far he or she feels able to control that threat may be influential,[52] as it appears that individuals who are active rather than passive in their response to cancer may adjust more successfully. The concept of self-efficacy,[53] defined as belief in one's own ability to influence events or master challenges,[54] is relevant here. Bandura's model suggests that an individual's sense of self-efficacy is strengthened by four main sources of influence as shown in Box 6.2.[55]

Box 6.2 Key influences on self-efficacy

1. *Experiencing success* – when a person achieves something that is important to them despite having some setbacks, their belief in their own ability to get through difficult times is likely to be strengthened.
2. *Vicarious experience through social role models* – seeing other people succeed is encouraging, particularly when their situations are similar. Interestingly, Bandura does not discuss the potential benefits of comparing one's situation with someone who appears to be 'worse off', although many people with cancer talk about the sobering effect that this has in helping to put their situation into perspective. Neither does Bandura raise the issue that vicarious experience through the media can sometimes be *unhelpful*. Although some patients gain considerable motivation from media stories about people who have survived cancer against all the odds, or achieved remarkable success despite having terminal disease, others can find such stories discouraging if they perceive themselves as having failed because they have not been able to match up.
3. *Social persuasion* – self-efficacy can be strengthened through an encouraging relationship, e.g. with a health professional. Acknowledging a person's achievements and strengths and encouraging them to believe in themselves is a key component of this relationship. In addition, the 'persuader' can help to structure and facilitate situations in which the person is likely to feel successful and unlikely to feel they have failed.
4. *Reduction in stress reactions and negative thought processes* – the experience of anxiety, tension and physical symptoms can all signify to a person that he or she is ill or not coping with the situation. Strategies that help to reduce stress reactions and/or challenge negative thoughts can be very helpful in improving the person's sense of self-efficacy.

The way in which a person appraises the magnitude or consequences of the threat of cancer may depend on their perception of the timeline of their cancer. Studies show that patients who conceptualise their cancer as a chronic illness are more anxious, depressed, and worried about recurrence than those who perceive their disease as acute and short-lived.[56] Other situational factors are also influential, including expectations about prognosis, physical health, emotional and social support, ability to find benefit in the situation, and previous mental health and life experiences.

Psychodynamic theorists believe that early developmental processes influence personality resources and thus the defence mechanisms employed in adjusting to life with cancer. When faced with the loss of control and threat of dependence imposed by cancer, attempts at retaining control are unconsciously made through enacting defences learned in childhood. Common defence mechanisms include:

- *denial*
- *projection* – attributing own unacknowledged feelings onto someone else
- *displacement* – redirecting energy into something other than the cause of the distress
- *sublimation* – channelling primitive emotions into something creative, for example anger or art
- *regression* – return to childlike behaviour
- *intellectualisation* – at the expense of emotional expression
- *conversion* – expression of emotional anxiety through a physical symptom.[4]

Most nurses will recognise at least some of these defence mechanisms as common manifestations of patients' emotional responses to cancer. Psychodynamic theorists believe that these defences help to protect against unbearable anxiety and that it is therefore important not to destroy them. It has been suggested that nurses have a crucial role in containing and holding this unbearable anxiety in order to make it feel more manageable for the person with cancer.[57]

If someone has experienced previous traumatic events in their life that are unresolved in some way, it is probably more likely that they will have difficulty dealing with the reality of having cancer.[58] Often, the emotional response evokes memories of difficult past experiences, for instance childhood sexual abuse, and this can lead to negative ways of behaving.[59] A study of holocaust survivors with cancer found that compared with others who had not experienced a traumatic life event, the holocaust survivors had significantly higher psychological distress scores.[60]

Identifying patients who are at high risk of experiencing real difficulties in adjusting to a diagnosis of cancer is clearly important. However, this is not straightforward, as oncology staff are known to be poor at identifying psychological distress,[61] and patients themselves may perceive that they do not need help or that there is nothing that can be done to help anyway.[62] Screening patients for psychological distress using validated assessment tools such as the hospital anxiety and depression scale (HADS),[63] or the Mental Adjustment to Cancer questionnaire,[64] may be helpful, provided that adequate psychological support is available. Unfortunately few oncology departments have sufficient access to psychological services, although the growth in information and support facilities such as Maggie's Centres (www.maggiescentres.org.uk) has enabled many more people to benefit from skilled psychological support.

Emotional support,[65] defined as 'spending time with another person, listening and talking about problems and concerns in a way that is helpful and reassuring' (p.1275) is clearly extremely important. However, the findings of a questionnaire study of 431 patients from seven different outpatient clinics raise serious questions about whether or not nurses are seen to fulfil this need.[65] Patients were given a list including doctors, family/friends, nurses, information resources, and support groups, and were asked to indicate the most important overall sources of emotional support. Senior doctors were rated as most important, followed by friends and family. Nurses were chosen by less than 10% of respondents.

In recent years, there has been a growing interest in the potential for psychological interventions to enhance emotional well-being, quality of life and even survival, but consistent evidence for the effectiveness of such interventions is limited. One systematic review concluded that only tentative recommendations could be offered for and against most intervention strategies.[66] Some evidence of medium- and long-term benefits from group therapy, education, counselling, relaxation, and cognitive-behavioural therapy was found but the results were not overwhelmingly positive. Another systematic review recommended that behaviour therapy is beneficial for people with advanced cancer.[67] However, there are a number of real difficulties with evaluating psychological interventions, with systematic reviews in this area being especially problematic (see Box 6.3).[68]

Although more objective evidence for the effectiveness of psychological interventions is required, there is no doubt that many patients benefit from learning strategies that enable them to manage the stress and disruption caused by cancer. Probably one of the most commonly used approaches is the use of adjuvant psychological therapy (APT),[52] in

which therapy is orientated towards problem solving, reappraisal and 'cognitive restructuring' (reality testing). The components of this structured approach include the following:

- enabling the patient to air their feelings
- teaching behavioural techniques such as relaxation, distraction, and activity scheduling, to maximise the patient's sense of control and ability to feel pleasure during daily life
- the use of cognitive techniques, which assist the patient to recognise any automatic or negative thoughts and learn to challenge them. The patient is helped to consider the evidence for any negative fears and to search for more constructive or alternative explanations. A process of 'decatastrophising' encourages the patient to confront their fears in a safe environment and to consider whether these are realistic. Simple distraction techniques that 'break into the spiral of increasing anxiety' (p.117) can be useful.[52] Patients can also be taught to say certain positive things to themselves whenever they feel anxious or have negative thoughts
- working with couples – partners can be effectively involved in this process by reminding the patient of their strengths, remembering previous ways that the couple have coped with stressful events. While working with the couple, the therapist can facilitate and enhance their communication skills through the use of behavioural and cognitive techniques.

This approach is essentially a joint problem-solving exercise, which is flexible enough to be tailored to an individual's needs. The application of these techniques can help to develop more constructive coping strategies, which can positively change the ways of responding and adjusting to living with cancer.

Frank is critical of the emphasis in the psycho-oncology literature on adjustment, and suggests that people also need to mourn in order to move on:[3]

> I want to emphasise mourning as affirmation. To mourn what has passed, either through illness or death, affirms the life that has been led. To adjust too rapidly is to treat the loss simply as an incident from which

---

Box 6.3   Difficulties in conducting systematic reviews of psychological interventions

- Heterogeneity of psychological interventions, e.g. group therapy facilitated by a trained therapist, individual counselling and self-help cognitive therapy are all very different.
- Publication bias may exist, with negative studies less likely to be published.[49]
- Quality of studies is variable – many are small, do not adjust for important predictors of survival, and have short follow-up periods, therefore give no information about long-term effects.
- Criteria used to assess the quality of studies may be inappropriate for psychological interventions.
- Outcome measures are variable – difficult to compare outcomes on several different scales.
- Randomised controlled trials may not be the best way of assessing psychological interventions and trials need to be comprehensively planned using a framework such as the Medical Research Council (MRC) framework for the evaluation of complex interventions.[69]
- Measuring overall coping styles and applying blanket findings to individual patients is problematic, due to the fact that patients' emotional responses are not usually linear or static.
- There are more studies of women with breast cancer than any other cancer, therefore it is difficult to apply findings universally.

one can bounce back; it devalues whom or what has been lost. When an ill person loses the body in which she has lived, or when a caregiver suffers the death of the person he has cared for, the loss must be mourned fully in its own time. Only through mourning can we find a life on the other side of loss [p.40].

Loss

The impact of cancer is largely felt through the losses experienced by the individual and family. Loss is felt in every aspect of life, perhaps most profoundly in terms of the loss of a sense of future. People often feel they cannot make plans, cannot allow themselves to have expectations or hopes for the future in case something goes wrong.

The loss of a sense of self is often deeply felt. The experience of being diagnosed with cancer seems to undermine a person's sense of who they are at a very fundamental level. In particular, people often lose a sense of being able to influence, control, or even engage in aspects of life which they have taken for granted – work, family relationships, home and social roles, sex, sport and leisure activities, eating and drinking, bodily functions, and appearance. As John Diamond so poignantly described:[70]

> When I told people that I was not quite myself I meant it almost literally: in the mirror I was somebody else. Precisely I was a little old man whom I imagine to be called Albert or Norman or George [p.191].

Another important dimension of loss is that of time, as life is largely taken over by the 'waiting culture of medicine'.[71] Imposed absence from work and home, attending hospital for clinic appointments and treatment, and waiting for results, all contribute to the loss of one's own routine, sense of time, and control over that time. The centralisation of services may make this worse, as people suffer the practical, physical, and psychosocial burden of travelling long distances for their treatment.[72]

Loss is often compounded by physical change. In a study of the experience of cancer of the head and neck, feelings of being embarrassed to go out showing any visible signs of cancer or its treatment, being embarrassed to eat in a restaurant for

fear of dribbling or needing to use a straw were reported.[13] Several of those interviewed explained how they held back from normal activities, preferring to do nothing, rather than be disappointed if they found they were unable to do what they had planned. Cancer and its treatment had knocked their confidence and caused withdrawal from many of the aspects of life that gave them their individuality, such as gardening, work, church, swimming, and going out socially. Withdrawal from these activities meant that these people experienced a loss of identity and loss of belonging. The following are excerpts from interviews with people following treatment for cancer of the head and neck.

> I dribble at the corner of my mouth and this upsets me, I've never got full control, the whole thing makes me feel as if I'm not functioning properly . . . I don't want to get into one to these things and then not be able to do it properly.

> I didn't want anyone asking me uncomfortable questions at the time . . . I felt I couldn't go out, people I knew I'd see and I didn't want to have to explain, that sort of thing.

> Didn't go to church – didn't want people surreptitiously looking at my burns.[13]

Life is disrupted by emotional, physical, and practical factors, which may include repeated hospital appointments for treatment or follow-up, the need for specialist clothing or food as a result of cancer surgery, or inability to work or care for children due to treatment side-effects. However, such disruption requires a re-evaluation of life in order to move towards wellness. This re-examination of life may be an enriching experience, resulting in a shift in self-image and perspective. Many people describe positive changes in their lives including closer relationships, changes in priorities, an enhanced sense of purpose, greater spirituality, and improved personal resources.[73]

One model of adjustment, which recognises that adapting to a cancer diagnosis is a dynamic process in which individuals struggle to make sense of changes imposed by the disease and its treatment and often manage to achieve some positive change, is the social–cognitive transition model of adjustment (SCT).[51] Brennan proposes that individuals hold a number of fundamental assumptions about themselves and the world, which are socially constructed and life-stage dependent. His model recognises that the way in which people respond to a diagnosis of cancer depends on three key factors:

- their 'assumptive world' – developed from their own life experiences about how the world functions. These assumptions are continuously revised as a person is challenged by life events
- the social context in which they experience cancer – gender, social class, culture and race, family, support, health care system
- the way in which they respond to information which is incompatible with their assumptions. For instance, people who have very rigid expectations or views about the future may find it more difficult to adapt to such a life-changing event and may be more vulnerable to prolonged post-traumatic stress symptoms.

People adopt a number of different strategies in order to live with either the real or potential threat of cancer. Taylor believes that people create 'illusions' for themselves which help them to make sense of cancer, enhance self esteem and encourage them to feel in control.[74] Some of these illusions may not be realistic, but provide a framework for understanding what is happening. Two recent studies of patients with advanced disease have revealed that only a minority acknowledge the incurability of their cancer.[75,76] One of the studies found that patients who scored highly in terms of their need to control were more likely to believe their cancer was curable and were more likely to use alternative therapy.[75] These findings suggest that patients reshape information in order to suit their own illusions. Evidence also exists that an individual may adapt their expectations of themselves, their lifestyle, or personal philosophy in order to cope with the disruption brought to life by cancer.[77]

A phenomenological study of patients with chronic illnesses including cancer, found that patients used some or all of the following strategies in order to deal with the challenges they faced in maintaining and promoting their own health:[78]

- creating a sense of purpose (for example, making the day worth something)
- consciously attending to own attitude (for example, thinking positively, doing things for oneself)
- drawing on personal and family 'patterning' (ways of coping)
- setting and striving for goals
- talking (to oneself and others)
- allowing oneself to learn about and learn from experiences
- taking one step at a time
- maintaining control
- using friends to help out
- comparing oneself favourably with others
- creating alternative ways of being (for example, moving the bed downstairs to increase independence)
- reframing expectations of life and self.

Wells' study found that a number of these strategies was used during recovery from radiotherapy treatment.[13] Creating a sense of purpose, and taking one step at a time were combined with a tendency to monitor and mark recovery. Going to the post office, doing some gardening, visiting the dentist again, all signified the return of normality. The kinds of achievement described in the following extracts may seem small, but it is important that nurses acknowledge their significance and encourage the adoption of meaningful coping strategies:[13]

> As for getting back to normal, I've made a start, I've been out this weekend, bought a load of seeds, some compost.

> I shall know I'm back to normal once I've had my teeth done . . . just step by step really, isn't it?

Unfortunately, the biomedical model concentrates on the pathophysiology of disease and impact of illness on specific clinical outcomes such as 5-year survival and recurrence. Symptoms are mainly seen in terms of being indicative of underlying pathology. Although sociological and coping models pay more attention to the meaning of illness for individuals, they focus on the human behavioural response to the disease process, and may neglect the importance of physical aspects of illness.[79,80] A more integrated approach to understanding the impact of cancer is required.

Quality of life

Models of quality of life incorporate both the physical and psychosocial dimensions of illness and have thus contributed a great deal to our understanding of the way in which cancer disrupts all aspects of life. It is now unusual for studies evaluating new treatments *not* to consider their impact on quality of life, even if their main focus is to assess effects on disease-free survival. Numerous definitions of quality of life exist, and many different methods of assessing quality of life are in use. Most focus on key domains such as physical, psychological, functional and social well-being. Many quality-of-life measures include disease-specific modules detailing symptoms and concerns likely to be experienced by particular patient groups. Although these tools cover a broad range of relevant issues that have an impact on patients' quality of life, they do not provide any indication of what matters most to an individual. More recent quality of life measures such as the Patient Generated Index (PGI),[81] and the Schedule for the Evaluation of Individual Quality of Life (SEIQoL),[82] allow patients to create their own definition of quality of life, by asking them to identify the aspects of illness that have most impact on valued aspects of their lives. These tools reflect a concept of quality of life that embraces both the individual context and experience of illness. Kenneth Calman's definition of quality of life in cancer as the difference between the hopes and expectations of an individual and the actual experience of their present situation enables this crucial concept to be understood.[83]

One study found that patients who experienced a discrepancy between their perceptions of their 'ideal' self and their 'actual' self had poorer physical health and lower levels of psychological well-being.[84] If such perceptions can be adjusted, or supportive care can be directed towards bringing actual experiences and aspirations more closely together, it is likely to have a positive impact on the individual's quality of life.

The impact of treatment

Promoting quality of life during cancer treatment can be a real challenge, as the person has to deal not only with the emotional and psychological impact of the diagnosis but also the additional burdens of toxic and lengthy treatment. As already pointed out, the progression from diagnosis to treatment may not always be immediate, and the period of waiting for treatment to start can be extremely difficult. As David Izod recounts, it can be weeks before being seen by an oncologist and a treatment plan initiated, and is like being placed in a 'twilight zone . . . a time of suspicion, rumour and possibility, and feeling utterly powerless'.[85]

Cancer treatment has emotional, social, physical and economic costs,[86] and it is important that all these aspects are considered. Chemotherapy and radiotherapy require repeated visits to hospital, which are disruptive and costly. The side-effects of treatment can make people feel worse rather than better, producing 'an unacceptable transformation from active, attractive independence to physically unattractive dependence'.[39] The 'chronic' nature of cancer and the increasing use of combination therapies can mean that treatment can continue for months or even years.

Although one of the main aims of curative therapy is to minimise late effects such as damage to vital organs, certain treatments will inevitably cause lasting side-effects or bodily changes, which can have a considerable impact on that person's ability to lead the life they might otherwise have done (see Table 6.1). Table 6.1 does not contain a complete list of side-effects, but illustrates those that can continue beyond completion of treatment and that may compromise quality of life.

Many studies of patients undergoing cancer treatment tend to isolate the impact of a particular therapy, which, although important in understanding the particular treatment, does not take into account the impact on the illness experience in its entirety. There is a need for more research that takes account of the impact of a range of treatments, symptoms, and events in the context of a person's life.

Table 6.1 The physical and functional impact of cancer treatments

Treatment	Potential impact
Surgery	Changes in body image due to scarring, loss of a body part, change in body shape
	Changes in mobility following loss of function, compromised range of movement, development of lymphoedema, or removal of body part
	Changes in diet due to absorption problems, shortened digestive tract or stoma formation following gastrointestinal surgery, and difficulties chewing or swallowing following head and neck surgery
	Changes in ability to communicate following head and neck surgery
	Changes in sensation following damage to nerves, including chronic pain
	Changes in elimination following pelvic surgery involving genitourinary or gastrointestinal tract
	Changes in sexual function following pelvic surgery, or body image change
Chemotherapy	Fertility problems or infertility
	Cognitive impairment; memory loss, concentration[a]
	Alopecia[a]
	Generalised aches and pains[a]
	Weight changes[a]
	Weakness and fatigue[a]
	Renal or cardiac dysfunction[a]
	Bone marrow depression[a] (particularly prolonged in patients who undergo high-dose chemotherapy)
	Food aversions and taste changes[a]
Radiotherapy	Dry mouth and/or throat following treatment to the head and neck[87]
	Skin and vascular changes
	Fatigue[a]
	Changes in sexual function after pelvic radiotherapy
	Visual impairment and dry eyes if the eye is included in the radiation field
	Respiratory or cardiac dysfunction following radiotherapy to the chest (depending on dose, field and fractionation)
	Osteoradionecrosis after treatment to the head and neck, particularly if dentition is poor
	Bowel problems such as urgency, strictures or fistulae after pelvic treatment
	Urinary problems such as urgency and frequency after pelvic treatment
	Secondary malignancies

NB: These symptoms and problems do not affect all patients and their occurrence or severity will depend on numerous factors including the characteristics of the cancer, drugs or dose of treatment, area treated etc.
[a]These symptoms are generally not permanent.

Surgery

The physical removal of a cancer through surgery can be reassuring, as it represents a cleansing and symbolic elimination of the evil within.[4] Izod explains that his retroperitoneal node dissection following chemotherapy was 'violent, purgative, cleansing and ... final'.[85] The impact of surgery is dependent on the significance of the site of surgery and individual effects it may have on body image and concept of self. Surgery for cancer often results in some kind of disfigurement or mutilation, and may threaten social and sexual identity. Removal of part of the body such as the breast, uterus, tongue, larynx, or limb induces a profound sense of loss as well as functional change, and the assault on body image and sexuality may also have an enormous impact on intimate relationships and the ability to interact socially.

The following is an excerpt from an interview with a patient and his wife following laryngectomy:

It must be very embarrassing when you first use the artificial voice . . . the noise, people sort of look down to see where it's coming from . . . a couple of our grand-daughter's friends, they both stood there and laughed . . . sometimes when he's eating, he can't help it, he makes [imitates a loud gulping sound] type of noise. If we wanted to start up a conversation, we would just say hello, whereas he can only gape . . . we don't go out much, I think he would be embarrassed if he was sitting in a restaurant and had to drink with a straw.[13]

Perhaps the most difficult aspect of cancer surgery is the sudden change it can produce. As John Diamond said:[70]

. . . the problem with major surgery – any surgery – is that there is no real way of anyone telling you how it will be when you come round . . . nobody can tell you how it feels to be that post-operative person, the person who is lying there waiting for the new chapter to start and with no idea of how that chapter will read [p.158].

Chemotherapy

Popular misconceptions about chemotherapy persist and many people still believe that severe vomiting and hair loss are inevitable. Although a range of debilitating side-effects are commonly experienced, sophisticated and effective drugs for managing these symptoms are now in widespread use. However, most people experience at least some of the following chemotherapy-related symptoms including nausea and vomiting, hair loss, mucositis, bone marrow depression, skin changes, diarrhoea, sterility, and damage to any of the major body systems. Alopecia appears to be one of the most distressing of these, symbolising cancer itself and stripping a person of their identity. A doctor who was being treated for leukaemia described this distress:[88]

I had four central lines, and I had two bouts of septicaemia, I lost every hair on my body, and it is the part of it that was really hard was the, the fact that you lose your identity. Because when I was at the hospital, and I would go down in the lift and up in the lift, and I would meet some of my colleagues after and had to introduce myself. People I had known for twenty or thirty years [p.1331].

As well as causing overt side-effects, chemotherapy removes the ability to take pleasure in everyday aspects of life. David Izod remembers:[85]

I didn't feel like drinking, smoking, had no sex and ate only to stop myself from vomiting. I didn't laugh much and went to bed at 8 o'clock.

Studies have shown that the daily disruption and cumulative effect of having chemotherapy is significant and that patients and health care professionals underestimate the burden of side-effects, particularly tiredness.[89] Patients in this study were more likely to report distress in diaries than in conversation with nurses and doctors, and nearly half had thought about discontinuing treatment, although few had discussed this with their doctor.

Continual communication throughout treatment is clearly necessary, but there is evidence that nurses and doctors are not good at identifying the concerns of patients undergoing chemotherapy. A cross-sectional study of 33 women receiving treatment for breast, ovarian, cervical or uterine cancer found that nurses were much more likely to identify physical or treatment-related problems than psychosocial concerns, and that they were unable to identify the women's three main concerns in 70% of cases.[90]

As well as causing significant emotional and physical disruption, chemotherapy has been associated with an increase in psychiatric morbidity. One study found that the incidence of anxiety, depression, and sexual difficulty was significantly higher in women who had undergone adjuvant chemotherapy after mastectomy, and that this was directly related to the degree of toxicity experienced.[91] Some people find the concept of toxic drugs entering their body particularly difficult, and some develop phobic reactions to chemotherapy; in particular, anticipatory nausea and vomiting, characterised as a learned or conditioned response to chemotherapy. This syndrome develops when certain events or stimuli are associated with treatment; for example, the journey to the chemotherapy clinic or the smell of alcohol wipes, inducing nausea and vomiting *before* the chemotherapy is actually given. Teaching progressive muscle relaxation and imagery can reduce anxiety and nausea, and can help people to overcome or control fears of the chemotherapy itself or the means by which it is administered.

Radiotherapy

The technical and invisible nature of radiotherapy and the popular understanding that exposure to radiation actually causes cancer inevitably produces fear and misconception in patients who require radiotherapy. Departments of radiotherapy are usually housed in the basement or outbuildings of cancer centres, and for some patients this emphasises concerns about danger and isolation.

Neither the experience of radiotherapy nor the development of supportive care strategies has received much attention in the literature.[92] Studies have generally focused on symptoms, by measuring distress experienced at specific time points during and after radiotherapy. Diaries have also been used successfully by patients undergoing treatment, often revealing intimate detail about the individuality of the experience, which helps to create a picture of the impact of cancer and its treatment on everyday life.[89,93–95]

Attempts have been made to assess the emotional impact of radiotherapy using quantitative measures, but there have been few qualitative studies exploring patients' own expressions of the experience of treatment. Although many patients describe radiotherapy as 'a doddle' compared with chemotherapy, the cumulative physical and emotional distress experienced with radiotherapy can be considerable. The daily disruption of attending for treatment for up to 6 weeks is compounded by an often insidious build-up of symptoms, which cause a gradual deterioration, not always noticed by health professionals, or even by those undergoing treatment themselves. Radiotherapy symptoms tend to develop towards the end of treatment, or may develop after treatment is finished. As a result, there may be insufficient access to expert help, leaving many to try and cope on their own with extremely debilitating side-effects. The following is an excerpt from an interview with a 42-year-old man with parotid cancer.[13]

It happens so gradually that it sort of infiltrates slowly and you don't realise how ill you are actually feeling . . . you don't realise it's waiting for you to say . . . it's not bad enough to tell anyone about, and when it's bad enough to tell anyone about, the pills you're given aren't good enough to do anything about it . . . you think they should be working and if they're not working you must be doing something wrong because the doctor knows what he's doing and he's given you these pills, they're not having any effect but they must be helping the pain because he's given them to you.

Most specialist nursing roles and thus research and practice development have, up until recently, been concentrated in the area of chemotherapy rather than radiotherapy, perhaps because its side-effects tend to be more obvious and immediate. Those undergoing radiotherapy have been perceived as 'self-caring' or 'walking wounded', and have not been seen to require the same level of expert nursing attention as those undergoing toxic drug therapy. This is a misconception, and has led to the neglect of the development of nursing interventions in this area.[96]

Recovery from treatment

Patients consistently report that the period after treatment is over can be particularly difficult. Although finishing treatment is often a huge relief and many patients will face the prospect of a full 'recovery', returning to normal is far from easy. As one patient said:[13]

It's really hard when you have to start functioning normally again. You just aren't the same person as you used to be. You'd like to get well as soon as possible and start working again, but you just can't cope you know [p.150].

Far too little attention is paid to the immediate period following the end of treatment, when side-effects may continue to be experienced, but also where there is loss of contact with the specialist treatment centre, which for many may have been a lifeline. Alby concludes that 'discharge is feared just as much as it is wanted', and describes the fear and uncertainty associated with this transition as due to a combination of factors:[97]

• the fear of leaving a protected environment with skilled, supportive staff

- the fear of facing life with a different body (for example, as a result of weight loss, scars, loss or alteration of a body part, alopecia)
- the constraints of treatment and diet (for example, immunosuppressive therapy following allogeneic bone marrow transplantation, steroid therapy, changes in diet following oesophagectomy, gastrectomy, or head and neck surgery).[97]

Frank and Izod both describe the importance of 'ceremonies' and 'boundaries', which provide some structure to life *after* cancer.[3,85] Frank describes how difficult it was for him to 're-enter' his world after the end of his treatment for testicular cancer.[3] He believes that rituals are necessary to mark the end of treatment because they enable the process of re-entry to occur more easily. Even after 'cure' he described that his 'consciousness remained suspended between the insulated world of illness and the healthy mainstream'. When cancer treatment ends, it is some considerable time before a person can know with any certainty whether treatment has been successful or that they have been 'cured'. This is somewhat similar to the experience of having a chronic illness that is in remission. It may mean that people have no 'socially sanctioned position on the health–illness continuum; they are neither sick nor well'.[98]

> The period after treatment can be terribly hard for the cancer patient. For the previous six months, cancer, the treatment, and particularly the staff at the hospital had been the dominant factor in my life. And then all of a sudden nothing. I had been sucked in by the system as an ill person, treated by it and now it was spitting me out as a healthy person, but I was left with a very big hole. Although I hadn't been discharged, indeed I won't be for another 5 years, the intimacy had gone, there were other people more important than me, people whose treatment had just begun. And I didn't know what the hell to do with myself.[85]

Considerable difficulty may be experienced at the end of successful treatment, since an individual's 'share of attention has been used up',[27] and they may feel that their problems are no longer legitimate. This may lead to self-doubt, a crisis of credibility, and the feeling that problems are not worthy of mentioning; a reluctance that may be reinforced by health professionals who make light of them.[79] In an interview study of women with breast cancer, at or around the time of recurrence, Robinson revealed that women felt supported up until the end of primary treatment, but they then experienced a lack of continuity of care and lack of interest in their case during outpatient consultations.[99] They no longer felt treated as individual people, and expressed an unfulfilled desire to talk about the future.

A review of psychological functioning in patients undergoing radiotherapy found that the completion of treatment can be a difficult time.[100] Many patients experience emotional distress, unexpected side-effects and a lack of information and support after treatment ends. Wells found that despite the level of distress at this time, there was also a reluctance to ask for help – as one woman said:

> You don't like to ring because there are other people still having treatment . . . you've finished your treatment, you ought to be fine.[101]

One problem for people completing radical treatment is that 'routine follow-up' practice does not always permit them to talk about their experiences, except in relation to the physical effects of therapy. The space and opportunity to explore meaning and the experience of cancer treatment appears to be reserved for those who are dying of their disease, rather than those who are in the recovery phase of illness. Nurse-led care may provide a more holistic approach to follow-up, and studies have shown that such models are safe and acceptable to patients.[102,103]

Many patients describe very mixed feelings about follow-up appointments. On the one hand, they want to be told that they are well and that there is no sign of disease, but on the other hand, they do not want to be reminded about their cancer by having to attend the clinic. This type of ambiguity and uncertainty often remains a persistent feature of living with cancer. A phenomenological study carried out in Iceland explored the 'lived experience' of nine men and women in remission from their cancer.[35] An overriding theme of this experience was 'experiencing existential changes' encompassed by the five themes of uncertainty, vulnerability, isolation, discomfort, and redefinition.

Uncertainty was experienced at all stages of the disease, about either the cancer itself, the efficacy of treatment, the threat of recurrence, or uncertainty about the likelihood of imminent death. Other studies have also revealed the pervasive nature of uncertainty. The following is an extract from an interview with a 41-year-old man receiving phase I trial chemotherapy for metastatic cancer of the parotid gland following disease progression after radical radiotherapy:

> The uncertainty's the most difficult bit to deal with because there's uncertainty about whether or not the treatment you're having is doing any good, there's uncertainty about basically how long you've got . . . there'll always be uncertainty about how long I've got, I suspect, until I start getting symptoms that are very clearly demonstrating things . . . I don't know whether . . . I'm going to be able to work next week . . . I never know how I'm going to feel . . . I'm getting myself a second hand car to do up as a project but to be perfectly honest I don't know whether I'm going to be able to do it. . . .[13]

In Halldorsdottir and Hamrin's study, vulnerability was another feature of having lived with cancer.[35] The impact of communications with health professionals at this vulnerable time was identified, in particular, the necessity for the latter to offer respect, warmth and understanding. Isolation and loneliness had been experienced by most at some point during their cancer, either because they perceived or actually experienced rejection by others, or because they had shut themselves off or withdrawn from normal life. As one explained, 'we cancer patients shut ourselves inside, draw the curtains, avoid people and feel poisonous'.[35]

All identified changes in themselves following the experience of cancer. Often these involved physical discomfort or an alteration in their perception of the world around them or of emotional relationships. Many felt they had become stronger or closer to those closest to them. Some did not feel so positive, regretting the incapacity imposed by the disease, or lamenting their changed role or position in society. The authors of the study recognise the limitations of generalising from a small interview study beyond the cultural and social group of Icelanders represented in their research. However, it does demonstrate the need for security, certainty, care, and respect, as well as support to maintain a feeling of control over their situation and finding ways of redefining themselves or their lives.

Recurrence

The threat of recurrence is ever present, and the uncertainty it causes is central to the experience of cancer.[104] Lee-Jones *et al.* argue that fear of recurrence is a neglected area, and offer a model for understanding the way in which patients construct such fear.[105] This model proposes that internal stimuli (e.g. symptoms) and external stimuli such as hospital appointments, family concerns, and media can work together to fuel personal worries and perceptions of risk. These personal cognitions, beliefs and emotions are also influenced by past experiences of cancer and its treatment, and are likely to lead to behavioural responses such as body checking, seeking advice, limited planning for the future, and a range of psychological symptoms. The dread that the disease may return is continuous, and if it does, anxiety and distress can be greater than at initial diagnosis, because the threat of death is 'more real'.[106,107] Many people have difficulty regaining their belief in the future,[108] and if recurrence is diagnosed, this belief is explicitly challenged. Not only is the diagnosis devastating, but it also brings disillusionment that attempts at prevention or detection have failed.[99]

The identification of recurrent disease causes the future to be viewed in terms of uncertainty, death and dying, and loss. The psychological impact of recurrence is often compounded by a reduction in activity and stamina due to pain, weakness, or debilitating symptoms.

The discovery of recurrent disease often evokes memories of the initial diagnosis and produces feelings of anger, injustice, fear, emotional volatility, and the need to regain control.[109] It is important not to make assumptions that levels of understanding, treatment preferences, or support networks remain the same as before. Careful assessment is needed of an individual's current condition, emotional or physical concerns, and support available.

Rehabilitation and survivorship

There is increasing recognition of the importance of rehabilitation in helping people to live as normal a life as possible after a diagnosis of cancer. Surviving cancer may be a mixed experience; while cancer survivors often say that they lead more fulfilling, meaningful lives through experiencing life-threatening illness,[110] they may also find it difficult to come to terms with the feeling that they do not deserve to be alive, or that they are not coping in the way they feel they should. This 'survivor guilt' may reflect a sense of unfulfilled desires and expectations, as described by a man who had apparently been cured of bowel cancer:[88]

> Well I feel like it is, I feel like it is a weakness or you know, a thing that I should be able to control, be, be in charge of, my moods and be able to rise above them, you know, and just go ahead and do what I have to do, you know [p.1335].

In a British study, survivors of lymphoma described survival as a process through which stages of adjustment took place and changes had to be accepted.[111] Although many felt that the experience of cancer had produced positive outcomes, several had found it very difficult to forget and move on from the experience, and had flashbacks in which aspects of their life as a cancer patient were continually recalled. The authors concluded that although survival may be adequate reward for some, others may seek to improve, change, or adjust their lives, struggling with the effects of cancer long after cessation of treatment.

A survey of 687 cancer survivors who were members of the National Coalition for Cancer Survivorship in the US collected demographic and quality-of-life data.[112] Although they were clearly a self-selected group – over three-quarters of the sample were women, and nearly half had breast cancer – the survey still provides an insight into the factors influencing quality of life in survivors. Psychological well-being was found to be lower than functional, social, or physical well-being, and this appeared to be affected by recall of initial diagnosis and treatment as well as fear of recurrence. Family distress and sexuality were reported as having the most negative influences on quality of life. Physical well-being was most severely affected by fatigue and aches and pains.

Given that survivors appear to have more difficulty living with the psychological, social, and sexual consequences of cancer, it is unfortunate that the primary focus of cancer rehabilitation in the UK tends to be on regaining physical function or adapting to physical changes. Although vitally important, this is not the only aspect of rehabilitation that deserves attention. Many people need practical and emotional support in order to regain a sense of self-worth and purpose, and in order to resume social relationships and work. Employment and insurance difficulties have mainly been studied in the US, and there is evidence that people with cancer experience difficulties obtaining work and promotion.[113–115] However, a recent study of colorectal survivors found that most people in their sample did in fact return to work, illustrating a more hopeful picture.[116]

Whether working or not, the financial burden of cancer and its treatment can be considerable. An interview study of people with lung cancer revealed that many patients lacked knowledge of the financial benefits they were entitled to, or experienced a struggle in obtaining advice and help.[117] Difficulties obtaining affordable holiday insurance can cause significant worry and concern to people who have had a diagnosis of cancer. Resources produced by Cancerbackup on work, travel, and financial benefits are an invaluable source of practical and useful information as are those from Macmillan Cancer Support (www.cancerbackup.org.uk, www.Macmillan.org.uk).

Although considerable controversy exists as to the extent to which psychological factors can influence survival, research studies of patients who have survived far beyond medical expectations provide compelling insights into the characteristics of 'remarkable survivors'.[118] A qualitative study found that nearly all of the 10 patients interviewed described three major qualities:

- *authenticity* – a clear understanding of what was important in their lives
- *autonomy* – perceived freedom to shape their life around valued activities and people
- *acceptance* – perceived change in self-esteem, tolerance for others, closeness to others, and a more peaceful and joyous outlook.

The authors of this study advocate a programme of psychological therapy aimed at enabling people to develop and fulfil these fundamentally important aspects of survival.[118]

Dying

Inevitably, many patients will die of their cancer. When chronic illness becomes terminal illness, yet another adaptation is faced. Glaser and Strauss conceptualise the experience of dying using four 'dying trajectories':[119]

1. certain death at a known time
2. certain death at an unknown time
3. uncertain death but a known time when the question will be resolved
4. uncertain death and an unknown time when the question will be resolved.

Many people want to know exactly when they are going to die, and ask direct questions such as 'How long have I got?'. If death is inevitable, having some idea of when and how to expect it may feel preferable in such a distressing and uncertain situation. However, it is unlikely to be possible to identify the trajectory of certain death at a known time until the last few days or perhaps weeks of life and, rightly, few doctors are prepared or able to make such precise predictions. If they do, it can produce a feeling of marking time and waiting for disaster to strike, which may limit the ability to enjoy the life that is left, as the following excerpt from an interview with a 42-year-old man with metastatic parotid cancer illustrates:

> I was told that I've got between 4 and 12 months, so you think, right, when was I told? So 6 months from then is then, therefore I've got to make sure this month I'm going to feel all right, this month I'm going to be in bed all the time, this month I've had it.[13]

Other personal experiences of death may give rise to expectations or preconceptions. This may make it difficult to face the prospect of one's own death. As one man who had been in the RAF explained: 'I've always been rather accustomed to sudden death . . . quite, quick bang, just like that . . . sudden not drawn out, I can't stand that . . . I don't like this at all',[13] Thus he knew that he would die of his disease, but admitted that he was 'scared stiff ', waiting for it to happen.

The fears of the dying have been described, and the importance of eliciting individual experiences of death so that such fears can be understood has been highlighted.[120] Most are understandably afraid of the unknown, of being separated from the people that they love, and of suddenly ceasing to exist. Fears of dying in pain, or alone, losing control of bodily functions or mind, dying suddenly or violently, or being rejected by friends and family are all common. If these fears can be discussed, and preferences about death are taken into account, including where the person wants to die, this can at least give back some control and enable care to be focused on preventing these fears from becoming a reality. Unfortunately, a plethora of studies illustrate that health care professionals do not do this successfully. Rogers and coworkers surveyed bereaved relatives who had experienced a cancer death, and they reported that their loved ones' negative experiences of hospital care had arisen as a result of feeling devalued as individuals, not being treated with dignity, and being disempowered.[121]

The concept of a 'good death' has received increasing attention in recent years, and the development of hospice and palliative care services has transformed the care of dying patients. However, as Ellershaw and Ward point out, too many patients die an undignified death with uncontrolled symptoms.[122] One of the key problems is in diagnosing dying. There are many opportunities for ambiguity and it is vital that the key signs and symptoms of dying are recognised and explicitly communicated to patients and relatives who wish to know. The Liverpool care pathway for the dying patient has been adopted by many hospitals and palliative care units, and provides a valuable framework for the care of people who are dying (see Box 6.4).[123]

Box 6.4 The Liverpool care pathway for the dying patient – goals of care

- *Comfort measures* – assessment of current medication and discontinuation of non-essentials, as-required subcutaneous drugs prescribed, inappropriate interventions discontinued and avoided (including writing up do not resuscitate orders).
- *Psychological and insight issues* – assessment of ability to communicate in English and translator organised if necessary, assessment of insight into condition.
- *Religious and spiritual support* – needs assessed with patient and family.
- *Communication with family or others* – identification of how family and others are to be informed of patient's impending death, communication of relevant hospital information.
- *Communication with primary health care team* – communication with general practitioner about patient's condition.
- *Summary* – plan of care explained and discussed with patient and family and understanding of plan of care shown by patient and family.

Adapted from Ellershaw and Wilkinson (2003).[123]

Providing sensitive care that addresses all the above issues is clearly very much dependent on a full assessment of the individual's needs and also on the flexibility and creativity of the caring team. If a person does have to die in hospital, nurses can do a great deal to integrate rather than separate the experience into the life of that person. Too often we stick to the rules and try to constrain the experience, or imagine that we can protect families from some of the realities of death. Sometimes families prefer not to be involved, but it can make a huge difference to both the dying person and their family if they are permitted to be part of the experience.

Conclusion

This chapter began with an acknowledgement of the overwhelming disruption that a diagnosis of cancer causes, and a recognition that every person with cancer is different and will have a different experience. Adequate recognition of these differences is essential to understanding the impact cancer has on that individual. Examples have shown that the personal meaning of cancer and the context in which cancer is experienced may strongly influence a person's adjustment and adaptation to their diagnosis. Life can be profoundly disrupted at any stage of the cancer trajectory, disturbing physical, emotional, financial, social, and spiritual equilibrium. Fear and uncertainty can suspend any sense of future, and 'normal' life takes on a different interpretation. Living with cancer, however, is not always an overwhelmingly negative experience; for many, it precipitates a re-evaluation of priorities and relationships that may greatly improve life.

Many opportunities exist for nurses to contribute towards improving the experience of cancer. At every stage of the cancer trajectory, nurses can provide support and care that will enhance quality of life in its widest possible sense. This chapter has illustrated potential times of vulnerability during the trajectory, and demonstrated some of the many problems faced when living with a cancer diagnosis.

Nurses are in a unique position to anticipate and respond to these problems, and to develop care strategies that will help to reduce the impact of cancer in whatever sense it is felt. Assessing and understanding differences between individuals – their responses, support systems and interpretations of their illness – must be the starting place.

References

1. Clark R.N., Jeffries N., Hasler J. and Pendleton D. (2002). *A Long Walk Home.* Oxford: Radcliffe Publishing Limited.
2. Keswick Jencks M. (2003). *A View from the Frontline.* London, Expedite Graphic Ltd.
3. Frank A.W. (1991). *At the Will of the Body. Reflections on Illness.* Boston, MA: Houghton Mifflin.
4. Guex P. (1989). *An Introduction to Psycho-oncology.* London: Routledge.
5. Barraclough J. (1995). *Cancer and Emotion: A Practical Guide to Psycho-oncology,* 2nd edition. Chichester: John Wiley.
6. Patterson J.T. (1987). *The Dread Disease. Cancer and Modern American Culture.* Cambridge, MA: Harvard University Press.
7. Dorsett D.S. (1991). The trajectory of cancer recovery. *Scholarly Inquiry for Nursing Practice: An International Journal* **5**, 177–184.

8. Sontag S. (1991). *Illness as Metaphor.* London: Penguin Books.

9. Benner P. and Wrubel J. (1989). *The Primacy of Caring: Stress and Coping in Health and Illness.* Menlo Park, CA: Addison–Wesley.

10. Tritter J. (2002). Cancer as a chronic illness? Reconsidering categorization and exploring experience. *European Journal of Cancer Care* **11**, 161–165.

11. Little M. (2004). Chronic illness and the experience of surviving cancer. *Internal Medicine Journal* **34**, 201–202.

12. Saegrov S. and Halding A. (2004). What is it like living with the diagnosis of cancer? *European Journal of Cancer Care* **13**, 145–153.

13. Wells E.M. (1995). *The Impact of Radiotherapy to the Head and Neck: Patients' Experiences During and After Completion of Treatment.* University of London: Institute of Cancer Research, unpublished MSc thesis.

14. Kirk P., Kirk I. and Kristiansen L.J. (2004). What do patients receiving palliative care for cancer and their families want to be told? A Canadian and Australian qualitative study. *British Medical Journal* **328**, 1343–1349.

15. Buckman R. (2005). Breaking bad news: the S-P-I-K-E-S strategy. *Community Oncology* **2**, 138–142.

16. Ziebland S., Chapple A., Dumelow C. *et al.* (2004). How the internet affects patients' experience of cancer: a qualitative study. *British Medical Journal* **328**, 564–569.

17. Jones R., Pearson J., McGregor S. *et al.* (1999). Randomised trial of personalised computer based information for cancer patients. *British Medical Journal* **319**, 1241–1247.

18. Jenkins V, Fallowfield L. and Saul J. (2001). Information needs of patients with cancer: results from a large study in UK cancer centres. *British Journal of Cancer* **84**, 48–51.

19. McNamara S. (1999). Information and support: a descriptive study of the needs of patients with cancer before their first experience of radiotherapy. *European Journal of Oncology Nursing* **3**, 31–37.

20. Macleod U., Ross S., Fallowfield L. and Watt G.C.M. (2004). Anxiety and support in breast cancer: is this different for affluent and deprived women? A questionnaire study. *British Journal of Cancer* **91**, 879–883.

21. Leydon G., Boulton M., Moynihan C. *et al.* (2000). Cancer patients' information needs and information seeking behaviour: in depth study. *British Medical Journal* **320**, 909–915.

22. Taylor E.J. (1995). Whys and wherefores: adult patient perceptions of the meaning of cancer. *Seminars in Oncology Nursing* **11**, 32–40.

23. Loeshcher L.J., Clark L., Atwood J.R., Leigh S. and Lamb G. (1990). The impact of the cancer experience on long term survivors. *Oncology Nursing Forum* **17**, 223–229.

24. Cassel E.J. (1982). The nature of suffering and the goals of medicine. *New England Journal of Medicine* **306**, 639–645.

25. Kleinman A. (1980). *Patients and Healers in the Context of Culture: An Exploration of the Borderland between Anthropology, Medicine and Psychiatry.* Berkeley, CA: University of California Press.

26. Good B.J. and DelVecchio Good M. (1980). The meaning of symptoms: a cultural hermeneutic model for clinical practice. In Eisenberg L. and Kleinman A. (eds.) *The Relevance of Social Science for Medicine.* Dordrecht: Reidel, pp. 165–196.

27. Bury M. (1991). The sociology of chronic illness: a review of research and prospects. *Sociology of Health and Illness* **13**, 451–468.

28. Wenger A.F.Z. (1993). Cultural meaning of symptoms. *Holistic Nursing Practice* **7**, 22–35.

29. Saillant F. (1990). Discourse, knowledge and experience of cancer: a life story. *Culture, Medicine and Psychiatry* **14**, 81–104.

30. Williams G.H. (1984). The genesis of chronic illness: narrative reconstruction. *Sociology of Health and Illness* **6**, 174–200.

31. Mathieson C.M. and Stam H.J. (1995). Renegotiating identity: cancer narratives. *Sociology of Health and Illness* **17**, 283–306.

32. Carlick A. and Biley F. (2004). Thoughts on the therapeutic use of narrative in the promotion of coping in cancer care. *European Journal of Cancer Care* **13**, 308–317.

33. Chelf J., Deshler A., Hillman S. and Durazo-Arvizu R. (2000). Storytelling: a strategy for living and coping with cancer. *Cancer Nursing* **23**, 1–5.

34. Atwood M. (1997). *Alias Grace.* London: Virago Press.

35. Halldorsdottir S. and Hamrin E. (1996). Experiencing existential changes: the lived experience of having cancer. *Cancer Nursing* **19**, 29–36.

36. Corner J., Hopkinson J., Fitzsimmons D. *et al.* (2005). Is late diagnosis of lung cancer inevitable? Interview study of patients' recollections of symptoms before diagnosis. *Thorax* **60**, 314–319.

37. Monfardini S. and Yancik R. (1993). Cancer in the elderly: meeting the challenge of an ageing population. *Journal of the National Cancer Institute* **85**, 532–538.

38. Edlund B. and Sneed N.V. (1989). Emotional responses to the diagnosis of cancer: age related comparisons. *Oncology Nursing Forum* **16**, 691–697.

39. Naysmith A., Hinton J.M., Meredith R., Marks M.D. and Berry R.J. (1983). Surviving malignant disease: psychological and family aspects. *British Journal of Hospital Medicine* **30**, 22–27.

40. Priestman T. (1986). In Stoll A.B. (ed.) *Coping with Cancer Stress*. Dordrecht: Matginus Nijhoff, pp. 21–27.

41. Finerman R. and Bennett L.A. (1995). Guilt, blame and shame: responsibility in health and sickness. *Social Science and Medicine* **40**, 1–3.

42. Rowe D. (1987). *Beyond Fear*. London: Faber.

43. Kubler-Ross E (1970). *On Death and Dying*. London: Tavistock.

44. Weisman A. and Worden J.W. (1976–1977). The existential plight in cancer: significance of the first 100 days. *International Journal of Psychiatry in Medicine* **7**, 1–15.

45. Greer S., Morris T. and Pettingale K.W. (1979). Psychological response to breast cancer: effect on outcome. *Lancet* **ii**, 785–787.

46. Pettingale K.W., Morris T. and Greer S. (1985). Mental attitudes to cancer: an additional prognostic factor. *Lancet* **i**, 750.

47. Greer S., Morris T., Pettingale K.W. and Haybittle J.L. (1990). Psychological response to breast cancer and 15 year outcome. *Lancet* **335**, 49–50.

48. Watson M., Haviland J., Greer S., Davidson J. and Bliss J.M. (1999). Influence of psychological response on survival in breast cancer: a population based cohort study. *Lancet* **354**, 1331–1336.

49. Petticrew M., Bell R. and Hunter D. (2002). Influence of psychological coping on survival and recurrence in people with cancer: systematic review. *British Medical Journal* **325**, 1066.

50. Greer S. (2002). Psychological intervention. The gap between research and practice. *Acta Oncologica* **41**, 238–243.

51. Brennan J. (2001). Adjustment to cancer – coping or personal transition? *Psycho-oncology* **10**, 1–18.

52. Moorey S. and Greer S. (1989). *Psychological Therapy for Patients with Cancer*. Oxford: Heinemann Medical Books.

53. Bandura A. (1977). Self efficacy. Toward a unifying theory of behavioural change. *Psychological Review* **84**, 191–215.

54. Schulz U. and Mohamed N. (2004). 'Turning the tide: benefit finding after cancer surgery. *Social Science and Medicine* **59**, 653–662.

55. Bandura A. (1994). Self-efficacy. In Ramachaudran V.S. (ed.) *Encyclopedia of Human Behavior*. New York: Academic Press. **4**, 71–81.

56. Rabin C., Leventhal H. and Goodin S. (2004). Conceptualization of disease timeline predicts posttreatment distress in breast cancer patients. *Health Psychology* **23**, 407–412.

57. Bailey C. (1995). Management of breathlessness. *European Journal of Cancer Care* **4**, 184–190.

58. Futterman A.D. and Wellisch D.K. (1990). Psychodynamic themes of bone marrow transplantation: when I becomes thou. *Haematology Clinics of North America* **4**, 699–709.

59. Freir V. (2004). Childhood trauma. *Cancer Nursing Practice* **3**, 17–19.

60. Baider L., Peretz T. and Kaplan De-Nour A. (1992). Effect of the holocaust on coping with cancer. *Social Science and Medicine* **34**, 11–15.

61. Sollner W., DeVries A., Steixner E. *et al.* (2001). How successful are oncologists in identifying patient distress, perceived social support, and need for psychosocial counselling? *British Journal of Cancer* **84**, 179–185.

62. Van Halteren H., Bongaerts G. and Wagener D.J. Th. (2004). Cancer and psychosocial distress: frequent companions. *Lancet* **364**, 824–825.

63. Zigmond A. and Snaith R. (1983). The Hospital Anxiety and Depression Scale. *Acta Psychiatrica Scandinavica* **67**, 361–370.

64. Watson M., Greer S., Young J. *et al.* (1988). Development of a questionnaire measure of adjustment to cancer: the MAC scale. *Psychological Medicine* **18**, 203–209.

65. Slevin M., Nichols S.E., Downer S.M. *et al.* (1996). Emotional support for cancer patients: what do patients really want? *British Journal of Cancer* **74**, 1275–1279.

66. Newell S.A., Sanson-Fisher R.W. and Savolainen N.J. (2002). Systematic review of psychological therapies for cancer patients: overview and recommendations for future research. *Journal of the National Cancer Institute* **94**, 558–584.

67. Uitterhoeve R., Vernooy M., Litjens M. *et al.* (2004). Psychosocial interventions for patients with advanced cancer – a systematic review of the literature. *British Journal of Cancer* **91**, 1050–1062.

68. Bredart A., Cayrou S. and Dolbeault S. (2002). Re: Systematic review of psychological therapies for cancer patients: overview and recommendations for future research. *Journal of the National Cancer Instititue* **94**, 1810–1811.

69. Medical Research Council (2000). *A Framework for Development and Evaluation of RCTs for Complex Interventions to Improve Health*. London: Medical Research Council.

70. Diamond J. (1998). *Because Cowards Get Cancer Too*. London: Vermilion.

71. Frankenberg A. (1993). *Time, Health and Medicine*. London: Sage.

72. Payne S., Jarrett N. and Jeffs D. (2000). The impact of travel on cancer patients' experiences of treatment: a literature review. *European Journal of Cancer Care* **9**, 197–203.

73. Carver C. and Antoni M. (2004). Finding benefit in breast cancer during the year after diagnosis predicts better adjustment 5 to 8 years after diagnosis. *Health Psychology* **23**, 595–598.

74. Taylor S.E. (1983). Adjustment to threatening events. A theory of cognitive adaptation. *American Psychologist* **November**, 1161–1173.

75. Beadle G., Yates P., Najman J.M. *et al.* (2004). Beliefs and practices of patients with advanced cancer: implications for communication. *British Journal of Cancer* **91**, 254–257.

76. Koller M., Lorenz W., Wagner K. *et al.* (2000). Expectations and quality of life of cancer patients undergoing radiotherapy. *Journal of The Royal Society of Medicine* **93**, 621–628.

77. Heidrich S.M. and Ward S.E. (1992). The role of the self in adjustment to cancer in elderly women. *Oncology Nursing Forum* **19**, 1491–1496.

78. McWilliam C.L., Stewart M., Brown J.B., Desai K. and Coderre P. (1996). Creating health with chronic illness. *Advances in Nursing Science* **18**, 1–15.

79. Waxler N.E. (1980). The social labelling perspective on illness and medical practice. In Eisenberg L. and Kleinman A. (eds.) *The Relevance of Social Science for Medicine.* Dordrecht: Reidel, pp. 283–306.

80. Morse J.M. and Johnson J.L. (eds.) (1991). *The Illness Experience: Dimensions of Suffering.* London: Sage.

81. Ruta D., Garratt A., Leng M. *et al.* (1994). A new approach to the measurement of quality of life. The Patient-Generated Index. *Medical Care* **32**, 1109–1126.

82. Waldron D., O'Boyle C., Kearney M., Moriarty M. and Carney D. (1999). Quality of life measurement in advanced cancer: assessing the individual. *Journal of Clinical Oncology* **17**, 3603–3611.

83. Calman K.C. (1984). Quality of life in cancer patients – an hypothesis. *Journal of Medical Ethics* **10**, 124–127.

84. Heidrich S.M., Forsthoff C.A. and Ward S.E. (1994). Psychological adjustment in adults with cancer: the self as mediator. *Health Psychology* **13**, 346–353.

85. Izod D. (1996). The patient's perspective. Plenary paper given at the *9th International Conference on Cancer Nursing,* 12–18 August, 1996, Brighton, UK.

86. Pearce S., Kelly D. and Stevens W. (2001). More than just money – widening the understanding of the costs involved in cancer care. *Journal of Advanced Nursing* **33**, 371–379.

87. Khoo V. (2003). Other late effects. In Faithfull S. and Wells M. (eds.) *Supportive Care in Radiotherapy.* Edinburgh: Churchill Livingstone, pp. 348–371.

88. Little M. and Sayers E. (2004). While there's life. Hope and the experience of cancer. *Social Science and Medicine* **59**, 1329–1337.

89. Love R., Leventhal H., Easterling D.V. and Nerenz D.R. (1989). Side-effects and emotional distress during cancer chemotherapy. *Cancer* **63**, 604–612.

90. Farrell C., Heaven C., Beaver K. and Maguire P. (2005). Identifying the concerns of women undergoing chemotherapy. *Patient Education and Counseling* **56**, 72–77.

91. Maguire P., Tait A., Brooke M., *et al.* (1980). Psychiatric morbidity and physical toxicity associated with adjuvant chemotherapy after mastectomy. *British Medical Journal* **281**, 1179–1180.

92. Wells M. and Faithfull S. (2003). The future of supportive care in radiotherapy. In Faithfull S. and Wells M. (eds.) *Supportive Care in Radiotherapy.* Edinburgh: Churchill Livingstone, pp. 372–382.

93. Faithfull S. (1992). The diary method for nursing research: a study of somnolence syndrome. *European Journal of Cancer Care* **1**, 13–18.

94. Wells M. (1998). The hidden experience of radiotherapy to the head and neck: a qualitative study of patients after completion of treatment. *Journal of Advanced Nursing* **28**, 840–848.

95. Sharp L., Laurell G., Tiblom Y., Anderson A. and Birkjsö R.M. (2004). Care diaries: a way of increasing head and neck cancer patients' involvement in their own care and the communication between clinicians. *Cancer Nursing* **27**, 119–126.

96. Wells M. (1998). What's so special about radiotherapy nursing? *European Journal of Oncology Nursing* **2**, 162–168.

97. Albi N. (1991). Leukaemia bone marrow transplantation. In Watson M. (ed.) *Cancer Patient Care: Psychosocial Treatment Methods.* Cambridge: British Psychological Society/Cambridge University Press.

98. Kagawa-Singer M. (1993). Redefining health: living with cancer. *Social Science and Medicine* **37**, 295–304.

99. Robinson L. (1994). *Cancer Recurrence: a Phenomenological Study.* London: King's College, London, unpublished MSc thesis.

100. Steigelis H., Ranchor A. and Sanderman R. (2004). Psychological functioning in cancer patients treated with radiotherapy. *Patient Education and Counseling* **52**, 131–141.

101. Wells E.M. (1994). *The First Few Weeks at Home: Patients' Experiences of Finishing Radiotherapy to the Breast.* London: University of London, Institute of Cancer Research, unpublished care study.

102. Moore S., Corner J., Haviland J. *et al.* (2002). Nurse-led follow-up and conventional medical follow-up in management of patients with lung cancer: randomised trial. *British Medical Journal* **325**, 1145–1147.

103. Corner J. (2003). The role of nurse led care in cancer management. *The Lancet Oncology* **4**, 631–636.

104. Nelson J.P. (1996). Struggling to gain meaning: living with the uncertainty of breast cancer. *Advances in Nursing Science* **18**, 59–76.

105. Lee-Jones C., Humphris G., Dixon R. and Hatcher M.B. (1997). Fear of cancer recurrence – a literature review and proposed cognitive formulation to explain exacerbation of recurrence fears. *Psycho-oncology* **6**, 95–107.

106. Mahon S., Cella D. and Donovan M. (1990). Psychosocial adjustment to recurrent cancer. *Oncology Nursing Forum* **17**, 47–52.

107. Hall A., Fallowfield L. and A'Hern R. (1996). When breast cancer recurs: a 3-year study of psychological morbidity. *Breast Journal* **2**, 197–203.

108. Breaden K. (1997). Cancer and beyond: the question of survivorship. *Journal of Advanced Nursing* **26**, 978–984.

109. Mahon S. (1991). Managing the psychosocial consequences of cancer recurrence: implications for nurses. *Oncology Nursing Forum* **18**, 577–583.

110. O'Connor A.P. and Wicker C.A. (1995). Clinical commentary: promoting meaning in the lives of cancer survivors. *Seminars in Oncology Nursing* **11**, 68–72.

111. Wallwork L. and Richardson A. (1994). Beyond cancer: changes, problems and needs expressed by adult lymphoma survivors attending an out-patients clinic. *European Journal of Cancer Care* **3**, 122–132.

112. Ferrell B.R., Dow K.H., Leigh S., Ly J. and Gulasekaram P. (1995). Quality of life in long-term cancer survivors *Oncology Nursing Forum* **22**, 915–922.

113. Hoffman B. (1989). Cancer survivors at work: job problems and illegal discrimination. *Oncology Nursing Forum* **16**, 39–43.

114. Mundy R., Moore S. *et al.* (2001). A missing link: rehabilitation counseling for persons with cancer. *Journal of Rehabilitation* **April/May/June**, 47–49.

115. Spelten E.R., Sprangers M.A.G. and Verbeek J.H.A.M. (2002). Factors reported to influence the return to work of cancer survivors: a literature review. *Psychooncology* **11**, 124–131.

116. Sanchez K., Richardson J. and Mason H.R.C. (2004). The return to work experiences of colorectal cancer survivors. *AAOHN Journal* **52**, 500–510.

117. Chapple A., Ziebland S., McPherson A. and Summerton N. (2004). Lung cancer patients' perceptions of access to financial benefits: a qualitative study. *British Journal of General Practice* **54**, 589–594.

118. Cunningham A. and Watson K. (2004). How psychological therapy may prolong survival in cancer patients: new evidence and a simple theory. *Integrative Cancer Therapies* **3**, 214–229.

119. Glaser B. and Strauss A. (1965). *Awareness of Dying.* Chicago, IL: Aldine.

120. Stedeford A. (1994). *Facing Death: Patients, Families and Professionals*, 2nd edition. Oxford: Sobell.

121. Rogers A., Karlsen S. and Addington-Hall J. (2000). 'All the services were excellent. It is when the human element comes in that things go wrong': dissatisfaction with hospital care in the last year of life. *Journal of Advanced Nursing* **31**, 768–774.

122. Ellershaw J. and Ward C. (2003). Care of the dying patient: the last hours or days of life. *British Medical Journal* **326**, 30–34.

123. Ellershaw J. and Wilkinson S. (2003). *Care of the Dying: a Pathway to Excellence.* Oxford: Oxford University Press.

CHAPTER SEVEN

The impact of cancer on the family

Hilary Plant

The impact of cancer on an individual is invariably a profound and life-changing experience, with the consequences frequently continuing long beyond the initial period of treatment. The impact of this disease on the family and friends of someone with cancer may be equally disturbing, but perhaps harder to recognise or know how to support.

'Family' is not easy to define, holding a different meaning for each individual according to their personal history. The concept of family may hold inherent connotations of its 'nuclear' form. The Canadian Palliative Care Association defines a family as, 'those closest to the patient in knowledge, care and affection. This includes the biological family, the family of acquisition (related by marriage/contract), and the family of choice and friends (not related or by marriage/contract)'.[1] For the purpose of this discussion, the term 'family' will be broad and inclusive; the focus is on the defining relationships in a person's life, those with whom there is a degree of emotional attachment, however complex this might be. Thus the terms 'family' or 'relatives' are used to refer to those who are close to a person who has been diagnosed with cancer, and includes partners, parents, offspring, siblings, and close friends.

Family relationships are dynamic, and the diagnosis of cancer in one member will resonate throughout the whole social group, changing the relationship with the person who has cancer and relationships with one another. This will be influenced by the stage each individual has reached in their own developmental process and their social circumstances – their own health, financial circumstances, sex, and any co-existent events or stressors. The experience of cancer is also mediated by factors such as the relationship an individual has with the person who has cancer, their own perceptions and understanding of cancer, and the site and stage of the cancer involved.[2–4]

The major themes concerning the impact of cancer on families are interrelated and surround:

- the experience of cancer for families
- communication within the family
- living with cancer in the family
- interacting with health care professionals
- approaches to caring for families.

Each of these will be illustrated by comments made by individuals who took part in a study undertaken with the families of people diagnosed with lung or colorectal cancer.[5] These experiences were explored through in-depth interviews, undertaken over a period of 18 months. Participants who took part in the study were from diverse although ethnically similar social backgrounds, and all had established relationships with the person with cancer. Cancer is predominantly a disease of middle and older age, and the focus of this chapter is on the impact that it has on adults. The experiences of young children whose parents have cancer, or those affected by childhood cancer itself are also included through their experiences as reported in the literature, as are those of individuals from culturally diverse backgrounds.

The experience of cancer for families

The close family and friends of someone with cancer will experience distress. However, the extent of such distress is difficult to gauge. For many there is a deep 'existential' element to this, which can be hard to understand or talk about, but that is in essence a fundamental loss of one's bearings and a sense of unreality created by the threat to the life of someone close. This is often accompanied by a tangible change in outlook – for example, in life's priorities or direction.

The news of a cancer diagnosis in a partner, friend or relative can cause intense emotional disturbance in the form of sadness, depression, anxiety, or anger.[6] This may also manifest in a range of physical problems such as fatigue, weight loss, or insomnia.[7] Just as for the person with cancer, the experience for families evolves over time as the illness progresses. Individual family members will feel the impact of cancer differently. This is illustrated by the comments of the following woman whose husband was newly diagnosed with cancer of the lung:

> But of course, when anybody sort of says the word cancer, the first thing you think about is, that's it, you've not got a chance in hell . . . you can't imagine the feeling until it actually happens . . . a very good friend of mine had cancer . . . so I mean I've been through the stages of it and it was pretty horrendous, but then it was a friend, not my husband . . . [now] it's like a blood relation . . . whatever Arthur was going through I was going through, I was going through the same with him.[5]

The threatened loss precipitated by a cancer diagnosis in the family causes the onset of grief since 'part of the social context for understanding, organising, validating, and defining feeling, action, values, and priorities is removed . . .'.[8] Thus grief can be seen as arising not only because of a loss of a person but also because of losing a part of the foundation for dealing with loss and with all of

experience,[8] as Anna Quindlen's fictionalised account of a daughter's experience of her mother's cancer illustrates:

> I remember that the last completely normal day we ever had in our lives, my brothers and I, was an ordinary day much like this one, a muggy August-into-September weekday. Afterward I wondered why I hadn't loved that day more, why I hadn't savoured every bit of it like soft ice cream on my tongue, why I hadn't known how good it was to live so normally, so everyday. But you only know that, I suppose, after it's not normal and everyday any longer. And nothing ever was after that day.[9]

A feeling of loss of security following the diagnosis of cancer in a partner can be experienced as the woman below expresses. She yearns for the time in her life when she felt safe and cared for:

> . . . the mental torture of it all. But I suppose it would be nice to have someone like your mum, it's stupid isn't it, but it's the comfort. You know when you are ill at home and you've been a young child, and your mum's there and it's lovely, but as you get older unfortunately you haven't got these people around you anyway. You *are* the person. It's the security you miss.[5]

Much of this loss of security must stem from the fact that for most, the immediate thought on hearing the diagnosis of cancer is that the person they love is going to die.[10,11] Partners may in fact express more fear of death than the person with cancer themselves,[12] as one husband describes when his wife was in hospital having surgery for bowel cancer. He was frightened for her but also very frightened for his own world without her. Many express the wish that it was they themselves who had the cancer, since this might make them feel more in control, or prevent them facing the prospect of being left alone:

> . . . at the time I was really scared . . . of her dying, because again . . . it's self . . . it's giving way to yourself . . . just because somebody else is dying, you should be sorry for them, but no if you're honest, you're worried about yourself.[5]

Life may change quite fundamentally as a result of the diagnosis of cancer – for example, giving up work to care for the person with cancer, moving to live nearer them, or taking on additional household tasks. Important aspects of family lifestyle may be lost, for example, holidays no longer planned, or there may be financial difficulties, sometimes to the extent of losing one's home if there is a substantial loss of earnings. In other instances there might be a less obvious change in daily life creating more of a sense of uncertainty and confusion about plans and hopes for the future. For example, a man whose wife had colorectal cancer reflected that:

> . . . you come to a sort of junction and you change . . . you go off a different way . . . it changes your whole life . . . there's no two ways about that.[5]

A young woman who had only recently left home, described her thoughts about how the loss of practical and emotional support from her mother would change her life:

> . . . all I could think of was . . . what's going to happen to me, who's going to look after me . . . she was going to organize my wedding and look after me when I have children.[5]

This may be reflecting the view of a teenager or young adult affected by cancer in a parent. Adult children may perceive that their parent has changed because of the cancer and they may find this difficult and wish that it had not happened.[13] The relationship between parent and child is an important source of security throughout life, and disruption to this in childhood creates a vulnerability to psychiatric disorder in adulthood. Anxiety levels experienced by a child who has a parent with cancer are decreased when they have an understanding about the illness and are able to communicate well with their parents.[14] The parents of a child with cancer will invest everything in the child during the illness in the hope of recovery and all other aspects of life may become neglected.[15]

Several studies indicate that distress in family members is as great or greater than in the person who has cancer themselves.[16] One study that attempted to identify the pattern of crisis experienced following discharge after surgery for bowel cancer found that there were few differences in the intensity of distress between the person with cancer and their spouse.[17]

Attempts have been made to assess the levels of anxiety and depression experienced amongst families where one member is diagnosed with cancer.[18] Helplessness, fear, and anger are reported as the most stressful emotions encountered amongst those who have family or friends undergoing chemotherapy.[19]

A man whose wife was in hospital with colorectal cancer and who was himself disabled commented:

> I could have gone off the deep end, one hears about people in hospitals who go and rush into the casualty and thump the doctors, I can sympathize with them . . . because to them why isn't somebody doing something, they don't know what is happening, they see you calm and quiet, I sympathize with them. When you don't know . . . this is . . . animal instinct. If you don't know you bite it or hit it or something, and I'm prepared to accept that . . . that when you're reduced to the minimum, all you do is act like an animal.[5]

Many relatives appear to find it hard to reflect on their own emotional distress. Sometimes it is easier to describe the physical manifestations of the emotional upheaval than more abstract emotions. For example, when relatives describe hearing the diagnosis they may recall reactions such as feeling 'dizzy', having a 'dry mouth', feeling 'cold', or unable to speak for some time. If these coincide with the moment when important information regarding the diagnosis or treatment is being communicated by doctors, or when they are asked if they have any questions, this may act as a barrier to full understanding of the news. One man who found it hard to express his worries described how he felt when he heard his wife's cancer had spread:

> I felt as though something had been stuck inside me . . . a knife or something, I don't know. That was the piercing blow I think . . . It was as though I had a sword stuck in me. It was like . . . that sort of feeling you get when . . . going to pass out . . . the hot feeling that goes right inside.[5]

These acute physical reactions experienced at times of stress such as on hearing the diagnosis or the news of recurrence, are usually short-lived, but they can contribute to longer-term difficulties in functioning by causing fatigue, anorexia, or insomnia. The husbands of women with breast cancer have been found to report increased moodiness, loss of energy, and growing fears about their own illness and death. This has been attributed to the fact that these men deny their own feelings and place those of their wives at the foreground of their thoughts, intensifying deeper anxieties.[10]

During the course of her father's lung cancer, a woman commented on her own deterioration:

> . . . but I suppose really your health does deteriorate, you feel tired, you feel irritable, in my case you lose weight, you find it hard to put back on, you're tired, but you can't sleep, and it does catch up with you in the end.[5]

A man describing his home when his wife was in hospital with lung cancer commented:

> What was it like? Like a mortuary . . . fed up, I hardly ate, I hardly cooked anything. Well I didn't fancy it, know what I mean? . . . Even the whisky there, one night I had a good dose of it, it didn't make no difference.[5]

In brief, those close to a person diagnosed with cancer will experience a wide range of reactions to the illness. Their feelings will be complex and often difficult to express. They themselves may become unwell. These issues may not be readily apparent to the health professionals whose acknowledgement of the relative's situation, particularly around the time of diagnosis, might provide support and ease the strains that can exist between patient, relative, and professional.

Communication within the family

The social consequences of cancer on the family are many and varied, and are exacerbated by the commonly experienced difficulties of talking about cancer. Communicating about the illness, changes in roles and coping strategies employed by different family members all have important social implications for family dynamics and functioning. The diagnosis of cancer in a family will have an impact not only on the internal world of each family member, but also on their relationships with the person who has cancer, and with others in their circle of acquaintances. Where relationships are strained, for example with an ex-partner or work colleagues, the tension may be heightened. People report that some (usually more distant) relationships are terminated entirely.

In Personal account 7.1, a young woman with ovarian cancer describes the impact on her relationship with her husband Paul,[20] illustrating how cancer may cause a slight but significant 'turning away', even in the most supportive relationships. Anne describes how she and her husband are adjusting together to the painful process they are going through. After 4 years of illness, it had become impossible to sustain the emotional

Personal account 7.1

Paul was so reluctant to tell me but I knew anyway. Fatigue has worn him down. The constant uncertainty, the ever present threat that I am going to die, has turned him away from me a little. It is so hard to remain committed to someone, not knowing whether they will be there in a few months or a few years time. I can understand that. And the uncertainty goes on and on. The tenderness when I was first diagnosed couldn't possibly be sustained without a break for nearly four years. I didn't expect or want it to. It would have been easier if I had either died or been cured quickly but it just isn't like that.

In a sense Paul is going through the same painful process of adjusting to this latest progression that I have had. The same resentment to the sharp cutting off of a relaxed attitude to life and an indefinite future. Anger at the possibilities we can't choose anymore . . .

It would be easier if I was less demanding, more oblivious, but I can't be. I have to be myself. More so perhaps now that I am under threat. I don't have the time, the patience to be untrue. That is part of the problem too. It hasn't been all bad. Cancer has given me opportunities for self development and I have taken them with both hands . . .

But Paul has been holding back, simply because I have cancer. I was angry when he said that, how could he be so patronising. I felt a little guilty too. I hadn't seen what was my advantage not to see.

closeness created at the time of diagnosis in the face of the prolonged uncertainty Anne's cancer had caused both of them.

While studies have shown that the reactions to cancer and the adjustment process are remarkably similar in both the person with cancer and family members, there are also important differences.[21] As in the case of Anne and Paul, cancer may confer some (albeit possibly unwanted) benefits to the person with the disease. However, this is less likely for the relative. Anne feels that Paul is 'holding back' or putting her first, attempting to protect her.

Talking about cancer and its implications and uncertainties is difficult. Much of this difficulty arises from a desire (for all parties) to protect each other from any additional hurt or pain. In a study of the husbands of women with breast cancer,[18] few (less than 7%) were found to have discussed their worries with anyone, and an interview study with the families of people with lung cancer found that most spouses were not sharing their concerns with them.[16] Even couples who profess a very close relationship or who have similar coping styles can be set apart by cancer, however much they attempt to share their feelings about the illness. This will ultimately lead both to feel a sense of loneliness.

Many people with cancer and those close to them declare and practise a philosophy of being open about the illness and of talking about it together. Nevertheless, there are invariably some things that are very difficult to share. Communication may be open for the person with the disease, but not for the relative in terms of expressing emotions such as anger, fear, or disappointment. Relatives may not have a place to vent their own emotions and sometimes find that they are becoming the 'butt' for the emotions of the person with cancer, with nowhere to take them or pass them on themselves.

The following comments illustrate the difficulties of being a 'cancer relative'.

One man describes the week after his wife's diagnosis with breast cancer:

> I think almost every time after she had gone out and I was on my own doing something I would quite often break down and cry, but she didn't realize that.[5]

Another man explains how his wife complains about her treatment in hospital:

> I mean she comes home and she shouts off . . . spouts off at me so then I take the deflect on that, you know, I feel the same as she does then . . . in fact more.[5]

If there is a decision as a family that the illness will not be discussed, a wall of unexpressed emotion between the person with the disease and their family can be created. The exclusion of friends or family can be engendered by the person who has cancer if they refuse to talk about their illness, which may be very hard to bear. The implications of the cancer for siblings, adult children, or friends, those who are less publicly involved in the daily life of the person with cancer, may not be acknowledged by other social acquaintances or work colleagues or by health professionals. Friendships sustained by infrequent meetings are vulnerable, and can be disrupted or lost altogether, since the illness may make keeping in contact very difficult.

A sister comments on the distancing of her brother through cancer:

> You feel you've done everything you can and then you're just shut off from it when you feel you want to be there. And you want to say something but you're not being given the opportunity to sort of say the right words . . . I think one of the hardest things is that when you feel you could be there for somebody they put up a barrier against you . . .[5]

Changes in roles at home, work, or socially have been found to occur in families, such as altered employment, household schedules, or curtailed social activities.[16,22] Recreational activities, finances if the person who is ill is the main source of income, and career plans may be severely disrupted. Sexual difficulties are common between partners where one has cancer. Fear and anxiety can decrease libido, as do many cytotoxic drugs. The fatigue experienced as a result of the disease or its treatment decreases interest in sex. Changed appearance may also cause embarrassment or physical difficulties.

Many relatives and friends have a conscious or unconscious desire to protect someone they love who has cancer from any additional hurt, both real and imagined. However well-meaning, this can add to problems in communicating. Wortman and Dunkel-Schetter hypothesise that other people's reactions to a person's cancer are as a result of conflict between the essentially negative feelings about cancer and their beliefs about appropriate behaviours to display towards the person who has the disease, such as optimism and cheerfulness.[23] They believe that this conflict results in responses that may be unintentionally damaging to the person with cancer, such as physical avoidance, and avoidance of open discussion. While social support is potentially beneficial to well-being, those closest to someone with cancer may be unable to give it in the most helpful way. Anxiety and tension can result among family members who are constantly worried that they will say the wrong thing. Buffering or shielding the person who has cancer from painful information and experiences is common. The most extreme form of this might be for the family to try to prevent the individual from knowing their diagnosis. This now happens infrequently, although families may still wish to protect the person from knowing the full extent of the severity of their illness and may not pass on any additional information that they have gleaned from health professionals. Hiding the full extent of the emotional distress the illness is causing and behaving in ways that they believe will be reassuring is also common, and reflects the ways in which families deal with illness. Protecting the person with cancer from painful situations also allows the relative to avoid facing difficult emotions. However, this may create a barrier or distance between the person with cancer and those close to them.

A woman whose husband was concerned about how she would cope after his death comments:

> I try to hold it in . . . I suppose what I try to do a lot is make him feel that I can manage, 'cos that's what he worries about.[5]

A daughter who wants to protect her mother from distress about her son's illness comments:

> . . . when you are close to people you tend not to want to worry or upset them, there is this barrier, between close relationships.[5]

One relative may attempt to shield others in the family whom they feel are vulnerable, an elderly mother, for example. Nevertheless, even those perceived as most vulnerable, such as children or the elderly, are usually better prepared to cope if they are aware of what is happening. As a 14-year-old girl whose mother died from ovarian cancer told her therapist:

> I can cope with honesty I can't cope with secrecy.
> Sophie aged 14 (Dreamcatchers, Dorset (2005).
> Personal communication)

While parents of children with cancer may want to protect the sick child, other relationships between family members may become neglected. Siblings in particular may feel resentful about the increased closeness between their parents and the child with cancer.[15] The child's experience and ability to understand what is happening will obviously be dependent on their developmental stage.[24] Separation from a parent who is sick in early childhood will be followed by protest, despair and detachment, accompanied by possible bedwetting, constipation and sleeping difficulties. In later childhood the loss of a parent may commonly cause emotional and behavioural problems.[24]

Relatives may attempt to monitor the person's environment to ensure that they do not encounter something untoward to upset them; for example, avoiding media coverage of cancer that may include survival statistics. They also monitor the person themselves, checking for subtle changes in their well-being, such as in their eating or energy levels. The families of people undergoing radiotherapy have been found to monitor symptoms closely even though this was not requested by health professionals,[25] and this can be overprotective and frustrating for the person undergoing treatment. Others attempt to keep the sick person from 'dwelling' on their cancer, encouraging them to take up an activity and think about other things. Thus, when cancer occurs within a family, adjustments in communication result – some conscious, some unconscious. Frequently these arise because open discussion of the disease and all its consequences is too difficult. The protection strategies employed by both the person with cancer and their relatives can sometimes exacerbate the problems consequent on opaque communication.

Living with cancer in the family

The social impact of the cancer and its effect on family relationships become part of day-to-day living with cancer. For example, the protection strategies just described are both a way of caring and a way of coping with the fear and uncertainty created by the illness.

There are many ways of defining care, and the amount and nature of caring undertaken, both practical and emotional, by families and friends will be variable.[4] The extent to which families provide care for the person with cancer is dependent on their relationships, perceptions of the illness, degree of physical problems, and level of dependency caused by the disease. Offering and giving care can be an important means of coping for some families, although other family groups may be so distant or dysfunctional that they will not take part in the course of the illness. Current research about care given by informal carers reflects both these contradictory, but closely interwoven elements of being both burdensome and rewarding.[4]

Many families will not actually perceive themselves as carers; rather they see themselves as dealing with changes in their daily routine brought about by the illness. Indeed, frequently people with cancer are quite well and are able to look after themselves. A study of people with cancer and their families during chemotherapy found that the people with cancer 'often vigorously resisted receiving help from others and strongly desired to maintain their self-care' (p.263).[26] Nevertheless, some additional practical tasks are invariably required even in the early stages of the illness. For example, for some people the biggest single problem may be fatigue, which can necessitate the family taking on extra practical duties.[7] In the face of terminal illness, the family caring for their relative at home will have great demands placed upon them, and a large resource of emotional and practical support is likely be required:[27–30]

. . . it's the watching, it tears you apart inside, because you can only do a certain amount for him, and sometimes I know I get on his nerves, I say 'Can I get you a drink?' . . . 'Can I get you this?' 'Shall I do that for you?' . . . 'What if you had this?' 'What if you have that?' And I know sometimes it does get on his nerves . . . but it's my way of trying to do something for him, and when I see him sitting there . . . really surviving as it were, and struggling, I just . . . I think 'Oh lord what are you doing . . . take him home now at the suffering.'[5]

'Standing by' and 'watching' as the disease progresses is an active process requiring emotional energy. The need to care and do something to help, even if this is not required, is intense. The physical demands of providing care while also struggling to make sense of the suffering observed are immensely demanding for families.[28,30] Adult children of people diagnosed with cancer may experience their family role abruptly changing to that of a support person in which they might feel more like parents themselves, and they might feel unprepared for this.[13]

The term 'caregiving burden' has been used to describe the caring activities of families of people with cancer.[28] McCorkle and coworkers conducted an interview study on the caregivers of people discharged from hospital who had complex care problems.[29] Caregivers were interviewed three times over a 6-month period. Even though the person's condition stabilised or improved over the 6 months, caregivers continued to report high levels of burden. Caregivers of those whose mental state was poor and who had greater responsibilities for physical care experienced greater impact on their daily life, finances, and health. Other studies have shown that caring for someone undergoing radiotherapy results in substantial time spent providing transport, undertaking extra household tasks, and giving emotional support.[25] For those caring for the terminally ill, the most frequently reported demand has been managing physical care, and this is made more difficult by the family carer's lack of expertise in this role.[30] The 'emotion work' involved in caregiving particularly around the management of emotions – both of the patient and those close to them – is key.[4,25,28,31]

The difficulties of caring increase with time, and in the case of cancer this may be prolonged over several years. The negative effects of caregiving have primarily been reported after the responsibility for care has continued for 2 years or more.[27] A sister describes the long-term emotional drain of caring in the following terms:

> You do feel guilty and I suppose really if you are very honest with yourself after a while (and this is the hardest thing in the world to say) you resent illness. And this sounds awful but . . . when someone's ill for a long time like that you do somewhere deep inside you begin to think, you know, you're never going to get better or . . . It's hard to explain, I suppose it's almost an intolerance after a while which you then feel terribly guilty about.[5]

Caring is not always perceived as a burden by the relatives. In some instances caring is 'internally related' to self-identity (Cribb A. (1999). Personal communication). The need to care is inherent within the person and is not something that is thought out or planned. Relatives may not comprehend any other option but to care.[32] The person concerned will not necessarily want to relinquish any of their caring role to outsiders and this may create problems for those who might believe that the family needs help, and would like to offer support.

A man who takes unpaid leave from work after his wife is diagnosed with cancer describes the following situation:

> And some people at work for instance have said, you know one person said 'You're being very unselfish about this'. And I said 'Well it's nothing to do with that', and somebody else said 'You know it's very good of you to give up work rather than trying to bury yourself in the work'. And it was no more like that than flying to the moon. I thought about it over that night and there was no way I could vaguely think about going to work.[5]

One woman described her feelings about caring for her husband:

> What kind of a burden is it? If it is classed as a burden . . . I don't class him as a burden, not at all. I don't class it as a duty, not at all. I do it because I love him, I love him.[5]

Observers of such care may see this as 'heroic' but for the caregiver themselves, they are doing the only thing they can in the circumstances.[33] It has been suggested that 'caring allows the person to focus on the event or the one cared for rather than on personal threat' (p.3).[33] For example, 'doing' things for the person to ensure their comfort can help to ameliorate feelings of grief about their illness. Concern to feed and nourish the person with cancer can be central to this for some. Large amounts of energy may be expended on searching out and cooking food, and attempting to present it in a way that is enticing. The activity of preparing and cooking food is a way of trying to do something constructive, bringing some normality to life and countering anxiety and deeper concerns, but this can also cause strain in the relationship. Cleaning and other household activities are also a means of maintaining order during times of stress for some people. Sustaining this level of caring over time, however, may become difficult. The relatives themselves may not perceive that they have needs of their own, which may be amenable to outside help. Women continue to undertake the majority of care at home.[34] They have been described as 'invisible',[35] or 'forgotten',[34] and the considerable time spent caring or even just being available for the person with cancer may often compromise other aspects of their life. Sisters rather than brothers, and daughters before sons become the closest support for the patient.[5] Place within the family, relationships and allegiances in childhood, personal circumstances and geographical distance are likely to play a part in who takes on the caring role. Teenagers may find it particularly difficult to provide support.[36] Their desire for independence may not fit easily with a possible requirement to take on more responsibility at home, and they may find it hard openly to acknowledge their feelings about the situation.

Caring does not necessarily involve practical activity. Parents have been described as 'keeping vigil' over their hospitalised child. This is more than simply being in close proximity to the child at their bedside; it is 'more often an intense bearing witness with the child's plight'.[37] The parents of a child with cancer have been described as functioning as a 'protective filter' through which experiences may filter both ways.[38] The parent filters what goes through to the child, and the child's experience of distress may be filtered back to the caring team through the father or mother. Although parents of sick children experience a particularly intense need to share their child's affliction, the need to be there and to be part of the experience applies to the families of adults as well.

Tension may also arise in the parents' relationship when a child has cancer because of the different roles and the separation that may occur during the illness. Women who tend to spend more time with the child appear better placed to cope with the illness than fathers, who are more likely to try to maintain life as it was.[15] Families are made up of diverse individuals with their own explanations and coping styles, and some families as a whole will create their own way of coping with the illness and its meaning.[39] Nevertheless, it is the individual diversity within the same family group that may create the most stress.

For both the person with cancer and family and friends, cancer disrupts the way they see their life and future. In order to cope with the uncertainties brought by the disease, their view of the future may need to be reconstructed. In terms of organising the family's lives it is most often the desire of the person with cancer that is adhered to. Some (quite appropriately) begin to make plans for their death and the family's life after death; but this may be distressing for families. Sometimes cancer precipitates a review of life, and a heightened awareness of mortality, or the decision to realise long-held ambitions. This is hard for a relative who has no such excuse and may not be included in the plans, who has to adjust their own to fit in with those of the person with cancer. It may no longer be possible for the family members to make plans of their own. This may create tension. For many, communicating the feelings of uncertainty that illness has brought, or the feelings surrounding the knowledge that there will come a time when they will be living alone, may be impossible.

Making sense of the illness is difficult. The cancer itself may be explained by factors such as lifestyle, smoking or diet, but there is invariably little attempt by the relatives to make sense of why this disruption has happened to their own lives. The lack of opportunity to talk about and work through their own experience of the cancer may

make it hard for the relatives to come to terms with it.

A diagnosis of cancer usually introduces into a family an onus to provide physical and emotional support. This may fall unevenly on the various members. For some it is accepted unquestioningly and the provision of physical care may be integral to a relative's coping mechanisms. Those close to the person with cancer may rarely spend time reflecting on their own needs, and contemplation of their own future may become difficult.

Interactions with health professionals and the health care system

Research studies indicate that although the distress of the family and friends of someone with cancer is invariably high, it is inadequately addressed by health professionals, who frequently exclude them from care.[18,22,40] In Personal account 7.2 there are two extracts from interviews conducted in the same week with a brother and sister who share a house. They were recorded 18 months after the brother was diagnosed with advanced colorectal cancer. The sister's life revolves around her brother's illness and she considered later in her

Personal account 7.2

When you're faced with an illness you can do nothing about and it has the potential to kill you, it's not like a broken leg which is going to get better, you are wholly in the hands of the doctors and their attitude is of paramount importance to your own feelings about what you're going through . . . And the attitude at the hospital was superb, it was all hopeful and you know, things to be done, and of course they were carrying on the treatment.

Brother

I still think the doctors and nurses are treated as if they're almost God, I still think that there is that feeling, although we're meant not to be impressed by these things . . . we are. You still tend not to think . . . of them as another human being who I can talk to . . . like you might talk to the ticket collector at the tube station . . . you do still tend to have this feeling that you should be looking up to them, you know they've descended from dizzy heights.[5]

Sister

interview when she would have to give up work to look after him full-time. Their attitudes towards the professional carers are strikingly different. The brother perceives the care he is receiving as good, but in effect this excludes his closest relative.

The sister does not find the professionals either approachable or accessible. She has a need for information and later in the interview expressed the need for support for herself, although this is prevented by her situation. She is not married to the person with cancer, she is his sister, thus the professionals may not anticipate her needs to be great. She has at times a strained relationship with her brother who neither informs her of what is happening nor likes her to come with him to the hospital. Indeed, he does not want her to know very much. She, like many relatives, also has a full-time job and an elderly mother to care for. She thus remains on the margins of the medical care that her brother receives.

Most studies show that, whatever their own needs, relatives want good clinical care to be provided above all else, and where care is good most will declare themselves satisfied.[41] This overwhelming concern for the well-being of the person with cancer means that it is difficult for the family to consider or declare their own requirements for help as distinct from those of their sick relative.

Professional carers profoundly influence families' experience of cancer, for good or bad. For some, contact with health professionals is a key focus for the whole experience and there is great appreciation where care is perceived as good. However, distress may be high for those who have no contact with health professionals, and where staff are difficult to approach or information giving is poor.

Hull interviewed family caregivers at home in the weeks before their relative died, to examine caregiving behaviours among people who were part of a hospice home care programme.[41] Families identified four essential aspects of good care: 24-hour accessibility, effective communication, a non-judgemental attitude, and clinical competence. These are likely to be equally important to families at earlier stages of the disease. Several studies report that the telephone is an important means of maintaining contact when the person has been discharged from hospital.[11] The follow-

ing comments from the wife of a man undergoing chemotherapy show how reassuring a telephone link to health professionals can be:

> It's that sort of relationship there   to know that you can actually phone them and you know who you are talking to . . . by face, is very important . . . particularly this problem, because you want to relate it to somebody that you know.[5]

A woman caring for her sick husband at home comments:

> So I found myself reaching for the phone . . . getting ready to phone for the district nurse, but then thinking, 'Should I? Shouldn't I?' . . . I was worried, can I be doing any more for him? So if somebody had just like come or phoned, and said . . . 'how are things . . . It's three weeks since I last came. I know you said you don't need help, but how are things? Right?' and then I could say . . . 'Oh well by the way . . . he's got such and such thing at the moment, is that all in order' . . . Do you see what I mean?[5]

Lack of information or understanding of the care and treatment can be agonising. Parents of children with cancer have been described as experiencing 'heightened cue awareness', where the need for information creates a 'tendency to attribute meaning and significance to just about anything that is said or done by professionals'.[11] This 'over-interpretation' of the comments or behaviour of health care professionals is born out of a need for information and reassurance and is also likely to be experienced by all of those close to someone with cancer.

In the first 30 000 calls to the cancer information service of the British Association of Cancer United Patients (Cancerbackup), more calls were received from relatives than from people with cancer themselves.[42] They required information in two key areas: medical information and support services. The need for honest, sensitively delivered information given at the appropriate time is crucial yet beset with potential difficulties, and the need to 'have questions answered honestly' has been ranked as the highest need amongst relatives.[42]

The family make themselves known to professional carers by their bedside vigil, attendance at hospital appointments, or requests for information. The contact with the professionals is likely to be couched in terms of how best to fulfil the patient's needs, with the relative possibly perceiving that they have no 'right' to make any request for themselves. Relatives who, because of work or other demands, have difficulties in making themselves accessible to the health care system, remain invisible to health carers. In addition, relatives may not behave in a way that is expected by others, particularly health professionals who may have no knowledge of the histories and motivations of those involved. Furthermore, the strategies patients use for living with their cancer may inhibit communication between their families and health professionals. If someone is coping by knowing as little as possible about their illness, their relatives may also be denied information. Below, a woman describes how her husband prevented her from knowing that he was to be discharged following a thoracotomy, even though she would need to care for him and change his dressings:

> . . . the doctor told him he could come home, but he didn't tell me. I was going in three times a day, going in the morning, and then going in the afternoon and coming back and going in the evening . . . sometimes my daughter came in with me, but most times I was there, and he didn't say anything . . . and all of a sudden . . . The nurse came up to do something . . . and said, 'Oh anyway, you're going home tomorrow'. So I looked at him, you know . . . 'I knew three days ago' [he said] . . . he was frightened to say about it.[5]

It is not uncommon for someone to desire privacy about their disease and refuse to be accompanied on visits to the hospital. Just as relatives and friends attempt to protect the person with cancer from anxiety about the illness, the person themselves may desire to protect family from difficult news or from witnessing them being unwell; for example, while having chemotherapy. This is particularly pronounced for parents who wish to protect their children, even when they may be adults themselves. Alternatively, a relative's own anxiety about the situation may prevent them from attending hospitals and clinics. This can also hinder the recognition of their need for help. Some people do not want what they regard as interference from outsiders in their homes, and this can also create barriers to the provision of adequate support.

Cancer is predominantly a disease of older adults and therefore close family and friends may also be elderly, with their own health problems, which prevent them from attending the hospital. For example, the daughter of a man with lung cancer described anticipating the day when her father would be taken into a hospice, which would mean that her mother who was housebound with cardiac failure would never able to see him again.[5] For a relative with a serious chronic illness or disability who is dependent on the person diagnosed with cancer, the consequences are likely to be serious since they risk losing the person who has supported and cared for them.

Lack of familiarity with the health care system can preclude the family from being able to speak to professional carers. A study in Britain revealed a lack of cultural sensitivity, which created deficiencies in access and provision of palliative care services to the black and minority ethnic communities.[43] For those who do not have English as a first language, information about services and diagnosis in the language of their choice was found to be unavailable.[43] The need for accessible support at diagnosis and information about symptoms was particularly emphasised. Close family and friends may react to the illness in a way that professionals might not expect. Furthermore, contact with professionals may be inhibited by various factors such as longstanding, unresolved differences with the person who has cancer resulting in an apparent lack of concern, or non-attendance at the bedside of a dying relative, or by refusals of help offered by professionals. Complicated relationships within the family may obscure the distress of some of those affected from the professionals – for example, ex-partners who share children. The difficulties of ensuring that adequate support is given to the whole family may be compounded by the geographical spread of modern families who live many miles apart.

Approaches to caring for families

Family distress is both substantial and complex.[44] The role of the health professionals in providing support for the family is much less well defined than when providing care for the person with cancer. Early discharge and the increasing use of high-technology treatment at home is increasing the level of care expected from family and friends.[29] Independently of any care they offer themselves, families require support. However, family members can be difficult to identify, and many relatives are unable to express what their own needs or requirements from nurses might be. Caring for the person with cancer is sometimes a crucial part of managing the illness for families, therefore well-intentioned but insensitive outside support risks causing key coping mechanisms to collapse. For many reasons it is not straightforward to assess the needs of the family.[45,46] A recent literature review of support for informal carers in cancer and palliative care identified few targeted interventions with only a very small number of these being evaluated.[47] The challenges of introducing new interventions directed at family caregivers in palliative care have been identified in a further review of the literature and these are described in three broad categories: challenges related to the family, their relationships, and ways of living with the illness; barriers in the communication process, both within the family and with the health professionals; and health system barriers including insufficient resources and lack of health professional skills.[48]

In addition, since family members are not usually physically ill there may be a further issue about where the responsibility lies for providing them with support. In cases of more severe distress, hospital health professionals need to be prepared to refer them for specialist counselling.[44,49] Nurses who know the person with cancer and who come into contact with the family are well placed to be able to offer support, although it is not currently always clear what the best form of such support might be. National Guidance produced for England and Wales in 2004 highlights family and carers' need for support and the issue that it is not always available to them.[50] While acknowledging that there is currently no clear evidence to suggest just how this should be implemented, the guidance recommends, amongst other things, that family members and carers should be offered the opportunity for their needs for support and information to be assessed separately from those of the patient. Carers should be

made aware of, and have easy access to, culturally sensitive sources of local information, advice and support.[50]

Care strategy 7.1

- Do not prejudge the situation.
- Identify key people who might constitute 'family'.
- Provide a contact telephone number.
- Listen to the relative's own story and acknowledge what is important for them.
- Be sensitive to the level of adjustment.
- Provide a supportive environment for the expression of distress.
- Be aware of the possible need to facilitate family communication.
- Be sensitive to individual requirements for information.
- Prepare for what might happen during the course of the illness.
- Attend important consultations with the family.
- Facilitate practical and financial support when required.
- Refer on to appropriate professionals where necessary.
- Assist attendance at support group if required.

Having the opportunity to talk about the experiences of having a member of the family with cancer, and acknowledgement of these is helpful for families.[51] The most commonly cited concern for relatives has been reported as 'dealing with the symptoms'. While relatives may acknowledge the need for information, the need to express their fears and other emotions is often identified as a low priority.[52] A dilemma revealed in a number of studies of the needs of families has been:

> . . . related to whether families wanted to share their feelings. If families needed to maintain control of their emotions and if the nurses encouraged them to ventilate their feelings, this was distressing and unsupportive. In contrast, if families wanted to discuss problems and share their feelings, the nurses' ability to explore these feelings was perceived as caring. The nurses needed to be sensitive enough to take the cue from what families were comfortable doing.[41]

Relatives need a calm unhurried approach by nurses, since it takes time to form a relationship of trust with individuals who may be anxious and frightened.

Children of people with cancer benefit from open and honest communication about illness. Parents will need support from early in the course of the disease about how to deal with their children's feelings, reactions and questions about the cancer.[14] Judd describes the role of the 'involved witness' in psychotherapeutic intervention with teenagers with cancer, a role that nurses may fulfil, even if intensive psychotherapy is not planned:

> During the initial stage of the family's attempt to survive the shock of diagnosis, the therapist's usefulness is in being an involved witness: to feel, to hear, to register, and attempt to 'contain' the immediate as well as the far-reaching implications. This early position is important to subsequent work with the family or individual, without which it is difficult for the sufferer to feel understood or be believed.[45]

It is important that professionals are knowledgeable about and sensitive to racial and cultural issues for the family.[43] If time and attention have been given to establishing a relationship with the family as well as with the person with cancer, some of these issues will become easier and nurses will be more attuned to the appropriate moment and style for communicating with an individual family. Confidentiality for the patient creates dilemmas when working with families. Relatives may want to speak with nurses without the person with cancer being present, in order to glean more information, and to protect them from difficult news. Families need their own time to allow communication; however, in most circumstances they should not be given information that the person themselves does not know, and if they are this should be discussed with the person and family together. Some may want information withheld from the person. If this is an issue, the opportunity to explore feelings surrounding the desire not to communicate openly is important, as is the facilitation of more open discussion about the disease in families. The need to have accurate and accessible information given sensitively at the appropriate time is clear. However, this may be a difficult task; Ball *et al.*

describe what was helpful to the parents of children with cancer:

> Skilled communicators are able to convey a sense of 'ifs and buts' and medical realism, while still holding out the possibility of a successful outcome to treatment.[11]

Families need the opportunity to prepare them as much as possible for what may ensue. A recent audit of contact between family and carers of people with lung cancer and lung cancer nurse specialists in the UK found that there was a significant amount of contact with those close to the person with cancer, with 78% of this occurring by phone and about half initiated by the family.[53] Both the person who has cancer and their family may need to know how future events might unfold, perhaps to make them less frightening. 'Therapeutic emplotment' has been described as a technique used by physicians whereby an attempt is made to provide continuity in discussions about illness; by agreeing together the likely course of the disease, this reduces uncertainty.[54]

The need for information and emotional support has provided the impetus for the establishment of self-help and voluntary organisations over the last few years. While these organisations play a vital part in supporting families, they do not excuse health professionals from providing information and explanation in the most appropriate way.[55]

One of the most frequently expressed unmet needs for families is a place to discuss their fears.[56] Long-term intensive psychotherapy is unlikely to be sustainable for families facing the trauma of cancer; instead, a supportive relationship, especially in the early days following diagnosis, is possibly the best solution:

> . . . therein, the therapeutic ingredients are empathy, attempts at understanding the confusions around crisis (some of which may echo earlier infantile traumas), understanding the ensuing losses, giving words to feelings and the facilitation of grief.[38]

A study comparing death in a hospital with death in a hospice found that following death in the hospice where more open communication had been facilitated, surviving family members were less anxious and depressed, more involved socially, and less likely to be using tranquillisers.[57] An environment that allows the family open expression of grief, a resolution of unfinished business, and times for the person and family to talk about their life after the anticipated death is ideal.[57]

Support groups either exclusively for the family or that include the person with cancer are one way of enhancing the support available, and in some instances have been shown to improve communication within the family. A study of a support group offered to the male partners of women with breast cancer using 'sex role therapy' reported that the group members became significantly more communicative with their spouses about issues to do with mastectomy than members of a control group did.[10] Wellisch *et al.* describe a group initially set up specifically for the families of people with cancer.[58] Among the aims were to enhance communication between people with cancer and their families, and to enable them to deal with intrapsychic conflicts concerning serious illness. This group was led by a clinical psychologist, but had a nurse as part of the team. After a few months the group was extended to include the person with cancer as well, and attendance by family members increased markedly. The authors found the group a safe arena for the expression of powerful emotions such as fear, rage, and sadness.

Support groups by no means suit everybody, and the availability of a support group does not necessarily mean that those invited will automatically attend and be supported. An evaluation of a support group for people with cancer and their families and friends at a London hospital showed that only a small number of those invited attended. For the people with cancer who attended, 80% felt happier and more relaxed, compared with only 46% of relatives who attended the group. A majority said that talking about cancer was easier after attending the group.[59]

Wortman and Dunkel-Schetter discuss a family therapy programme which:

> . . . makes cancer patients and their family members aware of the complicated social environment in which they may be trapped, and which encourages more

open communication . . . family members could be taught that their feelings of anger and guilt towards the patients are normal under the circumstances.[23]

Despite the challenges of supporting a loved one through cancer, there is increasing evidence of how, in the right circumstances, the caring can have a positive impact on the experiences. An interview study of family caregivers in advanced cancer revealed that 60% could readily identify positive aspects of their role, which for some appeared to provide some meaning to the experience, for example through becoming closer to the person with cancer, or stronger as an individual.[60] Information, access to resources and symptom-management education were some of the key factors which it was proposed might lessen the stress for people giving care.[60] As in all aspects of health care these issues are increasingly being addressed by people with cancer and carers themselves. Deborah Hutton, an English journalist diagnosed with lung cancer, responded to her experience of the desire of her family and friends to do something to help her, by writing an anthology of practical examples of the ways in which this need to support someone you care about who has been diagnosed with cancer might be galvanised into action.[61] Detailed practical advice for carers about issues such as symptom management and communication is provided by a physician who is both cancer patient and carer himself,[62] highlighting and hopefully strengthening the partnership between the professional carers and those doing the caring at home.

Relatively little attention has been paid to the impact of cancer on those close to a person with cancer, by either health professionals or researchers. It is apparent that a complex alteration in the emotions and patterns of communication between family members follows a diagnosis of cancer. These changes will accompany, and sometimes conflict with, the practical adjustments that might of necessity be made.

Health care professionals should view the needs of other family members as integral to those of the person with cancer. Acknowledgement that the illness will impact on relatives, and assuring that their individual needs for support and information are recognised are key first steps. Nurses are often well placed to initiate and facilitate the process of meeting these needs.

One woman's feelings about her need for support was as follows:

> People need it . . . I mean not to sort of go there for counselling, we had each other for that and I wouldn't have wanted anyone to invade our privacy, but just to sort of understand . . . what they're saying to you, for them to sort of talk to you in English . . . So people could . . . begin to understand, begin to think that there's more than this . . . and hope . . . things like that.[5]

References

1. Canadian Palliative Care Association. (1998). *Standards for Palliative Care Provision.* Ottowa: Canadian Palliative Care Association. www.chpca.net/home.htm (accessed 24 July 2007).
2. Given B., Dwyer T., Vredevoogd J. and Given B. (1988). Family caregivers of cancer patients: reactions and assistance. In Pritchard P. (ed.) *Fifth International Conference on Cancer Nursing.* London: Macmillan Press, pp. 39–43.
3. Rolland J. (1989). Chronic illness and the family life cycle. In Carter B. and McGoldrick M. (eds.) *The Changing Family Life Cycle. A Framework for Family Therapy,* 2nd edition. Boston, MA: Allyn and Bacon.
4. Thomas C., Morris S. and Harman J. (2002). Companions through cancer: the care given by informal carers in cancer contexts. *Social Science and Medicine* **54**, 529–544.
5. Plant H. (2000). Living with cancer: understanding the experiences of close relatives of people with cancer. Unpublished Ph.D. thesis, University of London.
6. Pitceathly C. and Maguire P. (2003). The psychological impact of cancer on patient's partners and other key relatives: a review. *European Journal of Cancer Care* **39**, 1517–1524.
7. Krishnasamy M. and Plant H. (2004). Carers, caring and cancer-related fatigue. In Armes J., Krishnasamy M. and Higginson I. (eds.) *Fatigue in Cancer.* Oxford: Oxford University Press, pp. 157–175.
8. Rosenblatt P. (1988). Grief: the social context of private feelings. *Journal of Social Issues* **44**, 67–78.
9. Quindlen A. (1996). *One True Thing.* London: Arrow.
10. Sabo D., Brown J. and Smith C. (1986). The male role and mastectomy support groups and men's adjustment. *Journal of Psychosocial Oncology* **4**, 19–31.
11. Ball S., Bignold S. and Cribb A. (1996). Death and the disease: inside the culture of childhood cancer. In Howeth

G. and Jupp P. (eds.) *Contemporary Issues in the Sociology of Death, Dying and Disposal.* London: Macmillan Press.
12. Gotay C. (1984). The experience of cancer during early and advanced stages: the views of patients and their mates. *Social Science and Medicine* **18**, 605–613.
13. Germino B. and Funk S. (1993). Impact of a parent's cancer on adult children: role and relationship issues. *Seminars in Oncology Nursing* **9**, 101–106.
14. Kroll L., Barnes J., Jones A. and Stein A. (1998). Cancer in parents: telling children. *British Medical Journal* **316**, 880.
15. Bignold S., Cribb A. and Ball S. (1996). *Families After Cancer: The Psychosocial Context of Surviving Childhood Cancer.* London: Cancer Relief Macmillan Fund and The Department of Health.
16. Cooper E.T. (1984). A pilot study on the effects of the diagnosis of lung cancer on family relationships. *Cancer Nursing* **August**, 301–308.
17. Oberst M. and Scott D. (1988). Post-discharge distress in surgically treated cancer patients and their spouses. *Research in Nursing and Health* **11**, 223–233.
18. Maguire P. (1981). The repercussions of mastectomy on the family. *International Journal of Family Psychiatry* **1**, 485–503.
19. Hart K. (1986). Stress encountered by significant others of cancer patients receiving chemotherapy. *Omega* **17**, 151–167.
20. Dennison A. (1996). *Uncertain Journey.* Newmill: Patten Press.
21. Cassileth B., Lusk E., Strouse B. *et al.* (1985). A psychological analysis of cancer patients and their next-of-kin. *Cancer* **55**, 72–76.
22. Oberst M. and James R. (1985). Going home: patient and spouse adjustment following cancer surgery. *Topics in Clinical Nursing* **April**, 46–57.
23. Wortman C. and Dunkel-Schetter C. (1979). Interpersonal relationships and cancer: a theoretical analysis. *Journal of Social Issues* **35**, 120–155.
24. Black D. (1998). Bereavement in childhood. *British Medical Journal* **316**, 931–933.
25. Oberst M., Thomas S., Gass K. and Ward S. (1989). Caregiving demands and appraisal of stress among family caregivers. *Cancer Nursing* **12**, 209–215.
26. Schumacher K. (1996). Reconceptualising family caregiving: family-based illness care during chemotherapy. *Research in Nursing and Health* **19**, 261–271.
27. Gaynor S. (1990). The long haul: the effects of homecare on caregivers. *Image: Journal of Nurse Scholarship* **22**, 208–212.
28. Carey P., Oberst M., McCubbin M. and Hughs S. (1991). Appraisal and caregiving burden in family members caring for patients receiving chemotherapy. *Oncology Nursing Forum* **18**, 1341–1348.

29. McCorkle R., Shegda Yost L., Jepson C. *et al.* (1993). A cancer experience: relationship of patient psychosocial responses to care-giver burden over time. *Psycho-oncology* **2**, 21–32.

30. Stetz K. (1987). Caregiving demands during advanced cancer. *Cancer Nursing* **10**, 260–268.

31. James N. (1989). Emotional labour: skill and work in the social regulation of feelings. *Sociological Review* **15**, 4.

32. Rose K.E., Webb C. and Waters K. (1997). Coping strategies employed by informal carers of terminally ill cancer patients. *Journal of Cancer Nursing* **1**, 126–133.

33. Benner P. and Wrubel J. (1989). *The Primacy of Caring. Stress and Coping in Health and Illness.* Menlo Park, CA: Addison–Wesley.

34. Hicks C. (1988). *Who Cares: Looking After People at Home.* London: Virago.

35. James V. (1998). Unwaged carers and the provision of health care. In Field D. and Taylor S. (eds.) *Sociological Perspectives on Health, Illness and Health Care.* Oxford: Blackwell Science.

36. Larson P. and Dodd M. (1990). Caring – issues and patterns for the family experiencing cancer. *Sixth International Conference on Cancer Nursing,* Amsterdam, pp. 177–180.

37. Darbyshire P. (1994). Parenting in public: parental participation and involvement in the care of their hospitalized child. In Benner P. (ed.) *Interpretive Phenomenology.* London: Sage, pp. 185–210.

38. Judd D. (1994). Life-threatening illness as psychic trauma: psychotherapy with adolescent patients. In Erskine A. and Judd D. (eds.) *The Imaginative Body.* London: Whurr, pp. 87–112.

39. Thorne S. (1985). The family cancer experience. *Cancer Nursing* **8**, 285–291.

40. Northouse L. (1988). Social support in patients' and husbands' adjustment to breast cancer. *Nursing Research* **37**, 91–95.

41. Hull M. (1991). Hospice nurses. Caring support for caregiving families. *Cancer Nursing* **14**, 63–70.

42. Slevin M., Terry Y., Hallett N. *et al.* (1988). BACUP – the first two years: evaluation of a national cancer information service. *British Medical Journal* **297**, 669–672.

43. Iqbal H., Field D., Parker H. and Iqbal Z. (1995). The absent minority: access and use of palliative care services by black and minority ethnic groups in Leicester. In Richardson A. and Wilson-Barnett J. (eds.) *Nursing Research in Cancer Care.* London: Scutari Press, pp. 83–96.

44. Harrison J., Haddad P. and Maguire P. (1995). The impact of cancer on key relatives: a comparison of relative and patient concerns. *European Journal of Cancer* **31A**, 1736–1740.

45. Hileman J. and Lackey N. (1990). Self-identified needs of patients with cancer at home and their home caregivers: a descriptive study. *Oncology Nursing Forum* **17**, 907–913.

46. Wingate A. and Lackey N. (1984). A description of the needs of noninstitutionalized cancer patients and their primary care givers. *Cancer Nursing* **12**, 216–225.

47. Harding, R. and Higginson I. (2003). What is the best way to help caregivers in cancer and palliative care? A systematic literature review of interventions and their effectiveness. *Palliative Medicine* **17**, 63–74.

48. Hudson, P., Aranda S. and Kristjanson L. (2004). Meeting the supportive needs of family caregivers in palliative care: challenges for health professionals. *Journal of Palliative Medicine* **7**, 19–25.

49. Fallowfield L. (1995). Helping the relatives of patients with cancer. *European Journal of Cancer* **31A**, 1731–1732.

50. National Institute for Clinical Excellence (NICE). (2004). *Guidance on Cancer Services. Improving Supportive and Palliative Care for Adults with Cancer. The Manual.* London: NICE.

51. Plant H. (1995). The experiences of families of newly diagnosed cancer patients – selected findings. In Richardson A. and Wilson-Barnett J. (eds.) *Nursing Research in Cancer Care.* London: Scutari Press, pp. 137–150.

52. Wright K. and Dyke S. (1984). Expressed concerns of adult cancer patient's family members. *Cancer Nursing* **October**, 371–374.

53. Moore S., Sherwin A. and Plant H. (2006). Caring for carers: a prospective audit of nurse specialist contact with families and carers of people with lung cancer. *European Journal of Oncology Nursing* **10**, 207–211.

54. DelVecchio Good M., Munakata T., Kobayashi Y., Mattingly C. and Good B. (1994). Oncology and narrative time. *Social Science and Medicine* **38**, 855–862.

55. Cull A.M. (1991). Studying stress in care givers: art or science? *British Journal of Cancer* **64**, 981–984.

56. Hinds C. (1985). The needs of families who care for patients with cancer at home: are we meeting them? *Journal of Advanced Nursing* **10**, 575–581.

57. Ransford H. and Smith M. (1991). Grief resolution among the bereaved in hospice and hospital wards. *Social Science and Medicine* **32**, 295–304.

58. Wellisch D., Mosher M. and Van Scoy C. (1978). Management of family emotion stress: family group therapy in a private oncology practice. *International Journal of Group Psychotherapy* **28**, 225–231.

59. Plant H., Richardson J., Stubbs L., Lynch D., Ellwood J. and Slevin M. (1987). Evaluation of a support group for

cancer patients and their families and friends. *British Journal of Hospital Medicine* **38**, 317–322.

60. Hudson P. (2004). Positive aspects and challenges associated with caring for a dying relatives at home. *International Journal of Palliative Nursing* **10**, 58–65.

61. Hutton D. (2005). *What Can I Do to Help?* London: Short Books.

62. Finnegan W. (2005). *Being a Cancer Patient's Carer: A Guide.* Oxford: Radcliffe Publications Ltd.

CHAPTER EIGHT

The impact of cancer on health care professionals

Anne Lanceley

The study of the impact of cancer and cancer care on health care professionals and the nature of nurses' strategies for working with people who have cancer shares a theoretical literature with other established investigations of therapeutic work, occupational development, and stress. However, these texts, concerned with professionalisation, role, competencies, and strategies, share a history of limitations. For researchers and practitioners alike, nurses' therapeutic work needs to be understood in the context of the workplace and in terms not only of what the nurse practitioner does (forms of practice) but also of why (professional and individual purpose).

Exploration of roles and functions, communications skills and competencies provides a useful starting point for understanding nurses' therapeutic work in cancer care. However, models of therapeutic practice need to be developed, not only to allow for the integration of different perspectives from other involved professional groups, but also to offer an integrated social and psychological reconstruction of the nature of therapeutic nursing practice that take account of conscious and unconscious processes.

This discussion is, in part, the product of research that began in 1991.[1] The verbatim accounts and care strategy commentaries are based largely on transcripts of tape recordings collected for this research, of cancer nurses talking with people they were caring for in acute and home care settings, and nurses' own reflections on these conversations.

The organisation of the chapter also owes a debt to this research, which acknowledges conscious and unconscious processes at work in nurses' encounters with cancer, and explores fundamental issues about cancer nursing, such as what the distinctive aspects of interpersonal work are, how nurses use their personality on behalf of people they are caring for, what the role imposes, what the irrational elements are, the ways nurses communicate with patients and colleagues, what the nurse and patient may represent to each other, and how nurses manage their anxiety in the face of relentless psychic pain and suffering.

The use and effectiveness of various nursing care strategies and approaches are considered alongside an evaluation of the impact the strategy may have on the nurse. This chapter deals with the theoretical, professional, and organisational context of cancer nurse–patient relationships. Drawing on examples from the UK and the US, it is concerned with the contentious issue of how far the concept of 'therapeutic nursing' is useful and appropriate to describe nurses' work with people who have cancer, and their families. It explores the relationship between 'nursing as therapy', 'counselling', and more circumscribed ideas of cancer nurses' work, reflected in specific health-promotional or support goals. Health care professionals' attitudes and defences to cancer are introduced as a way of understanding communication patterns in cancer care settings. Methodological issues in researching and evaluating the nature and impact of the nurse–patient relationship in cancer care are considered.

The theoretical context of nursing in cancer care

Within contemporary cancer nursing, the relationship between nurse and patient is perceived to be of central importance to emotion-focused interventions and the overall provision of quality care.[2,3]

This has not always been so and it is generally accepted that until recently the potential of nurse–patient relationships was limited. Medical diagnosis and treatment dominated cancer nursing's ideology, and a person's physical body represented the primary focus of nursing work.[4]

Peplau was perhaps the first to emphasise the potential therapeutic value of the nurse–patient relationship, maintaining, in particular, that nursing is 'educative and therapeutic when nurse and patient come to know and respect each other, as persons who are alike and yet different; as persons who share the solutions of problems'.[5]

Her account conceives of the nurse as detached from the person being cared for, and although she suggests that professional closeness shares some features with the physical closeness and interpersonal intimacy found in non-professional relationships, its focus is exclusively on the interests and needs of the patient. Effectively, she distinguishes 'professional closeness' as non-reciprocal, demonstrated by the nurse who can 'put herself aside and can bring all of her capacities and talents to bear upon the life of another person to the end that that person will grow a little, learn something new and, in effect, be strengthened in a favourable direction.'[6]

As Savage notes, the closeness that Peplau refers to is 'not so much a matter of being closer to the person who is ill, but rather one of being "closer to the truth" of that person's possible life-threatening dilemma'.[7] The cultivation of a special kind of detachment, demonstrating concern, competence, and interest, while maintaining an emotional distance, is the hallmark of Peplau's model.

More recently, there is evidence of an alternative view, and the themes of the patient knowing the nurse as a person and working in partnership have received considerable attention by nurses as part of effective cancer nursing practice.[8–11]

In 1991, McMahon and Pearson published their important book *Nursing as Therapy*.[11] This did not offer a definitive explanation of what nursing as therapy is, since the role of the nurse depends on many societal and health care factors that are far from static. Instead, the authors set out their developing ideas, founded on the belief that a certain form of nursing, which involves deliberate nurse decision making, has a powerful effect on the patient and promotes adaptation, healing, and health.

Areas in which nursing was considered to have therapeutic potential were:

- the nurse–patient relationship
- the interpersonal care environment
- providing comfort
- conventional and unconventional nursing interventions
- patient teaching.

The first two areas are the subject of this chapter.

MacMahon and Pearson believe that the ideal nurse–patient relationship involves mutuality or reciprocity. They consider the ideas of Muetzel, who focused on three elements that coalesce in the encounter between nurse and patient: partnership, intimacy, and reciprocity.[12] As key ingredients of a therapeutic nursing process, interaction between each pair of concepts generates three further concepts of atmosphere, spirit, and dynamics with concomitant defining characteristics.

What Muetzel is attempting to clarify through her therapeutic practice descriptors is the nature of the nurse's use of 'self ' within the relationship. It is valid for the nurse and the patient to disclose their feelings and benefit from the relationship, and she argues that the nurse who is 'self-aware' has a special contribution to make in the relationship, and that this self-awareness is a necessity for the achievement and evaluation of a subjectively therapeutic encounter. As Muetzel puts it:

'Being there' is that intangible and paradoxically difficult and very simple essence of the dimension of reciprocity and intimacy. It is simple because it is in the desire for closeness of the philanthropic vocation 'to help people'; difficult because a closeness that is mutually beneficial in a therapeutic relationship requires mature confrontation by the nurse . . . of the vulnerability of her own humanness [pp.106–107].

People with cancer demand and help to evoke a particularly sensitive use of the self by nurses.[13]

The value of 'being with' the patient or providing 'existential presence' has been explored by other writers. Halldorsdottir considers that there are five modes of being with another, each representing a qualitatively different degree of caring (Box 8.1).[14]

Box 8.1 Halldorsdottir's 'Five modes of being with another'[14]

- *Life-giving* – affirming the personhood of the other
- *Life-sustaining* – acknowledging the personhood of the other
- *Life-neutral* – where there is no effect on the life of the other
- *Life-restraining* – which is detached from the true centre of the other
- *Life-destroying* – which depersonalises the other.

Kitson[15] and Ersser[16] both explore the therapeutic dimension of nursing in their research, while Campbell describes the companionship that nurses offer as a 'closeness' that is neither sexual nor deep personal friendship, but a bodily presence; it involves a 'being with' and not just a 'doing to'.[17]

A therapeutic nurse relationship

The work of Carper[18] and Benner and Wrubel[19] helps in establishing a working definition of what a therapeutic nurse–patient relationship may be. Carper describes fundamental patterns of nursing knowledge (Box 8.2).[18]

Box 8.2 Carper's patterns of nursing knowledge[18]

- The scientific knowledge of human behaviour
- The aesthetic perception of significant experiences
- A personal understanding of the unique individuality of the self
- The capacity to make choices within concrete situations involving particular moral judgements.

She stresses that none of the patterns is sufficient in itself and that if:

. . . the design of nursing care is to be more than habitual or mechanical, the capacity to *perceive and interpret* the subjective experiences of others and to imaginatively project the effect of nursing actions on their lives, becomes a necessary skill.[18]

The capacity of nurses to perceive and interpret the subjective experiences of others is the central tenet of the 'helping role' of the nurse as defined by Benner, who makes the fundamental point that 'the ability to interpret concerns enables the health care provider to help people deal with their illnesses'.[19] Since, in order to understand how someone feels, you must understand what they say, comprehending the meaning of the spoken word is a vital part of therapeutic nursing practice.

It is worth making a distinction between an identical expression of anxiety to a close friend during a 'heart-to-heart' and that which can take place between a nurse and the person being cared for. The difference lies in the imaginative, purposeful, and strategic use the nurse makes of the 'data' the person has offered. The nurse may use this information to facilitate further disclosure or, if necessary, delay it. The heart-to-heart with the friend may be enormously helpful but is very different from a professional relationship, in which data 'about' the person and the experience of 'being with' them endorse each other and help the nurse to structure her interventions. The nurse practising therapeutically will create an emotional climate that will enable the person to explore their thoughts and feelings about their cancer illness progressively, to review problems and difficulties, and to have a sense of self-mastery.[20,21]

These theoretical ideas concerning the ideal therapeutic relationship are helpful in conceptualising the nature and range of relationships that may exist for nurses and the association between these and the experience or expertise of individual nurses. However, they do not consider the impact of the workplace organisation and ethos on nurses' professional relationships. Since they also overlook the collective nature of nursing work, any identified failure of the nurse to create a therapeutic relationship would rest firmly with the individual nurse.

Professional and policy context

UK health policy over the last 15 or 20 years can be seen as the bringing in of successive waves of rationality, with the government aim of calling various groups of health care professionals to account.[22] Rational approaches to managing health care were sought from within private sector organisations, a search that culminated in the introduction of general management and the 'internal market' into the health service,[23] ideas which underpin recent cancer and palliative care policy.[24]

Some claim that the impact of these changes on nurses' professional activity is minimal,[25] while others consider that moves such as the incorporation of professionals into management roles is an effective way of controlling their activity and thinking. The professional is a member of a team, and beyond that an employing organisation, and so subject to the rules, plans, and priorities of that organisation.

That accounting system initiatives, such as resource management, may have far-reaching effects upon both the practice and values of nurses has been noted by Bloomfield *et al.*[26] These systems develop standards of behaviour such that 'normal' practice can be not only defined, but also measured, and deviations and outcomes noted. What is also implied is that what is rendered visible, measured, and rewarded gains legitimacy. Conversely, that which is not recognised by the formal system may not be considered legitimate and consequently not rewarded. This is exactly the conclusion James reached about the lack of value attributed to emotional care by nurses.[27]

This raises several problems for the emotion-focused work of nurses where there can be no unequivocal answer about 'success' or about whether a particular intervention is 'good'. The nursing strategy will be based on value and choice – without the freedom of that choice, no therapy based on self-mastery could ever hope to succeed. The very nature of the intervention makes it problematic to evaluate.

The emotion-focused work of cancer nurses received a significant policy boost with the National Institute of Clinical Excellence guidance on cancer services, particularly the document *Guidance on Cancer Services: Improving Supportive and Palliative Care for Adults with Cancer.*[28] The aim of this 200-page document is to define a service model to ensure that patients with cancer, their families, and other carers receive support to help them cope with the diagnosis of cancer and its treatment.

While not wishing to detract from the overall benefits of the guidance, it is important to our discussion that the guidance outlines services that are designed to *react* to psychological distress when it is identified. In other words clinical care is provided as a reactive service. In such a model, varying interventions are provided in relation to the level of distress identified in the person with cancer. There is little room in such service models of care for the prevention of psychological distress in people affected by cancer or for fostering ways in which individuals may be actively supported to manage their worry and distress. Once again, what is rendered visible and can be measured gains legitimacy. A reorientation of thinking is needed to recognise this, also that the type of service provided may in fact be a significant determinant of the level of distress that patients experience.

The roots of the managerialism described above are traced to the growth of bureaucracies by Davies who comments upon the way that formality and distance are not only valued within bureaucracies but seen as the only route to rational decision making.[29]

Traynor examines the impact of this managerial rationality on nurses' work.[30] In his research study he explores the value systems of the new general managers and the nursing workforce of

Commentary 8.1 A possible reading of the nurse's comment (after Traynor[30])

The nurse sets the scene, telling of the intrusion into nursing of a contrasting and alien set of values. While the way she lists the characteristics of this new value system – 'customer, computer, audit and budget' – are not intrinsically undesirable, we experience them as such, particularly when contrasted with the traditional and human terms 'empathy', 'bedside manner' and 'care'.

Perhaps by her use of the verb 'replace' and the words 'being replaced by' rather than 'are replaced', the nurse is enacting in words a passivity and powerlessness that she feels with her profession. As a consequence, we are encouraged to see the nurse as the victim in this situation.

'Coming in' identifies the business orientation as a fad and reinforces the idea of an inappropriate intrusion, with the nurse as the victim.

The third sentence can be understood in a number of ways. Its metaphor is one of the body. A possible reading is as a plea for a body (nursing), which is at the moment divided against itself to become integrated; for eye and hand to work together. Upper body organs are traditionally associated with rationality and so they are here, with 'thoughtful eyes' needing to combine with the lower organs, hands. Atypically these lower organs are given a privileged position in the nurse's account as they are associated with the physical world of practical action, 'caring for our patients'. This is, at once, the end purpose of nursing and of her statement. The whole may be regarded as a desire for balance and integration; to reconnect and reground the rational, non-physical aspects of the organisation and profession that are becoming dominant and disconnected from physical, practical concerns.

These words are being replaced by customer, computer, audit, budget. Why don't we start looking down at our hands with our thoughtful eyes and using common sense and intelligence; use those hands practically, to care for our patient?[30]

Traynor's view is that organisational strategies, which have emphasised continuity of care, camouflage extensions to the power of management control over the professional activity of nurses. However, the profession has responded positively to these developments. One response may reflect nursing's unique version of professional autonomy, characterised by moral agency and self-sacrifice.

The commitment to continuity of care is clearly expressed in what has been referred to as 'the new nursing',[31] typified by primary nursing, which explicitly aims to transform relationships with patients and promote their participation in care. As such, primary nursing is one example of an organisational mode in which communication is viewed as a central and legitimate aspect of nurses' work.[32] Underlying the 'new nursing' is a belief that the relationship between nurse and patient has the potential to be therapeutic and central to the process of recovery.

Professional debate about specialist and advanced practice roles also drives theoretical discussion and practice initiatives concerning the therapeutic nature of cancer nursing. Questions that have arisen include whether it is possible for all nurses in cancer care to develop therapeutic relationships with the people in their care; what sort of environment or 'culture' is most conducive and supportive of this way of working; and what part might be played by an advanced nurse practitioner.

The role of advanced practitioner in cancer care encompasses more than expert nursing practice. Although there is no consensus view of such posts, they are generally considered to be multidimensional.[33] The final results of Manley's action research project identified the subroles of the consultant nurse as: nursing practice; consultancy; management processes; and leadership. Manley argues that an integration of these roles is needed to promote and develop clinical nursing from clinical to stategic and policy levels, while

four first-wave NHS community-based trusts through analysis of their talk. The managers' talk emphasises quantities, levels, numerical patterns; in short, it is disembodied knowledge, while embodied meaning and a language of closeness and human values haunt the nurses' talk. The conflict experienced by the nurses is distressingly evident, as illustrated by the comments of one staff nurse in a community hospital:

I'm dissatisfied with 'simple is best' attitude in nursing being replaced by 'let's communicate', 'high tech' attitude coming in. Empathy, bedside manner, care.

simultaneously creating and sustaining a culture in which nurses and nursing strive for more effective patient-centred services.[34]

Manley highlighted not only the knowledge, skill, and expertise needed within identified subroles, but also the personal qualities and processes by which the advanced practitioner/consultant nurse fulfils each subrole (see Figure 8.1). These bear remarkable resemblance to qualities attributed to counselling relationships.[21]

Corner takes up the debate and recasts the dimensions of the advanced practitioner role into 'cancer nursing as therapy'.[2] This, Corner suggests, has the potential to operate on four levels to effect radical reconstruction of care, cancer services, and wider health care environments, so that they are more patient focused and offer 'nursing as therapy' as an integral part of cancer care. These levels include:

- fundamental knowledge and theory generation for therapeutic practice

- therapeutic interventions for individuals or problems
- developing and changing health systems or environments
- critique and reconstruction of care from a societal perspective.

Crucial to the accounts of Manley and Corner is the idea of radical change and facilitation of a 'transformational culture', which enables the therapeutic work of nurses.

The broad idea of 'cancer nursing as therapy' outlined above, is offered as a contemporary vision of the necessary professional and organisational context for the concerns of this chapter, which are the emotion-focused interventions of cancer nurses working in one-to-one relationships with patients. It is for a variety of reasons that the nurse–patient relationship has come to be redefined. However, the extent and nature of the change required to realise the vision are likely to be immense.

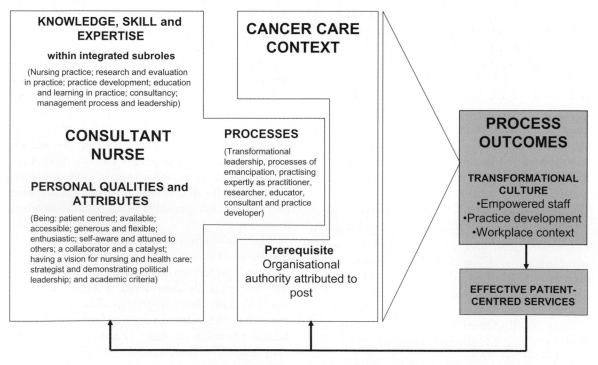

Figure 8.1 Framework for the concept of the consultant nurse and its relationship between context and outcomes. Adapted with permission from Manley K. (2002). Refining the consultant nurse framework: commentary on critique. *Nursing in Critical Care* **7**, 84–87, Blackwell.[34]

Organisational context

Glaser and Strauss were the first to expose the profound emotional basis for the social organisation and context of care in relation to people with cancer and the dying.[35] In their important study they not only identified the troubling reality of awareness categories in relation to a dying person but also described ways in which knowledge about diagnosis and prognosis was used to disallow or control feelings.

James develops this theme of emotion management in her examination of the disclosure of a cancer diagnosis.[36] She describes the management of emotions at this time by lay and professional carers, noting that many manage by denying rather than engaging with emotions. She attributes differences in emotion management to different levels of involvement with the feelings associated with the cancer and competing forms of status and knowledge. These then influence the organisational and interpersonal mechanisms used to manage the feelings, such as the use of particular kinds of space and time, more or less public encounters, denial of the emotion, limiting the information released, formal and informal disciplinary rules, gender-divided labour and, most significantly, senior staff setting the context, routines, and rituals within which other staff and clients can express their anxieties and feelings.

In her study of nursing practices in a London teaching hospital, Isabel Menzies noticed that, far from responding in contextually sensitive ways to particular patients, nurses were task centred and, for example, awoke people in their care to give them drugs, regardless of need. Also, finding that nurses rotated frequently between wards, Menzies argued that these organisational procedures and practices became an end in themselves. They were rituals that were not designed to help people who were hospitalised, but rather enabled the nurses to contain the anxiety of working with the sick and dying.[37] The nurses did not have to think about what they were doing and, by not thinking, they could avoid feeling anxious. Menzies called such rituals social defences.

Menzies felt that 'although by the very nature of her profession the nurse is at considerable risk of being flooded by intense and unmanageable anxiety', the nature of nursing did not, by itself, account for the high levels of anxiety apparent in nurses. The very techniques used by nurses to contain and modify the anxiety appeared to constitute part of the problem. Not recognising the individual needs of people helped detachment, and led to minimising the mutual interaction of nurses with people in their care, since this might lead to 'attachment'. This trend was reinforced by an implicit operational policy of 'detachment', where the assumption was that a nurse would not mind moving from ward to ward, or hospital to hospital, without notice. The pain and distress of the moving, of breaking stable and continuing relationships, are implicitly denied by the system, although often stressed personally by people (including senior nurses who initiate such moves) within the system. In addition, nurses were encouraged to deny any disturbing feelings that arose within relationships. Those nurses facing difficulties were reprimanded rather than supported.

It is arguable that these social defence systems do not exist in cancer care today. If task allocation protected the nurse from anxiety, new organisational modes stressing continuity of care have stripped this defence away and pose new, personal challenges for nurses. There is compelling evidence to suggest that cancer nurses and their professional colleagues have generated various new 'systems' to organise their own work, the care environment, and cancer services in ways that may reflect a spectrum of techniques to defend against, contain, or modify what Menzies calls 'the unmanageable anxiety' of their work.

Lawton's detailed ethnographic study of the care of dying patients in hospices and day care provides complex examples of this.[38] Lawton describes how the suffering that patients actually experience is masked and can be hidden away in inpatient facilities and professional idealism that elevate the dying to heroic status. A study of hopelessness and how it is represented on a leukaemia ward is another example of a defensive system. This study revealed that 'hope work' was conducted within an objectifying medical frame as opposed to the person's own frame of reference. Not only was the legitimacy and credibility of the medical version of reality maintained, but emotionally charged conversations were largely avoided.[39]

Another interesting example is research that was carried out on two wards where a high proportion of people with gastrointestinal cancers were nursed.[40] One ward used a primary nursing approach and the other patient allocation. The aim of the study was to explore ways in which nurses managed interactions and, in particular, their 'closeness' or intimacy while caring for people.

Data revealed that nurses managed deep, close, and consistent relationships with them, not only by expressive behaviours including the use of touch, body posture, and humour, but by transforming the ward into a symbolic space in which the relationship became analogous with family relationships. Savage deduces that reconstructing the context of care in domestic rather than institutional terms enabled the nurses to deal better with the many anxieties and ambiguities of emotional closeness inherent in the 'new nursing'. The 'family' or the 'home' were not the only observed models for providing a context of care. It seemed that 'camaraderie' in the nurse team offered an alternative.

Another relevant finding from Savage's study is that the realisation of contexts for care deemed to have a therapeutic potential is less dependent upon the organisational mode of nursing on the ward than on the interrelationship of this with specific local conditions of the hospital infrastructure including resource allocation, the approach of general management, and the attitudes of other members of the health care team. The work of Smith supports this.[41]

The point is that feelings and how they are managed contribute to and reflect the structure and culture of the cancer care setting.[42] It is useful to consider communication patterns in this light.

Communication patterns in cancer care settings

Communication in cancer care settings is characterised by the avoidance of difficult or painful topics and misunderstandings that arise between the person who has cancer, their family, and the involved health care professionals.[43–45]

Sociologists attribute the cause of avoidance and misunderstandings to the nature of health care professional–patient relationships, which are largely dependent upon the power inherent in professional expertise and specialised knowledge.[46]

A considerable amount of the research on doctor–patient and nurse–patient communication in cancer care has been conducted specifically to analyse and to criticise the means, methods, asymmetry, and humaneness of the relationships.[47] The language doctors use in encounters with people with cancer has been shown repeatedly to reflect the non-egalitarian nature of the relationship.[48,49]

There is recognition from within the professions of the huge complexity of communicating with people who have cancer and their families.[50,51] Almost 30 years ago Souhami highlighted the particular difficulties for doctors who often have to deal with probability rather than certainty of treatment outcome, and repeatedly may be the bearers of bad news. The doctor also has to contend with the high expectations of team members, that these encounters will be good and that he or she will 'get it right'.[52]

It is suggested in this book that cancer illness in Western biomedical culture is itself dependent upon this relationship, the encounter with the expert medical oncologist, radiotherapist, or cancer geneticist, for its definition. This emphasises the point that, whatever else it is, cancer illness exists as a social phenomenon, constructed through the interaction of the person with his or her relatives, the doctor, the nurse, and society at large.

Some studies of doctor–patient interaction have focused in recent years on problems of communication often caused by conflicting notions concerning the nature of this relationship.[53]

Mishler considers the root cause of these difficulties to lie in the asymmetrical nature of medical consultations and presents the analogy of a struggle between *voices*: on the one hand, the 'voice of medicine' and on the other, the 'voice of the life-world' representing, respectively, the 'technical–scientific' assumptions of medicine and the natural attitudes of 'everyday life'.[54]

According to this model, the doctor is seen as pursuing a line of talk determined almost exclusively by biomedicine, which is often at odds with the person's own view, representing what Mishler terms 'life-world contexts'. Since the talk is dominated by the voice of medicine, argues Mishler, any contribution from the voice of the life-world is regarded by the doctor as an interruption. Conversely, any interruption by the voice of medicine when the person is speaking is not an interruption at all, but a return to reality, that is to the dominant medical techno-rational reality. The medical voice is clearly indicated within consultations by the typical patterns of:

Doctor: question
Patient: response
Doctor: assessment/next question.

The tendency of doctors to use closed rather than open-ended questions serves further to maintain the doctor's control of talk. This in turn strengthens the biomedical model as the framework of the talk and permits the doctor to carry out the medical tasks of diagnosis and prescription, while avoiding discussion of the person's feelings and individual response to their cancer illness.[53]

This bias towards the 'voice of medicine' prevails in cancer care today, which is surprising considering the emphasis since the 1970s on the emotional needs of people with cancer, influenced in particular by the pioneering work of Kubler-Ross,[55] and also the beliefs about the ultimate benefits of:

- adopting a client-centred approach of open-ended questions
- explaining medical agendas
- the use of the person's own words in asking further questions
- listening with minimum interruption

to engender collaborative models of care based on desired right choice and self-determination for people with cancer.[56]

It may be that the coercive strength of medically orientated styles of talk is so entrenched in social attitudes that the style has become naturalised. Indeed, when ill, many people would feel uncomfortable without the asymmetry of the relationship with their doctor.

Silverman suggests that despite their pleas for humanism and equality, proponents of the client-centred approach are unwittingly reinforcing the central strategy of power in the doctor–patient relationship.[46] Attempts to conduct the relationship along the lines of an equal partnership would only be a simulation and would leave intact the essential nature of the power imbalance, which is based upon professional expertise and specialised knowledge. This situation is further complicated by the fact that recent technological advances mean that often oncologists and radiotherapists are working at the fringes of their own knowledge, and the consultation is therefore forever threatened with becoming the domain of 'another expert', in which any progress towards interactional symmetry would have to begin again.

Other sociologists, in assessing the power relation within the medical interview, have been heavily influenced by the work of Foucault,[57] and perceive the client-centred approach that has come to dominate first progressive and now mainstream thinking in cancer care, as little more than a placebo designed to obscure the real 'treatment' of an all-encompassing form of surveillance in which the medical gaze can roam freely.[58] They regard the arguments of the supporters of this approach as tenuous, relying as they do on the belief that liberation from the tyranny of conflicting and unequal power relationships can somehow be achieved by an incitement of the person to talk and by encouraging the doctor to listen.

These writings and research evidence present health care professionals with an impasse that must be negotiated if any meaning or credibility is to be salvaged. Silverman suggests that there is a way out and that it lies in individual practitioners rejecting pre-established roles and evading stereotyped talk with people, but instead constructing their own dialogues with them.[46]

Nevertheless, stereotyped interprofessional relationships account for some of the patterns of communication in cancer care. Nurses perceive that they often do not have sufficient clinical information to respond to the questions that are posed by people who are anxious about their illness, and that, even if they had, their own and others' expectations of their role may preclude further discussion.

According to some researchers, the positive effects of a good communication climate, in which there is open communication within the team, stimulate the 'therapeutic' interventions of individual practitioners, lead to an attitude of openness to feelings and have a beneficial effect on team members' mental health.[59] Earlier work revealed that individual nurses take fewer risks in emotionally hazardous one-to-one conversations with people they are caring for than as members of groups.[60] Certain characteristics of the group facilitate risk taking and these include:

• the extent to which risk taking is a norm of the group
• the extent to which exchange of feelings is possible
• the extent to which members of the group support each other
• the extent to which responsibility can be shared.

Results from these studies caution against solutions aimed at improving the emotional focus of cancer care which are confined to the organisation of the nursing team or interventions solely reliant upon nurses. Improvement will depend on changes in working methods and working relationships between nurses, doctors, and management.

There is growing evidence not only that the expression of feelings may affect someone's ability to adjust to their diagnosis of cancer and cope with treatment, but also that such disclosure may also influence recurrence and progression of disease.[61] Cancer nurses acknowledge this and also recognise the power of communication to arouse or assuage the fear that often accompanies cancer.[62] Yet numerous studies reveal that patterns of nurses' communication are dominated by routinised, stereotyped and overtly controlling forms of communication, which serve to maintain the conversation at a superficial level.

Avoidance of potentially difficult and emotional discussions of poor prognosis and death was identified by Glaser and Strauss in the seminal work, *Awareness of Dying*, as being surrounded by a 'conspiracy of silence'.[35] They identified various forms of this, each dominated by secrets and silence: 'closed awareness' existed when health care professionals chose not to tell someone of their poor prognosis and impending death; 'suspected awareness', was where the patient has a hint of the truth; and in 'mutual pretence', both parties, the health professionals and the patient, knew but chose to remain silent.[35]

Although there have been dramatic changes in the behaviour of health professionals with regard to telling someone their cancer diagnosis and prognosis, so that by the late 1970s most doctors said that they informed patients,[63] the reality is that uncertainty often exists about what has been said to whom and when. This affects team communication and requires constant vigilance by all members of the team.

Parkes recognised that questions may be asked of nurses that would not be asked of a doctor because a nurse can be more easily disbelieved if the information about the illness is given when someone is not ready to know.[64] He acknowledged that the systematic investigation of such 'defended talk' is very difficult.

The idea of 'defended' talk introduces an additional explanation for the patterns of communication existing in cancer care settings. This concerns the attitudes and levels of anxiety and the stress experienced by health care professionals working with cancer patients, and includes the patient as one who can avoid and deny distressing thoughts and feelings as effectively as a nurse or doctor, thus 'blocking' professional help.

Health care professionals' attitudes and defences to cancer

Repeated reports to the health ombudsman of insensitive, inattentive treatment, particularly of people who are dying and their families, have led to investigations into the importance of health care professionals' attitudes in the care of cancer patients and also to investigations of the levels of stress experienced by staff.

Attitudes
There is reliable evidence that nurses hold stereotyped, negative attitudes to cancer, which

significantly affect their behaviour and communication with people who have cancer,[65,66] Some more experienced trained nurses hold a more optimistic view of cancer, but they are in the minority. Elkind found that most nurses considered it at least sometimes true that cancer treatment can do more harm than good and that they were pessimistic regarding the number of deaths caused by cancer, sharing the same fears as the general population.[67]

The association of cancer with death and suffering held by many individuals is carefully analysed by Stacey, who explores the cultural meanings of cancer.[68] From her analysis, cancer emerges as a symbol of death and suffering, and the societal battle against cancer is then seen as the struggle to resist acceptance of the inevitability in life of death, decay, and decomposition. These overall trends play a significant role in the development of attitudes amongst individuals.

One well-documented danger in negative-attitude, stereotype-governed health care professional behaviours is that people who have cancer may 'become' the stereotype.[69] For example, nursing staff guided by a strong prior belief that a diagnosis of cancer is hopeless and that all who have it suffer and die from their disease may, through their conversational approach, instill that belief in the person themself.

A study by Mood and Lick designed to examine nurses' attitudes to the terminally ill provides some evidence for this.[70] In their study, increased use of negative words (e.g. no, not, never, nothing, none), and substitution of the impersonal pronoun 'it' for death, were found in discussions of death as opposed to other topics. They concluded that such subtle encoding of the nurses' own fear, anxiety, and negative attitudes to death significantly altered the quality of the message communicated to dying people and their families, and would confirm feelings of helplessness and hopelessness.

Stress

Since the early work of Vachon et al.,[71] there has been a recognition that health professionals who work closely with people who have cancer can experience stress from their work, arising from the deterioration and death of patients, and from dealing with the emotional distress.[72] In a recent Delphi study to identify cancer nursing research priorities in Northern Ireland, the top priority areas were psychosocial issues, and professional issues relating to nurse burnout, and stress.[73]

Reviews and research studies over the last 15 years, focusing on stress and burnout in those caring for people with cancer, have used quasi-experimental designs to attempt to delineate the specific variables of stress within predetermined categories, using a variety of measurement scales.[74–76] For example, Kent et al. examined the relationship between oncology staff's perceived success in helping patients and their levels of stress using the Maslach Burnout Inventory (MBI), the Hospital Anxiety and Depression Scale (HADS), and intention to leave their current post.[77] Isikhan et al. relied on self-report questionnaires, a Job Stress Inventory and a Ways of Coping Inventory in their study to determine in health care professionals working with cancer patients the factors influencing stress and the strategies used to cope with it.[78]

Sources of stress consistently identified are:

- feeling overloaded with work and the effect of this on home life
- poor management support and resource/staffing limitations
- dealing with patients' suffering
- death and dying
- relationships with other health professionals
- lack of experience.

Working with cancer may force health professionals to face their own mortality and that of their family and friends. In addition, the conflict between the curative goals of medicine and the reality that many people will not respond to treatment in the long term, can lead to tensions between cancer care team members, as well as death being seen as a personal failure.[79] In palliative care, working with people who have incurable disease and who are dying is thought to barrage health professionals daily with suffering and tragedy.[80]

As a result of the particular demands made of them, cancer health professionals are perceived to experience high levels of job stress and to be at risk of developing work-related distress or compassion fatigue.[81] As highlighted earlier this may have repercussions for interprofessional work relations and organisational efficiency within the cancer care setting.[82]

However, according to this body of research, levels of distress do not appear to be uniquely high for those working with cancer compared to other health care professionals. Two large surveys conducted by Ramirez' research group interestingly contradict these results. In 1995 Ramirez *et al.* conducted a survey to assess the mental health of UK hospital consultants.[83] A 27% prevalence of psychiatric morbidity among 882 repondents from five specialties: gastroenterology, radiology, surgical oncology, clinical oncology, and medical oncology, was reported. This prevalence was markedly higher than the 18% of the general population. Ramirez decided to re-assess the situation in 2002 because much had changed in the NHS.[84] Additional funding for health care had been committed and the consultant workforce had expanded. However, patients' expectations regarding their care have risen and clinicians face new pressures, which include: implementation of new policies to drive service improvement, including the *NHS Cancer Plan*,[85] and associated National Service Framework; introduction of targets; formal procedures for consultant appraisal; and changes in clinical governance. In essence Ramirez *et al.* resurveyed their initial study cohort and added a new cohort, from the same five specialties, of consultants who were new to the grade since 1994. Psychiatric morbidity was estimated with the 12-item General Health Questionnaire (GHQ-12), emotional exhaustion, the principal component of burnout, was assessed by the MBI, and job stress and satisfaction were measured by a study-specific questionnaire. The proportion of consultants with psychiatric morbidity rose from 27% in 1994 to 32% in 2002. The prevalence of emotional exhaustion increased from 32% in 1994 to 41% in 2002. Multivariate analysis showed that increased job stress without a comparable increase in job satisfaction accounted for the decline in mental health, which was especially marked in clinical and surgical oncologists. Ramirez *et al.* conclude that the reconfiguration of cancer services driven by the *Calman–Hine Report* and *NHS Cancer Plan*, while

benefiting patients, might contribute to the increased job stress without similar, and thereby protective, increased job satisfaction for clinical oncologists and surgical oncologists. The implications of these findings for care, in addition to the personal suffering of health professionals, point to the need for action to reduce burnout and stress among those professional groups, and to support them and enhance their job satisfaction.

It is difficult to know what to make of the counter-intuitive findings of research that fails to identify dealing with fatal illness and death as a major source of job stress among cancer professionals.[86–88] Perhaps the explanation lies in the way in which stress is conceptualised by these researchers and the influence this has on study design.

Though it is often not explicit, in most cases a psychological approach to stress underpins research studies. Lazarus is the main exponent of this.[89] He maintains that stress occurs when there are demands on the individual that he or she cannot cope with or adjust to. Stress arises when the individual perceives and evaluates this situation as threatening. The model incorporates the concept of appraisal and reappraisal, together with the transactional view that stress can only be defined by the relationship between the individual and his or her environment. The premise of this model is that there is a 'right' way to cope and manage thoughts and feelings, and a range of 'appropriate' responses to stress.

What this model largely omits, argue Benner and Wrubel, is the view that stressful experiences and coping options are constituted by a person's unique involvement in a situation and their skills, concerns, meanings, particular history, and anticipation and projection of themselves into the future.[19]

One explanation for the counter-intuitive results could lie therefore in the mechanistic approach to the experience of stress in which an individual's stress is measured by a variety of tools at a single point in time without thought for the changing nature of stress or the societal or organisational context of it.

Irrational processes highlight another possible limitation of classic stress theory. Theorists such as Lazarus or the more sociologically orientated

Pearlin[90] have argued that all individuals face continuing stressors and that coping strategies and cognitive reappraisals are mechanisms for reducing stress. But because these theorists do not link the experience of stress to people's feelings of anxiety, they may have posed the issue of stress too narrowly and focused their solutions too narrowly on rational means.

When anxiety intrudes, rational thinking is distorted by irrational processes. For example, nurses in many oncology units 'fight' chronically with doctors over treatment policy, each blaming the other for the gap between expectation and treatment outcome. Because they feel anxious, they project their sense of blame and failure outwards, often scapegoating the person they need to work closely with, to reduce the stress they face.

Psychodynamic concepts, which highlight how people use one another to stabilise their inner lives and feelings and then how these psychodynamic processes within people help to shape the relationships between them, may be particularly helpful in understanding the stress health care professionals experience when working with cancer patients.[91] The ideas may go some way to providing an explanation for the low levels of communication identified in some research studies between cancer care professionals and patients, and the apparent endemic verbal 'blocking' behaviours.

Defences

Sometimes aspects of ourselves and our experience conflict with our consciously held ideals. These aspects of ourselves and our experiences cannot be easily assimilated into our conscious view of ourselves because of the anxiety or psychic pain they arouse. We may find it easier to function by suppressing and denying difficult or painful experiences and memories.[92,93]

When our work brings us into contact with cancer, it can be a very powerful experience because those in our care may be attempting to relieve their internal pains and distress by externalising them, and requiring us to contain and carry aspects of these. The difficulty for us is that we too have our own internal processes to contend with, such as our own unresolved conflicts and impulses, particularly those to do with death and destructiveness.

For brief periods we may be able to tolerate considerable anxiety and bear considerable mental pain and depression, for instance following a bereavement. Alternatively, we may try to ward off such emotional discomfort by employing a number of defence mechanisms (see Table 8.1). The defences work through the processes of *splitting, projection*, and *introjection*.[94,95]

Menzies' interpretation of how nurses protect themselves against the anxiety caused by primitive feelings and impulses elicited by physical and psychological closeness to people in their care illustrates these processes.[96]

Menzies observed that nurses feel the anxiety and stress of helping sick people who might die and that they often engaged in physical care that by 'ordinary standards is distasteful, disgusting and frightening'. The nurses are unable to balance and integrate powerful and opposing feelings of compassion for the ill person and revulsion at their physical state. Unconsciously, the nurses welcome depersonalised care practices as a way of relieving themselves of contradictory feelings and of keeping the good feelings separate from the bad ones. By *splitting off* their sense of personal authority and agency from their own experience and *projecting* it outside – onto the ritual of drug administration, for example – they relieved themselves of the anxiety of the patient's experience. The nurses also psychologically took in, or *introjected*, the new authority of the rituals to justify their depersonalised relationship to the people in their care. Thus, through the linked processes of splitting, projection, and introjection, the nurses lent their individual and collective authority to ritual care, which in turn authorised them to behave in a depersonalised way. The milieu and thrust of present-day cancer care challenges the defences of health care professionals by ever-increasing complex combination treatments, long illness trajectories, new technologies, increased specialisation and possible fragmentation, consumer expectations, and competition for patient contracts and research funds. As the risks of work grow, anxiety increases as well.

Menzies' work and other studies by psychoanalysts suggest that health care professionals may be deeply 'defended' against the stresses and anxieties of caring for people who have cancer. In a classic

Table 8.1 Defences against anxiety commonly encountered in everyday clinical work

Denial	A defence mechanism by which either an aspect of the self is denied or some painful experience is denied.
Suppression	A conscious attempt to forget or deny and to avoid thinking about something.
Repression	An idea may be unconsciously repressed owing to its unthinkable nature. It may be an idea or feeling that conflicts with our view of ourselves and what is acceptable. It is prevented from coming to consciousness.
Splitting	Involves separation of good and bad aspects of the self and others, or between good and bad feelings.
Projecting	Externalising unacceptable feelings and then attributing them to others or an object.
Projective identification	Projecting not only feelings but important aspects of the self onto others so that that person feels and owns qualities and impulses that are otherwise not their own.
Reaction formation	Going to an opposite extreme to obscure unacceptable feelings, e.g. excessive calm to hide panic.
Rationalisation	Justifying an unconscious impulse or giving a good reason for something but it is not applicable to the situation.
Psychosomatic reactions	Unacceptable feelings may be converted into physical symptoms.
Phobic avoidance	Avoiding situations that arouse unpleasant feelings.
Displacement	Being too afraid to express feelings to the person who provoked them and deflecting them elsewhere.
Regression	If we feel unable to cope we may regress to more childlike and dependent ways of behaving.
Sublimation	Unconscious drives are allowed partial expression in modified, socially acceptable, even desirable ways.

paper entitled 'The ailment', Main considers that our choice to work with cancer has deep personal reasons and that it has abiding unconscious determinants, such as the need to heal sick parts of ourselves.[97] There is therefore a range of feelings that may invade us as we work, including anxiety, guilt, depression, and compulsive reparative wishes.

Rather than being aware of our defences, which are developmentally normal and protect us from excessive anxiety, and ensuring they are reasonably flexible to enable us to remain open to distress, our defences can become immovable barriers to thoughtful, responsive practice. Institutional cancer care settings may actively contribute to this, since to keep the institution functioning and individual cancer care professionals functioning within it, time and other constraints only permit working at a superficial level.

This provides an alternative reading to the mainstream studies of stresses and burnout among cancer care professionals, in which the comparatively low levels of stress found may be an indicator of the extent and effectiveness of staff's defences against the anxiety of their work, rather than an accurate indicator of their stress.

Methodological issues in researching and evaluating the nature and impact of the nurse–patient relationship in cancer care

Research is needed that will not only enhance understanding of the complex processes of communication between nurses and people with cancer, but also provide evidence of the value claimed, and indicate the nature of support and education required, to facilitate this therapeutic opportunity.

Almost all nurse–patient communication research to date has been carried out with a positivist psychological orientation. One consequence of this has been the focus on quantitative approaches concerned with the attributes of nurses or an enumeration of their communication skills (see Table 8.2). There has been a tendency in this research to

Table 8.2 Examples of research exploring cancer nurses' practice in comprehending and responding to patients' concerns

Study	Method	Findings
Hunt (1989)[99]	Extended case study within an ethnographic framework. Tape recordings of nurse–patient conversations over 3 months.	Patients did not express wishes to discuss their feelings. Processes that promoted expression of feelings, the meaning of death or spiritual need were limited.
Wilkinson (1991)[47]	Tape-recorded nurse–patient interactions followed by semi-structured interviews with the nurses. Coding frame used to categorise 'blocking' or 'facilitating' interventions by the nurse.	54% of nurses' verbal behaviours found to be 'blocking'; psychological and emotional needs assessment largely ignored by nurses.
Lanceley (1995)[1]	Tape-recorded nurse–patient conversations. Nurse–participant reflective interviews. Discourse analysis, including analysis of figurative language.	Patients expressed their feelings to nurses. Conversations were jointly constructed. Nurses' response to patients' emotional expression was highly variable. The impact on nurses of cancer patients' expressions of feelings has been underestimated. Study revealed a depth and range of emotional expression to nurses.
Heaven and Maguire (1996)[100]	Pre-test tape recordings of an assessment interview and nurses' list of patient concerns. Researcher–patient interview and administration of HADS and self-assessment scale; 10-week training programme; 9-month nurse post-test.	Communication workshops based on 'skills' model provide necessary but not sufficient training to achieve sustained changes in nurses' behaviours.
Booth et al. (1996)[98]	Prospective study of nurse–patient taped interactions before and after training and 9 months later. Researcher–nurse semi-structured interviews; questionnaire re nurses' perceived level of support.	Blocking behaviours most evident when patients disclose feelings. These behaviours were less when nurses felt practical help and support was available.
Jarrett and Payne (2000)[101]	Ethnomethodological study. Tape-recorded nurse–patient interactions. Nurse and patient participant accounting interviews. Communication skills analysis.	Patients valued 'ordinary' conversation with nurses as well as talk about their illness. Optimistic cheerful conversation is a jointly produced feature of nurse–patient interaction in cancer care.

establish operational definitions of 'facilitative' or 'blocking' nurse communications, which are then considered in relation to some idealised normative standard, or 'good' communication checklist.[47,98] Though these works have provided invaluable insights into nurses' communication practices, the focus of such research has had adverse spin-offs. It has meant that linguistic and sociological issues such as language use, social context, and the conversation as a joint construction between nurse and patient have been downplayed. The therapeutic effectiveness of the communication has not been evaluated, and the role of nurse researcher, attempting to understand the complexities of nurses' therapeutic work and the stress of health care professionals in the field of cancer care, rather than exposing failures, has not been fully realised.

The challenges facing researchers are immense for it is proving difficult to establish ways to evaluate therapeutic work in health care.[102,103] Studies are required that will explore the nature and effectiveness of nurses' therapeutic work, as well as studies that go beyond individuals' communicative practice to address systemic and institutional influences. Such research will complement existing studies and reveal the limits of theoretical accounts of nurses' therapeutic potential, highlighting the education and support needs for practice.

A spectrum of research methods is necessary to explore fully the processes and impact of nurses' therapeutic strategies in cancer care. Interpretative, figurative analysis needs to be incorporated into the more formulaic discourse analytical approaches, which have been used by some researchers to reveal the structures and general patterns of communication within therapeutic encounters. This innovation would reveal people's idiosyncratic, metaphoric ways of understanding and attributing meaning to their cancer illness, and offer practitioners insights into how they might respond and work with these.

Put another way, therapeutic work, with its emphasis on feelings and motivations, as a subject of enquiry, invites research approaches that cross disciplinary boundaries.

Geertz[104] sees this 'blurring of genres' in research as part of a wholesale tendency towards decategorisation:

What we are seeing is not just another redrawing of the cultural map . . . but an alteration in the principles of mapping. Something is happening to the way we think about the way we think.[104]

This blurring of genres means that the dividing lines between the humanities and the human sciences is less clear,[105] and that more than one disciplinary or theoretical 'map' may be needed to explore the emotional 'territory' of cancer care. It is tantalising to speculate how far the assumptions of conscious intention and the transparency of language can be set aside, and research approaches that examine metaphor and personal imagery used to produce sociologically and psychologically intelligible, clinically relevant findings.

References

1. Lanceley A. (1995). Emotional disclosure between cancer patients and nurses. In Richardson A. and Wilson-Barnet J. (eds.) *Nursing Research in Cancer Care*. London: Scutari Press, pp. 167–188.
2. Corner J. (1997). Beyond survival rates and side-effects: cancer nursing as therapy. *Cancer Nursing* **20**, 3–11.
3. Smith M.E. and Hart G. (1994). Nurses' responses to anger: from disconnecting to connecting. *Journal of Advanced Nursing* **20**, 643–651.
4. Armstrong D. (1983). The fabrication of nurse–patient relationships. *Social Science and Medicine* **17**, 457–460.
5. Peplau H. (1952). *Interpersonal Relationships in Nursing*. New York: GP Putnam.
6. Peplau H. (1969). Professional closeness. *Nursing Forum* **8**, 342–360.
7. Savage J. (1995). *Nursing Intimacy: An Ethnographic Approach to Nurse–Patient Interaction*. London: Scutari Press.
8. Bailey C. (1995). Nursing as therapy in the management of breathlessness in lung cancer. *European Journal of Cancer Care* **4**, 184–190.
9. Davis B. and Oberle K. (1990). Dimensions of the supportive role of the nurse in palliative care. *Oncology Nursing Forum* **17**, 87–94.
10. Froggatt K. (1995). Nurses and involvement in palliative care work. In Richardson A. and Wilson-Barnett J. (eds.) *Nursing Research in Cancer Care*. London: Scutari Press, pp. 151–164.
11. McMahon R. and Pearson A. (1991). *Nursing as Therapy*. London: Chapman and Hall.
12. Muetzel P. (1988). Therapeutic nursing. In Pearson A. (ed.) *Primary Nursing: Nursing in the Burford and*

Oxford Nursing Development Unit. London: Croom Helm.

13. Judd D. (1995). *Give Sorrow Words: Working with a Dying Child,* 2nd edition. London: Whurr Publishers.

14. Halldorsdottir S. (1991). Five basic modes of being with another. In Gaut D. and Leininger M. (eds.) *Caring: The Compassionate Healer.* New York: National League for Nursing Press, pp. 37–50.

15. Kitson A. (1986). *Steps toward the identification and development of nursing therapeutic functions in the care of hospitalised elderly.* PhD thesis, University of Ulster, Coleraine.

16. Ersser S.J. (1990). A search for the therapeutic dimensions of nurse–patient interaction. In Pearson A. and McMahon R. (eds.) *Nursing as Therapy.* London: Chapman and Hall.

17. Campbell A.V. (1984). *Moderated Love: A Theology of Professional Care.* London: SPCK.

18. Carper B. (1978). Fundamental patterns of knowing in nursing. *Advances in Nursing Science* **1**, 13–23.

19. Benner P. and Wrubel J. (1989). *The Primacy of Caring: Stress and Coping in Health and Illness.* Menlo Park, CA: Addison–Wesley.

20. Cox M. (1988). *Structuring the Therapeutic Process: Compromise with Chaos.* London: Jessica Kingsley.

21. Burnard P. (1994). *Counselling Skills for Health Professionals,* 2nd edition. London: Chapman and Hall.

22. Pollitt C. (1991). *The Politics of Quality: Managers, Professionals and Consumers in the Public Services.* London: Royal Holloway and Bedford New College, Centre for Political Studies.

23. Griffiths R. (1983). *Report of the NHS Management Inquiry.* London: Department of Health and Social Security.

24. Calman K. and Hine D. (1995). *A Policy Framework for Commissioning Cancer Services.* London: Department of Health and Welsh Office.

25. Harrison S., Hunter D., Marnock G. and Pollit C. (1989). General management and medical autonomy in the National Health Service. *Health Services Management Research* **2**, 38–46.

26. Bloomfield B., Coombs R., Cooper D. and Rea D. (1992). Machines and manoeuvres: responsibility accounting and the construction of hospital information. *Accounting, Management and Information Technologies* **2**, 199–205.

27. James N. (1992). Care = organization + physical labour + emotional labour. *Sociology of Health and Illness* **14**, 488–509.

28. National Institute for Clinical Excellence. (2004). *Guidance on Cancer Services: Improving Supportive and Palliative Care for Adults with Cancer.* London: National Institute for Clinical Excellence.

29. Davies C. (1995). *Gender and the Professional Predicament in Nursing.* Buckingham: Open University Press.

30. Traynor M. (1996). A literary approach to managerial discourse after the NHS reforms. *Sociology of Health and Illness* **18**, 315–340.

31. Salvage J. (1990). The theory and practice of the 'New Nursing'. *Nursing Times* **86**, Occasional Paper, 42–45.

32. Pearson A. (ed.) (1988). *Primary Nursing: Nursing in the Burford and Oxford Nursing Development Units.* London: Chapman and Hall.

33. Manley K. (1997). A conceptual framework for advanced practice: an action research project operationalizing an advanced practitioner/consultant nurse role. *Journal of Advanced Nursing* **6**, 179–190.

34. Manley K. (2002). Refining the consultant nurse framework: commentary on critique. *Nursing in Critical Care* **7**, 84–87.

35. Glaser B. and Strauss A.L. (1965). *Awareness of Dying.* Chicago, IL: Aldine.

36. James N. (1993). Divisions of emotional labour: disclosure and cancer. In Fineman S. (ed.) *Emotions in Organizations.* London: Sage, pp. 94–117.

37. Menzies Lyth I. (1988). The functioning of social systems as a defence against anxiety (1959, 1961,[1961b], 1970). In Menzies Lyth I. (ed.) *Containing Anxiety in Institutions: Selected Essays.* London: Free Association Books, pp. 43–94.

38. Lawton J. (2000). *The Dying Process: Patient's Experiences of Palliative Care.* London: Routledge.

39. Peräkylä A. (1991). Hope work in the care of seriously ill patients. *Qualitative Health Research* **1**, 407–433.

40. Savage J. (1992). *Implications of New Nursing Initiatives for the Nurse–Patient Relationship: An Ethnographic Study of Two Wards.* London: Bloomsbury and Islington College of Nursing and Midwifery.

41. Smith P. (1992). *The Emotional Labour of Nursing: How Nurses Care.* Basingstoke: Macmillan.

42. Obholzer A. and Roberts V.Z. (eds.) (1994). *The Unconscious at Work: Individual and Organizational Stress in the Human Services.* London: Routledge.

43. Di Giacomo S.M. (1987). Biomedicine as a cultural system: an anthropologist in the kingdom of the sick. In Baer H. (ed.) *Encounters in Biomedicine: Case Studies in Medical Anthropology.* New York: Gordon and Breach, pp. 315–346.

44. Hak T.A.-M., Koeter T. and van der Wal G. (2000). Collusion in doctor-patient communication about imminent death: an ethnographic study. *British Medical Journal* **321**, 1376–1381.

45. Knight M. and Field D. (1981). A silent conspiracy: coping with dying cancer patients on an acute surgical ward. *Journal of Advanced Nursing* **6**, 221–229.

46. Silverman D. (1987). *Communication and Medical Practice: Social Relations in the Clinic.* London: Sage.

47. Wilkinson S. (1991). Factors which influence how nurses communicate with cancer patients. *Journal of Advanced Nursing* **16**, 677–688.

48. Stead M., Brown J.M., Fallowfield L. and Selby P. (2003). Lack of communication between health care professionals and women with ovarian cancer about sexual issues. *British Journal of Cancer* **88**, 666–671.

49. Dowsett S.M., Saul J.L., Butow P.N. *et al.* (2000). Communication style in the cancer consultation: preferences for a patient-centred approach. *Psycho-oncology* **9**, 147–156.

50. Maguire P., Faulkner A., Booth K., Elliot C. and Hillier V. (1996). Helping cancer patients disclose their concerns. *European Journal of Cancer* **32A**, 78–81.

51. Fallowfield L., Jenkins V., Farell V. *et al.* (2000). Efficacy of a Cancer Research UK communication skills training model for oncologists: a randomised controlled trial. *Lancet* **359**, 650–656.

52. Souhami R. (1978). Teaching what to say about cancer. *Lancet* **ii**, 935–936.

53. Rogers M.S. and Todd C.J. (2000). The 'right kind' of pain: talking about symptoms in outpatient oncology consultations. *Palliative Medicine* **14**, 299–307.

54. Mishler E.G. (1984). *The Discourse of Medicine: Dialectics of Medical Interviews.* New Jersey: Norwood Publishing Company.

55. Kubler-Ross E. (1970). *Death: The Final Stage of Growth.* London: Tavistock.

56. Leydon G.M., Boulton M., Moynihan C. *et al.* (2000). Cancer patients' information needs and information seeking behaviour: in depth interview study. *British Medical Journal* **320**, 909–913.

57. Foucault M. (1973). *The Birth of the Clinic.* London: Tavistock.

58. Armstrong D. (1984). The patient's view. *Social Science and Medicine* **18**, 737–744.

59. Haward R., Amir Z., Borrill C. *et al.* (2003). Breast cancer teams: the impact of constitution, new cancer workload, and methods of operation on their effectiveness. *British Journal of Cancer* **89**, 15–22.

60. Teger A.I. and Pruitt D.G. (1967). Components of group risk taking. *Journal of Social Psychology* **5**, 189–205.

61. Lewis C., O'Brien R. and Barraclough J. (2002). *The Psychoimmunology of Cancer.* Oxford: Oxford University Press.

62. Moorey S., Greer S., Watson M. *et al.* (1994). Adjuvant psychological therapy for patients with cancer: outcome at one year. *Psycho-oncology* **3**, 39–46.

63. Cassileth B.R. (1980). Information and participation preferences among cancer patients. *Annals of Internal Medicine* **92**, 832–836.

64. Parkes C.M. (1978). Psychological aspects. In Saunders C.M. (ed.) *The Management of Terminal Diseases.* London: Arnold, pp. 44–64.

65. Baider L. and Porath S. (1981). Uncovering fear: group experiences of nurses in a cancer ward. *International Journal of Nursing Studies* **18**, 147–152.

66. Hanson E.E. (1991). *The Cancer Nurse's Perspective: Stress and the Person with Cancer.* Lancaster: Quay Publishing.

67. Elkind A.K. (1982). Nurses' views about cancer. *Journal of Advanced Nursing* **7**, 43–50.

68. Stacey J. (1997). *Teratologies: A Cultural Study of Cancer.* London: Routledge.

69. Word C.O. (1974). The nonverbal mediation of self-fulfilling prophesies in interaction. *Journal of Experimental Social Psychology* **10**, 109–120.

70. Mood D. and Lick C.F. (1979). Attitudes of nursing personnel toward death and dying: linguistic indicators of denial. *Research in Nursing and Health* **2**, 95–99.

71. Vachon M., Lyall W. and Freeman S. (1978). Measurement and management of stress in health professionals working with advanced cancer patients. *Death Education* **1**, 365–375.

72. Delvaux N., Razavi D. and Farvacques C. (1988). Cancer care–stress for health professionals. *Social Science and Medicine* **27**, 159–166.

73. Mcilfatrick S.J. and Keeney S. (2003). Identifying cancer nursing research priorities using the Delphi technique. *Journal of Advanced Nursing* **42**, 629–636.

74. Ullrich A. and Fitzgerald P. (1990). Stress experienced by physicians on the cancer ward. *Social Science and Medicine* **13**, 213–218.

75. Whippen D.A. and Canellos G.P. (1991). Burnout syndrome in the practice of oncology: results of a random survey of 1000 oncologists. *Journal of Clinical Oncology* **9**, 1916–1920.

76. Cull A. (1991). Staff support in medical oncology: a problem solving approach. *Psychology and Health* **5**, 129–136.

77. Kent F.G., Wills G., Faulkner A. *et al.* (1994). The professional and personal needs of oncology staff: the effects of perceived success and failure in helping patients on levels of personal stress and distress. *Journal of Cancer Care* **3**, 153–158.

78. Isikhan V., Comez T. and Zafer Danis M. (2004). Job stress and coping strategies in health care professionals

working with cancer patients *European Journal of Oncology Nursing* **8**, 234–244.

79. McNamara B., Wadell C. and Colvin M. (1995). Threats to the good death: the cultural context of stress and coping among hospice nurses. *Sociology of Health and Illness* **17**, 222–244.

80. Miller D. and Gillies P. (1996). Is there life after work? Experiences of HIV and oncology health staff. *AIDS Care* **8**, 167–182.

81. Weisman A.D. (1981). Understanding the cancer patient: the syndrome of the caregiver's plight. *Psychiatry* **44**, 161–168.

82. George J. (1990). Why stress is a management issue. *Health Manpower Management* **December**, 17–19.

83. Ramirez A.J., Graham J., Richards M.A., Cull A. and Gregory W.M. (1996). Mental health of hospital consultants: the effects of stress and satisfaction at work. *Lancet* **347**, 724–728.

84. Taylor C., Graham J., Potts H.W.W. *et al.* (2005). Changes in mental health of UK hospital consultants since the mid-1990s. *Lancet* **366**, 742–744.

85. Department of Health (2000). *The NHS Cancer Plan: A Plan for Investment, a Plan for Reform.* London: Department of Health.

86. Wilkinson S.M. (1994). Stress in cancer nursing: does it exist? *Journal of Advanced Nursing* **20**, 1079–1084.

87. Bruneau B.M. and Ellison G.T. (2004). Palliative care stress in a UK community hospital: evaluation of a stress reduction programme. *International Journal of Palliative Nursing* **10**, 296–304.

88. Papadatou D., Anagnostopouros F. and Mouros D. (1994). Factors contributing to the development of burnout on oncology nursing. *British Journal of Medical Psychology* **67**, 187–199.

89. Lazarus R. (1966). *Psychological Stress and the Coping Process.* New York: McGraw-Hill.

90. Pearlin L.I. (1989). The sociological study of stress. *Journal of Health and Social Behaviour* **30**, 241–256.

91. Hirschorn L. (1988). *The Workplace Within: Psychodynamics of Organizational Life.* Cambridge, MA: MIT Press.

92. Freud A. (1993). *The Ego and the Mechanisms of Defence.* London: Karnac Books.

93. Klein M. (1937). *Love, Guilt and Reparation and Other Works*, 1975 edition. London: Hogarth.

94. Brown D. and Pedder J. (1991). *Introduction of Psychotherapy: An Outline of Psychodynamic Principles and Practice.* London: Tavistock/Routledge.

95. Jacobs M. (1998). *The Presenting Past: the Core of Psychodynamic Counselling and Therapy.* Buckingham: Open University Press.

96. Menzies Lyth I. (1988). *Containing Anxiety in Institutions*, Vol. 1. London: Free Association Books.

97. Main T. (1968). The ailment. In Barnes E. (ed.) *Psychosocial Nursing: Studies from the Cassel Hospital.* London: Tavistock Publications, pp. 33–60.

98. Booth K., Maguire P.M., Butterworth T. and Hillier V.F. (1996). Perceived professional support and the use of blocking behaviours by hospice nurses. *Journal of Advanced Nursing* **24**, 522–527.

99. Hunt M. (1989). *Dying at Home: its Basic 'Ordinariness' Displayed in Patients' Relatives' and Nurses' Talk.* PhD thesis, University of London.

100. Heaven C.M. and Maguire P. (1996). Training hospice nurses to elicit patients' concerns. *Journal of Advanced Nursing* **23**, 280–286.

101. Jarrett N. and Payne S.A. (2000). Creating and maintaining 'optimism' in cancer care communication. *International Journal of Nursing Studies* **37**, 81–90.

102. Silverman D. (1997). *Discourses of Counselling: HIV Counselling as Social Interaction.* London: Sage.

103. Savage J. (2004). Researching emotion: the need for coherence between focus, theory and method. *Nursing Inquiry* **11**, 25–34.

104. Geertz C. (1983). *Local Knowledge: Further Essays in Interpretive Anthropology.* New York: Basic Books.

105. Denzin N.K. (1970). *The Research Act: A Theoretical Introduction to Sociological Methods*, 3rd edition. Englewood Cliffs, NJ: Prentice Hall.

CHAPTER NINE

Therapeutic strategies in cancer care

Anne Lanceley

There is an increasing awareness among health care professionals and consumers of the painful issues surrounding cancer treatment and care. Receiving the diagnosis and negotiating subsequent treatment constitutes a psychic trauma, and in this case professionals need to look into their own feelings, as well as attempting to be aware of those of the people in their care. An understanding of the need for not only quality medical care but also emotional care and support, including the right to express every sort of emotion as a response to the trauma of cancer illness, is well established.[1,2]

This interest and awareness has been driven, in part, by the idea that the way feelings are expressed, and in particular active holding back from expressing feelings, not only may render a person 'cancer prone' but may affect the progress of the cancer illness.[3,4] This has been a powerful theme in the cancer literature and in the minds of some people who have cancer, judging by patients' own accounts of their illness experience.[3-7] It continues to be a high research priority.

What is striking in this context is that cancer nurses, though generally accepting of the therapeutic potential of their role at some level, and while acknowledging that the people for whom they care may use the trusted relationship with them to explore their own feelings, in practice are pragmatic in their approaches to managing individual concerns. Put another way, nurses' actual practices are not generally theory driven and do not involve an explicit, mutually negotiated therapeutic plan.

Much of what follows is theoretical. This is not as a way of avoiding the feelings of uncertainty and the sense of vulnerability nurses experience when working with cancer but as a way of providing a variety of lenses through which the practice can be viewed. The use of theory and alternative frameworks for understanding this work enables us to see when processes are 'stuck'. It is hoped that the verbatim accounts will allow for contemplation and the pursuit of the reader's personal meanings in the light of their own clinical experience.

No essential right or wrong theories or practical ways of managing the concerns of people with cancer are advocated here. There are numerous texts describing ways of managing these practically.[8-12] At one level everything depends on how the particular nurse is attempting to work with an individual. There are, however, fundamental beliefs and questions that run throughout the chapter. They concern:

- the relative importance of nurses sharing awareness of their intent when working with someone with cancer
- how unconscious thoughts and feelings may influence work with cancer
- different levels and ways of helping individuals express and understand their feelings, deal with problems, adjust and make treatment decisions

- the ways nurses define themselves as 'listener', 'counsellor', or 'therapist'
- the belief that contact with the nurse is beneficial or 'therapeutic' if an individual feels understood and is thus helped to understand himself better.

The understanding alluded to in the last point may take an unspoken form in the case of a nurse who sits and bears silent witness to someone who is dying. Being with the person is an opportunity for them to 'be'. Allowing the person to be dying validates them, whereas to deny the person's dying life would be to deny their life. The nurse is communicating understanding and acceptance of the person's life and impending death.[13]

There are two styles of relating to someone with cancer, which can be placed along a continuum of therapeutic strategies: the first is concerned with the deciphering of meaning, whereas the second is in the nature of 'holding' and 'containing' the experience. The cancer nurse needs to strike a balance within these two broad types of functioning.

Structuring the nurse–patient relationship

In order for the nurse to do this and remain sensitive to the often chaotic emotional experiences during cancer treatment, as well as recognising and helping with their information needs, Cox advocates structuring the relationship.[14] The dimensions of time, depth, and mutuality, if thought about by the nurse, can help to locate her use of herself on behalf of the person, and offer a means of monitoring the changing course of what happens in the relationship. Cox makes a useful analogy with the built-in range finder on a camera and the nurse's initiative in bringing what the person is saying into focus so that they are both operating at the same focal point. Like the personal qualities considered essential for nurses to relate and respond effectively – acceptance, warmth, genuineness, and empathy – the dimensions of time, depth, and mutuality are independent of any particular theoretical approach and are relevant, however brief or extended the encounter may be.

Time

The significance of time as a dimension is intensified for someone with a life-threatening illness and there is a shared awareness of this as the uncertainty of a limited prognosis is tolerated. This uncertainty gives an added poignancy to the maxim from counselling psychology: if the patient does not know when the end is, he cannot know when 'just before the end' is. This is important for thinking about the timing of someone's disclosures, and particular moments of insight within a talk, when feelings are expressed and may be acknowledged and understood for the first time. The maxim is also relevant for a series of conversations and encounters that a person may have with a nurse over many months or years. It prompts the nurse to consider the beginning of her relationship with them and its likely duration, which may coincide with a treatment regime or commence at the palliative phase of the illness, ending with their death; it focuses attention on the length of time available for any single encounter, and on how boundaries may be set so that the time available can be used constructively. Holidays and other absences may become increasingly important and require managing.

A more subtle aspect of the time dimension is how aspects of the person's past, their present, and their plans and hopes for the future may be acknowledged and balanced so that there is momentum and sense of continuity in the relationship.

Depth

The second dimension concerns depth. This is related to levels of patient disclosure from surface to hidden aspects of their lives and themselves. It brings into play the complex interaction between unconscious and conscious levels of awareness, which has been one of the major contributions of psychoanalytic theory to the understanding of human behaviours and experience. Linked to this are the skills and activity of the nurse responding to different levels of personal disclosure. Cox distinguishes between three levels of self-disclosure and offers them as a useful conceptual tool for practice, also suggesting that they can be used to assess the depth of the relationship.[14]

First-level disclosures are safe and relatively unimportant and act as 'feelers' in the relationship. Level two disclosures involve the disclosure of personal information but tend to be emotionally neutral. They are an indication that the relationship has developed to the point where the person feels confident and trusting with the nurse. Third-level disclosures give insight into the personal, deep, existential concerns, and by definition are unique to the individual. Things from the person's own private world that they may not have revealed before may be disclosed. The three levels can be used to assess the depth of the relationship, both on a session-by-session basis and within a longer term relationship.

While attempting to integrate depth and time structuring into a cohesive therapeutic strategy, the nurse must also be aware of the crucial significance of the place of mutuality and reciprocity within the nurse–patient relationship.

Mutuality

The third dimension of structure is mutuality, which describes the potential significance of the shared relationship. Mutuality refers to how much the nurse discloses about herself in order to share with the person the experience he is disclosing. This is not primarily about how much the nurse reveals about her own problems, which could be perceived as overburdening. It is about a mutuality of disclosure grounded in the here-and-now of the talk and physical care. The nurse may be very open in expressing her feelings in relation to this shared experience, which is very different from disclosing her own personal life experiences. Rather than emotionally withdrawing and hiding behind a professional mask, the nurse acknowledges the person's distress and the shared pain and distress inherent in the situation. This involves acceptance, warmth, genuineness, and empathy and, in addition, may develop through the nurse actively using transference and countertransference.

Empathy is the ability to enter the perceptual world of another person and convey this identification of feeling to them.[8] As well as an empathetic 'looking in' through an exploration of inner feelings and meanings, empathy also involves 'looking out' on behalf of someone else; seeing the world, the context in which they live, work, and receive their treatment, through their eyes.

Some nurses have greater intuitive awareness than others, and a question that taxes nurse educators is how far empathy can be both taught and learned.[15] What seems clear is that it is the nurse's use of her own personality that sustains empathy. The quality that enables people who have cancer to risk what may amount to further reduction of self-esteem and distress, by emotionally exposing themselves still further, is if the nurse is empathetic and not only listens, but hears, understands and, most difficult of all, is able to convey that she understands. How is this done? Can one nurse do this for all those in her care?

One of the essentials for empathy is that of showing by word, gesture, and expression a detrivialising, unconditional concern. The person believes that what concerns him is not trivial and he may to some extent test out the nurse, who may be presumed to adopt a 'trivialising' attitude to them by the very fact that he has become, and is labelled, a 'cancer patient'.

Therefore, mutuality is a measure of the depth of the relationship and of the nurse's commitment to the relationship.

Developing communication skills

The personal qualities of empathy, a nonjudgemental attitude and even genuineness are considered essential for nurses to respond effectively to patients, and the use of communication skills enhances the nurse's ability to relate and to work confidently across the spectrum of functioning. The use of communication skills is independent of theoretical approach or the way in which the nurse and patient agree to structure their relationship.

Active listening
- Attending and being physically 'present'
- Questioning: closed
                      open
                      leading
                      value-laden
                      'why', 'how', and 'what'
                      questions
                      confronting questions

- Allowing expression of feelings
- Prompting
- Probing
- Focusing
- Clarifying
- Reflecting
- Paraphrasing
- Challenging
- Self-sharing
- Summarising
- Monitoring transference and counter-transference.

As this chapter is more a contextual exploration of nurses' strategies for managing cancer patient's concerns, knowledge and understanding of the skills needed to communicate effectively are not described in detail. A great deal has been written on this, and numerous texts explain and give practical examples of the skills summarised above.[8,16–20]

Alternative frameworks for understanding nurses' work with cancer patients

Knowledge of a range of theoretical approaches (see Table 9.1) will open up a spectrum of possibilities for managing a person's concerns, and is necessary if the nurse is to understand and work comfortably across the spectrum of functioning described at the beginning of the chapter, from 'holding' and 'containing' to helping to decipher the meaning of cancer illness.[12,21–35]

The meaning of illness and its therapeutic use

Cancer can disrupt virtually all aspects of a person's life. Everyday activities are affected, as well as short-term and long-term goals. A person is forced to reassess what is meaningful and to scrutinise values that have hitherto governed their life.

Silver and Wortman suggest that a person's ability to find meaning or purpose in a crisis is

Table 9.1 Theoretical approaches for managing a person's concerns

Psychological approach	Theorist
Personal construct approach	Kelly (1955)[22]
Gestalt therapy	Perls (1969)[23]
Transactional analysis	Berne (1964)[24]
	Harris (1973)[25]
Person-centred therapy	Rogers (1951)[26]
Rational emotive therapy (RET)	Ellis (1962)[27]
Behavioural therapy	Krumboltz and Thorenson (1969)[28]
Neuro-linguistic programmes (NLP)	Bandler (1985)[29]
Reality therapy	Glasser (1965)[30]
Psychosynthesis	Ferrucci (1982)[31]
Psychotherapy	Freud (1938)[32]
	Klein (1937)[21]
	Bion (1962)[33]
Cognitive therapy	Beck (1976)[34]
Adjuvant psychological therapy for patients with cancer (APT)	Moorey and Greer (1989)[12]
Logotherapy	Frankl (1959)[35]

associated with the ability to adjust to it.[36] People need to see their lives as essentially meaningful, and as Brody noted, 'suffering is produced and alleviated primarily by the meaning that one attaches to one's experience'.[37]

The primary mechanism for attaching meaning to particular experiences is to tell stories about them. It is through hearing and telling stories that human beings have always come to organise and understand their experiences.[38] There are numerous important testimonies of personal struggles with cancer illness: *Diary of a Breast*, written by a woman with breast cancer,[39] *Cancer Through the Eyes of Ten Women*,[7] *Cancer in Two Voices*, co-written by partners facing cancer,[40] the intense descriptions by Ruth Picardie,[41] first in a series of newspaper articles and later in a book of the progress of her breast cancer, or *And When Did You Last See Your Father?* about a son's understanding of his father's cancer,[42] and the elegiac accounts of the experience of ovarian cancer treatment and illness by Anne Dennison,[43] to quote but a few. They provide crucial insight into work in the field and contribute forcibly to our clinical thinking. Stories and testimonies of illness are no different from other descriptions; we construct an understanding of illness by comparing it to things other than itself, to things found in the realm of our personal experience. It is all but impossible to conceive of illness without recourse to metaphor, if only because 'the objective world is not directly accessible but is constructed on the basis of the constraining influences of human knowledge and language'.[44] Lakoff and Johnson's seminal work provided evidence that metaphor was responsible for an individual's method of making sense of things.[45]

The metaphorical potency of cancer illness stories has been explored in the writings of Sontag,[46] and is evidenced in recent studies.[47] By examining professional and lay expressions of cancer illness, Sontag revealed just how prevalent certain metaphorical descriptions are: 'cancer is war' and 'cancer is invasion' are two examples that sustain a host of other metaphorical expressions, such as 'they attacked it with chemotherapy', or 'his natural defences were low'. It is only recently that these ideas have begun to influence ideas for practice in cancer care.[48–50] Attention to the metaphors and personal imagery used by individuals is important, in the therapeutic sense that an illness conceived of metaphorically might be coped with and responded to in the same way.[51]

There is a substantial literature concerned with narrative analysis of health and illness, much of it influenced by the seminal work of Kleinman and Mishler.[52,53] Kleinman suggests that individuals' explanatory models of illness originate in biomedicine but also from the construction of sustaining fictions that can make sense of the illness for the individual experiencing self.[52] Kleinman insists that the patient's personal narrative does not merely reflect illness experience but rather it contributes to the experience of symptoms and suffering.

A nurse's ability to facilitate someone to find meaning in their illness and to help someone with cancer to arrive at explanations that sustain them are research and practice themes in cancer care.

This interest comes from an interweaving of various threads:

- an acknowledgement of the psychodynamic processes in which the patient comes to tell and then re-author his or her individual life story, thus throwing light upon their inner life
- the application of social constructionist philosophy and politics to health care, which places a sense of the person as a story-making, story-consuming, social being embedded in social, cultural, and historical conditions, at the centre of its conceptual framework
- the movement towards post-modern forms of clinical practice where the key characteristics are:
  - reflexivity
  - local knowledge replacing 'grand narratives'
  - multiplicity of meanings
  - patient empowerment
  - commitment to pluralism and multiplicity of meaning
  - deconstruction of the idea of a singular entity
  - the 'true self'
  - in favour of the self as a construction.

How an individual nurse listens to a person's story and interprets it will depend on the broad theoretical approach of the nurse and decisions about the structuring of the relationship. There are many different ways in which a nurse and patient can work together to tell and then retrieve meaning from the story. If the nurse has a psychodynamic orientation, the interpretation of the story will be in terms of unconscious emotional processes, the functioning of psychological defences, and how the person's core life story repeats itself in different relations at different points in his or her life. If the nurse has a behavioural orientation, then the story may be used to identify behavioural routines, and if the nurse works cognitively, telling the story may be viewed as an act of problem solving and management. These broad approaches are summarised here:

Care strategy 9.1 Preliminary nurse strategies for narrative change

- Nurse listens for patient stories.
- Nurse uses communication skills to elicit the stories the person lives by.
- Nurse listens to *how* the story is told:
  - pauses
  - voice quality
  - phrasing
  - control of emotional distance by:
    - use of objectifying language, e.g. 'it', 'one'
    - absence of experiential detail and colour
  - emotional immediacy by:
    - descriptions of place
    - direct speech
    - present tense.
- Nurse gives close attention to the symbolisation of feelings in the stories and to the metaphors used as indicators of implicit meaning.
- Nurse has a sensitive ear for differences and incongruities in story construction and telling.

Though it is recognised that there may be intrinsic value in the person telling their story to give voice to areas of experience that have previously been silenced, there is a difference between the nurse simply hearing the story, and therapeutic storytelling described in Care strategy 9.1. In the former, the person may tell and retell the same story in the same way throughout their treatment experience and for years afterwards, and derive comfort and support from this. With therapeutic storytelling, the shared expectation for patient and nurse would be that the story can change. Through careful listening and sensitive interpretation of what the patient says, the nurse facilitates the ability of the patient to make sense of their illness, with the possible emergence of a more satisfying and personally meaningful narrative.

Psychodynamic approach

An emphasis on the existence of unconscious processes and their role in communication lies at the heart of psychodynamic understanding, which differs from other theories concerned primarily with the conscious mind.

The approach focuses on early memories and feelings from the past that usually remain hidden from our conscious mind but that can be triggered by something in the present. The impact of past memories on present behaviour patterns can be a powerful one. A process of transference occurs when thoughts, feelings, emotions, and expectations belonging to a person in the past are transferred to a person in the present. That person is then reacted to *as if* they were the person from the past, which is often inappropriate.[53] An understanding of this process of transference may be an important tool for the nurse working to understand someone with cancer and other relationships within the work setting.

Behind the psychodynamic approach is the idea that meaning and the key to understanding a person's response to illness and ourselves lie beneath the surface and in the past, and that what we are is the result of the dynamic interplay between past and present experience, between our conscious and unconscious, between our external and internal reality and our developing personality.

Internal reality, the part of the mind referred to as our 'internal world', contains many parts or representations of ourselves, as well as representations of relationships with important others and between parts of ourselves, i.e. our child self may be in conflict with our parent self. The nature of these representations is influenced not only by our early external relationships with mother and father, but also by fantasies fuelled by impulses such as aggression, hate, and love, with which children try to make sense of the world, when there is no way to check their perceptions against reality.[21]

These early imaginings are gradually modified, because we test them against reality as we progress through life. However, it is to these perceptions of people, ourselves, and the world that we often fall back or regress, when under stress. It is this inner world that informs and colours our perception of the outer world.[54]

When cancer strikes, usual ways of coping may not help, and the person becomes vulnerable and regresses to reacting in more primitive ways. This might show itself through someone trying to cope with the severe anxiety of having cancer by temporarily transferring onto the role of the nursing staff qualities of an all-giving, warm, protective maternal figure.[54] Futtermen and Wellisch provide some evidence for this.[55] In their study, they observed how patients on a bone marrow transplant unit experiencing extreme distress and anxiety regressed to emotional levels of early childhood, relating to staff in the transference much as they did to their own parental figures.

Alternatively, the person with cancer may avoid struggling with ambivalent feelings by splitting them. They may need to keep hope and goodness separate so they do not get spoiled by more negative feelings such as rage and despair. In these circumstances when experience cannot be integrated, a nurse may be either idealised or denigrated.[54]

Another example of this is the kind of psychic splitting that facilitates the person's acceptance of impending death. Two opposite ideas are verbalised. One reflects a full realisation of the closeness of impending death, the other a faith in surviving, often expressed in vivid fantasies about the future.[54]

If nurses remain open to distress, holding onto feelings for a person until they can be made sense of or borne, broadly speaking they would be fulfilling the function a mother performs quite unconsciously for her baby. The mother allows herself to experience her baby's distress, to think about it and process it, so that she can think about and respond to the baby in a sensitive way. Our capacity to do this depends on the quality of our own mothering and the confidence we feel in our 'mother' institution to contain us.[54]

The idea of container/contained is another powerful idea for framing clinical work in which nurses may be needed to offer containment to cancer patients who cannot make sense of their experience for themselves, and feel overwhelmed with anxiety as a consequence.[56]

In Bion's theory of container/contained, the capacity to think about emotional experience and develop emotional resilience to cope with difficulties in later life depends on a baby's earliest experience of being thought about and someone being attentive to him or her.[57]

Emmanuel describes what happens according to this theory.[58] A baby is bombarded by sense data that threaten to overwhelm him or her. The baby's mind is not developed enough to contain the powerful feelings and the baby is therefore totally dependent on the availability of an object into whom the powerful feelings can be put in order to get rid of them. Bion calls this object the 'container' and the incomprehensible painful feelings the 'contained'. The container, the mother or caregiver, then has to try and make sense out of the baby's experience by thinking about whatever the baby has made her feel. The mother has to decipher what the baby is communicating. By receiving the baby's feelings, i.e. the contained, and making sense of them, the mother can respond to the baby with understanding. The baby feels immediately more comfortable and is also able to take inside himself the idea that his mother has space in her mind for him and he feels understood. The baby begins to develop his own capacity to reflect on his experience and think. The relevance of this theory to nurses caring for cancer patients who may not be able to make sense of their experience for themselves, and feel overwhelmed with anxiety as a consequence, is clear: the nurse may be needed to offer containment to the person with cancer.

A nurse may gain crucial clues as to how far a person is requiring her to act as a container, and an understanding of the communication by the feelings aroused in him or her by the person. Counter-transference is the name given to the nurse's emotional response to the person, i.e. the conscious thoughts and feelings the nurse has when she is with them. This form of communication from the person can provide the nurse with valuable information as to their state of mind. When thought about by the nurse it can also inform him or her as to the most appropriate response to the person, since it prompts the question: 'What sort of feelings am I being asked to hold for this person?'

They may be feelings of vulnerability or feelings of anger, defeat, or overwhelming depression. When nurses have contact with a person's own unconscious in this way it is usually a very powerful experience. It is powerful because the person is attempting to relieve internal distress by externalising it and giving the nurse responsibility to contain aspects of the self.[54]

If the nurse can allow the person's feelings to sink in, this helps the person to explore the feelings in a personality powerful enough to contain them and perhaps to face something they previously viewed as unbearable. A further therapeutic skill lies in acknowledging the person's anxiety, naming it, and then deciding when and if to hand the feeling back to the person in a form that they can manage.

Cognitive approach

This approach relies on an understanding that behaviours and emotions are intimately linked with beliefs about the world. While beliefs influence feeling responses, they are rarely questioned; they lie beyond normal awareness but are not unconscious. In this approach it is not the appraisals, interpretations, and evaluations that the individual makes about their cancer symptoms or the effects of treatment *per se*, but the meanings they hold for the person involved. How a person *thinks* about the illness and his or her life is consequently central to their mental adjustment to cancer. As Moorey and Greer note, if loss is the predominant meaning a person attributes to their cancer then the person is likely to feel depressed.[12] If cancer primarily represents a threat to health, security, or life itself, the person is more likely to feel anxious.

In practice this approach aims to help people identify the relationship between cognitions, emotions, and behaviours, to increase their awareness of what seem like dysfunctional thoughts and alter them (see Care strategy 9.2). This means challenging and confronting the person's beliefs and negative automatic thoughts. Negative thoughts may be enhanced and perpetuated by distortions in thinking and appraisal: for example, people may focus on only one part of their memory of a diagnostic consultation – the negative aspects – even though other parts contradict this. Habitual thinking increases a person's vulnerability to hearing certain information: someone whose usual style of thinking is very 'black and white' may think they face imminent death when they have been told that all diagnostic tests indicate that the cancer they have has a good prognosis.

Care strategy 9.2 Cognitive strategies

- Facilitation of emotional expression
- Elicitation of automatic thoughts associated with the person's problems
- Person is taught to identify his or her own negative thoughts
- Person set task of monitoring own thoughts
- Distorted, negative thinking is challenged by reality testing and examining evidence for a particular thought and belief. Searching for an alternative, decatastrophising and helping the person to think about what they fear to see
- The use of more constructive thoughts and behaviours as a response to distressing thoughts is practised and reinforced.

The work is conceptualised as a joint problem-solving exercise in which the nurse collaborates with the person, seeking primarily cognitive or rational explanations in order to develop and try out strategies for coping with cancer. Therapeutic strategies are primarily educational and designed to foster a positive attitude so that insights gained will extend to future events. They are used extensively with people with cancer to reduce emotional distress and improve coping.[12]

Behavioural approach

This approach is based on the idea that since all human behaviour is learned through processes of positive reinforcement it can, if necessary, be unlearned.[28] The nurse working within this framework will be interested to identify with the person what they see as undesirable behaviours. Once these behaviours have been identified, the next step is to organise a scheme of reinforcement whereby more positive behaviours will be encouraged. No attempt is made in the behavioural approach to understand the cause of behaviours or to understand current behaviours in relation to the person's past. Instead the focus is learning, unlearning, and relearning.

Cancer robs patients of a sense of control of their own bodies, and behavioural techniques are considered to help give a sense of mastery or control over the person's life and environment.

Behavioural assignments can help the person to develop a sense of control over the illness through encouraging co-operation with treatment or self-help techniques such as visualisation and relaxation, distraction, graded task assignments, and activity scheduling. These behavioural assignments can also develop control in areas unrelated to cancer, and indirectly foster a fighting spirit. The techniques are used in cancer to help with symptom distress, anxiety, and depression, and notably as part of cognitive therapies, including Moorey and Greer's 'adjuvant psychological therapy'.[12]

Humanistic approach

Drawing heavily on the field of existential philosophy, humanistic psychology argues that people are essentially free and responsible for their own condition. We are not driven by an unconscious mind, nor are we simply the product of what we have learned. Essentially, we are agents. It is the fact of consciousness that gives us the ability to determine our own course of action through life and we are the best arbiters of what is and is not good for us. It was out of the humanistic school that the client-centred approach to counselling developed. The aim of working with the person, according to Rogers,[26] was not necessarily to explore their past, or to modify their behaviour or thinking, but to accept them and to help them progress through their difficulties by their own route, accompanying them on their own personal search for meaning.

Charting the work with cancer patients

Tschudin[10] and Burnard[8] argue that nurses need to make explicit the possible nature of their helping relationships with the person with cancer, based on the individual's needs. This is essential for the relationship to be consensual and collaborative. It may be that the nurse and patient explicitly agree to enter into a counselling relationship in which the nurse agrees to act in the capacity of 'counsellor'. Alternatively, the nurse and patient may agree to work on certain concerns

while the nurse will continue to perform within her functional role as nurse. In this case, she will be using counselling skills to enhance her communication with the person. In either situation, a model for practice allows both the nurse and the individual to chart where the relationship is going and how it is progressing. As a result, work is likely to be more focused and more satisfying, and goals will be identified, agreed and reached.

Different models for helping are presented in Table 9.2. They are broadly problem-management models, which are underpinned by cognitive-behavioural approaches to helping people with cancer. The primary sources give more information on these models.

How a nurse eventually does help a person to manage their concerns, how they incorporate a range of theoretical approaches into a personal repertoire of strategies for helping, and how they structure and model the progress of their work will depend on a number of things, including:

- skill level
- what he or she feels comfortable doing
- beliefs and value systems concerning people
- level of self-awareness
- mood at the time
- present life situation
- perception of what is 'wrong' with the person
- current workload
- nature of support and supervision available
- the context for the work
- lay and professional expectations of the therapeutic potential of the nurse–patient relationship.

Some of these influences will be evidenced in the extracts chosen to explore strategies for managing concerns below.

Managing concerns

This section of the chapter describes work with four people with cancer, using verbatim accounts of their experiences and how the nurse responded to their concerns. It is recognised here that there are times when the most important communication from the person is unspoken and that people

Table 9.2 Different models for helping the nurse–patient relationship

Egan (1994)[17]	Carkhuff (1987)[59]	Nelson-Jones (1993)[20]	Burnard (1994)[8]	Tschudin (1995)[10]
Three-stage open systems model	**Developmental model**	**Lifeskills helping model**	**Eight stage map**	**Four questions model**
I Problem definition story: Present scenario Indentify blind spots	Attending Responding to clients' feelings, thoughts	Developing the relationship, identifying and clarifying problems Accessing problem(s) and redefining in terms of life-skills	1. Meeting the person	1. What is happening?
			2. Discussion of surface issues	2. What is the meaning of it?
	Personalising the experience Meaning		3. Revelations of deeper issues	3. What is your goal?
II Goal development possibilities: Preferred scenario Goals Objectives	Goals	Stating working goals and planning interventions	4. Ownership of feelings and emotional release	4. How are you going to do it?
			5. Generation of insight	
			6. Problem-solving future planning	
III Action strategies plan	Initiating action	Interventions to develop self-helping skills	7. Action by person	
		End and consolidate	8. Disengagement from the relationship	

with cancer often stir up feelings in the nurse. Nurses' own accounts of their interactions will be used to identify this unconscious dimension of their communication.

It is hoped that the clinical cases will provide useful learning material. All too often clinical examples either show the health professional in a good light or denigrate their skills. Nurses do not so readily share their difficulties but more can be gained if we are prepared to do so. The selection and permissions gained for the clinical material that follows keep faith with this.

Helping with fear and anxiety
Case examples
Joyce is a 58-year-old single woman who lives alone. The palliative care nurse who visits her on this occasion has known her for 2 years, since her breast cancer was first diagnosed. The nurse

has been seeing Joyce weekly, for 3 months, either at home or at the hospital, after it was discovered that she had metastatic spread of her cancer. Joyce has been undergoing a course of chemotherapy but has become increasingly breathless, as the nurse discovers during this planned visit to her home the day before she is due to be seen by the doctor in the hospital clinic. This extract occurs 10 minutes into their half-hour conversation:

195 P. I'm really bad aren't I mmm . . . mmm . . .

196 N. I don't know Joyce I don't think you're getting better

197 P. No [long pause] oh God oh it's alright darling [long pause] sorry about this [sounding distressed]

198 N. That's alright

199 P.   What is it the doctor thinks I should do really?

200 N.   Uhm I don't think she's made a decision at the moment and I think she's waiting to see . . .

202 P.   No, alright

203 N.   . . . what the X-ray shows tomorrow . . .

204 P.   Okay

205 N.   . . . Joyce

206 P.   But I'm getting worse

207 N.   Mmm I think so . . . what does it feel like to you Joyce?

208 P.   It's very tight I know it's worse it's the breathing that worries me like I feel as if I'm never going to breathe again

210 N.   Mmm

211 P.   They will be able to help me won't they . . . I can't go round like this you see not breathing [long pause]

213 N.   I hope we'll be able to relieve the tightness in your chest but I can't promise that we'll be able to take the breathlessness away altogether

215 P.   No

216 N.   I think we'll be able to make it a bit better than it is at the moment

217 P.   Moment

218 P.   [long pause] but my life is limited isn't it . . . from the point of view of longevity [long pause]?

220 N.   I think so . . .

221 P.   . . . Months years [long pause]

222 N.   That's a really difficult thing . . .

223 P.   Mmm

224 N.   . . . to answer Joyce I think probably the person to talk to about that with would be the doctor

Joyce's breathlessness is a new and frightening feeling for her and induces fear of impending death. This prompts Joyce to seek reassurance from the nurse that something can be done to relieve her breathlessness. The nurse gives Joyce time to voice her fears (line 198) and gently explores the catastrophic understanding of her impending death (lines 196, 207, 213–214 and 220–224). Unbeknown to Joyce and the nurse the cancer has spread to the bones in Joyce's rib cage and shoulders and these have collapsed in on her lungs, causing her current breathing difficulties. In the next extract, Joyce gives a vivid description of her embodied experience of the metastatic spread of her cancer:

380 P.   I can't can't unbend my shoulders either that's another thing I, why's that?

381 N.   I'm not sure about that

382 P.   . . . My shoulders are all hunched up and I can't

383 N.   . . . Yeh I noticed that

384 P.   I can't get them straight I have to do like a little old . . . hunch back. It doesn't straighten out that doesn't help either . . . it's uncomfortable for me . . . radiotherapy wouldn't help me really any more would it?

387 N.   On your lungs

388 P.   No well on my sort of try to do something to my back

389 N.   I'm not sure . . . possibly that's something else you could talk to doctor about tomorrow I really don't know what that is

391 P.   You see I go like this [hunches her shoulders]

392 N.   Mmm

393 P   I can't straighten out can I [long pause] I can't get straight

394 N.   Mmm [long pause]

395 P.   Oh God I don't know what to do [tearful]

396 N.   Come Joyce [long pause]

397 P.   I just want to lead my life

398 N.   Mmm [pause]

399 P.   So *simple* I don't want I don't want to ask for very much you see [pause] just want to lead a (. . .) simple life go to I mean I've got it's a very mundane little job but I like it and [pause] and a nice little flat I mean it needs a lot of money spent on it but I like it and

I've got what I want and . . . and now all this happens [long pause] it's my mouth's so sore I can't eat properly [long pause] I mean I suppose some of these ulcers are on my throat as well probably . . . which doesn't help

405 N. Mmm mmm

406 P. Mmm

407 N. That *will* get better

408 P. Mmm

409 N. I . . . can assure you that erm yeh [long pause], mmm, [long pause] know this is really hard for you [long pause]

410 P. I don't know what to do [pause] or say or think, [long pause] sorry it's uncomfortable for you here [leaning on the window ledge] . . . but it's the only way I can

412 N. . . . I'm fine . . . no don't worry I'm fine [long pause]

413 P. They'll probably give me something tomorrow do you think [pause] mmmm

414 N. Yeh I hope so . . . try something [long pause] it might be that they could try some radiotherapy [long pause] I don't know whether they'd be able to do that tomorrow . . .

416 P. . . . No . . .

417 N. . . . Its probably unlikely but erm that might help.

At first the nurse takes her cue from Joyce's description and considers with Joyce different treatment possibilities (lines 387 and 389). There is then a qualitative shift in the nature of Joyce's expression. From not being able to get her shoulders straight (line 384), she conveys very accurately her all-encompassing anxiety of not being able to 'straighten out' and understand her situation (line 393). This reading of the conversation is borne out in Joyce's explanation that she just wants to lead her life (lines 399–404). It seems that here, Joyce is attempting to reconcile wants for a 'simple life' with what is happening to her. Her anxiety and fear overwhelm her and unconsciously she wishes to rid herself of these feelings and for them to be 'contained' by the nurse. Joyce cannot bear speaking of her anxieties directly for very long and perhaps not surprisingly returns to

describing her worries about her mouth ulceration and sore throat (lines 399–404).

This raises an interesting point about how far the nurse limits or engages her interpretive energy and skills in the face of the symptoms of cancer illness and treatment. In describing her sore mouth at this point Joyce is perhaps giving further voice to her overwhelming anxiety by associating primitive feelings and needs from childhood for feeding and being held. It appears very difficult for the nurse to receive Joyce's anxious communication at this point and she responds by acknowledging the symptoms Joyce is experiencing and reassures Joyce that these can be alleviated. It is distressing being with someone who is really upset and, just like the people we care for, we have ways of reducing the emotional discomfort. In her own reflection on the conversation the nurse described:

> The overriding thing is of erhm feeling absolutely helpless in the face of this extreme breathlessness and just and you know hoping against hope that they would actually be able to do something tomorrow but thinking probably they wouldn't. Poor Joyce. Poor woman, just lying there going 'huh huh' and it's just awful, you can't do anything.

The nurse continues to discuss the management of Joyce's symptoms and avoids directly addressing her anxiety. She fears causing Joyce additional distress and perhaps taking away hope. Joyce herself returns to her anxious thoughts after 5 minutes:

473 P. I don't know what to think I don't know what to do (34.0) miserable isn't it [laughs]

474 N. Mmm [long pause] you're doing really well Joyce

475 P. I'm not really it's it's just a miserable life I want no I'll get there [long pause] to sort to breathe [long pause] if I could just breathe a little is that *too* much?

476 N. [long pause] Mmm . . . the tongue I think won't get better straight away but it *will* get better *that* I can assure you it won't always be like this . . . your breathing we might not be able to get back to normal but I hope that we'll be able to get it significantly better than it is now

480 P.   Mmm [long pause] but the tight there isn't it

482 N.   The tightness yeh . . .

483 P.   The bones is it in the bones?

484 N.   No it's inside the lungs themselves

485 P.   Oh

486 N.   Some sort of plaques

487 P.   Yes tumour things [pause]

488 N.   Yeh

489 P.   It won't go away will it?

490 N.   No they were hoping that they would be able to erase them with the chemotherapy . . .

491 P.   . . . But I've only had two chemos so far

492 N.   I know yeh there is a possibility that

493 P.   I mean are you saying now that maybe the chemo's not going to do it

495 N.   That's what they don't know

496 P.   Mmm . . .

497 N.   . . . but that's why doctor wanted to see you straight away with an X-ray so she can . . .

498 P.   Mmm mmm

499 N.   . . . Have a good look at what's happening and see *you* at the same time

500 P.   I mean it's only two weeks since I saw the consultant could it happen in such a space of time I suppose it could anything can can't it

502 N.   Mmm [long pause]

503 P.   I'll just have to hope that tomorrow I can breathe [pause] because if I can't I don't know what I'm going to do [long pause]

505 N.   With regards to getting there

506 P.   Oh no no no I mean just from the point of view of just being able to breathe again . . . oh no I'll get there

508 N.   But tomorrow they'll be able to do something is that what you're saying?

509 P.   Mmm uhm mmm [long pause]

510 N.   I think it's quite important that you emphasise that to the doctor when you see her

512 P.   Mmm uhm

513 N.   That actually . . . the situation as it is right now is . . . not something that you can live with.

In her long pauses and statements Joyce clearly gives the nurse an experience of what it is like 'not to know what to think or do'. The nurse's responses (lines 474, 476–479) indicate perhaps that she is at a loss to know what to do or think as well, in the uncertain context of Joyce's sudden deterioration. Joyce clearly wants the nurse to perform some thinking function for her. The nurse responds in practical ways and with clinical solutions, leaving unanswered Joyce's question, 'Is it too much to ask, to just breathe a little?'

It is important to consider the nature of reassurance in helping with fear and anxiety and whether, in the face of worrying evidence to the contrary, reassurance can leave the person feeling unsafe, and at risk of losing confidence in the nurse. It is also important to consider ways in which the nurse might have communicated more strongly her understanding of Joyce's predicament and feelings. The nurse recognised that the ability to receive the feelings that Joyce engendered in her was the key to future work in helping Joyce with her fear and anxiety. This led the nurse to communicate her understanding of Joyce's predicament and feelings more effectively than demonstrated in these extracts.

This example vividly demonstrates the dynamics of container and contained in attempts to understand.

Helping with guilt

Clarrie is 28 years old and has leukaemia. She is married and has three young children. Clarrie has been in hospital for 8 weeks because her disease relapsed after treatment. The nurse has been closely involved with Clarrie throughout her treatment. This extract is taken from an hour-long conversation they had together after Clarrie indicated to the nurse that she was feeling particularly 'fed up':

200 P.   My mum scares me . . . she's the one really upsets me [cries]

201 N.   She's your mum

202 P.   Mmm [crying]

203 N.   It's just her way of is she angry do you think that it's happened?

204 P.   I don't know . . . she's not saying [pause] I mean she has said to me before that 'why why you' . . .

I mean I could ask the same question [giggles] I would not ask myself that . . . 'cos things like that happen all the time and you . . . just because you are not in it you don't know about it . . . you hear about it like on telly and things [pause] and yeh you think I won't ask that I think I dread to ask that not towards me but towards other people . . . 'cos you're made to feel like rot . . . I think I've done this to them [her family]

301 N.   You haven't done anything to them, Clarrie

302 P.   What do you . . . ?

303 N.   You have got leukaemia through no fault of your own . . . through nothing you've . . .

305 P.   No you know what my sister-in-law said to me . . . she said to me that it was my fault

307 N.   Why would it be your fault?

308 P.   . . . I don't know

309 N.   . . . How could it possibly be?

310 P.   I told my sister that [cries] I thought why . . . and I couldn't understand . . . I *couldn't* understand why she said it I think thinking that I'd done something that's why I'd got it

313 N.   There's nothing you could have done to make you get leukaemia, little children get leukaemia

315 P.   I know I kept thinking . . . what I kept thinking 'why'

316 N.   Well believe me . . .

317 P.   If she'd told my husband that can you imagine what he would then start thinking you know [pause] I probably caused it [sobbing]

319 N.   Please believe me you've got nothing to reproach yourself about you didn't cause this leukaemia it just happened to you, you had no say in the matter

321 P.   A grown woman telling me that it's my fault if I had known something maybe I would have acted sooner

323 N.   But that maybe wouldn't have altered anything anyway but *Clarrie* you didn't know you DIDN'T KNOW you had this last year and you didn't know when you just felt tired and unwell but . . .

326 P.   Do you [long pause] [cries] when I think about that at the time [cries] I think about that and I'm trying to work out why it was my fault

Clarrie is focusing on the consequences of what she has or has not done to get leukaemia and thus 'hurt' her family (lines 204, 311–312). Her sister-in-law personifies the persecutory, blaming part of herself that tells her that she is guilty of bringing the disease on herself and her family. The nurse recognises this self-blaming as a negative and faulty cognition (lines 301, 303) and wants to help Carrie see that her thinking is being fuelled by irrational beliefs and feelings, perhaps of excessive responsibility in relation to the cause of the cancer. The nurse directly challenges Clarrie's thinking (lines 307, 309) and reinforces less negative, 'right' thinking about the onset of her leukaemia (lines 313, 319).

It appears from the extract that the illness re-evokes painful needs in Clarrie's family relationships, which are mentioned but not fully articulated or discussed (lines 200, 204–300). Clarrie gives an indication that she is not experiencing her mother as supportive or nuturing and that she resents having to carry the emotional burden of her illness for her mother as well as for her own children. The nurse considered that Clarrie's negative thoughts had had a strange hold for some time and that she needed to work with Clarrie and some members of her family on this and a number of related issues over a period of several weeks. Together they decided to explore:

- how Clarrie first suspected she was unwell
- her partner's and family's immediate reaction to her diagnosis, including how they had been told and what they each now understood of the diagnosis
- what had changed for Clarrie and her partner and Clarrie and her mother, and what they

had discovered about each other since her diagnosis

- the impact of these discoveries on their relationships and parenting
- what they now wanted from each other.

Helping with anger and hostility

This is an example of low-key verbal aggression by a 45-year-old woman, Susan, in hospital for chemotherapy to treat a recurrence of her breast cancer. Susan's anger is directed first at the nurses caring for a dying woman on the ward and then at doctors, who she does not perceive consider the individual communication needs of people in their care. She tells the nurse:

64 P. I've been a bit sort of upset at the way erhm . . . she's looked after very well in terms of being cleaned and turned and whatever but there's not an *awful* lot of time erhm that's devoted to all the little things I think she's very abrupt but then she has a right to be hasn't she . . . I mean if you're on your way out you can be any way you like [pause]

69 N. It's not just . . .

70 P. . . . I sometimes think some people don't know how to approach someone they are very cheerful and 'how are you today' you know and 'those are nice flowers' but that's not what I think someone wants to hear, they want to get down to the nitty gritty you know and talk about what's happening you know and I think the consultants are not very good at that either . . .

75 N. Some aren't always perhaps er I mean *you* saw Dr Thorn this morning and were you able to get down to the nitty gritty?

77 P. Well it was all very cheerful in that he said I wouldn't expect it to come back and he said I'd be very unlucky if it did but I still don't know whether he's actually saying that because of all the years of experience or whether he's saying it because it's cheerful [laughs] you know and I would like him to talk to me as if he were talking to another doctor

82 N. What do you think he might have said about you to another doctor?

83 P. And I think consultants are so erhm used to being jolly that sometimes they forget you want to talk you know brass tacks really

85 N. Yeh yeh.

86 P. You know I don't know everyone is different . . . but I think erhm maybe they should try and gauge what kind of a person you are

88 N. Yes . . .

89 P. . . . If you want to hear or not [pause] I'm sure they do try but I think there's a lot of 'be better for her if I didn't' which makes me cross 'cos of the sort of person I am . . . I think when they are ill erhm they need special treatment and I think they need to be *really* asked how they are feeling

93 N. Yes . . . yes

94 P. You know and not just say 'oh how are you?' . . . 'good, fine' you know

95 N. Well how are *you* feeling Susan?

96 P. Well I you know still have seeds of doubt in my head thinking there must be people here who've had treatment like I've had and then they've come back and that's why I'd like the doctor to be frank because I hate that sort of feeling of of er you don't have all the facts and I well I think I wanted to sort of make my feelings apparent . . . I was frightened I would appear grumpy and ungracious but if someone's ill I think then you have to sort of with . . . your yard's measure of people's behaviour has to go out of the window.

103 N. My yard stick is away so can you tell me what sort of feelings you wanted . . . ?

104 P. . . . You know without being rude or anything I did I am very I'm made [pause] I feel very grumpy and cross

What is immediately striking in this extract is how the language Susan uses portrays her self-identity. She is reluctant to describe herself in the first person, preferring to use phrases like 'some people', and the words 'someone' and 'everyone' to distance herself from her experience and her feelings of anger, but also perhaps her uncertainty, fear, and anger in relation to the cancer itself. It may be that her anger is emerging, as denial and numbness of the news of her recurrence fade. Anger is often suppressed, perhaps unconsciously, by hospital staff in their attempts to make the environment as positive and cheerful as possible as this woman describes (lines 70–74, 77–81). It is then difficult for the person to express anger or negative thoughts and feelings, especially when staff are doing so much for them. Susan believes that more attention should be given to people's need and right to be angry and she is critical of false cheerfulness. Susan also seems to have mixed feelings of anger and dependency towards the doctors and nurses, and this can make the role of carers more difficult, as it seems to here.

The challenge for the nurse attempting to help Susan to understand her angry feelings is first to help her to verbalise and own them in relation to her own situation. The nurse does this successfully (lines 75–76, 82, 95, 103) and clearly provides a setting in which Susan feels secure enough to voice her dissatisfaction and angry feelings. The nurse does this by hearing her criticisms of care, not being defensive, and by channelling the energy of Susan's anger into asking for what she needs from professionals, all of which augurs well for Susan's emotional well-being.

Helping with a depressive response

An example of a nurse helping with a depressive response occurs when Tony, a 52-year-old man with myeloma, has been describing the problems he has been having walking with crutches and then using a wheelchair, and remarks to the nurse that 'I have to keep trying, I'm afraid, that's me'. He follows this with:

674 P.   I suppose in a way I'm worse off [long pause] I'm my own worst enemy in a way [pause] well I don't know sometimes I ought to rest more than I do erhm I don't I keep getting into this model where I rest like I use the wheelchair and I stay in it all day long faithfully and then I try and walk . . . I've got stiff and stuff so I think well try being out of the chair a bit more and then you get tired and you want to sit in the chair and I don't know which end of the candle to put out

700 N.   Mmmmm I see

701 P.   It's very difficult er whether it's just me getting worse this is what I was saying I get depressed I'm getting worse and worse and I don't know which way to go [sighs] erhm what I'd like to do is just sort of ignore the whole thing and just get on with life but I

can't do that erhm [long pause] I'm no use to the kids or Dorothy [wife] I'm not sure whether I should just stay in bed I mean I've stayed in bed longer since I've been in hospital for the last two days erhm and I've never felt more tired than I do now I feel really strange so I'm not winning that either

708 N.   Yes

709 P.   I'm getting a bit tired of it all [pause] I just want to be made better

710 N.   Yes

711 P.   I can't do much at all at the moment and I'm quite an active person normally in fact I'm supposed to be organising a camp in two weeks' time

713 N.   Are you? Where are you going to?

714 P.   In Sussex but I am getting quite stupified with all these pills I have been taking [pause] it doesn't look as if I'll get there [pause] and I feel very tired and well . . .

716 N.   . . . Do you think it would be wise to have a period when you're resting and also a time when you get up and potter around?

718 P.   Mmm

719 N.   Because then when you are resting it would be proper rest instead of just lying in bed

721 P.   I've thought of that but what happens is my staying vertical is that my legs start to swell up and all my stockings start to cut in

723 N.   But the other thing is you can sit out in the garden for a little while as long as you keep your feet up and er I can sort out a footstool

725 P.   Oh . . . that yes would be helpful

Tony uses the image of a candle (line 684) to represent the essence of his experience and his pronounced feelings of unhappiness. Instead of burning the candle at both ends, with its youthful connotations, Tony does not know which end of the candle to put out. The balance between fighting the illness and yielding to its implications has become dysfunctional for him. The nurse needs to work at Tony's own pace as much as possible, while being prepared to shift this balance when what is happening seems to be inappropriate.

Tony is 'still trying' and the nurse encourages this (lines 716, 723–724) but perhaps does so by denying the seriousness of how Tony feels. It is the physical humiliation of the illness that disempowers Tony as he struggles to manage his pain and fatigue. For Tony to hold in his mind the incompatible images of his current state and his previous health is painful, and the temptation for both him and the nurse is to switch the focus of attention onto something else or fail to take the implications on board, which avoids the distress (lines 715–716).

In this excerpt, the nurse recognised that he found it uncomfortable to confront what the physical changes of the illness meant for Tony's self-image, in terms of the value Tony placed on himself as a father of three young adults setting out on their careers, and as a husband. The nurse also recognised just how much Tony had revealed of his underlying concerns and sadness in this 45-minute talk. It is important to be aware of the ways we screen out pain and ask ourselves whether we inhibit the person exploring uncomfortable ideas by the methods we use to reduce our own exposure. In his future work with Tony, the nurse planned to empathise with Tony's concerns and to provide a comforting and supportive context so that Tony could be upset if he wished. Through more careful listening the nurse thought that, although he could not take away Tony's sadness and loss, he could work with Tony to shift the emphasis in his narratives from one of dependency to one of greater agency and sense of control. Tony placed considerable value on his expertise as an engineer, husband and father, and felt that helping strategies about acceptance and accepting his continuing responsibilities as a father and husband (his responsibility to help his wife and children face his illness, for example) may help to increase his sense of self-worth. The nurse considered how some of this work might take place with another family member, intrinsic to Tony's sense of self-worth.

Understanding how gender constructs our lives and our understanding of the meaning of care is growing. In this clinical example, a male nurse is talking with Tony and it is to this nurse that Tony is able to voice some of his worries. Tony's illness and incapacity presents an enormous challenge to his gendered identity. Bringing thoughts about gender overtly into discussions with Tony, and his preconceptions about providing and receiving care, might provide an alternative lens through which to explore his situation. Therefore, it may be useful for the nurse to explore with Tony how being a man influences his response to cancer.

Helping when treatment fails

Phyllis is a 75-year-old woman with endometrial cancer. Phyllis suspects that the cancer might have spread:

442 P.　I suppose I will find out when I'll get sorted out in the end

443 N.　. . . Yes [pause] but what would I mean what if they turned around and they said there's nothing really we can do about it?

445 P.　There's nothing I can do about it is there

446 N.　No . . . 'cos I mean 'cos that 'cos that could be a possibility I mean 'cos you have been in a week and if there was anything they were going to do

448 P.　That's what I mean yeh

450 N.　They'd erhm [pause]

451 P.　I mean if I've got it somewhere else then it's

452 N.　You've obviously thought about that

453 P.　Yeh well you 'ave to don't ya [long pause] [clears throat] I mean it's hard

454 N.　[long pause] Oh dear I know

455 P.　[pause] It's not that I'm frightened I *am* frightened but I'm not frightened if you know what I mean

457 N.　[long pause] Yes

458 P.　Err

459 N.　What are you frightened of?

460 P.　Oh I don't know

461 N.　It's the *not* knowing it's

462 P.　I don't know what I am frightened of I mean . . . I mean I don't know if it's er [pause] I don't know I really don't know

464 N.　The uncertainty or

465 P. Well yeh in one way [pause] erm but erm [long pause] depends what I am you know . . .

466 N. Yeh

467 P. . . . I think it's more that [pause] *if* it has gone inside somewhere else

468 N. Yes

469 P. . . . How am I gonna feel how am I gonna get you know what I mean?

470 N. Yes it's . . .

471 P. You know am I goin' to be *really* ill and in *pain* or you know what I mean?

472 N. Yes

473 P. You know the things you you the things you you know what I mean?

474 N. [long pause] There are things that we can deal with when they come

475 P. Yes yes I mean you know I think to myself I'm just going to end in a wheelchair that's it . . . a nice wee chat [laughs]

478 N. [laughs]

479 P. Your little machine [referring to the tape-recorder]

In this extract the nurse introduces bad news, i.e. news that materially alters Phyllis's view of her future. She does this in a supportive way (lines 443–444, 446–447). A person may temporarily block news they cannot take, but at least the information is made available so that they can use it constructively when they are ready. Here the nurse gives time for the idea she has raised to sink in and is not frightened of unleashing a reaction that might be difficult to deal with in the conversation. Phyllis does not block out the news by lightening the mood and changing the topic of the conversation until line 477. Up to this point she explores some of her thoughts about treatment failure. Even though the nurse tries to anticipate what Phyllis might be feeling (lines 461, 464), Phyllis does express her own particular concerns and uncertainty within the context of the supportive conversation with the nurse. Phyllis sets the agenda for subsequent conversations with this particular nurse. She wanted to talk more fully about what might happen to her as she got closer to death and how the family and friends could help her at home. The nurse agreed to do this in three half-hour conversations before Phyllis was discharged the following week.

Conclusion

Despite the urgency of the possibility of death for some cancer patients, it is important that nurses' therapeutic strategies proceed at a pace that feels safe, a pace dictated by the person and the nurse. Decisions about what feels safe to share rest with the individual and their family, and this also influences the timing and pacing of the work. Creating space for the person to gain some understanding of their own response to cancer can help them to retain competence and integrity.

The extracts above are powerful reminders of the fear, anxiety, guilt, and humiliation that can disempower people as they struggle to manage pain, discomfort, fatigue, and disfigurement from cancer. It is therefore essential that we all examine what we can do in our different contexts to help and empower the people we meet in our work. This includes ensuring that our own authority and 'knowingness', manifest in a dogmatic application of our knowledge about cancer illness, do not lead to sterile, unhelpful interpretations of experience that unwittingly undermine the dignity of individuals.

All too easily we can find ourselves responding to people in terms of our familiarity with a certain theory or our clinical experience. We then attach to the person the understanding that we have gleaned elsewhere, even though it may not apply to this particular individual. We are most likely to engage in clichéd thinking about people when we feel insecure about our clinical understanding. By prematurely believing we recognise what the person is communicating, even if we don't, we can preserve the appearance of being competent. There is a danger in this: that we identify worries on the sole basis of similarity rather than from a genuine process of collaborative, consensual working with an individual.

The pitfalls of preconceptions are a hazard, and not only for the inexperienced nurse. A similar danger lies in wait for the experienced nurse who might have got into a rut with his or her thinking, or be a bit too sure. It is so tempting to use short cuts to insight based on what has made sense with other patients, particularly when we are working in very busy clinical settings.

Effective clinical supervision is an essential venue for prompting us to re-orientate our thinking and question assumptions we might hold about a person with cancer, so that we remain receptive and responsive to them and feel supported in our work.

References

1. Cooper C.L. and Watson M. (eds.) (1991). *Cancer and Stress: Psychological, Biological and Coping Studies*. Chichester: Wiley.
2. Barraclough J. (1994). *Cancer and Emotion: A Practical Guide to Psycho-oncology*, 2nd edition. Chichester: Wiley.
3. Greer S. and Watson M. (1987). Mental adjustment to cancer: its measurement and prognostic importance. *Cancer Surveys* **6**, 439–451.
4. Kreitler S., Chaitchik S. and Kreitler H. (1993). Repressiveness: cause or result of cancer. *Psycho-oncology* **2**, 43–54.
5. Doan B.D. and Gray R.E. (1992). The heroic cancer patient: a critical analysis of the relationship between illusion and mental health. *Canadian Journal of Behavioral Science* **24**, 253–266.
6. Zorza R. and Zorza V. (1980). *A Way to Die: Living to the End*. London: Deutsch.
7. Duncker P. and Wilson V. (eds.) (1966). *Cancer Through the Eyes of Ten Women*. London: Harper Collins.
8. Burnard P. (1994). *Counselling Skills for Health Professionals*, 2nd edition. Campling J. (ed.) *Therapy in Practice Series*. London: Chapman and Hall.
9. Jacobs M. (1988). *Psychodynamic Counselling in Action*. London: Sage.
10. Tschudin V. (1995). *Counselling Skills for Nurses*, 4th edition. London: Baillière Tindall.
11. Altschuler J. (1997). *Working with Chronic Illness: A Family Approach*. London: Macmillan.
12. Moorey S. and Greer S. (1989). *Psychological Therapy for Patients with Cancer: A New Approach*. Oxford: Heinemann.
13. Judd D. (1995). *Give Sorrow Words: Working with a Dying Child*, 2nd edition. London: Whurr.
14. Cox M. (1988). *Structuring the Therapeutic Process: Compromise with Chaos*. London: Jessica Kingsley.
15. Gregory J. (1996). *The Psychosocial Education of Nurses: The Interpersonal Dimension*. Aldershot: Avebury.
16. Casement P. (1985). *On Learning from the Patient*. London: Routledge.
17. Egan E. (1994). *The Skilled Helper: A Systematic Approach to Effective Helping*, 5th edition. Belmont, CA: Brooks/Cole.
18. Murgatroyd S. (1985). *Counselling and Helping*. London: Routledge.
19. Mearns D. and Thorne B. (1988). *Person-centred Counselling in Action*. London: Sage.
20. Nelson-Jones R. (1993). *Practical Counselling and Helping Skills*, 3rd edition. London: Cassell.
21. Klein M. (1937). *Love, Guilt and Reparation and Other Works*, 1975 edition. London: Hogarth.
22. Kelly G. (1955). *The Psychology of Personal Constructs*, Vols 1 and 2. New York: Norton.
23. Perls F. (1969). *Gestalt Therapy Verbatim*. Lafayette, CA: Real People Press.
24. Berne E. (1964). *Games People Play*. Harmondsworth: Penguin.
25. Harris T. (1973). *I'm OK You're OK*. London: Pan.
26. Rogers C.R. (1951). *Client-centred Therapy*. Boston, MA: Houghton Mifflin.
27. Ellis A. (1962). *Reason and Emotion in Psychotherapy*. New York: Lyle Stuart.
28. Krumboltz J.D. and Thorenson C.E. (1969). *Behavioural Counselling: Cases and Techniques*. New York: Holt, Rinehart and Winston.
29. Bandler R. (1985). *Using Your Brain – For a Change*. Moab, UT: Real People Press.
30. Glasser W. (1965). *Reality Therapy*. New York: Harper and Row.
31. Ferruci P. (1982). *What We May Be*. Wellingborough: Thorson.
32. Freud S. (1938). An outline of psychoanalysis. In Strachey J. (ed.) *The Standard Edition of the Complete Psychological Works of Sigmund Freud*, Vol. 23. London: Hogarth.
33. Bion W.R. (1962). A theory of thinking. *International Journal of Psycho-analysis* **43**, parts 4–5.
34. Beck A.T. (1976). *Cognitive Therapy and the Emotional Disorders*. New York: International Universities Press.
35. Frankl V.E. (1959). *Man's Search for Meaning*. New York: Beacon Press.
36. Silver R.L. and Wortman C.B. (1980). Coping with undesirable life events. In Garber J. and Seligman M.E.P. (eds.) *Human Helplessness: Theory and Application*. New York: Academic Press, pp. 279–340.
37. Brody H. (1987). *Stories of Sickness*. New Haven, CT: Yale University Press.
38. Linde C. (1993). *Life Stories: The Creation of Coherence*. Oxford: Oxford University Press.

39. Segrave E. (1995). *Diary of a Breast.* London: Faber and Faber.

40. Butler S. and Rosenblum B. (1994). *Cancer in Two Voices.* London: Women's Press.

41. Picardie R. (1998). *Before I Say Goodbye.* London: Penguin.

42. Morrison B. (1993). *And When Did You Last See Your Father?* London: Granta Books.

43. Dennison A. (1996). *Uncertain Journey: A Woman's Experience of Living with Cancer.* London: Patten Press.

44. Ortony A. (1993). Metaphor, language and thought. In Ortony A. (ed.) *Metaphor and Thought.* Cambridge: Cambridge University Press, pp. 120–207.

45. Lakoff G. and Johnson M. (1980). *Metaphors We Live By.* Chicago, IL: University of Chicago Press.

46. Sontag S. (1991) *Illness as Metaphor.* Harmondsworth: Penguin Books (first published in 1978).

47. Stacey J. (1997). *Teratologies: A Cultural Study of Cancer.* London: Routledge.

48. Savage J. (1995). *Nursing Intimacy: An Ethnographic Approach to Nurse–Patient Interaction.* London: Scutari Press.

49. Bailey C. (1996). *Derrida, de Man, Habermas: Implications for Qualitative Analysis of Interviews in Cancer Care Research. A Methodological Study.* MSc thesis, University of London.

50. Froggatt K. (1998). The place of metaphor and language in exploring nurses' emotional work. *Journal of Advanced Nursing* **28**, 332–338.

51. Lanceley A. (1995). Emotional disclosure between cancer patients and nurses. In Richardson A. and Wilson-Barnett J. (eds.) *Nursing Research in Cancer Care.* London: Scutari Press pp. 167–188.

52. Kleinman A. (1988). *The Illness Narratives: Suffering, Healing and the Human Condition.* New York: Basic Books.

53. Mishler E.G. (1986). *Research Interviewing – Context and Narrative.* Cambridge, MA: Harvard University Press.

54. Gilbert A. (1994). *Personal Communication of Transference and Counter Transference.* London: Tavistock Centre.

55. Futterman A.D. and Wellisch, D.K. (1990). Psychodynamic themes of bone marrow transplant. *Haematology/Oncology Clinics of North America* **4**, 699–709.

56. Emanuel R.B. (1990). Counter-transference: a spanner in the works or a tool for understanding. *Journal of Educational Therapy* **3**, 3–12.

57. Bion W.R. (1962). *Learning from Experience.* New York: Jason Aronson.

58. Emanuel R.B. (1992). *Personal Communication on Containment, Cure, Care or Control.* London: Tavistock Centre.

59. Carkhuff R.R. (1987). *The Art of Helping,* 6th edition. Amherst, MA: Human Resource Development Press.

Part 3

The Experience
of Treatment

Introduction

Cancer, its construction, and society's response to it, has been highlighted as pervasive and problematic. Characterised by fear and uncertainty, this response shapes the very environment in which people with cancer find themselves, and has been explored in the preceding chapters. The experience of having cancer treatment is much less evident in the cancer literature than the events surrounding being given a diagnosis of cancer. Instead, the focus has been on the efficacy of cancer treatment, measured as the proportion of people who will survive 5 years from the point at which they were diagnosed.

When oncology emerged as a medical specialty in the 1950s, survival from cancer of any type was relatively poor; few people would expect to survive their illness. A number of critical developments in cancer treatment have transformed the chances of surviving a number of cancers – from a situation of near-certain death, to the possibility of cure. This has been particularly evident in childhood cancers, some of the leukaemias, and testicular teratoma. Early diagnosis, accurate staging, and multimodal therapy (the use of multiple cancer treatments: surgery, chemotherapy, radiotherapy; and multiple-agent rather than single-agent chemotherapy) have made progress in cancer treatment possible. In other situations, cancer treatment is increasing in sophistication so that some of the side-effects and difficulties of treatment have been reduced. More recently, developments in molecular biology and genetics have made a vast new range of treatments possible. These new treatments, and in particular issues around cancer genetics, are already presenting challenges and dilemmas to those working in cancer treatment settings.

Advances in molecular biology have led to the understanding of cancer as a genetic disease (not to be confused with an inherited disease); although inherited cancers are the focus of a large research effort, these probably only account for about 5–10% of all cancers and are discussed in Chapter 16. The genetic basis of cancer suggests a model whereby cancer initially develops from cells that have undergone a series of genetic mutations or alterations. As a result, cells become unable to respond to intra- or extracellular signals that control proliferation, differentiation and cell death. According to Hill, cancer treatment can be thought of as adding negative signals to the cellular environment, and thus arresting or inhibiting tumour cell growth and multiplication.[1] It is hoped that these will prevent the development of further cancer cells at the originating site, or sites of metastatic growth at any other site in the body. The object of cancer science is to develop new and better methods of preventing the growth of cancer cells. The reality for people in cancer clinics is rather different, since it is impossible to detect cancer cells within the body once a tumour has been removed; cancer treatment is inevitably sometimes given where little is known about whether it is needed for any given individual. This can only be projected through estimates of risk, based on studies of cancer populations. Here lies a dilemma for the treatment team that is difficult to convey to people facing the devastating news of a cancer diagnosis; the personal accounts presented throughout this section convey the difficulty for people of living with this uncertainty.

Cancer treatment is an uncertain venture and is often experimental. The extent to which treatment will be effective in preventing future cancer spread is often unknown, yet it involves many side-effects both at the time of treatment, or in the long term, such as infertility or the risk of developing a second cancer, or permanent disfigurement or disability. Little is known about how people with cancer make choices about treatments in the light of their own risk of developing progressive cancer at some future date. This, when accompanied by the fear engendered by cancer, creates a cocktail of anxiety mixed with various personal and professional agendas, and makes genuine partnership in planning care and treatment difficult.

Studies of the quality of life of people undergoing cancer treatment have used questionnaires to evaluate the impact of treatment on the individual. The effects of cancer treatment on an individual's ability to function, the physical and emotional symptoms they may experience, and the social and psychological sequelae of cancer are reported by the patient, usually through a series of rating scales. These studies have documented the many effects of cancer and its treatment but, unfortunately, they have tended to be seen as simply an adjunct, or additional piece of data to be collected alongside survival data, for monitoring the side-effects of cancer therapies. By being combined with side-effect data, the relevance and impact of these data have been reduced in importance, so that insufficient information exists regarding the problems and difficulties that accompany cancer treatment. Studies of quality of life in people undergoing cancer treatment have offered little insight into the turmoil and confusion surrounding cancer treatment, or the sheer difficulty of living through the devastating effects that it can have on daily life.

The purpose of this section is to provide insights into the experience of cancer treatment through the use of personal accounts. Information is also presented on different treatment modalities and strategies for managing the problems people face while undergoing treatment. Nursing is presented as central to managing the experience of treatment, both emotionally and physically. An increasing number of nursing research studies are being undertaken into the problems caused by cancer treatment, and findings from these studies are presented throughout. Nurses are making contributions to the science of cancer treatment – in particular, in exposing the need for a more person-focused culture in cancer treatment.

Reference

1. Hill R.P. and Tannock I.F. (2005). Introduction to cancer biology. In Tannock I.F. and Hill R.P. (eds.) *The Basic Science of Oncology*, 4th edition. New York: McGraw Hill.

CHAPTER TEN

The experience of treatment

Lynne Colbourne

'Treatment' refers to the therapies that are used with the aim of eradicating cancer cells, such as radiotherapy and chemotherapy. However, the experience of cancer treatment cannot be explored in isolation, it needs to be considered alongside the process of obtaining a diagnosis, undergoing staging investigations, follow-up and aftercare, as each of these are also part of the treatment experience and together are often described as the 'cancer journey' or treatment pathway.

The treatment pathway (see Figure 10.1) is not always straightforward, and may involve a number of investigational tests, and single, or more often combined or sequential, treatments. This chapter will explore the treatment pathway by drawing on the direct experience of people with cancer and detailing clinically relevant aspects of therapy and care. The text boxes containing personal accounts provide excerpts from the narrative of men (diagnosed with prostate or testicular cancer) and their spouse/partners, who participated in a qualitative, prospective case study.[1]

Diagnosis and staging

Michele Angelo Petrone was diagnosed and treated for Hodgkin's lymphoma, and expressed in words and paintings his experience of cancer and treatment. This work is available as a book and presents a powerful insight of the emotional impact of the cancer journey. A brief excerpt from this book is presented in Box 10.1.

Box 10.1 The beginning of the cancer experience

Between night and day
As time goes by, night follows day, and day follows night – a natural cycle without beginning, without end and without gaps. Life's cycle continues without interruption, or at least it should do. Suddenly illness arrives, uninvited, unexplained. I found myself caught between life and death, light and dark, banished to an unknown place – between night and day. The illness forced itself into my life where there was no place for it. The arrival of illness stole a place and time that should have been destined for better things (p.6).

Reproduced with permission from Michele Angelo Petrone (2003) *The Emotional Cancer Journey.* Brighton: MAP Foundation. www.mapfoundation.org.[2]

The period leading to confirmation of a cancer diagnosis and subsequent staging investigations is a time of oscillating emotions, fear and uncertainty, where normality and control are lost and there is shock that an apparently 'normal' body has malfunctioned in some way.

Each person has an individual perception of what cancer means to him or her, a mental, socially constructed interpretation that is brought to the cancer experience.[3,4] Some may have previous knowledge of cancer (commonly negative) through someone close to them. Previously

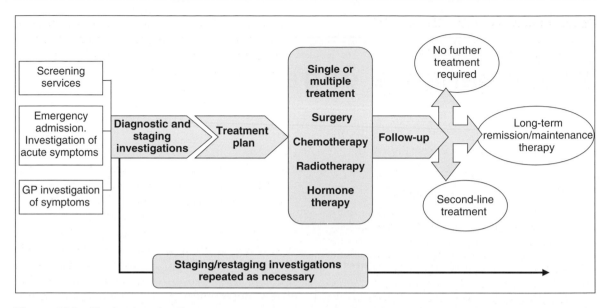

Figure 10.1 The treatment pathway.

constructed thoughts and beliefs surrounding cancer can affect the degree of emotional impact cancer has. This is a key point of the pathway where the person affected by cancer and those close to them may need an opportunity to talk through their fears of cancer and to clarify understanding of their situation to resolve any potential misconceptions.

The management of the pre-diagnostic phase, cancer diagnosis, and staging can be critical in shaping the view and perceptions of people facing cancer, and their family members throughout treatment and beyond.[1,4,5] Some will be satisfied with the care and information they receive. However, if the opposite is the case, expressions of frustration, anger and a wariness of being let down by the health care system or health professionals can arise, and may persist throughout the pathway or with time.[1,6,7] Difficulties can arise during the process of diagnosis or staging if:

- an individual considers symptoms they experienced before diagnosis were not taken seriously or investigated appropriately
- investigations were requested by clinical staff but there was in delay in investigations or tests commencing, or unacceptable waiting times were experienced

- there is poor management of this phase of the pathway because of lack of information, communication, explanation, or co-ordination of care.

Without appropriate management and planning of the staging process, diagnostic tests can seem disjointed events, isolated instances of investigation of different parts of one's body. The personal accounts illustrated in Personal account 10.1 provide differing experiences of obtaining diagnostic test results. These narratives highlight the importance of health professionals understanding the emotional implications of diagnostic tests and the need people facing a diagnosis of cancer have for information. Not knowing what is wrong and feelings of uncertainty dominate at this phase, and staff based in radiology and pathology departments need to deal empathetically with people undergoing tests and investigations where cancer is suspected.

When exploring the experience of men diagnosed with testicular cancer Jones and Payne offered the hypothesis that people under stress seek safety signals.[8] The study identified that a lack of opportunity for positive reinforcement of such safety signals increases anxiety levels. Attempting to assert oneself in a crisis situation to gain control is well known.[9–14] From the point of

Personal account 10.1 Diagnosis[1]

1. Luke was 30 years old when he noticed a lump on his breast.

> . . . he [breast surgeon] said that it looked like a hormone imbalance [and then he said] 'but we'll have an ultrasound scan on the breast and testicles, just you know [to be sure]' but he didn't explain why, and I went back to work, I thought 'fine I'm sorted . . .'.

Luke then attended for an ultrasound scan:

> . . . I had my ultrasound scan and they examined my testicles first, and they went to my left breast, and my right breast, and he did my stomach . . . and I'm thinking he's not doing my stomach, I'm not down for that, I remember that letter! So I said 'Is there a problem here?' And he said, 'Oh yes you've got a tumour', and I thought 'a tumour?' I thought 'oh God major panic', he stopped and he said, 'Oh, no need to worry, it's the best type, erm, go and get changed . . .'.

The radiologist returned and took blood tests and apologised that the consultant couldn't see Luke until later that week, but Luke was confused:

> . . . I said, 'So I've got a tumour in my left breast?' . . . and he said, 'No, no, no it's in your testicle, it's in your testicle', and that was it! He walked away, and I was, I thought, 'oh shit I've got a tumour'.

> . . . I had three nights and two days thinking 'I've got a tumour, isn't cancer a tumour? is it a malignant tumour? is it a large one? is it a small one? . . .' I went on to NHS Direct and the opening sort of paragraph, on the internet, is, this is the biggest killer between the ages of 15 and 30!

At a time when this man desperately needed explanations there appeared to be no one knowledgeable to contact.

2. Colin was 53 years of age when he attended for a well man's check at his general practitioner (GP) surgery. Blood tests suggested prostate cancer, and this was confirmed with a prostate biopsy. The following excerpt was taken from Colin's description of one of his staging investigations:

> . . . I had a wonderful man who was in charge of the [bone] scan, and when I'd finished, 'cos he obviously knows how worried people are, when I'd finished, he said 'You haven't heard this from me', he said 'but it's clear'. So I was able to walk out of that hospital and I felt good.

diagnosis, individuals may search for positive information to resolve negative preconceptions of cancer, for example seeking reassurance from information that reinforces the potential of successful cancer treatment.[1,8,12] How a person seeks and attempts to gain control over their situation is variable. People with cancer, and family members, can have different practical, emotional, and supportive needs and require varying levels of control/empowerment over the situation. People tend to 'box off' the cancer experience into manageable parts (for example by focusing on the immediate challenge of 'getting through' treatment) to cognitively deal with the experience.[1,3,4] Early access to a knowledgeable health professional can assist individuals in making sense of their situation, and in clarifying understanding of staging and prognostic information as results become available. Nurses are in an ideal position to help individuals and families by providing opportunities for reassurance and optimising coping strategies and this can include:

- offering information in 'chunks' at appropriate and regular time points
- initiating referral as appropriate to members of the multiprofessional health care team
- providing awareness of the benefits of sharing or learning about the cancer experience with others (for example via support groups or 'phone buddy programmes).

Taylor and Lobel describe this form of coping strategy as social comparison.[15] Comparison is sought with a person in a similar situation or someone considered a survivor to provide inspiration or hope. Gray *et al.* identified this process occurring with men diagnosed with prostate cancer, and refer to it as 'providing models of recovery'.[16]

Diagnostic tests

Formal diagnosis requires the collection of data through a series of tests, investigations, tissue specimens obtained from biopsy or needle aspiration to provide histology, and different scans for radiological reports. For some cancers the diagnostic pathway is simple with limited investigations, while for others a clear diagnosis is not always easy to determine. The primary site of a tumour may be confirmed quickly, but confusion and delay might occur as staging investigations are carried out. Diagnostic tests are frequently managed on an outpatient basis, and performed at various hospital sites by different health professionals. Over the last 10 years, greater coordination of this pathway has occurred through diagnostic and treatment planning being undertaken by cancer site-specific multidisciplinary teams. However, this does not include pre-diagnostic tests undertaken in primary care or people being investigated for potentially rare tumours (where initial investigations will be performed locally, but ongoing referral and cancer treatment will be administered by multidisciplinary teams at a regional/tertiary cancer centre).

As cancer can develop from any organ in the body and present as one of more that 100 different histological types, accurate diagnostic data are essential in offering the appropriate treatment. Before any test, a detailed physical examination and medical history is undertaken. The purpose of medical investigation is to locate the primary cancer and to classify its histology and locate any spread (and, if present, the extent of metastases). Staging of cancer normally follows the internationally recognised TNM system (see Box 10.2).

The TNM staging system is a common predictor of prognosis but each cancer will have other prognostic indicators in addition to the TNM system. For example in prostate cancer the biopsy histology findings are graded and calculated as a Gleason score (4 or below low grade; 5–7 intermediate; 8–10 high grade and poor prognostic factor).[18] The level of the serum tumour marker, prostate-specific antigen (PSA), is also an essential addition to the TNM information.

At specific intervals during treatment, staging investigations are commonly repeated (as identified by treatment protocols) to measure the cancer response to treatment, to inform decisions regarding the need for additional therapy, and

---

Box 10.2 TNM staging/classification of solid malignant tumours

The classification describes the anatomical extent of the disease by using three components:

- T – the extent of the primary tumour
- N – the absence or presence (and therefore extent) of regional lymph node involvement
- M – the absence or presence of distant metastases.

Each of the above is assigned a number to indicate the extent of local and distant spread of a particular tumour: T1, T2, T3, T4, N0, N1, N2, N3, M1 (for some cancer types these classifications will be subdivided even further, e.g. T2a, T2b).
Other categories include:

- Tis – carcinoma *in situ*
- T0 – no evidence of primary
- Tx – primary cannot be assessed
- Nx – nodes cannot be assessed
- M0 – no evidence of metastases
- Mx – metastases cannot be assessed
- G1 – well differentiated.

Adapted from Neal and Hoskin (1994).[17]

---

post-treatment to monitor tumour absence or to investigate signs of cancer progression or recurrence.

To obtain the information required to complete a patient's TNM staging, various clinical investigations will be performed. These investigations provide greater visibility of the internal workings of the patient's body to clinical staff. The patient and their family will also attempt to use the findings as a means of interpretation of the seriousness of the situation, to monitor the effectiveness of therapy, and interpret the body for signs of metastases.[10,19–21] When exploring the experience of men with prostate cancer, Kelly illustrated how a man's cancer experience was lived through the response of their tumour to cancer treatment.[19] Information gleaned through clinical investigations is a primary way of making sense of the situation, and health professionals can use these findings to explain, inform, and 'cancer educate' patients in relation to their particular situation.

Making decisions about treatment

Accurate diagnosis and staging is important in the management of cancer, by informing treatment options and decisions. With advances in cellular science and imaging technology the level of information available from staging investigations is increasingly complex. Health professionals often have a superior knowledge of the disease process, and intentionally or unintentionally may use technical/medical language when discussing treatment options with people with cancer. The risk is that people with cancer can become excluded from treatment decisions because of this complexity. Silverman suggests that the problem is not simply solved by developing a more open dialogue between doctor and patient or creating a more straightforward language – the issues are much more involved.[22] Increasingly the costs of health care and particular treatments drive decision making, and the availability of particular treatments may be determined not only by evidence of their effectiveness but also by issues such as affordability within the health care system.[23]

Deciding upon a treatment plan can be more complex with certain tumour types. Clinical trials have determined ideal therapeutic regimes (for maximum disease-free survival) in the treatment of testicular teratoma or seminoma, and therefore choices that need to be made in relation to prognosis are potentially less complex. However, this is not the case for other tumours such as breast or prostate cancer where research data are less prescriptive. For example with prostate cancer, although staging, prognostic indicators, and performance status might direct treatment options to a degree, a man will still be offered a multitude of treatment choices and these are depicted in Figure 10.2. To illuminate this situation further, Personal account 10.2 provides a personal account of the difficulties experienced in being offered a treatment choice.

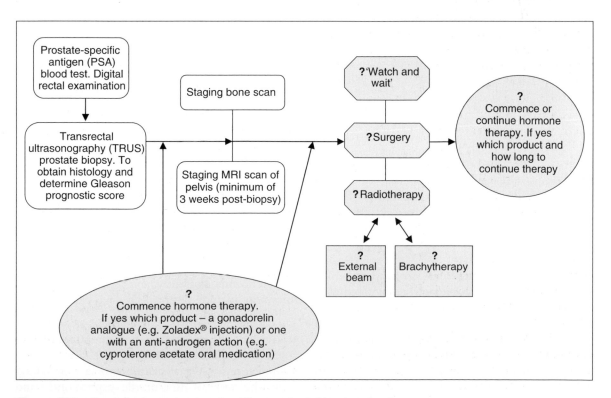

Figure 10.2   Prostate cancer treatment pathway: potential treatment options.

Personal account 10.2   Treatment choices[1]

At the age of 57 Julian had been diagnosed with prostate cancer after attending a routine health check. Julian and his wife had sought several second opinions and had desperately tried to seek the treatment Julian considered personally appropriate. Julian had finally located a consultant oncologist he had faith in and had commenced a three-month course of hormone therapy in preparation for external beam radiotherapy.

> . . . the other thing I heard a few times, that, what I got in the very early stages is, it's your choice as to how the treatment is, and in hindsight it's wrong. You know I'm an [states profession], and I don't go along to my clients and say 'What do you want and I will [produce it] for you', I am not a parrot, and I expect the consultants to lead you, a lot of them said 'No, it's your choice' and I defy you, I defy anybody to be in a rational mind and make choices, you can't do it, I couldn't do it, and it's just I'm trying to think, I've got to make a choice here, on this most monumental, you know, treatment . . . I need to be guided, but my reaction was, what would you do in my circumstances, but it's [left as] your job, it's a load of cobblers quite honestly, the best they could say is 'I strongly recommend, you know, in these circumstances everything points to, you should go this route' you know.

> In hindsight I could have gone into brachytherapy, 'cos we pushed very hard for it, and thank God, I mean it was a low point going up to [that centre], but in hindsight with that PSA I shouldn't have been having brachytherapy and the guy wouldn't do it . . . so yes I would make a very strong recommendation that people aren't asked or told it's their choice and what do you want to do, 'cos the only thing you want to do is, go backwards or get out you know, tell me I am cured, but how do you get cured, I would defy anyone to choose . . . you look to be advised, and directed in a certain route, I accept in the end that you can't tell them that you must have this . . .

A number of studies have been undertaken to explore the desire of people newly diagnosed with cancer to be involved in making decisions about their treatment.[23–28] Degner and Sloan developed a tool for evaluating such preferences, and identified a continuum of scenarios from the desire to play an active role in decision making, through the desire for a collaborative or shared role, to the preference for a passive role, where the physician or other health professionals or carer is the primary or sole decision maker.[23] The scenarios of this continuum were evident in the findings of a study exploring the experience of women newly diagnosed with breast cancer. Beaver *et al.* suggest an important distinction between participation and a desire to make decisions about treatment, and the need for information.[25] In their study of women with breast cancer they reveal that women express a high desire for information but not necessarily for active participation in decisions about which treatment they should have.

There is obviously an immense challenge for health professionals in providing support for people with cancer in relation to treatment choices. An awareness of the potential roles people with cancer and family members might adopt should inform this process. Additionally, time, information and repeated opportunity for discussion (and possibly second opinions) need to be factored into the treatment pathway.

Improving diagnostic care provision

In the UK since 1995 when the first comprehensive report recommending how cancer services should be organised was published,[29] there has been a series of guidelines published for the clinical management of specific cancers, and numerous government reports that dictate the implementation of initiatives and targets to rectify deficiencies in cancer care provision. A key focus has been to reduce waiting times for diagnostic/staging investigations and also the time from urgent referral for investigation to commencement of treatment (this is specified to be no more than 62 days) in order to deliver faster diagnosis and treatment, and reduce delays in diagnosis and the commencement of treatment. Extended nursing roles are being developed as part of initiatives to meet targets for waiting times for diagnosis and the commencement of treatment. Increasingly nurse roles now include performing diagnostic tests.

For example:

- advanced nurse practitioners are undertaking screening flexible sigmoidoscopy[30,31]
- clinical nurse specialists in breast care are taking on the task of fine-needle aspiration,[32] and including this service within previously established nurse-led outpatient clinics offering

symptom management, prosthetics, information, and emotional support

- clinical nurse specialist roles have been developed to provide one-stop clinics to perform colposcopy and provide treatment.[33,34]

A focus of research studies investigating these new roles is to evaluate potential cost savings and the ability of nurses to obtain accurate tissue samples for diagnosis, comparable to that of medical colleagues.[30,31,35] These evaluations, although indicating positive outcomes from the implementation of such roles, may not capture other potential benefits these nurse roles could deliver. In 2000, Doyal and Cameron suggested nurses as a substitute for doctors as a solution for manpower issues.[36] The previous examples illustrate that nurses are expanding their roles by undertaking tasks previously the province of medical staff. However, the evidence for nurse-led care in cancer (effectiveness or acceptability) has not been thoroughly evaluated.[37,38] After reviewing the current evidence, Corner concluded that to improve cancer service provision, the best results may not necessarily be gained through nurses substituting directly for doctors, but through investment in nurse-led care by providing new professional roles and new services in areas of need, and thereby wider benefits in the experience of treatment and care may be realised.[37] Box 10.3 details the introduction of a nurse-led service that includes the nurse/doctor substitution of the task of skin biopsy but moves beyond this by providing a nursing assessment of patient need and access to an 'oncology-knowledgeable' key worker at an important phase of the treatment pathway.

From 1995 the focus of directives from the Department of Health centred primarily on the organisation of cancer care provision and medically orientated treatment delivery. This agenda widened with the publication of the National Institute for Clinical Excellence (NICE) guidance, *Improving Supportive and Palliative Care for Adults with Cancer* in 2004.[43] This document emphasised supportive, emotional, and rehabilitation care as a priority and equal to diagnostic investigations and treatment. Deficits in care were acknowledged and models offered to address care shortfalls. Important aspects of this guidance included:

- the need for a service model that recognises the central role of families/carers in providing support to patients
- the separate assessment of the needs of the carer, family, and patient at key points in the pathway
- recognition that care is managed across health care settings and specialties, and new models of working are needed to deliver planned, integral care for those receiving curative, palliative, or end-of-life care, from pre-diagnosis throughout the treatment pathway and beyond.

To promote continuity of care, the nomination of a person to take on the role of 'key worker' for individual patients was the preferred model.

The immediate response to the last point has been that nurses would be in the ideal situation to take on the role of key worker. Commonly the person undergoing investigations for suspected cancer receives this care as an outpatient. Access to a key worker at this stage of the treatment pathway would ideally be to an oncology outreach nurse or nurses already based in primary care. To ensure all patients have such an oncology-knowledgeable key worker, this will require changing models of care to increase cross-boundary working of acute oncology teams and/or increasing availability and access of oncology-related education and experience for nurses and health professionals based in primary care.

THE EXPERIENCE OF UNDERGOING TREATMENT

Specific oncology treatments are explained and discussed in detail in the following chapters. This section will provide an overview of the experience of receiving treatment.

Obtaining a cancer diagnosis, a treatment plan, and relevant information can afford some relief from anxiety. A treatment plan provides positive information that something can be done to deal with the cancer. However, the emotional

Box 10.3 Nurse-led service – one-stop skin biopsy clinic

By responding to patient, legislative and service need, a skin cancer nurse specialist changed the pattern of health care service delivery locally. The following are the steps and observations taken from a paper by Gill Godsell that described introducing a one-stop skin biopsy service to a cancer centre.[39]

Aim of the nurse biopsy role

. . . to improve care delivery for the patient with suspected skin cancer by reducing the wait for a biopsy and providing continuity and a complete package of care from pre-diagnosis to treatment and discharge [p.50].

Steps

1. Develop a professional framework for practice, in line with Nursing and Midwifery Council guidance (this should include identification of need, rationale for change, proposed benefits for patients, consideration of issues of safety, nurse skill competence, education/training and validation).
2. Utilise legislation/government targets to support proposed change in service delivery and to facilitate funding if additional resources are required for role expansion. In this example Godsell cited the following documents: *Making a Difference*,[40] *The NHS Plan*,[41] and *The Cancer Plan*.[42]
3. Undertake skin biopsy training programme.
4. Employ an audit tool to measure efficacy of nurse biopsy role in (i) technique in obtaining adequate samples, and (ii) the impact of service on waiting times. In Godsell's experience, diagnosis was obtained on 100% of specimens and waiting times for a skin biopsy showed a reduction from 8 to 0 weeks.
5. Regularly undertake a patient and GP satisfaction survey to evaluate acceptability of service and to gain user and service commissioner opinion.
6. Inform others of this initiative and disseminate useful guidance and protocol documents.
7. Continue to develop the role and service. Future projects: development of a national skin biopsy training course to include guidelines and competencies; production of a handbook for nurses to perform skin biopsy including the theory of dermatology surgery.

Additional outcomes of introduction of this nurse-led service

- The reduction in waiting time for biopsy can lead to a reduction in anxiety level for those confirmed with, or without cancer.
- By reducing the biopsy workload from the doctors' list, the time for removal of the cancer can be reduced (in Godsell's experience from 8 weeks to 3 weeks).
- Provision of a patient-centred service; more time for the nurse to establish a rapport with the patient, to answer questions, allow expression of anxiety, assess psychosocial and information needs, and in addition offer sun protection/wound care advice, and information about possible diagnoses.
- At the diagnostic/staging phase the skin biopsy nurse specialist is in an ideal position to function as the patients' 'key worker'.

roller-coaster does not cease, and anxiety occurs waiting for treatment to commence. There are fears of what side-effects will occur, to what degree they will impact, and the likelihood of treatment success or failure. A frustration for those receiving treatment and for family members is a lack of definites. Treatment plans often change due to scheduling difficulties, overwhelming toxicity, and on occasions poor response of the cancer to treatment. As a result estimated end dates of therapy may be put back and a life post-treatment cannot be planned for with certainty.

The equipment and personnel required for treatment administration often dictate where therapy can be provided (although service user pressure can often challenge current service arrangements). Cycles of treatment can be multiple and involve more than one modality; courses of treatment can be scheduled over weeks or months, and maintenance therapy can continue for years. Each cancer therapy brings with it specific side-effects. Attempting to maintain elements of normality during active treatment can help to exert some control. Where possible, patients may continue working even if this means reducing their hours. Families will often try to create routine to incorporate treatment in an attempt to make children feel secure. The cycles of attending for treatment can become a routine of normality. The risk of trying to maintain normality (and possibly a brave face) is that anxieties and queries may not be aired. As many treatments are delivered in an outpatient or ambulatory setting, opportunities for people with cancer and family members to locate someone to talk to may be limited.

Treatment side-effects

The nature of external beam radiotherapy tends to result in acute side-effects becoming cumulative and occurring towards the latter portion of treatment, and for several weeks after completion. The type and severity are dependent upon the specific area of the body being treated, the size of the radiotherapy field and the number of treat- ments. Acute side-effects from chemotherapy have the potential to occur within minutes of administration but usually begin to resolve before the next cycle of treatment is administered. The effects are dependent on the specific cytotoxic agents used and their toxicity profile, single or, more commonly, multiple drug combinations, dose, and the number and frequency of cycles within a course of treatment. Personal account 10.3 provides personal accounts of the cancer treatment phase. These accounts demonstrate the individuality of the impact of cancer treatment for the patient and the spouse/partner.

A medical aim of cancer treatment is to destroy cancer cells and optimise the possibility of disease-free survival. Fear of cancer and death is such that people with cancer are often willing to accept treatment toxicity even for a slim chance of treatment response.[44] People may have to deal with alterations in body shape, image and function, some of which might be temporary or permanent such as hair loss, weight gain/loss, gynaecomastia, sexual dysfunction, infertility, skin pigmentation, surgical scarring, lymphoedema, tinnitus/hearing loss, colostomy formation. It could be argued that as such outcomes of treatment are not life threatening, less attention is given to them in comparison to maximising the

Personal account 10.3   The impact of chemotherapy/radiotherapy administration[1]

The patient perspective

1. Ian was 27 years old when he was diagnosed with a testicular teratoma. The following extracts are taken from an interview that was undertaken after he had received the second of three cycles of inpatient chemotherapy (each inpatient episode was interspersed with an outpatient injection of chemotherapy).

I started the first round of chemo, got a bit knocked around, I was a bit poorly, came out, it took me a few days to get over it, returned to normal for the best part of a week, doing normal things . . . then about a week later I picked up an infection, which obviously put me straight back into hospital again, um, I was quite poorly, in hospital for three and a half days, out on Sunday then straight back in for the second round of chemo then . . . that's really knocked me around.

I was supposed to go back in on the Monday [for treatment], and I was delayed, my results [blood counts] were too low, and I was having this problem all the time, anyway because of what I had, that bad infection, the first time, they decided they'd leave it three days so I went back in on the Thursday [to start second cycle] . . . and then on the Saturday I did nothing but throw up, all day, all day there was nothing they could do for me, I was as sick as a dog . . . at about seven o'clock in the evening, I was I just felt my stomach, I thought there was nothing more to come up, I was just retching, they managed to give me my next lot of anti-sickness stuff, and I seemed to settle down then. I got home settled down and the stomach settled down, erm, still had the 'manicness', I mean that was just horrendous, usual thing, you know just staring at the walls, not really knowing what to do with myself, I was quite weak actually as well so I didn't really have much energy to do anything, everything was a real effort . . .

. . . towards the end of the week I started getting quite rough, I mean, I wasn't throwing up but I got, it was just my brain wouldn't work, I was just sat here, and just stringing sentences together was so difficult, and the actual effort of actually trying to think about something to say and I really didn't actually speak probably for the best part of two days, because I really, really did not have the energy at all, or the inclination, I just spent most of my time watching telly or sleeping to be honest . . . it's almost like, I'm awake but I am asleep, and I know things are going on around me, but I can't interact . . . I am just completely detached, in a world of my own, and I get quite agitated as well . . . if I am sat watching telly, and if Jane is just looking through the paper, that really irritates me, it just really, I notice every little thing around me, and I just get very irritated and I just take myself off and go and lie down.

I go for my booster tomorrow, and when I get to six o'clock I will start feeling a bit rough, and I take a couple of paracetamol and I feel all right. I mean I feel rough all day Wednesday but Thursday morning I will be all right, you know, so I know the cycles now, and like now when I go for the next chemo I will feel a little bit rough on Tuesday but I will be throwing up all day Wednesday, it's just one of those things now, but I know it's coming now.

2. Graham was 65 years old when diagnosed with prostate cancer. He had requested a PSA test after hearing about prostate cancer screening on a radio programme. The following extracts are taken from two interviews, (one when Graham was mid-radiotherapy treatment and the other on completion of this treatment). Graham often read directly from his diary annotations during his interview. The effects of treatment that Graham describes appear less acute than in the previous case but they had an immense impact on his quality of life.

Graham had commenced hormone therapy three months prior to radiotherapy. This had caused erectile dysfunction. During interview Graham acknowledged the impact of this had been devastating but he found it difficult to talk about (this topic of conversation was usually raised after the taped interview). Graham also developed gynaecomastia as a side-effect from hormone therapy. Graham's wife believed he was terribly embarrassed about his altered body image and he would not initiate any discussion of it during medical consultations. However during interview this issue was discussed:

My breasts ache here [indicates all breast tissue] which when you lie over [in bed], oh gosh it's uncomfortable, and it's, I comment that I'll need a new bra soon [laughs] but hopefully this will cease when I finish with the Casodex. It's when you, you're in bed and you perhaps turn over, it, you know, it just feels uncomfortable, when I pour the tea in the morning, golly it aches, it's that sort of feeling you know . . .

Graham began to experience side-effects from pelvic radiotherapy halfway into 6 weeks of daily treatments. Due to the action of radiotherapy on cells these reactions continued for several weeks post-therapy. The following excerpts illustrate issues identified by Graham who completed radiotherapy on 3 February:

. . . on the 24th [January] I've got an upset tummy, 25th the same, 26th took two Imodium, plus one later . . . then the 30th I'd got a sore bottom, feeling very poorly and I took Fybogel, I'd asked the doctor about this and he said it's a finely balanced thing with the Imodium, anyway I took that . . . so, then the 31st that was the same still feeling poorly, and when I look back on this [the diary] yea gods! I went through the mill! . . . on the 2nd [February] I went to church, still sore, I had a slight [rectal] bleed then, but that cleared up . . .

Alteration in bowel and urinary function, seeking methods of control, and the social restrictions resulting from increased toileting was a constant feature:

. . . there were times when I got on that [radiotherapy machine] table and, the worst part about it was getting and holding a full bladder, I got on the table and she [radiographer] said 'I'll be another 10 minutes', and I said 'I can't wait', and of course you've lost your [treatment] slot, then you've got to have some more water and they fetch you back later . . .

Off-tape Graham explained that his radiotherapy-induced tiredness was compounded by lack of sleep. The radiotherapy was causing irritation to the bladder mucosa, which resulted in frequency of micturition. Some nights Graham was passing water on an hourly basis, which resulted in sleep-deprived exhaustion. A month after completing radiotherapy Graham read from his diary:

. . . I'm starting to feel good again, another milestone, slept right through the night without getting out to the loo, absolutely wonderful . . .

On 7th and 9th [February] still diarrhoea I was suffering from, I normally go to church but this particular day I didn't go, 10th not feeling very well drinking more fluid . . . I made an appointment to see the doctor [GP] on the 13th, still having trouble with going to the loo . . . years ago I suffered from a fissure, a tear in the anal canal, and this problem had re-occurred, so I had a word with the doctor, and he recommended Proctosedyl which is an ointment and I used that and it was absolutely wonderful, ah what a blessing that was, and I started to feel better.

. . . I can go out and when I see a toilet I'll never pass them by! but another thing I meant to tell you, when I was feeling very, very tired, I took some glucose, vitamin C powder, and just put a spoonful of that in with me drink and that gives you energy, that little bit of a boost, and that helped me overcome my tiredness quite a bit really, you still had to rest from it all when really tired but glucose has always worked well . . . I'm using it occasionally now [three months post-treatment] but I'm not dependent on it now, where the first few days you were crawling around on your hands and knees, but no, I can't believe how much sleeping I did.

The carer perspective

3. At the age of 34 years, Kevin had been diagnosed with a testicular tumour. From diagnosis Kevin had hidden his cancer diagnosis from all family and friends except his wife, best friend and his employer. The couple had four young children. Kevin's wife (Stacy) was finding it difficult to cope financially while Kevin was not working. All of these factors intensified the impact of Kevin's treatment experience (three cycles of inpatient chemotherapy). The following are extracts from interviews with Stacy:

Stacy found it hard dealing with the extra pressure of the deceit:

I thought 'Oh my God, don't keep putting this pressure on me' . . . I was having to cope with going backwards and forwards from [the cancer centre], cope with the kids, I had his mum up here every day, I thought I can't cope with this much longer . . .

Stacy was continually having to lie and field questions concerning Kevin's absence. During the first course of chemotherapy Stacy was visiting and taking food to Kevin twice a day (600 miles in one week), co-ordinating child care, and dealing with all household issues. Stacy admitted 'I'm absolutely knackered'.

Stacy wanted to be with Kevin and support him. The unknown of the first course of chemotherapy was scary for Stacy as well as Kevin. Stacy had to deal with her own fears for Kevin's safety and described an instance:

. . . you don't know what to expect, the thing that got to me was . . . he was fine sat up talking, then they give him some tablets, they said they were anti-sickness tablets, and then 15 minutes later it's like somebody had given him an anaesthetic, he just lay there and he was slurring . . . going home I started crying, I thought 'What the hell are they giving him?' . . .

A major difficulty for Stacy was not being able to access ongoing information about Kevin's treatment and progress, and ask questions. Due to school runs and child care Stacy was unable to visit the hospital when doctors were routinely available and she described feeling left out. The following quote illustrates the stress Stacy was experiencing:

. . . it's weird, you know, you're going through it as well but you seem pushed back, it's all at the hospital . . . and you think you never get to see a doctor, you don't know what's happening, he's too ill, you know, he can't tell you . . . 'cos I had to take her [youngest child] with me every day . . . you come home, you know you are going through it but you sort of hold back yourself and you put all your efforts into somebody else . . . it's like you've got the kids to think of, got to protect the kids and, you go to the hospital, you've got to concentrate on him . . .

and:

. . . I think it's having the kids as well, you just sort of go on, automatic, and you just get up and you know what you've got to do and you do it and you just sort of put yourself on the back burner, you've got to get up, you've got to get the kids done, you've got the meals to cook, you've got the washing to do . . . so everybody comes first.

Stacy acknowledged that the nurse specialist was available and approachable but didn't want to bother this nurse unless there was an emergency. Stacy was concerned that the nurse would be busy with other patients and she didn't want to interrupt this work.

For the first few days after treatment Stacy became a nursemaid. Kevin's incapacity resulted in him lying in bed or on the sofa. Tasks included encouraging Kevin to take medication, cajoling him to eat and drink, and clearing receptacles that were used to collect vomit and urine. Stacy also had to contend with Kevin's mood swings, he had become irritable and short tempered and often snapped at Stacy and the children. Kevin recognised Stacy's strength and the supportive/ carer role she provided, but an awareness of the depth of emotional trauma was not openly acknowledged.

Stacy indicated that although the experience was really stressful, trying to maintain normality for the children was a diversion but also surreal:

. . . it's really weird the things that go through your head, 'cos, you go home [from the hospital] and everything's normal, and I go over to the supermarket, and you go over and everything's normal, you're out with the kids, you are doing the shopping and you come home, it's right, it's time to go up the hospital, see him attached to that drip and it's weird . . .

Stacy developed panic attacks several weeks earlier and they continued during this phase. Stacy turned to her GP who offered antidepressants, to which Stacy responded 'I'm not depressed, I'm stressed!'. Four of the five interviews undertaken with Stacy illustrated a woman cut off from emotional and practical support. Stacy had often become upset when talking of her isolation. The pressure to juggle finances, family, and Kevin's illness were immense.

potential of life extension through trials of anti-cancer agents.

If the philosophy of care is 'cure at all costs' acceptance of unnecessary toxicity or physical impairment may be an outcome. It is an important role of health professionals to help patients recognise the reality of their situation, to balance decisions concerning the level of treatment-induced toxicity, potential permanent impairment, and potential tumour control, with an acceptable degree of quality of life.

Needs assessment and patient-/ family-focused care

Receiving cancer treatment can be physically debilitating, and cause emotional difficulty, social problems and financial hardship. It is therefore worrying that a number of recent studies have identified a general lack of proactive assessment of patient and carer needs, and co-ordination of appropriate care.[1,3,45–49] Bottomley suggests this is compounded by the absence of consideration of informal social support that patients have access to.[48,49] This may be a result of:

- inadequate manpower
- lack of appropriately trained personnel

- deficient partnership arrangements between health and social care services and the voluntary sector
- health professionals concentrating primarily on the immediate administering of treatment and monitoring physical side-effects.

Colbourne found that where the person with cancer and their spouse/partner were introduced to chemotherapy nurse teams, clinical nurse specialists, or therapeutic radiographers, these health professionals were identified as beneficial and supportive providers and co-ordinators of care.[1] However, these staff generally met patients well along the diagnostic/treatment pathway and this might be considered too late in the treatment pathway. Schou and Hewison explain that the availability of key staff during treatment is a result of the acute illness model dominating cancer care provision, with treatment delivery and institutional management of 'the treatment calendar' taking precedence.[4]

There is evidence of nursing initiatives that have been shown to enhance patient-focused care (two examples are highlighted in Table 10.1). However, for some reason this work does not seem to be impacting universally across cancer care delivery. Greater investigation is needed to identify the barriers preventing the comprehensive

Table 10.1 Examples of patient-focused initiatives applicable to the treatment phase

Reference	Role/initiative	Main benefits/comments
Dennison and Shute (2000)[45]	Feasibility project and audit of a 'concerns checklist' to identify patient problems/issues when attending a general oncology treatment and follow-up clinic.	The checklist directed health professionals to areas of patient concern/need and increased patient referral to appropriate agencies. Patient and staff evaluation of the initiative indicated improved quality of the visit through greater communication/transfer of information and improved staff/patient relationships. An additional observation during the project resulted in the recommendation that the outpatient oncology nurse role/function needs development to maximise skill and minimise clerical/administration duties.
Faithfull (2000)[50]	A three-phase investigation to explore the experience of men receiving pelvic radiotherapy, and to develop, introduce and evaluate a nurse-led intervention compared with conventional care.	Protocol development for nurse-led support, information and practical care. The nurse role included 'medical' monitoring of treatment side-effects but also a health promotion model aimed at addressing the more subjective nature of symptoms such as urinary incontinence, diarrhoea, pain and reduced libido. To encourage self-reporting, patients were prepared in advance for potential problems and provided with options for preventative and early management strategies. This nurse-led, on-treatment management resulted in: • a reduction in medication to control symptoms • increased reporting of issues (that patients originally considered a by-product of treatment which they would just have to live with) • greater patient satisfaction with care.

introduction of innovative and beneficial models of nursing care during the treatment phase.

It could be argued that the needs of the carer or family members are as important as those of people with cancer themselves. In researching the impact of cancer on the family, Plant identified that caring and putting the well-being of the person with cancer first was a practical necessity but caring activities also fulfilled the carer's need to be useful.[51] Often carers 'need to be needed' and want to understand the experience from the person's perspective. During the 'merry-go-round' of treatment, the focus is on the individual receiving treatment. Whether the person is receiving treatment with palliative or curative intent the role of the spouse/partner is considered that of carer by the patient and spouse/partner.[16,52–55] Research by Northouse,[54] and Schou and Hewison[4] identifies that commonly the role of carer is not acknowledged or validated by health professionals. This narrow view of the impact of cancer therapy must be rectified to reduce the stress of the treatment experience for the carers.

Role expansion of the chemotherapy nurse

Intravenous administration of chemotherapy is undertaken by nurses, and over 60% of cancer patients in the UK receive chemotherapy.[56] Although cancer centres and units in the UK employ nurses to administer chemotherapy, an investigation by Fitzsimmons et al. identified little evaluation of nurse-led models of chemotherapy service delivery.[57] It was found that particular components of service provision, such as patient information needs and technical aspects of administration, were investigated rather than evaluation of a whole nurse-led service. It could be argued that although chemotherapy is administered by a nursing workforce, in the majority of cases this is not a total nurse-led service, as prescribing chemotherapy and symptom-relieving drugs and the non-protocol-driven requesting of clinical investigations remain the province of medical staff.

The focus of the research by Fitzsimmons *et al.* (a qualitative, interview study) was to explore user and health professional perspectives of medical consultant-led ambulatory chemotherapy service provision and the acceptability of a nurse-led service.[57] The findings identified that concern was raised by health professionals and users regarding a nurse–doctor substitution model; people with cancer wanted to know that doctors were taking overall responsibility for their treatment. A proposition was a 'mixed economy-model, with nurses working in an enhanced therapeutic role, reflecting the centrality of a multidisciplinary approach to cancer care delivery' (p.9). This would involve treatment planning by consultant medical staff but enhanced roles of nurses in relation to physical assessment skills and prescribing chemotherapy according to local protocols. Since the publication of the study by Fitzsimmons *et al.*, the situation in relation to nurse prescribing has moved on. In the UK, as of May 2006, qualified nurse independent prescribers are able to prescribe any licensed medicine for any medical condition within their competence. Implementation of this legislation has enabled the realisation of the 'mixed economy-model' in a growing number of cancer centres and units.

Post-treatment

The completion of an episode of treatment can bring mixed emotions – feelings of elation that therapy is finished but also the realisation that the unknown of treatment success and the potential for recurrence will remain. Instances of individuals describing feelings of abandonment and vulnerability on completion of treatment, and also a perception of no longer being a priority within the system are documented.[11,58–62] After treatment

people need to be advised that side-effects can continue to impact or new problems may manifest; however, the intensity of these effects (such as reduced physical fitness and energy levels or cognitive difficulties) and the length of time these may take to resolve (if at all) can often be underestimated. The physical impact of treatment is compounded by the need to come to terms with the feelings of uncertainty that accompany a cancer diagnosis and the difficulties of living with the psycho-emotional repercussions of the cancer experience and treatment. This is explored by Little *et al.*, who investigated the experience of cancer survivors and highlight that people undergo an adaptive process of regaining a post-treatment life.[10] This study is described in Research study 10.1. It appears that people are faced with the challenge of assimilating the cancer experience, and the physical, emotional and social effects of cancer into their post-cancer life. Achieving or attempting to accept the continuing impact of cancer appears to be an essential component of the adaptation process.

Follow-on care

Care from the oncology team who have administered treatment is traditionally offered through follow-up. As a minimum this includes regular surveillance with the aim of monitoring cancer absence or detecting cancer recurrence in its early stages. Co-ordinated and timely management of clinical investigations used in cancer monitoring is as important at this point in the treatment pathway as during diagnosis and staging.

There is debate and varying opinion surrounding the purpose, and benefit versus disadvantage of follow-up monitoring, including:[65–68]

- concern over the degree of anxiety compared with the reassurance gained
- the lack of cost/benefit analysis of specific imaging investigations
- the resources allocated to cancer monitoring compared to the lack of evidence of survival benefit.

Follow-up is contested as recurrence is frequently detected through the person seeking

Research study 10.1

Little M., Paul K., Jordens C.F.C. and Sayers E. (2002). Survivorship and discourses of identity. *Psycho-oncology* **11**, 170–178.[10]

Aim of study
To explore the post-treatment personal identity and life continuity of cancer survivors. Definition of cancer survival, living at any time after diagnosis and treatment have finished, apparently free of cancer.

Design
Qualitative cross-sectional design. Grounded theory approach.

Sample
Seven women, six men (diagnosed with colon cancer, liver cancer or lymphoma) and three lay carers. Age range: 18 to 89 years. Six months to 25 years post-treatment.

Method
Face-to-face unstructured interviews to explore how participants managed the post-treatment experience. Two lay carers interviewed with their spouses and one alone. Interviews lasted 50–90 minutes and were conducted by two non-medical research workers.

Inter-rater reliability coding of data. Findings tested and modified through focus groups/workshops involving cancer survivors, lay and professional carers.

Results
A core concept: an extreme illness experience can threaten an individual's life continuity and personal identity.

Analysis of data and discussion of findings provides a model of discourses of survival. The central theme of this model relates to cancer survivors having to restore or preserve 'personal continuity' and a disrupted 'future continuity' that they had expected before diagnosis. People manage the illness and survival discontinuity by reference to stable 'anchor points'. The anchor points are strong values and beliefs that are not affected by the turmoil of illness, e.g. gaining strength from religious belief, or maintaining identity through work. Giving meaning to the experience creates post-treatment identity, continuity, and acceptance. Those who cannot achieve a sense of continuity or meaningful future may feel alienated from themselves and their social world, uncertain and unsettled about the direction and purpose of their life.

It was identified that accommodation and resolution were factors that assisted resumption of life continuity, i.e. accommodating any residual aspects of the cancer experience and incorporation of the experience into everyday life (one way to assist this was by helping others who were experiencing a cancer diagnosis). Resolution of the 'discontinuities' of the cancer experience occurred through establishing an identity as a 'cancer survivor' and using survival as a new anchor point. The survivor is confronted with assimilating the cancer experience into a post-treatment identity. It was stressed that an 'extreme experience' is extreme because it leaves no aspect of identity untouched and that bouncing back (if at all) from such an event takes time and effort. The paper concluded by suggesting that the survivor has as yet no defined status and can only try to fit into models of the sick or chronically ill.

On completion of treatment people often closely observe their bodies for indications of treatment success or failure. The increased visibility of the internal workings of the body that clinical tests provide can encourage 'body watching',[1] and create a dependency on regular clinical investigations that are often part of cancer follow-up care. Several studies researching the experience of cancer patients cite the theory of embodiment to explain this type of behaviour;[1,19,21,63,64] embodiment refers to the experience of both being and living through a body. Lawton identified that embodiment is not an issue until the body cannot be controlled by the self as a result of serious or chronic illness.[63] From the point of diagnosis an individual's physical vulnerability is exposed and the body's inability to control cancer cell proliferation is evident to the person. Post-treatment, regaining faith in the body is a slow process. Although a double-edged sword that creates both anxiety as tests and investigations and their results are anticipated, and reassurance once the 'all clear' is given, seeking evidence through clinical investigations can offer a feeling of control. Personal account 10.4 contains personal accounts of this phase of the treatment pathway.

Personal account 10.4   Post-treatment experiences[1]

1. The following excerpts are taken from an interview with Jay, a 31-year-old man who had completed three cycles of chemotherapy for a testicular tumour 3 months previously.

I've tried to be like, work as normal but I, I just ain't as fit as I used to be now, I try to get back into the normal routine, the heavy lifting and that, an' it's my body aches and that, I suffer with a bit of back pain an', nothing on the old cancer side, the opposite side, it's a bit funny and tender at the moment, but my feet seem to like, it's the circulation, I don't know if it's because I didn't do nothing for a long time and sort of getting back into it, I think me body's took that much of a shock to the system and that stuff, it's just trying to, I suppose trying to get back into your normal routine, it ain't as easy as I thought it would be, you know 'cos I don't feel 100%.

Jay described his first CT scan post-treatment:

. . . waiting, going for me scan, that was quite, I was lay on that bed like, me fingers crossed and me legs crossed, you feel the loneliest person in the world when you are in that room, cos everyone comes in, wires you up and puts that thing in your arm for the dye, and, and it's quite cold in there like, and you lie there in your gown and you've got your bald head, you look like you're on death's door, with your white bald head, you look a right mess, you look like something out of a concentration camp, and they [staff] just look at you, you know, and they might do you a hello, and that, they all go out of that room and they're all talking, and you're thinking, 'Are they all talking about me? What, have they seen something?' You know what I mean, so, so it's the old [cancer] paranoia like, you know, I felt like the loneliest person in the world for that scan, well weird . . .

And at the first follow-up appointment waiting to hear the CT scan results:

. . . when she [registrar] got the results and we sat there like, oh me heart was going at 100 mile per hour . . . and she got it [scan report] and there was this stony silence and she was reading it, and it was yep, yep, yep, it's all right, and I went 'Ahhhh!', oh, I felt like really like, I could fly, it was just like . . . if they give, like there was a million pounds there.

And about other appointments attended:

. . . and my results, I'd go, and it was like, gone through the roof like, you know it's, really, really, good, and I still want, now, like I'm worried about the next one now . . . you know that's what's doing my head in, the next scan, you know, from the high of feeling, and like 'Yes!', to 'Oh no', down, it was like, the thing is I feels good, but I think, the worry at the moment, I really am like . . . I think once I've got this one [scan] over, I will, and then you know if it's still all right then I think I'll stop worrying, and er, get on with me life.'

2. Derek was 70 years of age when diagnosed with prostate cancer, he had completed a 6-week course of external beam radiotherapy 3 months previous to the interview from which these excerpts were taken.

. . . it's slowly getting better, it goes up and down, one week it can go the up and you're on the way, but then the next week you can have all sorts of things happen like water trouble, bowel trouble, and that lasts a week or so, and, that sort of puts you back a little and also, takes a bit away from your confidence as well . . . you tell yourself it's all over and of course you don't really know, the doctor told us afterwards that it could take quite a long time . . . and the other thing is I'm waiting for a bone scan, to see if it's gone into my bones or not, which they're not sure about, that's the only way to tell, but there's such a long waiting list . . . but that's a little bit frustrating 'cos obviously I can't make plans years ahead anyway but at least if you knew the results of a bone scan, you'd have a better idea.

. . . the backup when you've left the hospital for some time, isn't as good as when you are actually attending it, I rang, I had trouble with my bowels, and I rang up and, they were sort of putting me off from seeing the doctor . . . it was reception, I couldn't get through to the secretary, they just said 'Well when is the next time [outpatient appointment]?', I told them the dates and she said 'Well are you ill?' and I said 'Well I'm not ill but I'm not well' . . . this is the reason I asked you about your other patients [the other research participants], how it affected them, because I don't know, I mean we don't know one another, myself and your other patients, and you don't talk to anyone so it's hard knowing, I would have liked to have had a word with the doctor of the symptoms I was getting because I didn't know if it was right or not, if I should be having them . . .

investigation of symptoms that they have identified themselves rather than as a result of formal cancer surveillance protocols.[65] An exception to this is testicular cancer where detection of relapse is possible through routine follow-up investigations and where metastatic recurrence is responsive to treatment that can deliver survival benefit.[65,69] The arguments against follow-up appear to be considered in relation to cancer-recurrence detection. This neglects the potential for follow-up to include rehabilitative care for residual physical effects, and opportunities to assist with psychosocial and emotional issues which may involve the patient and carer/family.

Studies of alternative schedules of cancer surveillance have been undertaken. The following three randomised controlled studies compared different models of follow-up for women who were in remission after completing breast cancer treatment.

1. Grunfeld *et al.* compared conventional, hospital-based follow-up with follow-up in primary care with the GP.[70] No differences were found in the effectiveness of the two models. Of the 26 out of 269 women who developed a recurrence during the study, nine had experienced delays of more than 28 days in the diagnosis of recurrence. These were largely due to administrative errors, in particular delays in obtaining outpatient appointments when the case was not considered to be urgent. The majority of women with signs of recurrence visited their GP in the first instance, regardless of whether they were in the hospital or primary care follow-up system. An important finding was that 36% of women refused to participate in the study, suggesting that at least one-third of women with breast cancer want the reassurance of ongoing care by a specialist. Unfortunately no information regarding satisfaction with the two models of care was collected.
2. Gulliford *et al.* explored the follow-up experience of women by comparing the conventional schedule of clinic visits with reduced frequency of appointments (i.e. visits only after mammography).[71] The preference of participants was for reduced frequency of visits but with

open access if difficulties or symptoms were experienced. However, 118 of the 196 women recruited to the study were more than five years post-treatment with no evidence of recurrence. Findings might be different if the study were repeated with a sample of women who had just commenced follow-up.

3. Brown *et al.* assessed two types of follow-up for women previously treated for stage 1 breast cancer who were in remission: standard clinic follow-up and patient initiated follow-up.[72] The latter group was given written information on the signs and symptoms of recurrence and instructions to contact the breast nurse specialist if problems were encountered. There were no major differences in quality of life or psychological morbidity between the two models. More women in the standard care group reported reassurance and being checked as an advantage, while more women in the patient-initiated follow-up group reported convenience as an advantage. As in the first study, participant refusal rate was high at 50%, suggesting that women with breast cancer prefer conventional follow-up appointments. Women recruited to this study were at low risk of recurrence, women diagnosed with high-risk disease may have a greater preference for standard follow-up.

An interview study of attitudes to follow-up among people with colorectal cancer in the Netherlands found a high level of satisfaction with the conventional follow-up system;[73] a similar level of satisfaction was found in a UK study of 252 people attending a general oncology follow-up clinic.[74] Also, a reluctance to accept a system based on follow-up outside the hospital setting was expressed.

The previous examples illustrate that there are no definitive answers or a single participant preference for a model of follow-up. However, these studies indicate that replacing a hospital-based system with a less intensive model of care will not necessarily address the ongoing need for information and support following cancer treatment. In the last decade, alternative models of follow-up have been evaluated with the aim of enhancing the experience beyond cancer surveillance monitoring. Pre-appointment checklists of symptoms/issues/concerns have been used to guide health professionals to relevant areas of patient need or difficulty and increase appropriate referral to support agencies.[45,46,75,76] Nurse specialists are increasing their role in managing ongoing support and follow-up, and examples are provided in the following paragraphs.

Nurse-led telephone follow-up has been suggested as a potentially efficient and economical way of providing post-treatment interventions and support. Cox and Wilson conducted a literature search to draw together the evidence relating to follow-up for people with cancer delivered by nurse-led services and telephone interventions.[77] This literature review suggested nurse-led follow-up met needs for psychological support and information, and the telephone was an acceptable route of providing elements of this service.

Protocol-driven nurse-led clinics running parallel to consultant clinics have proved successful. They offer reduced waiting times, and increased throughput of patients, while continuity of contact is maintained that can lead to a trusting long-term relationship.[78] Fitzgerald-Smith *et al.* highlight that an additional benefit is increased access, as patients can obtain telephone advice or book appointments directly with a nurse specialist who can see the patient outside clinic times to deal with symptoms or other issues.[78]

Introduction of the role of an outreach oncology nurse practitioner in rural Ireland aimed to deliver a post-treatment service sympathetic to local need.[38] Evaluation of this new role identified that it provided three main functions, a post-treatment review clinic, services for other people who had cancer, and a link between the consultant oncologist, patient and local clinicians. The emphasis was on assessment, examination, support, education, and continuity of care. The local clinics were viewed by users as more convenient with the benefit of longer appointments. Satisfaction with the model of care was high.

It seems apparent that one model of follow-up care will not suit the preferences of all or fit the particularities of certain populations. Box 10.4 suggests service provision that could enhance post-treatment care.

Box 10.4 Post-treatment care – suggested service improvements

- Individuals need opportunities and explanation to understand implications of clinical surveillance investigations. Health professionals need to be aware of the potential reliance on clinical tests and turn it into an opportunity for reassurance and anxiety reduction.
- Cohesive 'calendar management' of follow-up to include physical, psychosocial assessment of patient and carer/family need.
- Provide patient, carer/family and generalist health professionals with access to oncology-knowledgeable key worker from diagnosis.
- Reconfigure services for oncology teams/key worker to cross traditional care boundaries.
- Increase availability of easily accessible/innovative oncology education opportunities for generalist health professionals.
- Networked IT to assist communication transfer.
- Enhance nurse roles to provide, develop and evaluate innovative models of cancer care delivery.
- Offer a variety of evidence-based options (models, settings) of follow-up that cater for individual preferences and needs, i.e. a continuum from disease surveillance to more therapeutic, emotion-focused consultations.

Final comment

Advances in cancer treatment have equated to increasing numbers of people living with cancer for longer. Services need to change to accommodate the needs of this group. The role of nursing in relation to cancer treatment is essential, and is not simply about being a participant in the team making decisions about treatment, and then taking responsibility for administering and monitoring the effects of treatment. Nurses are central to determining the level of care and support required for individuals, and to establishing a package of care strategies. Such supportive care is distinct from cancer treatment, and since it relates to emotional, practical and functional problems, it may be more difficult to identify the most appropriate responses required or how these may need to alter as individuals progress through the treatment pathway. The pathway through cancer treatment is difficult, and insufficient attention has been given to how to manage problems caused

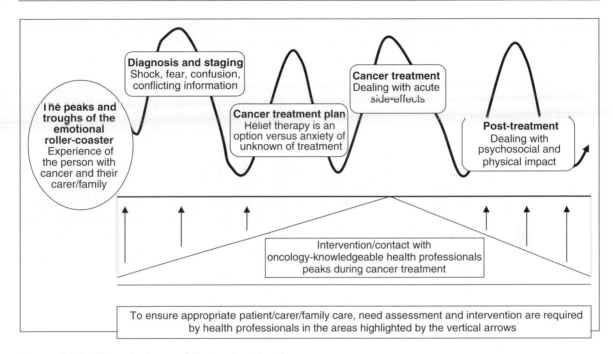

Figure 10.3   The experience of the treatment pathway.

by therapies or how to help people sustain them through it and beyond. Figure 10.3 illustrates the experience of the treatment pathway. The greatest involvement of oncology-knowledgeable health professionals surrounds the administration of cancer treatment. It is evident that the individual with a cancer diagnosis, and their carers/family, require assessment of their needs and supportive care earlier than at present and that this should be ongoing beyond completion of chemotherapy or radiotherapy. The role of nursing will be pivotal in developing efficient, innovative models of care to rectify the current deficit.

References

1. Colbourne L.C. (2005). *Testicular and Prostate Cancer: Explaining the Treatment and Post Treatment Experience of Couples*. PhD thesis, University of Southampton.
2. Petrone M.A. (2003). *The Emotional Cancer Journey*. Brighton: MAP Foundation. www.mapfoundation.org (accessed 27 July 2007).
3. Kelsey S.G., Owens J. and White A. (2004). The experience of radiotherapy for localized prostate cancer: The men's perspective. *European Journal of Cancer Care* **13**, 272–278.
4. Schou K.C. and Hewison J. (1999). *Experiencing Cancer*. Buckingham: Open University Press.
5. Mcilfatrick S., Sullivan K. and McKenna H. (2003). Exploring the patient's experience of a day hospital chemotherapy service: preliminary fieldwork. *European Journal of Oncology Nursing* **7**, 197–199.
6. Leydon G.M., Bynoe-Sutherland J. and Coleman M.P. (2003). The journey towards a cancer diagnosis: the experiences of people with cancer, their family and carers. *European Journal of Cancer Care* **12**, 317–326.
7. Stacey J. (1997). *Teratologies: A Cultural Study of Cancer*. London: Routledge.
8. Jones G.Y. and Payne S. (2000). Searching for safety signals: the experience of medical surveillance amongst men with testicular teratomas. *Psycho-oncology* **9**, 385–394.
9. Leventhal H., Leventhal E.A. and Contrada R.J. (1998). Self-regulation, health, and behaviour: a perceptual-cognitive approach. *Psychology and Health* **13**, 717–733.
10. Little M., Paul K., Jordens C.F.C. and Sayers E. (2002). Survivorship and discourses of identity. *Psycho-oncology* **11**, 170–178.
11. Pelusi J. (1997). The lived experience of surviving cancer. *Oncology Nursing Forum* **24**, 1343–1353.
12. Taylor S.E. (1983). Adjustment to threatening events: a theory of cognitive adaptation. *American Psychologist* **38**, 1161–1173.

13. Woolley N. (1990). Crisis theory: a paradigm of effective intervention with families of critically ill people. *Journal of Advanced Nursing* **15**, 1402–1408.

14. Salander P., Bergenheim T. and Henriksson R. (1996). The creation of protection and hope in patients with malignant brain tumours. *Social Science and Medicine* **42**, 985–996.

15. Taylor S.E. and Lobel M. (1989). Social comparison activity under threat: downward evaluation and upward contacts. *Psychological Review* **96**, 569–575.

16. Gray R.E., Fitch M., Phillips C., Labrecque M. and Fergus K. (2000). To tell or not to tell: patterns of disclosure among men with prostate cancer. *Psycho-oncology* **9**, 273–282.

17. Neal A. and Hoskin P. (1994). *Clinical Oncology: A Textbook for Students.* London: Edward Arnold.

18. Otto S.E. (1997). *Oncology Nursing.* London: Mosby.

19. Kelly D.M. (2002). *In the Company of Men: Embodiment and Prostate Cancer.* 2002. PhD thesis, University of London.

20. Gordon D.R. (1990). Embodying illness, embodying cancer. *Culture, Medicine and Psychiatry* **14**, 275–297.

21. Nettleton S. and Watson J. (1998). *The Body in Everyday Life.* London: Routledge.

22. Silverman D. (1987). *Communication and Medical Practice: Social Relations in the Clinic.* London: Sage.

23. Degner L. and Sloan J.F. (1992). Decision making during serious illness: what part do patients really want to play? *Journal of Clinical Epidemiology* **45**, 944–950.

24. Degner L. and Russell A. (1988). Preferences for treatment and control among adults with cancer. *Research in Nursing and Health* **11**, 367–374.

25. Beaver K., Luker K., Glynn Owens R., Leinster S.J. and Degner L. (1996). Treatment decision making in women newly diagnosed with breast cancer. *Cancer Nursing* **19**, 8–19.

26. Henman M.J., Butow P.N., Brown R.F., Boyle F. and Tattersall M.H.N. (2002). Lay constructions of decision-making in cancer. *Psycho-oncology* **11**, 295–306.

27. O'Rourke M.E. (2001). Decision making and prostate cancer treatment selection: a review. *Seminars in Oncology Nursing* **17**, 108–117.

28. O'Rourke M.E. and Germino B.B. (1998). Prostate cancer treatment decisions: a focus group exploration. *Oncology Nursing Forum* **25**, 97–104.

29. Calman K. and Hine D. (1995). *A Policy Framework for Commissioning Cancer Services.* London: Department of Health.

30. Maule W.F. (1994). Screening for colorectal cancer by nurse endoscopists. *The New England Journal of Medicine* **330**, 183–187.

31. Schoenfeld P., Lipscomb S., Crook J. *et al.* (1999). Accuracy of polyp detection by gastroenterologists and nurse endoscopists during flexible sigmoidoscopy: a randomized trial. *Gastroenterology* **117**, 312–318.

32. Garvican L., Grimsey E., Littlejohns P., Lowndes S. and Sacks N. (1998). Satisfaction with clinical nurse specialists in a breast care clinic: questionnaire survey. *British Medical Journal* **316**, 976–977.

33. Smith T. (2000). Colposcopy. *Nursing Standard* **15**, 47–52.

34. Jolley S. (2004). Quality in colposcopy. *Nursing Standard* **18**, 39–44.

35. Hillier A. (2001). The advanced practice nurse in gastroenterology: identifying and comparing care interactions of nurse practitioners and clinical nurse specialists. *Gastroenterology Nursing* **24**, 239–245.

36. Doyal L. and Cameron A. (2000). Reshaping the NHS workforce. *British Medical Journal* **320**, 1023–1024.

37. Corner J. (2003). The role of nurse-led care in cancer management. *The Lancet Oncology* **4**, 631–636.

38. McKenna H., McCann S., McCaughan E. and Keeney S. (2003). The role of an outreach oncology nurse practitioner: a case study evaluation. *European Journal of Oncology Nursing* **8**, 66–77.

39. Godsell G. (2003). Introducing a nurse biopsy role in a skin cancer clinic. *European Journal of Oncology Nursing* **7**, 50–52.

40. Department of Health. (1999). *Making a Difference: The New NHS.* London: HMSO.

41. Department of Health. (2000). *The NHS Plan.* London: HMSO.

42. Department of Health. (2000). *The Cancer Plan.* London: Department of Health.

43. National Institute for Clinical Excellence. (2004). (NICE) guidance, *Improving Supportive and Palliative Care for Adults with Cancer.* London: NICE.

44. Slevin M.L., Strubbs L. and Plant H.J. (1990). Attitudes to chemotherapy: comparing views of patients with cancer with those of doctors, nurses, and general public. *British Medical Journal* **300**, 1458–1460.

45. Dennison S. and Shute T. (2000). Identifying patient concerns: improving the quality of patient visits to the oncology out-patient department – a pilot audit. *European Journal of Oncology Nursing* **4**, 91–98.

46. Wright E.P., Selby P.J., Gould A. and Cull A. (2001). Detecting social problems in cancer patients. *Psycho-oncology* **10**, 242–250.

47. Wright E.P., Kiely M.A., Lynch P., Cull A. and Selby P.J. (2002). Social problems in oncology. *British Journal of Cancer* **87**, 1099–1104.

48. Bottomley A. (1995). The development of the Bottomley Cancer Social Support Scale. *European Journal of Cancer Care* **4**, 127–132.

49. Bottomley A. and Jones L. (1997). Social support and the cancer patient – a need for clarity. *European Journal of Cancer Care* **6**, 72–77.

50. Faithfull S.C. (2000). *Supportive Care in Radiotherapy: Evaluating the Potential Contribution of Nursing.* PhD thesis, University of London.

51. Plant H, (2001) *Understanding the Experiences of Close Relatives of People with Cancer.* PhD thesis, University of London.

52. Baider L., Cooper C. and Kaplan de Nour A. (1996). *Cancer and the Family.* London: John Wiley and Sons.

53. Lavery J.F. and Clarke V.A. (1999). Prostate cancer: patients' and spouses' coping and marital adjustment. *Psychology Health and Medicine* **4**, 289–302.

54. Northouse L.L., Mood D., Templin T., Mellon S. and George T. (2000). Couples' patterns of adjustment to colon cancer. *Social Science and Medicine* **50**, 271–284.

55. Matthews B.A. (2003). Role and gender differences in cancer-related distress: a comparison of survivor and caregiver self-reports. *Oncology Nursing Forum* **30**, 493–499.

56. Cancer Care in England & Wales Commission for Health Improvement and Audit Commission. (2001). *National Service Framework No.1.* London: Audit Commission.

57. Fitzsimmons D., Hawker S.E., Simmonds P. *et al.* (2005). Nurse-led models of chemotherapy care: mixed economy or nurse-doctor substitution? *Journal of Advanced Nursing* **50**, 244–252.

58. Belec R. (1992). Quality of life: perceptions of long term survivors of bone marrow transplantation. *Oncology Nursing Forum* **19**, 31–37.

59. Davies M. and Sque M. (2002). Living on the outside looking in: a theory of living with advanced breast cancer. *International Journal of Palliative Nursing* **8**, 583–590.

60. Ferrell B.R., Dow K.H., Leigh S., Ly J. and Gulasekaram P. (1995). Quality of life in long term cancer survival. *Oncology Nursing Forum* **22**, 915–922.

61. Loescher L., Clark L., Attwood S. and Lamb G. (1990). The impact of the cancer experience on long term survivors. *Oncology Nursing Forum* **17**, 223–229.

62. McCaffrey D. (1991). Surviving cancer. *Nursing Times* **87**, 26–30.

63. Lawton J. (2000). *The Dying Process: Patients' Experiences of Palliative Care.* London: Routledge.

64. Copp G. (1999). *Facing Impending Death: Experiences of Patients and their Nurses.* London: NT Books.

65. Brada M. (1995). Is there a need to follow-up cancer patients? *European Journal of Cancer* **31A**, 655–657.

66. Butow P.N., Brown R.F., Cogar S., Tattersall M.H.N. and Dunn S.M. (2002). Oncologists' reactions to cancer patients' verbal cues. *Psycho-oncology* **11**, 47–58.

67. Loprinzi C, (1995) Follow up testing for curatively treated cancer survivors: what to do? *Journal of the American Medical Association* **273**, 1877–1878.

68. MacBride S.K. and Whyte F. (1999). Attendance at cancer follow-up clinic: does it increase anxiety or provide reassurance for men successfully treated for testicular cancer? *Cancer Nursing* **22**, 448–455.

69. Ellis M., Hartley L. and Sikora K. (1984). Value of follow up in testicular cancer. *British Medical Journal* **289**, 1423.

70. Grunfeld E., Mant D., Yudkin P. *et al.* (1996). Routine follow-up of breast cancer in primary care: randomised trial. *British Medical Journal* **313**, 665–669.

71. Gulliford T., Opumu M., Wilson E., Hanham I. and Epstein R. (1997). Popularity of less frequent follow-up for breast cancer in randomised study: initial findings from the hotline study. *British Medical Journal* **1314**, 177.

72. Brown L., Payne S. and Royle G. (2002). Patient initiated follow up of breast cancer. *Psycho-oncology* **211**, 346–355.

73. Stiggelbout A.M., de Haes J., Van de Velds C. *et al.* (1997). Follow-up of colorectal cancer patients with quality of life and attitudes towards follow-up. *British Journal of Cancer* **75**, 914–920.

74. Thomas S., Glynne-Jones R. and Chait I. (1997). Is it worth the wait? Survey of patient's satisfaction with an oncology outpatient clinic. *European Journal of Cancer Care* **6**, 50–58.

75. Velikova G., Booth L., Smith A.B. *et al.* (2004). Measuring quality of life in routine oncology practice improves communication and patient well-being: a randomized controlled trial. *Journal of Clinical Oncology* **22**, 714–724.

76. Rogers M. and Todd C. (2002). Information exchange in oncology outpatient clinics: source, valence and uncertainty. *Psycho-oncology* **43**, 336–345.

77. Cox E. and Wilson E. (2003). Follow-up for people with cancer: nurse-led services and telephone interventions. *Journal of Advanced Nursing* **43**, 51–61.

78. Fitzgerald-Smith A.M., Srivastava P. and Hershman M.J. (2003). The role of the nurse in colorectal cancer follow-up. *Hospital Medicine* **64**, 344–347.

CHAPTER ELEVEN

Surgery

Stephen O'Connor

Introduction

Surgery has been the mainstay of cancer treatment since the Egyptian physician Imhotep, later deified as the god of healing, developed procedures for the surgical excision and cauterisation of breast tumours in 2650 BC.[1] Similar interventions were used throughout the classical world, the Persian physician Asclepiades regularly performing tracheotomies on patients with an impaired airway by 100 BC, and his countryman Democedes being attributed with the first successful 'cure' for breast cancer when operating on the wife of the Persian King Darius.[2] In later centuries the Byzantine physician Aetius of Amida was to advocate the cutting back of sufficient healthy tissue when excising tumours in 502 AD, but much of this knowledge was lost to mainland Europe after the fall of the Western Empire in 476 AD, where surgery had little basis in science or the knowledge of earlier civilisations and was carried out by monks, barbers, and poorly trained 'surgeons',[3] until it was expressly forbidden to all 'decent physicians' on religious and moral grounds by the Council of Tours in 1163 AD. Notwithstanding this, surgery continued to develop and was regarded with increasing eminence in the East, the first recorded colostomy being formed by an unnamed surgeon in Shiraz (Iran) at this time, and the Moorish physician Abu Al-Zahravi (930–1013 AD), otherwise known as Albucasis advocating that surgical excisions be 'wide and bold', and

include any veins running to and from the tumour, which he regarded as responsible for the spread of the disease. Ambrose Paré (1510–1590) realised the importance of lymphatic spread when operating on small breast lesions in 16th century France, and the following century found his countryman Bernard Peyrilhe developing the first radical mastectomy to include the pectoralis muscle and axillary lymph nodes in 1773.[2]

The Renaissance saw the rehabilitation of surgery as a legitimate province of medicine in Western Europe, Johann Schultes of Ulm carefully describing the instruments and procedures required for mastectomy in his treatise *Armamentum Chirurgicum* published in 1645,[1] although little real progress in the management of the disease was made in the two centuries that followed, William Marsden declaring that physicians knew 'absolutely nothing' about it when founding his London hospital (now the Royal Marsden Hospital) for the treatment and study of cancer in 1851. By the end of that century, William Halsted (1894–5) had perfected Peyrilhe's procedure to include the supraclavicular lymph nodes, and surgical interventions for the treatment of cancer grew apace following the first public demonstration of inhaled anaesthesia for the removal of a jaw tumour by William Morton at the Massachusetts General Hospital on 16 October 1846, a landmark event which was to be replicated in the same hospital just one day later by the surgeon George Hayward who rendered a female patient into a 'state of insensibility' prior to the removal of a large tumour on the arm using Morton's 'Letheon' gas inhaler. Abdominal surgery remained a rare event until Christian Billroth, a German-born Professor of Surgery in Vienna, undertook the first successful partial gastrectomy for the removal of a cancerous pylorus in 1881. Billroth had already pioneered a number of procedures for head and neck cancer, including the first successful resection of an oesophagus in 1872, laryngectomy in 1873, and the first successful resection for carcinoma of the rectum in 1876, rendering gastrointestinal surgery a much safer and more commonplace phenomenon that it had hitherto been.[4]

Advances in surgical techniques since then have been at the leading edge of scientific enquiry,[3] and have led to dramatic improvements in the management of many cancers.[5,6] These include the 'laparoscopic revolution',[7] which has improved outcomes, recovery times and morbidity associated with the treatment of prostate, colorectal, gynaecological, renal, and gastric cancers to name but a few,[8–14] the minimally invasive treatment of breast, renal, and prostate cancers with cryosurgical ablation,[15–21] and the use of intra-operative radiotherapy to deliver a single therapeutic dose of ionising radiation during surgery.[22–26] These developments have enabled surgeons to engage in tissue-sparing surgery in those with early disease, which has better cosmetic results. An additional advantage of such developments is the reduction in hospitalisation and recovery time for such patients, Holub *et al.*'s (2002) multicentre comparison of laparoscopy versus open laparotomy for endometrial cancer showing a mean of 3.9 as opposed to 7.3 days to discharge.[10]

Other developments have included the growing use of sentinel lymph node biopsies in cancer surgery. These are based upon the realisation that the disease status of the axillary lymph nodes in breast cancer patients could be anticipated by the pathological status of the first lymph node to receive lymphatic drainage from the breast – otherwise termed the sentinel lymph node.[27] This allowed surgeons to omit axillary lymph node dissection in women with disease-negative sentinel lymph nodes, and considerably reduced the incidence of post-operative pain, lymphoedema, numbness, and restricted arm movement associated with complete axillary lymph node dissection.[28,29] Sentinel lymph node lymphoscintigraphy is, furthermore, a more accurate indicator of disease spread than surgical examination alone, one study demonstrating positive lymph node involvement in 89% of cervical cancer cases whereas the intra-operative detection rate was only 70%.[30] Sentinel lymph node biopsy is now used extensively in many types of cancer surgery including lung, gastrointestinal, genitourinary, oropharyngeal, and head and neck cancers in addition to breast cancer, where it may be used to give an indication of post-operative recurrence as well as determining the extent of surgery required.

Principles of surgical oncology

While the use of ionising radiation and cytotoxic chemotherapy is virtually synonymous with cancer care, surgery remains the primary treatment modality for the majority of solid tumours and offers the greatest hope of cure.[31] It has been estimated that surgery is responsible for complete remission of the disease in 43% of cases, as opposed to 18% for radiotherapy and only 6.5% for chemotherapy;[31,32] its success rising considerably when the disease is discovered in its earlier stages, or when it is used in conjunction with radiotherapy and/or chemotherapy.[5] The scope of surgery has expanded considerably in the last few decades and does not simply include definitive treatment.[5] Most individuals with cancer will undergo some form of surgical procedure at some time during the disease process, whether it be a biopsy taken to assist with their diagnosis,[33,34] the insertion of a central venous line for the administration of cytotoxic chemotherapy,[35,36] the formation of a colostomy or jejunostomy to reduce the impact of advanced disease or its treatment,[37,38] decompression laminectomy for spinal cord compression, or the insertion of an expandable metal stent for superior vena cava syndrome in an oncological emergency.[39,40] Further treatment may be required in the aftermath of definitive surgery to overcome the physical or psychosocial impact of treatment and improve quality of life.[41] This may include reconstruction of the breast or voicebox after the radical excision of a tumour,[41,42] or the insertion of prostheses or implants in children following surgery for sarcoma.[43] The indications for surgery are manifold therefore, and include:

- prophylactic surgery
- diagnostic surgery
- definitive (or curative) surgery
- rehabilitative (or reconstructive) surgery
- palliative surgery.

Surgery may also elicit considerable benefit in disseminated disease so long as metastases remain isolated and resectable,[31] and its role in the palliation of advanced symptoms such as bowel obstruction, spinal cord compression and superior vena cava obstruction has long been recognised.[40,44,45] Meanwhile, developments in our understanding of molecular oncology, the endocrine system and cancer genetics have given rise to the notion of prophylactic or pre-neoplastic surgery,[46] for certain types of breast, ovarian, and colorectal cancers as well as cryptorchidism, ulcerative colitis and multiple endocrine neoplastic syndrome.[5,6]

Tumour-related factors indicating whether a solid tumour is amenable to surgery include its location, histology, growth rate, invasiveness, and metastatic potential.[5,6,31] Slow-growing tumours with a long cell cycle, low growth fraction and low metastatic potential are the most amenable to definitive surgical treatment, although as many as 70% of tumours will have metastasised by the time that a primary tumour is diagnosed, requiring systemic chemotherapy or locoregional treatment with radiotherapy in addition to surgery if an acceptable outcome is to be achieved.[5,6] In making such decisions, it is vital that the surgeon be provided with an accurate histology, staging, and grading for the tumour since this will impact directly upon the nature and extent of the surgery undertaken. In early breast or bladder cancer, the extent of surgery required to effect a cure may be limited, a simple lumpectomy or transurethral resection of the bladder tumour being sufficient to remove the disease, whereas a more radical approach may be required in advanced disease.[31] In addition, the surgeon will need to consider the age, functional status and anticipated quality of life for the individual after surgery, and the appropriateness of adjuvant therapies that may further complicate the individual's post-operative recovery such as impaired secondary wound healing, infection or electrolyte imbalance caused by prior exposure to ionising radiation, the concomitant use of anti-metabolite drugs, or the systemic side-effects of cytotoxic drugs more generally.[31]

Post-operative morbidity and mortality are also important considerations that will be borne in mind when deciding upon an appropriate choice of treatment. Prospective scoring systems such as POSSUM (the Physiologic and Operative Severity Score for the enUmeration of Mortality and morbidity),[47] and the Association of Coloproctology of Great Britain and Ireland's (ACPGBI) risk score for malignant large bowel obstruction[48] are becoming more prevalent in the decision-making process.[49–51] POSSUM takes into account physiological measures such as an individual's age, Glasgow score, electrolytes, respiratory and cardiovascular status, as well as the stage of the cancer and number of operations previously performed,[47] while the ACPGBI risk assessment scale uses morbidity and mortality data from 10 613 procedures conducted in 93 different hospitals together with the Duke's staging system and the American Society of Anesthesiologists (ASA) functional status scale (see Table 11.1) to calculate the risks associated with surgery for large bowel cancer.[48] However, even large datasets such as those in the ACPGBI study represent only a small proportion of the entire cancer population, and the lack of prospective randomised controlled trials and a clear evidence base for specific surgical interventions continues to frustrate the development of a more empirical approach to surgical oncology.[31,52] This is particularly relevant when one considers the impact that consultant training, preference, and the frequency with which procedures are performed have upon surgical outcomes, there being a marked contrast between the performance of individual surgeons, hospitals, and even nations where surgery for many common cancers is concerned.[31,53,54]

Table 11.1 Duke's staging system and the American Society of Anesthesiologists' status scale

Duke's staging	Criteria
A	Tumour confined to the innermost lining of the colon or rectum and does not extend beyond the muscularis propria
B	Tumour has grown beyond the muscle layer and extends into the subserosa or the serosa but has not spread to the lymphatic system
C	One or more of the regional lymph nodes is disease positive (C1) or one or more of the apical lymph nodes is disease positive (C2)
D	Distant metastases are present beyond the original limits of surgical resection

ASA score	Criteria (with mortality risk expressed as a percentage)
I	Normal health (0.05%)
II	Mild systemic disease that does not inhibit activity (0.4%)
III	Severe systemic disease that inhibits activity but is not incapacitating (4.5%)
IV	Incapacitating systemic disease which is constantly life threatening (25%)
V	Moribund. The patient is not expected to survive more than 24 hours without surgery (50%)

However, no one study can possibly control for the myriad variables faced by individual surgeons in their daily practice that could impact upon the outcomes of treatment. These include individual differences in the staging and grading of cancers at presentation, functional status, the presence or absence of co-morbidity, and differences in the disease trajectory and treatment histories experienced by individuals by the time that surgery is attempted. Similarly, international and regional variations must take account of local culture, health beliefs and socio-economic factors, since these too play an important role in the development, presentation and outcomes for certain types of cancer such as gastric, breast, colorectal, and bladder disease, which may have completely different aetiologies and presentation patterns in some settings or minority groups.[5] Considerable progress has been made in the UK and other countries, since the introduction of subspecialties within surgical oncology, although the benefit of this may be offset by the need for individuals with less common cancers to travel greater distances for treatment by a site specialist.[5] A small number of studies question the need for the establishment of surgical subspecialties within oncology,[31,55] overall standards of training and competence assessment appearing more important in the promotion of clinical effectiveness than the frequency with which procedures are performed by any one individual.[55]

Prophylactic surgery

Prophylactic surgery may involve the excision of non-cancerous or pre-cancerous cells or tissues in order to avoid their becoming malignant, or the surgical correction of an anatomical, developmental or genetic defect which may subsequently give rise to cancer. It may be considered for a number of conditions or 'at-risk' groups, including cryptorchidism or undescended testis which is associated with a 10- to 40-fold increase in the incidence of testicular cancer.[5,6] About 10% of men developing testicular germ cell cancer have a history of testicular maldescent,[5] and orchidopexy during infancy may reduce, although it may not entirely remove the risk of testicular cancer later in life. The incidence of testicular cancer is actually quite low within the general population, with a reported incidence of between 2 and 5.7 per 100 000 of the population in the West and lower still in those of South-East Asian and African descent,[5,6] but it remains the commonest malignancy and, until recently, the commonest cause of cancer deaths in young men between the ages of 25 and 35 years, warranting the surgical correction of cryptorchidism as early in infancy as possible.

Hereditary non-polyposis colorectal cancer
Hereditary non-polyposis colorectal cancer (HNPCC) is the most common form of hereditary colorectal cancer and accounts for approximately

20% of all colorectal cancers, most families having three or more instances in their family history.[6] Those affected by the syndrome have an 80% lifetime risk of developing the disease,[56] which may not become apparent until the affected person is in his or her early 40s, HNPCC lacking many of the systemic manifestations of familial adenomatous polyposis coli.[6] Family history is therefore the main method for identifying an individual's susceptibility to HNPCC, followed by genetic counselling and testing. Although primarily affecting the gastrointestinal system, some women are also at increased risk of developing precocious ovarian and endometrial cancers at a young age,[6] and the aggressive nature of the colorectal adenomas associated with the condition lead many to undergo a prophylactic colectomy rather than endure a lifetime of uncertainty.[56]

Trials are also currently being undertaken into the efficacy of cyclo-oxygenase enzyme (COX-2) inhibitors and the non-steroidal anti-inflammatory drug (NSAID) sulindac for HNPCC, since these have been demonstrated to reduce the conversion of arachidonic acid into prostaglandins and reduce both the size and incidence of colorectal tumours.[57–59] Sulindac carries significant risk of gastric disturbance, particularly with long-term use, and recent controversy around the clinical use of the COX-2 inhibitors make it likely that endoscopic surveillance with or without colonoscopy and ileoanal pouch formation is likely to remain the most important risk-reducing intervention for the condition. These same surgical interventions have also been used for the treatment of ulcerative colitis,[60,61] which predisposes the individual to both bile duct and colorectal cancer.[6] Those diagnosed at a young age,[5] or with disease beyond the splenic flexure are most at risk,[6] and were previously recommended surgical intervention although surveillance is now more common, as dysplastic changes to the mucosal lining of the gut tend to provide adequate warning of malignancy so that surgery can be undertaken.[5]

Familial adenomatous polyposis coli

Prophylactic surgery may also be performed in those diagnosed with the rare autosomal dominant condition familial adenomatous polyposis coli (FAP), which results from a mutated gene on chromosome 5.[5] Those affected by the gene mutation begin to develop multiple benign polyps from puberty and have a high lifetime risk of developing colorectal cancer if these are allowed to develop unabated. Annual colonoscopy is commonly used to screen the affected individual from the age of 19 or 20 years, and an oesophagogastric duodenoscopy may be indicated to observe for lymphoid hyperplasia, gastric, and duodenal adenomas.[60,62] If polyps appear, a prophylactic colectomy with ileo-rectal anastamosis is likely to be performed.[62–64] Complications associated with the establishment of an ileo-anal pouch or reservoir after colectomy may require frequent contact with members of the health care team, and provide the basis for the development of an ongoing therapeutic relationship which will vary according to the vicissitudes of the individual's condition.[60] Those living with an ileo-anal pouch face many difficulties, one study suggesting that they may live in a world of restricted opportunity, where uncertainty and the fear of malignant disease are common, the individual having to come to terms with an altered body image and cope with unpredictable periods of ill-health on a continuing basis.[61] Strategies used to cope with the uncertainty of the condition and the complications of treatment include a need to maintain control, to give and receive help from others, and a heightened appreciation for life and relationships – though an individual's capacity to achieve all of these varies according to their health status.[61]

Multiple endocrine neoplasia

Prophylactic surgery may also be used in the treatment of multiple endocrine neoplasia (MEN), a series of rare inherited autosomal dominant conditions that affect both sexes equally and show no racial or geographical distinction in their prevalence.[65,66] Each cause the proliferation of benign, and if uncorrected, malignant tumours with advancing age.[5] The first, MEN1 or Wermer's syndrome, affects the pituitary, parathyroid and pancreatic islet cells giving rise to hyperparathyroidism, which causes kidney stones and renal problems from young adulthood onwards, and the development of gastrin-secreting gastrinomas associated with Zollinger–Ellison syndrome. Ninety per cent of gastrinomas occur in the pancreas, 5% in the duodenum and others in the stomach, though local spread to adjacent nodes, the liver, and distal metastases occurs in 60% of cases making pancreatectomy unsuitable.[5] Medical management using histamine antagonists,[5] or proton pump inhibitors is now being advocated as a first line of treatment for this condition in preference to surgery,[65] which may still be required for the removal of prolactinomas, benign tumours occurring as a result of an overactive pituitary gland. These affect sex-drive or fertility in men and women respectively, but may also give rise to visual disturbance because of their proximity to the optic nerves and require surgical intervention when dopamine agonists fail to correct the condition.[65] Harmless fatty lipomas may also form under the skin, which may be removed surgically for cosmetic reasons, but insulinomas and, less frequently, glucagonomas may form in the pancreas giving rise to hypoglycaemia or diabetes. These require surgical excision wherever possible since they metastasise to the liver and adjacent nodes and cause premature death in about 10% of cases.[5] Gauger *et al.* recommend aggressive screening using endoscopic ultrasonograpy in order to elicit prompt surgical intervention in such cases.[67]

Adenomas of the parathyroid glands are also common in the second type of multiple endocrine neoplasia (MEN2 or Sipple's syndrome),[6] which has a penetrance rate of 70% by age 70 years.[68] Although most carriers are diagnosed on the basis of their clinical signs by the age of 30 years, this figure is falling with the advent of calcitonin assays and improved understanding of the genetic nature of this condition which allows specific gene testing in the children of affected adults.[5,64] MEN2 individuals have a 100% likelihood of developing medullary thyroid tumours which have a high metastatic potential via both the lymphatic and venous routes,[5] and while their prognosis depends upon the stage of the disease at presentation, prophylactic thyroidectomy is advocated in children as young as 5 years if they carry the genetic mutation,[64] and younger in those carrying the *RET* proto-oncogene because of its more aggressive nature in these individuals.[68,69] Phaeochromocytomas, vascular tumours of the adrenal gland which cause excessive secretion of the catecholamines

adrenaline and noradrenaline, leading to weight loss and hypertension, commonly occur in MEN2 individuals. These may be excised surgically, although careful clearance of the excision margins is required.[5] Small to medium-sized tumours can also be removed using laparoscopic techniques,[70,71] which may prove advantageous as the relatively small number of studies to date show a decrease in both the length of hospital stay and post-operative complications, making it a preferable option to open surgery although tumour-mediated irregularities in blood pressure and cardiac rhythm will require intensive medical management in the pre-operative period using both α- and β-blockers.[5]

Hyperparathyroidism occurs less often in MEN2 than MEN1, although its incidence increases with age. Hypocalcaemia may result from too aggressive an excision, subtotal parathyroidectomy and cervical thymectomy being advocated in such cases because of the formation of supernumerary parathyroid glands,[68,72] dietary supplementation of both vitamin D and calcium being required in those undergoing a complete thyroidectomy.[66] Newer recommendations for treatment, emanating from the Netherlands and elsewhere, advocate prophylactic thyroidectomy and parathyroidectomy with the re-implanation of one or more parathyroid glands into the neck or non-dominant forearm for MEN2 individuals carrying the causative *RET* mutation.[73] A small number of individuals present with mucosal neuroma syndrome, which contains features of both MEN1 and MEN2, most notably phaeochromocytoma and medullary carcinoma of the thyroid, although the most important distinguishing feature is the early development of mucosal neuromas in the lips, tongue, mouth and gut which may require definitive surgery followed by surgical reconstruction.[5]

Psychological and ethical considerations of prophylactic surgery

The impact of surgery on an individual depends upon a complex array of factors, including the real or perceived sense of threat they feel themselves to be under as a result of their cancer risk, personality traits, and the psychological morbidity that a strong family history of cancer engenders.[74] These concerns may be unalleviated by medical surveillance or counselling, and lead them to seek radical surgery in the absence of actual disease.[75,76] The psychological impact of mastectomy has been well documented,[75,77] but women with the breast/ovarian cancer syndrome attributed to germ-line mutations in the *BRCA1* and *BRCA2* tumour suppressor genes may also opt for prophylactic laparoscopic oophorectomy which may lead to a loss of fertility and additional body image and sexuality problems, the impact of which has been little studied.[64,78] Individuals may inherit germ-line mutations in these genes which normally repair damaged cellular DNA prior to mitosis, or the genes may themselves become damaged, rendering them less effective at preventing the replication of mutated DNA during cell division, and hence cancer. The development of predictive genetic tests for these mutations means that lifetime risk for FAP and MEN as well as many breast and ovarian cancers is increasingly diagnosed in young children or adolescents who will subsequently live with both the knowledge and consequences of their diagnosis for the rest of their lives. The psychological and emotional impact of regular invasive screening for these potentially life-threatening conditions has been little studied, but its effects should not be underestimated, thus prophylactic surgery may be offered in an attempt to limit cancer risk and the psychological impact of regular surveillance in such individuals.[63,79,80]

One longitudinal study of 48 children at risk from FAP found that positive children who also had an affected older sibling demonstrated significantly higher, though subclinical, increases in depressive symptoms in comparison to those who tested negative and whose siblings did not have the condition. Children found not to have the gene mutation, but who nevertheless had an affected brother or sister also had higher depression scores than those without, and one should not underestimate the significance of either result on children submitted to such tests, since relief may soon give way to feelings of guilt and remorse for their afflicted sibling.[63] Altered body image, alienation, isolation from friends and peer groups, and the fear of death or medical interventions has been well documented among children and adolescents with cancer, one strategy to overcome

this being their inclusion in decision making and the negotiation of desired care outcomes,[81] but decisions about the appropriateness of genetic testing and prophylactic surgery may cause friction among parents, grandparents and older siblings at a time when the child is incapable of making a legally autonomous decision on an issue that will affect them for the rest of their life. It would appear that the psychological risk of a positive test result is greater in the young and those portraying higher premorbid anxiety traits than older adults,[82] but young probands (the affected individual through whom a family with a genetic disorder is first identified) may, in addition, be confronted with a loss of sexual function, changes in body image and ongoing surgical interventions which may affect self-esteem and psychosexual development for the rest of their lives.[61,83,84] Furthermore, research into the impact of genetic testing for MEN suggests that a negative result does not necessarily equate with a reduction in anxiety for either the proband or their family, since mutation-positive parents frequently demand further screening on the basis that the test result may be wrong or unreliable.[85] Nurses engaged in the care and support of those undergoing such tests should adopt an approach to care that elicits the concerns of the whole family therefore,[63,79] since anxiety, uncertainty and an irrational fear of cancer may persist irrespective of the test result.[86–88]

The evidence base for prophylactic mastectomy

Individuals with breast cancer who carry a *BRCA1* gene mutation have a 64% lifetime risk of developing a second primary breast cancer and a 44–60% chance of developing primary ovarian cancer during their lifetime.[64] Thus the decision to undergo prophylactic bilateral mastectomy and oophorectomy in order to reduce their lifetime risk of either disease is a reasonable one in women with a good prognosis. A number of papers suggest that bilateral prophylactic mastectomy may also reduce the lifetime cancer risk in disease-negative breast cancer gene mutation carriers,[89–91] although it does not completely eradicate the possibility of it occurring.[76] The authors of one study calculated on the basis of the literature reviewed, that prophylactic bilateral mastectomy reduces the 50–80% lifetime risk for *BRCA1* and *BRCA2* carriers by as much as 80–95%, and report a 74% decrease in breast cancer anxiety in such women.[91] Their analysis shows that on average, 70% of respondents were satisfied with the physical outcome of their mastectomy, particularly if nipple-sparing surgery had been performed, one unanticipated finding being that a small number of women were happier with post-operative reconstruction of their breast than their pre-operative state. These conclusions are broadly consistent with the results of other studies which posit both survival and psychosocial benefits of prophylactic mastectomy in such women,[89,92–95] but prophylactic mastectomy in women who do not show evidence of the disease remains controversial.[64] One Cochrane systematic review has identified serious methodological limitations,[76] including a lack of suitable control groups,[96] follow-up times of less than 5 years,[95] and the use of unvalidated patient satisfaction tools in many of these studies, while many carried out in the 1970s and 1980s included women who would not now be considered at high risk of developing breast cancer. Notwithstanding this, reported levels of satisfaction with the physical, emotional, and psychological outcomes of prophylactic bilateral mastectomy cited in recent studies using tools such as the General Health Questionnaire and the Body Image Scale is high,[92,93] though many retrospective studies rely heavily upon respondent recall – often over several months – and frequently lack baseline data by which to make a comparison.[76]

One problem inherent in advocating prophylactic mastectomy is the inability – even amongst *BRCA1* and *BRCA2* gene mutation carriers – to judge with any accuracy which of them may or may not go on to develop breast cancer. The picture is even more confused in those lacking a gene mutation but, nevertheless, faced with a strong family history of the disease.[76] The decision whether or not to undergo prophylactic mastectomy is rarely made lightly,[97] though a heightened sense of vulnerability and the presence of psychological anxiety has been positively correlated with a decision to undergo mastectomy in the absence of breast disease.[98] A substantial number of individuals may return to their general practitioner

(GP) or the cancer genetics service with cancer anxieties in the aftermath of prophylactic surgery,[64] whilst cancer-related distress, quality of life and body image problems associated with surgery may persist for many years after surgery.[96] An over emphasis on individual responsibility for treatment decisions is occasionally correlated with poorer satisfaction outcomes in the aftermath of surgery, and it would seem vital, therefore, that the decision to undergo prophylactic mastectomy is not made in isolation.[99] Many making the decision will have been personally affected by the death of a close friend or relative, and several studies highlight the importance of psychosocial support at such a time.[92,95] Lostumbo *et al.* (2004) draw an important distinction between prophylactic and curative mastectomy, arguing that the former does not constitute a medical emergency and should only be made after careful explanation of both the real and relative risks has been given, and sufficient time allowed for reflection on the information provided.[76]

While there is strong evidence to support the value of prophylactic oophorectomy in women with pre-existing breast disease, the evidence base for contralateral prophylactic mastectomy remains contentious.[64] Some studies suggest that it may decrease the risk of a second primary cancer occurring in the remaining breast,[100,101] although Lostumbo *et al.* again point out the methodological limitations inherent in these studies, most notably, the lack of control for confounding variables such as concomitant cancer therapies.[76] Moreover, a reduction in contralateral spread by such means does not necessarily equate with improved survivorship, the risk to the individual from metastatic disease being much greater than that for a second breast cancer occurring – even in *BRCA* gene mutation carriers.[76] If, however, a decision is taken to remove the contralateral breast, this should always be preceded by sentinel lymph node biopsy in order to reduce the need for complete axillary node dissection and thus spare the individual from common problems such as lymphoedema, numbness and restricted movement in her second arm.[102] It will also indicate whether adjuvant treatment with cytotoxic chemotherapy is warranted prior to the removal of the sentinel node,[103] an important consideration given that up to 5%

of prophylactically excised breasts contain occult disease which may already have metastasised by the time of surgery.[104]

Diagnostic surgery

Major surgical procedures are becoming less common in the diagnosis of cancer, and it is becoming rarer for a cancer to be diagnosed on the basis of a laparotomy alone.[5] Minimally invasive procedures such as fine needle aspiration are increasingly used in conjunction with computed tomography (CT) or magnetic resonance imaging (MRI) in order to establish the presence and extent of a tumour,[31] though diagnostic laparoscopy has also helped to reduce the need for laparotomy. Open surgery may still be used where laparoscopic investigation is not possible, or is unlikely to identify the presence of disease (e.g. in a retroperitoneal mass), or a large tissue sample is required to establish the histology of a tumour.[31] It may also be necessary in soft tissue sarcomas or lymphomas where an accurate grading of the disease is essential in establishing the most appropriate treatment plan.[31]

The collection of cancer cells for cytological and morphological diagnosis now primarily involves the use of 'minimally invasive' sampling techniques such as exfoliative cytology or aspiration cytology.[105] In the former, a selection of cells that are normally desquamated are collected or detached from the underlying tissue by mechanical means such as a spatula or brush. A Papanicolaou or 'pap' smear which identifies early changes in cervical cells before they become cancerous is one example of an exfoliative cytological sample,[106,107] as is bronchial or pleural lavage.[108] Other examples of exfoliative diagnostic tests include lumbar puncture, the collection of voided urine or a bladder wash, thoracocentesis, and laparocentesis. The collection and inspection of spontaneously voided cells from body cavities in the latter instances may indicate the presence of neoplastic cells within the sample, but they may not give conclusive information as to the location or extent of the disease.[105] Similarly, cells collected via this means may have undergone a degree of deterioration in the time since they were voided

or detached from their original site, or have been damaged in the process of collection, making it difficult for the histopathologist to examine important attributes such as the number and ratio of nuclei to cell size, shape and structure, or the cells' chromatin content.[105] Further investigations such as cervical colposcopy or cystoscopy may therefore be required in order to obtain a definitive diagnosis that also give a clear indication of the site, size and extent of tumour spread. Additional procedures such as an intravenous venogram or urogram may be used to assess the function of any vital organs that may be affected by the tumour, and provide important information about the degree of tumour infiltration. Some tests such as a sputum or bronchial lavage sample may need to be repeated in order to provide a more accurate diagnosis; thus the individual undergoing diagnostic tests to establish whether or not they have cancer may require any number of separate procedures and may become frustrated at the apparent repetition of such tests or the tardiness of medical staff in providing them with a definitive diagnosis. Careful explanation of the need for such tests and the likely time scales required for the completion of each is important therefore, and should be communicated to the individual in a sensitive and supportive manner prior to their being undertaken.

Other minimally invasive techniques used in the diagnosis of cancer include biopsies, fine needle aspiration cytology, needle core biopsy, incisional biopsy, and excisional biopsy, which will now be discussed separately and are illustrated in Figure 11.1. Each have their advantages and disadvantages and may be used in different circumstances, but it is important to remember that while these are often regarded by health care professionals as minor or routine procedures, they are far from routine for the individual concerned and may elicit a great deal of anxiety notwithstanding the significance of their result once known. Health care professionals frequently regard diagnosis as the first stage in the cancer journey, but for the individual, these tests may come at the end of an indeterminate period of anxiety, somatic preoccupation and any number of distressing signs such as weight loss, haemoptysis, changes in body function, or pain.[5] Discussion of the need

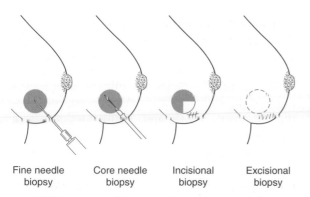

Fine needle biopsy | Core needle biopsy | Incisional biopsy | Excisional biopsy

Figure 11.1 Types of biopsy. Reproduced with permission from Love S.M. (1995). *Dr Love's Breast Book*. New York: Perseus Book Publishers.[113]

for, and likely outcomes of any diagnostic tests may provide the first point of contact with the world of clinical oncology, while others may have formed strong opinions about cancer and its treatment from the prior experience of friends or family members. Lay perceptions of cancer are also informed by portrayals of cancer and cancer 'patients' in the media and, increasingly, by personal research on the internet and other means,[29,110–111] so it is advisable to ascertain what they feel is wrong with them and their understanding of the disease so that an appropriate level of support can be given. Open questions such as, 'what do you feel may be wrong with you?' or 'what in particular is worrying you at the current time' may help to elicit personal concerns and give one a good idea of the individual's insight into their condition.[5] Moreover, it will reassure them that their fears and anxieties matter to the team caring for them and are an appropriate matter for discussion, encouraging honest communication from the outset of their cancer journey,[29] and providing important information on their coping strategies so that an appropriate explanation of the different diagnostic tests that they are about to undergo can be given.[112]

Fine needle aspiration biopsy

A variety of biopsies are used to diagnose cancer, each varying in the amount and type of tissue taken. The least invasive procedure is the fine needle biopsy which involves the aspiration of

tissue cells for cytopathology. It has a number of advantages over other biopsy techniques in that it can be performed in an outpatient setting and is least likely to cause tissue damage. This is important as cancers will invariably grow along a weakened tissue plane, and fine needle biopsy limits both tissue damage and the risk of malignant cells being spread by a more cumbersome instrument.[105] Great care should be taken when undertaking a biopsy that the incision site and any subsequent drains are placed appropriately, so that tumour seeding does not occur beyond the surgical field which will require additional excision of healthy tissue in the procedure that follows. Initially developed for the aspiration of palpable masses such as breast lumps and enlarged lymph glands, the advent of improved imaging and laparoscopic techniques means that samples can now be taken from almost any area of the body, including the lungs, liver, pancreas, kidneys, spleen, and bone tissue.[105] A successful cytology sample obtained by such means will include a mixture of dispersed cells, cell clusters, and possibly small pieces of the tumour known as 'microbiopsies', which will identify not only the histopathology of the tumour, but its grade as well.[105]

A positive cytology report provides the rationale for surgery without additional biopsy in a growing number of cancers, including breast, thyroid, lung, renal, pancreatic, and liver cancers, although the accuracy of such tests varies depending upon the skill of the person undertaking the biopsy or fixing the specimen, and the type of tumour aspirated. It has been estimated that an experienced cytologist is able to distinguish malignant from non-malignant cells in 70–80% of biopsy samples, the most amenable to diagnosis being breast, bone, and soft tissue cancers, while non-Hodgkin's lymphoma, non-follicular thyroid cancer, primary lung cancer, and breast disease can be successfully classified in the majority of cases from a sample obtained via such means.[105] There remains the possibility for a false-negative or a false-positive test result in a small number of cases, a false positive being least likely in all except thyroid cancer,[105,114–116] although the use of additional tests such as histochemistry, electron microscopy, immunohistochemistry, and chromosomal and DNA analysis significantly improve the accuracy of a cancer diagnosis in the majority of cases.[105]

Histochemistry may indicate the presence of osteosarcoma and eliminate other possible causes of bone pain, while immunohistochemistry can be used to indicate the hormone receptor status of breast cancer or differentiate between benign lymphoid hyperplasia and indolent non-Hodgkin's lymphoma in haematological disease.[105] Electron microscopy may be used to identify structural differences in cancers that do not stain successfully, or to differentiate between leiomyosarcoma, malignant peripheral nerve sheath tumour, or osteosarcoma in the presence of osteoid, collagen-rich uncalcified bone matrix which may accumulate where there is inadequate osteoblast activity or insufficient mineralisation of bone tissue.[105] Electron microscopy is indicated in such cases, as the clinical and radiographic appearance of bone tumours may be atypical and resemble non-malignant conditions such as local or systemic infection (osteomyelitis) or mineral, and specifically vitamin D deficiencies (osteomalacia). The side-effects of fine needle aspiration biopsy are relatively few, but include the possibility of swelling, tenderness and slight haemorrhage where this is performed on palpable tumours, and pneumothorax in fine needle biopsies of the breast, axillary lymph nodes, lung, mediastinum, and thoracic wall.[105]

Psychological preparation and impact of biopsy
The propensity of patients to experience these side-effects is mitigated by the considerable advantages that fine needle aspiration offers over other biopsy methods, but should again remind the professional that these are far from routine experiences for the majority of people seeking a differential diagnosis for the complex array of signs they may have been experiencing, and reinforce the need for full explanation of the post-operative risks so that informed consent can be obtained prior to the procedure taking place.[5] This is particularly important as numerous studies have indicated the paucity of information given by medical staff – particularly in a busy outpatient setting where physical examination and the elicitation of the individual's medical history may dominate proceedings in a time-constrained consultation.[29]

There is also evidence that medical staff overestimate the level of medical knowledge among the general public, or amend the amount of information that they give on the basis of subjective evaluations about the socioeconomic or educational status of their clients.[29,117,118] Appropriate information given in a timely and sensitive fashion is an important means of reducing anxiety and promoting active participation in the decision-making process,[118,119] and nurses play a vital role in establishing what the individual understands about the procedure and ensuring that informed consent has been obtained,[118] while reinforcing the positive contribution that a negative result or the proper histology, staging, and grading of a tumour will make to the treatment of their cancer if that is what is diagnosed.[120] Similarly, information on where, when and by whom the results will be communicated is important, particularly in the outpatient or short-stay setting where there may be a time-lag between the procedure and discussion of its outcome, since the intervening period may be a time of considerable anxiety.[121] Nurses can also greatly assist the individual by encouraging them to bring a friend or family member to the consultation since they will provide important psychological support in the event that a positive diagnosis has to be relayed, and may be in a better position to recall or reinforce what was said in the aftermath of the consultation.

Other types of biopsy
A core needle (or course needle) biopsy involves the removal of a 1.0–1.2 mm core of tissue through a hollow needle under local anaesthetic. It is more invasive than a fine needle aspiration, but provides a larger specimen for histopathological investigation and is adequate for the diagnosis of most types of tumour.[33] Unfortunately, with the exception of a frozen section, the results of a core needle biopsy take longer to report upon, as the sample requires fixing and mounting in wax which takes several days,[6] while multiple sampling may not be feasible because of its greater invasiveness.[105] It does allow better evaluation of the tissue pattern however, as a greater quantity of both malignant and non-malignant cells will be present in the sample, giving a lower number of false-negative results, but the tissue samples may be less amenable to

ancillary diagnostic tests once fixed.[105] As with all biopsies, the quality of the sample does depend upon the skill of the individual taking it, and there is the possibility, especially with a movable lump or focal disease, that the physician may miss the tumour completely, which limits the usefulness of the procedure. For this reason, only a positive result is regarded as clinically significant since a negative biopsy does not necessarily indicate the absence of disease,[5] which may require an incisional or 'punch' biopsy to obtain a useful tissue sample.[6]

Incisional biopsy requires the removal of an elliptical tissue sample from a larger tissue mass, using a scalpel or punch biopsy instrument. It is the preferred method for diagnosing soft tissue and bone tumours, but great care should be taken to ensure that the needle track or incision sites are appropriately placed to avoid the possibility of tumour seeding and the need to excise more tissue than necessary during the subsequent surgical procedure.[31] Excisional biopsy involves the removal of an easily accessible tumour in its totality, together with a healthy tissue margin, and may be curative for benign tumours and non-melanoma skin cancers such as basal cell carcinomas when the microscopic margins are clear.[6] It is also indicated for melanoma of the skin providing that it is anatomically, functionally, and cosmetically acceptable,[122] and preferable to other forms of biopsy given the propensity of the disease to spread both locally and systemically. In this case excisional biopsy allows accurate calculation of the tumour depth (Breslow thickness) and its invasiveness, which provides important prognostic information for the surgeon,[122] and determines the clearance margin required; several large-scale studies demonstrating that a 1 cm margin is adequate for tumours less than 2 mm deep, and a 2 cm margin for those greater than 2 mm deep.[122] Prophylactic lymph node dissection, once routinely undertaken as part of the excisional biopsy, is no longer considered appropriate since systemic spread is already likely to have occurred in tumours greater than 2 mm deep,[123] five-year survival rates ranging from 25% to 40% in those requiring full regional lymph node dissection at the point of diagnosis.[122]

Notwithstanding developments in the above methods, it may on occasions be necessary to perform an examination under anaesthetic, or an open laparotomy, to establish the nature and extent of the tumour although their use is diminishing. Laparotomy may be undertaken in ovarian cancer where laparoscopic examination under anaesthetic or peritoneal washings have failed to identify residual disease, in a process known as a 'second look laparotomy', although its effectiveness is debatable, Souhami and Tobias (2005) suggesting that its benefit for anything other than staging purposes remains uncertain.[5] A number of recent studies have reported beneficial outcomes following second-look laparotomy for ovarian cancer, where this was used to stage patients for salvage whole abdominal radiotherapy,[124] and in primary peritoneal mesothelioma,[125] where patients with residual disease were treated with cytotoxic chemotherapy following laparotomy and omentectomy, but such cases remain rare, and in the latter case experimental; patients derive significant palliative benefit from cytotoxic chemotherapy, particularly the newer antifolate agents pemetrexed and raltitrexed in such circumstances.[5,126–129] Similarly, laparotomy and splenectomy, once common in the staging and treatment of Hodgkin's disease have now been replaced by percutaneous biopsies including marrow trephine, which may indicate the need for chemotherapy – though the disease foci may be missed in a percutaneous liver biopsy and consequently provide a false-negative result.[5]

Nurse-led endoscopy services

Endoscopy is increasingly used in the diagnosis of a great many cancers and has dramatically reduced both the hospitalisation time and costs previously associated with laparotomy (see Research study 11.1).[130] Its effectiveness in reducing the pain, infection, and post-operative complications associated with open surgery has been well documented and many types of endoscopic investigation now take place on a regular basis.[131] These include laryngoscopy, bronchoscopy, colonoscopy, and gastroscopy to name but a few, and a brief discussion of their benefits is of direct relevance to the small but growing number of nurses undertaking laparoscopy as part of their regular employment.[132,133] Early anxiety about nurses and other non-medical staff undertaking diagnostic endoscopies seems still to exist,[132,134,135] one study demonstrating that GPs were more likely to request follow-up barium enemas from a nurse-led than a physician-led endoscopy service.[136] However, there was little difference in the total number of cancers detected or the number of false-positive and false-negative diagnoses detected by nurse-led and physician-led services; suitably qualified nurses appear as capable of detecting malignant disease as medically trained practitioners, and provide a more cost-effective service, particularly for screening services where the unit cost of a nurse-led service for each cancer detected will be considerably lower than for a medically led service.[137]

Nurse-endoscopists are now leading services for FAP and a variety of other 'at-risk' groups,[138] including capsule endoscopy for bleeding disorders,[139] and an increasing number of hospitals in the UK are training nurses in the competencies required to undertake flexible sigmoidoscopy and oesophago-gastroduodenoscopy as part of the government's drive to improve the detection rates for cancer as part of *The NHS Cancer Plan*.[140] Colorectal cancer in particular remains a significant cause of cancer-related morbidity and mortality in the UK, but has been resistant to early detection and, consequently, curative surgical treatment.[5,133,141] Nurse endoscopists were found to provide a valuable service in one national survey of hospitals employing nurse-endoscopists,[141] with the benefits including cost, patient acceptability, and improved care. Nurses are now involved in sedated and unsedated techniques including flexible sigmoidoscopy, colonoscopy, and oesophago-gastroduodenoscopy in addition to capsule endoscopy,[132,141] but there is to date, very little literature on the additional contribution that nurse-endoscopists make to the care of individuals undergoing such anxiety-inducing procedures; one study suggests that there was little difference between nurses' and medical endoscopists' ability to accurately assess the comfort of those undergoing gastroscopy, both rating their comfort higher than did the individuals themselves. There can be no doubt that the number of unsedated procedures undertaken will continue to rise, but it is salutary to note that while these are generally safe and well tolerated, a significant number of individuals find them uncomfortable and distress-

ing. Interpersonal communication skills are paramount in this setting therefore,[29] and pre-operative education may be of some benefit in both preparing the individual and reducing the need for a repeat procedure.[130] The preparation of nurse-endoscopists should therefore include the acquisition of advanced assessment and communication skills in addition to the competencies required to undertake an endoscopy, if patient satisfaction with such services is to be maintained.[133]

Definitive (or curative) surgery

Factors indicating the use of definitive surgery include the histology of the tumour, its growth rate, location, invasiveness, and capacity to metastasise. The presence of metastases may indicate the need for systemic or locoregional therapy, although surgery may be used for symptom control or cosmetic purposes in such instances.[6] The surgical team will also want to consider the performance status of individuals about to undergo surgery (see below), but the primary course of action for the majority of solid tumours is the removal of visible, palpable masses which remain limited to the tissue of origin.[142] The goal of treatment in such circumstances is complete resection of the tumour together with a margin of healthy tissue, and resection of regional lymphatic drainage to prevent local recurrence. Thus radical bowel excision with end-to-end anastamosis and removal of lymphatic drainage remains the only curative treatment modality for colorectal cancer, but this may also involve removal of the mesorectum or the formation of a temporary colostomy which will be reversed at a later date.[5,6] Similarly, a radical or modified radical (Patey) mastectomy facilitates clearance of a large primary breast tumour but may also require breast reconstruction using a Becker's prosthesis, gluteal, latissimus dorsi, or a pedicled transverse rectus abdominis myocutaneous (TRAM) flap in which the rectus muscle is separated in the lower abdomen and tunnelled under the skin to form a breast mound at the mastectomy site (see Figure 11.2),[142] extending the original extent of definitive surgery and potentially requiring further procedures at a later date.

Research study 11.1

Abuksis G., Mor M., Segal N. *et al.* (2001). A patient education program is cost-effective for preventing failure of endoscopic procedures in a gastroenterology department. *American Journal of Gastroeneterology* **96**,1786–1790.[130]

Aim of study

This was a prospective, randomised, controlled study to determine the cost-effectiveness of a patient education programme in 142 adults referred for an endoscopic procedure.

Method

Ninety-one patients (64%) participated in a targeted educational programme conducted by a nurse specially trained to discuss the indications, choice, possible side-effects, and complications of endoscopic procedures on an individual basis. This was followed up with specific written information on the procedure to be undertaken and advice on colonic preparation together with an invitation to call the nurse with any last-minute questions prior to admission. All patients completed a questionnaire covering background data, endoscopy-related variables, anxiety level, and satisfaction before endoscopy.

Results

The mean interval between the educational interaction and endoscopy was 22.9 days (range 1–90 days) and there were no significant differences between patients in the intervention group (91 patients) and those in the control arms, consisting of 38 persons (27%) receiving leaflets but no instruction and 13 (9%) who were given telephone instructions and an information leaflet. No significant relationship was found between the intervention and control groups in relation to anxiety, which was reported to be quite low in this study, although the benefits of the educational programme were negatively correlated in those undergoing a repeat procedure. Satisfaction with the procedure booklets was high in all groups, but there was a statistically significant relationship between attendance on the educational programme and the success of the procedure undertaken (95.6% versus 73.6% and 62.3% respectively) when clinical causes for failure were taken into account. Failures in the pre-procedural education group were positively correlated with an increase in time between the intervention and the endoscopy.

Conclusions

Previous research indicating that patient adherence and the success of endoscopic procedures increases with patient education was supported by the study; those not attending the teaching sessions showed a six-fold increase in the number of procedural failures. Calculations based upon nursing costs alone showed a 5.5–8.8% reduction in the cost of endoscopy in the intervention group – the greatest saving being for colonoscopies. This supports many other studies that demonstrate the value of educational preparation on patient satisfaction, co-operation, anxiety, and the success of endoscopic procedures, but adds a new and increasingly important consideration to the equation – that of cost-effectiveness. The study clearly demonstrated the benefits accrued from pre-procedural education and posits an important role for nurses engaged in the care of patients undergoing investigative procedures of this type.

Limitations

The study comprises a good number of participants but the uneven distribution of patients between the intervention groups is a limitation of the study. It is interesting to note that patients who called the service for advice were automatically transferred to group 3 and that these had the lowest success rate for their investigation. The reasons why they telephoned were not fully reported but may have had a bearing upon their performance on the day of the procedure.

Definitive surgery in lung cancer

Lobectomy or pneumonectomy are the most effective treatments for non-small-cell lung cancer and offer the best chance of cure for individuals although surgery will only be suitable in about 25–30% of individuals,[5] and the cure rate for node-positive stage IIA non-small-cell lung cancer is low, with only 7–16% of individuals surviving to their fifth year.[144] Surgery following induction with neoadjuvant radiotherapy and/or cytotoxic chemotherapy offers moderate survival benefit and slightly reduces recurrence,[144,145] as does the use of

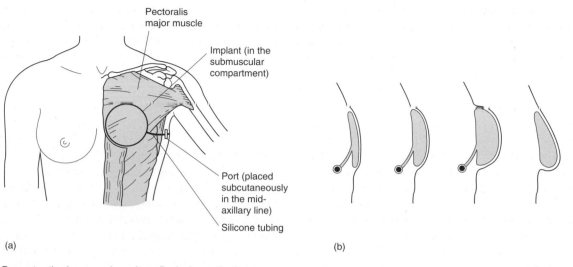

(a)

Pectoralis major muscle

Implant (in the submuscular compartment)

Port (placed subcutaneously in the mid-axillary line)

Silicone tubing

(b)

Reconstruction by expansion using a Becker's prosthesis.

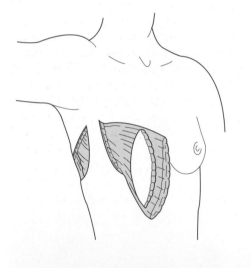

(c) Latissimus dorsi flap reconstruction. The myocutaneous flap is delivered through the mastectomy wound.

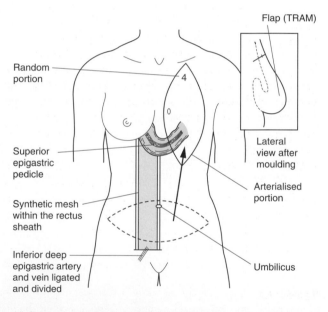

Flap (TRAM)

Random portion

Superior epigastric pedicle

Synthetic mesh within the rectus sheath

Inferior deep epigastric artery and vein ligated and divided

Lateral view after moulding

Arterialised portion

Umbilicus

(d) Conventional (pedicled) TRAM reconstruction.

Figure 11.2 Types of breast reconstruction surgery. Reproduced with permission from Baum M., Saunders C. and Meredith S. (1995). *Breast Cancer: A Guide for Every Woman.* Oxford: Oxford University Press, p. 70.[143]

specialist thoracic surgical teams,[146] although the outcomes of lung cancer resection tend to be worse in the UK than elsewhere in the developed world.[147] The comparative benefits of lobectomy versus limited resection for individuals with stage I–II non-small-cell lung cancer and those with resect-

able stage IIIA disease have been the subject of a recent Cochrane systematic review, which found that lobectomy with mediastinal lymph node dissection provided a modest survival advantage over tumour resection and lymph node sampling alone,[148] though the limited size and number of clinical trials available for review limits the strength of the conclusions that can be drawn from data in these studies as do their methodological limitations. It has been argued that extensive surgery that removes more tissue than is absolutely necessary is of little value, one aim of surgery being to retain healthy lung tissue so as to maximise pulmonary function,[149] thus pneumonectomy may be avoided in individuals with tumours in the descending bronchial tree by performing a sleeve resection or segmentectomy in those with limited pulmonary reserve.[147,149] It is clear that even in early disease, limited resection increases the likelihood of recurrence and potentially reduces the individual's survival chances in comparison to lobectomy or (less commonly) pneumonectomy, further underlining the argument that if non-small-cell lung cancer is to be resected at all, it should be as complete a resection as possible.[108] One factor limiting comparative analysis of different studies has been the lack of a clear and unambiguous definition of what is meant by 'complete resection', different interpretations being used in different settings and between different studies making accurate comparison of survival advantage between different techniques difficult. The International Association for the Study of Lung Cancer Staging Committee (IASLC) has therefore suggested new criteria for the definition of complete, incomplete, and unsuccessful resections in an attempt to facilitate international comparisons and provide predictive prognostic indicators for surgical resection.[108] These may be seen in Table 11.2.

Pneumonectomy is normally indicated for tumours in the main stem of the bronchus or when more than one lobe is affected,[5] although the post-operative mortality rate for pneumonectomy is approximately twice that for lobectomy, variously reported as 5–10% as opposed to 2–5%.[5,6] There is a lack of clear criteria for the surgical management of advanced disease, the outcomes of surgery alone in node-positive individuals being quite poor and demonstrating little difference in survival than for those being treated with radiotherapy and/or cytotoxic chemotherapy.[150] Given the morbidity and mortality associated with surgery and the high metastatic potential of the disease, locoregional radiotherapy with or without systemic cytotoxic chemotherapy is now the treatment of choice for stage IIIa non-small-cell lung cancer,[151] although the majority of individuals with superior sulcus involvement in one study enjoyed disease-free survival in excess of 18 months with a combination of pre-operative radiotherapy, surgery, and intra-operative radiotherapy,[152] making surgery a viable option for individuals presenting with this condition.[5,153] There is no proven role for surgery in the management of small-cell lung cancer, and the 20–30% mortality rate associated with pleuropneumonectomy (excision of the lung, pleura, hemidiaphragm, and the ipsilateral pericardium) for mesothelioma favours the use of less radical surgery (pleurectomy) in the small percentage of individuals with resectable disease, often in combination with radiotherapy.[154,155]

Table 11.2 International Association for the Study of Lung Cancer (IASLC) Staging Committee's definition of complete, incomplete and unsuccessful resection for non-small-cell lung cancer (after Rami-Porta *et al.* (2005))[108]

Level of resection	Criteria
Complete resection	No extracapsular nodal extension of the tumour seen
	Complete systematic nodal dissection or lobe-specific nodal dissection undertaken
	Highest mediastinal node removed must be disease negative
	Microscopically proven disease-free resection margins
Incomplete resection	Extracapsular nodal disease remains
	Disease-positive lymph nodes left *in situ*
	Resection margin contains evidence of disease
	Disease-positive pleural or pericardial effusions present
Unsuccessful resection	No residual tumour left and resection margins disease free but one or more of the additional criteria above are not met

Pre-existing co-morbidity is a significant problem in lung cancer and may impact upon the individual's ability to undergo or gain significant survival advantaged from lung surgery.[156] Smoking remains without doubt the primary cause of both lung cancer and a number of common co-morbidities associated with it such as ischaemic heart disease, hypertension, and carotid stenosis,[157] which pose additional health problems for many undergoing surgery.[149] Assessment of cardiac function and exercise tolerance will therefore be undertaken in addition to lung function tests prior to the procedure, and the need to improve cardiac function, treat hypertension, or resolve pre-existing cardiac arrhythmias with drug therapy may cause a delay in definitive surgery while the individual's functional status is optimised preoperatively.[149] Post-operative morbidity includes the risk of thrombus formation, respiratory infection, and cardiac dysrhythmias such as atrial fibrillation, particularly in older individuals,[149] but relatively little is known about the experience or quality of life of those surviving beyond this period,[156,158] one seminal study being reported in more detail in Research study 11.2. Reported 30-day post-operative mortality for pneumonectomy is in the region of 7%, approximately twice that for lobectomy, although this may be an underestimate, many deaths being ascribed to pneumonia or multi-organ failure rather than lung injury or adult respiratory distress syndrome which can be directly attributable to surgery.[149] Handy *et al.* (2002) suggest that as many as 12% may die in the first 6 months after surgery though few surgical studies follow individuals up for this length of time.[156]

Of more importance is the apparent dissonance between surgeons' expectations of 'cure' and the long-term or 'fixed functional outcomes' of lung surgery which may be debilitating for the individual and members of their family.[159] These include pain caused by disturbance of the intercostal nerves at the time of surgery, which may take 6–18 months to resolve,[160] dyspnoea and fatigue which interfere with activities of daily living such as walking, personal cleansing and dressing, work, and the expression of sexuality.[156,161,162] Cachexia is another distressing symptom which may not be alleviated by surgery,[163] while symptom distress may be compounded by psychosocial issues such as anxiety, role change, a shrinking of the individual's social world, and depression.[164] One large-scale ($n = 4496$) study looking at the psychological distress caused by different cancers found that lung cancer elicited ongoing symptom distress in 43.4% of individuals, the largest proportion of any site-specific cancer and considerably higher than the overall prevalence of 35.1%.[165] Oxygen dependence is another 'fixed functional outcome' which may have both a psychological and physiological cause post-pneumonectomy, although its incidence is lower in those receiving parenchymal sparing surgery such as lobectomy or segmentectomy.[156,166] Some have argued that reports about the poor quality of life experienced by those receiving lung surgery should be balanced against poor pre-operative functioning and the low rates of cure obtained with other treatment modalities such as radiotherapy and cytotoxic chemotherapy for unresectable disease, which are not themselves without risk.[160]

Additional psychological issues such as guilt or self-blame may also have a deleterious impact on perceived quality of life and mental health, smoking being the most common cause of most lung cancers,[157] although as many as 50% may have stopped smoking by the time of diagnosis.[158] The provision of smoking-cessation advice may appear belated to some and may worsen guilt or anxiety in others, but considerable benefit may accrue from smoking cessation following surgery; long-term complications such as infection, cough, wheeze and dyspnoea are less common in ex-smokers than in those continuing to smoke.[161] Non-smokers and ex-smokers also demonstrate lower levels of anxiety and depression after surgery although the reasons for this are unclear.[161] This may be related to ex-smokers perceiving themselves to have a higher locus of control over the treatment process,[167] though it should be remembered that smoking is a deeply embedded behaviour with both physiological and psychological antecedents,[167,168] with some individuals continuing to smoke even after lung surgery. Smoking may form an important coping mechanism for many, and has strong links with ruminative coping styles,[169,170] thus it may be difficult to break such

Research study 11.2

Sarna L., Evangelista L., Taskin D. *et al.* (2004). Impact of respiratory symptoms and pulmonary function on quality of life of long-term survivors of non-small cell lung cancer. *Chest* **125**, 439–445.[158]

Aim of study

This cross-sectional survey sought to describe the long-term symptom experience of non-small-cell cancer patients in relation to their respiratory symptoms, pulmonary function and quality of life.

Method

Symptom distress, respiratory function and quality of life were assessed in 142 individuals between 5 and 22 years after treatment for non-small-cell lung cancer using repeated physiological measures such as the forced expiratory volume (FEV), forced expiratory vital capacity (FVC), and forced expiratory flow (FEF). The American Thoracic Society questionnaire and the Short-form Quality of Life Questionnaire (QOL SF-36) were also administered. The average age of respondents was 71 years and the majority (74%) had received lobectomy. Fifty-four per cent of the sample were women.

Results

Analysis included frequency of self-reported respiratory symptoms such as cough, phlegm, wheezing, and breathlessness and repeated objective measures of lung function such as FEV, FVC, and FEF. The study demonstrated that 66% had at least one respiratory symptom, 26% had two, 10% had three, and 5% had four or more symptoms which impacted upon their quality of life and functional status. Breathlessness was the commonest symptom (39%) followed by wheezing (31%), phlegm (28%), and cough (25%). Eleven per cent of respondents were too breathless to leave the house and 21% reported that they had spent most of the day in bed in the 12 months preceding the study because of their respiratory symptoms, though co-morbidities such as unstable angina appeared more important than the extent of cancer surgery in determining the severity of this problem. Symptom burden, rather than ventilatory impairment, appeared to contribute most to a diminished quality of life in these and the remainder of the sample, although 36% had a moderate-to-severe obstructive and/or restrictive ventilatory disorder on spirometry. Survivors exposed to second-hand smoke (28%) were more than three times as likely to report respiratory symptoms as those living in a smoke-free environment.

Conclusions

Spirometry successfully predicted the presence of respiratory impairment although the severity of respiratory function measured by such means did not correlate with any of the QOL dimensions tested or the subjective reporting of symptom severity by respondents. Survivors' perceptions of symptom severity provided a more important indicator of physical, role, social, and psychological functioning as well as their general health and vitality, although symptom severity was greater in the presence of second-hand smoke, indicating an important health-promotion role for nurses working with long-term lung cancer survivors and their carers. The authors concluded that further studies are needed to fully understand the nature and extent of symptom distress in long-term non-small-cell lung cancer survivors so that effective management strategies can be designed to combat these and the accumulated effects of other co-morbid conditions.

Limitations

Few studies have considered the long-term symptom experience of lung cancer patients beyond a relatively short post-operative period but the elective nature of this study may have prevented those with more serious impairments from participating in the study. Furthermore, the disease-free status of respondents was not independently verified and disease recurrence may have been a confounding variable in some cases. Notwithstanding this, the study identifies the need for further research into the impact of total symptom burden on diminished quality of life, and a better understanding of the effect that co-morbidity has on breathlessness, which remains the most troubling symptom in this client group and correlates most closely with self-reported quality of life.

an embedded habit, especially in those with a history of depressive symptoms,[169,170] and nurses should attempt to understand the seemingly inexplicable reasons why an individual might continue to smoke in the aftermath of lung surgery, offering advice and support to the individual in respect of smoking cessation without increasing the burden of guilt or self-blame that may already exist in this highly stigmatised client group.

Definitive surgery for gastric cancer

As with lung cancer, surgery remains the only treatment for gastric cancer that holds out a reasonable hope of cure,[171] several Japanese and South Korean studies showing excellent cure rates in those diagnosed with early carcinomas as a result of greater awareness of the disease and national screening programmes.[172–175] In comparison, up to 80% of those diagnosed in the UK have unresectable disease,[5,6] many presenting with large intra-abdominal masses, disease-positive lymph nodes, malignant ascites, or liver metastases as a result of late presentation. The incidence of stomach cancer in the UK and US has declined considerably in the last 50 years although it remains the second most common cancer in the world,[5] but in spite of this it remains a significant cause of cancer-related mortality in the UK, the presence of 15 or more positive lymph nodes or a disease-positive peritoneal cytology being important indicators of increased recurrence and early mortality after curative surgery.[171,176] It has been estimated that up to 67% of those treated with surgery alone fail to achieve long-term survivorship or improvements in their quality of life,[177] although this rate is improved significantly when surgery for resectable disease is aligned with other modalities such as radiotherapy and chemotherapy.[178]

The surgical management of gastric cancer involves either a total or partial gastrectomy, the extent of the procedure depending upon the size, location and local spread of the tumour.[5] Preoperative staging involves physical examination, chest X-ray, a CT scan and ultrasound of the liver to determine hepatic spread, and endoscopic ultrasound of the gastric wall to determine the extent of tumour infiltration and local damage.[179] A laparoscopy is a more reliable means of staging

the tumour than CT scanning and will show peritoneal disease and liver metastases which may remain unrecognised on a CT scan, thus preventing many with unresectable disease from undergoing an unnecessary laparotomy.[179] The 5-year survival rate for individuals with unresectable disease is extremely low at just 5%, although the 11–12% 5-year survival rate for those treated with curative intent in the UK is only half the European average and far short of the 90% 5-year survival rates reported in Japanese studies, where the diagnosis of early resectable tumours as a result of screening dramatically improves treatment outcomes.[5] Total gastrectomy involves the complete removal of the stomach and greater omentum, and may also involve the removal of the lower oesophagus or spleen, depending upon the location of the tumour.[5] A partial or subtotal gastrectomy may also involve resection of part of the omentum, and possibly part of the oesophagus or duodenum depending upon the tumour's location.[5,180,181] Total gastrectomy is a long and complicated procedure requiring anastomosis of the oesophagus with the jejunum, or oesophagojejunostomy. Leakage from the site of the anastomosis is common, occurring in 5–20% of those undergoing surgery, while malabsorption, diarrhoea, weight loss, and indigestion increase the postsurgical morbidity associated with the procedure.[179] Loss of the stomach may lead to feelings of satiety after a relatively small meal and some individuals may also suffer from a chronic iron deficiency and macrocytic anaemia caused by vitamin B_{12} deficiency.[5]

'Dumping syndrome' is a particularly unpleasant experience for individuals following total gastrectomy and is caused by the arrival of carbohydrates (particularly refined sugars) that have not previously been broken down by gastric acid or proteases in the stomach, into the proximal section of the small bowel.[182] The sudden and irregular arrival of large volumes of hyperosmolar sugars into the small bowel after a meal draws fluid from the intravascular compartments and gives rise to bloating, cramping and diarrhoea within an hour of eating.[179,182] The ensuing hypovolaemia leads to tachycardia, lightheadedness, and palpitations which may last for 15 minutes or more, whilst the too-rapid absorption of glucose may lead to an increase in insulin production and precipitate reactive hypoglyaemia 1–3 hours after the meal in a 'late dumping' syndrome.[182,183] Hypoglycaemia associated with 'late dumping' leads to decreased concentration, shakiness, perspiration, acute hunger and potentially coma unless it is recognised immediately.

Attempts at the pharmacological management of reactive hypoglycaemia using the somatostatin analogue octreotide to reduce gut motility and acarbose to inhibit carbohydrate digestion and reduce plasma glucose levels after eating, have proved successful,[184] but many individuals find the post-prandial effects of dumping syndrome distressing and may be deterred from maintaining an adequate nutritional intake.[185] One small study into gastrectomy patients' experiences of eating and drinking after surgery found that individuals struggled to maintain an adequate oral intake and found it difficult to adapt to dietary changes made necessary by their surgery,[186] thus the role of nurses in providing information and referring individuals for further nutritional advice is paramount if the neccesary adjustments to diet and lifestyle are to succeed and the impact of surgery is to be minimised. The individual should be advised that the effects of dumping syndrome will normally recede with time, but that they should try to eat several small, energy-dense meals a day and avoid taking fluids (including soup) within half an hour of eating, as this will potentiate the too-rapid passage of food in the jejunum and excacerbate bloating or satiety. Carbohydrate intake should be restricted and refined sugars avoided completely, complex carbohydrates or starches (such as wholemeal bread, pasta, and cereals) being preferable in small portions as these release glucose more slowly than their processed counterparts. Milk and milk products will also need to be restricted,[183] and the individual should try to increase their fat and protein intake in order to compensate for a reduction in carbohydrates, one study demonstrating that individuals undergoing gastrectomy are particularly susceptible to a loss of body protein mass.[187] Relief of the short-term symptoms may be achieved by advising the individual to eat in a semi-recumbent position or to lie down after a meal in order to slow down the transit of food in the small bowel.

The morbidity and mortality associated with radical surgery in advanced disease have been a source of grave concern, with many individuals struggling to maintain an adequate nutritional intake and suffering nutritional deficiencies – particularly of iron and vitamin B_{12} – which causes post-operative complications such as impaired wound healing and immune function.[187,188] These long-term effects are often made worse by traditional approaches to gastric surgery in which the individual may remain 'nil by mouth' for anything between 8 and 12 days so that the anastamosis can heal sufficiently. In such circumstances, post-operative feeding via a percutaneous jejunostomy tube will minimise weight loss and promote a swifter post-operative recovery allowing continuous feeding to take place in a pattern which is more redolent of normal digestion as the fundal sphincter normally releases small amounts of liquified chyme into the small bowel on a near-continuous basis after eating. A number of studies have also looked at jejunal pouch formation as a means of creating additional gastric reservoir function thus slowing down the entry of foodstuffs to the small bowel,[189,190] though Bonenkamp et al. (2002) question the value of such pouches in improving nutritional status,[179] and Scholmerich (2004) advocates nutritional rather than surgical approaches for the problem of malabsorption and dietary deficits.[185] The formation of jejunal pouches normally requires the retention of at least part of the stomach, making them less feasible for those receiving total gastrectomy although a Roux-en-Y oesophagojejunostomy (a procedure allowing removal of the stomach and anastomosis of the lower oesophagus with the jejunum while maintaining pancreatic drainage/function via the newly isolated duodenum and formation of a jejunojejunostomy at its lower end) may be indicated following both partial and complete gastrectomy for persistent oesophagitis caused by non-gastric alkaline reflux, as this may cause intestinal metaplasia leading to secondary malignancy in the small intestine and the oesophagus if uncorrected.[5,179,191]

Since the introduction of laparoscopic surgery for gastric cancer by Kitano and Shiraishi in 1991,[192] much emphasis has been placed upon the comparative benefits of laparoscopic interventions for stomach cancer and there is a broad body of evidence to support the use of minimally invasive techniques such as endoscopy and laparoscopy in both the diagnosis and management of gastric cancers.[171,193] Dulucq *et al.* (2005)[180] argue that laparoscopic surgery has proven benefit in the treatment of gastric cancer, reducing intraperative blood loss, pulmonary and post-operative complications, the time required for the resumption of oral intake, and hospital stay, and improving cosmetic outcomes while maintaining cure rates.[13,194,195] The role of lymphadenectomy remains controversial, some Japanese studies demonstrating better outcomes for larger invasive tumours although the tendency is growing for sentinal lymph node biopsy as a precursor to such extensive surgery.[196–198] In a review of the literature, Brennan (2005) found that there was very little survival benefit from extensive lymph node dissection which is likely to be offset by the additional peri- and post-operative stress of such extensive surgery.[171]

Treatment outcomes for gastric cancer are also improved with multimodality treatments.[178] The use of chemoradiotherapy is controversial, many of the organs adjacent to the stomach, such as the kidneys, small bowel and transverse colon being extremely sensitive to the effects of ionising radiation and tissue repair being compromised in previously irradiated sites;[5] one study demonstrated the increased likelihood of wound dehiscence at thoracotomy sites previously exposed to radiotherapy.[199] Consequently, post-operative chemoradiotherapy is increasingly being used as the standard treatment for the management of gastric cancer in the US, based largely upon the results of one randomised controlled trial,[200] although a stronger evidence base has yet to be established for this practice by large, multicentre prospective randomised controlled trials.[171]

Definitive surgery for oesophageal cancer

As with stomach cancer, surgery remains the single most important treatment modality for carcinomas of the oesophagus and gastric cardia, the incidence of which is rising in the developed world. This is particularly apparent for adenocarcinoma which now matches squamous cell carcinoma in its incidence.[201,202] Squamous cell carcinoma of the oesophagus has been associated with lifestyle factors such as tobacco and alcohol consumption, whereas recent increases in the number of adenocarcinomas has been linked to a parallel rise in the incidence of chronic gastro-oesophageal reflux and Barret's metaplasia in the developed world.[5,201] Surgical resection of the tumour together with an adequate disease-free margin and lymph node dissection is the treatment of choice for localised tumours in the lower third of the oesophagus, while radiotherapy is the treatment of choice for unresectable tumours and those in the upper third of the oesophagus, which are less accessible for surgical resection.[6] The choice of surgical procedure depends in addition upon the pre-operative staging and the performance status of the individual, tumours in the middle third of the oesophagus frequently being resected by means of a two-stage (Ivor-Lewis) procedure via an abdominal incision and the right fifth intercostal space.[6]

Approximately 50% of individuals present with resectable disease, but cure can only be achieved by *en bloc* resection of the tumour together with the regional lymph nodes, and any procedure failing to do this remains palliative, the individual's prognosis being less than 12 months in the majority of cases.[201] An exploratory laparotomy may be indicated, particularly for a total or radical oesophagectomy to facilitate the creation of a colonic interposition between the pharynx and stomach, although the stomach is most commonly used to replace the resected oesophagus, with the fundus being drawn up to anastamose with remaining tissue above the resected portion (see Figure 11.3). This may be contraindicated if there has been previous gastric surgery or other gastric problems, in which case a section of the colon or jejunal loop may be used, though these procedures carry additional operative risks.[201] Until recently, it was thought that adjuvant therapies added little survival benefit to those capable of undergoing surgery, though one large-scale study recently conducted by the Medical Research Council has indicated that neoadjuvant therapy using cisplatin and 5-fluorouracil combinations together with radiotherapy may provide additional survival advantage over surgery alone.[203]

The quality of life of individuals following surgery for oesophageal cancer varies depending

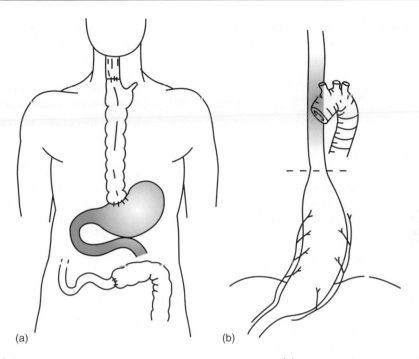

(a) (b)

Figure 11.3 (a) Colonic interposition following total oesophagectomy; (b) gastric mobilisation and pull-through for carcinoma of the lower third of the oesophagus. Reproduced with permission from Blackwell Publishing, from Souhami R.L. and Tobias J. (2005). *Cancer and its Management*, 5th edition, p. 240.[204]

upon the surgery undertaken, one study suggesting that total gastrectomy with Roux-en-Y oesophagojejunostomy had fewer and less frequent symptoms than oesophagogastrectomy alone, though few individuals undergo such radical surgery.[205] Several studies on the impact of oesophagectomy have found that hoarseness, gastric reflux, diarrhoea, and dysphagia were the commonest long-term side-effects of treatment, the latter being by far the most prominent in most individuals' recollection,[206–208] with dysphagia remaining the most enduring problem requiring intensive multiprofessional interventions by the speech and language therapist, dietician and the physician in order to guarantee sucessful rehabilitation.[209] Dysphagia is a distressing symptom which affects the individual's ability to eat and enjoy food, or engage in many important aspects of social interaction such as celebrating an anniversary or enjoying a drink with friends, and limiting the individual's oral intake of food and fluids.[210] Individuals may become bored with the limited soft diet that they are able to tolerate and frustrated by the effort of trying to speak with a painful or hoarse voice, so patience, empathic listening and the use of closed questions that allow simple answers will be appreciated by the individual thus affected. Individuals should be encourged to eat acceptable foodstuffs little and often and may require nutritional support in the immediate post-operative period.

Definitive surgery for prostate cancer

The surgical management of prostate cancer has elicited a great deal of debate and controversy in recent years, several options being available to the individual but few experts agreeing on the most appropriate course of treatment for a condition which is the third-largest cause of cancer-related mortality in the UK,[5] with a death rate of 1520 per 100 000 men.[211] The use of radical prostatectomy, consisting of resection of the prostate together with the prostatic urethra and seminal vesicles has grown in recent years, largely due to the widespread use of prostate-specific antigen (PSA) testing, which has led to earlier diagnosis and a consequent increase in the number of cases that remain confined to the prostate capsule and with node-negative disease,[5,212] although some surgeons are now undertaking prostatectomy for stage III cancers following the use of hormonal treatments to reduce tumour mass prior to surgery.[5] Lymph node metastases are a poor prognostic indicator but the percentage of men presenting with disease-positive lymph nodes has fallen from 20–30% to less than 7% since PSA testing became commonplace,[213] and radical retropubic or perineal prostatectomy is therefore usually carried out with curative intent, though its use is more widespread in the US than the UK and mainland Europe, where hormonal approaches to management are more commonly employed.[211]

Proponents of early prostatectomy suggest that it can achieve excellent control of the disease with minimal morbidity and impact on the individual's quality of life,[214] although erectile dysfunction and urinary incontinence are significant causes of postoperative morbidity,[5,215] which can have a negative impact upon self-esteem, emotional and social well-being, and sexual relationships in the aftermath of treatment.[216,217] Horwich et al. (2002) suggest that the clinical indications for radical prostatectomy are proportionate to the tumour grade and inversely proportional to the age of the individual,[213] those with low grade tumours and advanced age being likely to attain their normal lifespan and enjoy a better quality of life without prostatectomy than younger men with high-grade tumours that are likely to metastasise and cause premature death. There is no conclusive evidence that radical prostatectomy prolongs life or reduces disease-related morbidity in those with localised non-metastatic disease, but it may be indicated in those with an anticipated lifespan of 15 years or more, age being an important determining factor since those over the age of 70 years are also more likely to experience urinary and erectile problems in the aftermath of their surgery.[213,216]

Attempts to develop nerve-sparing surgical techniques have met with varied success, as the visualisation and preservation of cavernous nerves during radical prostatectomy may not always be possible.[212] These techniques do not always ensure the retention of sexual function therefore,[219] and may only be effective in 30–60% of individuals depending upon their age and the extent of the tumour.[220] These figures may be overly optimistic, individuals themselves consistently reporting a much higher incidence of erectile dysfunction than those carrying out the procedure;[220–223] 96% of men complained of inadequate erectile function 3 months after surgery in Talcott et al.'s (1998) study.[222] Sexual function may take a great deal longer than this to return to acceptable levels,[220] particularly where nerve-grafting rather than nerve-sparing surgery has taken place. Kim et al. (2001) performed wide bilateral neurovascular bundle resection and nerve grafting during radical prostatectomy where nerve-sparing surgery was not possible, but long-term follow-up of their sample showed that sexual function did not return to a satisfactory level until the fifth post-operative month and much longer in some instances.[224]

It has been estimated that only 25% of men are sexually active at the start of treatment for prostate cancer although much of the research has been done on those receiving hormonal treatments with anti-androgens or radiotherapy rather than surgery,[225] where the long-term effects of treatment may be equally debilitating.[220,226–229] It is likely that surgery will become more commonplace for younger men with encapsulated disease identified by PSA testing, and assumptions about the sexual activity of these men cannot be made from historical antecedents. Kelly (2004) points out that male sexuality is a complex phenomenon which is shaped by personal, cultural, and social factors that go beyond the remit of physical potency and may, additionally, require men to renegotiate the sexual terrain of their relationships.[230] Men undergoing radical prostatectomy have to learn to live with embodied changes and emotional, social, and sexual vulnerability, which they may not always have considered (or been informed about) at the outset of treatment when the main focus of their attention is upon the efficacy rather than the consequences of their treatment.[230] One study by Gray et al. (2002) found that sexual issues were rarely mentioned in the immediate aftermath of surgery but surfaced as a major consideration in the months that followed;

71% of their sample of 34 men continued to experience impotence while the remainder continued to have problems a full year after surgery.[221] Erectile dysfunction and lack of orgasm negatively influenced the quality of life of half the men studied in one report,[227] and prospective studies are required to further evaluate the true impact of prostatectomy on male sexual function and quality of life, particularly as early drug treatment with phosphodiesterase-5 (PDE-5) inhibitors decreases the risk of post-operative erectile dysfunction and promotes recovery in those with some degree of nerve patency.[212,220] Recent studies have demonstrated the efficacy of the selective PDE-5 preparations sildenafil, vardenafil, and tadalafil and found them to be effective in the treatment of surgery-related erectile dysfunction after nerve-sparing radical prostatectomy,[231] where they are thought to provide a measure of neuronal protection, reducing the apoptosis of cavernosal smooth muscle, improving endothelial function, stimulating neuronal regeneration, and eliciting a sevenfold improvement in the return of spontaneous erectile function within 2 months of treatment cessation.[232]

Nurses caring for individuals undergoing radical prostatectomy with or without nerve-sparing procedures should be aware, therefore, of the likely impact of surgery on the physical, psychosexual, and social functioning of the individual, the strategies available to overcome these problems, and the importance that men attribute to sexual functioning.[223,230] Some suggest that greater emphasis should be placed upon the 'healing work' that men and their partners are engaged in to overcome the deleterious effects of their surgery, helping them come to terms with the biotechnical remedies required for the management of their impotence,[221] while some argue that nurses should encourage a partnership approach to rehabilitation that encompasses the individual, their partner, and health professionals.[233] Some studies have found that men are generally reluctant to discuss their feelings, or downplay the impact of their illness experience with health care professionals, fearing that they would 'lose face' or be regarded as unmasculine by admitting their anxieties,[221,223] and there is no doubt that many find themselves vulnerable in

this situation,[230] fearing that relationships may suffer as a result of their impotence.[234] Many find it easier to talk to an empathic health care professional about sexual issues, with the possible exception of older men who may be embarrassed at discussing such issues with members of the opposite sex.[234]

Men may need reassurance about their partners' understanding and the long-term recovery of sexual function, particularly with newer drug therapies, while partners may need advice and support in dealing with their husband's insecurity, anxieties and frustration at the slow progress of treatment. Nurses may greatly assist this process by giving positive affirmation, information, and time for discussion while identifying those couples who may benefit from further psychosexual counselling. Great sensitivity is required in this respect since many men appear to prefer pharmacological and physical solutions to the problem rather than counselling,[234] the aim of information giving being to stress the normality and predictability of the problem rather than to pathologise it unnecessarily. Similarly, urinary incontinence, another common problem associated with radical prostatectomy needs to be dealt with sensitively, many men reporting anxiety about wetness, odour and body image changes which can restrict social activity and self-concept,[215,235] while others demonstrate the impact of urinary incontinence on the daily lives, sleep patterns, and quality of life of those affected (see Research study 11.3).[236] As with erectile dysfunction, there is a significant difference between individuals' and health care professionals' evaluation of its incidence,[215] which appears to depend as much upon the definition or measurement used as any other factor, making comparison across different studies difficult.[237,238]

There is evidence that, as with erectile dysfunction, men about to undergo radical prostatectomy and their partners are ill-informed about the likelihood of urinary incontinence occuring,[217] with many failing to remember it being mentioned pre-operatively.[215] Information giving prior to surgery is crucial if the individual is to be prepared and equipped to deal with the impact that urinary incontinence will have.[235] A role for the urology nurse specialist in pre-operative assessment and information giving, in which both the 'best-case'

Research study 11.3

McGlynn B., Al-Saffar N., Begg H. *et al*. (2004). Management of urinary incontinence following radical prostatectomy. *Urologic Nursing* **24**, 474–515.[215]

Aim of study

The study evaluated the impact of a new, nurse-led histology clinic and pre-operative teaching programme for men undergoing radical prostatectomy, provided by a newly appointed urology oncology nurse specialist.

Method

Prostate symptoms in individuals undergoing radical prostatectomy were evaluated before and after surgery using the International Prostate Symptom Score (IPSS), in order to evaluate the effectiveness of educational interventions provided by a newly appointed urology oncology nurse specialist. The initiation of a nurse-led histology clinic enabled the newly appointed urology oncology nurse specialist to share the patient's diagnosis, arrange further staging investigations, and discuss possible treatment options in a half-hour consultation which included the provision of written information and advice about pelvic floor training and self-management strategies. Patients were provided with a contact telephone number for the urology oncology nurse specialist who saw them a further two or three times prior to surgery to discuss the implications of their diagnosis and treatment, at which the issue of urinary incontinence was also discussed. The nurse specialist initiated a pre-operative referral to the continence and physiotherapy teams for a full continence assessment and pelvic floor training[239] at that time. Advice concerning the avoidance of stimulants such as tea, coffee and carbonated drinks was also given so as to reduce frequency and urgency in the post-operative period,[240] and a joint appointment with each of these services arranged for the day on which the patient's urinary catheter was to be removed. Post-intervention follow-up was conducted via telephone interview using the IPSS, and results were compared with data from those who had undergone surgery prior to the introduction of the new service.

Results

The initiation of a nurse-led histology clinic reduced waiting times from an average of 3 months to 1 month prior to the new service being introduced, and significantly increased the length of time available for individual consulation with a health care professional (30 minutes as opposed to an average of 8 minutes previously). Patients had previously reported that they felt poorly prepared for surgery after the shorter medical consultation, in which their diagnosis, further investigations, treatment options, side-effects, and likely prognosis were discussed. Ninety-nine per cent of the men expressed satisfaction with the way in which the results of their histology were given in the new nurse-led histology clinic, these patients being fully staged, better prepared, and having already commenced hormonal therapy (where appropriate) by the time that they met with the surgical team. Pre-operative review of patients by the continence team increased from 32% to 100%, 85% being taught pelvic floor exercises as outpatients at least 2 weeks prior to surgery, and the rest on the day of their admission for surgery. Incontinence following removal of the urinary catheter fell from 72% to 49% with most men discharged as continent within 2 months as opposed to an average of 8 months prior to the service starting. Ninety seven per cent of patients reported that they were delighted, happy or pleased with their bladder control in comparison to only 68% treated prior to the introduction of the new service.

Conclusions

The study, while relatively small, demonstrated how the introduction of an innovative nurse-led service, the provision of pre-operative education, pelvic-floor exercise training and a collaborative approach to patient care improved treatment outcomes, self-management and quality of life in patients undergoing radical prostatectomy. It suggests that the introduction of the urology oncology nurse specialist role had made a significant impact on post-operative continence rates and overall satisfaction with service provision.

Limitations

While the study demonstrates a correlation in the increased amount of time spent by the urology oncology nurse specialist and clinical outcome measures such as post-operative urinary continence and time to incontinence-free discharge from the hospital's continence service, these findings could have been anticipated given their comparison to data collected about the routine (but inferior) service provided before the introduction of the changes to service delivery described. The conclusion that these 'significant' improvements are solely attributable to the educational intervention of the urology oncology nurse specialist are unfounded however. Timely access to a variety of services including pre-operative review of patients by physiotherapists and the continence team had increased dramatically as a result of the changes, and while it may be true that the urology oncology nurse specialist fulfilled an important patient-education role, this cannot be divorced from the increased support and education provided by other members of the health care team. The study does not take adequate account of these 'counfounding variables', and thus the claim that the urology oncology nurse specialist's educational interventions played a 'significant' role in improving overall patient satisfaction with oncology-related care may be unwise. It could be argued instead, that improvements in patient satisfaction and outcomes accrue from the interventions of each of these individuals. It may have been more appropriate to focus on the co-ordinating rather than the educational role of the urology oncology nurse specialist therefore, as this appears to have been strategically more important. Claims about the undoubted benefits of longer and more frequent pre-operative consultations with the urology oncology nurse specialist may have been easier to substantiate, but it seems unlikely that education was the sole intervention provided during these sessions. The study highlights the dangers inherent in evaluating changes to any service given the complex interplay between individuals, disciplines, and services engaged in the provision of patient care, the impact of multiple variables affecting patient outcomes, and the absolute necessity of drawing tentative conclusions from the data in such circumstances; however, it does describe an innovative and beneficial change in surgical services which merits further evaluation using a more rigorous methodological approach.

and 'worst-case' scenarios are discussed and realistic targets set for the recovery of urinary continence, has been described by one group of writers,[215] and the urology nurse specialist may also be engaged with other members of the multidisciplinary team in teaching pelvic floor exercises as a means of reducing stress incontinence after surgery,[239] or providing advice about the avoidance of caffeine-containing beverages which may cause frequency and urgency of micturition.[240] Teaching the individual how to void their bladder completely, and co-ordinating input by other members of the health care team when urinary function does not return to normal is also an important nursing role.[215] As with erectile dysfunction, there is also an important role for the partner as they will often be involved in assisting the individual with changes to their normal routine in order to accommodate urinary incontinence, and may themselves require support in making adequate adaptation to changes in activities of daily living that may mean changes in sleeping, travelling, and dressing arrangements to name but a few. The man will also need constant reassurance and encouragement to persist with self-care activities, and may feel himself reduced to a child-like status when unable to control such basic physiological functions, so positive affirmation is crucial in developing and maintaining the therapeutic relationship.[235]

Definitive surgery in colorectal cancer

Surgery is the main treatment modality for colorectal cancers, although there has been little improvement in 5-year survival rates for those treated with surgery alone over the last 50 years; long-term survival depends largely upon the use of appropriate adjuvant therapies such as chemotherapy and intra-operative radiotherapy.[241–243] Unlike gastric cancer, the vast majority (80%) of colorectal cancers are resectable,[6] radical surgery with resection of local lymphatic drainage being more common than simple excision of the tumour, as the propensity of colorectal cancers to spread to other organs is great.[5] In the absence of metastatic disease, the tumour is resected *en bloc* and bowel function restored as well as possible.[241] Surgery may also be indicated in advanced disease – even in the the presence of hepatic or peritoneal metastases as it is the most effective means of debulking the tumour, external beam radiotherapy being too damaging to many of the vital organs lying in the vicinity of the bowel. Brachytherapy and intra-operative radiotherapy to the tumour bed are increasingly used as an adjunct to surgery,[242–245] avoiding as they do the linear transfer loss of energy to surrounding tissues that may be mechanically shielded during the intra-operative procedure. Hahnloser *et al.* (2003)[245] argue that intra-operative radiotherapy may elicit disease responses and an increase in long-term survival even in advanced or recurrent disease although, as with all locoregional treatments, distal relapse remains problematic and systematic treatment with cytotoxic chemotherapy, most notably 5-fluorouracil and leucovorin, may also be indicated for patients with incomplete resection or advanced disease.[246]

One large audit of 374 procedures demonstrated that there is little difference in the surgery performed in individuals with early or advanced disease, and very little difference in the peri-operative morbidity or mortality between each group.[247] Surgical resection of colon cancer is also likely to prevent intestinal obstruction and other distressing symptoms such as pain, nausea, and vomiting, and is warranted even in advanced disease as a palliative intervention.[241] Significantly more important in terms of the procedure undertaken is the site of the tumour, a right hemicolectomy being used for cancers of the caecum, ascending colon, and hepatic flexure, a transverse colectomy for tumours in the transverse colon, and a left hemicolectomy or sigmoid colectemy for tumours of the splenic flexure, descending colon, or sigmoid colon.[241] In the majority of cases, hemicolectomy is completed by the re-anastomosis of the remaining healthy bowel tissue, but on occasions, a temporary colostomy may be formed for closure at a later date.[6] The creation of a defunctioning colostomy prior to tumour resection may be indicated for those who have previously suffered from obstruction, perforation, or cachexia, and may be performed even in those with unresectable tumours in order to maintain bowel function in those receiving radiotherapy to other parts of the colon.[5]

In comparison to colorectal disease, rectal cancers pose a more difficult challenge to surgeons because of their relative inaccessibility within the lower two-thirds of the rectum.[6] Prior to the introduction of laparoscopic techniques and the circular stapling gun, the vast majority of cancers in the lower two-thirds of the rectum were treated with abdominoperineal or anterior resection of the rectum, resulting in numerous post-operative consequences for the individual as a result of wide excision margins and the loss of the anal sphincter which led to incontinence and sensory deficits.[241] It is now known that microscopic tumour spread occurs for the most part circumferentially, particularly in the mesorectum, so total mesorectal excision is now carried out irrespective of the surgical technique used. This has reduced the need for wide clearance margins elsewhere,[241] and sphincter-sparing surgery now constitutes 75% as opposed to 25% of all procedures performed, with an ensuing reduction in post-operative incontinence.[241] Notwithstanding this, many individuals still experience the need to defaecate frequently and urgently as a result of a reduction in the size of the rectal reservoir, and there is also a risk of bladder and sexual problems if the pelvic nerves are damaged during the mesorectal excision.[241] Abdominoperineal excision is still frequently used for tumours in the upper third of the rectum and for those occurring within 5 cm of the anal verge, sphincter-sparing surgery being unnecessary in the former case and contraindicated in the latter because of the paucity of tissue that will remain.

It has been argued that colorectal surgeons have been slow to make use of the minimally invasive surgical techniques that have become commonplace in other surgical specialties,[248] but their restriction to clinical trials has been due largely to concerns about port site recurrences, and difficulties inherent in forming intracorporeal anastomoses and ensuring the total, safe dissection of the tumour via such means.[248] Early evidence suggests that laparoscopic colectomy may be as safe as open procedures and elicit recurrence and survival rates similar to traditional procedures while minimising post-operative pain, ileus, and hospital admission time.[248,249] The clinical picture is far more certain in rectal surgery where transanal endoscopic surgery for rectal adenomas overcomes the problem of accessibility and is said to have 'revolutionised' procedures for the resection of early rectal cancers, with insufflation of the rectum with CO_2 gas allowing clear visualisation and easy access to the upper and middle sections of the rectum.[248] Transanal endoscopic microsurgery does not allow lymph node sampling or clearance during surgery,[248] and its use tends to be restricted to those individuals unlikely to require conversion to open surgery, the more radical abdominoperineal excision of the rectum being more appropriate for those with advanced disease.[241]

The formation of a colostomy or ileostomy in the aftermath of a colectomy or resection of the rectum may impact upon the individual's real or perceived quality of life in a number of ways, including eating and drinking, elimination, working, sleeping, body image and sexuality, travel, and self-esteem.[250] Great care should be taken in the positioning of any stoma therefore (Figure 11.4), and nurses undoubtedly have a role to play in discussing the impact and location of this opening, particularly where lifestyle issues such as sports or leisure activities, or religious and cultural beliefs which define which hand should be used to deal with bodily waste or clean bodily orifices may indicate a better alternative site than that originally planned.[251] Post-operatively, they will require total parenteral nutrition until adequate healing of the bowel has taken place, and sips of fluid will only be recommended once normal bowel sounds have returned and the ostomy shows signs of activity in the form of flatus. The individual will be commenced on a very light diet for some time and may be disturbed by the appearance of the ostomy site, which some find visually offensive. Others may be reticent to touch it for fear of infecting or damaging it in some way, particularly in the initial stages when it may appear red or inflamed. Many will be fearful of eating a normal diet and anxious about their inability to control defaecation, and wary that the ostomy pouch may burst or become disconnected from the flange when mobilising, sleeping, or engaged in other social activity. Several authors have noted the relationship between bowel control and attainment of maturity or 'adulthood',[252,253] and fear of embarrassment may curtail some from normal social and sexual activity until they have gained confidence in both the ostomy and their ability to care for it. In the initial stages of management, many may feel themselves

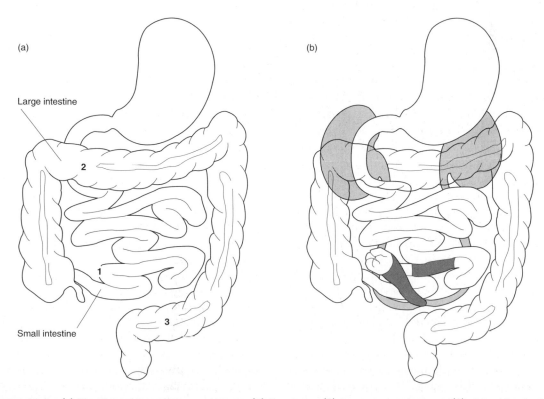

Figure 11.4   (a) Position of bowel cancer stomas: (1) ileostomy, (2) transverse colostomy, (3) sigmoid colostomy; (b) ileal conduit. Reproduced with permission from Salter M. (1997). *Altered Body Image: The Nursing Role*, 2nd edition. London: Ballière Tindall, p. 181.[251]

infanticised by their inability to control their own defaecation or manage their stoma effectively, particularly when concomitant disability such as poor vision, arthritis, or poor manual dexterity accentuates their reliance upon others.[254,255] Some may curtail social activites such as visiting friends, family, or public locations unless they know that discrete toileting facilities for the care of their stoma are available, while others may be fearful of partners' or childrens' reactions to the presence of a permanent or temporary colostomy, or of discussing taboo subjects such as death, sexuality, and elimination problems with those closest to them.[252,256,257]

One qualitative study found that 80% of respondents reported negative lifestyle changes in the aftermath of colorectal cancer treatment with ostomates, ranking changes in physical function, and spouses' social roles and relationships as having been most deleteriously affected.[257] This early finding is confirmed by later studies which found that social restrictions caused by the stoma extended beyond the individual to the whole family.[258] The impact of colorectal surgery upon sexual functioning is rarely considered by health care professionals, who may regard a limited reduction in quality of life as a worthwhile trade-off for survivorship – though evidence is mounting that the opinions of those affected by colorectal cancer and those caring for them are not always in alignment.[259] Abdominoperineal resection in particular may occasionally cause males to have dry or retrograde ejaculations and, less frequently, impotence or a loss of sensuality, while pelvic exenteration in younger women with locoregional disease will cause loss of fertility and premature menopause. Stoma formation may cause changes in the individual's social roles, body image, and sexuality requiring empathy, understanding, and open communication by nurses and other health professionals if such problems are to be overcome.[260] Regrettably, there is evidence that communication deficits are common in this respect, with both individuals and family members reporting disatisfaction with the level of information provided by health carers.[261,262] Practical help in particular is appreciated by individuals and their carers, which may include information about what foodstuffs might cause gas or malodorous

stool, those that may help to thicken watery stool or diarrhoea, and those helping to loosen stool in the aftermath of stoma formation.

Surgery in the elderly

Sixty per cent of all cancers and two-thirds of all cancer deaths in the developed world occur in individuals over the age of 65 years,[263,264] the median age at presentation for all cancers being 69 for men and 67 for women.[263] Historically, age has been used by clinicians to deny surgery to elderly individuals on the basis that the risks are too great or the benefits too little in this age group to merit the discomfort and dangers associated with it, and despite evidence to the contrary, discrimination on the basis of an individual's age continues to persist.[265,266] Some have attempted to defend this practice on the basis of economic, moral, and philosophical grounds using the 'equal worth', 'fair innings' and 'prudential lifespan' arguments,[267] but while these may well hold credence for some, the incontrovertible evidence in cancer care is that older individuals can and do gain substantial benefit and a better health-related quality of life from cancer surgery when other factors such as co-morbidity and social dependence are taken into account.[268] Moreover, there is evidence that in the long-term, older people report either stable or better outcomes throughout their cancer experience than either an age-matched non-cancer population or younger people (<65 years) who do have the disease.[269] Older people are likely to benefit both physically and socially from surgical interventions for their cancer therefore,[270] and should not be denied the favourable long-term outcomes that it offers in the majority of cases.[271]

Several studies demonstrate that while older individuals are less likely to be treated with surgery for head and neck cancer, there are no statistical differences in the outcomes of treatment between older (>70 years) and younger (<70 years) individuals, the rate of surgical and systemic complications being similar for each group.[272] Thus head and neck surgery may be carried out in older people so long as meticulous assessment of both the individual's functional status and any pre-existing disease is made, and surgical stress reduced to a minimum.[273] Studies of breast cancer treatment in the elderly have demonstrated similar outcomes, with both older and younger women experiencing similar survivorship patterns following breast-conserving surgery,[274] axillary dissection and radiotherapy to the breast or chest wall being safely excluded in such women in favour of tamoxifen and tumour excision or simple mastectomy.[275] Laparoscopic colorectal resection has been demonstrated to be a safe surgical option for older individuals with colorectal disease, reducing the length of hospital stay, ensuring a swifter return of bowel function, and eliminating some of the cardiopulmonary risks associated with open laparotomy,[276] the Duke's or TNM staging (see Tables 11. 1 and 11.3), and the presence of distant recurrence being better prognostic indicators of long-term surgical outcome than age alone,[270] hence the decision as to whether or not to operate on an older person should focus upon the same prognostic indicators as for a younger person, including an evaluation of the individual's functional status and physiological – rather than chronological – age.[277]

Surgery remains the treatment of choice for early-stage non-small-cell lung cancer irrespective of the individual's age,[263] the outcomes of complete surgical resection being comparable to those of younger cohorts,[278,279] even in octogenarians in whom non-cancer health status and tumour stage are more important in determining the appropriateness of surgery than chronological age.[280] Individuals with an adequate predicted post-operative lung function, a good performance status, and adequate social support should therefore be offered surgical resection for early-stage non-small-cell lung cancer, particularly as the morbidity and mortality rates associated with these procedures have fallen dramatically in recent years.[266] Notwithstanding this, treatment outcomes for any surgical procedure are far from predictable and it may be appropriate in advanced disease not to treat the asymptomatic person where the impact of surgery may outweigh the benefits to be gained from it.[6] Quality rather than the quantity of life may be a more important consideration under such circumstances, and nurses, alongside medical staff, may be involved in the assessment of this. The challenges inherent in this are considerable,[268] not least in the elderly who may be particularly vulnerable to negative stereotyping.[281,282] Nurses may therefore be in a position to act as patient advocate, a situation which will be helped considerably by seeing that person as an individual with a unique history and aspirations for the future.[282] Given the demographic overlap between oncology and gerontological nursing in the presentation of many cancers, Ford and McCormack's (2000) exhortation that nurses should get to 'know the

Table 11.3 TNM staging for colorectal cancer

Staging	Criteria
TX	Primary tumour cannot be assessed
T0	No primary tumour identified
Tis	Tumour *in situ* (limited to mucosa)
T1	Tumour has invaded the submucosa but has not penetrated the muscularis propria
T2	Tumour has invaded but not penetrated beyond the muscularis propria
T3	Tumour has penetrated beyond the muscularis propria into the subserosa (if present) or pericolic fat but not into the peritoneal cavity or adjacent organs
T4	Invasion of adjacent organs or the peritoneal cavity
NX	Nodal metastases cannot be assessed
N0	No nodal metastases
N1	1–3 pericolic/perirectal nodes involved
N2	4 or more pericolic/perirectal nodes involved
MX	Distant metastases cannot be assessed
M0	No distant metastases
M1	Distant metastases

patient' is especially pertinent and should help nurses to work in partnership with them, their carer or partner, and the medical team in making such decisions.[283] Many have advocated that nurses should take a biographical approach, encouraging the individual and family members to locate the disease process and treatment experience in relation to their life-journey, hopes, and fears for the future so that a full understanding of its significance and impact can be established,[283–285] and such an approach is equally appropriate to the surgical oncology setting when caring for older people with cancer.[270]

Rehabilitative (or reconstructive) surgery

Despite the increasing use of tissue-sparing surgery, radical procedures such as mastectomy, mandilectomy or laryngectomy may still be required to remove a primary tumour because a tissue-sparing procedure is not possible or local recurrence has taken place.[2] The role of reconstructive surgery is a vital part of the surgical team's portfolio, enabling surgeons to undertake radical curative surgery where necessary in the knowledge that functional or cosmetic deficits can be minimised or reversed in its aftermath. Reconstructive surgery in cancer care is therefore concerned with the restoration, reconstruction or correction of tissues that are damaged by either the disease or its treatment, although it may also be undertaken in the aftermath of prophylactic interventions in 'at-risk' individuals or for cosmesis alone. Many individuals will undergo reconstructive surgery either during or after definitive surgery, the extent of which will depend upon the nature of the restoration, reconstruction or correction required. Reconstructive and cosmetic surgery is an important component of comprehensive cancer care,[41] and offers significant benefits to the person affected by cancer since altered body image, and sexuality and the maintenance of normative physical functioning rank highly amongst the concerns of those faced with cancer surgery.[230,286,287] Changes in the nature or quality of an individual's voice following head and neck surgery may be very distressing, and necessitate

both psychosocial and physical interventions.[288,289] Surgical insertion of a vocal prosthesis such as a Blom–Singer valve, an airflow-sensitive valve that remains open during respiration but avoids the need for manual closure during speech rehabilitation, may be required by individuals who are unable to develop adequate oesophageal speech following laryngectomy, in order to improve communication – an essential activity that is fundamental to psychosocial well-being and quality of life. Similarly, the impact of incontinence following surgery for prostate or colorectal cancers may be significantly reduced by reconstructive measures such as those previously discussed.[215,236] Reconstructive surgery serves both a physical and a psychological function therefore, minimising deformity or functional deficit, and optimising psychosocial well-being in a great many cancers including gynaecological, colorectal, prostate, and urinary tract cancers to name but a few.[41]

One obvious example of this is in head and neck cancer, the psychological sequelae of which have been well documented in numerous studies.[290] While the impact of facial disfigurement can be ameliorated by family understanding and intensive psychosocial support,[291] individuals subjected to anatomical changes to their face or neck as a result of cancer or its treatment may experience profound psychological distress:[290] low self-esteem, depression, impaired psychosocial functioning, and isolation are more common amongst these individuals than other cancer cohorts.[291–293] In addition to this, many will have physiological problems such as dysphagia and difficulty masticating their food, which may be exacerbated by adjuvant treatments such as chemotherapy or radiotherapy.[209,210,294] Reconstructive procedures are a vital component of head and neck surgery, where they serve important functional and psychological as well as cosmetic purposes.[288,290,295] Individuals being considered for head and neck surgery should therefore receive a careful and detailed pre-operative assessment of their needs and preferences so that appropriate reconstructive measures can be undertaken during or after the procedure. These range from a number of relatively common procedures such as the creation of a permanent tracheostomy,[296] or the insertion of a Blom–Singer valve to aid voice rehabilitation after surgery or radiotherapy, to more unusual or experimental procedures.

Several authors have described a variety of reconstructive procedures such as the formation of a rectus abdominis free flap for individuals undergoing total glossectomy in advanced carcinoma of the tongue, and a free radial forearm flap to reconstruct the floor of the mouth or upper lip after resection of an oral tumour or malignant melanoma.[297,298] Others include the removal of the eyelid and its reconstruction using autogenous cartilage or achilles tendon in a Cutler–Beard procedure for recurrent basal cell carcinoma of the eyelid,[299] and a variety of buttressing techniques used to provide support for dental prostheses, prevent maxillofacial deviation, and maintain the anatomical position of features such as the eye, buccal cavity, and nasopharynx following various head and neck procedures.[300]

Reconstructive surgery in breast cancer

As with head and neck surgery, mastectomy results in a deformity that completely changes both the body contour and body image of women undergoing the procedure. Reconstructive surgery in breast care may include the insertion of a prosthesis containing either silicone gel or normal saline at the time of surgery if adequate skin flaps are available, or as a delayed procedure following tissue expansion if greater volume is desired. A tissue expander is a silicone shell which can be gradually inflated with normal saline via a subcutaneous filler port over a period of 4–6 weeks,[301] to create a sack into which a prosthesis may be inserted at a later date (see Figure 11.2(b)). In order to achieve the desired ptosis (sagging), this may need to be inflated slightly more than required for a period of time before reducing the tissue expander to match the volume of the contralateral breast. A prosthesis may then be inserted under the skin or muscle to provide an acceptable shape and size of breast, while some modern tissue expanders may simply be left *in situ* with the removal of just the filler port and line if further surgery is not desired.[2] Silicone gel implants give the most natural feel and consistency to the reconstructed breast, although capsule contraction, infection and rupture are reported in 10%, 5% and 1% per cent of cases respectively.[2] Fears that

rupture or seepage of silicone from the prosthesis may cause connective tissue disease or secondary malignancy appear to be unjustified:[2] an authoritative review by the United States Institute of Medicine's Committee on the Safety of Silicone Breast Implants failed to establish a relationship between silicone implants and either of these problems,[302] though women may have to undergo further surgery to remove or replace a faulty implant on occasions.[301]

Singletary (2001) argues that whilst breast implants may be less technically demanding for the surgeon, autologous reconstructions involving the mobilisation of skin, muscle or fat from one part of the body to the chest wall offer fewer complications and better cosmetic outcomes in the long term, whether performed as part of the mastectomy or as a delayed procedure.[301] One of the commonest forms undertaken is the transverse rectus abdominis myocutaneous or 'TRAM' flap, which relocates abdominal skin, fat and muscle to the mastectomy site.[2,143] In a pedicled TRAM flap reconstruction, the entire rectus abdominis muscle and the superior epigastric artery are tunnelled under the skin to the mastectomy site where the latter continues to provide a blood supply for the prosthetic breast mound. Weakening of the abdominal wall poses the slight risk of abdominal herniation, and the tunnelled tissue may cause a discernible bulge when the flap is left attached.[301] A 'free' TRAM flap involves the complete removal of the rectus muscle, fat, and skin from both the donor site and its blood supply, in a procedure similar to an abdominoplasty or 'tummy tuck'.[301] This is then shaped and applied to the chest wall, microvascular anastomosis being used to connect the donor tissue to the thoracodorsal and inferior epigastric vessels in the axilla to provide an adequate blood supply to the grafted tissue. The need for vascular microsurgery makes it a more complex procedure, but it generally gives a better surgical and cosmetic outcome as less rectus abdominis muscle is removed, thereby maintaining abdominal strength, and eliminating abdominal bulging.

While a pedicled TRAM flap has an intact blood supply from the superior epigastric artery, microvascular surgery in a free flap formation has an extremely high success rate and offers an improved blood supply to the grafted tissue.[303] The combination of retained abdominal strength and a more robust blood supply makes the free TRAM flap a more suitable procedure for larger women, smokers, or those with other predisposing risk factors such as cardiovascular or respiratory disease or diabetes,[143] although smoking is likely to predispose the woman to more postoperative complications, the reported rate in one large study being 71% in smokers as opposed to 50% in non-smokers.[304] Women with low abdominal scars such as those from caesarian section may still be able to undergo TRAM flap procedures,[143] though a latissimus dorsi or gluteal free flap may be performed in those who are very thin, have already undergone cosmetic abdominoplasty, or have extensive abdominal scarring from previous surgery.[143,301] These procedures will also be used in women who have, or are at risk from contralateral breast disease, or are undergoing elective bilateral mastectomy (such as those with the *BRCA* germline mutation), as TRAM flap procedures entail significant anatomical changes to the abdominal wall and the procedure cannot be repeated at a later date if cancer occurs in the contralateral breast.[143] Latissimus dorsi or gluteal free flaps may require the insertion of a prosthesis between the chest wall and the muscle flap in order to achieve adequate breast volume,[2] as the removal of sufficient tissue for these procedures may result in donor-site deformity.[301]

It is important when women are undergoing breast reconstruction that they are fully informed of the additional scars that the removal of tissue for breast reconstruction is likely to cause, since these considerations should be borne in mind when evaluating the advantage of surgical reconstruction over externally worn prostheses (see Research study 11.4). Insertion of a tissue expander or prosthesis is usually carried out through the mastectomy scar, so that additional scarring is avoided, but reconstruction using endogenous tissues is likely to result in changes to appearance elsewhere on the abdomen in the case of a free or pedicled TRAM flap, the back with a latissimus dorsi flap, or the buttocks in the case of a gluteal free flap. Ideally, women will be fully informed of the benefits and disadvantages of each approach, but this is seldom the case, with clinical exigencies

and surgeon preference taking precedence in the majority of cases. This may be particularly pertinent where reconstruction is desired in the aftermath of prophylactic mastectomy where the extent of physical scarring elsewhere may be a deciding factor in whether or not to undergo the procedure in the absence of clear clinical need.[91]

Once the reconstruction of the breast volume is complete, additional cosmesis may be achieved through the reconstruction of a nipple with groin tissue, although it is best to wait until the reconstructed breast has attained its final shape before nipple reconstruction is completed as it cannot be relocated easily once formed.[143] The reconstructed nipple will lack the sensitivity of the old one, although its visual appearance can be further improved with micropigmentation (tattooing) in order to create visual symmetry and the appearance of a normal nipple and areola.[143,306] Interest in nipple and areola, together with skin-sparing surgery is now growing, with a number of recent papers considering the benefits of each both in prophylactic and curative mastectomy.[306–310] There is little evidence that skin-sparing mastectomy increases the risk of locoregional recurrence,[307] and one study found that the aesthetic results of surgery were rated as excellent or good in 91% of individuals undergoing skin-sparing mastectomy, although satisfaction increased with the retention of the nipple–areola complex.[308] These authors stress the need for intra-operative inspection of frozen sections prior to nipple or areolar sparing surgery, to eliminate the risk of their containing malignant cells.

Results from a 2-year follow-up study published in 2004 suggest that while skin-sparing surgery which maintains the areola provides excellent aesthetic results without recurrence at the 2-year period, this should be restricted to women with ductal carcinoma *in situ*, or small, early-stage tumours; all of the women with stage III breast cancer demonstrated areolar disease, while nipple involvement was also considerably higher in this group.[310] Notwithstanding this, the number of studies to date is relatively small and there is a lack of consensus about the use of such techniques in all but the most limited of cancers. They do, however, provide women undergoing prophylactic mastectomy with the considerable advantage

Research study 11.4

Wolf L. (2004). The information needs of women who have undergone breast reconstruction. Part II: Information giving and content of information. *European Journal of Oncology Nursing* **8**, 315–324.[305]

Aim of study

To elicit greater understanding about the information needs of women undergoing reconstructive breast surgery.

Method

A qualitative descriptive design was used which presented data from two focus groups (*n* = 8).

Results

Findings show that the tendency to overload women with information on the same day that they are told their diagnosis and treatment plan may be inappropriate, most suggesting that information giving should be staggered over several appointments with medical or nursing staff. Many participants described their limited recall, even when fully informed about the procedure, and valued advice to list their questions, take notes and be accompanied by another during consultations. Women in the study indicated that they wanted realistic information about the length of time that initial surgery would take, and some indication of how long it would be before they got back to 'normal again', many indicating that they had vastly underestimated the time that full recovery from their surgery would take. Many were surprised at the loss of sensation in their reconstructed breast/nipple and changes in sensation (such as tightness or pulling) at the donor site, while others complained that the implant felt foreign or strange and wished that they had been given more warning about these changes prior to surgery. Realistic information about the time (and number of procedures) required to elicit an acceptable cosmetic outcome was also needed, together with advice about practical issues such as suitable clothing, bras and swimwear that would enable them to retain some sense of normality. Advice about self-care strategies such as massage and skin care for the affected area was also required. Fears about the potential risks associated with breast implants were less prevalent than had previously been feared, while the opportunity to touch and feel an implant prior to surgery was valued by many. One particularly interesting finding was the fear expressed by some that mammography implants may mask the development of recurrent disease. The need for better information about future surveillance, risk of recurrence and breast monitoring was evident therefore. Respondents perceived that male surgeons tended to disregard the importance of the nipple, focusing instead upon the recreation of a satisfactory breast mound to the detriment of women's body image, psychosocial, and sexual needs.

Conclusions

Those involved in imparting information to women about such surgery should be aware of the type of information that is considered relevant, the manner in which it should be delivered, and when to deliver that information. Women require information in a manner and at a time that is appropriate to their needs, and getting back to normal is a key concern. Practical advice about how they could look and feel normal again is particularly important, and greater sensitivity and forewarning about the deleterious effects of breast surgery, particularly in respect of changes in nipple sensation, are required.

Limitations

This exploratory study highlights some interesting findings which may be of relevance to many women undergoing reconstructive surgery, but the number of women participating in each focus group was quite small and, given the limitations of this, one wonders why an interview study was not conducted instead. The strength of focus groups is that they quickly reveal the nature and range of participants' views, but do not necessarily indicate the strength of those convictions or their durability. As such, the comparatively small size of each group (at the lower end of the 4–8 respondents generally recommended) could be considered a limitation of the study as larger focus groups may have revealed a greater number and range of opinions. Moreover, the degree to which women perceived male surgeons to be insensitive to their feelings about nipple reconstruction and the durability of those views may have become more explicit within the context of an interview study. It is difficult therefore, to ascertain whether the phenomenon described is truly representative of the collective experience (even within this small sample), or whether the opinions of a few vocal members may have shaped the perceptions or recollections of others in the group on this matter. It would be unwise therefore, on the basis of this particular study, to conclude that male surgeons are generally insensitive to this issue as is suggested, given the relative weakness of the study design.

of maximising the cosmetic appearance of a reconstructed breast should they decide to undergo bilateral prophylactic mastectomy in response to their cancer risk.

Palliative surgery

In general, any surgical intervention intended to alleviate a distressing symptom in an individual for whom there is no hope of cure and no deliberate intent to lengthen their lifespan is a palliative one, although this is not always understood by the individual, family members, and, ocasionally, those in the health care team.[311] This is not surprising, for the scope of procedures meeting these criteria is vast, ranging from obvious palliative interventions, such as neurolytic blockade of the mandibular or sphenopalatine nerves in head and neck disease, or coeliac plexus and splanchnic nerve blockade for intractable pancreatic cancer pain,[312–314] to radical mastectomy or surgical debulking for a fungating malodorous breast lesion, or salvage cystectomy or pelvic exenteration for advanced prostate, cervical, vaginal, or vulval cancers.[315–317] Often termed 'salvage' procedures, these are frequently undertaken with palliative intent, even when the chances of eliciting 'cure', or at best a reasonable remission from the disease, is unlikely,[311] but they are no less valuable from the perspective of the individual's quality of life in the time that remains to them. Other procedures are recognised as palliative because they are undertaken towards the end of an individual's life,[39,40] such as decompression laminectomy or the insertion of a self-expanding vascular stent for the alleviation of spinal cord compression and superior vena cava obstruction, each of these being indicative of a poor prognosis, but nevertheless amenable to successful palliation with such interventions.[5,6]

In spite of their immense number and variety, Feig (2003) suggests that palliative surgical procedures tend to have five main purposes: evaluation of the extent of the disease; control of locoregional spread; control of a fungating tumour, discharge, or haemmorhage; control of pain; and surgical reconstruction (or rehabilitation) which will enable the individual to enjoy a better quality of life.[311] The extent of some palliative surgical procedures becomes greater as the disease worsens, with relatively minor interventions for the drainage of malignant ascites using thoracentesis or paracentesis giving way to pleurodesis or peritonenous shunting as the disease accelerates and ascites become more pronounced,[311] or the insertion of nasogastric tubes and octreotide infusions giving way to laparoscopic bypass surgery, cholecystojejunostomy, adhesiolysis, or open colectomy when the bowel becomes completely obstructed and the individual's situation worsens to such a degree that surgery becomes a desirable intervention.[318,319] On occasions, the palliative nature of treatment only becomes apparent after a staging laparotomy in circumstances where occult disease may remain hidden from the most sophisticated imaging techniques as happens occasionally in breast, colorectal, or pancreatic disease and intra-abdominal lymphoma.[103,104,320] Surgery may well continue in such circumstances, but the intent of the intervention at this point has become palliative rather than curative in the absence of other effective treatment modalities such as hormonal, cytotoxic therapy, or radiotherapy, though an individual's family members and members of the health care team may still construe it as curative on occasions.

It would be wrong to assume that palliative surgery is always or only reactive to the disease process. Much of the surgery undertaken with palliative intent is proactive and intended to prevent problems from occuring in the first place, hence knowledge of the disease and its likely trajectory is a necessary attribute for the therapeutic team caring for the individual with advanced cancer. The prophylactic fixation of weight-bearing bones in metastatic disease is a commonly used measure to alleviate bone pain or prevent pathological fracture in those with advanced bone metastases,[321] as is the removal or debulking of a tumour pressing against the spine or a major blood vessel in order to prevent spinal cord compression or a fatal haemmorhage from occuring. Spinal metastases may be treated with decompression laminectomy and stabilisation, but occasionally, reconstructive surgery to the anterior column may be considered, particularly if the individual has an expected lifespan greater than 6–12 months so that he or she can continue to live life to the full.[322] Ureteral stenting or the formation of an ileal conduit, while not healing the cancer or necessarily extending the individual's lifespan, may be undertaken to improve the quality of life and functional status of individuals with ureteral blockage or renal insufficiency.[311,323] Procedures such as these have been made easier and safer by the introduction of laparoscopic techniques that reduce the impact of surgery in those who may already have a complex symptomatology and impaired quality of life. Similarly, endoscopic cryo-ablative treatments may be used for a wide variety of cancers such as recurrent soft tissue tumours, prostate, and renal carcinomas, with the sole purpose of improving distressing symptoms.[311,324] This is an important development, as one fundamental tenet of palliative care is that the intervention should always improve, rather than worsen, an individual's symptoms; any intervention which is likely to do this being contraindicated in this case.

The transition from curative to palliative care is often a difficult one, and the delineation between the two may be blurred by conflicting messages received by the individual and his or her family from members of the health care team.[311] Good communication is vital therefore in eliciting the individual's views and evaluating the therapeutic benefits of any proposed intervention.[325] The individual requires adequate information to consider the implications of any proposed procedure, since information provides an important coping mechanism and may signifiantly alter their perception of control in very difficult circumstances.[326] There is a growing expectation that individuals will be fully involved in decisions affecting their care, and it is important that their needs and wishes are elicited and discussed prior to the procedure taking place. Nurses have a valuable role to play in this respect, and are in a privileged position to discuss the desired outcomes of treatment with the individual and their family so that they can play an active role in the decision-making process. This is particularly important in advanced or terminal illness where the individual or members of their family may require additional support in order to engage fully in the decision-making process, or in facilitating the inclusion of others, such as a minister of religion, counsellor or social worker in such discussions depending upon the individual's expressed wishes, culture and life-view.[325]

Conclusion

Cytotoxic chemotherapy and radiotherapy figure highly in most individuals' conceptions of cancer and its treatment, but surgery has been and remains the mainstay of cancer therapy, offering the most versatile range of interventions for the diagnosis, treatment, rehabilitation and palliation of cancer and its sequelae. Surgery elicits more cures for cancer than all other treatment modalities combined, and has a significant role to play in the management of cancer care. It is the most effective treatment for early, locoregional disease, and may also be used to stage a cancer so that appropriate non-surgical modalities may be used when a tumour is unresectable. The value of surgery as a cancer treatment modality has increased tremendously in the last few decades, with the advent of laparoscopic interventions in particular reducing the intra- and post-operative morbidity and mortality rates formerly associated with many radical procedures, and allowing unhindered access to tissues that were once considered inaccessible to the surgeon without a great deal of tissue damage or disfigurement. Improvements in our knowledge of physiological mechanisms such as lymphatic drainage and tumour spread have led generally to a reduction in the number of potentially disfiguring procedures, and widespread introduction of tissue-sparing techniques which render surgery a more acceptable form of cancer treatment. These advances have made the risks associated with surgical prophylaxis in 'at-risk' groups of individuals more acceptable, and reduced the complex array of symptoms associated with advanced disease in those for whom cure is not possible.

Nurses too have an important role to play in the promotion of successful surgical outcomes, whether this is in the development of new and innovative roles such as the nurse-endoscopist or genetic counsellor, or enabling individuals to reduce their cancer risk through the provision of health advice and education as part of their nursing care. Increasingly, nurses are becoming site-specialist practitioners and perform an invaluable service to a great many individuals whether it be in the counselling and supportive role of a breast care nurse specialist, or as a colostomy nurse specialist, helping an individual to become competent in the management of a functioning colostomy. As part of the multiprofessional surgical team, nurses are also increasingly engaged in a number of minor surgical procedures such as the insertion of peripherally inserted central-venous catheters (PICC lines), or the assessment of likely post-operative outcomes, and it is incumbent upon all those engaged in the care of those affected by cancer to understand the therapeutic intentions of a given procedure so that they may explain these to the individual concerned and alleviate anxiety and any misunderstandings. Similarly, nurses plays a crucial role in assessing the physical, psychosexual, and social impact of surgery on their patients, and referring the individual to other members of the multiprofessional team where specialist interventions may be required. Thus surgery is, and will doubtless remain for a long time to come, an exciting and rewarding area of practice for those engaged in the care of people with cancer.

References

1. Lee H. *Dates in Oncology*. (2000). London: Taylor and Francis.
2. Rayter Z. (2003). History of breast cancer. In Rayter Z. and Mansi J. (eds.) *Medical Therapy in Breast Cancer*. Cambridge: Cambridge University Press, pp. 1–28.
3. Chitwood W.R. and Sabiston D.C. (1997). Selected historical perspectives on the evolution of surgical practice. In Spitzer W.O., Mulder D.S., McPeek B. *et al.* (eds.) *Surgical Research*. New York: Springer, pp. 23–38.
4. Kazi R.A. and Peter H.E. (2004). Christian Albert Theodor Billroth: Master of Surgery. *Journal of Postgraduate Medicine* **50**, 82–83.
5. Souhami R.L. and Tobias J. (2005). *Cancer and its Management*, 5th edition. Oxford: Blackwell Scientific.
6. Neal A.J. and Hoskin P.J. (2003). *Clinical Oncology: Basic Principles and Practice*. London: Arnold.
7. Underwood R.A. (2004). The laparoscopic revolution. In Jones D.B., Wu J.S. and Soper N.J. (eds.) *Laparoscopic Surgery*. New York: Marcel Dekker.
8. Trabulsi E.J. and Guillonneau B. (2005). Laparoscopic radical prostatectomy. *Journal of Urology* **173**, 1072–1079.
9. Alvarez N.R., Lee T.M. and Solorzano C.C. (2005). Complete androgen insensitivity syndrome: the role of the endocrine surgeon. *The American Surgeon* **71**, 241–243.
10. Holub Z., Jabor A., Bartos P. *et al.* (2002). Laparoscopic surgery for endometrial cancer: long-term results of a multicentric study. *European Journal of Gynaecology and Oncology* **23**, 305–310.
11. Bollens R., Sandhu S., Roumeguere T., Quackels T. and Schulman C. (2005). Laparoscopic radical prostatectomy: the learning curve. *Current Opinion in Urology* **15**, 79–82.
12. Slim K. (2005). Laparoscopic surgery for colorectal cancer. *British Journal of Surgery* **92**, 896–897.
13. Lee J.H., Han H.S. and Lee J.H. (2005). A prospective randomized study comparing open vs laparoscopy-assisted distal gastrectomy in early gastric cancer: early results. *Surgical Endoscopy* **19**, 168–173.
14. Johnston W.K. 3rd and Wolf J.S. Jr. (2005). Laparoscopic partial nephrectomy: technique, oncologic efficacy, and safety. *Current Urology Reports* **6**, 19–28.
15. Asimakopoulos G., Beeson J., Evans J. and Maiwand M.O. (2005). Cryosurgery for malignant endobronchial tumors: analysis of outcome. *Chest* **127**, 2007–2014.
16. Agnese D.M. and Burak W.E. Jr. (2005). Ablative approaches to the minimally invasive treatment of breast cancer. *Cancer Journal* **11**, 77–82.
17. Huston T.L. and Simmons R.M. (2005). Ablative therapies for the treatment of malignant diseases of the breast. *American Journal of Surgery* **189**, 694–701.
18. Prepelica K.L., Okeke Z., Murphy A. and Katz A.E. (2005). Cryosurgical ablation of the prostate: high risk patient outcomes. *Cancer* **103**, 1625–1630.
19. Ahmed S., Lindsey B. and Davies J. (2005). Salvage cryosurgery for locally recurrent prostate cancer following radiotherapy. *Prostate Cancer and Prostatic Diseases* **8**, 31–35.
20. Gill I.S., Remer E.M., Hasan W.A. *et al.* (2005). Renal cryoablation: outcome at 3 years. *Journal of Urology* **173**, 1903–1907.
21. Jang T.L., Wang R., Kim S.C. *et al.* (2005). Histopathology of human renal tumors after laparoscopic renal cryosurgery. *Journal of Urology* **173**, 720–724.
22. Herskind C., Steil V., Kraus-Tiefenbacher U. and Wenz F. (2005). Radiobiological aspects of intraoperative radiotherapy (IORT) with isotropic low-energy X rays for early-stage breast cancer. *Radiation Research* **163**, 208–215.

23. Veronesi U., Orecchia R. and Luini A. *et al.* (2005). Full-dose intraoperative radiotherapy with electrons during breast-conserving surgery: experience with 590 cases. *Annals of Surgery* **242**, 101–106.

24. Merrick H.W. 3rd, Hager E. and Dobelbower R.R. Jr. (2003). Intraoperative radiation therapy for breast cancer. *Surgical Oncology Clinics of North America* **12**, 1065–1078.

25. Arthur D.W., Morris M.M. and Vicini F.A. (2004). Breast cancer: new radiation treatment options. *Oncology* **18**, 1621–1629; discussion 9–30, 36–38.

26. McPherson C.M. and Warnick R.E. (2004). Results of contemporary surgical management of radiation necrosis using frameless stereotaxis and intraoperative magnetic resonance imaging. *Journal of Neurooncology* **68**, 41–47.

27. Cody H.S. (ed.) (2001) *Sentinel Lymph Node Biopsy*. London: Taylor and Francis.

28. Osborne M.P. and Rosenbaum-Smith S.M. (2001). The historic background of lymphatic mapping. In Cody H.S. (ed.) *Sentinel Lymph Node Biopsy*. London: Taylor and Francis, pp. 3–10.

29. Poole K. and Fallowfield L.J. (2002). The psychological impact of post-operative arm morbidity following axillary surgery for breast cancer: a critical review. *Breast* **11**, 81–87.

30. Angioli R., Palaia I., Cipriani C. *et al.* (2005). Role of sentinel lymph node biopsy procedure in cervical cancer: a critical point of view. *Gynecologic Oncology* **96**, 504–509.

31. Gunther K., Dworak O., Remke S. *et al.* (2002). Prediction of distant metastases after curative surgery for rectal cancer. *Journal of Surgical Research* **103**, 68–78.

32. Rosenberg S.A. (2001). Principles of cancer management: surgical oncology. In Rosenberg S.A., DeVita V.T., Hellman S.A. and Rosenberg S.A. (eds.) *Cancer: Principles and Practice*, 6th edition. Philadelphia, PA: Lippincott, Williams and Wilkins, pp. 253–264.

33. Katz M.H., Savides T.J., Moossa A.R. and Bouvet M. (2005). An evidence-based approach to the diagnosis and staging of pancreatic cancer. *Pancreatology* **5**, 576–590.

34. Mozzillo N., Chiesa F., Botti G. *et al.* (2001). Sentinel node biopsy in head and neck cancer. *Annals of Surgical Oncology* **8(9 suppl)**, 103S–5S.

35. Josephson D.L. (2003). *Intravenous Infusion Therapy for Nurses: Principles and Practice*. Clifton Park, NY: Thomson Delmar.

36. Finlay T. (2004). *Intravenous Therapy*. Oxford: Blackwell Science.

37. Liu J., Bruch H.P., Farke S., Nolde J. and Schwandner O. (2005). Stoma formation for fecal diversion: a plea for the laparoscopic approach. *Techniques in Coloproctology* **9**, 9–14.

38. Riediger H., Makowiec F., Schareck W.D., Hopt U.T. and Adam U. (2003). Delayed gastric emptying after pylorus-preserving pancreatoduodenectomy is strongly related to other postoperative complications. *Journal of Gastrointestinal Surgery* **7**, 758–765.

39. Ryken T.C., Eichholz K.M., Gersten P.C. *et al.* (2003). Evidence-based review of the surgical management of vertebral column metastatic disease. *Neurosurgical Focus* **15**, 1–10.

40. Rowell N.P. and Gleeson, F.V. (2005). Steroids, radiotherapy, chemotherapy and stents for superior vena caval obstruction in carcinoma of the bronchus. *The Cochrane Library*, Issue 3. Oxford: Update Software.

41. Hasen K.V., Few J.W. and Fine N.A. (2002). Plastic surgery: a component in the comprehensive care of cancer patients. *Oncology* **16**, 1685–1698; discussion 98, 702–705, 708.

42. Kim K.H., Sung M.W., Chang K.H. and Kang B.S. (2000). Therapeutic dilemmas in the management of thyroid cancer with laryngotracheal involvement. *Otolaryngology and Head and Neck Surgery* **122**, 763–767.

43. Gudas S.A. (2000). Rehabilitation of pediatric and adult sarcomas. *Rehabilitation Oncology* **18**, 10–13.

44. Miner T.J. (2005). Palliative surgery for advanced cancer: lessons learned in patient selection and outcome assessment. *American Journal of Clinical Oncology* **28**, 411–414.

45. Gonzalez R., Smith C.D., Ritter E.M. *et al.* (2005). Laparoscopic palliative surgery for complicated colorectal cancer. *Surgical Endoscopy* **19**, 43–46.

46. Gunther K., Braunrieder G., Bittorf B.R., Hohenberger W. and Matzel K.E. (2003). Patients with familial adenomatous polyposis experience better bowel function and quality of life after ileorectal anastomosis than after ileoanal pouch. *Colorectal Disease* **5**, 38–44.

47. Tekkis P.P., Kessaris N., Kocher H.M. *et al.* (2003). Evaluation of POSSUM and P-POSSUM scoring systems in patients undergoing colorectal surgery. *British Journal of Surgery* **90**, 1021.

48. Smith J.J., Tekkis P.P., Thompson M.R. and Stamatakis J.D. (2004). *Report of the ACPGBI Bowel Cancer Study*. London: Association of Coloproctology of Great Britain and Ireland.

49. Kaneko H., Takagi S., Otsuka Y. *et al.* (2005). Laparoscopic liver resection of hepatocellular carcinoma. *American Journal of Surgery* **189**, 190–194.

50. Menon K.V. and Farouk R. (2002). An analysis of the accuracy of P-POSSUM scoring for mortality risk assessment after surgery for colorectal cancer. *Colorectal Disease* **4**, 197–200.

51. Metcalfe M.S., Norwood M.G., Miller A.S. and Hemingway D. (2005). Unreasonable expectations in emergency colorectal cancer surgery. *Colorectal Disease* **7**, 275–278.

52. Spitzer W.O., Mulder D.S., McPeek B. *et al.* (1997). *Surgical Research*. New York: Springer.

53. Parry J.M., Collins S., Mathers J., Scott N.A. and Woodman C.B. (1999). Influence of volume of work on the outcome of treatment for patients with colorectal cancer. *British Journal of Surgery* **86**, 475–481.

54. Hillner B.E., Smith T.J. and Desch C.E. (2000). Hospital and physician volume or specialization and outcomes in cancer treatment: importance in quality of cancer care. *Journal of Clinical Oncology* **18**, 2327–2340.

55. Porter G.A., Soskolne C.L., Yakimets W.W. and Newman S.C. (1998). Surgeon-related factors and outcome in rectal cancer. *Annals of Surgery* **227**, 157–167.

56. Yu A.H.J., Lin K.M., Ota D.M. and Lynch H.T. (2003). Hereditary nonpolyposis colorectal cancer: preventive management. *Cancer Treatment Reviews* **29**, 461–470.

57. Ishikawa H. (2004). Chemoprevention of carcinogenesis in familial tumors. *International Journal of Clinical Oncology* **9**, 299–303.

58. Ishikawa H. (2005). [Prevention of carcinogenesis in familial tumors.] *Gan To Kagaku Ryoho* **32**, 973–976.

59. Sinicrope F.A., Lemoine M., Xi L. *et al.* (1999). Reduced expression of cyclooxygenase 2 proteins in hereditary nonpolyposis colorectal cancers relative to sporadic cancers. *Gastroenterology* **117**, 350–358.

60. Onaitis M.W. and Mantyh C. (2003). Ileal pouch-anal anastomosis for ulcerative colitis and familial adenomatous polyposis: historical development and current status. *Annals of Surgery* **238(6 suppl.)**, S42–48.

61. Beitz J.M. (1999). The lived experience of having an ileoanal reservoir: a phenomenologic study. *Journal of Wound Ostomy and Continence Nursing* **26**, 185–200.

62. Knudsen A.L., Bisgaard M.L. and Bulow S. (2003). Attenuated familial adenomatous polyposis (AFAP). A review of the literature. *Familial Cancer* **2**, 43–55.

63. Codori A.M., Zawacki K.L., Petersen G.M. *et al.* (2003). Genetic testing for hereditary colorectal cancer in children: long-term psychological effects. *American Journal of Medical Genetics* **116**, 117–128.

64. Eeles R. (2002). Familial cancer. In Souhami R.L., Tannock I., Hohenberger P. and Horiot J.C. (eds.) *Oxford Textbook of Oncology*, 2nd edition. Oxford: Oxford University Press, pp. 33–47.

65. Marx S.J. and Jensen R.T. (2002). *Multiple Endocrine Neoplasia Type 1*. Bethesda, MD: National Institute for Diabetic, Digestive and Kidney Diseases, National Institutes for Health.

66. Marx S.J. (2001). Multiple endocrine neoplasia type 1. In Scriver C.S. (ed.) *Metabolic Basis of Inherited Diseases*. New York: McGraw Hill, pp. 943–966.

67. Gauger P.G., Scheiman J.M., Wamsteker E.J. *et al.* (2003). Role of endoscopic ultrasonography in screening and treatment of pancreatic endocrine tumours in asymptomatic patients with multiple endocrine neoplasia type 1. *British Journal of Surgery* **90**, 748–754.

68. Richards M.L., Carter S.M., Gross S.J. and Freeman R. (2005). Multiple endocrine neoplasia, Type 2. In Pourmotabbed G., Talavera F., Khardori R., Cooper M. and Griffing G.T. (eds.) *emedicine: World Medical Library* www.emedicine.com/med/topic1520.htm (accessed 6 September 2007).

69. Van Heurn L.W., Schaap C. and Sie G. (1999). Predictive DNA testing for multiple endocrine neoplasia 2: a therapeutic challenge of prophylactic thyroidectomy in very young children. *Journal of Pediatric Surgery* **34**, 568–571.

70. Kercher K.W., Novitsky Y.W., Park A. *et al.* (2005). Laparoscopic curative resection of pheochromocytomas. *Annals of Surgery* **241**, 919–926; discussion 26–28.

71. Del Pizzo J.J., Schiff J.D. and Vaughan E.D. (2005). Laparoscopic adrenalectomy for pheochromocytoma. *Current Urology Reports* **6**, 78–85.

72. Evans D.B., Fleming J.B. and Lee J.E. (1999). The surgical management of medullary thyroid carcinoma. *Seminars in Surgical Oncology* **16**, 50–63.

73. Lips C.J., Hoppener J.W., van Nesselrooij B.P. and van der Luij B.P. (2005). Counselling in multiple endocrine neoplasia syndromes: from individual experience to general guidelines. *Journal of Internal Medicine* **257**, 69–77.

74. Geirdal A.O., Reichelt J.G., Dahl A.A. *et al.* (2005). Psychological distress in women at risk of hereditary breast/ovarian or HNPCC cancers in the absence of demonstrated mutations. *Familial Cancer* **4**, 121–126.

75. Van Dijk S., Otten W., Zoeteweij M.W., Timmermans D.R., Van Asperen C.J., Breuning M.H. *et al.* (2003). Genetic counselling and the intention to undergo prophylactic mastectomy: effects of a breast cancer risk assessment. *British Journal of Cancer* **88(11)**, 1675–1681.

76. Lostumbo L., Carbine N., Wallace J. and Ezzo J. (2004). Prophylactic mastectomy for the prevention of breast cancer (Cochrane Review). *The Cochrane Library*, Issue 3. Oxford: Update Software.

77. Hatcher M., Fallowfield L. and A'Hern R. (2001). The psychological impact of bilateral prophylactic mastec-

tomy: prospective study using questionaires and semistructured interviews. *British Medical Journal* **13**, 76–79.

78. Levine D.A. and Gemignani M.L. (2003). Prophylactic surgery in hereditary breast/ovarian cancer syndrome. *Oncology* **17**, 932–941.

79. Grosfeld F.J., Lips C.J. and Beemer F.A. (1997). Psychological risks of genetically testing children for a hereditary cancer syndrome. *Patient Education and Counselling* **15**, 217–225.

80. MacDonald D.J. and Lessick M. (2000). Hereditary cancers in children and ethical and psychosocial implications. *Journal of Pediatric Nursing* **15**, 217–225.

81. Hedstrom M., Skolin I. and von Essen L. (2003). Distressing and positive experiences and important aspects for adolescents treated for cancer. Adolescent and nurse problems. *European Journal of Oncology Nursing* **8**, 6–17.

82. Grosfeld F.J., Lips C.J. and Beemer F.A. (2000). Distress in MEN2 family members and partners prior to DNA test disclosure. Multiple endocrine neoplasia type 2. *American Journal of Medical Genetics* **91**, 1–7.

83. Gallagher M.C., Sturt N.J. and Phillips R.K. (2003). Female fecundity before and after operation for familial adenomatous polyposis. *British Journal of Surgery* **90**, 761.

84. Olsen K.O., Juul S., Buelow S. *et al.* (2003). Female fecundity before and after operation for familial adenomatous polyposis. *British Journal of Surgery* **90**, 227–231.

85. Grosfeld F.J., Beemer F.A. and Lips C.J. (2000). Parents' responses to disclosure of genetic test results of their children. *American Journal of Medical Genetics* **94**, 316–323.

86. Giarelli E. (2002). Bringing threat to the fore: participating in lifelong surveillance for genetic risk of cancer. *Oncolology Nursing Forum* **30**, 945–955.

87. O'Brien M. (2001). Living in a house of cards: family experiences with long-term childhood technology dependence. *Journal of Paediatric Nursing* **16**, 13–22.

88. Woodgate R.L. and Degner L.F. (2002). 'Nothing is carved in stone': uncertainty in chidren with cancer and their families. *European Journal of Oncology Nursing* **6**, 191–202.

89. Brinton B., Persson I., Boice J.D., McLaughlin J.K. and Fraumeni J.F. (2001). Breast cancer risk in relation to amount of tissue removed during breast reduction operations in Sweden. *Cancer* **91**, 478–483.

90. Goodman A. (2005). Bilateral prophylactic mastectomy dramatically decreases incidence of breast cancer in mutation carriers. *Oncology Times* **27**, 22.

91. Spear S.L., Carter M.E. and Schwarz K. (2005). Prophylactic mastectomy: indications, options, and reconstructive alternatives. *Plastic and Reconstructive Surgery* **115**, 891–909.

92. Hatcher M.B., Fallowfield L. and A'Hern R. (2001). The psychosocial impact of bilateral prophylactic mastectomy: prospective study using questionnaires and semistructured interviews. *British Medical Journal* **322**, 76–79.

93. Hopwood P., Lee A., Shemon A. *et al.* (2000). Clinical followup after bilateral risk reducing (prophylactic) mastectomy: mental health and body image outcomes. *Psycho-oncology* **9**, 462–472.

94. Frost M.H., Schaid D.J., Slezak J.M. *et al.* (2000). Long-term satisfaction and psychological and social function following bilateral prophylactic mastectomy. *Journal of the American Medical Association* **284,** 319–324.

95. Meijers-Heijboer H., van Geel B., van Putten W.L. *et al.* (2001). Breast cancer after prophylactic bilateral mastectomy in women with a BRCA1 or BRCA2 mutation. *New England Journal of Medicine* **345**, 159–164.

96. Hartmann L.C., Sellers T.A., Frank T.S. *et al.* (2001). Efficacy of bilateral prophylactic mastectomy in BRCA1 and BRCA2 gene mutation carriers. *Journal of the National Cancer Institute* **93**, 1633–1637.

97. Ghosh K. and Hartmann L.C. (2002). Current status of prophylactic mastectomy. *Oncology* **16**, 1319–1325; commentary 29.

98. Metcalfe K.A., Esplen M.J., Goel V. and Narod S.A. (2005). Predictors of quality of life in women with a bilateral prophylactic mastectomy. *Breast Journal* **11**, 65–69.

99. Lantz P.M., Janz N.K., Fagerlin A. *et al.* (2005). Satisfaction with surgery outcomes and the decision process in a population-based sample of women with breast cancer. *Health Services Research* **40**, 745–767.

100. Peralta E., Ellenhorn J., Wagman L. *et al.* (2000). Contralateral prophylactic mastectomy improves the outcome of selected patients undergoing mastectomy for breast cancer. *American Journal of Surgery* **180**, 439–445.

101. McDonnell S.K., Schaid D.J., Myers J.L. *et al.* (2001). Efficacy of contralateral prophylactic mastectomy in women with a personal and family history of breast cancer. *Journal of Clinical Oncology* **19**, 3938–3942.

102. Dupont E.L., Kuhn M.A., McCann C. *et al.* (2000). The role of sentinel lymph node biopsy in women undergoing prophylactic mastectomy. *American Journal of Surgery* **180**, 274–277.

103. Frizelle F.A., Hemmings C.T., Whitehead M.R. and Spigelman A.D. (2003). Familial adenomatous polyposis and duodenal lymphoma: report of a case. *Diseases of the Colon and Rectum* **46**, 1698–1701.

104. Dupont E., Cox C.E., Nguyen K. *et al.* (2001). Utility of internal mammary lymph node removal when noted by intraoperative gamma probe detection. *Annals of Surgery and Oncology* **8**, 833–836.

105. Akerman M. (2002). Cytology and minimal sampling techniques. In Souhami R.L., Tannock I., Hohenberger P. and Horiot J.C. (eds.) *Oxford Textbook of Oncology.* Oxford: Oxford University Press, pp. 241–254.

106. Benedet J.L., Bertrand M.A., Matisic J.M. and Garner D. (2005). Costs of colposcopy services and their impact on the incidence and mortality rate of cervical cancer in Canada. *Journal of Lower Genital Tract Disease* **9**, 160–166.

107. Newman C. and Finan M.A. (2003). Hysterectomy in women with cervical stenosis. Surgical indications and pathology. *Journal of Reproductive Medicine* **48**, 672–676.

108. Rami-Porta R., Wittekind C. and Goldstraw P. (2005). Complete resection in lung cancer surgery: proposed definition. *Lung Cancer* **49**, 25–33.

109. Dowdall J.F., Maguire D. and McAnena O.J. (2002). Experience of surgery for rectal cancer with total meso-rectal excision in a general surgical practice. *British Journal of Surgery* **89**, 1014–1019.

110. Graydon J., Galloway S., Palmer-Wicham S. *et al.* (1997). Information needs of women during early treatment for breast cancer. *Journal of Advanced Nursing* **26**, 59–64.

111. Luker K.A., Beaver K.A., Leinster S.J. and Owens R.G. (1996). Information needs and sources of information for women with breast cancer: a follow-up study. *Journal of Advanced Nursing* **23**, 487–495.

112. Parle M., Jones B. and Maguire S. (1996). Maladaptive coping and affective disorders in cancer patients. *Psychological Medicine* **26**, 735–744.

113. Love S.M. (1995). *Dr Love's Breast Book.* New York: Perseus Book Publishers.

114. Willis S.L. and Ramzay I. (1995). Analysis of false results in a series of 835 fine needle aspirates of breast lesions. *Acta Cytologica* **39**, 858–864.

115. Atula T., Grenman R., Laippala P. and Klemi P. (1996). Fine needle biopsy in the diagnosis of parotid gland lesions. Evaluation of 438 biopsies. *Diagnostic Cytopathology* **15**, 185–190.

116. Bondeson L. and Lindholm K. (1997). Prediction of invasiveness by aspiration cytology applied to non-palpable breast carcinoma and tested in 300 cases. *Diagnostic Cytopathology* **17**, 315–320.

117. Veronesi U., von Kleist K., Redmond K. *et al.* (1999). Caring about women and cancer (CAWAC): a European survey of the perspectives and experiences of women with female cancers. *European Journal of Cancer* **35**, 1667–1675.

118. Sainio C. and Eriksson E. (2003). Keeping cancer patients informed: a challenge for nursing. *European Journal of Oncology Nursing* **7**, 39–49.

119. Sainio C., Eriksson E. and Lauri S. (2001). Patient participation in decision making about care. *Cancer Nursing* **24**, 172–179.

120. Yarbro C.H., Frogge M.H. and Goodman M. (2002). *Clinical Guide to Cancer Nursing.* Boston, MA: Jones and Bartlett.

121. Saares P. and Suominen T. (2005). Experiences and resources of breast cancer patients in short-stay surgery. *European Journal of Cancer Care* **14**, 43–52.

122. Eggermont A.M.M., Autier P. and Keilholz U. (2002). Cutaneous malignant melanoma. In Souhami R.L., Tannock I., Hohenberger P. and Horiot J.C. (eds.) *The Oxford Textbook of Oncology.* Oxford: Oxford University Press, pp. 1175–1211.

123. Cady B. (1988). 'Prophylactic' lymph node dissection in melanoma: does it help? *Journal of Clinical Oncology* **6**, 24.

124. Dowdy S.C., Metzinger D.S., Gebhart J.B. *et al.* (2005). Salvage whole-abdominal radiation therapy after second-look laparotomy or secondary debulking surgery in patients with ovarian cancer. *Gynecologic Oncology* **96**, 389–394.

125. Taub R.N., Keohan M.L., Chabot J.C. *et al.* (2000). Peritoneal mesothelioma. *Current Treatment Options in Oncology* **1**, 303–312.

126. Anonymous. (2002). Brachytherapy for accelerated partial breast irradiation after breast-conserving surgery for early stage breast cancer. *TEC Bulletin (Online)* **19**, 6–9.

127. Vogelzang J.N., Rusthoven J.J., Symanowski J. *et al.* (2003). Phase III study of pemetrexed in combination with cisplatin versus cisplatin alone in patients with malignant pleural mesothelioma. *Journal of Clinical Oncology* **21**, 2636–2644.

128. Vogelzang N.J. (2004). Multimodality treatments in mesothelioma: role of chemotherapy. *Thoracic Surgery Clinics* **14**, 531–542.

129. Andreopoulou E., Ross P.J., O'Brien M.E. *et al.* (2004). The palliative benefits of MVP(mitomycin C, inblastine and cisplatin) chemotherapy in patients with malignant mesothelioma. *Annals of Oncology* **15**, 1406–1412.

130. Abuksis G., Mor M., Segal N. *et al.* (2001). A patient education programme is cost-effective for preventing failure of endoscopic procedures in a gastroenterology department. *American Journal of Gastroenterology* **96**, 1786–1790.

131. Jones D.B., Wu J.S. and Soper N.J. (2004). *Laparoscopic Surgery.* New York: Marcel Dekker.

132. McCallum J. (2003). The role of the nurse endoscopist. *Hospital Medicine* **64**, 337–339.

133. Kneebone R.L., Nestel D., Moorthy K. *et al.* (2003). Learning the skills of flexible sigmoidoscopy: the wider perspective. *Medical Education* **37(suppl. 1)**, 50–58.

134. Basnyat P.S., West J., Davies P. and Davies P.S. (2000). The nurse practitioner endoscopist. *Annals of the Royal College of Surgeons* **82**, 331–332.

135. Chapman W. (2005). Lay endoscopy: concerns not laid to rest. *Gastrointestinal Nursing* **3**, 14.

136. Arumgan P.J., Rao G.N., West J., Foster M.E. and Haray P.N. (2000). The impact of open access flexible sigmoidoscopy: a comparison of two services. *Journal of the Royal College of Surgeons* **40**, 366–368.

137. Douglass H.O. (1993). Current approaches to multimodality management of advanced pancreatic cancer. *Hepatogastroenterology* **40**, 433–442.

138. Man R. (2004). Nurse-led endoscopy for familial adenomatous polyposis. *Gastrointestinal Nursing* **2**, 22–24.

139. Schofield G., Thapar C. and Vance M. (2004). Capsule endoscopy and the development of a nurse-led service. *Gastrointestinal Nursing* **2**, 25–29.

140. Department of Health. (2000). *The NHS Cancer Plan.* London: Department of Health.

141. Pathmakanthan S., Murray I., Smith K.R., Heeley R. and Donnelly M. (2001). Nurse endoscopists in United Kingdom health care: a survey of prevalence, skills and attitudes. *Journal of Advanced Nursing* **36**, 705–710.

142. Dow K.H. (2004). *Contemporaray Issues in Breast Cancer.* London: Jones and Bartlett.

143. Baum M., Saunders C. and Meredith S. (1995). *Breast Cancer: A Guide for Every Woman.* Oxford: Oxford University Press.

144. DeCamp M.M. Jr., Ashiku S. and Thurer R. (2005). The role of surgery in N2 non-small cell lung cancer. *Clinical Cancer Research* **11**, 5033s–5037s.

145. Depierre A., Milleron B., Moro-Sibilot D. *et al.* (2002). Preoperative chemotherapy followed by surgery compared with primary surgery in resectable stage I (except T1N0), II, and IIIa non-small-cell lung cancer. *Journal of Clinical Oncology* **20**, 247–253.

146. Martin-Ucar A.E., Waller D.A., Atkins J.L. *et al.* (2004). The beneficial effects of specialist thoracic surgery on the resection rates for non-small cell lung cancer. *Lung Cancer* **46**, 227–232.

147. Martin-Ucar A.E., Chaudhuri N., Edwards J.G. and Waller D.A. (2002). Can pneumonectomy for non-small cell lung cancer be avoided? An audit of parenchymal sparing lung surgery. *European Journal of Cardiothoracic Surgery* **21**, 601–605.

148. Manser R., Wright G., Hart D., Byrnes G. and Campbell D.A. (2005). Surgery for early stage non-small cell lung cancer (Cochrane Review). *The Cochrane Library*, Issue 1. Oxford: Update Software.

149. Arriagada R., Goldstraw P. and Le Chevalier T. (2002). Management of non-small cell lung cancer. In Souhami R.L., Tannock I., Hohenberger P. and Horiot J.C., (eds.) *Oxford Textbook of Oncology*, 2nd edition. Oxford: Oxford University Press, pp. 2089–2110.

150. Turrisi A.T. (2005). A case against surgery for most I.I.Ia non-small cell lung cancer. *Seminars in Oncology* **32(2 suppl. 3)**, S6–8.

151. Eberhardt W.E., Hepp R. and Stamatis G. (2005). The role of surgery in stage IIIA non-small cell lung cancer. *Hematology/Oncology Clinics of North America* **19**, 303–319, vi–vii.

152. van Geel A.N., Jansen P.P., van Klaveren R.J. and Van Der Sijp J.R. High relapse-free survival after preoperative and intraoperative radiotherapy and resection for sulcus superior tumors. *Chest* **124**, 1841–1846.

153. Feins R.H. and Watson T.J. (2004). What's new in general thoracic surgery? *Journal of the American College of Surgeons* **199**, 265–272.

154. Gupta V., Mychalczak B., Krug L. *et al.* (2005). Hemithoracic radiation therapy after pleurectomy/decortication for malignant pleural mesothelioma. *International Journal of Radiation Oncology Biology Physics* **63**, 1045–1052.

155. Lee T.T., Everett D.L., Shu H.K. *et al.* (2002). Radical pleurectomy/decortication and intraoperative radiotherapy followed by conformal radiation with or without chemotherapy for malignant pleural mesothelioma. *Journal of Thoracic and Cardiovascular Surgery* **124**, 1183–1189.

156. Handy J.R., Asaph J.W., Skokan L. *et al.* (2002). What happens to patients undergoing lung cancer surgery? Outcomes and quality of life before and after surgery. *Chest* **122**, 21–30.

157. Rudd R. and Rabbitts P. (2002). Lung cancer: epidemiology, causation, genetics. In Souhami R.L., Tannock I., Hohenberger P. and Horiot J.C. (eds.) *Oxford Textbook of Oncology*, 2nd edition. Oxford: Oxford University Press, pp. 2067–2076.

158. Sarna L., Evangelista L., Tashkin D. *et al.* (2004). Impact of respiratory symptoms and pulmonary function on quality of life of long-term survivors of non-small cell lung cancer. *Chest* **125**, 439–445.

159. Rocco G. and Vaughan R. (2000). Outcome of lung surgery: what patients don't like. *Chest* **117**, 1531–1532.

160. McManus K. (2003). Concerns of poor quality of life should not deprive patients of the opportunity of curative surgery. *Thorax* **58**, 189.

161. Myrdal G., Gustafsson G., Lambe M., Horte L.G. and Stahl E. (2001). Outcome after lung cancer surgery:

factors predicting early mortality and major morbidity. *European Journal of Cardiothoracic Surgery* **20**, 694–699.

162. Tanaka K., Akechi T., Okuyama T., Nishiwaki Y. and Uchitomi Y. (2002). Impact of dyspnea, pain, and fatigue on daily life activities in ambulatory patients with advanced lung cancer. *Journal of Pain and Symptom Management* **23**, 417–423.

163. Bedor M., Alexander C. and Edelman M.J. (2005). Management of common symptoms in advanced lung cancer. *Current Treatment Options in Oncology* **6**, 61–68.

164. Cooley M.E., Short T.H. and Moriarty H.J. (2002). Patterns of symptom distress in adults receiving treatment for lung cancer. *Journal of Palliative Care* **18**, 150–159.

165. Zabora J., Brintsenhofeszcoc K., Curbow B., Hooker C. and Piantadosi S. (2001). The prevalence of psychological distress by cancer site. *Psycho-oncology* **10**, 19–28.

166. Cykert S., Kissling G. and Jansen C.J. (2000). Patient preferences regarding possible outcomes of lung resection: what outcomes should preoperative evaluations target? *Chest* **117**, 1551–1559.

167. Cohen L.M., McChargue D.E. and Collins F.L. (2003). *The Health Psychology Handbook: Practical Issues for the Behavioural Medicine Specialist.* London: Sage.

168. Booth-Butterfield M. (2003). Embedded health behaviours from adolescence to adulthood: the impact of tobacco. *Health Communication* **15**, 171–184.

169. Richmond M., Spring B., Sommerfeld B.K. and McChargue D.E. (2001). Rumination and cigarette smoking: a bad combination for depressive outcomes? *Journal of Consulting and Clinical Psychology* **69**, 836–840.

170. Glassman A.H., Covey L.S., Stetner F. and Rivelli S. (2001). Smoking cessation and the course of major depression: a follow up study. *Lancet* **357**, 1929–1932.

171. Brennan M.F. (2005). Current status of surgery for gastric cancer: a review. *Gastric Cancer* **8**, 64–70.

172. Kim M.C., Kim H.H. and Jung G.J. (2005). Surgical outcome of laparoscopy-assisted gastrectomy with extraperigastric lymph node dissection for gastric cancer. *European Journal of Surgical Oncology* **31**, 401–405.

173. Kitagawa Y., Fujii H., Kumai K. *et al.* (2005). Recent advances in sentinel node navigation for gastric cancer: a paradigm shift of surgical management. *Journal of Surgical Oncology* **90**, 147–151; discussion 51–62.

174. Noh S.H., Hyung W.J. and Cheong J.H. (2005). Minimally invasive treatment for gastric cancer:

approaches and selection process. *Journal of Surgical Oncology* **90**, 188–193; discussion 93–94.

175. Yokota T., Kunii Y., Saito T. *et al.* (2002). Prognostic factors of gastric cancer tumours of less than 2 cm in diameter: rationale for limited surgery. *European Journal of Surgical Oncology* **28**, 209–213.

176. Bentrem D., Wilton A., Mazumdar M., Brennan M. and Coit D. (2005). The value of peritoneal cytology as a preoperative predictor in patients with gastric carcinoma undergoing a curative resection. *Annals of Surgical Oncology* **12**, 347–353.

177. Glehen O., Peyrat P., Beaujard A.C. *et al.* (2003). Pattern of failures in gastric cancer patients with lymph node involvement treated by surgery, intraoperative and external beam radiotherapy. *Radiotherapy and Oncology* **67**, 171–175.

178. De Paoli A., Buonadonna A., Boz G. *et al.* (2003). Combined modality treatment for locally advanced gastric cancer. *I Supplementi di Tumori* **2**, S58–62.

179. Bonenkamp J.J., Van Krieken H., Kuipers E. *et al.* (2002). Gastric cancer. In Souhami R.L., Tannock I., Hohenberger P. and Horiot J.C. (eds.) *Oxford Textbook of Oncology.* Oxford: Oxford University Press, pp. 1517–1535.

180. Dulucq J.L., Wintringer P., Perissat J. and Mahajna A. (2005). Completely laparoscopic total and partial gastrectomy for benign and malignant diseases: a single institute's prospective analysis. *Journal of the American College of Surgeons* **200**, 191–197.

181. Dulucq J.L., Wintringer P., Stabilini C. *et al.* (2005). Laparoscopic and open gastric resections for malignant lesions: a prospective comparative study. *Surgical Endoscopy* **19**, 933–938.

182. Hasler W.L. (2002). Dumping syndrome. *Current Treatment Options in Gastroenterology* **5**, 139–145.

183. Aldrich C.M. and Barker H.M. (2002). *Nutrition and Dietetics for Health Care.* London: Elsevier.

184. Imhof A., Schneemann M., Schaffner A. and Brandle M. (2001). Reactive hypoglycaemia due to late dumping syndrome: successful treatment with acarbose. *Swiss Medical Weekly* **131**, 81–83.

185. Scholmerich J. (2004). Postgastrectomy syndromes – diagnosis and treatment. *Best Practice and Research. Clinical Gastroenterology* **18**, 917–933.

186. Olsson U., Bergbom T. and Bosaeus I. (2002). Patients' experiences of their intake of food and fluid following gastrectomy due to tumour. *Gastroenterological Nursing* **25**, 146–153.

187. Kiyama T., Mizutani T., Okuda T. *et al.* (2005). Postoperative changes in body composition after gastrectomy. *Journal of Gastrointestinal Surgery* **9**, 313–319.

188. Farreras N., Artigas V., Cardona D. *et al.* (2005). Effect of early postoperative enteral immunonutrition

on wound healing in patients undergoing surgery for gastric cancer. *Clinical Nutrition* **24**, 55–65.

189. Liedman B., Hugosson I. and Lundell L. (2001). Treatment of devastating postgastrectomy symptoms: the potential role of jejunal pouch reconstruction. *Digestive Surgery* **18**, 218–221.

190. Ikeda M., Ueda T., Yamagata K. *et al.* (2003). Reconstruction after distal gastrectomy by interposition of a double jejunal pouch using a triangulating stapling technique. *World Journal of Surgery* **27**, 460–464.

191. Peitz U., Vieth M., Ebert M.A. *et al.* (2005). Small bowel metaplasia arising in the remnant esophagus after esophagogastrostomy: a perspective study in patients with a history of total gastrectomy. *American Journal of Gastroenterology* **100**, 2062–2070.

192. Kitano S. and Shiraishi N. (2004). Current status of laparoscopic gastrectomy for cancer in Japan. *Surgical Endoscopy* **18**, 182–185.

193. Carboni F., Lepiane P., Santoro R. *et al.* (2005). Laparoscopic surgery for gastric cancer: preliminary experience. *Gastric Cancer* **8**, 75–77.

194. Huscher C.G., Mingoli A., Sgarzini G. *et al.* (2005). Laparoscopic versus open subtotal gastrectomy for distal gastric cancer: five-year results of a randomized prospective trial. *Annals of Surgery* **241**, 232–237.

195. Kim M.C., Kim K.H., Kim H.H. and Jung G.J. (2005). Comparison of laparoscopy-assisted by conventional open distal gastrectomy and extraperigastric lymph node dissection in early gastric cancer. *Journal of Surgical Oncology* **91**, 90–94.

196. Tonouchi H., Mohri Y., Tanaka K. *et al.* (2005). Laparoscopic lymphatic mapping and sentinel node biopsies for early-stage gastric cancer: the cause of false negativity. *World Journal of Surgery* **29**, 418–421.

197. Kitagawa Y. and Kitajima M. (2002). Gastrointestinal cancer and sentinel node navigation surgery. *Journal of Surgical Oncology* **79**, 188–193.

198. Kinami S., Miwa K., Ishii K. *et al.* (2005). [Limited surgery for early gastric cancer using lymphatic basin dissection – a sure method of sentinel node biopsy for gastric cancer]. *Gan To Kagaku Ryoho* **32**, 405–410.

199. Torre W. and Sierra A. (2002). Postoperative complications of lung resection after induction chemotherapy using Paclitaxel (and radiotherapy) for advanced non-small lung cancer. *Journal of Cardiovascular Surgery* **43**, 539–544.

200. MacDonald J.S., Smalley S.R., Benedetti J. *et al.* (2001). Chemoradiotherapy after surgery compared with surgery alone for adenocarcinoma of the stomach or gastroesophageal junction. *New England Journal of Medicine* **345**, 725–730.

201. Benhidjeb T. and Hohenberger P. (2002). Oesophageal cancer. In Souhami R.L., Tannock I., Hohenberger P. and Horiot J.C. (eds.) *Oxford Textbook of Oncology*, 2nd edition. Oxford: Oxford University Press, pp. 1484–1515.

202. Wu P.C. and Posner M.C. (2003). The role of surgery in the management of oesophageal cancer. *The Lancet Oncology* **4**, 481–488.

203. Medical Research Council Oesophageal Cancer Working Group. (2002). Surgical resection with or without preoperative chemotherapy in oesophageal cancer: a randomised controlled trial. *Lancet* **359**, 1727–1733. www.mrc.ac.uk/OurResearch/Recent-Advances/2002-

204. Souhami R.L. and Tobias J. (2005). *Cancer and its Management*, 5th edition. Oxford: Blackwell Publishing, p. 240.

205. Spector N.M., Hicks F.D. and Pickleman J. (2002). Quality of life and symptoms after surgery for gastroesophageal cancer: a pilot study. *Gastroenterology Nursing* **25**, 120–125.

206. Sweed M.R., Schiech L., Barsevick A., Babb J.S. and Goldberg M. Quality of life after esophagectomy for cancer. *Oncology Nursing Forum* **29**, 1127–1131.

207. Chan K.P.W., Eng P., Hsu A.A.L., Huat G.M. and Chow M. (2002). Rigid bronchoscopy and stenting for oesophageal cancer causing airway obstruction. *Chest* **122**, 1069–1072.

208. Watt E. and Whyte F. (2003). The experience of dysphagia and its effects on the quality of life of patients with oesophageal cancer. *European Journal of Cancer Care* **12**, 183–193.

209. Bailey K. (2004). Management of dysphagia in patients with advanced oesophageal cancer. *Gastrointestinal Nursing* **2**, 18–22.

210. Camp-Sorrell D. (2003). Dysphagia. In Yarbro C.H., Frogge M.H. and Goodman M. (eds.) *Cancer Symptom Management*. Boston, MA: Jones and Bartlett, pp. 168–186.

211. Greenlee R.T., Hill-Hamon M.B., Murray T. and Thun M. (2001). Cancer statistics 2001. *CA: A Cancer Journal for Clinicians* **51**, 15–36.

212. Feneley M.R., Thompson P.M. and Kirby R.S. (2004). Radical surgical treatment of prostate cancer: evolution of the techniques. *Cancer Topics* **12**, 6–9.

213. Horwich A., Waxman J., Abel P., Laniado M. and Dearnaley D.P. (2002). Tumours of the prostate. In Souhami R.L., Tannock I., Hohenberger P. and Horiot J.C. (eds.) *Oxford Textbook of Oncology*, 2nd edition. Oxford: Oxford University Press, pp. 1939–1972.

214. Walsh D. (2000). Radical prostatectomy for localized prostate cancer provides durable cancer control with excellent quality of life: a structured debate. *Journal of Urology* **163**, 1802–1807.

215. McGlynn B., Al-Saffar N., Begg H. *et al.* (2004). Management of urinary incontinence following radical prostatectomy. *Urologic Nursing* **24**, 475–515.

216. Colley W. (2003). The assessment of continence problems in adults. *Nursing Times* **99**, 50–51.

217. Butler L., Downe-Wamboldt B., Marsh S., Bell D. and Jarvi K. (2000). Behind the scenes: partners' perceptions of quality of life post radical prostatectomy. *Urologic Nursing* **20**, 254–258.

218. Albertsen P., Gleason D. and Barry M. (1998). Competing risk analysis of men aged 55 to 74 years at diagnosis managed conservatively for clinically localised prostate cancer. *Journal of the American Medical Association* **280**, 975–980.

219. Holzbeierlein J., Peterson M. and Smith J.A. (2001). Variability of results of cavernous nerve stimulation during radical prostatectomy. *Journal of Urology* **165**, 108–110.

220. Fossa S.D. (2002). Sexual dysfunction following pelvic malignancy in men. In Souhami R.L., Tannock I., Hohenberger P. and Horiot J.C. (eds.) *Oxford Textbook of Oncology*, 2nd edition. Oxford: Oxford University Press, pp. 2057–2063.

221. Gray R.E., Fitch M.I., Phillips C. *et al.* (2002). Prostate cancer and erectile dysfunction: men's experiences. *International Journal of Men's Health* **1**, 15–29.

222. Talcott J.A., Reicker P., Clark J.A. *et al.* (1998). Patient-reported symptoms after primary therapy for early prostate cancer: results of a prospective cohort study. *Journal of Clinical Oncology* **16**, 275–283.

223. Chapple A. and Ziebland S. (2002). Prostate cancer: embodied experience and perceptions of masculinity. *Sociology of Health and Illness* **24**, 820–841.

224. Kim E.D., Nath R., Kadmon D. *et al.* (2001). Bilateral nerve graft during radical retropubic prostatectomy: 1-year followup. *Journal of Urology* **165**, 1950–1956.

225. Schroder F.H., Collette L., De Reijke T.M. and Whelan P. (2000). Prostate cancer treated by anti-androgens: is sexual function preserved? *British Journal of Cancer* **82**, 283–290.

226. Porpiglia F., Ragni F., Terrone C. *et al.* (2005). Is laparoscopic unilateral sural nerve grafting during radical prostatectomy effective in retaining sexual potency? *BJU International* **95**, 1267–1271.

227. Helgason A.R., Adolfsson J., Dickman P. *et al.* (1996). Waning sexual function – the most important disease-specific distress for patients with prostate cancer. *British Journal of Cancer* **73**, 1417–1421.

228. Merrick G.S. and Butler W.M. (2003). The dosimetry of brachytherapy-induced erectile dysfunction. *Medical Dosimetry* **28**, 271–274.

229. Dubocq F.M., Bianco F.J. Jr., Maralani S.J., Forman J.D. and Dhabuwala C.B. (1997). Outcome analysis of penile implant surgery after external beam radiation for prostate cancer. *Journal of Urology* **158**, 1787–1790.

230. Kelly D. (2004). Male sexuality in theory and practice. *Nursing Clinics of North America* **39**, 341–356.

231. Setter S.M., Iltz J.L., Fincham J.E., Campbell R.K. and Baker D.E. (2005). Phosphodiesterase-5 inhibitors for erectile dysfunction. *Annals of Pharmacotherapy* **39**, 1286–1295.

232. Padma-Nathan H., McCullough A. and Forest C. (2004). Erectile dysfunction secondary to nerve sparing radical prostatecomy: comparative phosphodiesterase-5 inhibitor efficacy for therapy and novel prevention strategies. *Current Urology Reports* **5**, 467–471.

233. Maliski S.L., Heilemann M.V. and McCorkle R. (2001). Mastery of postprostatectomy incontinence and impotence: his work, her work, our work. *Oncology Nursing Forum* **28**, 985–992.

234. Mick J. (2003). The lived experience of men with erectile dysfunction was reflected in the themes of loss and being alone with it. *Evidence Based Nursing* **6**, 32.

235. Fan A. (2002). Psychological and psychosocial effects of prostate cancer. *Nursing Standard* **1**, 33–37.

236. Powel L.L. (2000). Quality of life in men with urinary incontinence after prostate cancer surgery. *Journal of Wound Ostomy and Continence Nursing* **27**, 174–178.

237. Moore K.N. and Dorey G.F. (1999). Conservative treatment of urinary incontinence in men – a review of the literature. *Physiotherapy* **85**, 77–87.

238. Bates T.S., Wright M.P.J. and Gillat D.A. (1998). Prevalence and impact of incontinence and impotence following total prostatectomy assessed anonymously by the ICS-Male questionnaire. *European Urology* **33**, 165–169.

239. Wille S., Sobottka A., Heidenreich A. and Hofmann R. (2003). Pelvic floor exercises, electrical stimulation and biofeedback after radical prostatectomy: results of a prospective randomized trial. *Journal of Urology* **170**, 490–493.

240. Bryant C.M., Dowell C.J. and Fairbrother G. (2002). Caffeine reduction education to improve urinary symptoms. *British Journal of Nursing* **1**, 72.

241. Nortover J.M.A., Arnott S., Jass J.R. and Williams N.S. (2002). Colorectal cancer. In Souhami R.L., Tannock I., Hohenberger P. and Horiot J.C. (eds.) *Oxford Textbook of Oncology*, 2nd edition. Oxford: Oxford University Press, pp. 1545–1589.

242. Moore H.G., Shoup M., Riedel E. *et al.* (2004). Colorectal cancer pelvic recurrences: determinants of resectability. *Diseases of the Colon and Rectum* **47**, 1599–1606.

243. Valentini V., Balducci M., Tortoreto F. *et al.* (2002). Intraoperative radiotherapy: current thinking. *European Journal of Surgical Oncology* **28**, 180–185.

244. Strassmann G., Walter S., Kolotas C. *et al.* (2000). Reconstruction and navigation system for intraoperative brachytherapy using the flab technique for colorectal tumor bed irradiation. *International Journal of Radiation Oncology Biology Physics* **47**, 1323–1329.

245. Hahnloser D., Haddock M.G. and Nelson H. (2003). Intraoperative radiotherapy in the multimodality approach to colorectal cancer. *Surgical Oncology Clinics of North America* **12**, 993–1013, ix.

246. Patel K., Anthoney D.A., Crellin A.M. *et al.* (2004). Weekly 5-fluorouracil and leucovorin: achieving lower toxicity with higher dose intensity in adjuvant chemotherapy after colorectal resection. *Annals of Oncology* **15**, 568–573.

247. Isbister W.H. (2002). Audit of definitive colorectal surgery in patients with early and advanced colorectal cancer. *Australian and New Zealand Journal of Surgery* **72**, 271–274.

248. Makin G.B., Breen D.J. and Monson J.R.T. (2001). The impact of new technology on surgery for colorectal cancer. *World Journal of Gastroenterology* **7**, 612–621.

249. Hartley J.E., Mehigan B.J., MacDonald A.W., Lee A. and Monson J.R.T. (2000). Patterns of recurrence and survival after laparoscopic and conventional resections for colorectal carcinoma. *Annals of Surgery* **232**, 181–186.

250. O'Brien B., Baddi L. and Benson A. (2005). Ostomy care: the added considerations for cancer patients. *Journal of Supportive Oncology* **3**, 71–72.

251. Salter M. (1997). *Altered Body Image: The Nursing Role*, 2nd edition. London: Ballière Tindall.

252. Rozmovits L. and Ziebland S. (2004). Expressions of loss of adulthood in the narratives of people with colorectal cancer. *Qualitative Health Research* **14**, 187–203.

253. Kelly D. (2004). Patients with colorectal cancer expressed a loss of adulthood related to a loss of professional and sexual identity, dignity, privacy, independence and ability to socialise. *Evidence Based Nursing* **7**, 126.

254. Burch J. (2005). Caring for the older person with a stoma. *Nursing and Residential Care* **7**, 1624–1626.

255. Plant C. and Brierley R. (2001). Helping residents live with a colostomy. *Nursing and Residential Care* **3**, 320–323.

256. Black P.K. and Hyde C. (2002). Parents with colorectal cancer: 'what do I tell the children?' *British Journal of Nursing* **11**, 679–685.

257. Northouse L.L., Schafer J.A., Tipton J. and Metivier L. (1999). The concerns of patients and spouses after the diagnosis of colon cancer: a qualitative analysis. *Journal of Wound Ostomy and Continence Nursing* **26**, 8–17.

258. Persson E., Severinsson E. and Hellstrom A.L. (2004). Spouses' perceptions of and reactions to living with a partner who has undergone surgery for rectal cancer resulting in a stoma. *Cancer Nursing* **27**, 85–91.

259. Solomon M.J., Pager C.K., Kesheva A. *et al.* (2003). What do patients want? Patient preferences and surrogate decision making in the treatment of colorectal cancer. *Diseases of the Colon and Rectum* **46**, 1351–1371.

260. Black P.K. (2004). Psychological, sexual and cultural issues for patients with a stoma. *British Journal of Nursing* **13**, 692–697.

261. Persson E., Gustavsson B., Hellstrom A.L. *et al.* (2005). Information to the relatives of people with ostomies: Is it satisfactory or adequate? *Journal of Wound Ostomy and Continence Nursing* **32**, 238–245.

262. Persson E., Gustavsson B., Hellstrom A.L., Lappas G. and Hulten L. (2005). Ostomy patients' perceptions of quality of care. *Journal of Advanced Nursing* **49**, 51–58.

263. Makrantonakis P.D., Galani E. and Harper P.G. (2004). Non-small cell lung cancer in the elderly. *The Oncologist* **9**, 556–560.

264. Yancik R. and Ries L.A. (2000). Aging and cancer in America. Demographic and epidemiologic perspectives. *Hematology/Oncology Clinics of North America* **14**, 17–23.

265. Rotter N., Wagner H., Fuchshuber S. and Issing W.J. (2003). Cervical metastases of microcystic adnexal carcinoma in an otherwise healthy woman. *European Archives of Otorhinolaryngology* **260**, 254–257.

266. Dexter E.U., Jahangir N. and Kohman L.J. (2004). Resection for lung cancer in the elderly patient. *Thoracic Surgery Clinics* **14**, 163–171.

267. Clarke C.M. (2001). Rationing scarce life-sustaining resources on the basis of age. *Journal of Advanced Nursing* **35**, 799–804.

268. Fitzsimmons D. (2004). What are we trying to measure? Rethinking approaches to health outcome assessment for the older person with cancer. *European Journal of Cancer Care* **13**, 416–423.

269. Bowman K.F., Deimling G.T., Smerglia V., Sage P. and Kahana B. (2003). Appraisal of the cancer experience by older long-term survivors. *Psycho-oncology* **12**, 226–238.

270. Bailey C.M. and Gilbert J.M. (2002). Avoiding inappropriate surgery for secondary rectal cancer. *European Journal of Surgical Oncology* **28**, 220–224.

271. Smith T.J., Rothenberg S.S., Brooks M. *et al.* Thoracoscopic surgery in childhood cancer. *Pediatric Hematology and Oncology* **24**, 429–435.

272. Derks W., De Leeuw J.R., Hordijk G.J. and Winnubst J.A. (2003). Elderly patients with head and neck

cancer: short-term effects of surgical treatment on quality of life. *Clinical Otolaryngology and Allied Sciences* **28**, 399–405.

273. Zabrodsky M., Calabrese L., Tosoni A. *et al.* (2004). Major surgery in elderly head and neck cancer patients: immediate and long-term surgical results and complication rates. *Surgical Oncology* **13**, 249–255.

274. Papadopoulos S.M., Selden N.R., Quint D.J. *et al.* (2002). Immediate spinal cord decompression for cervical spinal cord injury: feasibility and outcome. *Journal of Trauma* **52**, 323–332.

275. Odendaal J.V. and Apffelstaedt J.P. (2003). Limited surgery and tamoxifen in the treatment of elderly breast cancer patients. *World Journal of Surgery* **27**, 125–129.

276. Law W.L., Chu K.W. and Tung P.H. (2002). Laparoscopic colorectal resection: a safe option for elderly patients. *Journal of the American College of Surgeons* **195**, 768–773.

277. Conti B., Brega M.P.P., Lequagli C., Magnani B. and Cataldo I. (2002). Major surgery in lung cancer in elderly patients? Risk factors analysis and long-term results. *Minerva Chirurgica* **57**, 317–321.

278. de Perrot M., Licker M., Reymond M.A., Robert J. and Spiliopoulos A. (1999). Influence of age on operative mortality and long-term survival after lung resection for bronchiogenic carcinoma. *European Respiratory Journal* **14**, 419–422.

279. Sakayama K., Kidani T., Fujibuchi T. *et al.* (2003). Definitive intraoperative radiotherapy for musculoskeletal sarcomas and malignant lymphoma in combination with surgical excision. *International Journal of Clinical Oncology* **8**, 174–179.

280. Brock M.V., Kim M.P., Hooker C.M. *et al.* (2004). Pulmonary resection in octogenerians with stage I non-small-cell lung cancer: a 22 year experience. *Annals of Thoracic Surgery* **77**, 271–277.

281. Hahn E.A. and Cella D. (2003). Health outcomes assessment in vulnerable populations: measurement challenges and recomendations. *Archives of Physical Medical Rehabilitation* **84(suppl. 2)**, s35–s42.

282. Nolan M., Davies S., Brown J., Keady J. and Nolan J. (2002). *Longitudinal Study of the Effectiveness of Educational Preparation to Meet the Needs of Older People and Carers. The AGEIN (Advancing Gerontological Education in Nursing) Project Final Report*. London: English National Board.

283. Ford P. and McCormack B. (2000). Keeping the person in the centre of nursing. *Nursing Standard* **14**, 40–44.

284. Roth T.M., Secord A.A., Havrilesky L.J., Jones E. and Clarke-Pearson D.L. (2003). High dose rate intra-operative radiotherapy for recurrent cervical cancer and nodal disease. *Gynecologic Oncology* **91**, 258–260.

285. Poen J.C., Ford J.M. and Niederhuber J.E. (1999). Chemoradiotherapy in the management of localized tumors of the pancreas. *Annals of Surgical Oncology* **6**, 117–122.

286. Hewitt M., Herdman R. and Holland J. (2004). *Meeting Psychosocial Needs of Women with Breast Cancer*. Washington, DC: National Academies Press.

287. Hendren S.K., O'Connor B.I., Liu M. *et al.* (2005). Prevalence of male and female sexual dysfunction is high following surgery for rectal cancer. *Annals of Surgery* **242**, 212–223.

288. Happ M.B., Roesch T. and Kagan S. H. (2004). Communication needs, methods, and perceived voice quality following head and neck surgery: a literature review. *Cancer Nursing* **27**, 1–9.

289. Semple C.T., Sullivan K., Dunwoordy L. and Kernohan W.G. (2004). Psychosocial interventions for patients with head and neck cancer: past, present, future. *Cancer Nursing* **27**, 434–441.

290. Callahan C. (2004). Facial disfigurement and sense of self in head and neck cancer. *Social Work in Health Care* **40**, 73–87.

291. Katz M.R., Irish J.C., Devins G.M., Rodin G.M. and Gullane P.J. (2003). Psychosocial adjustment in head and neck cancer: the impact of disfigurement, gender and social support. *Head and Neck* **25**, 103–112.

292. Chen M. and Chang H. (2004). Physical symptom profiles of depressed and non-depressed patients with cancer. *Palliative Medicine* **18**, 712–718.

293. Tesch R.S., Denardin O.V.P., Baptista C.A. and Dias F.L. (2004). Depression levels in chronic orofacial pain patients: a pilot study. *Journal of Oral Rehabilitation* **31**, 926–932.

294. Rogers S.N., Lowe D., Fisher S.E., Brown J.S. and Vaughan E.D. (2002). Health-related quality of life and clinical function after primary surgery for oral cancer. *British Journal of Oral and Maxillofacial Surgery* **40**, 11–18.

295. Schliephake H. and Jamil M.U. (2002). Prospective evaluation of quality of life after oncologic surgery for oral cancer. *International Journal of Oral and Maxillofacial Surgery* **31**, 427–433.

296. Mishra S., Bhatnagar S., Jha R.R. and Singhal A.K. (2005). Airway management of patients undergoing oral cancer surgery: a retrospective study. *European Journal of Anaesthesiology* **22**, 510–514.

297. Ito O., Igawa H.H., Suzuki S. *et al.* (2005). Evaluation of the donor site in patients who underwent reconstruction with a free radial forearm flap. *Journal of Reconstructive Microsurgery* **21**, 113–117.

298. Eguchi T., Nakasuka T., Mori Y. and Takato T. (2005). Total reconstruction of the upper lip after resection of a malignant melanoma. *Scandinavian Journal of Plastic Reconstructive Surgery* **39**, 45–47.

299. Holloman E.L. and Carter K.D. (2005). Modification of the Cutler–Beard procedure using donor achilles tendon for upper eyelid reconstruction. *Opthalmic Plastic Reconstructive Surgery* **1**, 267–270.

300. Yamamoto Y. (2005). Mid-facial reconstruction after maxillectomy. *International Journal of Clinical Oncology* **10**, 218–222.

301. Singletary S.E. (2001). New issues in surgical management. In Bonadonna G., Hortobagyi G.N. and Gianni A.M. (eds.) *Textbook of Breast Cancer*, 2nd edition. London: Taylor and Francis, pp. 99–118.

302. Committee on the Safety of Silicone Breast Implants (CSSBI). (1999). *Safety of Silicone Breast Implants*. Washington, DC: Institute of Medicine.

303. Schusterman M.A. (1998). The free TRAM flap. *Clinical Plastic Surgery* **25**, 191–195.

304. Deutsche M.F., Smith M.R., Wang B., Ainsle N. and Schusterman M.A. (1999). Immediate breast reconstruction with the TRAM flap after neoadjuvant therapy. *Annals of Plastic Surgery* **42**, 240–244.

305. Wolf L. (2004). The information needs of women who have undergone breast reconstruction. Part II: Information giving and content of information. *European Journal of Oncology Nursing* **8**, 315–324.

306. Rayter Z. (1998). Early experience of the nipple/areaola tattoo after breast reconstruction. *European Journal of Surgical Oncology* **24**, 629–630.

307. Cunnick G.H. and Mokbel K. (2004). Skin sparing mastectomy. *American Journal of Surgery* **188**, 78–84.

308. Gerber B., Krause A., Reimer T. *et al.* (2003). Skin-sparing mastectomy with conservation of the nipple-areola complex and autologous reconstruction is an oncologically safe procedure. *Annals of Surgery* **238**, 120–127.

309. Simmons R.M., Brennan M., Christos P., King V. and Osborne M. (2002). Analysis of nipple/areolar involvement with mastectomy: can the areola be preserved? *Annals of Surgical Oncology* **9**, 165–168.

310. Simmons R.M., Hollenbeck S.T. and Latrenta G.S. (2004). Two-year follow up of areola-sparing mastectomy with immediate reconstruction. *American Journal of Surgery* **188**, 403–406.

311. Feig B.W. (2003). Principles of palliative surgery. In Fisch B.M. and Bruera E.D. (eds.) *Handbook of Advanced Cancer Care*. Cambridge: Cambridge University Press, pp. 22–25.

312. Suleyman O.N., Talu G.K., Camlica H. and Erdine S. (2004). Efficacy of coeliac plexus and splanchnic nerve blockades in body and tail located pancreatic cancer pain. *European Journal of Pain* **8**, 539–545.

313. Mercadante S., Catala E., Arcuri E. and Casuccio A. (2003). Celiac plexus block for pancreatic cancer pain: factors influencing pain, symptoms and quality of life. *Journal of Pain and Symptom Management* **26**, 1140–1147.

314. Varghese B.T., Kishy R.C., Sebastian P. and Joseph E. (2002). Combined sphenopalatine ganglion and mandibular nerve neurolytic block for pain due to advanced head and neck cancer. *Palliative Medicine* **16**, 447–448.

315. Hockel M. (2003). Surgical treatment of locally advanced and recurrent cervical carcinoma: overview on current standard and new developments. *Onkologie* **26**, 452–455.

316. Arroyo C., Andrews H., Rozet F., Cathelineau X. and Vallancien G. (2005). Laparoscopic prostate-sparing radical cystectomy: the Montsouris technique and preliminary results. *Journal of Endourology* **19**, 424–428.

317. Ward J.F., Sebo T.J., Blute M.L. and Zincke H. (2005). Salvage surgery for radiorecurrent prostate cancer: contemporary outcomes. *Journal of Urology* **173**, 1156–1160.

318. Al-Rashedy M., Issa M.E., Ballester P. and Ammori B.J. Laparoscopic surgery for the management of obstruction of the gastric outlet and small bowel following previous laparotomy for major upper gastrointestinal resection or cancer palliation: a new concept. *Journal of Laparoendoscopic and Advanced Surgical Techniques. Part A* **15**, 153–159.

319. Cummins E.R., Vick K.D. and Poole G.V. (2004). Incurable colorectal carcinoma: the role of surgical palliation. *American Surgeon* **70**, 433–437.

320. Asoglu O., Porter L., Donohue J.H. and Cha S.S. (2005). Laparoscopy for the definitive diagnosis of intra-abdominal lymphoma. *Mayo Clinic Proceedings* **80**, 625–631.

321. Ampil F.L. and Sadasivan K.K. (2001). Prophylactic and therapeutic fixation of weight-bearing long bones with metastatic cancer. *Southern Medical Journal* **94**, 394–396.

322. Olerud C. and Jonsson B. (1996). Surgical palliation of symptomatic spinal metastases. *Acta Orthopaedica Scandinavica* **67**, 513–522.

323. Shaaban A.A., Mosbah A., Abdel-Latif M., Mohsen T. and Mokhtar A.A. (2003). Outcome of patients with continent urinary reconstruction and a solitary functioning kidney. *BJU International* **92**, 987–992.

324. Beland M.D., Dupuy D.E. and Mayo-Smith W.W. (2005). Percutaneous cryoablation of symptomatic extraabdominal metastatic disease: preliminary results.

AJR American Journal of Roentgenology **184**, 926–930.

325. Jarrett N. and Maslin-Prothero S. (2004). Communication, the patients and the palliative care team. In Payne S., Seymour J. and Ingleton C. (eds.) *Palliative Care Nursing: Principles and Evidence for Practice*. Maidenhead: Open University Press, pp. 142–162.

326. Sawyer H. (2000). Meeting the information needs of cancer patients. *Professional Nurse* **15**, 244–247.

CHAPTER TWELVE

Chemotherapy

Lisa Dougherty and Christopher Bailey

The term 'chemotherapy' was originally coined at the beginning of the 20th century to refer to the theoretical possibility of utilising substances with specific toxicity towards micro-organisms such as bacteria.[1] Cancer chemotherapy – the administration of antineoplastic agents either alone or in combination – frequently makes use of drugs that disrupt cellular replication by inhibiting the synthesis of new genetic material or causing irreparable damage to DNA itself.[2]

> *Cyto-* (or *-cyte*) = cells or a cell
> *chemo-* = chemical
> *neoplasm* = new or abnormal growth of tissue in some part of the body, especially a tumour

Chemotherapy in cancer may be used in the expectation of achieving a cure, when all cancer cells are destroyed and life expectancy is similar to the life expectancy of a person who does not have cancer. It may be used to achieve control over the disease by preventing or slowing down the growth of a malignant tumour, and thus prolonging survival, and it may be used palliatively in the management of symptoms such as pain or breathlessness. Chemotherapy used for the palliation of symptoms is not expected to achieve either cure or control.

- *Definitive chemotherapy* is chemotherapy given as the sole treatment of a disease; the term *salvage chemotherapy* is sometimes used to denote treatment given to patients who have relapsed following initially successful treatment with another modality (such as surgery or radiotherapy). Experimental chemotherapy is given to investigate the usefulness of a new drug whose role is not proven at the time of treatment.
- *Adjuvant chemotherapy* refers to the use of antineoplastic drugs after removal of the primary tumour to eliminate as many remaining cancerous cells or micrometastases as possible.
- *Neoadjuvant chemotherapy* refers to the use of chemotherapy or radiotherapy before surgery to 'debulk' or reduce the size of the primary tumour and to maximise the effectiveness of subsequent therapies. In the treatment of rectal cancer, for example, neoadjuvant radiotherapy may be given to patients with resectable tumours, to destroy microscopic tumour cells that could not be surgically removed without increasing the risk of major post-operative complications. If the tumour is not resectable (which may be the case if it has become attached to adjacent organs such as the bladder), pre-operative radiotherapy may be given to shrink the tumour and 'downstage' the disease.[3]

When evaluating the response to chemotherapy, it remains remarkably difficult to define 'cure' reliably in cancer care. One definition is that cure is achieved when the life expectancy of a person with cancer is the same as for a person of the same age and sex who has not been affected by cancer.[4]

Many research trials use duration of survival as a measure of the success of treatment. The aim of treatment is to prevent cancer cells from 'multiplying, invading, metastasizing and ultimately killing'[5] the patient, and in general, survival is likely to be longer with treatment than if treatment had not been given, but shorter than it would have been had the person not developed cancer. Objective criteria are needed, based on the immediate response of the tumour and a patient's physiological status, to evaluate the effects of treatment. Tumour regression often occurs early and can be expressed in terms of tumour size. To summarise some key definitions of response:

- *complete response* (CR) – disappearance of all known disease
- *partial response* (PR) – a decrease in total tumour of 50% or more
- no change (NC) – neither a 50% decrease nor a 25% increase in tumour size can be demonstrated
- *progressive disease* (PD) – increase in tumour size of 25% of more.

(Adapted from Horwich A. (ed.) (1995). *Oncology: A Multidisciplinary Textbook*. London: Chapman and Hall, p. 136.)[6]

Patients' own accounts and reflections are also extremely valuable to clinicians, and often help the patient to understand and make sense of their illness and treatment. Measures of performance status are sometimes used to assess response to treatment (e.g. Karnofsky Performance Status Scale,[7] visual rating scales, verbal rating scales, and patient diaries). Measurement tools such as these often reflect one aspect of function rather than multidimensional function,[8] and may not give a comprehensive picture of the effects of illness or treatment.

The cell cycle

The sequence of phases through which cells must pass as they replicate (the *cell cycle*) is the fundamental biological context for many of the anticancer drugs.

The term 'cell cycle' refers to the process through which cells, both normal and malignant, grow and replicate (see Figure 12.1). The cycle comprises five phases: G_0, G_1, S, G_2, and M. The 'G' phases are gap phases, in which cells are preparing for active DNA (deoxyribonucleic acid) synthesis and mitosis (division), or are resting.

- G_1 is the first gap or growth phase (also known as the intermitotic phase), in which cells prepare for DNA synthesis by producing RNA (ribonucleic acid) and protein. Cells in G_0 are resting (that is, not preparing for cell division), though they remain viable and are capable of division if suitably stimulated. G_0 is considered a subphase of G_1.
- S is the synthesis phase, in which cells double their DNA content (DNA is the coded genetic information required for the growth, repair, and reproduction of cells). Many cytotoxic drugs work by disrupting genetic codes during DNA synthesis.
- G_2 is the second gap or growth phase (premitotic phase). Synthesis of RNA and proteins continues in preparation for mitosis.
- M is the mitotic phase, in which cell division (mitosis) takes place. The cell divides into two daughter cells, each containing the same number and type of chromosomes as the parent cell. At the end of the M phase, cells either rejoin the cell cycle at G_1, or enter the resting subphase G_0.

Cytotoxic drugs affect both normal and malignant cells by altering activity during one or more phases of the cell cycle. Though both types of cells are destroyed by chemotherapy, normal cells have a greater ability to repair minor damage and remain viable than malignant cells. The susceptibility of malignant cells to irreparable damage is utilised to achieve the therapeutic effects of cytotoxic chemotherapy.

Schwarz and Yarbro (in Perry[1]) describe the delicate balancing act of cytotoxic chemotherapy in this way:

> The metabolism of the cancer cell has been thought to be so similar to that of the normal cell that investigators have been forced to use rather minute differences through which drugs might exert a differential effect. Traditionally, the most important such

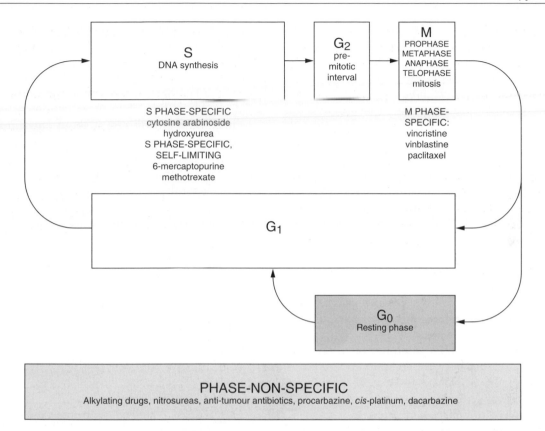

Figure 12.1   The cell cycle and the relationship of anti-tumour drug action to the cycle. Reproduced with permission from Brunton L.L., Lazo J.S. and Parker K.L. (eds.) (2006) *Goodman and Gilman's The Pharmacological Basis of Therapeutics*, 11th edition. New York: McGraw Hill, p. 1320.[2]

difference has been considered to be the rapid rate of division of the cancer cell relative to most other body tissues . . . this small difference allowed chemotherapeutic cures in rapidly proliferating animal tumours such as the L1210 mouse leukaemia [p.1].

Human tumours, however, are more complex, and follow a 'Gompertzian' growth curve (see Figure 12.2) in which there are resting, non-proliferating cells that are resistant to chemotherapy.

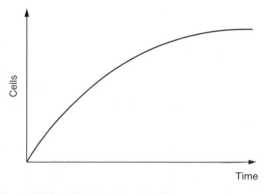

Figure 12.2   Gompertzian growth curve.

Tumour growth

Tumour growth is affected by *cell cycling time* and *growth fraction*.

Cell cycling time

Originally tumours were thought to grow because they consisted of cells that multiplied more rapidly than cells in the surrounding tissue. In fact, the average cell cycle of 48 hours for human tumour cells is slightly longer than the cycle of non-malignant cells. If the rate of cell division were the only factor to determine tumour growth, cancers would grow at the same rate as or more slowly than normal tissue and cause no problems.

When a normal cell divides, it does so only to replace a cell that has been lost and in this way a constant cell population is maintained. In tumour cells the control mechanism appears to have been lost: as the cell divides it adds to existing numbers of cells and increases the total population. The cause of this phenomenon remains unclear.

A measure of the rate of tumour growth is the time taken for a given population of malignant cells to double in size (*doubling time*). If the cell cycle takes between 15 and 120 hours, the doubling time can be between 96 hours and 500 days, depending on the histological type of the tumour, its age, and whether it is a primary or metastatic growth. A shorter doubling time (less than 30 days) is seen with teratomas, non-Hodgkin's lymphomas, and acute leukaemias; common solid tumours such as squamous cell carcinoma of the bronchus and adenocarcinoma of the breast and bowel have doubling times in excess of 70 days. In any patient the growth of a cancer is only detectable and observable during the last 10–14 of its 35–40 doubling times.

Growth fraction

In the early stages of development tumour volume is low, but the proportion of viable cells in the active division cycle at any one time (the *growth fraction*) is high.[9] However, most malignant neoplasms are only detected at a later stage. By this time, poor tumour vascularity and consequent hypoxia, or poor nutrient supply together with other factors, mean that the rate of growth is decelerating, and the tumour contains a high fraction of slowly dividing or non-cycling (G_0) cells (i.e. the growth fraction is low).[10] Studies of adenocarcinoma in mice have shown that as the tumour increases in size, the mass doubling time (time taken for the tumour mass to double)

increases many-fold, while the growth fraction is drastically reduced (that is, the mass doubling time is inversely proportional to the growth fraction).[11] This pattern of growth is close to what is known as a *Gompertzian* growth curve: cells accumulate slowly at first, then more rapidly, achieving a maximum growth rate at about one-third of maximum tumour volume.[1] The rate of growth then slows gradually and almost levels out (the 'plateau phase') (see Figure 12.2).

Most chemotherapeutic agents are most effective against rapidly dividing cells, i.e. when tumours are still in the proliferating stage. Some are phase specific, and are most effective against cells in a particular phase of the cell cycle. Therefore, at the point at which most tumours are detected clinically, the situation is not immediately best suited for intervention with cytotoxic therapy. However, reducing the number of malignant cells with surgery, radiotherapy or non-cycle-specific drugs may lead to an increase in the rate of cell division and may induce (or 'recruit') resting cells to re-enter the cell cycle, where they are more vulnerable to cycle-specific agents. The proportion of malignant cells destroyed may therefore increase over repeated courses of treatment.

First-order kinetics

Cancer cells appear to be destroyed by chemotherapy according to first-order kinetics, that is, a certain dose of drug will destroy a constant proportion of malignant cells, rather than a constant number. Pratt *et al.*[12] explain some of the implications of 'first-order kinetics':

> . . . it will take just as much drug to lower the tumour cell number from 10^6 to 10^3 (a loss of less than 1 mg of tissue) as to lower the tumour cell number from 10^9 to 10^6 (a loss of 1 g of tissue) . . . at the time of diagnosis of a number of disseminated malignant diseases, as many as 10^{12} tumour cells may be present. This may be close to the fatal number for certain tumours. Successful chemotherapy may kill 99.9% of the cells . . . and still leave 10^9 cells in the patient. This number is barely detectable, and clinically, the patient may appear to be 'in remission'. But it is necessary to continue therapy even in the face of an apparent remission to eliminate the many malignant cells that are still present . . . to produce a cure, therapy must be

continued until the last tumour cell is killed. There is ample experimental evidence that one viable tumour cell can produce a tumour that will kill a susceptible host animal [pp.29–30].

Pharmacology

The way that cancer chemotherapy is selected, calculated, and administered depends on a variety of pharmacological factors. Knowledge of the *pharmacodynamic* properties of a drug ('what drugs do and how they do it') is 'essential to the choice of drug therapy' and 'the basis of intelligent use of medicines'.[13] Doses have to be set to achieve neither too much nor too little of the right effect. Too much may cause unwanted and dangerous toxic effects; too little may not achieve any therapeutic goals.

Pharmacokinetics is about achieving:

> . . . the right effect at the right intensity, at the right time, for the right duration, with minimum risk of unpleasantness or harm . . . [and] . . . is concerned with the rate at which drug molecules cross cell membranes to enter the body, to distribute within it and to leave the body, as well as with the structural changes [metabolism] to which they are subject within it [p.83].[13]

The therapeutic effect of a drug thus rests on achieving a balance between what the drug does, its action or its pharmacodynamic properties, and its behaviour within the body, or its pharmacokinetic properties, to achieve the right kind of effect with the right intensity and duration.

Route of administration
The route of administration is dictated by the characteristics of individual drugs and is chosen to optimise drug availability. Careful selection of an appropriate route of administration can improve the anti-cancer effect of a drug by enabling a higher concentration to reach the tumour.

Drug distribution
The distribution and transport of drugs within the body can significantly influence the effects of chemotherapy. After they have been administered, drugs can bind to serum albumin, which affects the proportion of free or pharmacologically active drug in the bloodstream. When free drug leaves the bloodstream (for example, when it is metabolised or excreted), it is replaced by drug that was previously protein bound. Drugs sometimes compete for binding sites: one drug can displace another from a binding site, which can lead to toxic levels of the drug that is displaced. Methotrexate is displaced by aspirin and probenecid and possibly by other non-steroidal anti-inflammatories in this way, causing severe toxicity.[13]

Biotransformation
Cytotoxic drugs undergo a wide range of metabolic transformations, including oxidation, reduction, hydrolysis, or configuration, most of which take place in the liver.

Excretion
Drugs are commonly excreted via the kidneys or the liver. The function of these organs is crucial to successful treatment, as impaired clearance may cause increased toxicity.

Drug interactions
Interactions between drugs are not uncommon. One drug may either inhibit or potentiate the action of another, thus modifying its therapeutic or toxic effects, or its enzyme inhibition or induction.

Drug resistance
The value of any cytotoxic agent can be severely limited by tumour resistance. There are two main types of tumour resistance. *Primary resistance* occurs when tumours show no response when drugs are administered; it is thought to be a major factor in the failure of chemotherapy drugs. *Secondary resistance* is said to occur when tumour regression is initially seen following administration of a drug, but is temporary, with the tumour reappearing and the patient relapsing. Factors contributing to secondary resistance include:

- variations in drug bioavailability
- drug metabolism or elimination
- tumours possibly located in 'sanctuary sites'
- changes in cell kinetics
- drug-related toxicity in the recipient
- reduced blood supply to the tumour.

There are four main categories of drug resistance:

1. *kinetic resistance* – anti-cancer drugs may be cell cycle or cell cycle phase specific, so cells can be less sensitive to particular agents by virtue of their position in the cell cycle
2. *biochemical resistance* will occur if drugs are not transported across the cell membrane, if they are not activated within the cell, if they are confronted with an excess of their target substance within the cell, or if cells possess an enhanced ability to repair their DNA[1]
3. *pharmacological resistance* – tumour cells may be located in areas where it is difficult to achieve the required drug concentration, and may therefore in effect be less sensitive. The central nervous system is one such area. Changes in the way a drug is metabolised in an individual patient may also make it more difficult to achieve adequate concentration of a drug[1]
4. *selected/induced resistance* – one possible explanation of the biological reasons for drug resistance (or reduced sensitivity) in tumours is that it is due to genetic factors. This type of resistance is known as *selected resistance*. However, it is also possible that resistance is a direct result of exposure to an anti-cancer drug. This type of resistance is known as *induced resistance*. Resistance may also be *intrinsic*, as opposed to *acquired*: that is to say, it is present in cells that have not previously been exposed to a particular drug.

Multidrug resistance (MDR) is now a well-recognised phenomenon: exposure to a single drug is followed by cross-resistance to other apparently unrelated drugs. Impaired drug transport appears to be a critical factor in MDR, resulting in reduced or altered drug accumulation in the cell. Two mechanisms have been proposed to account for this: (a) drug enters the cell at the normal rate but is removed by a biochemical 'pump'; (b) a biochemical barrier controls entry to the cell. Evidence suggests that a cell surface glycoprotein (P-glycoprotein) acts as a pump, removing toxins from the cell. Drugs are thought to become bound to P-glycoprotein, and are subsequently moved across the cell membrane and

out of the cell. Tumour cells appear to be able to increase the amount of P-glycoprotein on their surface membrane.

Effects of cytotoxic drugs

All cytotoxic drugs share two properties: an ability to inhibit the process of cell division and an inability to distinguish between normal and malignant cells. The effects of cytotoxic drugs are most obvious in normal tissues where cells are dividing most rapidly, and it is the appearance of toxicity in these tissues that limits their usefulness as anti-cancer agents.

Tissues that are rapidly and continuously proliferating include the following:

- *bone marrow* – here there is continuous cellular repair and replacement of two types of cell: *stem cells* (progenitor cells from which all other cells are derived) and *differentiated* (mature) cells
- *gastrointestinal tract* – the mucosal epithelium that lines the gastrointestinal tract is composed of cells that frequently divide to repair the day-to-day damage caused by nutrients and waste on their way through the gut
- *hair follicles* – between 60% and 90% of hair follicles are actively dividing at any one time. Cytotoxic drugs can damage the epithelial cells of the hair follicle: stem cells at the base of the shaft atrophy, hairs become thinner and more fragile, and can break off or fall away[14] (see Research study 12.1)
- *testicular germ cells* – the germinal epithelium of the seminiferous tubules of the male testicles replicates continuously throughout adult life and is therefore highly sensitive to the effects of anti-cancer agents.[4]

Some tissues proliferate slowly and continuously (e.g. tracheobronchial and vascular epithelium), some proliferate in a cyclical fashion (e.g. glandular female breast cells and the endometrial lining of the uterus), some possess the capacity to proliferate after injury (e.g. liver and bone tissue), and some do not proliferate at all (e.g. skeletal and cardiac muscle, cartilage, and neurones).

Research study 12.1

Batchelor D. (2001). Hair and cancer chemotherapy – consequences and nursing care: a literature study. *European Journal of Cancer Care* **10**, 147–163.[15]

In this study, Diane Batchelor discusses the psychological, social, cultural, and political importance of our hair and relates this to the hair loss that occurs with some types of anti-cancer chemotherapy. She points out, for example, that:

Loss of hair symbolizes the destruction of personality, diminution of self or lowering of status, either in the course of nature, such as ageing, or artificially by an act of man, such as shaving the head. Natural hair loss whether temporary or permanent is usually deplored, as opposed to hair that is voluntarily removed [p.147].

She includes personal accounts of the experience of hair loss as a result of treatment for cancer, and refers to evidence that for some women with breast cancer, hair loss may be more difficult to manage than the loss of a breast. Although hair loss is usually reversible, Batchelor refers to reports of people declining treatment for fear of its disfiguring effects (p.148).

The paper discusses the underlying mechanisms and incidence of chemotherapy-induced hair loss, and provides a list of drugs that cause it, while acknowledging that the literature is not unanimous about which drugs can be categorised as 'mild', 'moderate', or 'severe' in this respect (p.150). A number of potentially preventative measures are identified, including hypothermia (application of cold to the scalp), and mechanisms of action and evidence of effectiveness are discussed (pp.152ff). The possibility of developing scalp metastases as a result of hypothermia to prevent hair loss is recognised, and measures to minimise the risk of it are identified from the literature. Camp Sorrell notes that while scalp hypothermia was used until the early 1990s to minimise hair loss,[16] it is no longer recommended because of the risk of scalp micrometastasis. This places heightened importance on psychologically supportive measures and imaginative management of appearance and self-image.

Alopecia from anti-cancer chemotherapy may be unavoidable and Batchelor emphasises the importance of understanding its meaning as a prerequisite for nursing care. Patients appreciate knowing what to expect, and specific information can have a positive effect. Batchelor helpfully summarises the key categories of information that may be required (p.157). Many people will need to manage treatment-related hair loss at home, which makes self-management strategies especially important. Strategies to minimise hair loss include: adopting a shorter hair style, avoiding daily shampooing, advice on washing and combing techniques, changing to satin pillow-cases, and avoiding hair clips, hair dryers, dyes, and so on (pp.157ff). Batchelor also helpfully discusses how people may be supported to cope with the experience of hair loss when it occurs. She concludes that information and self-care strategies can help people to 'move through a potentially devastating experience to a renewed sense of well being' (p.160).

Giving anti-cancer chemotherapy

Single-agent continuous cytotoxic therapy

Priestman[4] notes that in the early period of anti-cancer chemotherapy the principles of antimicrobial chemotherapy were used as the basis for single-agent continuous therapy, the object being to produce and maintain a constant level of cytotoxic agent in the patient until:

. . . unacceptable toxicity, drug resistance, or cure resulted. Toxicity determined the amount of drug that could be given. As it was considered that the blood level of the drug should be as high as possible, the dose was adjusted upwards until toxicity was apparent and then maintained at a level which caused minimal side-

effects (such as slight nausea or a small depression in the white cell count) [p. 55].

It is now recognised, however, that with a few exceptions, single-agent chemotherapy does not lead to cure.[17]

Continuous infusional chemotherapy

Anti-cancer chemotherapy is often most effective when tumour cells are cycling, or when they are in a specific phase of the cell cycle. When chemotherapy is given by continuous infusion, the anti-cancer agent is present when a sensitive phase of the cycle is reached, irrespective of the length of the cell cycle. The transport of the agent across the tumour cell membrane may depend not only on drug concentration but also on the length of time the drug is available to the cell membrane. Most chemotherapeutic agents have a short pharmacological half-life and may be more effective if tumour cells are exposed to them for prolonged periods, which cannot be achieved if they are given by intermittent bolus injection. When given continuously, the concentration of drug in the plasma may be lower than levels reached immediately following bolus injection or intermittent bolus infusion, and some of the toxicities associated with a drug may thus be avoided. Perry[1] notes, for example, that:

> The antitumour efficacy of some chemotherapeutic agents appears to be related to delivered dose intensity. Because of diminished toxicity, some chemotherapeutic agents, such as 5-fluorouracil, may be given in more dose-intense schedules if delivered by continuous infusion. However, measured dose intensity between differing schedules of administration may not relate to antitumour activity [p. 145].

Intermittent chemotherapy

Populations of normal cells are diminished by treatment with anti-cancer chemotherapy, but initially recover far more rapidly than malignant cells. Because restoration is achieved more quickly in normal tissue than in malignant tissue, if a series of treatments is given with intervals to allow normal tissue to recover, it may be possible to eradicate a tumour without jeopardising the population of normal cells. Timing of the treatments is very important. If the interval between treatments is too short, normal stem cells will not have recovered sufficiently, and cumulative toxicity will result, preventing adequate treatment. If the interval between treatments is too long, tumour cell recovery will be complete, and tumour size will remain static or increase between treatments. Dividing chemotherapy regimens into short, intensive treatments followed by intervals is known as intermittent chemotherapy. Intermittent chemotherapy has enabled combinations of drugs to be used to increase response rates without irreversible toxicity.

Combination chemotherapy

Chemotherapeutic agents have a variety of actions on the dividing cell. A tumour cell that is resistant to one drug with a particular mode of action may well be sensitive to a different agent with an alternative form of cytotoxicity. Combining drugs with different mechanisms of action should reduce the likelihood of resistance, increase the fractional cell kill, and improve response rates. All drugs used in combination chemotherapy should be of proven value in the disease they are intended to treat; they should have different modes of cytotoxic action and, if possible, the dose-limiting toxicities of the chosen agents should be different, so that the additive toxicity does not limit the dose intensity of the treatment.

High-dose chemotherapy

A few drugs (those that principally cause toxicity to the bone marrow) may be used in very high doses if bone marrow is taken from the patient prior to treatment and returned later (autologous bone marrow transplantation or 'autografting'). In this way doses of a drug that are very toxic to the bone marrow may be given, as the autograft of bone marrow or stem cells is not exposed to the chemotherapeutic agent. Following re-infusion of the autograft, the patient's blood count will gradually return to normal. Autografting of bone marrow does not, however, reduce the toxicities of high-dose chemotherapy that affect tissues other than the bone marrow.

Drug dosage and scheduling

There is a definite relationship between drug dose and response in sensitive tumour cell populations. Therapeutic effect may be compromised by an inadequate dose of chemotherapy, and commonly results from a reduction of the prescribed dose. Three parameters are used to define the dose component of treatment: size, total amount delivered, and rate.

Care settings

While some systemic chemotherapy can be provided in the home, most is now administered in an outpatient setting or in day-care units.[18] Despite the introduction of new and more intensive forms of chemotherapy, relatively few people require hospital admission for administration of their chemotherapy, unless they are acutely ill or require close monitoring.[19] Allwood *et al.* point out that the wards in which many patients receive routine chemotherapy serve a broad range of cancer patients, which may be inappropriate given the different needs of, for example, people receiving treatment for early-stage cancer and those receiving palliative care.[18] It may be difficult for staff to balance the needs of short-stay patients with the longer-term needs of others, and they suggest that separate nursing teams may be needed to care for different groups of patients. They argue that most patients in the UK will continue to receive their chemotherapy as outpatients, but that facilities are often less than ideal, leading to delays and other problems. They call for both better resourcing and better organisation of outpatient chemotherapy services.[18]

Development and assessment of new anti-cancer chemotherapy

Clinical evaluation of new drugs has developed into a standard pattern of three clearly defined phases:

- *phase I* – assessment of the maximum tolerated dose of drug with a given schedule and route of administration, and definition of the toxicity profile of the compound. This involves identifying the side-effects and whether they are predictable, tolerable, and reversible in patients who would potentially benefit from the drug
- *phase II* – assessment of the efficacy of a drug in a group of patients with a single tumour type. The number of patients depends on the expected response rate. Often patients have not received previous treatment or they have malignancies that have shown little or no benefit from chemotherapy. Information is collected about tumour activity, techniques for administering the drug, precautions to be taken, possible dose modifications, acute toxicities, and necessary supportive care (see Research study 12.2)
- *phase III* – the drug is tested in clinical trials against existing agents or other forms of treatment known to be of value. Measures of efficacy involve demonstrating one or more of the following: improved cure rates, improved survival times, improved response rates, improved palliation, and improved quality of life.

Informed consent

In health care, informed consent has been defined as giving patients sufficient information to allow them to make the decision to undertake, or not, the proposed procedure or treatment, and to give or withhold consent.[23] Informed consent is intended to ensure that patients are in possession of comprehensive information about the treatment or research process they are about to undergo. Thompson *et al.*[24] point out that doctors and nurses have a fiduciary duty:

> not only to protect the interests of and to care for people who have entrusted themselves into their care, but they also have an obligation to give patients relevant information in return for their cooperation (concerning the diagnosis of their problem and the proposed methods of care and treatment), and to enable them to make an informed choice about whether they wish to continue with treatment. In this, health professionals have a fundamental duty to ensure that the consent to treatment given by patients is both 'fully informed' and 'voluntary' [pp.139–140].

Before administering chemotherapy it is important to obtain valid informed consent: this will help to maintain the autonomy of the individual involved and ensure their involvement in treatment decisions.[25,26] Although there is a great deal of literature on the ethical principle of informed consent, there are only a few examples that discuss it in the context of anti-cancer chemotherapy.[25] It is possible that too little information is given about the risks and difficulties of the side-effects of chemotherapy. Nurses may infer from this that they have an ethical and a professional responsibility to engage in a caring way in the process of informed choice. There are real and valid reasons why patients may want to decline, and do decline, to be treated.

Routes of administration

Intrapleural

Pleural effusions are a frequent complication of a number of cancers, including lung, breast, and prostate cancer, and cancers of the gastrointestinal tract and ovary, and can cause severe breathlessness. Chemotherapeutic agents such as bleomycin and cisplatin, and other agents (such

Research study 12.2

Cox K. (2000). Enhancing cancer clinical trial management: recommendations from a qualitative study of trial participants' experiences. *Psycho-oncology* **9**, 314–322.[20]

In this study, Karen Cox interviewed people with advanced cancer to record their perceptions of participating in early-phase anti-cancer drug trials. She points out that the type of research and the nature of this group of patients is such that few will receive any benefit at all. Difficult ethical and practical issues are raised, emphasising the importance of 'hearing, interpreting and acting on patients' views' (p.314). Cox believes that prior to her study, little research had been done in this area, with the result that the 'trial participants' voice' was 'largely ignored', and little was understood about 'how patients make sense of the total experience of trial participation' (p.315). This is just one in a series of papers aimed at providing a more comprehensive understanding of the experience of taking part in early phase anti-cancer drug trials.[20–22]

Method
Fifty-five patients taking part in phase I or II anti-cancer drug trials were interviewed about their experiences at four different time points: just after the decision to participate in the trial, after two cycles of treatment, upon withdrawal from or completion of the trial treatment, and after the end of the trial. Topics included: recruitment process, information received, reasons for taking part, experiences of the trial, support, quality of life, and satisfaction with care. Two quality-of-life questionnaires were also used to collect and compare pre- and post-trial information.

Results
Entering the trial seemed like a turning point, a 'light at the end of the tunnel', or a miracle cure. It made patients feel uncertain, but sometimes also lucky or special, with a chance to fight their illness (p.316). Most of the patients in the study felt that the trial had been presented to them in a positive way, but only 16 out of the 55 were able to say what the purpose of the trial was. Reasons for participating included being in expert hands, helping others, having no choice, and having nothing to lose (p.317).

As the trial went on, people reflected a growing sense of being 'burdened' by their involvement. They began to feel disillusioned, or that the harm of being in the trial was too great. One patient commented, 'I'm frightened I am not going to be able to make the course' (p.317). However, stopping the trial would mean having to face the fact that there was nothing else on offer. Feelings of disappointment that the new drug or treatment regime had not worked, and fear of abandonment, followed when people withdrew from or completed the trial. The end of the trial, says Cox, was a distressing time when high hopes were seen to have not been fulfilled. At the same time, a feeling of altruism, that they had been given a chance to help others as well as themselves, seemed to persist.

Discussion
Karen Cox believes that the altruism shown by patients like those in her study needs to be supported and acknowledged. It may be part of the search for meaning in life-threatening illness, and this has been shown to contribute to psychological well-being. Patients should be informed of the 'real' benefits of participation (the effects on feelings of self-worth, for example): benefits in terms of tumour response are likely to be 'limited' (p.320). Cox believes that people running trials like the ones featured in her study should acknowledge that people participating in their research are dying and 'need support during and beyond the trial to deal with this' (p.320). They should have the right, she says, to influence the choices available to them, and research is beginning to explore ways that patients' views can be incorporated into clinical trial design and treatment follow-up:

> There is a need to mobilise and engage with public opinion, and ensure that special interest groups – such as consumers, carers and researchers – have a voice, and that their views are taken into account [p.321].

as tetracycline or sterilised talc) have been administered into the pleural cavity following aspiration of fluid to prevent or delay recurrence of an effusion. After aspiration alone, some 60% of pleural effusions will recur.[27]

Traditionally, the prescribed agent is administered into the pleural space through the chest wall using a large-bore chest tube, causing the two pleural surfaces to sclerose and adhere. This procedure can be repeated daily for several days if required. Local pleural pain for 24–48 hours after instillation is the most common side-effect. More recently, a small-bore 'pig-tail' catheter has been used as a less restrictive alternative method.[28] Recurrent pleural effusions can be treated using an implantable port.[27,29] Sterman et al. describe the role of a pleuroperitoneal shunt in the drainage of reaccumulating pleural fluid in patients with pleural mesothelioma.[30]

Intravesical

Direct instillation of anti-cancer chemotherapy into the bladder can be a simple and effective means to treat superficial cancer of the bladder.[19] The most widely used agents include doxorubicin, epirubicin, mitomycin C, mitozantrone, thiotepa, and bacillus Calmette-Guérin (BCG). Schedules vary, but may include combinations of weekly and/or monthly instillations over differing periods of time.[18] Administration involves insertion of a urinary catheter, drainage of the bladder, and instillation of the drug, which is retained for 1–2 hours and dispersed throughout the bladder by frequent changes of position. The bladder is emptied of the chemotherapeutic agent by either unclamping the urinary catheter, or voiding. Leucopaenia and thrombocytopaenia have been associated with the use of mitomycin C and thiotepa, and most agents can cause irritation of the bladder.[18] It is important that patients practise careful personal hygiene, including hand washing and cleansing of the genitalia after voiding, and the toilet should be flushed at least twice after use. Following treatment patients may experience a number of local effects including dysuria and occasional haematuria, and there is a possibility of urinary tract infection. Increased intake of fluids after the 'dwell time' of the chemotherapy in the bladder will dilute the drug and can reduce side-effects.[27]

Intrathecal

Drugs can be administered into the central nervous system via the cerebrospinal fluid, usually by means of a lumbar puncture (the intrathecal route).[27] The only proven value of anti-cancer drugs administered in this way is as prophylaxis in leukaemia or lymphoma, where the central nervous system provides a 'sanctuary' site for malignant cells.[18] Drugs used in intrathecal chemotherapy include cytarabine and methotrexate. Allwood et al.[18] note that this route is unpleasant for the patient, technically difficult, and has been associated with a number of fatal drug errors. There is a risk of infection or trauma, and only drug formulations suitable and preferably licensed for this route should be used.[18] It is essential that drugs delivered by this route are prepared under strictly sterile conditions, and that drugs and their diluents are preservative free.[19,27] Updated national guidance from the Department of Health on the safe administration of intrathecal chemotherapy was published in 2003,[31,32] and includes a series of key requirements to be implemented by trusts. An Ommaya reservoir can be used to instil a drug directly into the ventricle of the brain. The reservoir is located beneath the skin and a catheter extends from it into the ventricle. The placement of the reservoir and catheter involves a degree of risk, but provides permanent access and offers an alternative to repeated lumbar puncture.[19]

Intraperitoneal

Direct instillation of drugs such as bleomycin, carboplatin, cisplatin, 5-fluorouracil (5-FU), mitomycin C, mitozantrone, and paclitaxel into the peritoneal cavity has been performed with two different objectives: control of ascites following aspiration, and control of tumour growth. The use of platinum-based agents (cisplatin and carboplatin) delivered by the peritoneal route has been most extensively explored; intraperitoneal 5-FU has been tested as an adjuvant therapy in small-volume residual gastrointestinal disease; and intraperitoneal paclitaxel has been administered in trials as treatment for microscopic residual ovarian cancer.[1] The intraperitoneal route allows 'bathing' of ovarian or colorectal tumours with proportionately high concentrations of chemotherapeutic agents.[18]

Prior to delivery by the intraperitoneal route, anti-cancer agents are mixed with large volumes of fluid to maximise distribution within the peritoneal cavity, exposing as much of this area as possible to the effects of the drug. Lower concentrations enter the bloodstream, and consequently systemic side-effects are mild or delayed. The peritoneal space can be accessed in three ways:

1. a temporary indwelling catheter for short-term/intermittent use, for example in symptom relief or palliative care
2. a Tenckhoff external catheter, used when treatment is planned for several months, and requiring more extensive care and maintenance by the patient. There is a greater likelihood of infection and leakage around the catheter, but rapid flow rates can be achieved
3. an implantable peritoneal port, which is internal and requires no care when not in use. It therefore carries a lower risk of infection, and may be more acceptable to patients. Flow rates may be relatively low, and there is the potential for extravasation.[19,27,33]

Problems associated with intraperitoneal chemotherapy include respiratory distress, abdominal pain, pyrexia, and diarrhoea, and may result from increased intra-abdominal pressure, mechanical difficulties with the catheter, infection, or electrolyte imbalance. Allwood *et al.* note that peritonitis (chemical and/or infective) can develop, which is both painful and, if allowed to progress, potentially fatal.[18]

Oral

A variety of anti-cancer agents can currently be administered orally, and use of these drugs is likely to increase. The oral route has a number of advantages in terms of quality of life, including shorter treatment time, greater independence, and improved tolerability.[34] There are also disadvantages, including less-intensive monitoring by health care professionals, potential lack of concordance, risk of over/underdosing, and inconsistency of absorption from the gastrointestinal tract.[19] It is therefore important for patients to understand the need for careful dosing and scheduling, and the importance of following the prescribed regimen correctly. Hayden and Goodman point out, for example, that compliance is necessary to maximise the goals of therapy, and that, in the case of therapy in which methotrexate is followed by leucovorin, for example, non-compliance may have fatal consequences.[19] Effective management of side-effects such as nausea is crucial, as the difficulty these may cause can impact on adherence to the prescribed treatment regimen.[27]

Intramuscular/subcutaneous

Only a few chemotherapies can be administered by the intramuscular or subcutaneous route, owing to the irritant nature of the drugs involved, the risk of tissue damage, bleeding caused by thrombocytopenia, and pain or discomfort.[27] Allwood *et al.* suggest that some small-volume subcutaneous injections (α-interferon, for example) may be appropriate for self-administration if toxicity is not a barrier and the drug is a non-vesicant.[18] Specific guidelines for the administration of drugs intramuscularly or subcutaneously should be followed, including rotation of sites, use of large muscles, and the 'Z-track' technique to prevent leakage into the skin. The smallest needle that will allow passage of the solution should be selected, to minimise discomfort and scarring.[27]

Intravenous

Of all the routes of administration, intravenous (IV) delivery is most frequently used for anti-cancer agents and ancillary drugs (e.g. antiemetics) and supportive therapy (e.g. antibiotics, blood transfusions). The means of gaining venous access should be considered before treatment starts: nursing assessment of the patient's physical status and needs plays an important part in this process. Venous access is either peripheral, using a winged infusion device or IV cannula, or central, involving the insertion of an indwelling catheter or implanted port.

Peripheral venous access

The veins of the lower arm (e.g. the large veins of the forearm[35]) are the preferred site for peripheral venous access as they are more numerous, cause fewer complications, and are more convenient to use than the peripheral veins of the lower limbs, for example. Using specific criteria in the selection of veins for peripheral access helps to ensure that the best vessel is chosen for the given purpose on each occasion. This is important as vein status may change in accordance with the patient's clinical condition: for example, anaemia or dehydration may reduce the circulating volume and cause veins to become flaccid. Choice of a vein for peripheral access is influenced by the type of medication to be used (e.g. vesicant or non-vesicant), the volume to be injected or infused, the rate of administration desired, and the duration of therapy (e.g. minutes, hours, or days).[36]

Hayden and Goodman[19] stress the importance of taking time to find the most appropriate vein:

> All too often the nurse fails to assess the veins properly, fails to distend the veins sufficiently prior to attempting venepuncture, and fails to apply adequate traction to the vein to prevent the vein from rolling [p.361].

For a variety of reasons it is advisable to administer vesicant drugs first.[18,27] At the beginning of the procedure:

- the integrity of the vein is greater
- the nurse's assessment skills and the patient's level of awareness are more acute
- veins may become irritated by other drugs given first.[19]

Winged infusion devices. Commonly known as 'butterflies', winged infusion devices consist of a short section of tubing attached to a steel needle. They can be used to administer bolus injections into a peripheral vein. Steel needles are not used in the administration of vesicant drugs because they are associated with a greater risk of extravasation.[32]

Peripheral cannulae and midline catheters. Peripheral cannulae consist of a flexible tube containing a disposable needle or stylet used during insertion. They are intended for short term use (3–5 days), either for bolus injections or short infusions. Midline catheters are peripheral devices inserted into and advanced along the antecubital vein, but not beyond the axilla. They are particularly useful for patients who have few accessible peripheral veins.[32] Peripheral cannulae can cause inflammation of the vein (phlebitis) and often require frequent resiting.[32,35]

Factors to consider when choosing a means of venous access include the following:

- *the condition and accessibility of the peripheral veins* – there are many reasons why the choice of vein may be limited. In children and obese patients veins may be obscured by subcutaneous fat. In the elderly they may be fragile and inelastic. Previous surgical procedures (for example,

amputation or axillary node dissection) may restrict the available vessels or compromise venous return. Lymphoedema may be present and other clinical conditions such as arthritis may reduce the number of available sites. The most common cause of reduced venous access is previous IV therapy, resulting in scarred or thrombosed veins

- *the nature and duration of therapy* – the length and nature of treatment may be difficult to predict but with most cancers a fairly reliable estimate is possible. Differences in the nature and duration of therapy can make different demands upon patients and their veins. Regimens vary, from the injection of a single agent twice a month, to continuous infusion of large volumes for 5 days every 3 weeks, a combination of three or more drugs given cyclically and requiring weekly venepuncture, or high-dose single-agent regimens delivered over a few hours but producing acute toxicity lasting several weeks and during which intensive supportive therapy is required

- *the type of chemotherapy prescribed* – some anti-cancer drugs are thrombo-irritants, and cause chemical phlebitis; some are vesicants with the potential to cause tissue necrosis. Diluents with which the drugs are mixed may be alkaline (pH > 7) or acidic (pH < 7) and cause extra irritation and scarring of the venous pathway. Supportive therapy, involving intensive use of antibiotics or other drugs, may limit the availability of veins for future IV therapy

- *patients' feelings about repeated venepuncture* – this is perhaps the single most important factor to be considered. Repeated venepuncture for blood sampling and administration of chemotherapy is at best uncomfortable, but may be the cause of considerable anxiety as treatment progresses and peripheral venous access diminishes. This anxiety may be influenced by the relationship between IV therapy and underlying illness. Fear of needles may develop and occasionally become phobic in nature. This additional stress compounds the problem. Veins disappear and each venepuncture becomes an ordeal for all concerned. Ways to minimise this include: establishing and maintaining a relationship of trust; explanation of procedures and involvement of patients in decision making; careful preparation to achieve maximum dilation of veins, together with skilful technique when placing or accessing the device; reducing discomfort by careful maintenance of the IV device once established; and consideration of patients' thoughts, fears, and previous experiences.[36]

Venous access deteriorates over time, and it is important that technically proficient staff are available to reduce the likelihood of both physical and psychological trauma for patients, and the incidence of local toxicity and complications such as infection. Nurses are well placed to extend their caring role into this field of practice.

Central venous access
The advantage of central venous access is the absence of repeated venepuncture and reduction of the risk of local toxicities such as extravasation or phlebitis. McLure[37] emphasises the importance to patients of secure long-term venous access:

> Patients with cancer often undergo repeated assaults on their venous system as part of their treatment. Multiple stabs must be endured to collect samples of blood, place IV cannulae for the infusion of clear fluids, antimicrobials, chemotherapy, blood and blood products. Many chemotherapeutic agents have a high osmolality, so are intensely toxic to vein endothelium. They must be administered via a central vein where they are diluted rapidly. Infusions of these agents may be given continuously or intermittently over a prolonged period of time. Without a long-term central venous catheter, the patient would be exposed to the risks of central venous cannulation with each course of treatment. Even with less toxic chemotherapy, peripheral venous access is often unsustainable and a central vein is the only reliable route of access. For both humanitarian and technical reasons, a long-term central vascular access solution is desirable [p.159].

Careful discussion of the management of central venous access devices with a patient is essential, as they are often asked to take on aspects of the maintenance of the device themselves. Infection is a major hazard, and home circumstances and personal hygiene are of prime importance. Dexterity and quality of eyesight also have to be taken into consideration when assessing someone's ability to manage a central venous device. Family members or friends may need to be taught the basic skills and principles involved in caring for the catheter at home. Written information should be provided to guide procedures, though these must be performed successfully both with and without supervision before a patient leaves hospital. Nurses have a responsibility to educate patients and others in the care of their device, and whenever possible should allow them to continue to manage the device when readmitted to hospital.[38]

Current technology and materials make it possible to maintain long-term central venous access effectively. There are a number of different methods and devices, including the following:

- *PICCs (peripherally inserted central catheters)* are a group of single- or dual-lumen central venous access devices inserted in the cephalic or basilic veins at the antecubital fossa, and threaded along the veins in the upper arm until the tip rests in the superior vena cava.[36] They do not require a surgical procedure to place them, and are well-suited for short-term central venous access. PICCs can be inserted at the bedside by a physician or a suitably trained and qualified nurse, provided that the patient has suitable veins in the antecubital fossa. This is an advantage for patients, but they must be able to care for the catheter effectively themselves. Rates of infection, clotting and malfunction are similar to those for other vascular access devices[19,39,40]
- a *skin-tunnelled catheter* provides safe and reliable long-term access with a low rate of infection. The most well-known catheter of this type is the Hickman catheter, developed by Robert Hickman in the mid-1970s. The catheter is made of an inert material such as silicone, which is sufficiently rigid at room temperature to allow insertion, but soft and flexible at body temperature.[37] Its tip lies at the junction of the superior vena cava and right atrium, within the superior vena cava, or in the upper right atrium; it exits the skin midway from the exterior chest wall.[32] The subcutaneous channel in which the catheter lies acts as a barrier to bacteria entering the vein from the skin.[19,32] This type of catheter incorporates a Dacron cuff, which lies under the skin. Fibrous tissue forms around the cuff,

keeping it in place and inhibiting tracking of micro-organisms along the outside of the catheter.[41] Insertion can now be carried out percutaneously by anaesthetists and nurses,[42] as well as surgeons, with advantages in terms of length of procedure and morbidity.[37] Skin-tunnelled central venous catheters are the preferred option for long-term parenteral nutrition, vesicant infusion therapy, and continuous infusions[19]

Skin-tunnelled catheters are available with a single, double, or triple lumen, and are either open or closed (e.g. Groshong type with a slit valve) at the tip. Pneumothorax can occur during insertion, and once in place catheters can become occluded or infected, or provide a site for thrombus formation. There is a risk of infection at the exit site of the catheter, and the sight of the catheter coming out from the skin may be a reminder to some patients of their illness and need for treatment. Surgical procedures, weight loss, and hair loss from chemotherapy may add to the effect on body image and self-esteem. The presence of the catheter may be seen as another insult and can affect sexual function. Although the catheter may not be in use at home it may still be regarded as an intrusion in intimate situations. In one study, patients felt that long-term central venous access adversely affected their body image, affected their partner, and reminded them of their disease[43]

- *Implantable port* – a silicone catheter leading to a central vein is attached to a port implanted under the skin of the chest wall, which acts as a barrier to infection. Single and double ports are available.[19] The advantage of an implanted port over a skin-tunnelled catheter is that when not in use, the port requires a minimum of care or maintenance. Access is provided by inserting a non-coring needle through the skin into a silicone septum in the port. The needle is cushioned by gauze and covered by a transparent dressing to reduce the risk of it becoming dislodged and leading to extravasation.[32] Inserting the needle correctly, and avoiding the use of small syringes that create high pressure within the catheter, are also important factors in minimising the risk of extravasation.[32] Implantable ports are ideal for intermittent therapies and for

patients who are unable or unwilling to care for an external device, who are concerned about altered body image, and who are particularly active physically (for example, patients who swim frequently).[19] The disadvantage of an implanted port is that it involves using a needle, although local anaesthetic cream can reduce the discomfort of inserting the needle. Needles can be left in place for up to 7 days,[19,32] after which time they must be replaced if treatment is to continue. After a course of therapy, the port is heparinised and the needle removed. Most port manufacturers state that ports should be flushed with sterile heparinised saline every month, however Hayden and Goodman indicate flushing every 3–4 months.[19] A recent German study of patients with breast and gynaecological cancer showed that the majority were satisfied with their port, were able to work, and did not feel disturbed during general activities.[44] Arm mobility was minimally affected, and more than half found that the port gave them a feeling of security. One-third of patients were not satisfied with the care they received after leaving hospital, possibly due to the inexperience of family doctors in the management of implantable ports.

Infusional ambulatory chemotherapy

Cancer chemotherapy has traditionally been administered using a schedule of intermittent doses, requiring patients to be admitted to hospital or to attend as day cases and separating them from home, family and work.[45] Home-based chemotherapy is now possible as a result of technological innovation and the introduction of continuous and portable infusion devices. It is claimed that these devices offer advantages in terms of maintaining lifestyle and minimising disruption of day-to-day activities.[46] However, the benefits of home chemotherapy and the cost of changing the way services are delivered in the UK has yet to be conclusively determined,[46] and its precise role therefore remains unclear.[47] Cancer care provided in the home setting is expanding to include high-tech interventions, and community nurses are increasingly involved in providing support.[48] In their small study of district nurses' experiences with continuous ambulatory chemotherapy, Turner and Pateman identified the need for further research into the management of ambulatory chemotherapy to support the development of best practice recommendations.[48]

Home chemotherapy is thought to enhance patients' independence and sense of control, particularly if it is self-administered.[18,49] The opportunity for patients to be actively involved in their treatment can encourage a positive attitude, and patients receiving treatment at home have reported psychological benefits because they are among people and possessions that are important to them.[50] Patients also appear to be more able to tolerate drug-related side-effects in this setting.[18] While the families of people with cancer can feel helpless and inadequate, home chemotherapy may enable them to become more involved and to give greater assistance and support. Chemotherapy at home reduces the risk of exposing immunocompromised individuals to the harmful pathogens found in hospitals.[18]

Overall, the benefits of home chemotherapy, including convenience, the opportunity for active participation, and cost-effectiveness, may well outweigh the disadvantages, though these must be considered carefully. In hospital, staff are always available to assist and support patients when needed, whereas this may not always be the case at home. In spite of recent increases in the number of community nurses who have the skills and knowledge to manage IV therapy in the home, it is not possible for them to be present round the clock. For this reason, it is vital to make careful decisions with patients about whether home chemotherapy is suitable and likely to be successful. Some patients may not be able to undertake the procedures necessary for maintaining treatment at home, either because they are confused by the instructions, because they are fearful, or because there is a physical reason why some part of the care of their drugs and infusion device may not be possible. Some people may prefer the feeling of security that being in hospital can give, and may not wish to take on a programme of treatment at home. Complications do occur, and can cause severe anxiety or stress for some patients.[38]

- *Catheter-related complications* include extravasation of drugs and clotting within the catheter, which may lead to occlusion. Loss of patency often occurs after failure to switch the pump on, during periods of malfunction, or if the catheter is not flushed using the correct solution or the recommended technique.[49] Patency can usually be restored with a fibrinolytic agent.[51]
- *Drug-related complications* can be caused by precipitation of a drug,[45] or by toxicities such as bone marrow suppression, mucositis, diarrhoea, or palmar-plantar erythrodysesthesia syndrome (i.e. 'hand–foot syndrome', where high-dose continuous infusion of 5-FU causes pain, tenderness, and erythema of the palms and soles). Such toxicities may necessitate a break in treatment.
- *Infusion device-related complications* can occur as a result of leakage or rupture of the drug reservoir,[49] pump malfunction,[49,50] or incorrect infusion rate. Depletion or failure of the pump battery can also be a problem.[45,52]

Consideration must also be given to the changes in body image caused by the location of the central venous catheter, which may be connected to an infusion pump for days or weeks at a time. Some patients find even a portable pump cumbersome, and day-to-day and sporting activities and holidays may become difficult or intolerable. Chemotherapy, which takes a considerable time to complete, may be difficult to tolerate for patients who prefer to get their treatment over and done with as quickly as possible.

When considering whether to begin a programme of home chemotherapy, a number of factors must be carefully weighed. Careful discussion with patients about the implications, and comprehensive teaching are essential. Hayward advocates a home visit before administering chemotherapy to assess a range of factors including the patient's condition, social circumstances, home environment, and vascular access.[53] Further key objectives of careful assessment of the patient and their environment include: safety of the patient and nurse, safe transportation of drugs, safe administration by suitable trained staff, preparations for emergency situations, and arrangements for follow-up care.[47]

Patients must be willing participants in their own care, and either they or their family and/or friends must be comfortable with and skilled in the operation of the infusion pump and venous access device, as well as able to respond to the effects of the chemotherapeutic agent in use.[49] From a medical point of view, disease stage and the patient's general health status must be such that home chemotherapy is appropriate and feasible.[54] Thought must be given to the choice of infusion device: given the effect of central venous catheters on lifestyle and activities, it is important to meet each individual's needs as closely as possible. A wide variety of ambulatory infusion pumps is now available, from external syringe drivers to totally implantable systems, including disposable pumps.[18] One type may be more appropriate than another, given a person's particular circumstances.[38]

Fernsler and Cannon point out that the objectives of a learning programme for patients include adherence to a therapeutic regimen, increased satisfaction, enhanced self-determination, increased ability to manage symptoms, and enhanced recovery from surgical procedures.[55] However, increased knowledge is possibly the outcome that is most often seen in nursing documentation. Before conducting a programme of learning it is important to consider the process of learning and the factors that affect a person's ability to learn, both in everyday situations, and in potentially more stressful health care-related situations.

Patients facing the possibility of a central venous catheter, continuously or intermittently infused medications, the need to become familiar with and operate infusion equipment, as well as the likelihood of drug-related side-effects, are not in an easy situation for learning. Initially they may find it difficult to become motivated, as it is likely that they are feeling frightened and anxious, powerless and out of control. Sometimes the amount of information to be absorbed about their illness and their treatment can be overwhelming. They may also be anxious about personal issues, and the environment in hospital is often intimidating and stressful.[38] Patients may not share a common language with hospital staff, there may be an organic obstacle to communication such as dysphasia, and literacy may be limited. Culturally,

patients may feel ill at ease with the organisation of Western hospitals and treatment, and may be suffering from the effects of their illness and/or its treatment.

Studies have shown that patients receiving chemo- or radiotherapy can use targeted information to learn about their treatment and carry out self-care activities, and want these to be presented in an organised and pragmatic way.[56] Dodd and Miaskowski describe the development of one self-care symptom management programme for people receiving aggressive chemotherapy that focuses on information about disease, treatment and side-effects, instruction in essential self-care skills, and ongoing supportive nursing care:

> self-care agency is enhanced through the provision of relevant information, the enhancement of self-care skills, and the provision of support . . . Nursing is needed when there is a deficit between the patient's self-care agency and the existing therapeutic self-care demands [p.302].[56]

Initial assessment of patients' needs should include information about their response to their diagnosis, their communication style, and their ability to read and understand written information. It may be useful for nurses to ask patients to explain their understanding of their situation in their own words, to provide a basis for further explanations. Supporting written information should be provided so that patients and their families are able to refer back to relevant points about the illness and treatment when they are at home. It may be necessary to begin with simple information or instructions, and to move towards more complex information gradually, as a relationship is established between nurse and patient.[38,57] Patients must feel able to ask for further instructions if they feel worried or unsure, and a contact number should be provided for this purpose. Listening and observing a patient's demeanour to become familiar with characteristic mannerisms and anxieties is always as important as giving explanations.

A successful learning programme depends on individualised and mutually identified goals and objectives. Verbal information ought be supported by clear and effective written information. Learning can be formal or informal, and can include videos, booklets, or audio tapes, or a combination of these. Learning about treatment can help to reduce fear, increase feelings of being in control, make treatment regimens more manageable, and make taking responsibility for one's own care a more positive experience.

Decision making and involvement

The multidisciplinary team plays an increasingly important role in identifying the most appropriate care and treatment for people with cancer. Under the terms of the *NHS Cancer Plan*,[58] surgeons, radiologists, pathologists, oncologists, nurse specialists, palliative care specialists, and others work together to provide appropriate investigations and treatment and deliver co-ordinated care.[59] Reports from practice reflect the strengths of flexible approaches where patients are able to initiate access to multidisciplinary team members quickly and according to their needs. Effective teams can help patients to remain involved in decision making:

> By having written protocols, guidance and regular communication between team members, the patient was given timely and appropriate information, allowing her to make informed decisions about her own care . . . Effective communication between team members, from primary care through to supportive care, is essential. But, despite these protocols being in place, the decision to access services ultimately remains in the hands of the patient.[60]

Discussions with patients about treatment choices should, it has been suggested, address two fundamental issues: preferences about the amount and type of information provided, and preferences about participation in decision-making.[61] Fallowfield argues that a clear distinction should be made between the desire for information and the wish to assume responsibility for decision making: her research suggests that improvements in quality of life for patients facing choices about treatment may be linked primarily to levels of satisfaction with information received.[61] She emphasises the importance of providing objective, patient-centred information supported by information booklets, audio and video tapes, and web-based resources such as Cancerbackup (www.cancerbackup.org.

uk), the National Library for Health (www.library. nhs.uk), and DIPEx (www.dipex.org).

Active involvement in care can enhance the patient's experience and make use of patients' knowledge of their own bodies. It helps to ensure patient satisfaction and a sense of control during treatment.[41] Patients should be informed of the early signs of extravasation of vesicant drugs, for example, or the sensations associated with anaphylaxis, so that they can alert health care professionals promptly. Weinstein[41] emphasises the importance of intuitive patient and family education, alongside skilled technical care, in the work of health professionals involved in IV therapy, and sets out some key teaching points, summarised below:

- assessment of patients' and families' need for knowledge about disease and treatment
- learning outcomes based on patients' needs
- participation in decision making
- appropriate selection of teaching and learning methods and materials
- ongoing evaluation of patients' and families' learning in relation to original learning outcomes
- documentation of teaching and learning process (p.491).

Handling cytotoxic drugs and disposal of waste

The actual or potential hazards of exposure to cytotoxic drugs are such that careful attention must be paid to safe handling and disposal of waste. Cytotoxic drugs are known to be potentially mutagenic (i.e. induce genetic mutations), teratogenic (i.e. produce physical defects in the fetus), and carcinogenic (i.e. induce tumours), and some studies of hospital staff have demonstrated an incidence of chromosomal abnormalities and excretion of mutagenic products.[1,18,62] Drugs may be inhaled when powder or liquid is 'aerosolised' or emitted in a fine airborne powder or spray during reconstitution, or if spillage occurs during preparation or administration. They may also be ingested or come into contact with the skin.[18] They therefore represent a health risk for staff regularly involved in their preparation and administration. The safest way of working with cytotoxic drugs is to develop and apply policies and guidelines to reduce the possibility of direct exposure to them. Studies have shown that relevant safety measures can reduce the level of exposure to potentially hazardous substances.[1,18]

Cytotoxic chemotherapy presents two levels of health risk: first, a definite risk arises from the fact that a number of chemotherapeutic agents are known to be extremely irritant and to produce harmful local effects after contact with the skin or eyes; second, a potential risk exists because such substances have been shown to cause changes in humans on the cellular or genetic level. Local effects of exposure to cytotoxic drugs include dermatitis, inflammation of the mucous membranes, excessive lacrimation (production of tears), pigmentation, blistering, and a range of other allergic reactions. Systemic effects include dizziness, hair loss, headaches, blurred vision, light-headedness, cough, pruritis, and general malaise.

The Health and Safety at Work Act (1974) and control of substances hazardous to health (COSHH) regulations published by the Health and Safety Executive (HSE) make it mandatory for employers to identify hazardous substances in use, people at risk, and measures to ensure safe handling and an effective response to accidental exposure and adverse events.[63,64] Guidelines for preparation, handling, and management of spillage must be in place before nurses handle chemotherapeutic agents.

In ideal conditions, safety cabinets provide a balance between protection for the operator and the necessity to handle equipment and products. Cabinets and isolators should be located in a designated area with restricted access. Adequate levels of safety must be provided for both patients and staff preparing and administering drugs, using, for example, vertical laminar flow cabinets or isolators.[18] Some form of protective clothing must be worn at all times when handling cytotoxic agents, though the degree of protection required depends on the type of preparation facility available, the nature of the agents being handled, and the extent of the exposure. The minimum requirement is for an overall and gloves of suitable quality; additional protection can be provided by non-absorbent armlets, plastic apron, eye protection, and face mask. Disposable gloves should be worn throughout preparation and checking of cytotoxic chemotherapy. Recommendations about the best type of glove material vary, but when selecting gloves the user must be certain that the material is of a suitable thickness and integrity to maximise protection.[65] Double gloving is recommended for dealing with spillages.[18]

The key to reducing the risk of exposure is good technique. The Health and Safety at Work Act[63] and COSHH regulations[64] (see www.hse. gov.uk/coshh/) provide important additional guidelines on safe working environments and handling hazardous substances, including management of spillage and disposal of waste. All possible precautions should be taken to avoid accidental spillage, though staff should be aware of the approved written procedure for managing spillage should it occur. Staff must receive education and training in procedures and guidelines, to a level appropriate to their level of involvement with the handling, preparation, or administration of cytotoxic drugs.[66,67]

A Dutch survey highlighted a number of issues related to the handling of cytotoxic chemotherapy.[68] Out of a total of 824 respondents in 10 hospitals, 750 (91%) wore gloves when administering drugs, but only 173 (21%) wore a gown or an apron; 634 (77%) were aware of the risk posed by 'aerosolisation', but 157 (19%) did not believe that opening a glass ampoule was accompanied by any risk; 775 (94%) felt that protective measures were adequate, though 280 (34%) attached bags or bottles to IV administration sets with the bag or bottle on the stand. Researchers concluded that nurses do not always follow safety guidelines or use recommended protective measures, because they may be perceived as inconvenient or unnecessary. Nurses may take their own safety less seriously than that of their patients.

Extravasation

A number of cytotoxic anti-cancer drugs are known to cause venous irritation; others, known as *vesicants*, can cause intense local tissue inflammation and pain, progressing to necrosis and ulceration if they leak from the vein during administration. The escape of a chemotherapeutic agent from a vessel into the surrounding tissues by leakage or as an involuntary injection of a drug into the tissues is known as *extravasation*.[69] Tissue damage following extravasation of a vesicant drug can be severe and long term. Incidence in adults is estimated at between 0.1% and 6%, although this may be an underestimate, and incidence may be higher, for example, with implantable ports.[32,69] It is essential that nurses know which of the drugs they are administering are vesicants, as well as how to recognise and manage extravasation should it occur. Extravasation can normally be avoided by using good administration techniques, but even with the greatest care and skill accidents can occasionally occur. The incidence of extravasation is low among experienced cancer nurses in specialised settings, but higher in general hospital settings.

A number of factors can increase the risk of extravasation:

- additional difficulties present during cannulation or administration of drugs (for example, if a patient is very young, elderly, debilitated, or confused)
- the IV cannula may be placed in an awkward position where monitoring of administration is more difficult (e.g. over a bony prominence or joint)
- some equipment (such as steel needles, including winged infusion devices or 'butterflies') is unsuitable: a plastic cannula should be inserted into a vein
- small and fragile veins should be avoided, and limbs affected by lymphoedema or neurological weakness
- vascular access devices (e.g. skin-tunnelled/non-skin-tunnelled catheter, implantable port) may be indicated if patients have small, fragile veins or require long-term administration/continuous infusion of vesicants
- optimal peripheral access is provided by the large veins of the forearm (e.g. posterior basilic vein)
- use of veins in the hand and wrist carries increased risk of damage to tendons and nerves should extravasation occur

- poor standard of practice (for example, incorrect amount or type of diluent, failure to observe the IV site correctly while drugs are administered, or use of inappropriate peripheral vein as opposed to central vein).[19,36,41,69,70]

Early recognition of extravasation is imperative to minimise potential tissue damage. The following signs and symptoms of extravasation can occur singly or in combination:

- swelling (most common)
- stinging, burning, or pain at the injection site (not always present)
- redness (not seen initially)
- lack of blood return into the syringe (though this is not always indicative of extravasation)
- pressure or resistance to syringe plunger or infusion.[27,41,69]

Implanted ports and skin-tunnelled catheters are considered to be safe and reliable means of drug delivery, but extravasation can also occur with these devices. The consequences in these circumstances are very serious, and careful note should be taken of any complaints of pain or change in sensation around the port or catheter during administration. If extravasation from a central venous catheter is suspected, the infusion or injection must be stopped immediately and medical staff notified.

Vesicants can be divided into non-DNA-binding vesicant drugs (e.g. vinblastine, vincristine, vinorelbine, docetaxel, paclitaxel) and DNA-binding vesicant drugs (e.g. nitrogen mustard, daunorubicin, doxorubicin, epirubicin, idarubicin, dactinomycin, mitomycin C).[69] Non-DNA-binding vesicants often cause immediate damage such as burning and ulceration, but are less likely to lead to erosion of deeper structures, and healing may take place within 3–5 weeks. DNA-binding vesicant drugs tend to cause both immediate damage and slower ongoing tissue necrosis.[32]

While there is agreement about the signs and symptoms of extravasation, its management remains controversial. However, if there is reason to believe that extravasation of a vesicant agent has occurred, it is essential that immediate action is taken to minimise tissue damage and prevent further serious consequences. An extravasation kit containing the materials and equipment (including all appropriate antidotes and diluents, and a copy of extravasation policy and procedures) should be available whenever vesicant drugs are administered.

Management of extravasation often includes the following steps:

1. stop administration of drug
2. stop fluid flow if drug is administered through side arm of free-flowing IV infusion
3. attempt to aspirate any residual drug
4. remove the IV access device (if peripheral)
5. apply heat with vinca alkaloids, or cold with anthracyclines, as recommended
6. prepare antidote and inject subcutaneously around the site of the extravasation using a 25G needle (according to institutional policy and procedure)
7. elevate the affected limb
8. notify medical staff
9. document the incident and if necessary photograph affected area
10. request advice from a plastic surgeon if necessary
11. instruct the patient in care of the affected area, ensure adequate systemic analgesia, and plan follow-up.[18,19,27,36,41]

Veins that have previously been punctured are not suitable for administration of vesicant drugs due to increased risk of leakage. Following an unsuccessful attempt at cannulation, a different vein in the opposite limb should be used. If this is not possible, a site in the same vein may be used, but should be proximal to the previous puncture site.[32] When using an existing peripheral site, it is essential to ensure that the site is adequate and appropriate (e.g. not over a joint or the wrist) and ideally less than 24-hours old. Drugs should not be administered if the site is red, swollen or painful, or if there is evidence of infiltration of fluids into the surrounding tissue.[32] Before administering vesicant drugs through a cannula or catheter, brisk blood return should be confirmed, and there should be easy flow of fluids. Observation of insertion sites should be continuous, and when

vesicants are administered peripherally, patients should never be left unattended.[19]

Caring for patients receiving chemotherapy

Patients' experiences

Cancer patients undergo numerous blood tests and are often required to have an IV cannula sited for chemotherapy or supportive therapy (for example, blood products or antibiotics). They are also subjected to a variety of diagnostic tests including bone scans, computerised tomography (CT) scans, lumbar punctures, and bone marrow aspirates, all of which require the insertion of a needle. Griffin *et al.* found that patients ranked having a needle inserted in the top ten most difficult psychosocial cancer-related symptoms, which gives an indication of how important this event is for many patients.[71] Cohn[72] writes:

> As my veins become increasingly scarce, mobile and collapsible, I sometimes had to be needled as many as five times, because laboratory technicians would not listen when I said that Vacutainers did not work any more [p.1008].

Technical skill is not the only requirement when inserting a peripheral venous access device. It is just as important to understand the fears and anxieties that surround the cannulation procedure, and the implications of the presence of the device during hospital admission. The intrusion and restriction caused by the siting of an IV cannula can affect a patient's body image, and the cannula can be a constant source of anxiety while it is in place.[73] Kaplan suggests that once an IV infusion is in progress, anxieties may change, but do not necessarily diminish: questions such as 'Will the drip stop or run dry?', 'Will the pump alarm and if so why?', and 'What if the cannula is dislodged or becomes occluded?' can still persist.[74] Concerns over a cannula being dislodged may not always relate to fear of having another device put in place; it is sometimes a matter of wanting to avoid inconvenience and delays in being treated.[75]

Patients also worry about the security of IV devices. One report describes how a patient needed a family member present during every infusion because a previous infusion had leaked into sub-cutaneous tissues.[76] Anxieties may focus on the contents of injections or infusions, in particular possible side-effects, or the fear that blood may be incompatible or infected.[75,77] Patients may be disturbed by changes in routine, for example if che motherapy is administered in a way with which they are not familiar.[74]

Nursing interventions play an important part in allaying patients' fears and in ensuring that treatment is correctly and efficiently given. The manner in which nurses undertake the care of IV sites, and the way in which drugs are administered has an important influence on whether patients feel safe or anxious. Patients like to feel that IV devices are secure and will remain in position:[75] a nurse may 'know' what should be done, but a patient knows what feels best, making it important that the two discuss the care involved in IV therapy.[78] Fear and anxiety stirred up by a painful experience can persist for some time: measures taken to comfort and reassure a frightened person may need to continue after the end of the procedure that caused the distress. Nurses often leave once a procedure has been completed, and do not realise the impact of post-event stress. Skill and familiarity on the part of nurses handling and using equipment, and regular checks to make sure that equipment is functioning correctly and that infusions are running properly and safely, can be emotionally supportive for patients and their relatives and reduce levels of anxiety.

Mobilising patients' strengths and coping strategies, using relaxation or distraction techniques, being able to listen and talk, paying attention to detail, and experience and confidence have been found to be highly valued approaches. Inexperienced nurses:[75,76]

> ... can produce fear in patients ... sensitive nurses who feel unsure of a particular procedure will ask someone with experience to assist them [p.105].[74]

Patients may feel more in control of their IV therapy if they are given the opportunity to become active participants, for example by choosing the site for their IV access device. One study suggested that patients who were able to choose the arm from which to donate blood experienced less discomfort and pain when compared with patients who were not given a choice.[79] Being able to care for oneself even in a small way is an important dimension of health care,[80] even when patients are faced with the emotionally difficult experience of being confined to bed with an IV infusion. Providing patients with options and choices may have an important influence on behavioural and physiological stress reactions.[79] Patients may feel a greater degree of control over their situation if they have a say in the scheduling of treatment. (For example, they may want to have treatment overnight to give them more freedom during the day.) Having a choice about where an IV device is placed may ensure that it remains effective and in place longer, and that treatment is completed with fewer interruptions.[81] It is important to have the opportunity to participate and to foster a sense of independence and control in a potentially difficult situation.

Loss of control

Nurses are constantly involved in helping patients to meet the challenges of daily living. Interventions focused on physical care are likely to be evaluated frequently, providing a means of monitoring the quality of this aspect of care. It is as important to understand the role of other non-physical factors in maintaining quality of life.

Control has been described as the belief that one has at one's disposal a response that can influence awareness of an event. Loss of control, a feeling that chemotherapy is 'done for you or done to you', is a frequent experience for cancer patients; having a blood sample taken can feel like 'relinquishing control over access to personal space'.[82] Feelings of loss of control, together with possible lack of understanding about the rationale and procedures related to chemotherapy, contribute greatly to anxiety.

Greater knowledge and understanding can help to restore part of the feeling of being in control. As one researcher with personal experience of treatment for Hodgkin's disease[83] puts it:

> I decided before being hospitalised ... that my best chance of staying sane lay in using my skills as a researcher and ethnographer to demystify my disease

and its treatment, and thereby to restore some sense of control. Treatments of indefinite length and uncertain outcome invariably inspire fear and rage, and rob the cancer patient of much of his personal autonomy. In such circumstances knowledge is the only kind of power available. It imposed order, pattern and meaning to a life that had suddenly taken on a frighteningly random character, and so made it possible to manage the fear [p. 316].

Research has shown that there is a positive relationship between people's sense of perceived control and health-related outcomes. There are two main types of perceived 'locus of control': internal and external. In the management of chronic pain, for example, internal locus of control, which reflects a belief in personal control over behaviour, has been related to the use of more effective coping strategies; external locus of control, in which the role of chance and powerful others are seen as more influential, has been related to maladaptive strategies.[84,85] Involvement in decision making and taking personal responsibility for aspects of health care can be constructive:

> . . . my relationship with my oncologist continued to change, involving more and more negotiation and compromise . . . as my understanding of the treatment processes expanded and my physical condition deteriorated. I brought all my capacities for identifying and analysing pattern to bear on my body's increasingly violent response to chemotherapy, using every treatment as an opportunity to try out my theories on my oncologist. He came to respect my ability to observe and report sensitively and accurately . . . as I began to negotiate more aggressively (and more successfully) for lower doses. This was no fiction of participation; it was based on a mutual understanding of chemotherapy . . . [p. 333].[83]

Patients may choose to adopt a lifestyle that helps them to foster the sense that they are 'fighting' their illness, the side-effects of treatment, or both.

Feelings associated with chemotherapy

Receiving chemotherapy has been likened to riding a roller-coaster: a study of women with breast cancer found that the rapid changes in physical state and psychological ups and downs that occurred with cycles of adjuvant chemother-

apy made 'normalisation' more difficult.[86] Chemotherapy can seem mysterious and frightening, both before and after it has been experienced at first hand:

> I've always said, all my life, even if I was dying, I would refuse chemotherapy because no way would I put myself through what I feel other people go through for all I didn't know what the process involved. You know, you can see people who've gone through it. The guy in church had, er, lung cancer, and he went through chemotherapy, but he was marvellous. I mean, he came every week until, towards the end, he couldn't stand up, he was so weak, and all his hair had dropped out and he had a gaunt expression. But that was probably the cancer because it overtook him and he died eventually. So I really knew very little about it, other than what people look like [p.317].[86]

> We were like robots . . . There is a kind of disassociation . . . you just know that you have to detach yourself . . . look aside . . . I would turn up for chemotherapy, put out my arm for them to do whatever they wanted; I tried persuading myself; they pricked me . . . but today I don't want to be touched . . . I don't want to undress . . . I don't want anybody to come near me. This is my trauma [p.61].[87]

Events that may seem trivial to health care professionals can assume major proportions for patients, from the frustration of waiting for blood results to indicate whether treatment can go ahead, to the exasperation and rage experienced when an injection has to be postponed. Events that have not been anticipated and prepared for are often traumatic, as are changes in routine: any event that occurs unpredictably, regardless of the cause, should be expected to produce feelings of helplessness and outrage.[72] Fear and anxiety are felt both before and after chemotherapy treatments, and have numerous causes, including the possibility of side-effects, venepuncture, feelings of isolation or loss of independence, just being in hospital, or conversely having to manage treatment and equipment at home. Conflicting emotions often arise when patients relapse after treatment, when either further chemotherapy is recommended, or treatment is halted. The end of chemotherapy can be viewed with both delight and fear. The feelings of security and opportunities to discuss worries that come with regular hospital visits can be lost. Patients sometimes experience the fear that without chemotherapy their illness will recur, and relapse can provoke intense feelings of vulnerability and mortality. It is also possible that some patients will feel better able to cope with chemotherapy the second time around.

Nurses need to be aware that chemotherapy evokes strong and varied emotions that need to be expressed and received with understanding and compassion. Buckalew[76] proposes three broad approaches to psychosocial care:

1. helping patients to identify and utilise sources of support to alleviate anxiety (for example, support from the family or from relaxation exercises or guided imagery)
2. providing the opportunity to ventilate or express feelings about treatment and side-effects freely and without judgement being passed: anxiety is a normal reaction to the stress and trauma of chemotherapy
3. referral to appropriate members of the multi-disciplinary team (for example, stoma thera-pists, breast care specialists, the palliative care team, cognitive therapists) or user support groups.

Isolation

Physical weakness, an inability to write or concen-trate, and forgetfulness can reduce a patient's ability to take part in social and recreational activi-ties. Kathy Charmaz describes suffering in chronic illness as much more than physical discomfort: it is a 'loss of self', a 'crumbling away of former self-images' without 'development of equally valued new ones' (p.168).[88] Many of the most valued parts of people's lives, including their social life, careers, relationships, outward appearance, and self-respect can be stripped away.

Patients may be apprehensive about the ability of family and friends to adjust to their illness and treatment, and sometimes initial attentiveness by families and others is followed by withdrawal at what is a crucial time. A study of the social and emotional effects of chemotherapy[89] emphasises the importance of family relationships as well as the difficulty with which these are sometimes sustained:

Family [members] who did not reside with partici-pants popped in and out of their lives . . . Mostly they acted as a distraction, and because they were not living with the cancer and chemotherapy . . . they were able to sustain detachment unlike spouses and partners [pp.4–5].

For the majority of participants, partners/spouses were a source of support, encouragement and great strength. Living with someone undergoing chemotherapy treat-ment was obviously a cause of distress, and intensity of emotion, anxiety and the possibility of an unpredict-able illness trajectory often resulted in tensions between participants and their spouses/partners [p.5].

A sense of isolation can be linked with a feeling of being unable to communicate with nursing staff, or that nurses are too busy to 'waste time' talking to them.[90] However, nurses are well placed to help patients to manage feelings of isolation. A willingness to listen, to identify needs and worries, and to collaborate to maintain physical and emo-tional well-being can contribute to feelings of being included, as opposed to being on the outside.

Personal growth

Cancer is distressing and disruptive, but there are aspects of the experience (for example, improved personal resources, enhanced sense of purpose, and changes in life priorities) that patients may find beneficial.[91] Research has shown that per-ceived social support and 'approach' coping strate-gies (positive reappraisal, planned problem-solving, confrontive coping, and seeking social support) can promote positive adjustment.[92] Among married women with breast cancer, perceived support from husbands and contact with breast cancer survivors who felt that their experience had benefits have been shown to be positive in terms of 'post-traumatic growth', including positive changes in views of self, sense of relationship with others, and philosophy of life.[93]

The opportunity for personal growth during chemotherapy can and should be conveyed to patients, because the heightened self-esteem that results from that growth will increase patients' stamina during treatment and diminish the likeli-hood of their discontinuing therapy prema-turely.[72] Nurses can offer guidance to patients searching for a way of regaining their self-esteem. One approach is jointly to set goals that are achievable and consistent with realistic expectations. Goals are sometimes therefore necessarily short term and based on a 'take each day as it comes' philosophy. It is often important to provide patients with encouragement to maintain their commitment, and achieving goals may not always become easier as time goes on. Side-effects may get worse, or new ones might appear, and if patients experience a deterioration in their overall situation, some goals may have to be reassessed. Steps taken and strategies agreed during an initial course of chemotherapy may positively influence a patient's ability to manage subsequent courses, and could explain why some people are better equipped and more assertive the second time around. Psychological well-being is often related to physical well-being, so efforts to prevent, minimise, or treat the physical effects of illness and treatment can play an important part in sustaining feelings of integrity, and help patients to adjust in periods of personal upheaval and disturbance.

Sexuality and body image

Sharing intimacy and giving pleasure to a partner is a major source of personal value. When diagnosed with cancer, some people do not experience any changes to their sexuality or sex lives, while others may choose this point to cease sexual activity. However, cancer and cancer treatment do sometimes affect frequency of sexual activity, sexual satisfaction, and sexual confidence and body image.[94] Anllo suggests that most couples adjust well,[95] although relationship difficulties may disproportionately affect women under 50 years. She adds that for women with breast cancer, for example, the

> diagnosis has a way of bringing pre-existing problems into sharper focus. Communication about the cancer is a common area of difficulty. Some women may find that their partners are uncomfortable with discussions about lingering fears of recurrence; the partners may be protective and afraid to reinforce negative thinking. Brief couples counselling can be useful for this type of problem. Research has shown that couples who have open communication have better marital adjustment following breast cancer [pp.241–242].

In a French survey of 100 people with a variety of cancers, both men and women ranked loss of sexual feeling in their top ten most severe side-effects. Younger people ranked this side-effect as more severe than older people, and it ranked fourth among married patients and patients who did not live alone.[93]

Indirect effects of illness such as anorexia, nausea, and vomiting can cause significant changes in appearance, body image, and feelings of well-being. Hair loss, pallor, malaise, and lethargy may exacerbate these effects. Emotional and psychological reactions to illness can potentiate fatigue. Understandably, sexual activity may be difficult to sustain for both partners in a relationship. This in itself may further reinforce disruptions to an already threatened body image.[96] Society remains uncomfortable with overt expressions of concern about sexual function, but nurses need to be able to discuss this aspect of our lives without being dismissive or getting embarrassed. It helps to be comfortable with the idea of your own sexuality and attitudes towards sex, and counselling skills may help.[97] If nurses lack the confidence to participate in discussions about sexuality or the possibility of modifying sex to take account of health care needs, referral to a counsellor or specialist with the appropriate skills should be considered.

Worries related to sexual function (for example, the effects of chemotherapy on future pregnancies) also need to be addressed. Advice on contraception during and for some time after chemotherapy should always be given to women of childbearing age, to avoid the possibility of teratogenic effects; the need for sperm banking should be considered for men before the start of chemotherapy. Treatment with chemotherapy does not preclude expressions of physical affection, though familiar activities like kissing can be difficult if, for example, someone is badly affected by stomatitis. Chemotherapy can cause hot flushes, vaginal dryness, amenorrhoea, and painful intercourse (dyspareunia), and may induce an early menopause. It is difficult to predict whether patients will become sterile or not as a result of chemotherapy, though in women the risk appears to be related to age. Perry points out that a proportion of adult men with Hodgkin's disease or testicular tumours have reduced fertility before treatment.[1] Older regimens for Hodgkin's disease cause permanent damage to sperm production in a high proportion of cases, although newer regimens are better tolerated. With treatment for testicular cancer, sperm production often recovers within 1–2 years, although there may be more permanent effects on the motility of sperm and volume of ejaculate.

Side-effects, toxicities, and nursing implications

Chemotherapy is a systemic treatment, which can produce a great number and variety of side-effects throughout the body. These effects depend upon the drug or the combination of drugs used, the dose, the schedule of administration, and the route of administration. Perhaps the greatest variable of all, however, is the reaction of individuals given their physical and/or emotional circumstances when they are given chemotherapy.

Medical and nursing assessment of patients, and the investigations carried out before starting chemotherapy, have three main objectives:

1. to assess each person's physical condition, including nutritional status, renal, liver, and cardiac function, bone marrow reserve, and performance status; to resolve problems where possible and to identify anyone at risk of specific short- or long-term toxicities
2. to determine the extent of a person's cancer to provide a baseline against which to measure response to therapy, for example, using X-rays, scans, or measurement of tumour markers
3. to calculate the correct dose of drug or drugs, avoiding unnecessary risk of toxicity; dosage is often based on body surface area in m², calculated from height and weight.

Assessment and investigations may be repeated at regular intervals to detect at an early stage toxicities that could lead to irreversible damage if not addressed. The information gathered, together with patients' descriptions of their usual level of function and activity, will assist medical and nursing staff to plan a safer course of chemotherapy, either preventing or minimising physical discomfort and distress. Anticipation of toxicities makes it possible to provide effective prophylaxis in some cases. It is essential to be familiar with protocols in use when taking responsibility for patients receiving chemotherapy or for administering the drugs; in addition to giving details of chemotherapy, protocols contain vital information about prophylactic medications such as antiemetics and antidotes given as part of a particular course of treatment.

Assessing the toxicities of anti-cancer chemotherapy in practice requires knowledge of the effect of cytotoxic drugs on the body in general, and familiarity with the effects of the specific drugs or combinations of drugs in use. It is important to observe the onset, severity, and duration of toxicities, to recognise any risk to patients, and to initiate interventions and make prompt referrals to ensure that chemotherapy-related problems are dealt with effectively. The World Health Organization and other bodies such as American National Cancer Institute (see http://ctep.cancer.gov/reporting/ctc.html) have developed systems of common toxicity criteria to facilitate the reporting of toxicities in clinical practice and clinical trials.[16]

The side-effects of chemotherapy can be divided into three categories according to their time of onset.[36] Immediate side-effects (Box 12.1) can be said to occur within 30 minutes of the start of treatment; short-term side-effects (Box 12.2) can be said to occur between 3 and 7 days after therapy begins; and long-term side-effects (Box 12.3), which are often cumulative, can be said to occur after 7 days.

Immediate side-effects

Local effects of chemotherapy, which are related to the venepuncture site and the venous pathway, are often transient. It is important to inform patients of what to expect so that they can provide the information nurses and clinicians need to help them to distinguish between events such as local allergic reaction, and extravasation. Doxorubicin and daunorubicin have been associated with a localised hypersensitivity reaction known as a *flare* reaction. In a flare reaction, urticaria (itching, 'hives') can occur at the injection site and along the vein. It may occur only with administration

Box 12.1   Immediate side-effects of chemotherapy

- Pain at insertion site
- Venous pain
- Cold sensation along the vein
- Red flush along the vein
- 'Nettle' rash along and adjacent to the vein
- Facial flushing
- Bodily flushing
- Hypotension
- Hypersensitivity reactions
- Anaphylaxis
- Abnormal tastes or smells

Box 12.2   Short-term side-effects of chemotherapy

- Anorexia
- Nausea
- Vomiting
- Stomatitis
- Possible recall of radiation skin reactions
- Pain at tumour site or jaw area
- Malaise
- Flu-like syndrome, including fever
- Chemical cystitis
- Haematuria
- Red urine/green urine
- Constipation
- Diarrhoea
- Cold-induced paraesthesia (oxaliplatin)

Box 12.3   Long-term and cumulative side-effects of chemotherapy

- Bone marrow depression
- Alopecia
- Skin reactions, including rashes, inflammation, pigmentation, photosensitivity, palmar plantar syndrome
- Nail ridging
- Pulmonary fibrosis
- Thrombophlebitis
- Pulmonary fibrosis
- Congestive cardiac failure
- Liver dysfunction
- Renal toxicity
- Sexual dysfunction, including amenorrhoea, sterility, possible chromosomal damage
- Neurological problems, including peripheral neuropathy, muscle weakness, high-frequency hearing loss, paralytic ileus, bladder atony
- CNS toxicity, including lethargy, fatigue, depression, headaches

of the first dose of the drug, or alternatively, on second and subsequent occasions.[14]

Short-term effects

Anorexia

Anorexia, a loss of the desire to eat, is frequently experienced by people with cancer and patients receiving chemotherapy. It can lead to reduced food intake, malnutrition, impaired quality of life, and increased morbidity.[98] Anorexia can be secondary to a number of factors, including fatigue, nausea and vomiting, dry mouth, stomatitis, constipation, and alterations in taste and smell. Taste alterations, which can vary in degree, type, and duration, are thought to be caused by the direct

effect of chemotherapeutic agents on the taste buds of the tongue, which are replaced every 5–7 days.[14] Patients may experience a metallic or bitter taste, and there may be an increased threshold or aversion to sweet food. Within the family, a disinclination to eat or participate in meal times can be seen as a rejection of caring feelings and actions, and may lead to uncomfortable pressures and tensions.[99] It is important that patients and their families understand this, and that they are given help to set realistic goals in terms of meeting nutritional requirements.

The first step is often nutritional assessment, which includes physical assessment, dietary history, what may have caused the loss of appetite, and specific measures such as weight, intake and expenditure of calories, or skin-fold thickness. It may be necessary to refer patients to a dietician for advice on nutritional supplements and on whether enteral or parenteral feeding is required. Patients and their families and friends should be assisted to maintain an interest in nutrition and the dietary choices available to them, and an awareness of the role of a well-planned diet in sustaining energy levels and physical and emotional well-being. It can be helpful to experiment with flavours, and strongly flavoured sweets to mask tastes or smells may make it easier to tolerate the administration of some drugs. Factors that contribute to the enjoyment of food, such as presentation, odour, texture, timing, social setting, and alcoholic drinks, can be discussed and taken into account when planning meals. Measures can be taken to prevent or minimise some of the conditions that impair sensation or perception and affect the intake of food and fluids, including scrupulous oral hygiene, and treatment of dry mouth, stomatitis, nausea, vomiting, and constipation. Alterations in taste are likely to be temporary, and it may help to reassure patients that their liking for favourite foods will return. In the meantime, regular, small meals can be offered, or alternatively, a good meal served at a time when a patient feels particularly able to eat.

Diarrhoea

Diarrhoea can be defined as an increase in stool volume and liquidity resulting in three or more bowel movements a day.[16] It may be accompanied by abdominal cramps and/or flatus. By inhibiting normal cell replication, chemotherapy can disrupt the process of cell replacement and disturb the integrity of the epithelial lining of the bowel, which becomes inflamed and oedematous. The overall size of the absorptive surface becomes smaller as villi and microvilli are flattened and become atrophic;[99] intestinal contents pass rapidly through the gut, with a consequent lessening in the absorption of nutrients. The degree and duration of diarrhoea depend on the chemotherapeutic agent in use, the dose, the timing of the nadir (lowest point in the peripheral blood count after chemotherapy), and the frequency of administration.[16] 5-FU is known to cause diarrhoea, as are actinomycin-D, arsenic trioxide, bortezomib, capecitabine, docetaxel, doxorubicin, gefitnib, irinotecan, and methotrexate. While diarrhoea is a less common complication with methotrexate, therapy must be halted if it occurs, to prevent serious gastrointestinal problems.[16]

Patients should be assessed to establish their normal bowel habit, ways of managing elimination, and nutritional status. Nutritional status, fluid balance, the frequency and characteristics of the diarrhoea, and the effectiveness of anti-diarrhoeal drugs (e.g. loperamide) in relieving diarrhoea and/or cramps should be frequently monitored. High-calorie, high-protein, low-residue, soft, bland, easily digested foods (e.g. fish, chicken, pasta, boiled or steamed vegetables) should be provided, and milk, milk products, high-fibre foods, and others that exacerbate diarrhoea avoided. Adequate fluid replacement is essential, as is careful perianal care. Octreotide acetate is suggested as a treatment for excessive diarrhoea following gastrointestinal resection or when chemotherapy-induced diarrhoea is not effectively controlled by other pharmacological interventions.[16]

Constipation

Constipation has been defined as infrequent, excessively hard and dry bowel movements resulting from a decrease in rectal filling or emptying.[16] The vinca alkaloids (e.g. vincristine and vinblastine) most commonly cause constipation, secondary to autonomic nerve dysfunction that is manifested as colicky abdominal pain and adynamic ileus.[14] Symptoms occur within 3–7 days after drug administration. Constipation is an uncomfortable and distressing side-effect, which can create nutritional problems and result in anal tears, bleeding, and infection.

The emphasis should be on prevention rather than treatment. The risk of constipation can be reduced through good knowledge of dietary measures such as adequate fibre and fluid intake, and through regular physical activity. Stool softeners and laxatives can be prescribed in conjunction with chemotherapeutic agents known to cause constipation. Early notification of medical staff when problems are developing, and appropriate use of prescribed medication, can help to prevent the more serious and distressing consequences of this condition. The use of laxatives and/or stool softeners such as lactulose is especially recommended for patients with a history of constipation. Choosing an appropriate medication from the range of enemas, suppositories, stimulants, and softeners available depends on what effect is required.

Stomatitis

Stomatitis is an acute inflammation of the oral and oropharyngeal mucous membranes, including the lips, tongue, gingiva (gums), buccal mucosa, palate, or floor of the mouth. The processes underlying the development of mucositis are complex and involve the interaction of a range of cellular, tissue, and oral factors. In the initial tissue injury phase, the cells of the basal epithelium are damaged. This is followed by the epithelial phase, in which there is epithelial atrophy, and then by the ulcerative/infective phase, and finally the healing phase.[100] Mucositis is very disabling and significantly affects quality of life, causing pain and difficulty with eating, drinking, and talking: research suggests that at least 40% and as many as 70% of patients receiving standard chemotherapy treatment will experience mucositis.[100,101] Many drugs, in particular bleomycin, doxorubicin, daunorubicin, docetaxel, 5-FU, and methotrexate, are known to induce stomatitis, in addition to high-dose therapy with busulphan, etoposide, melphalan, and thiotepa.

The mucosal lining of the mouth consists of non-keratinised squamous epithelium that regenerates every 10–14 days; the first symptoms of stomatitis, including pale, dry mucous membranes, can be seen as early as the third day after administration of the chemotherapeutic agent, and may be accompanied by a burning sensation. Diffuse ulceration may not appear for up to 7 days after treatment is given. A number of factors can influence the frequency and severity of oral complications, including drug type, dosage, nutritional status, oral health prior to treatment, and quality of oral care given during treatment.

Younger patients experience stomatitis more frequently than older patients, and the incidence of oral complications is two to three times higher in haematological malignancies than in solid tumours, possibly due to the immunosuppression that characterises haematological cancers. Good oral hygiene appears to reduce the severity of oral mucositis without increasing the risk of infection.[16,100] Both the more minor effects of chemotherapy on the mouth (for example, a burning sensation, intolerance to hot, spicy, or acidic foods, inflammation, and changes to saliva production), and the major effects, including sloughing, ulceration, bleeding, and bacterial, fungal, or viral infections, have profound effects on quality of life, and can undermine an individual's ability

and willingness to tolerate further chemotherapy. Stomatitis can indeed be so severe and painful that eating and drinking become extremely difficult, and it may be necessary to reduce the dose of chemotherapy or to delay subsequent courses.

Before the start of chemotherapy a baseline oral assessment is recommended, including a review of the patient's daily oral care routine. Effective oral hygiene and plaque control, with a soft toothbrush to prevent damage to delicate tissues, should be maintained. Specific nursing interventions depend on the extent of stomatitis, which may range from a potential problem to bleeding, ulceration, and an inability to take food or fluids (sometimes described as grade 4 stomatitis).[14] Measures include use of normal saline or antibacterial mouthwashes, and sodium bicarbonate solution or dilute hydrogen peroxide to remove thick secretions or debris.[14,16] The mouth should be rinsed with water after using hydrogen peroxide. A soft, bland diet with a smooth consistency is recommended; spicy or acidic foods (and tobacco) should be avoided. Topical analgesics for use before meals are available to control pain and dysphagia.[101] Application of emollients or medicated topical applications is often required to prevent cracking and drying of the lips and to treat infections, and antibacterial and antifungal oral suspensions to treat oral infections. In the most severe cases patients will require IV hydration, measures to control pain (which may include a morphine infusion), and on occasions enteral or parenteral feeding.

With some drugs (such as 5-FU) cryotherapy may be helpful in preventing stomatitis: patients start sucking ice chips 5 minutes before chemotherapy is given, and continue for 25 minutes afterwards.[100]

Nausea and vomiting
While clinicians often regard suppression of the bone marrow as being the major dose-limiting toxicity of chemotherapy, patients are likely to see nausea and vomiting as the most distressing side-effect:[70,102]

After the second course, I found that thinking about going there made me vomit, in fact it was almost as bad as when I was actually having treatment. Even now [2 years later] I start feeling sick when I pass the hospital.[103]

- *Nausea* is often experienced as the need to vomit, an unpleasant sensation of impending sickness focused on the stomach. Patients suffering from nausea often appear pale and sweaty; they may have a rapid pulse and feel cold and clammy.
- *Retching* is a rhythmic, often forceful, movement involving the diaphragm and abdominal muscles, which moves stomach contents in and out of the oesophagus.
- *Vomiting* occurs when the contents of the stomach, duodenum, or jejunum are expelled forcefully through the mouth. This is achieved by sudden powerful contractions of the respiratory muscles at the same time as relaxation of the upper oesophageal sphincter. Vomiting is often followed by lethargy and pronounced weakness of the muscles.

Chemotherapy-induced nausea and vomiting occurs at a variety of time points relative to the time that treatment was given. Nausea and vomiting occurring within 2 hours of treatment (and lasting up to 24 hours) is referred to as *acute*; *delayed* nausea and vomiting develops or persists 24 hours after chemotherapy; *anticipatory* nausea and vomiting occurs before or during administration as a result of operant conditioning from stimuli associated with chemotherapy.[16] Younger patients tend to experience more nausea and vomiting than older patients.[104] Chemotherapeutic agents can be described as having *mild, moderate,* or *severe* emetogenic potential, according to the severity of nausea and vomiting with which they are associated (see Table 12.1). Poor prophylaxis or control of nausea and vomiting has the potential to affect quality of life badly, by initiating a number of undesirable consequences, including anticipatory nausea and vomiting, unwillingness to continue with treatment, delays in treatment, dose reduction, dehydration, electrolyte imbalance, anorexia and aversion to food, oesophageal tears, dental erosion, muscular strain, and fatigue.

Mechanism of nausea and vomiting. The vomiting reflex in chemotherapy-induced nausea and vomiting is co-ordinated by the vomiting centre (VC) in the medullary reticular formation in the brain. The VC is located close to the chemoreceptor trigger zone (CTZ), which is sensitive to chemicals, drugs, and toxins, including chemotherapeutic agents, and radiation. The vomiting centre is sensitive to stimulation from the CTZ, afferent nerve fibres in the gastrointestinal tract, cerebral cortex, and vestibular apparatus.[16,105] Vomiting occurs when the vomiting centre is stimulated from the CTZ or other areas. Dopamine and serotonin receptors are located in the CTZ, and histamine and dopamine receptors in the VC.[16] Damage to the mucosa of the small intestine caused by chemotherapy releases sero-

Table 12.1 Emetogenicity of common chemotherapeutic agents

Mildly emetogenic	Moderately emetogenic	Highly emetogenic
Etoposide (oral)	Carboplatin	Cisplatin
Mitomycin C	Daunorubicin	Mustine
Methotrexate	Carmustine	Dacarbazine
Bleomycin	Lomustine	Cyclophosphamide (IV >1000 mg/m^2)
Chlorambucil	Doxorubicin	Melphalan (IV >100 mg/m^2)
5-FU (continuous infusion)	Dactinomycin	
Melphalan (oral)	Cytarabine	
Vincristine	Procarbazine	
Vinblastine	Mitoxantrone	
	5-FU (IV bolus)	
	Etoposide (IV)	

tonin (5-HT$_3$), which stimulates receptors on afferent nerve fibres, which in turn stimulate the vomiting centre. 5-HT$_3$ antagonists (e.g. ondansetron and granisetron) have shown considerable success in preventing and controlling acute nausea and vomiting in patients receiving chemotherapy, but have been less successful in treating delayed nausea and vomiting.[14,106]

Assessment of nausea and vomiting. Nausea and vomiting are distinct experiences, which are usefully assessed separately, though some studies appear not to distinguish between the two. The experience of nausea affects individuals in different ways, and assessment relies on eliciting patients' accounts. The word 'nausea' is not always understood: 'feeling sick' or 'feeling queasy' are more commonly used. It is possible to interpret the experience of nausea in terms of dimensions such as frequency, intensity, and duration, which can then be recorded by means of visual analogue scales (10 cm lines marked with a cross to indicate severity) or descriptive ordinal scales (where a choice is given between descriptors such as 'never', 'sometimes', or 'frequently', each of which is allocated a sequential score). However, patients' own accounts remain a fundamental source of information about nausea and/or vomiting, recorded in specially designed diaries or journals. Using a scale in conjunction with a diary or journal provides a simple means of comparing scores and assessments, though a scale necessarily omits much of the complexity of the experience.

Anticipatory nausea and vomiting. Although it occurs less frequently than post-treatment nausea and vomiting, anticipatory nausea and vomiting (ANV) can be just as distressing, and anti-emetic drugs do not appear to control it once it has developed. It is estimated that 25–30% of patients experience anticipatory nausea by their fourth cycle of chemotherapy, and that 8–20% of patients receiving chemotherapy experience anticipatory vomiting.[107]

ANV has been described as a learned or conditioned response:[107,108] neutral stimuli such as the odour or appearance of the treatment room or the sight of the nurse become strongly associated with the chemotherapy. They therefore lose their 'neutrality' and become 'conditioned stimuli'. Responses elicited by conditioned stimuli are known as conditioned responses. Conditioned responses (such as nausea and vomiting) may occur in the presence of conditioned stimuli (for example, the room, smell, or nurse), without the presence of the unconditioned stimulus (the chemotherapy itself).

Nausea and vomiting following chemotherapy are largely determined by the type of chemotherapy received, although other factors such as age (<50 years) and susceptibility to motion sickness may have an influence. Anxiety, severity, and duration of post-chemotherapy nausea, and pre-treatment expectations about developing nausea have been linked to an increased tendency towards ANV.[107]

Preventing ANV. It has been suggested that the development of anticipatory side-effects could be avoided, or at least significantly reduced, by better management of post-treatment nausea and vomiting. Allowing nausea and vomiting to develop before prescribing anti-emetics is a poor strategy in the management of the problem in general, and in the management of ANV in particular. Some research suggests that behavioural interventions (for example, deep relaxation or distraction) can be effective in controlling ANV:[109,110]

> During those chemotherapy treatments when the behavioural methods were implemented, no anticipatory vomiting occurred; however, during those chemotherapy treatments when the behavioural methods were not implemented, anticipatory vomiting occurred. Similarly dramatic results have been obtained with children using distraction through video game playing [pp.813–814].[109]

Nurses can take steps to reduce sounds and smells that may trigger ANV, and audio tapes, radios, and TV should be available in treatment areas to provide distraction.[16]

Choice of anti-emetic drugs. A number of factors may be relevant in determining the susceptibility of an individual to emesis following chemotherapy, including previous emesis during chemotherapy, a history of motion sickness, the emetic potential of chemotherapeutic agents (both singly and in combination), and the dose and schedule of anti-emetics. In practice, though, these factors do not usually influence the choice of anti-emetic drug, which is based on the emetic potential of the type of chemotherapy in use.

Anti-emetic agents. A variety of anti-emetic agents is in common use. No single drug has proven ideal, giving complete control of emesis and no toxicity. Combinations of different anti-emetics are frequently used to provide the most effective management. Phenothiazines (e.g. chlorpromazine and prochlorperazine) are useful in the treatment of motion sickness and other forms of emesis not related to chemotherapy; chlorpromazine has also been shown to give anti-emetic control in around 50% of patients receiving non-platinum-containing chemotherapy regimens.[111] Corticosteroids (e.g. dexamethasone) are widely used to provide control of emesis with moderately emetogenic chemotherapy, usually in high concentrations and in combination with metaclopramide or serotonin ($5-HT_3$) antagonists. Cannabinoids such as nabilone have an anti-emetic effect but also cause dysphoria, hypotension, and dizziness in up to 30% of patients. They are absorbed unpredictably when taken orally, and are not widely used in current anti-emetic practice. Butyrophenones (doperidol and haloperidol) have short plasma half-lives but are effective when given by IV or subcutaneous infusion. Their anti-emetic effect is dose dependent, and toxicity at therapeutic levels, including dystonia, dry mouth, and sedation, limits their use. Use of benzodiazepines such as lorazepam is also limited by their sedative effect, which precludes use in outpatients' departments for instance. However, their amnesic and anxiolytic properties may be useful in the treatment of anticipatory nausea and vomiting if given at least 24 hours before chemotherapy.[112]

Of the class of drugs known as substituted benzamides, metaclopramide is the most commonly used. Given by the oral route, it has little anti-emetic effect, but given over 15 minutes in higher doses by short IV infusion it is very effective in the treatment of acute emesis in moderately and highly emetogenic regimes, including platinum-based chemotherapy. Side-effects may occur, including akathesia and dystonic reactions; the overall incidence of extrapyramidal side-effects is between 10 and 15%.

The development of selective serotonin receptor antagonists has provided a class of drug that is very effective in controlling emesis without causing sedation or extrapyramidal effects.[1] Side-effects of $5-HT_3$ antagonists do include mild or moderate headache, flushing, fatigue, diarrhoea (1%), and constipation (3%). A number of $5-HT_3$ antagonists have been tested in clinical trials, including ondansetron, granisetron, and tropisetron. Ondansetron and granisetron have been shown to be effective in the prophylaxis of emesis caused by platinum compounds, with complete or major control of side-effects in around two-thirds of patients. They have been shown to be effective in the control of emesis caused by moderately emetogenic drugs, and in controlling emesis that has not responded to treatment with conventional agents such as dexamethasone or metaclopramide. Despite their role in the control of acute emesis, $5-HT_3$ antagonists are less effective in the management of delayed emesis.

Nursing interventions.

> The worst time was after the first chemotherapy. I was so frightened probably because I didn't know what to expect. It didn't seem so difficult after that, even though it was as bad, once I knew I'd survive it.[113]

Supporting patients who are coping with vomiting presents a challenge for nurses. Honesty and realism about the likelihood and duration of the problem must be combined with an explanation of why it is happening and a sensitive approach to the fears provoked. Patients are likely to benefit from opportunities to learn about the nature of the side-effects of chemotherapy and when they are likely to happen; exploring patients' expectations and previous experiences of vomiting with a particular chemotherapy regimen can help to identify care priorities. Knowledge and effective use of the range of pharmacological options for managing nausea and vomiting is essential, and written information on what to expect and how best to deal with it is often useful. Non-pharmacological measures are equally important. Advice on adjusting eating habits can help, including assessment of the most suitable timing, size, and content of meals. Small, frequent, low-fat meals, eaten cold to avoid cooking odours, and accompanied by fizzy drinks are often more easily tolerated. Sipping nourishing fluids regularly can assist in achieving the desired fluid and dietary intake. Nibbling on dry toast, crackers, or biscuits may help to settle a nauseous stomach. Relaxation and distraction exercises (some guidelines can be found in *Pain: Clinical Manual for Nursing Practice*[114]), therapeutic touch, massage, and aromatherapy can also have a positive effect.

It is important to pay careful attention to the patient's environment by using restful colours, and providing music, television, comfortable furniture including reclining chairs, and access to fresh air. It has been suggested that patients experience less severe nausea and vomiting when they are seated during administration of chemotherapy, rather than lying down.

Acupressure for nausea and vomiting is a noninvasive technique, which involves applying pressure to the P6 acupressure point located on the inner aspect of the wrist, three fingers' width above the distal skin crease of the wrist joint. It is easy to administer and safe to use. Patients can put commercially available bands in place as soon as chemotherapy has been administered, pressing the stud incorporated in the band at regular intervals. A recent systematic review of acupuncture-point stimulation for chemotherapy-induced nausea or vomiting for the Cochrane Collaboration[115] concluded that:

- electroacupuncture reduced first-day vomiting
- acupressure reduced first-day nausea (but there was no benefit for vomiting)
- acupuncture-point stimulation by any method is safe and has minimal rare side-effects.

Other side-effects

A recent review of research into the neuropsychological effects of adjuvant chemotherapy for breast cancer[116] concluded that there was a small effect on cognitive function, although findings did not suggest a clinically significant level of impairment:

> The cognitive domains most negatively affected were language, short term memory, and spatial abilities, with differences in mean scores ranging from about

one-quarter to one-half a standard deviation. Statistically significant, albeit lower deterioration, was also found in the domains of working and long-term memory, speed of processing, spatial and motor abilities – findings also consistent with previous reports suggesting that the effects of adjuvant chemotherapy on cognitive functioning were global in nature [p.84].

The less well publicised side-effects of chemotherapy, which may not be seen as priorities by nursing or medical staff, can trouble patients greatly. Patients may experience a great number and variety of effects which, without preparation and explanation, can seem to indicate a general deterioration in well-being that is not necessarily seen as relating to chemotherapy at all. Therefore, it is always important to take an inclusive approach to the subject of side-effects and to work together with patients so that as little as possible is unexpected, and a broad range of management strategies is made available.

Fatigue

This is a multidimensional concept including feelings of tiredness, lack of energy, and inability to continue, and is a common and distressing effect of both cancer and chemotherapy,[117] with research suggesting that between 60 and 90% of patients receiving chemotherapy experience it:[118]

> I'm exhausted all the time, both physically and mentally. I go to bed after lunch while my daughter sleeps and I just can't manage without that and then going to bed at night when she does. I'm doing nothing except existing.[113]

Acute fatigue can be seen as protective, in that it is an intermittent response to such things as overwork or a hectic timetable, and provides an opportunity to restore energy levels and preparedness. Chronic fatigue, in contrast, has been described as generalised, with extreme tiredness and very low energy, and is perceived as abnormal and excessive.[119] It affects the whole body, and is constant and difficult to resolve.

A number of theories have been put forward to explain chronic fatigue, though no conclusive explanation exists as yet. One theory is that fatigue is caused by an accumulation of waste products and metabolites; another is that muscular activity is impaired when the necessary 'materials' are not available. It has been suggested that increased energy expenditure, and changes in the production, utilisation, and distribution of hormones may influence feelings of fatigue, as well as having a functional effect. The neurophysiological model of fatigue suggests that it is due to alterations in the central nervous system,[120] and it has also been suggested that each of us has a specific amount of energy to aid adaptation to stressful situations and that once this is depleted, fatigue is inevitable.[121] Other factors, including the extent of tumour burden, physical symptoms, psychological stress, psychosocial changes such as isolation and boredom, and drugs such as antiemetics have also been put forward as possible explanations.

The time of onset, duration, pattern, and severity of chemotherapy-related fatigue may vary and appear to be related to the drug in use. In one study,[118] patients receiving 3–4-week cycles of chemotherapy experienced high levels of fatigue in the 4–5 days after treatment. Fatigue then decreased until the low point of the blood count (nadir) at around 15 days, when it increased again temporarily. Patients who received weekly injections, however, were found to experience moderate, cyclically fluctuating fatigue. It has been suggested that fatigue may be associated with disruption of neurotransmitters, and that drugs that cross the blood–brain barrier or cause neurotoxicities (for example, vinca alkaloids, 5-FU[122] or adjuvant chemotherapy for breast cancer[123,124]) are therefore more likely to cause it.

Rhodes has described how patients were able to care for themselves after chemotherapy,[125] but still found tiredness and weakness to be the symptoms that interfered most with self-care activities:

> I could not get out of bed and walk to the bathroom and would have to sit down and rest, then go to the shower . . . I would have to rest between each activity . . . because I had no energy left [p.191].

Objective assessment of fatigue is possible, but may be of less relevance practically than the patient's own assessment.[119]

Interventions. Tierney *et al.* found that patients felt that tiredness was one of the few side-effects of chemotherapy that they had any control over themselves, and most reported using specific measures to alleviate it.[113] In particular, coping with tiredness involved actions directed at conserving energy. Rhodes[125] has described how patients planned their activities to this end:

> . . . scheduling activities, stuff like that – became the most important thing for me . . . I had to figure out how far I could walk [p.191].

The aim is to alternate periods of activity with periods of rest, to build up or maintain levels of function:

> In the afternoon, I would be tired, so usually I would rest and then we would have to do any socialising we did in the evening [p.191].

Rest or sleep, in the form of naps or periods of inactivity, is frequently recommended to allow recuperation or conservation of energy, but extended periods of sleep do not always alleviate tiredness. Minimising boredom, and involving friends and relatives in household chores and food preparation, can prevent loss of focus and reduce the burden of unwanted activities. Exercise has been reported to have an influence on both perceptions and the experience of fatigue.

Recent work has focused on interventions specifically designed to alleviate fatigue in patients receiving chemotherapy. Adamsen *et al.*, for example, investigated the effect of multidimensional exercise on physical capacity, well-being, and quality of life in patients with a range of haematological and solid tumours.[126] Following the intervention, significant increases were found in a range of outcomes, including physical fitness and physical activity, alongside reductions in pain and fatigue. The authors suggest that further, large-scale trials of this type of intervention are warranted.

Hair loss (see also Research study 12.1)

Hair loss (alopecia) with anti-cancer chemotherapy is related to the cytotoxic effect of the drugs on rapidly proliferating cells in the hair matrix.[1]

Actively growing (anagen) hairs are affected by partial or complete disruption of cell division, leading to thin, fragile hairs or absence of growth. Hair loss due to chemotherapy is apparent 1–2 weeks after administration, and reaches a peak in 1–2 months.[1] The extent of hair loss can range from thinning of hair on the scalp to loss of all body hair.[16] Generally speaking, chemotherapy-related hair loss is reversible, although there are reports of permanent hair loss following administration of cyclophosphamide and busulphan prior to bone marrow transplantation.[1] Regrowing hair may be altered in colour and/or texture. Perry[1] suggests that anti-cancer agents associated with hair loss include: amsacrine, bleomycin, busulfan, cyclophosphamide, cytarabine, dactinomycin, daunorubicin, dacarbazine, doxorubicin, etoposide, 5-FU, hydroxyurea, ifosfamide, interleukin-2, methotrexate, nitrosureas, procarbazine, vinblastine, and vincristine.

Our hair plays an important part in the way we see or think of ourselves, and hair loss can badly damage our body image and self-concept,[127] particularly in view of current stereotypes of physical beauty.[128] Freedman[129] explains that:

> Embodied in the symbolism of hair is a concept of the whole self, a completed person, who has the possibility of expressing individualism through the design of her hair. If hair is seen as being associated with the person's identity, then the meaning of the loss of hair can be understood as symbolic of the devastating sense of the diminishing and eventual loss of the self. The loss of hair is an extremely traumatic experience precisely because it is the symbolic precursor to the loss of the self. This raises the psychological terror and consequent fear that the known self will no longer exist [p. 336].

Sudden changes in body image or alterations of body structure or function are perceived as threats and invariably cause anxiety. The hair loss caused by anti-cancer chemotherapy represents such a threat.[130] It has been suggested that of all the side-effects of chemotherapy, hair loss is the most distressing, and it may be the reason that some patients decline treatment.[128,131,132] A patient's own account[133] of hair loss expresses how distressing an experience it is:

> Mentally I had prepared myself for the likelihood of losing my hair and having to wear a wig; but the physical reality of the hair falling out posed emotional and practical problems which I had not anticipated. For two weeks I was in tears every morning, plucking the clumps of hair from all over the bedclothes . . . intellectually I understood what was happening, but emotionally it reinforced my feelings that I was losing part of myself [p.1022].

Hesketh et al.[134] point out that the impact of chemotherapy-induced alopecia (CIA) can be enormous:

> For some women, hair loss can have more of an impact than a mastectomy. Others are so distressed at the prospect of losing their hair that they may choose less effective therapies or opt for no treatment at all. CIA can cause anxiety, depression, negative body image, lowered self-esteem, and a reduced sense of well-being [p.545].

In one study of changes in self-concept and body image in women receiving chemotherapy for gynaecological cancers, however, all patients favoured the possibility of cure over loss of hair before treatment;[135] and while 13.3% of women felt, before chemotherapy, that their partners might reject them, only one patient actually felt rejected when hair loss had occurred.

Freedman[129] discusses the meaning or symbolism of hair loss:

> For many . . . the meaning of the shaved head can be symbolic of a state of disgrace, which becomes a stigmata of sin or wrongdoing. This symbolic meaning . . . may be part of the reason that women describe themselves as being in a state of shame when they lose their hair . . . 'Losing my hair was the most traumatic part of the cancer/chemo process for me. It makes it so obvious that you are sick. Under the wig I knew there was a shiny bald head. It really takes some getting used to. It's really hard to express how you feel when your hair is coming out in handfuls. Some words are panic, fear, hurt, and even shame for how you look, even though you know it is not your fault' [p. 337].

While the prospect of hair loss is a source of distress and anxiety for some (particularly if it occurs a second time),[136] not every patient will share this experience. It cannot be assumed that every patient will be distressed, and some may find that there are positive aspects to the situation.[135,137] An opportunity to talk about how you are feeling can be very helpful, and for nurses, developing an understanding of the meaning and importance of hair loss for different patients can lead to important insights into the caring process.[129] Nurses are well placed to provide support and information, and to highlight choices. They can offer realistic information about hair loss, details about what actually happens and when, and advice and assistance with practical problems (if and when to cut hair or choose a wig, for instance).[138,139] Scalp cooling, although it is not effective in all cases, can be offered in appropriate circumstances to prevent or reduce hair loss, though it may be a lengthy and uncomfortable procedure.[140–143] It should be carefully explained in advance, measures should be taken to minimise discomfort and anxiety, and patients' reactions should be carefully monitored.[144–146]

Long-term effects

Bone marrow suppression

Bone marrow suppression (myelosuppression) is the most frequent dose-limiting side-effect of cancer chemotherapy and is potentially life-threatening: when death occurs in the myelosuppressed patient it is most often due to infection or haemorrhage. Many of the agents used in cancer chemotherapy affect the rapidly dividing stem cells in the bone marrow: the red blood cells (erythrocytes), the white blood cells (leucocytes), and the platelets (thrombocytes). The onset of myelosuppression can be rapid: white blood cells divide every 6–8 hours, platelets every 7–10 days, and because chemotherapy interferes with dividing cells, these cells are most quickly affected by myelosuppressive drugs. Loss of white blood cells (neutropenia) is seen before loss of platelets (thrombocytopenia); and, generally speaking, neutropenia is more severe.[105] Red blood cells are replaced every 120 days or so and anaemia develops more slowly.

The lowest point to which the peripheral blood count of red and white cells and platelets falls is known as the 'nadir' (opposite of 'zenith'), which usually occurs 7–14 days after chemotherapy has been administered. As cells are replaced the nadir resolves; with high-dose chemotherapy, however, populations of stem cells may be unable to regenerate quickly, leading to a prolonged nadir period. Some of the alkylating agents, including nitrogen mustard (mechlorethamine), dacarbazine, busulfan, and the nitrosureas (e.g. carmustine and lomustine) are regarded as particularly myelosuppressive.[105] A number of newer drugs, including bortezomib, gemcitabine, imatinib mesylate, oxaliplatin, pemetrexed, and paclitaxel are also known to be myelosuppressive.[16] Several factors are cited as contributing to the degree of bone marrow suppression, including age (though some older people tolerate normal doses),[147] class of drug, combination of drugs, poor nutrition, reduced bone marrow reserve, poor renal or liver function, and previous treatment (for example, radiotherapy to sites of bone marrow production).[14]

Bone marrow suppression leading to loss of white cells, particularly neutrophils, increases the risk of patients experiencing severe bacterial infection. Neutrophils, which are one of three types of white cells known as granulocytes, are the largest group of white cells and act as phagocytes, playing a vital role in the body's inflammatory response and defence against micro-organisms. Neutropenia can be defined as an absolute neutrophil count (ANC) of less than 1500 cells/mm^3. Neutropenia can occur when the total white blood cell count (WBC) is within the range of normal. Chemotherapy is usually withheld if the patient's white blood cell count is between 1000 and 3000 cells/mm^3 or the ANC is below 1500 cells/mm^3.[16] Risk of infection increases proportionately as the neutrophil count decreases. Fever is often the first sign of infection, though when infection occurs in the neutropenic patient, signs such as inflammation or formation of pus at infected sites may be absent or less conspicuous. Infection with organisms such as *Pseudomonas aeruginosa*, *Staphylococcus aureus* and the fungus *Candida albicans* are common; sites include the blood, respiratory tract, and oral mucosa.

Thrombocytopenia, reduction of platelet counts below the normal level of 150 000–350 000 cells/mm^3, increases the risk of bruising, bleeding from the gums or nose, petechiae, and haemorrhage in the central nervous system or gastrointestinal tract.

Risk of bleeding increases in proportion to the decrease in numbers of platelets; the risk is regarded as moderate when counts fall below 50 000 cells/mm^3, and severe below 20 000 cells/mm^3.[14] Chemotherapy may be withheld if the platelet count falls below 75 000–100 000 cells/mm^5.[16]

Severe anaemia is less often seen with cancer chemotherapy; when it occurs it develops later than chemotherapy-induced neutropenia or thrombocytopenia, because of the longer half-life of red blood cells. Signs of anaemia include pallor of the skin, mucous membranes, conjunctiva, and nail beds, and hypotension, increased heart rate, breathlessness, headaches, and fatigue.

Patients should be asked to report any of the signs and symptoms associated with bone marrow suppression, and measures taken to reduce the risk of bleeding and infection. It is important to maintain the integrity of the skin and mucous membranes to provide a barrier against infection. Care should be taken to maintain personal hygiene, and to avoid cuts and bruises, for example by using a soft toothbrush for oral care, and an electric shaver in preference to a wet razor. The risk of constipation and straining can be reduced with the use of stool softeners, and adequate intake of fluids and dietary fibre.

Invasive procedures like injections and catheterisation, which breach the integrity of the skin and increase the risk of infection, should be kept to a minimum, and medications that interfere with clotting (such as aspirin) treated with caution. Patients may be asked to avoid crowded places or people with known infections; in severe cases of neutropenia, protective isolation and antibiotic and/or antifungal therapy are often required.

Anaemia may not prevent continuation of chemotherapy but has a significant effect on how patients feel about and cope with their treatment; blood transfusions may be required, especially if patients are symptomatic. Both anaemia and thrombocytopenia can be corrected by transfusions of blood or platelets.

In recent years the use of haematopoietic growth factors has had an impact on the management of chemotherapy-induced neutropenia. Colony-stimulating factors (CSFs) can be used to alleviate neutropenia, and have shortened the duration of neutropenia, thus alleviating infec-tion-related morbidity and mortality.[16] Erythropoietin can be used to reverse anaemia.[1]

Gonadal toxicity

In women, chemotherapeutic agents are known to affect ovarian function. Nitrogen mustard, cyclophosphamide, L-phenylalanine mustard (in adjuvant therapy for breast cancer), busulfan, and chlorambucil are known to be actually or potentially gonadotoxic. 5-FU, doxorubicin, and bleomycin (as single agents) are probably well tolerated. Menstrual irregularities are common in premenopausal women treated with tamoxifen for breast cancer. Infertility is an important consideration in some combination chemotherapies: the incidence of amenorrhea in women receiving MOPP, MVPP or COPP for Hodgkin's disease is reported to be between 15% and 80%.[1]

Women can experience amenorrhoea with hot flushes, insomnia, and vaginal dryness, as well as decreased fertility or permanent infertility. They may also experience decreased sexual interest and disruptions in self-confidence and close relationships. Menstruation sometimes recommences months or even years after treatment has finished. Damage to the ovaries appears to be age-related, with women aged over 30 years less likely to regain ovarian function:

> I went to my GP because my period was so late and also with these hot flushes I thought something might be up. He told me that chemotherapy can sometimes bring on the menopause. Well, I was really devastated. I could remember, after the mastectomy, that my period came and I thought to myself, well, that's good, at least I'm still a woman. I'd really be depressed if this treatment now finishes it off for me. I wouldn't be so upset maybe if I'd known this was possible . . . but no-one mentioned it.[113]

Clearly, it is important to work with women sensitively and supportively to enable them to discuss and consider the implications of chemotherapy on ovarian function, and to review, and if necessary adapt themselves sexually, with their partner, to changed sexual feelings. New approaches to sexual activity, including different positions for intercourse, alternatives to intercourse, and recognition that sex may be easier before rather than after a tiring day, may be helpful if previous approaches are now difficult or painful. Help from a specialised therapist or counsellor should be sought if necessary. Birth control measures should be continued for about 2 years after chemotherapy to avoid the potentially teratogenic or mutagenic effects of cytotoxic drugs (that is, their capacity to cause physical defects or genetic mutations in the fetus). Although data are scarce, recommendations for women who may be pregnant while receiving treatment for cancer include avoiding chemotherapy in the first trimester if possible. It is suggested that single-agent or combination chemotherapy using the least teratogenic regimens may be given in the second and third semesters with low risk of teratogenic effects.[1]

In men, alkylating agents can damage the testes, resulting in decreased or absent production of sperm. The extent and duration of damage is related to the patient's age and the amount of drug received. Recovery may be prolonged. Likewise, with cisplatin, vinblastine and bleomycin, sperm production can cease completely, but may recover over a period of years. Procarbazine appears to be particularly toxic, and has been associated with persistent azoospermia (e.g. in combination therapy for Hodgkin's disease). There are many reports of permanent infertility in men treated for Hodgkin's and non-Hodgkin's lymphomas, seminomas, and non-seminomatous testicular cancers.[1]

Cardiotoxicity
A number of chemotherapeutic agents have toxic effects on the heart. Doxorubicin has been most closely studied in this respect and is known to have the potential to cause changes to heart rate and rhythm during or shortly after administration, including supraventricular tachydysrhythmias and ectopic ventricular contractions. Early cardiac toxicity can also occur with daunorubicin.[1] Acute effects such as transient electrocardiogram (ECG) changes usually resolve quickly without complications.[16] Doxorubicin can also lead in the longer term (weeks and months) to chronic damage of the myocardial cells (cardiomyopathy) with heart failure. Up to 9% of patients receiving doxorubicin experience drug-induced cardiomyopathy; the condition is thought to be

fatal in over 60% of these cases.[105] Chronic cardiotoxicity can be difficult to detect, as patients may be asymptomatic before presenting with the signs and symptoms of congestive cardiac failure, including tachycardia, non-productive cough, distension of the neck veins, breathlessness, and ankle oedema. Clearly, the chronic cardiotoxic effects of anthracyclines such as doxorubicin are such that administration is discontinued as soon as signs and symptoms are detected.

Epirubicin, another anthracycline, has also been shown to be cardiotoxic, as has mitoxantrone, an anthraquinone. The cardiotoxicity of idarubicin has not been extensively investigated.[1]

Other anti-cancer agents with reported cardiotoxic effects include interferon-α, trastuzumab, bleomycin, cyclophosphamide (high dose), 5-FU, ifosfamide, mitomycin-C, and paclitaxel.[1,16]

Neurotoxicity
Neurological effects related to chemotherapy are not uncommon, but can be difficult to distinguish from the effects of cancer itself. In the majority of cases, neurotoxicity is temporary, although permanent neurological damage can occur. Severe neurotoxicity may lead to discontinuation of the drug involved or make it necessary to interrupt treatment to allow symptoms to resolve before dose modification or replacement of the drug.

When used in high doses, methotrexate can cause encephalopathy that is usually reversible.[16] Given intrathecally, it can lead to acute chemical arachnoiditis with severe headache, rigidity of the neck muscles, vomiting, and fever. Less acute, but serious toxicities include syndromes with effects such as motor paralysis of the extremities, seizures and coma, and (in children) dementia, limb spasticity, and coma.[10]

5-FU can cause a number of central nervous system effects, including acute ataxias, loss of muscle control, and speech and occulomotor disturbances. These effects are usually reversible following discontinuation of the drug. Serious complications, such as cognitive impairment, coma, and dementia have also been seen.[10]

Vincristine is known to cause peripheral neuropathy, which can be dose-limiting. Its effects include loss of the Achilles tendon reflex, sensory loss in the hands and feet, and weakness or atrophy of the muscles. Vincristine can also affect the autonomic nervous system, with effects such as constipation, urinary retention, and impotence.[16] Inadvertent intrathecal or intraventricular administration of vincristine is rapidly fatal.[1,10]

Neurotoxicity is a major side effect of cisplatin. Complications include hearing loss, tinnitus, and peripheral sensory disturbances (e.g. in the hands and feet), which may be experienced in the first instance as tingling and numbness, followed by proprioceptive disturbances. Barton Burke et al.[14] note that proprioceptive losses, which involve 'the loss of the ability to determine the position of body parts without visual cues' can be devastating. Effects may be dose-limiting and may not be reversible. Neurotoxicity is also a frequent side-effect of carboplatin and oxaliplatin.[10] Immediately after administration of oxaliplatin, patients may experience cold-induced paraesthesias (e.g. following cold drinks), muscle tightness (e.g. in the throat and jaw), and leg and arm cramps. Distal sensory loss may also occur with more prolonged treatment with oxaliplatin, and can lead to discontinuation of the drug.[148] A range of hypersensitivity reactions, some of them severe, are known to occur with cisplatin, carboplatin, and oxaliplatin.[1]

Paclitaxel has been reported to cause transient encephalopathies, and docetaxel with gemcitabine is neurotoxic in a proportion of cases. Paclitaxel is known to cause hypersensitivity reactions (e.g. breathlessness, bronchospasm, urticaria, and hypotension) within minutes of being administered, and can also cause peripheral neuropathy (e.g. numbness and paraesthesia of the hands and feet). Docetaxel is also associated with hypersensitivity reactions, and with peripheral neuropathy (although this is thought to be less severe and less common than the neurotoxicity associated with paclitaxel).[1]

Neurotoxicity has been reported with BCNU (e.g. optic neuroretinitis[1]), ifosfamide (e.g. seizures, extrapyramidal effects, somnolence[1,16]), and cytarabine (e.g. cerebellar dysfunction, more commonly in high-dose regimens[1,16]). Neurological effects, including difficulty with walking and standing, and mood and sleep disturbances, are common with corticosteroids. Some of the neurological effects of steroid therapy can be avoided or minimised by gradual dose reduction before discontinuation.

Pulmonary toxicity

Pulmonary toxicity, often in the form of pneumonitis or fibrosis, is a result of damage to the endothelial cells of the lungs. A large number of chemotherapeutic agents are known to cause pulmonary toxicity, including bleomycin (e.g. pulmonary fibrosis), BCNU and CCNU (e.g. pulmonary fibrosis), busulfan, carmustine (e.g. alveolitis and fibrosis), chlorambucil (e.g. pneumonitis), cyclophosphamide (e.g. pulmonary fibrosis), cytarabine (e.g. capillary leak syndrome), docetaxel, fludarabine, lomustine, melphalan (e.g. pneumonitis), methotrexate (e.g. interstitial fibrosis), mitomycin C (e.g. fibrosis), and paclitaxel.[1,10,16]

Hepatotoxicity

Liver damage as a result of cancer chemotherapy may become apparent through (sometimes transient) elevations in hepatic enzymes detected in liver function tests, or when the liver is found to be enlarged, or when a patient becomes jaundiced or experiences abdominal pain. Anti-cancer drugs reported to be hepatotoxic in varying degrees include chlorambucil, carboplatin, cisplatin, cytarabine, dacarbazine, 5-FU, dactinomycin, gefitnib, gemcitabine, imatnib mesylate, interferon-α, irinotecan, L-asparaginase, melphalan, methotrexate, mithramycin, oxaliplatin, paclitaxel, 6-mercaptopurine, trimetrexate, and streptozocin.[1,16] Because many chemotherapeutic agents are metabolised by the liver, dose modification may be necessary with impaired liver function. Hepatotoxicity is an uncommon but serious complication of chemotherapy, and it is important to monitor liver function through liver function tests throughout a course of treatment.

Haemorrhagic cystitis

This toxicity is associated with cyclophosphamide and ifosfamide; with these agents toxic metabolites are excreted in the urine. The complication varies in severity from transient cystitis to major damage to the bladder and life-threatening haemorrhage. MESNA (2-mercaptoethane sulfonate) is administered with ifosfamide and high-dose cyclophosphamide as prophylaxis against cystitis; adequate hydration, together with frequent voiding of the bladder, has an important role in protecting the bladder. Urine should be monitored for traces of blood.

Nephrotoxicity
Many chemotherapeutic agents are known to be nephrotoxic, including cisplatin, streptozocin, mitomycin C, ifosfamide, methotrexate, cyclophosphamide, and vincristine. With cisplatin, nephrotoxicity is dose-limiting. Its effects on renal function include both an acute form of renal failure (e.g. in patients who have not received adequate hydration during treatment) and more long-term effects on renal function.[1] Pre- and post-administration IV hydration with cisplatin to prevent or minimise impairment of renal function, and mannitol may be useful to improve urine flow.[10] Streptozocin causes nephritis and tubular atrophy, and nephrotoxicity is again dose-limiting. Renal failure due to streptozocin can be severe, necessitating dialysis, and may be fatal. Mitomycin C is associated with a syndrome comprising renal failure and microangiopathic haemolytic anaemia, usually with hypertension; mithramycin is known to cause necrosis of the renal tubules, and renal failure may occur in up to 40% of patients.[1] High-dose methotrexate can precipitate in the renal tubules, leading to impairment of the glomerular filtration rate; the nephrotoxicity of methotrexate can be minimised by simultaneous administration of sodium bicarbonate to maintain the alkalinity (pH > 7) of the urine. Hyponatraemia occurs in some patients receiving vincristine, and is associated with the peripheral and autonomic neuropathy occurring with this drug. The effect is clinically similar to inappropriate secretion of antidiuretic hormone.[1]

Common anti-cancer agents

Anti-cancer agents can be classified according to their mechanism of action.

The anti-metabolites
The anti-metabolites disrupt DNA synthesis, and are most active during the S phase of the cell cycle.

Examples of anti-metabolites include methotrexate, trimetrexate, raltitrexed, 5-FU, capecitabine, cytarabine (cytosine arabinoside/ara-C), gemcitabine, fludarabine, deoxycoformycin, hydroxyurea, 6-mercaptopurine, and 6-thioguanine.

- *Methotrexate* is an anti-folate/folate antagonist, which inhibits the enzyme dihydrofolate reductase, depleting the folates (derived from dietary folic acid) necessary for the synthesis of precursors of DNA (thymidylate and purines) and RNA (purines). Methotrexate is used in the treatment of acute lymphoblastic leukaemia, and choriocarcinoma. It is used in combination with other agents in the management of, for example, lymphoma, osteosarcoma, and breast, head and neck, lung, ovary, and bladder cancer. High-dose methotrexate is given in conjunction with folinic acid rescue to prevent excessive toxicity.
- *Trimetrexate* acts in a similar manner to methotrexate to inhibit DNA synthesis. It is active against malignant mesothelioma, and colorectal and bladder cancer.
- *Raltitrexed* directly inhibits the activity of the enzyme thymidylate synthase. In Europe, it is used in single-agent treatment for advanced colorectal carcinoma.
- *5-Fluorouracil (5-FU)* interferes with RNA synthesis and function. It has been used in the management of cancers of the breast, head and neck, gastrointestinal tract, bladder, cervix, and vulva.
- *Capecitabine* is an oral anti-cancer agent converted by the liver into 5-FU. It is used in the treatment of breast cancer that is resistant to paclitaxel and anthracycline-containing regimens.[1]
- *Cytarabine.* When activated, the anti-metabolite *cytosine arabinoside (ara-C)* is a potent inhibitor of DNA synthesis. To enable this sequence of events to take place, it is likely that cells must be exposed to ara-C during the S phase of the cell cycle (i.e. inhibition of DNA must continue for at least one complete cell cycle).[2] Administration schedules must be tailored to achieve this result: typically, ara-C is administered by bolus dose every 12 hours for 5–7 days, or by continuous infusion for

7 days.[2] Ara-C is used in the treatment of acute myelocytic leukaemia, and is a particularly important factor in the induction of remission.

- *Gemcitabine* inhibits DNA replication and repair. It is used in the treatment of locally advanced or metastatic non-small-cell lung cancer.[18]
- *Fludarabine* acts in a similar way to ara-C. Uses include chronic lymphocytic leukaemia and low-grade Hodgkin's lymphoma.[1]
- *Hydroxyurea* acts upon an enzyme (ribonucleoside diphosphate reductase) essential to the synthesis of DNA. It is cell cycle specific, acting upon cells in the S phase of the cycle. Hydroxyurea has been used as an anti-cancer treatment for a wide variety of tumours, including melanoma, chronic myeloid leukaemia, and ovarian, prostate, and head and neck cancer.
- The anti-metabolites *6-mercaptopurine* and *6-thioguanine* inhibit the action of enzymes required for the synthesis of DNA, and cause critical alterations in the synthesis of RNA.[2] Mercaptopurine is used in the treatment of acute lymphocytic leukaemia, and thioguanine in combination therapy for acute myeloid leukaemia.[1]
- *Deoxycoformycin (pentostatin)* disrupts DNA synthesis, replication and repair. It is used in the treatment of chronic lymphoid malignancies such as hairy cell leukaemia.[10]

Vinca alkaloids

Together with another vinca alkaloid, *vinblastine*, *vincristine* is derived from the pink periwinkle plant (*Catharanthus roseus*). *Vindesine*, a semi-synthetic derivative of vinblastine, has primarily investigational rather than therapeutic applications. The vinca alkaloids are cell-cycle-specific and have an anti-mitotic effect, blocking cells in mitosis. The microtubules of the mitotic apparatus (which are essential to the formation of the 'mitotic spindle') are disrupted, and cell division is arrested; chromosomes are free to disperse ('exploded mitosis') or clump within the cytoplasm.[2]

Vincristine is used in the treatment of childhood and adult acute lymphocytic leukaemias, lymphomas, and a range of solid tumours including Wilms' tumour, Ewing's sarcoma, and rhabdomyosarcoma.[1] Vinblastine is used in combination with other agents in the treatment of metastatic testicular tumours. *Vinorelbine*, a semi-synthetic derivative of vinblastine, is active against non-small-cell lung cancer and breast cancer, though its applications are still under evalauation.[1]

Taxanes: paclitaxel (taxol) and docetaxel (taxotere)

Paclitaxel was originally produced from the bark of the Pacific yew tree in 1971 but can now be produced semi-synthetically from products of the European yew. Docetaxel is synthesised from the same source materials. Taxanes disrupt many cellular activities by inducing abnormal stability in the microtubules, causing cells to arrest in mitosis. Paclitaxel and docetaxel have a wide range of applications, and are widely used in the treatment of metastatic cancer of the ovary, breast, lung, and head and neck.[2]

The alkylating agents

The alkylating agents disrupt DNA synthesis and cell division. They include: cyclophosphamide, ifosfamide, melphalan, and chlorambucil (nitrogen mustards); carmustine (BCNU) and streptozocin (nitrosureas); dacarbazine (DTIC) and temozolomide (triazenes); thiotepa, busulphan, and procarbazine.

- *Cyclophosphamide* is the most widely used of the alkylating agents. Following metabolic activation after administration, cyclophosphamide severely disrupts DNA molecules during the synthesis phase of the cell cycle. It is used in the management of lymphomas, chronic leukaemias and carcinomas (e.g. in combination with methotrexate or doxorubicin and 5-FU as adjuvant therapy for carcinoma of the breast).
- *Ifosfamide* is an analogue of cyclophosphamide. When metabolised, both agents produce alkylating compounds that destroy DNA. Ifosfamide is used in combination with other agents in the treatment of germ cell testicular cancer, as well as adult and childhood sarcomas.[2] Because ifosfamide causes urotoxicity, a 'uroprotector'

(MESNA) is administered concurrently during therapy.

- *Chlorambucil* is used in the treatment of chronic lymphocytic leukaemia; in combination with other agents, *melphalan* is used in regimens for multiple myeloma.
- *Carmustine* (BCNU) is a nitrosurea, which alkylates DNA and produces DNA–DNA and DNA–protein cross-links.[10] It is used with procarbazine in the treatment of malignant gliomas.[2] Chabner and Longo[10] note that:

> Currently, BCNU is used with HCT regimens for haematopoietic diseases. As predicted from the animal studies, the nitrosureas have shown significant activity against brain tumours. When used as an adjuvant to radiation therapy, they enhance survival modestly in patients with grade III and IV astrocytomas. The severe haematopoietic depression (especially thrombocytopaenia) and pulmonary toxicity produced by these agents are significant limiting factors in their use [p.287].

- *Streptozocin* is an alkylating agent that is a naturally occurring antibiotic methylnitrosurea derived from *Streptomyces*. Uses include treatment for carcinomas of islet cells in the pancreas.
- *Thiotepa* is one of a group of drugs thought to produce alkylation in a similar way to the nitrogen mustards. It has been used in the treatment of carcinoma of the bladder, breast, and ovary.[18]
- *Busulphan* is an alkylating agent that disrupts DNA synthesis and cell division. Before the introduction of imatinib, busulphan was used in the treatment of chronic myelogenous leukaemia;[1,2] it is used in high-dose regimens with cyclophosphamide prior to bone marrow transplantation.[2]
- *Dacarbazine* is a methylating agent that is metabolically activated in the liver following administration, and is active in all phases of the cell cycle. It has been used in the treatment of malignant melanoma, soft tissue sarcomas, and Hodgkin's disease.
- *Temozolomide*, like dacarbazine, kills cells in all phases of the cell cycle, and has demonstrated activity in recurrent and progressive high-grade gliomas.[2,10]

Other agents

Other agents that damage the DNA template through a variety of mechanisms include cisplatin and carboplatin (platinum analogues); doxorubicin, daunorubicin, mitoxantrone, idarubicin, epirubicin, and bleomycin (anti-tumour antibiotics); etoposide and teniposide (podophyllotoxins); dactinomycin and mithramycin (block RNA synthesis).

- The 'platinum co-ordination complexes'

> were first identified as potential anti-proliferative agents in 1965 by Rosenberg and co-workers. They observed that a current delivered between platinum electrodes produced inhibition of *E. coli* proliferation . . . (cisplatin) was the most active of these substances in experimental tumour systems and has proven to be of great clinical value . . . Carboplatin was approved for treatment of ovarian cancers in 1989, and *oxaliplatin* was approved by the FDA [Food and Drug Administration] for colon cancer in 2003 . . . As a group, these agents have broad neoplastic activity, and have become the foundations for treatment of testicular cancer, ovarian cancer, and cancers of the head and neck, bladder, oesophagus, lung, and colon [p.1332].[2]

- *Doxorubicin* is an anti-tumour antibiotic derived from the fungus *Streptomyces*. Its cytotoxic activity may result from an ability to cause breaks in strands of DNA. Perry[1] summarises the mechanisms of action of various anti-tumour antibiotics as follows:

> The focal point for the cytotoxicities of antitumour antibiotics is DNA . . . antibiotics can intercalate [i.e. bind] in between base pairs of DNA (doxorubicin, daunorubicin, dactinomycin, bleomycin), bind to DNA (mitomycin C, plicamycin) and generate toxic oxygen free radicals, which cause single- or double-stranded DNA breaks (doxorubicin, daunorubicin, idarubicin, bleomycin, mitomycin C). From this . . . DNA damage come some of the . . . cytotoxic actions of these agents, such as inhibition of DNA-directed RNA synthesis, protein synthesis . . . [p.229].

Doxorubicin is used in treatment of acute leukaemia, lymphomas, carcinoma of the breast and ovary, small-cell carcinoma of the lung, osteogenic and soft tissue sarcomas, and breast and lung carcinomas.[18]

- *Daunorubicin* is primarily used in the treatment of acute non-lymphocytic and acute lymphocytic leukaemias.[1] It has largely been replaced by *idarubicin*.[2]
- *Bleomycin* is an anti-tumour antibiotic originally produced by fermentation of *Streptomyces verticullus*. It is most commonly used in combination with other agents in the treatment of lymphomas,[1] and is effective in therapy for germ cell tumours of the testis and ovary.[2]
- *Mitoxantrone* is an anti-tumour antibiotic, which inhibits DNA and RNA synthesis. It has shown anti-cancer activity in acute leukaemias, breast cancer, and lymphomas.[1]
- The anti-tumour antibiotic *Dactinomycin (actinomycin D)* is primarily used in the management of childhood rhabdomyosarcoma and Wilms' tumour.
- *Mitomycin C* is an anti-tumour antibiotic derived from *Streptomyces*. Mitomycin C has been used in the treatment of carcinoma of the anus, bladder, breast, cervix, head and neck, lung, and stomach. Brunton *et al.* note that mitomycin has been replaced by less toxic and more effective agents in anal, colorectal, and lung cancers.[2]
- Together with *teniposide*, *etoposide* is derived from podophyllotoxin taken from the mandrake plant (*Podophyllum peltatum*). Etoposide and teniposide cause irreparable DNA breaks, which lead to cell death. Etoposide is most commonly used in the management of testicular cancer (with bleomycin and cisplatin) and small-cell carcinoma of the lung (with cisplatin and ifosfamide).[2] Other uses include treatment of non-Hodgkin's lymphomas, acute non-lymphocytic leukaemia, and Kaposi's sarcoma in AIDS. Teniposide is used in the management of acute lymphoblastic leukaemia in children, and acute monocytic leukaemia in infants.

Hormones

These include oestrogens, progestins, anti-oestrogens, and aromatase inhibitors.

- *Oestrogens* are useful in the treatment of metastatic breast cancer and prostate cancer. When a tumour is oestrogen-receptor positive, a response rate of about 60% can be achieved in metastatic breast cancer.[13] The most commonly used oestrogen in metastatic breast cancer is DES (diethylstilbestrol), although its toxicity means that its use in breast cancer use is generally limited to second- or third line therapy, after anti-oestrogens, progestins, and aromatase inhibitors.[1] Toxicities associated with DES in prostate cancer have affected the extent of its use.
- *Progestins* (e.g. megestrol acetate and medroxyprogesterone) have been used in breast and endometrial cancers. Toxicities associated with their use have led to their relegation to use as third-line therapies in breast cancer, following tamoxifen and aromatase inhibitors.
- *Anti-oestrogens* (e.g. tamoxifen) inhibit the action of oestrogen and are cytostatic rather than cytotoxic. Tamoxifen is used in post-menopausal women with advanced breast cancer, and as adjuvant therapy in all women with stage I or II oestrogen-receptor-positive breast cancer, to increase disease-free and overall survival.
- *Anti-androgens* (e.g. flutamide, nilutamide, bicalutamide) are used in combination therapy for carcinoma of the prostate.
- *Aromatase inhibitors* (e.g. aminoglutethamide, anastrozole/Arimidex, letrozole/Femara, exemestane/Aromasin) affect the function of the enzyme aromatase, leading to oestrogen deprivation.[2] Aminoglutethamide causes suppression of the adrenal gland and inhibits production of oestrogens and androgens. It has been used in the treatment of metastatic cancer of the prostate and breast. Patients receiving aminoglutethamide require corticosteroid supplements to avoid the symptoms of adrenal suppression. More modern aromatase inhibitors such as anastrozole, letrozole, and exemestane are more selective, and have an important role in the treatment of women with metastatic, oestrogen-dependent breast cancer, whose disease has progressed on tamoxifen.
- *Corticosteroids* (or *adrenocorticoids*) 'modulate DNA synthesis, mitosis, cell growth, differentiation, and . . . metabolism in normal and neoplastic target tissues' (p.313).[1] They are used in combination with other agents in the primary treatment of acute and chronic lymphocytic leukaemia, multiple myeloma, and Hodgkin's

and non-Hodgkin's lymphoma. Corticosteroids are also frequently used in anti-emetic therapy, as well as in the management of hypercalcaemia, the palliation of bone pain, to reduce cerebral oedema, and to alleviate breathlessness (e.g. in lymphangitis carcinomatosa).

Biological response modifiers

Biological response modifiers include interferons, interleukins, and monoclonal antibodies.

- The *interferons*, α- (alpha-), β- (beta-), and γ- (gamma-), were originally derived from leucocytes, fibroblasts, and T-cell lymphocytes, respectively; they cause inhibition of protein, DNA, and RNA synthesis. Perry notes that interferons activate natural killer (NK) and cytotoxic T-cells, in addition to their direct anti-proliferative activity.[1] Interferon-α is an important treatment for metastatic renal cell carcinoma, hairy cell leukaemia, and chronic myeloid (or myelogenous) leukaemia. It has also been used in the treatment of multiple myeloma.
- *Interleukin-2* has been most widely tested as a potential anti-tumour agent. Interleukins are, like interferons, produced by leucocytes. Interleukin-2 is derived from peripheral T-helper lymphocytes. Interleukin-2 stimulates immune responses, including cytotoxic T-cells, natural killer cells, other interleukins, and γ-interferon. Interleukin-2 has been used in the treatment of metastatic renal cell carcinoma and metastatic melanoma.
- *Rituximab* is a monoclonal antibody that attaches itself to CD-20 proteins on the surface of B-cell lymphocytes, stimulating the immune system to attack the targeted cells, and also, possibly, inducing cell cycle arrest or apoptosis. It is used in the treatment of B-cell non-Hodgkin's lymphoma.
- *Trastuzumab (Herceptin)* is a monoclonal antibody that attaches itself to HER2 proteins found on the surface of some breast cancer cells, preventing cell division. Around 20–30% of invasive breast carcinomas over-express the HER2 receptor.[2] Trastuzumab with paclitaxel is used in the treatment of metastatic breast cancer in women who over-express HER2. Trastuzumab has also been used in conjunction

Research study 12.3

Mitchell T. (2007). The social and emotional toll of chemotherapy – patients' perspectives. *European Journal of Cancer Care* **16**, 39–47.[89]

Mitchell presents the findings of a qualitative study, a key aim of which was to 'illuminate patients' journeys through the process of receiving chemotherapy treatment for cancer' (p.2). Participants were 19 men and women aged ≥18 years recruited from a pre-chemotherapy clinic, and the objective was to interview them at each time they received chemotherapy. Nine researchers conducted a total of 98 interviews, and met with participants on up to ten occasions. In addition to the interviews, participants were given the opportunity to keep written or audio diaries. Data from the study were analysed by generating common themes and categories. As a result, eight main themes were identified, including 'striving for normality', 'the role of significant others', 'feeling up, feeling down', and 'flagging'. Mitchell comments that

> Receiving chemotherapy appears to cause disruption in all dimensions of life, and the need to regain control, equilibrium, consistency and stability was paramount to feeling well again [p.4].

Participants provided some very vivid observations on the ups and downs of their experience. For example:

> I'm 42 today and part of me is gloomy that I'm most unlikely to reach 43 [p.6].
> I'm struggling to survive [p.6].
> I've lost my bubbly self [p.6].

The problem of sleeplessness is highlighted under the theme 'flagging', as are various manifestations of loss of concentration or feeling muddled:

> Mentally flagging – brain in low gear, can't think or retain thoughts [p.7].
> I feel cuckoo [p.7].
> My husband says I repeat myself over and over again [p.7].

Mitchell concludes that by using qualitative methods, including 'conversation-style interviews' (p.8), the study was able to reflect the private experiences of people undergoing chemotherapy, and that the insight into psychosocial issues it provides will assist nurses to reshape chemotherapy services to 'improve the experience of living with cancer' (p.8).

with other agents in early breast cancer to reduce the risk of recurrence. Recently, the National Institute for Health and Clinical Excellence (NICE) in the UK recommended that all women with early breast cancer should have HER2 testing. Women with primary invasive breast cancer who are HER2 positive, who meet a range of other clinical criteria and in whom certain contraindications are absent, should now be considered eligible for treatment with trastuzumab.[149]

Bacille Calmette-Guérin

BCG is derived from the live bacterium *Mycobacterium bovis*. BCG is administered intravesically to delay tumour progression and improve survival in patients with superficial bladder cancer.

L-Asparaginase

Asparaginase is an enzyme that can be isolated from many animal tissues, bacteria (including *Escherichia coli*), plants and the serum of some rodents. Asparaginase deprives leukaemia cells of asparagine, causing destruction of DNA and cell death; the cell cycle is arrested in G_1 phase.[150] It is used in combination with other agents in the treatment of acute lymphoblastic leukaemia.

References

1. Perry M.C. (ed.) (2001). *The Chemotherapy Source Book*. Philadelphia, PA: Lippincott Williams and Wilkins.
2. Brunton L.L., Lazo J.S. and Parker K.L. (eds.) (2006). *Goodman & Gilman's The Pharmacological Basis of Therapeutics*, 11th edition. New York: McGraw Hill.
3. Bleiberg H., Rougier P. and Wilke H.-J. (1998). *Management of Colorectal Cancer*. London: Martin Dunitz.
4. Priestman T.J. (1989). *Cancer Chemotherapy: An Introduction*, 3rd edition. London: Springer.
5. Skeel R.T. (2003). *Handbook of Cancer Chemotherapy*. Philadelphia: Lippincott Williams and Wilkins.
6. Horwich A. (ed.) (1995). *Oncology: A Multidisciplinary Textbook*. London: Chapman and Hall Medical.
7. Karnofsky D.A. and Burchenal J.H. (1949). The clinical evaluation of chemotherapeutic agents in cancer. In McLeod C.M. (ed.) *Evaluation of Chemotherapeutic Agents*. New York: Columbia University Press.
8. Fretwell D.F. (1990). Comprehensive functional assessment (CFA) in everyday practice. In Hazzard W.R., Andres R., Bierman E.L. and Blass J.P. (eds.) *Principles of Geriatric Medicine and Gerontology*. New York: McGraw Hill.
9. Mendelsohn M.L. (1960). The growth fraction: a new concept applied to tumors. *Science* **132**, 1496.
10. Chabner B.A. and Longo D.L. (2006). *Cancer Chemotherapy and Biotherapy: Principles and Practice*. Philadelphia, PA: Lippincott-Raven.
11. Schabel F.M. Jr (1969). The use of tumor growth kinetics in planning 'curative' chemotherapy of advanced solid tumours. *Cancer Research* **29**, 2384.
12. Pratt W.B., Ruddon R.W., Ensminger W.D. and Maybaum J. (1994). *The Anticancer Drugs*. New York: Oxford University Press.
13. Laurence D.R., Bennett P.N. and Brown M.J. (1997). *Clinical Pharmacology*. New York: Churchill Livingstone.
14. Barton Burke M., Wilkes G.M. and Ingwersen K. (1996). *Cancer Chemotherapy: A Nursing Process Approach*. Sudbury, MA: Jones and Bartlett.
15. Batchelor D. (2001). Hair and cancer chemotherapy – consequences and nursing care: a literature study. *European Journal of Cancer Care* **10**, 147–163.
16. Camp Sorrell D. (2005). Chemotherapy toxicities and management. In Yarbro C.H., Frogge M.H. and Goodman M. (eds.) *Cancer Nursing: Principles and Practice*. Sudbury, MA: Jones and Bartlett Publishers.
17. Scurr M., Judson I. and Root T. (2005). Combination chemotherapy and chemotherapy principles. In Brighton D. and Wood M. (eds.) *The Royal Marsden Hospital Handbook of Cancer Chemotherapy*. Edinburgh: Elsevier Churchill Livingstone.
18. Allwood M., Stanley A. and Wright P. (2002). *The Cytotoxics Handbook*. Oxford: Radcliffe Medical Press.
19. Hayden B.K. and Goodman M. (2005). Chemotherapy: principles of administration. In Yarbro C.H., Frogge M.H. and Goodman M. (eds.) *Cancer Nursing: Principles and Practice*. Sudbury, MA: Jones and Bartlett Publishers.
20. Cox K. (2000). Enhancing cancer clinical trial management: recommendations from a qualitative study of trial participants' experiences. *Psycho-oncology* **9**, 314–322.
21. Cox K. (2002). The hopes of the dying: examining patients' experience of participation in early phase cancer clinical trials. *NTResearch* **7**, 60–73.
22. Cox K. (2003). Assessing the quality of life of patients in phase I and II anti-cancer drug trials: interviews versus questionnaires. *Social Science and Medicine* **56**, 921–934.
23. Gillon R. (1986). *Philosophical Medical Ethics*. Chichester: John Wiley.
24. Thompson I.E., Melia K.M. and Boyd K.M. (2000). *Nursing Ethics*. Edinburgh: Churchill Livingstone.

25. Jefferies S. (2005). Ethical and legal issues. In Brighton D. and Wood M. (eds.) *The Royal Marsden Hospital Handbook of Cancer Chemotherapy*. Edinburgh: Elsevier Churchill Livingstone.

26. Department of Health. *Consent*. www.dh.gov.uk/PolicyAndGuidance/HealthAndSocialCareTopics/Consent/fs/en (accessed 30 July 2007).

27. Dougherty L. and Lister S. (2004). Drug administration: cytotoxic drugs. In Dougherty L. and Lister S. (eds.) *The Royal Marsder Hospital Manual of Clinical Nursing Procedures*, 6th edition. Oxford: Blackwell Publishing, pp. 228–258.

28. Saffran L., Ost D.E., Fein A.M. and Schiff M.J. (2000). Outpatient pleurodesis of malignant pleural effusions using a small-bore pigtail catheter. *Chest* **118**, 417–421.

29. Tsang V., Fernando H.C. and Goldstraw P. (1990). Pleuroperitoneal shunt for recurrent malignant pleural effusions. *Thorax* **45**, 369–372.

30. Sterman D.H., Kaiser L.R. and Albelda S.M. (1999). Advances in the treatment of malignant pleural mesothelioma. *Chest* **116**, 504–520.

31. Department of Health. (2003). *HSC 2003/010 – Updated National Guidance on the Safe Administration of Intrathecal Chemotherapy*. www.dh.gov.uk/PublicationsAndStatistics/LettersAndCirculars/HealthServiceCircularsArticle/fs/en?CONTENT_ID=4064931&chk = JA/pnL (accessed 30 July 2007).

32. Dougherty L. (2005). Intravenous management. In Brighton D. and Wood M. (eds.) *The Royal Marsden Hospital Handbook of Cancer Chemotherapy*. Edinburgh: Elsevier Churchill Livingstone.

33. Otto S.E. (1995). Advanced concepts in chemotherapy drug delivery: regional therapy. *Journal of Intravenous Nursing* **18**, 170–176.

34. Faithfull S. and Deery P. (2004). Implementation of capecitabine (Xeloda®) into a cancer centre: UK experience. *European Journal of Oncology Nursing* **8**, S54–S62.

35. Coward M. and Coley H.M. (2006). Chemotherapy. In Kearney N. and Richardson A. (eds.) *Nursing Patients with Cancer: Principles and Practice*. Edinburgh: Elsevier Churchill Livingstone.

36. Dougherty L. and Lamb J. (1999). *Intravenous Therapy in Nursing Practice*. Edinburgh: Churchill Livingstone.

37. McClure H.A. (2002). Hickman central venous catheters. *Current Anaesthesia and Critical Care* **13**, 159–167.

38. Dougherty L., Viner C. and Young J. (1998). Establishing ambulatory chemotherapy at home. *Professional Nurse* **13**, 356–358.

39. Gabriel J. (1996). Peripherally inserted central catheters: expanding UK nurses' practice. *British Journal of Nursing* **5**, 71–74.

40. Macrae K. (1998). Hand-held Dopplers in central catheter insertion. *Professional Nurse* **14**, 99–102.

41. Weinstein S.M. (2007). *Plumer's Principles and Practice of Intravenous Therapy*. Philadelphia, PA: Lippincott.

42. Boland A., Haycox A., Bagust A. and Fitzsimmons L. (2003). A randomised controlled trial to evaluate the clinical and cost effectiveness of Hickman line insertions in adult cancer patients by nurses. *Health Technology Assessment* 7(36). www.hta.ac.uk/project/1068.asp (accessed 30 July 2007).

43. Thompson A.M., Kidd E., McKenzie M., Parker A.C. and Nixon S.J. (1989). Long term central venous access: the patient's view. *Intensive Therapy and Clinical Monitoring* **10**, 142–145.

44. Kreis H., Loehberg C.R., Lux M.P. *et al.* (2006). Patients' attitudes to totally implantable venous access port systems for gynaecological or breast malignancies. *European Journal of Surgical Oncology* **33**, 39–43.

45. Lokich J., Bothe A. Jr, Fine N. and Perri J. (1982). The delivery of cancer chemotherapy by constant venous infusion: ambulatory management of venous access and portable pump. *Cancer* **50**, 2731–2735.

46. Kelly D., Pearce S., Butters E., Stevens W. and Layzelle S. (2004). Achieving change in the NHS: a study to explore the feasibility of a home-based cancer chemotherapy service. *International Journal of Nursing Studies* **41**, 215–224.

47. Wood M., Hyde L. and Salter M. (2005). Management of the adult patient with cancer receiving chemotherapy. In Brighton D. and Wood M. (eds.) *The Royal Marsden Hospital Handbook of Cancer Chemotherapy*. Edinburgh: Elsevier Churchill Livingstone.

48. Turner C. and Pateman B. (2000). A study of district nurses' experiences of continuous ambulatory chemotherapy. *British Journal of Community Nursing* **5**, 396–399.

49. Schulmeister L. (1992). An overview of continuous infusion chemotherapy. *Journal of Intravenous Nursing* **15**, 315–321.

50. Teich C.J. and Raia K. (1984). Teaching strategies for an ambulatory chemotherapy program. *Oncology Nursing Forum* **11**, 24–28.

51. Nanninga A.G., de Vries E.G., Willemse P.H. *et al.* (1991). Continuous infusion of chemotherapy on an outpatient basis via a totally implanted venous access port. *European Journal of Cancer* **27**, 147–149.

52. Koeppen M.A. and Caspars S.M. (1994). Problems identified with home infusion pumps. *Journal of Intravenous Nursing* **17**, 151–156.

53. Hayward T. (2002). Setting up a chemotherapy service at home. *Cancer Nursing practice* **1**, 22–25.

54. Garvey E. and Kramer R. (1983). Improving cancer patients' adjustment to infusion chemotherapy:

evaluation of a patient education program. *Cancer Nursing* **6**, 373–378.

55. Fernsler J.I. and Cannon C.A. (1991). The whys of patient education. *Seminars in Oncology Nursing* **7**, 79–86.

56. Dodd M.J. and Miaskowski C. (2000). The Pro-Self program: a self-care intervention program for patients receiving cancer treatment. *Seminars in Oncology Nursing* **16**, 300–308.

57. Butler M.C. (1984). Families' response to chemotherapy by an ambulatory infusion pump. *Nursing Clinics of North America* **19**, 139–143.

58. Department of Health. (2000). *The NHS Cancer Plan: a Plan for Investment, a Plan for Reform*. London: Department of Health. Available online at: www.dh.gov.uk/assetRoot/04/01/45/13/04014513.pdf (accessed 30 July 2007).

59. Department of Health. (2003). *The NHS Cancer Plan: Three Year Progress Report – Maintaining the Momentum*. London: Department of Health. www.dh.gov.uk/assetRoot/04/06/64/40/04066440.pdf (accessed 30 July 2007).

60. Steele S. (2002). A team approach to palliative chemotherapy. *Cancer Nursing Practice* **1**, 22–26.

61. Fallowfield L. (2001). Participation of patients in decisions about treatment for cancer. *British Medical Journal* **323**, 1144.

62. Valanis B.G., Vollmer W.M., Labuhn K.T. and Glass A.G. (1993). Acute symptoms associated with antineoplastic drug handling among nurses. *Cancer Nursing* **16**, 288–295.

63. *Health and Safety at Work Act (1974)*. London: HMSO.

64. Health and Safety Executive. (2005). *What you Need to Know about the Control of Substances Hazardous to Health Regulations 2002 (COSHH)*. London: Health and Safety Executive.

65. Laidlaw J.L., Connor T.H., Theiss J.C., Anderson R.W. and Matney T.S. (1984). Permeability of latex and polyvinyl chloride gloves to 20 antineoplastic drugs. *American Journal of Hospital Pharmacy* **41**, 2618–2623.

66. Goodman I. (1998). Development of national, evidence-based clinical guidelines for the administration of cytotoxic chemotherapy. *European Journal of Oncology Nursing* **2**, 43–50.

67. Baker E.S. and Connor T.H. (1996). Monitoring occupational exposure to cancer chemotherapy drugs. *American Journal of Health Systems and Pharmacy* **53**, 2713–2723.

68. Nieweg R.M., de Boer M., Dubbleman R.C. *et al.* (1994). Safe handling of antineoplastic drugs: results of a survey. *Cancer Nursing* **17**, 501–511.

69. Schrijvers D.L. (2003). Extravasation: a dreaded complication of chemotherapy. *Annals of Oncology* **14(suppl. 3)**, iii26–iii30.

70. Boyle, D.M. and Engelking C. (1995). Vesicant extravasation: myths and realities. *Oncology Nursing Forum* **22**, 57–67.

71. Griffin A.M., Butow P.N., Coates A.S. *et al.* (1993). On the receiving end V: patient perceptions of the side effects of cancer chemotherapy in 1993. *Annals of Oncology* **7**, 189–195.

72. Cohn K.H. (1982). Chemotherapy from an insider's perspective. *Lancet* **i**, 1006–1009.

73. Price B. (1992). Living with altered body image: the cancer experience. *British Journal of Nursing* **1**, 641–642, 644–645.

74. Kaplan M. (1983). Viewpoint: the cancer patient . . . being hospitalised on a cancer floor. *Cancer Nursing* **6**, 103–107.

75. Dougherty L. (1994). *A Study to Discover How Cancer Patients Perceive the Intravenous Cannulation Experience.* MSc thesis, University of Surrey.

76. Buckalew P.G. (1982). On the opposite side of the bed: a nurse clinician's experiences with anxiety during chemotherapy. *Cancer Nursing* **5**, 435–439.

77. Kaberry S. (1991). Blood simple? *Nursing Times* **87**, 56.

78. Messina S.M. (1989). The nurse with a central line: when the patient is you. *Journal of Intravenous Nursing* **12**, 29–30.

79. Mills R.T. and Krantz D.S. (1979). Information, choice, and reactions to stress: a field experiment in a blood bank with laboratory analogue. *Journal of Personality and Social Psychology* **37**, 608–620.

80. Richardson, A. (1992). Studies exploring self-care for the person coping with cancer treatment: an overview. *International Journal of Nursing Studies* **29**, 191–204.

81. Hudek J. (1986). Compliance in intravenous therapy. *CINA: Official Journal of the Canadian Intravenous Nurses Association* **2**, 7–8.

82. Kelly M.P. (1985). Loss and grief reactions as responses to surgery. *Journal of Advanced Nursing* **10**, 517–525.

83. DiGiacomo S.M. (1987). Biomedicine as a cultural system: an anthropologist in the kingdom of the sick. In Baer H.A. (ed.) *Encounters with Biomedicine*. New York: Gordon & Breach.

84. Coughlan A.M., Badura A.S., Fleischer T.D. and Guck T.P. (2000). Multidisciplinary treatment of chronic pain patients: its efficacy in changing patient locus of control. *Archives of Physical and Medical Rehabilitation* **81**, 739–740.

85. Gill K.M. (1984). Coping effectively with invasive medical procedures: a descriptive model. *Clinical Psychology Review* **4**, 339–362.

86. Cowley L., Heyman B., Stanton M. and Milner S.J. (2000). How women receiving adjuvant chemotherapy for breast cancer cope with their treatment: a risk management perspective. *Journal of Advanced Nursing* **31**, 314–321.

87. Feigin R., Greenberg A., Ras H. *et al.* (2000). The psychological experience of women treated for breast cancer by high-dose chemotherapy supported by autologous stem cell transplant: a qualitative analysis of support groups. *Psycho-oncology* **9**, 57–68.

88. Charmaz K. (1983). Loss of self: a fundamental form of suffering in the chronically ill. *Sociology of Health and Illness* **5**, 168–195.

89. Mitchell T. (2007). The social and emotional toll of chemotherapy – patients' perspectives. *European Journal of Cancer Care* **16**, 39–47.

90. Holmes S. and Dickerson J. (1987). The quality of life: design and evaluation of a self-assessment instrument for use with cancer patients. *International Journal of Nursing Studies* **24**, 15–24.

91. Carver C.S. and Antoni M.H. (2004). Finding benefit in breast cancer during the year after diagnosis predicts better adjustment 5 to 8 years after diagnosis. *Health Psychology*, **23**, 595–598.

92. Holland K.D. and Holahan C.K. (2003). The relation of social support and coping to positive adaptation to breast cancer. *Psychology and Health* **18**, 15–29.

93. Weiss T. (2004). Correlates of posttraumatic growth in married breast cancer survivors. *Journal of Social and Clinical Psychology* **23**, 733–746.

94. Lamb M.A. (1985). Sexual dysfunction in the gynaecologic oncology patient. *Seminars in Oncology Nursing* **1**, 9–17.

95. Anllo L.M. (2000). Sexual life after breast cancer. *Journal of Sex and Marital Therapy* **26**, 241–248.

96. Holmes S. (1990). *Cancer Chemotherapy*. London: Austen Cornish.

97. Yates A. (1987). Sexual healing. *Nursing Times* **83**, 20–30.

98. Wilcock A. (2006). Anorexia: a taste of things to come? *Palliative Medicine* **20**, 43–45.

99. Holmes S. (1987). Nutritional problems in the cancer patient. *Nursing* **3**, 733–735, 737–738.

100. Scully C., Epstein J. and Sonis S. (2003). Oral mucositis: a challenging complication of radiotherapy, chemotherapy, and radiochemotherapy: Part 1, pathogenesis and prophylaxis of mucositis. *Head and Neck* **25**, 1057–1070.

101. Scully C., Epstein J. and Sonis S. (2004). Oral mucositis: a challenging complication of radiotherapy, chemotherapy, and radiochemotherapy. Part 2: diagnosis and management of mucositis. *Head and Neck* **26**, 77–84.

102. Colbourne L. (1995). Patients' experiences of chemotherapy treatment. *Professional Nurse* **10**, 439–442.

103. Fallowfield L. and Clark A. (1991). *Breast Cancer*. London: Routledge.

104. Dodd M.J., Onishi K., Dibble S.L. and Larson P. (1996). Differences in nausea, vomiting and retching between younger and older outpatients receiving cancer chemotherapy. *Cancer Nursing* **19**, 155–161.

105. Perry M.C. and Yarbro J.W. (eds.) (1984). *Toxicity of Chemotherapy*. Orlando: Grune and Stratton.

106. Roscoe J.A., Morrow G.R., Hickok J.T. and Stern R.M. (2000). Nausea and vomiting remain a significant clinical problem: trends over time in controlling chemotherapy-induced nausea and vomiting in 1413 patients treated in community clinical practices. *Journal of Pain and Symptom Management* **20**, 113–121.

107. Hickok J.T., Roscoe J.A. and Morrow G.R. (2001). The role of patients' expectations in the development of anticipatory nausea related to chemotherapy for cancer. *Journal of Pain and Symptom Management* **22**, 843–850.

108. Pratt A., Lazar R.M., Penman D. and Holland J.C. (1984). Psychological parameters of chemotherapy-induced conditioned nausea and vomiting: a review. *Cancer Nursing* **7**, 483–490.

109. Redd W.H., Montgomery G.H. and DuHamel K.N. (2001). Behavioral intervention for cancer treatment side-effects. *Journal of the National Cancer Institute* **93**, 810–823.

110. Morrow G.R. and Morrell C. (1982). Behavioural treatment for the anticipatory nausea and vomiting induced by cancer chemotherapy. *New England Journal of Medicine* **307**, 1476–1480.

111. Cunningham D., Soukop M., Gilchrist N.L *et al.* (1985). Randomised trial of intravenous high dose metoclopramide and intramuscular chlorpromazine in controlling nausea and vomiting induced by cytotoxic drugs. *British Medical Journal* **295**, 250.

112. Lazlo J., Clark R.A., Hanson D.C. *et al.* (1985). Lorazepam in cancer patients treated with cisplatin: a drug having antiemetic, amnesic, and anxiolytic effects. *Journal of Clinical Oncology* **3**, 864–869.

113. Tierney A.J., Taylor J. and Closs S.J. (1992). Knowledge, expectations and experiences of patients receiving chemotherapy for breast cancer. *Scandinavian Journal of Caring Sciences* **6**, 75–80.

114. McCaffery M. and Pasero C. (1999). *Pain: Clinical Manual for Nursing Practice*. St Louis, MO: Mosby.

115. Ezzo J.M., Richardson M.A, Vickers A. *et al.* (2006). Acupuncture-point stimulation for chemotherapy-induced nausea or vomiting (Cochrane Review). *The Cochrane Library* Issue 2. Oxford: Update Software.

116. Stewart A., Bielajew C., Collins B., Parkinson M. and Tomiak E. (2006). A meta-analysis of the neuropsychological effects of adjuvant chemotherapy treatment in women treated for breast cancer. *The Clinical Neuropsychologist*, **20**, 76–89.

117. Tanghe A., Evers G. and Paridaens R. (1998). Nurses' assessment of symptom occurrence and symptom distress in chemotherapy patients. *European Journal of Oncology Nursing* **2**, 14–26.

118. Richardson A., Ream E. and Wilson-Barnett J. (1998). Fatigue in patients receiving chemotherapy: patterns of change. *Cancer Nursing* **21**, 17–30.

119. Piper B., Lindsey A. and Dodd M. (1987). Fatigue mechanisms in cancer patients: developing a nursing theory. *Oncology Nursing Forum* **14**, 17–23.

120. Grandjean E.P. (1970). Fatigue. *American Industrial Hygiene Association Journal* **31**, 401–411.

121. Selye H. (1974). *Stress without Distress*. Philadelphia, PA: J.B. Lippincott.

122. Nerenz D.R., Leventhal H. and Love R.R. (1982). Factors contributing to emotional distress during cancer chemotherapy. *Cancer* **50**, 1020–1027.

123. Knopf M.T. (1986). Physical and psychologic distress associated with adjuvant chemotherapy in women with breast cancer. *Journal of Clinical Oncology* **4**, 678–684.

124. Ehlke G. (1988). Symptom distress in breast cancer patients receiving chemotherapy in the outpatient setting. *Oncology Nursing Forum* **15**, 344–346.

125. Rhodes V.A. (1988). Patients' descriptions of the influence of tiredness and weakness on self-care abilities. *Cancer Nursing* **11**, 186–194.

126. Adamsen L., Quist M., Midtgaard J. *et al.* (2006). The effect of a multidimensional exercise intervention on physical capacity, well-being and quality of life in cancer patients undergoing chemotherapy. *Supportive Care in Cancer* **14**, 116–127.

127. Baird S.B. (1988). *Decision Making in Oncology Nursing*. Philadelphia, PA: BC Decker.

128. Baxley K.O., Erdman L.K., Henry E.B. and Roof B.J. (1984). Alopecia: effect on cancer patients' body image. *Cancer Nursing* **7**, 499–503.

129. Freedman T.G. (1994). Social and cultural dimensions of hair loss in women treated for breast cancer. *Cancer Nursing* **17**, 334–341.

130. Wagner L. and Bye M.G. (1979). Body image and patients experiencing alopecia as a result of cancer chemotherapy. *Cancer Nursing* **2**, 365–369.

131. Dean J., Salmon S.E. and Griffiths K.S. (1979). Prevention of doxorubicin-induced alopecia with scalp hypothermia. *New England Journal of Medicine* **301**, 1427–1429.

132. Love R.R., Leventhal H., Easterling D.V. and Nerenz D.R. (1989). Side-effects and emotional distress during cancer chemotherapy. *Cancer* **63**, 604–612.

133. Clement-Jones V. (1985). Cancer and beyond: the formation of BACUP. *British Medical Journal* **291**, 1021–1023.

134. Hesketh P.J., Batchelor D., Golant M. *et al.* (2004). Chemotherapy-induced alopecia: psychosocial impact and therapeutic approaches. *Supportive Care in Cancer* **12**, 543–549.

135. Münstedt K., Manthey N., Sachsse S. and Vahrson H. (1997). Changes in self-concept and body image during alopecia induced cancer chemotherapy. *Supportive Care in Cancer* **5**, 139–143.

136. Gallagher J. (1996). Women's experiences of hair loss associated with chemotherapy: longitudinal perspective. *Proceedings of 9th International Conference on Cancer Nursing*, Brighton, UK, 1996.

137. Tierney A.J. (1987). Preventing chemotherapy-induced alopecia in women treated for breast cancer: is scalp cooling worthwhile? *Journal of Advanced Nursing* **12**, 303–310.

138. David J.A. and Speechley V. (1987). Scalp cooling to prevent alopecia. *Nursing Times* **83**, 36–37.

139. Keller J.F. and Blausey L.A. (1988). Nursing issues and management in chemotherapy-induced alopecia. *Oncology Nursing Forum* **15**, 603–607.

140. Tierney A.J. (1991). Chemotherapy-induced hair loss. *Nursing Standard* **5**, 29–31.

141. Lemenager M. *et al.* (1998). Chemotherapy-induced alopecia: a controllable side-effect. *Oncology Nurses Today* **3**, 18–20.

142. Ron I.G., Kalmus Y., Kalmus Z., Inbar M. and Chaitchik S. (1997). Scalp cooling in the prevention of alopecia in patients receiving depilating chemotherapy. *Supportive Care in Cancer* **5**, 136–138.

143. Dougherty L. (2006). Comparing methods to prevent chemotherapy-induced alopecia. *Cancer Nursing Practice* **5**, 25–31.

144. Cavalli F., Hansen H.H. and Kaye S.B. (1997). *Textbook of Medical Oncology*. London: Martin Dunitz.

145. Crowe M., Kendrick M. and Woods S. (1998). Is scalp cooling a procedure that should be offered to patients receiving chemotherapy-induced alopecia for solid tumours? *Proceedings of the 10th International Conference on Cancer Nursing*, Jerusalem, 1998.

146. Dougherty L. (1996). Scalp cooling to prevent hair loss in chemotherapy. *Professional Nurse* **11**, 507–509.

147. Blesch K.S. (1988). The normal physiological changes of ageing and their impact on the response to cancer treatment. *Seminars in Oncology Nursing* **4**, 178–188.

148. Lehky T.J., Leonard G.D., Wilson R.H., Grem J.L. and Floeter M.K. (2004). Oxaliplatin-induced neurotoxicity: acute hyperexcitability and chronic neuropathy. *Muscle and Nerve* **29**, 387–392.

149. National Institute for Health and Clinical Excellence. *UK Clinical Guidelines for the Use of Adjuvant Trastuzumab (Herceptin®) with or Following Chemotherapy in HER2-positive Early Breast Cancer. NCRI Breast Clinical Studies Group 14th December 2005*. www.dh.gov.uk/assetRoot/04/12/63/84/04126384.pdf (accessed 30 July 2007).

150. Ueno T., Ohtawa K., Mitsui K. *et al.* (1997). Cell cycle arrest and apoptosis of leukaemia cells induced by L-asparaginase. *Leukaemia* **11**, 1858–1861.

CHAPTER THIRTEEN

Radiotherapy

Sara Faithfull

Radiotherapy plays a central role in the treatment of cancer. Over 50% of people with cancer will receive radiation therapy at some time. In the context of cancer therapy, its value lies in the local management of disease. Radiotherapy may be aimed at cure, may be palliative, or may be given as an adjunct to existing treatment. Its success depends on tumour bulk and the tumour's sensitivity to radiation, as well as the tolerance of surrounding tissues to radiotherapy. Radiotherapy is the use of ionising radiation. The ionisation damages DNA and consequently causes cell death, especially when the cell attempts to replicate. Radiation affects both normal and malignant cells; however, the goal of radiotherapy is to preserve normal tissue function, while damaging the tumour. This is possible owing to various factors. For example, more damage is caused to cancer cells than to normal cells. The kinetics of the cell usually favour the recovery of normal tissue over that of the tumour, and this is exploited by giving radiation in small daily doses (fractionated radiotherapy), over several weeks. Side-effects from treatment are a result of normal tissue damage and may continue long after radiotherapy has finished. Radiotherapy treatment is often seen as an acute event from which recovery is rapid. However, when side-effects of radiation therapy are superimposed on existing functional difficulties, morbidity can be significant.

Nurses are often unaware of the effects of radiotherapy or of how treatment works; with the advent of combined therapies nurses need to be more aware of the impact chemo-radiotherapy has on the severity of side-effects and their implications for resuming normal life. Radiotherapy is mainly organised as an outpatient treatment, and as a result nursing support may not be available routinely to people undergoing treatment.

Many people with cancer have the prospect of surviving their disease but can have side-effects of treatment in the short and long term that can be a debilitating sequel of radiotherapy.[1] Recent years have seen an increase in awareness of the morbidity and the impact of radiotherapy treatment. Radiotherapy may cause long-term physical effects and have consequences for body image, sexuality and physical functioning.[2] Much of the knowledge that exists as to how people react or cope with radiation treatment is focused on the physical effects, and much less on the psychological responses. However, radiation reactions can often exacerbate existing functional or emotional difficulties that can be as a result of the disease, or a combination of therapies.

Many studies have identified the emotional and physical distress associated with radiotherapy.[3–6] However, the proportion of people who experience distress or have psychological problems is unclear. In a study exploring the needs of radiotherapy patients, Fritzsche and colleagues found that over 50% of those assessed had adjustment disorders.[7] Maraste *et al.* identified that 15% of women undergoing adjuvant breast irradiation experienced distress as anxiety rather than as depression or other psychological states.[8] More recent work has identified that individuals still fear radiation and consider it negatively.[9] However, a small study by Hammick *et al.* does not identify whether this attitude influences people's experiences or distress more widely.[9] Young and Maher, in an audit of a counselling service, found that 44% of those attending a British radiotherapy centre had abnormal levels of anxiety.[10] Despite identifying that there is a need for psychosocial care in radiotherapy only 30–50% of those receiving treatment are motivated to accept an offer of counselling or psychosocial intervention.[7]

Nursing can play a major part, not only in understanding the treatment trajectory and side-effects of therapy, but also in bridging the gap between the technical aspects of treatment and in providing research-based interventions and support.[11]

The invisible and highly technical nature of radiotherapy contributes to the fact that 'few therapeutic modalities in medicine induce more misunderstanding, confusion and apprehension'.[12] Radiation therapy has been in existence since the 1900s. In the past the hazards and biological basis of it were little understood, but there is now a growing body of knowledge that provides new and exciting prospects for how the treatment is used, and of developments for the future.

Radiation is given in the form of X-rays, gamma-rays or electrons. Particles such as neutrons or protons are seldom used. Ionising radiation, by definition, is those types of radiation that produce ionisation of atoms and molecules with which they come into contact.[13] A simple understanding of atomic structure can help to explain the nature of these changes.

Atoms are essentially electric in nature. Ionising radiation has sufficient energy to cause atoms of cells in its path to lose orbiting electrons. When an electron is dislodged from its orbit the atom fragments acquire a positive electrical charge. These 'free' electrons interact with neighbouring atoms and hence these atom fragments acquire a negative electrical charge. When electrons are released from their orbit, energy in the form of free electrons is released at high speed and dis-

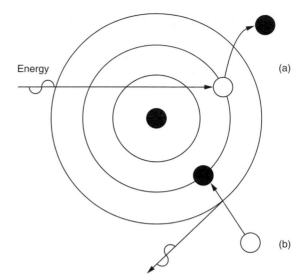

Figure 13.1 Ionisation and excitation of atoms. When an atom or molecule has too many electrons, it is called a negative ion. An atom with fewer electrons is called positive. The atom is said to be ionised when an electron is (a) completely removed, but (b) only excited when it moves from one orbit to another. This movement produces the emission of electromagnetic radiation or X-rays. (Based on Bomford CK., Kinkler I.H. and Sheriff S.B. (1993). *Walter and Millers Textbook of Radiotherapy: Radiation Physics, Therapy and Oncology*, 5th edition. Edinburgh: Churchill Livingstone.[15])

lodges more electrons from neighbouring atoms, which in turn release energy, and continue further ionisations until all energy is dissipated (see Figure 13.1).[14]

Although this process is hard to visualise, it is almost like playing marbles, where one marble may knock others in its path causing them to scatter, creating more movement in a cascade. The electrically charged particles are called ions and the process of their development is called ionisation. This ionisation is responsible for the chemical and biological changes that occur to tissues in the form of radiotherapy.

Ionising beams used in radiotherapy fall into two main types: (1) those that are electrically produced X-rays from a filament; and (2) those that are produced through the decay of radioactive isotopes, either naturally occurring or manufactured specifically in reactors.

Where do the rays come from?

The rays produced by radiotherapy machines are electromagnetic beams such as X-rays. These are similar to light but of a higher energy and shorter wavelength, consisting of photons (see Figure 13.2). The rays occur when speeding electrons hit high atomic weight targets such as tantalum. The early kilovoltage machines produced electrons from heated filaments. Modern megavoltage machines, known as linear accelerators, use a radiowave guide to accelerate further electrons produced in this way. These electrons bombard the target at high energy, producing X-rays in the range of 4–24 MeV (million electron volts). This form of radiotherapy is termed 'external beam' and is used for a variety of different treatments as outlined in Table 13.1.

At low energies the X-rays produced are absorbed to varying degrees by tissues dependent on their density, and this results in a clear

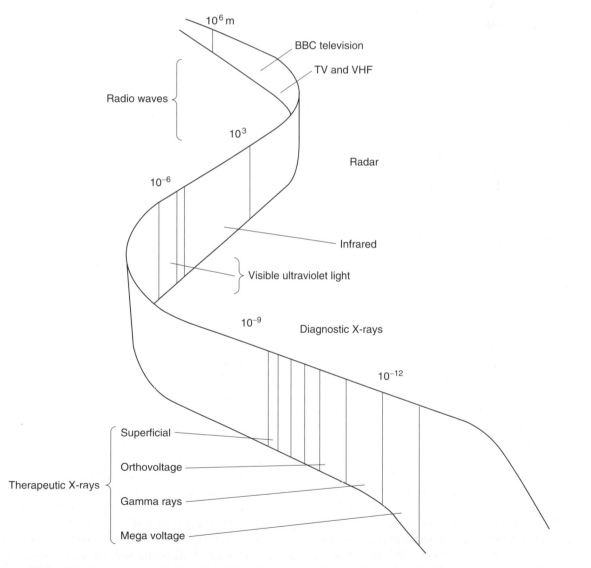

Figure 13.2 The electromagnetic spectrum. The electromagnetic spectrum extends from wavelengths of many kilometres (10^3) to less than 1 picometre (10^{-12}). These invisible waves are called X-rays and gamma (γ)-rays.

Table 13.1 Types of radiation

Type	Energy	Source	Clinical use
Oral or parenteral radiotherapy Radioactive isotopes administered orally or parenterally; their effect is targeted to tissues where they concentrate.		Iodine-131 Strontium-89	Thyroid tumours Multiple bone metastases
Brachytherapy Placing of radiation sources close to the tumour. A high dose is received by the tumour and less by surrounding normal tissues.		Iridium-192 (seeds or wires) Iodine-125 seeds Caesium-137	Sources can be implanted directly into small tumours such as the tongue, lip or breast. Intracavitary sources for cervical and uterine cancers.
External beam (teletherapy) Superficial Orthovoltage Low energy X-rays do not possess skin-sparing properties.	50–150 keV 250–500 keV	X-ray tube X-ray tube	Skin tumours Superficial sites, e.g. breast, rib, sacrum.
Megavoltage High energy and have skin-sparing effects.	>1 MeV (usually 4–16 MeV)	Linear accelerator	Main source of therapeutic beams for sites other than skin.
Gamma rays	2.5 MeV 4–30 MeV	Cobalt Linear accelerator	Superficial sites, e.g. skin, lymph nodes (depth depends upon electron energy).

distinction between bone, soft tissue, and air, which is visible on diagnostic radiographs (X-ray films). Irradiation to superficial layers occurs with photon energies of 150 keV and ortho-voltage at 300 keV. Deeper tissues are penetrated by megavoltage energies (4–25 MeV). These differences in photon energy levels are important, as increased energy of radiation produces a greater penetration of tissues. The different energy levels are often used for differing sites of radiotherapy treatments. Electrons created by removing the target travel only short distances so are limited in their therapeutic use, but are very good for superficial treatments such as basal cell skin cancers.

Radiation dose is defined as the amount of energy absorbed per unit mass of tissue.

Radiation dose is measured in gray (Gy): 1 gray = 1 joule/kg. For a conventional curative course of external beam radiotherapy the dose ranges from 55 Gy to 65 Gy and this is given in daily treatments of 1.6–2.5 Gy over 4–6 weeks dependent on radiotherapy centre. These treatments over time are termed fractionation. External beam radiotherapy utilises a beam from which the patient is placed at a defined distance (usually 100 mm). The isodose is the absorption of radiation in the tissues and varies at any point within the radiation field, depending on the distance of the tissue from the X-ray source. These isodose distributions often look like contours on a map and reflect changes in radiation concentration (see Figure 13.3). High-energy X-rays produced by the linear accelerator focus most of their energy at some distance from the skin surface, therefore leaving the surface skin relatively unaffected by radiation. This is known as the 'skin-sparing' effect.

Alternative radiation sources are those from naturally occurring radionucleotides; these elements have unstable nuclei, which release energy in the process of spontaneous disintegration. This may be in the form of gamma rays, high-speed electrons, or other particles. A variety of isotopes

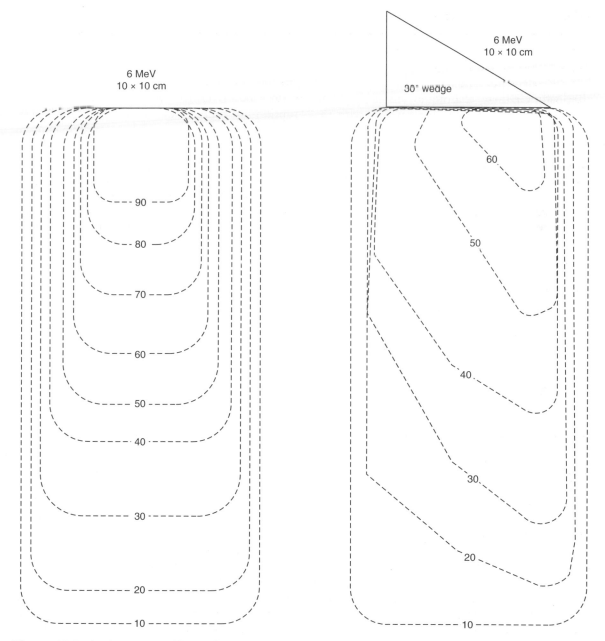

Figure 13.3 Isodose curves. The isodose is the distribution of absorbed X-rays from the individual beams. The maximum value is labelled 100% and lower dose values are drawn at 10% intervals. The isodose curve can be altered by insertion of 30° wedge into the beam.

is also used (see Table 13.1). These have a range of therapeutic uses that are continually being developed.

Brachytherapy involves the delivery of radiation by placing sources close to the tumour. The dose of radiotherapy decreases in proportion to the square of the distance from the source. Therefore the tumour receives a higher dose, with little radiation reaching the surrounding normal tissues. The most common example of brachytherapy is the insertion of interactive sources (see Table 13.1), for example in uterine or cervical carcinomas. Brachytherapy is often delivered by placing the radiation source in small catheters that can then be safely inserted and withdrawn, termed 'afterloading'; these techniques are designed to provide the ability to care for patients with the maximum radiation protection for staff.[16]

Radioactive isotopes for systemic treatments are administered orally. Localisation of the isotopes around tumours occurs when the chemical that is radioactive is metabolised. An example of this is iodine-131, which is used to treat cancer of the thyroid. Research into tagging of radioactive nucleotides to monoclonal antibodies has been progressing, and future therapies are being developed that combine both isotope technology and prevent normal tissue injury.[17]

Cells in action: radiobiology

The body's cells are affected by radiation in several ways through a series of molecular and genetic events.[18] This can be a direct or indirect interaction with tissues to produce short-lived ion radicals. These are associated with damage to deoxyribonucleic acid (DNA) and result in single- or double-strand breaks in its structure. This damage may lead to a chronic persistent alteration in the micro-environment and an aberrant tissue-healing response. Normal tissues have a greater ability to repair themselves than cancer cells.[19] Differences in how cells respond to irradiation are some of the reasons for the differences seen in the radiosensitivity of different cancers. The response to radiation is also affected by oxygenation, the number of cells actively dividing, and the rate at which cells grow within the tumour.[14] These changes are often termed the '4 Rs' and these steps are important in understanding the rationale behind how radiotherapy treatment works and why variation occurs in individual tissue damage and radiation side-effects.

The 'scattering marbles' effect described earlier has two modes of action. They interact directly or indirectly with the tissues. The direct damage is in the nucleus of the cell and affects the DNA, rather like chopping up spaghetti, and the cell is either unable to repair itself or does so inaccurately, resulting in cell death after several cell divisions. The indirect effects involve interaction of free radicals within the cells. These free radicals are OH^- ions and are oxidising agents. The mechanism is poorly understood but the result is a disruption in cellular and tissue function.[14] The direct effects are thought to be most damaging to cells (see Figure 13.4). This disturbance of DNA synthesis leads to abnormal mitosis. Cells that have a short mitosis (for example, mucosa and skin) will show signs of radiation damage more quickly than those whose cycle is long, and this explains why some of the symptoms experienced appear many months to years following treatment.

The considerable variation in radiosensitivity of different tissues is not fully understood. In experiments in the laboratory it is possible to analyse these differences and it is clear that cell survival after irradiation shows an initial curve of cell multiplication followed by rapidly declining cell numbers (see Figure 13.5). This curve represents the ability of cells in some way to repair themselves and this is termed 'sub-lethal damage'. Differences in this repair capacity between cancers may be part of the explanation for the different responses of tumours to fractionation regimes, especially when using low doses of radiation.[20]

A series of fractionated doses increases the difference in repair ability between normal tissue and tumour for several reasons. These are termed the '4 Rs' (see Box 13.1):

1. repair of injury
2. redistribution of cells within the cell cycle
3. repopulation
4. re-oxygenation.

Normal tissues surrounding the cancer also show different degrees of sensitivity in the extent of damage and the timing of the effect of this damage. These mechanisms are linked to the side-effects experienced: 'acute' reactions occur within 3 months of treatment, while 'late' reactions may occur up to several years after treatment. Tissues having a fast multiplication, such as skin and mucosal surfaces, show damage more quickly, whereas damage to slow-dividing cells may be responsible for many of the late complications of radiation.[21]

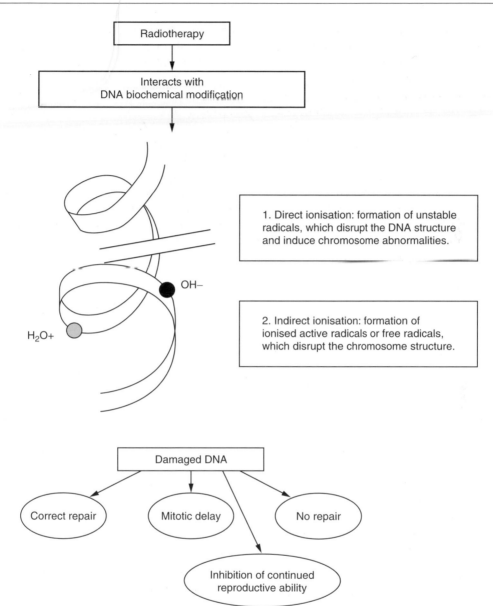

Figure 13.4 Effects of external beam radiation.

The dose of radiotherapy can have major implications for the response of tissues to irradiation. The dose–response curves both for normal tissues and cancer cells are similar. A relatively small change in the dose can have major implications both for tumour control and for the side-effects of treatment. The optimum dose is often balanced against the possible complications; however, some individuals appear to be more sensitive than others.[22,23] Certain tissues are very sensitive to radiotherapy (for example, eyes, lung, ovaries, and testes) and the dose that can safely be given to these areas is very limited. This tolerance to treatment is often the factor that limits the dose of radiation.[24] The relationship between dose and the probability of curing the cancer is shown in Figure 13.5. There is a threshold dose below which tumours are not controlled but above which

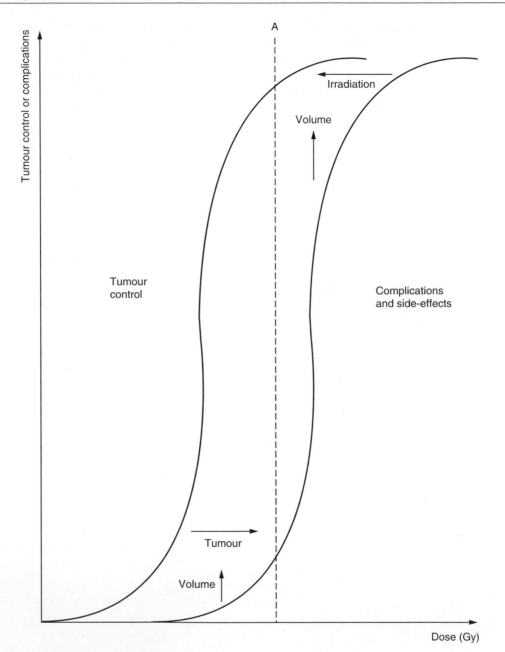

Figure 13.5 Dose–response curves for tumour control and complications. Small changes in radiation dose have major effects on the possible complications. A is the optimal dose giving high tumour control with a low complication rate. If you move to the right there is a significant increase in the number of side-effects. To the left there is a reduction in the tumour control.

control increases steeply. This also applies to normal tissue damage, but with fractionation it is displaced to the right. The greater the difference between the two curves, tumour control and complications, the greater the therapeutic ratio.[25] The link between acute and late effects of radiation is often disassociated in that a severe late reaction does not necessarily follow acute toxicity. Late tissue damage seems to be more related to fraction size than to acutely reacting tissues.

Fractionation is a technique that reduces the damage to normal tissues by giving the radiotherapy in smaller parts. Using smaller fraction sizes spares the normal tissue rather than the tumour, since small, frequent, sub-lethal damage allows normal cells to be repaired between the daily treatments. Many tumours have a poor blood supply and have regions of hypoxia that are relatively resistant to radiotherapy. Increasing the treatment time using a fractionated schedule allows hypoxic cells to re-oxygenate and redistribute themselves within the tumour so that more are in the radiosensitive phases of the cell cycle (see Figure 13.6).[26]

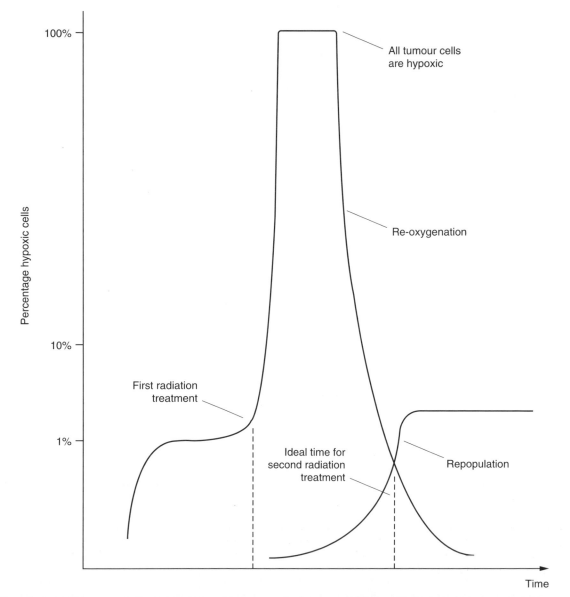

Figure 13.6   The pattern of oxygenated and hypoxic cells during radiotherapy. Radiotherapy is commonly given as a series of equal doses. Each daily dose or 'fraction' kills the same proportion of cells. When solid tumours grow, they often outstrip their blood supply and have areas of hypoxia. Hypoxic cells are two to three times as radioresistant. When multiple small doses of radiation are given, the oxygenated cells, being more sensitive, are killed first. During the interval between dose fractions, killed cells are eliminated and the previously hypoxic cells gain better access to oxygen. This process of re-oxygenation is utilised by giving the total radiation dose in many smaller doses.

Box 13.1 The '4 Rs' of radiotherapy

It is possible to think of the 4 Rs as being similar to the effects of a journey on a tube train in rush hour. The cancer cells are a group of people huddled together in the carriage. The train is packed, people are unable to move, you feel like a sardine if you are standing, but relieved if you have a seat. This is like the hypoxic cells in the tumour squashed together, with the surrounding cells having more space and being well oxygenated. The train pulls into a station and the train empties; those near the door now have more space so people spread out. This is rather like repopulation; the cells grow with the additional space and those that are hypoxic become better oxygenated. The train continues until at the end of the rush hour few standing people remain. The stops at the stations represent the fractions of radiation until there are no more viable cancer cells remaining.

Conventional fractionation is in 2 Gy treatment doses; however, there is very little consensus on optimal radiotherapy regimens.[27] Recent developments in radiotherapy have explored improving fractionation schedules and there are several regimens that are currently used. Accelerated treatment aims to overcome the problem of tumour cells repopulating as rapidly as the normal tissues, as this is a type of radioresistance.[28] Treatments are given twice per day to reduce the overall treatment time. Hyperfractionated treatment aims to improve the therapeutic ratio, reducing the dose given in each fraction.[29] This is to reduce late side-effects while also permitting an increased total dose to the tumour. Hypofractionated treatment, in contrast, gives a smaller number of radiation fractions, but the dose per fraction is increased. The total dose is lower than conventional treatments because of enhanced late side-effects. Hypofractionated regimens are often used for palliative treatments so that the course of treatment can be shorter.[30]

The homogeneity and accuracy of the radiotherapy are important, as the dose received by the target determines the outcome of the therapy and the probability of treatment side-effects.[20] Accuracy is achieved by using two or more radiation fields.[31] A composite isodose plan is drawn showing the isodose distributions from the individual beams. These beam characteristics may be altered with wedges or compensators when angled fields are used, or when there are changes in the patient's contour (see Figure 13.3). Most rectangular fields of radiotherapy are determined by thick collimators that are on the radiotherapy machine head, which, once set, determine the size of each field being given. Further shaping of the beams can be achieved by using shaped lead or alloy blocks, placed on trays in the path of the planned irradiation volume.

The volume of the tissue to be treated is determined by findings from diagnostic computed tomographic (CT) or magnetic resonance imaging (MRI) scans and knowledge of the usual patterns of spread of the cancer (see Figure 13.7). The target volume includes a margin of surrounding tissues, which might contain microscopic disease, but also allows for any inaccuracy of the treatment techniques – for example, patient movement or machine positioning.[31] The reproducibility of daily treatment is an important factor in delivering accurate radiotherapy.

Most radiotherapy is planned in two dimensions, but more sophisticated computer programs are used for shaping complex field arrangements for three-dimensional planned treatment. This type of planning requires reconstruction of tumour and target volumes from CT or MRI images so that the treatment volume can be localised and defined accurately for deep internal structures (see Figure 13.7).[32] During these procedures, localisation of the target volume is achieved with reference to the person's contours, as well as indelible skin markers such as tattoos or ink. Structures that may be at risk from toxicity of treatment can be identified and the field sizes and beam arrangements modified if appropriate. When sensitive tissues are adjacent to the treatment fields, fixation devices such as moulds or plastic casts are used to keep the person as still as possible (see Figure 13.8). The radiotherapy dose prescription and fractionation regime is then defined, detailing the dose to be delivered to target volume from each beam during radiotherapy. The standard dose is defined at the isocentre where the beams intersect. Once this plan of therapy has been devised, simulation of therapy is performed to verify the size, shape, and placing of the proposed beams (Figure 13.9).[33]

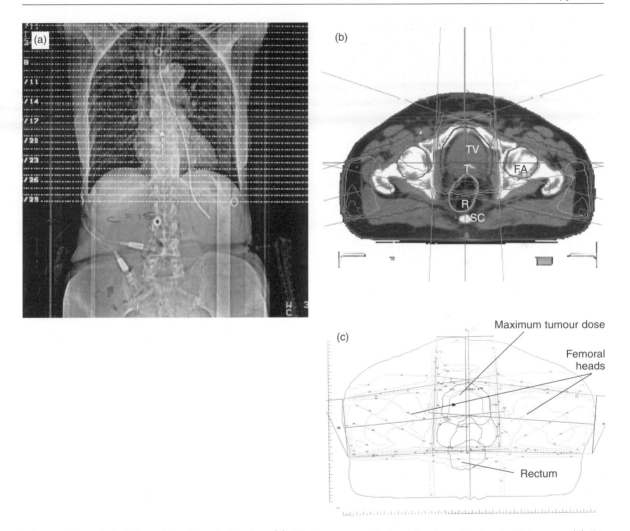

Figure 13.7   Principles of treatment planning. (a) CT topograms of chest to show levels of CT images. (b) CT image through the centre of the target volume. The target volume is drawn with a 1 cm margin. This example shows a pelvic treatment for carcinoma of the prostate. Sensitive normal tissues such as femoral heads and rectum are also outlined. TV, target volume; T, tumour; SC, spinal cord; FA, femoral heads; R, rectum. (c) The isodose distribution is outlined. This example is of a pelvic treatment for carcinoma of the prostate. Maximum tumour dose = 100%; minimum tumour dose = 95%. The femoral heads and rectum are identified to help avoid sensitive tissue as much as possible.

A simulator machine is identical to a therapy machine in its geometric specification and movements, but differs in that it emits diagnostic X-rays that produce an image of the tissue structures to be irradiated. At this time, the positioning of radiation beams can be checked and the reference markers on the skin used to set up the treatment (see Figure 13.10).

The treatment trajectory

The start of radiotherapy can be a lengthy affair, beginning with the planning of treatment, visits to the simulator and possibly a mould before starting radiotherapy. Although radiotherapy is given daily there are different stages of treatment, which can produce differing anxieties and fears. Anxieties

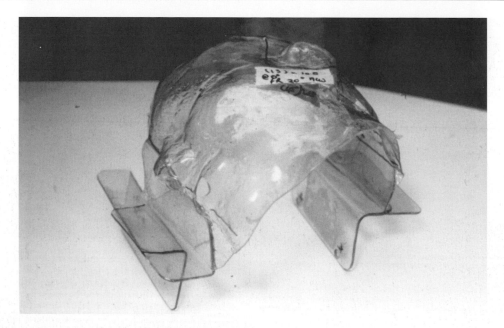

Figure 13.8 Mould for immobilisation for treatment of head and neck cancer.

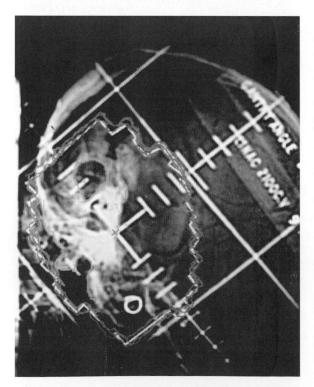

Figure 13.9 A simulator film shows the localisation of the target volume. The simulator is identical to a therapy machine but differs in that it emits diagnostic X-rays. The positioning of the radiation beams can be checked in relation to the tattoos used to set up treatment.

at the start of treatment may not necessarily become less as familiarity with treatment is gained. Studies have shown that emotional distress may be exacerbated by the completion of treatment, and unexpected physical side-effects may continue for many months after treatment is completed.[34] This trajectory of radiotherapy treatment can be thought of in three parts: the initial planning and preparation before starting treatment; the lengthy time of undergoing radiotherapy; and completion of treatment when visits to the treatment machine end.

Planning

The prospect of radiotherapy adds considerably to the fear and anxiety that may already be present following a diagnosis of cancer. Fear and misunderstandings of the use of radiation treatment, and negative attitudes regarding its effectiveness are known to be common.[35] In a study of women who were deciding whether to have either a mastectomy, or a lumpectomy with radiotherapy, concerns about the efficiency of radiation and its side-effects significantly influenced decisions.[36] Similar influences were found in communication in relation to palliative radiotherapy, and it has

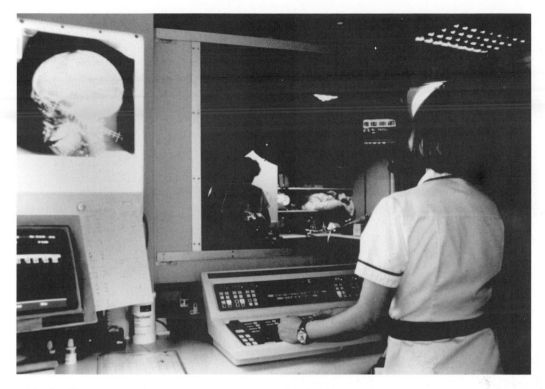

Figure 13.10   Planning radiotherapy.

been reported that patients who were receiving radiation with palliative intent were less involved in decision making than those receiving radiation with the purpose of cure.[37]

Radiation therapy machines are frequently situated in hospital basements and are therefore isolated. This may serve to create a mystique about the treatment and add to the apprehensions about having radiotherapy. The planning stage of radiotherapy is often perceived as taking a long time; this may be misconstrued as being on a waiting list for treatment, or having an indolent cancer as there appears to be no rush to provide therapy. People are often unaware that much of the preparation before treatment is essential for the accuracy and reproducibility of their radiotherapy. Planning and preparation for radiotherapy is 'behind the scenes', so that the extent of work required before treatment can proceed is not obvious. Once treatment has started it may take only a few seconds to deliver the therapy; however, checking the accuracy and

reproducibility of that radiotherapy is just as important. The feeling of delay, and CT or MRI tests can raise anxieties over the extent of disease or suggest that full information about the radiotherapy has not been given. Research study 13.1 reveals these to be central concerns of people undergoing radiotherapy.[38]

This can be a very lonely time; lots of investigations have to be undergone, but there is little contact with health professionals. Studies have identified the extent of fear and psychological morbidity associated with this stage of therapy. A controlled study using mock radiotherapy showed that 75% of people developed symptoms of nausea and fatigue following what they thought was therapy.[6] High levels of anxiety were found prior to treatment in a similar study.[39]

Restlessness, anxiety, apprehension, social isolation, unfounded pessimism over the likely outcome of treatment, and feeling withdrawn have been reported. This misapprehension about radiotherapy may be due to the lack of information

Research study 13.1

Eardley A. (1986). Expectations of recovery. *Nursing Times* **23 April**, 53–54.[38]

This study highlighted the general apprehension about treatment and misconceptions surrounding it. Thirty-nine patients were interviewed 1 week into their radiotherapy treatment and asked about how they felt about radiotherapy. One man described his wife's anxieties:

> She's not very happy because she's just hanging around – she thought she'd start straight away. She worried because she had those X-rays and no one's explained what they're for . . . it's not knowing what's going to happen . . . she was upset today after this X-ray, two doctors walked away from her whispering to each other, not saying a word to her. She got it into her head now that she's got something else.

Another had a fear that he would be crushed by the machine:

> I have a fear of machines, a fear of something coming on top of me.

It was clear from the interviews that the amount of knowledge and understanding of radiotherapy varied considerably:

> Even now, I don't know anything about the treatment – I just know I'm having preparation (mould room), not what the preparation is for.

Over half of those interviewed had worries about some aspect of treatment. Eighty-two per cent knew about their treatment and how long it would take; those remaining had little knowledge of what to expect. Thirty-six per cent were unaware that they might experience side-effects from the radiotherapy. Worries were expressed concerning cancer symptoms that had increased or arisen since radiotherapy referral.

given prior to the planning of treatment. Peck and Boland found that 60% of people were unprepared for the frequency, number of sessions, and prolonged course of therapy.[6] Most had received little information about the nature of radiotherapy and instead had gathered information from relatives and friends. Another study found that 52% of patients referred for radiotherapy felt that their referring physician had been no help in preparing them for radiation treatment,[40] and neither the referring doctor nor the radiotherapist was considered by patients as an individual to whom they would bring their fears or emotional problems. Educational interventions prior to start of radiotherapy are now more commonly provided, and structured information and visits to the radiotherapy centre are often encouraged. Significant benefits have been demonstrated by providing such educational packages, with patients demonstrating less anxiety and greater awareness of support services that are available.[41] Providing an orientation to the radiotherapy machines and an initial interview prior to radiotherapy is known to reduce anxieties and enhance compliance with therapy, which in turn contributes to better treatment.[42,43] Preparation for radiotherapy should include:

- provision of information about the treatment and the process of planning
- provision of information about practicalities such as car parking, driving and length of time of treatment
- prior to starting therapy, orientation to the machines and radiotherapy unit
- offering clear guidance on what to do prior to planning, such as to have a full bladder, and on how to care for radiotherapy skin marks
- assessment of levels of anxiety and depression prior to starting therapy.

During treatment

The fractionation for radiotherapy may differ depending on whether a palliative or curative regime is used, but may be completed in one day or last for several weeks. Radiotherapy is a difficult treatment modality to comprehend: 'being alone in a room and exposed to an invisible force that can destroy cells is an abstract experience that takes time and repeated information to become clear'.[44,45]

Individuals and families become used to the daily routine; however, of key focus and concern are the practicalities and costs of travel to the hospital. Travelling can be an additional burden for those who may be feeling unwell or frail due to their disease.[46] The experience of radiotherapy is physically demanding, and distress or anxiety may change during treatment, depending on how people feel but also on where radiotherapy fits into their wider cancer treatment plan. A study of 45 patients treated with external beam radiotherapy found significant changes in anxiety during the course of treatment.[47] Those who had an initially high level of anxiety reported a significant reduction as treatment progressed. Those with moderate anxiety reported no change, and those with low levels of anxiety reported significant increases as treatment progressed. It appeared that fear at the outset of treatment was predictive of adaptation to treatment. Radiotherapy side-effects, which may appear near the end of treatment, could have caused the increases in anxiety, particularly if these were interpreted as a sign of recurrent disease.

After treatment

The completion of radiotherapy treatment can be an extremely difficult time for patients. The day-to-day contact with radiotherapy staff and fellow patients may have provided informal support and reassurance. This is a time when nursing and medical support is, to some extent, withdrawn. Community care professionals may provide help, but they do not always have an expert knowledge of radiotherapy or its side-effects. Readjusting to 'normal life' at the end of treatment may not be easy. Loss of hope or confidence about the effectiveness of treatment, and depression, have been shown to feature at this time.[48] Ward *et al.*'s study of women's reactions to completion of treatment identified that the end of treatment did not always bring relief.[36] Out of the 38 women interviewed, 30% found termination of treatment upsetting, and this was frequently connected to a worsening of side-effects, not just a withdrawal of treatment. Women who were most anxious or depressed at the beginning of treatment were those who were most upset at treatment completion. Other studies suggest that emotional distress at the beginning of treatment is predictive of post-treatment functioning.[47,49] Eardley's longitudinal study of radiotherapy for head and neck cancer revealed that two-thirds of people felt that they had been inadequately prepared for discharge and were surprised at the length of time they took to recover from radiotherapy.[50]

There is an assumption on the part of health carers that the end of treatment will come as a relief. The loss of stability resulting from a cancer diagnosis may find temporary resolution in the routine of treatment but this can be shattered when it is completed.[4] 'Separation anxiety' may be seen at the end of treatment. Personal account 13.1 illustrates the extent of one person's anxiety.

Since completing treatment can be very difficult, it may be helpful to ask about feelings surrounding

Personal account 13.1 One woman's experience of radiotherapy

This account concerns a 65-year-old women with cancer of the right breast who, following surgery and wide axillary node clearance, was treated with 15 fractions of adjuvant radiotherapy. At interview prior to completing treatment, she was obviously well informed about her treatment and had supportive relationships with her family. She was keen to talk and had very mixed feelings about finishing her treatment.

> One part of me is pleased because I've begun to feel a bit unwell (on treatment) but . . . I also feel vulnerable . . . coming here, there are people I can talk to, people looking after me.

She wanted to regain control of her life, feeling that she had somehow 'lost her way'. She seemed unsure and fearful of both treatment and its cessation. She had found radiotherapy 'frightening' and 'alien'. Many of her fears had been fuelled by media publicity about damage caused by radiotherapy. At a subsequent interview, when she was beginning to feel better, most of the physical symptoms identified at the end of treatment were no longer a problem.

She felt that she had been keeping up appearances for her family and friends, who expected her to be relieved that treatment was over. Friends kept saying 'you must be so pleased it's all over':

> I was saying yes I am, it's great, but it was all lies really . . . the day after I finished my treatment, I felt quite awful . . . not well . . . and abandoned really . . . It seemed as though there is nothing. You get all this intensive treatment and then it's shut off . . . after the radiotherapy's finished, you shouldn't need to have any more contact but you do . . . I felt that everything had been taken away from me, although coming here had been a tiring routine I felt safe, I knew I could ask . . . what you need is a daily contact and a gradual weaning away from your dependency. I can't be isolated in feeling like this . . . a gradual weaning off and I wouldn't have felt so bereft.[33]

this, so that the insecurity over losing a 'safety net' can be acknowledged and discussed;[34,36] these feelings can be complex and may affect adjustment to cancer more generally. The feeling of needing to gain control after treatment and 'get back to normal' may be pressing, while for others the end of treatment is experienced as an anticlimax.

SIDE-EFFECTS OF RADIOTHERAPY

Radiotherapy treatment is limited by the severity and frequency of its side-effects. Adverse effects of treatment can be very debilitating and have a substantial impact on quality of life. Radiobiological data have revealed the mechanisms that cause side-effects, the immediate biological events trigger a series of genetic and molecular changes that lead to clinical injury. This process changes over time so that acute effects (occurring during and within the first 3 months of radiation) may be different from those experienced as late effects (3–12 months after radiation). Research has identified a number of pro-inflammatory cytokines that lead to damage to epithelial cells and subsequent fibrosis. Furthermore these events can develop over many months or years.[18] Because the events occur dynamically, the distinction between acute and late effects is not clear-cut. Therefore

these terms tend to be used for distinguishing management of symptoms rather than defining different biological effects. There are many assessment tools for the monitoring of radiation side-effects and cancer treatment toxicity. The result of this is that side-effect incidence data from patients who have received radiotherapy are often unreliable and difficult to compare between differing treatments and centres.[51] As clinical trials are becoming more extensive and radiotherapy treatments are revised, the documentation and assessment of side-effects is becoming clearer. One major problem is that, unlike many anti-cancer agents, the side-effects of radiotherapy develop in several stages. Late radiotherapy side-effects may take many years to develop and are often progressive and chronic, and therefore assessing and monitoring the toxicity of radiotherapy treatments is difficult.[23]

The link between total dose of radiation and its biological effect is well known, with the higher doses causing more adverse effects. The sensitivity of particular tissues to radiation also determines the side-effects of treatment. Those tissues with a high cell turnover often show more acute toxicity than tissues with a slow cell turnover.

Table 13.2 shows some of the treatment and biological characteristics that contribute to acute and late radiation reactions.

Table 13.2 Characteristics of early and late radiotherapy reactions in normal tissue

Property	Early responding tissue	Late responding tissue
Occurrence	Weeks to months, the latent time is independent of dose, but time for healing to occur is dose dependent.	6 months to 5 years. This is dose dependent.
Sensitivity for dose per fraction	Low	High
Fractionation timing	High	Low
Tissue characteristics	Rapidly self-renewing, stem cells or functional cells.	Slowly self-renewing.
Examples of tissues	Mucosa, skin, intestinal epithelia, urinary epithelia, bone marrow, lung alveolar, testes, and ovaries.	Muscle, liver, kidney, brain, spinal cord, nerves, and cartilage.
Response to radiation injury	Regeneration, resulting in stem cell depletion and functional breakdown.	Repair of sub-lethal damage, loss of parenchymal cells, fibrosis, and vascular damage.
Symptoms	Transient and usually reversible, but may continue into a late reaction.	Irreversible, progressive changes, but functional compensation may occur.

Often clear distinctions are made as to how different tissues respond to radiation; however, this is more complex than such simple classifications suggest. There are many exceptions, and tissues or organs proceed through several phases. For example, the urothelium is very sensitive to radiation. Symptoms are often described as acute, but injury can also become apparent after a long latent period because of the low cell turnover in the urothelium. Another example is that of lung tissue, where two waves of damage may be recognised, the first occurring 3–8 months after irradiation, and lung fibrosis, which develops after about 1 year.[23]

The extent and occurrence of symptoms is linked not only to the susceptibility of the tissue, but also to the innate susceptibility that the individual has to radiotherapy. Clinical and experimental studies are beginning to show that there is a genetic predisposition to hypersensitivity to radiation in normal tissues.[22] This would explain the range of side-effects occurring among those who receive similar radiotherapy treatments. Concurrent disease, age, and adjuvant therapy add to the predisposition to side-effects; however, these factors are not as yet clearly defined.

Symptoms occur as a result of tissue damage through the effects of radiation. In acutely responding cells, cell division may fail at some stage during mitosis. Non-proliferating cells may suffer apoptosis or cell death, or remain alive but be unable to perform their function. These biological effects result in tissue breakdown and inflammation. At the end of treatment the remaining cells repopulate and recover.

Late reactions in tissues often result from vascular changes as a result of the chronic inflammatory effects. This is seen in telangiectasia, where dilated capillaries appear on the skin surface.[52] The endothelial cells lining the capillaries are damaged, leading to irregular proliferation of surviving cells, changes in thickness, distortion, and thrombosis in the smaller vessels. This affects the blood supply to the tissue, leading to secondary damage.[51,53]

Radiotherapy side-effects can have enormous consequences if poorly managed, and can cause debilitating chronic problems, with a subsequent diminished quality of life.[54] This has led to litiga-tion and claims for compensation by people who have been badly affected, and may not have been warned of the possibility of late effects occurring.

The management of radiotherapy-induced side-effects is an important part of care; symptoms may be experienced during therapy but also many months to years after treatment.

Fatigue

Fatigue is recognised as a common symptom of radiotherapy, which not only occurs during treatment but also continues after the radiotherapy has ended. The incidence of moderate to severe fatigue following radiotherapy has been reported as between 32% and 59% of those undergoing treatment, and it is known to fluctuate over the treatment trajectory.[55–57] Although radiotherapy is a localised treatment with toxicity related to the specific site of the body being treated, fatigue can also be a systemic effect of radiotherapy and can significantly impact on quality of life.[58,59] The management of fatigue is often limited during radiotherapy, with an undue focus on anaemia-related problems rather than providing wider support.[60]

Possible causes of fatigue

The aetiology of fatigue may also be linked to certain sites of treatment. For example, in radiotherapy to the chest, such as in the treatment of breast cancer, the inclusion of sensitive lung tissue within the radiotherapy field may be linked to fatigue. The occurrence of radiation-induced pneumonitis or later fibrosis may also exacerbate fatigue.[61] The difference in incidence according to the site of treatment may be linked to the cell kinetics and ability of the tissues to repair themselves.

The pattern of fatigue

The pattern of fatigue following radiotherapy varies depending on the site and stage of therapy. Haylock and Hart first highlighted the changing pattern of fatigue symptoms during radiotherapy.[62] Fatigue is seen to increase over the course of radiotherapy treatment but has different incidence depending on the site and disease (see Figure 13.11). In a study of men receiving radiotherapy for prostate cancer, fatigue increased from 7% at baseline to 8% mid-radiotherapy and 32% at completion of treatment.[55] In a study of women with breast cancer, this weekly variation did not occur but fatigue decreased over the 3 weeks following completion of radiotherapy.[63] Fatigue has

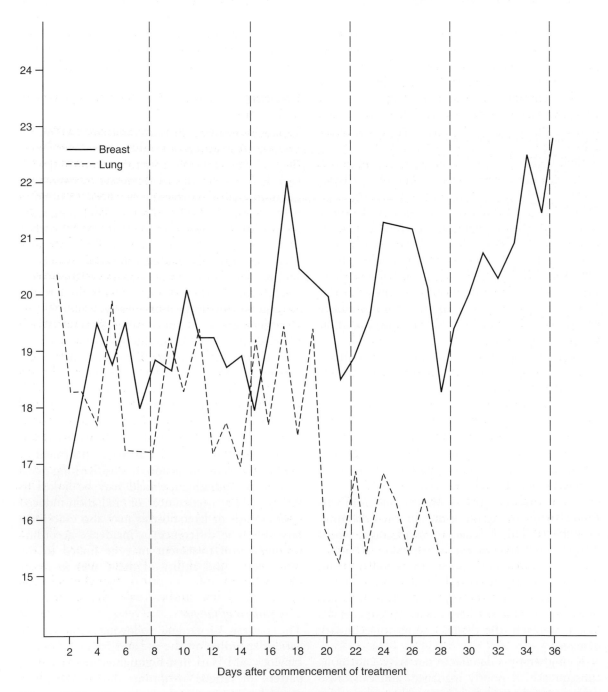

Figure 13.11 Mean fatigue scores during radiotherapy. Vertical lines indicate Sundays. Reproduced with permission from Haycock P. and Hart L. (1979). Fatigue in patients receiving localised radiation. *Cancer Nursing* **2**, 461–467.[62]

been shown to continue after completion of therapy; in one study up to 39% of patients were still experiencing fatigue at 3 months following radiotherapy treatment.[5] The severity of fatigue for patients undergoing radiotherapy has been defined by patient self-report;[57] in a study of 161 radiotherapy patients, symptom severity as mild to moderate fatigue was identified as occurring in 58.8% of patients, and severe and very severe fatigue was reported in 16.4% of patients.

The descriptions also give insight into the changing nature of the fatigue. Other studies have found that fatigue and skin problems were the most frequently reported side-effects of patients undergoing radiation for lung cancer, although levels of fatigue were higher at the start of treatment compared to women being treated with radiotherapy for breast cancer.[64] In head and neck cancer, the pattern of fatigue was at first periodic, but during the last 2 weeks of treatment became more continuous. An interview study ($n = 30$) of the experience of radiotherapy to the head and neck found that two-thirds said they still felt tired and weak 6–8 weeks after radiotherapy had been completed.[20] Men and women experienced different patterns of symptoms following radiotherapy to the pelvic area, men experiencing a lower incidence of fatigue. Women experienced increasing levels of fatigue over the course of the treatment and it was worse in the afternoons. Intracavitary treatment for gynaecological disease has been found to add to the extent of fatigue symptoms.[65] Fatigue is also a very debilitating symptom of cranial irradiation for brain tumours.

A longitudinal study of patients ($n = 19$) having cranial radiotherapy for primary brain tumours found that a specific pattern of incidence was experienced.[66] A daily diary was completed for 6 weeks after treatment and patients were interviewed 1 month and 3 months after treatment. The pattern of symptoms showed a peak of symptoms 2 weeks after therapy; patients complained of feeling fatigued, drowsy, and lethargic. This improved after several weeks but occurred again at 5–6 weeks and was exacerbated by feelings of lack of concentration, drowsiness and lethargy (see Figure 13.12).[67] This pattern of symptoms had not previously been identified, which may be because previous studies had used cross-sectional and retrospective research designs. The daily diary

enabled fluctuations in fatigue to be recorded. This pattern of symptoms appears distinct to that seen in patients undergoing cranial irradiation, and its aetiology may be due to the specific cells affected by the irradiation. The fluctuations demonstrated in these various studies may not be generalisable, as other researchers have not found similar patterns, but they highlight the need to look at subgroups in radiotherapy research.[63]

Factors that might influence the occurrence of fatigue

While fatigue is expected to accompany radiotherapy treatment, it is difficult to predict who may be most badly affected. Functional status may be an important factor in mediating cancer-related fatigue.[58,68] The physical complications of radiotherapy are linked not only to the cell types within the treatment field, but also to the volume and dose. The site of treatment is predictive, in that incidence of fatigue varies by site. Other factors that have been suggested are adjuvant therapy, hormone therapy chemotherapy, or surgery at the time of, or before, radiotherapy treatment. There is evidence for increased levels of fatigue with combined modality treatment. In a survey of 403 patients who were receiving a variety of adjuvant treatments, chemotherapy and radiotherapy (58%), radiotherapy (38%), and chemotherapy alone (5%), 90% reported that treatment had an effect on their energy levels.[69] For 37% this did not improve once treatment was completed. The younger patients (<34 years) fared best and felt that they had recovered within 12 months of finishing treatment, while older patients took longer to recover. Factors such as advanced disease, combined treatment modalities, and increased age were significant, although other studies have not shown fatigue and age to be related.[70] Fatigue may be more closely linked to frailty rather than chronological age as such; few studies make this distinction. Differing fractionation regimens may be a factor in the severity of fatigue experienced. In the study of somnolence syndrome, those patients having accelerated fractionation with twice-daily cranial radiotherapy had more fatigue than those patients having once-daily treatments.[67]

Factors influencing the occurrence of fatigue include:

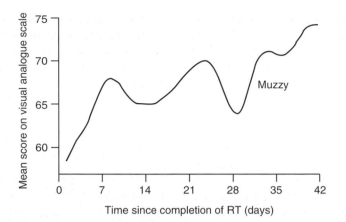

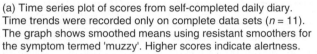

(a) Time series plot of scores from self-completed daily diary.
Time trends were recorded only on complete data sets (*n* = 11).
The graph shows smoothed means using resistant smoothers for
the symptom termed 'muzzy'. Higher scores indicate alertness.

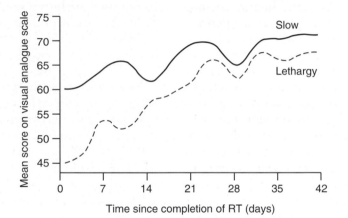

(b) Smoothed mean scores for the sensation of mental slowness
and lethargy. Higher scores indicate more vigour and lower
scores increased lethargy.

Figure 13.12 Fatigue after cranial radiotherapy. Reproduced with permission from Faithfull S. and Brada M. (1998). Somnolence syndrome in adults following cranial irradiation for primary brain tumours. *Clinical Oncology* **10**, 250–254.[67]

- adjuvant therapy:
  - hormone therapy
  - chemotherapy
  - recent surgery
- age
- frailty and functional status
- site of radiotherapy
- dosage of treatment
- fractionation regimen
- advanced disease.

Some individuals are more susceptible to the effects of radiation than others, although it is not, as yet, possible to identify those most at risk.[22] Depression may make fatigue symptoms worse; studies examining symptom clusters in cancer patients demonstrate that these symptoms influence severity.[71]

The experience of fatigue can cause great distress.[72] Munro *et al.*[1] explored the distress associated with radiotherapy by asking 72 patients to prioritise which symptoms or feelings were most distressing to them.[1] Fatigue was ranked second to worries about the success of therapy, but above other physical symptoms such as pain. The high levels of distress caused by fatigue could have been a somatic expression of anxiety, and not simply a physical effect of radiotherapy. It is clear that psychological distress is an important variable in fatigue, being linked with depression and anxiety, but it has also been linked to physical symptoms, such as pain.[73] Following radiotherapy, the experience of fatigue is so common that it is unlikely to be wholly a psychological manifestation. The distress of fatigue may be experienced in several ways, including the physical limitations of feeling exhausted and the social isolation that may result. Patients' accounts of what the fatigue is like give a clear picture of the lack of concentration, mental fogginess, and physical effects of experiencing fatigue as a result of radiotherapy treatment.

Feelings of fatigue during radiotherapy for many are an expected result of having cancer therapy, but not following treatment, where the expectation is to recover quickly. The long duration and severity of fatigue symptoms experienced after radiotherapy has been completed can be frightening and may not be understood to be a side-effect of radiotherapy treatment. It may be interpreted as a sign of the cancer progressing, as one man commented:

> I get worried that I'm not recovering. The whole time you think, 'Is it the tumour or is it the side-effect?'

Fatigue interventions is an area where much nursing research has developed. There are no clear ideas as to the aetiology and mechanism of radiotherapy-induced fatigue, and consequently interventions are mainly based on behavioural or psychosocial strategies. Fatigue is often an unexpected side-effect of treatment, and the severity and effects of fatigue symptoms can be a surprise.[66] By warning patients of the likelihood of fatigue occurring, and by providing information on strategies that may be helpful, the anxiety of unexpected symptoms can be prevented. However, there is little research evidence because at present fatigue interventions have not been adequately tested in cancer.[74] Exercise, stress-management

Personal account 13.2 The experience of fatigue following cranial radiotherapy

The accounts of 12 patients undergoing cranial radiotherapy interviewed for a qualitative study illustrate the pervasive nature of fatigue symptoms.[66]

The feeling of fatigue was described by one individual as 'I have felt like I had lead boots'. When asked to explain about how the fatigue affected them, they had difficulty in articulating what it was like:

> I just didn't want to do anything! I didn't feel I could do anything which was the worst thing.

Some described this feeling as lethargy.

> I felt lethargic. There were things which I had to think of doing, wanted to do and I just couldn't muster myself to do them you know.

Most described the effects of fatigue as influencing mental abilities but for those patients who experienced severe fatigue it had repercussions on physical activity:

> I mean physically. I knew I could walk across the kitchen and get myself a biscuit! But to get a biscuit! I would rather sit in a chair and think about it.

Others described how lack of mental concentration affected their lives:

> It felt like every day was a great effort and that just moving and doing anything was exceedingly hard, but not physically. It was more mentally than physically hard.

techniques and interventions aimed at reducing emotional distress may be effective ways to decrease feelings of fatigue (see Table 13.3).[75]

When experiencing fatigue, most people tend to rest, nap or sleep; however, this may not be the most appropriate strategy to reduce fatigue symptoms.[76,77]

In a study exploring which strategies were most effective in relieving fatigue associated with cancer treatment (chemotherapy: $n = 45$, radiotherapy: $n = 54$), sleep and exercise were found to be the most effective strategies.[78] The wide range of scores found between individuals for the different interventions suggests that fatigue management needs to be tailored to what works for each individual. A moderate walking exercise programme has been found to manage fatigue, but prevention

Table 13.3 Strategies for relieving fatigue

Assessment	Intervention strategy	Suggestions
Check for possible physical and psychological causes of fatigue, e.g. electrolyte imbalance or anaemia.	Reducing activity	Lie down, have a nap, sit and rest. Educate about the bad effects of too much rest.
Evaluate patterns of fatigue: encourage patients to maintain a diary.	Increasing activity	Encourage activity, walking programmes, exercise.
Forewarn patients of the occurrence of fatigue.	Distraction	Listen to music, read, socialise.
Differentiate fatigue from depression.	Schedule	Try different strategies, schedule important activities during times of least fatigue, and eliminate inessential activities.

through exercising during treatment may be more effective than managing fatigue once it has developed.[79]

Appropriate assessment is important in managing fatigue. Radiotherapy sites often involve bone tissue and this may affect the production of red cells in the bone marrow.[80] Anaemia, however, may cause fatigue symptoms and should be excluded in someone complaining of fatigue. Assessment of fatigue symptoms should be subjective: asking someone to rate their fatigue on a scale of 0 to 10 may be very useful.[81] Simply asking the person to express in their own words how they would describe their fatigue may be very valuable.

Quality-of-life issues in radiotherapy practice are only now beginning to be addressed with tools that reflect the extent of fatigue symptoms. Interventions for fatigue are now being tested in wider populations.[82] What is clear is that by taking the symptom seriously and offering support, information, and advice, the distressing nature of this symptom should be reduced.

Radiation enteritis

Radiation enteritis is a common side-effect of radiotherapy with fields that involve the pelvis or abdomen. Symptoms include nausea, diarrhoea, abdominal cramps, and proctitis. There may be acute as well as longlasting late effects, occurring in up to 70% of those whose treatment involves the gastrointestinal tract, while more than 80% of women being treated for gynaecological cancers suffer from diarrhoea during radiotherapy.[83,84] If symptoms are severe, they may interrupt or prolong the course of radiotherapy.

Modern techniques of radiotherapy using bowel-sparing techniques such as conformal treatment and computerised planning have reduced toxicity. There are distinct differences between acute and late side-effects with differing pathophysiology, symptoms, and management. The pathogenesis can mainly be attributed to the inherent sensitivity of the epithelial cells in the intestinal mucosa caused by rapid cell division.[85] Acute damage results in symptoms of nausea, diarrhoea, and abdominal cramps, which are often transient, and return to normal after completion of treatment. Secondary damage is more serious and may occur many months to years after the initial treatment, with signs of fibrosis, malabsorption, bleeding, and obstruction, which can be very debilitating (see Table 13.4). The assessment and management of radiation enteritis is an important clinical consideration when trying to balance the therapeutic benefit of treatment with potentially distressing side-effects.

Mechanisms causing radiation enteritis

Acute symptoms may start within the first 2 weeks of radiotherapy treatment. Damage is manifested in the stem cells, and the intestinal villi become shortened, reducing the tissue surface available for absorption.[83,86,87] The extent of mucosal abnormalities often correlates poorly with symptoms, and may persist after cells are seen to recover.[88]

Table 13.4 Side-effects of radiotherapy

Site	Acute (occurs from 18 to 22 Gy)	Late (many months to years)
Small intestine	Nausea, peptic ulcers Diarrhoea Cramps Distension	Peptic ulcers, stricture Diarrhoea Malabsorption, vitamin B_{12} deficiency, lactose intolerance Abdominal obstruction
Rectum and large intestine	Faecal incontinence Bleeding from rectum Anal pain Tenesmus	Fistula formation Bleeding from rectum Ulceration

The exact mechanism by which acute symptoms such as diarrhoea and discomfort arise, and what factors contribute to these, are still not known. Several causes have been suggested, such as malabsorption or neuroendocrine stimulation.

1. *Bile acid malabsorption* is considered a major factor contributing to the cause of diarrhoea. Bile salts in the normal gut are nearly totally reabsorbed; this is reduced in radiation enteritis.[89] The unabsorbed bile salts inhibit water reabsorption and stimulate peristalsis distally in the colon.[90] Normal bile salt absorption is thought to take place in the small intestine. Pelvic radiotherapy may include areas of terminal ileum, and may explain the differing incidence of bowel problems. Evidence for bile salt malabsorption comes from studies that have measured intraluminal fat content and abnormalities in bile salt metabolism. Fat absorption can be measured by faecal fat analysis but more easily by breath tests using a labelled triglyceride.[90] Forty-five per cent of women undergoing pelvic radiotherapy for gynaecological malignancies had abnormal breath tests during radiation treatment; abnormalities were still detected in 21% of these women 3 months following therapy, but returned to normal by 1 year.[91]
2. *Malabsorption of carbohydrate products* has also been suggested as a causative mechanism for enteritis symptoms. Carbohydrate, if not absorbed, also causes raised osmolarity, thereby increasing peristalsis. In the colon, bacterial fermentation of carbohydrate produces gas

and results in diarrhoea and discomfort. Few patients show demonstrable signs of malabsorption (for example, weight loss during treatment), but this may be a problem if they already have a pre-existing absorption or carbohydrate deficiency.[92] Malabsorption syndromes may be more of a problem in chronic radiation enteritis.

3. *Neuroendocrine changes* have also been suggested as a causative mechanism for radiation enteritis symptoms. Prostaglandins are released as a response to radiation cell damage. These are known to be stimulators of smooth muscle and have been shown to cause diarrhoea in animal experiments. A double-blind clinical trial using aspirin (a prostaglandin inhibitor) was able to reduce diarrhoea in women receiving treatment for uterine cancer.[93] However, contrary results from a study using olsalazine, a similar drug with minimal systemic absorption, increased symptoms rather than reduced them.[94]

There is evidence that all these mechanisms may play some part in radiation enteritis, but which mechanism is most prominent is not clear. Bile salt malabsorption has been shown to be a feature in most patients with diarrhoea following radiotherapy treatment. Differing sites of treatment may also influence the radiation enteritis.[88] Neuroendocrine changes may also contribute to symptoms but evidence is lacking as to the exact mechanism of action.

Late effects of radiation may occur from 6 to 18 months following completion of treatment and are considered among the most serious complications of radiation therapy. Symptoms can be insidious in onset, such as colicky abdominal pain, weight loss, or bleeding from the rectum, or diarrhoea. Late effects have been reported to occur in 5–21% of people and this variation may in part be due to the different doses of radiation used to treat different tumours, but may also relate to the way intestinal symptoms are defined and assessed. These late effects include proctitis, colitis, enteritis, ulceration, fistula formation, and obstruction. Chronic changes are often insidious, with progressive symptoms linked to vascular changes. Minor symptoms are often not well reported in the literature on toxicity following radiotherapy. Changes in bowel habit are often under-reported. Many women who have received pelvic radiotherapy for gynaecological malignancies report that they experience some bowel changes. Danielsson *et al.* ($n = 173$) found that 13% of women had diarrhoea 3–35 years (mean 9 years) after pelvic radiotherapy for gynaecological malignancies.[88] Intensive investigations showed that bile acid malabsorption was a common problem. Most studies have focused on gynaecological malignancies and the higher doses of intracavity treatment. These may over-represent the level and degree of late side-effects experienced more generally.

Although acute intestinal effects of radiation are well recognised and are usually transient, chronic enteritis may occur over a long time period and limit the effectiveness of radiation treatment by reducing the dose that can subsequently be delivered.[95]

Factors that might influence the occurrence of radiation enteritis

Factors that influence the occurrence of radiation enteritis symptoms have been studied in relation to the incidence of late effects. These factors can be divided into two types: patient characteristics and treatment factors.

Patient characteristics
- Age and gender are not considered important factors, but in studies older women are considered to have a higher incidence of radiation enteritis, possibly due to intracavitary therapy.
- Those who are underweight or have a thin physique are more at risk. This is linked to the anterior posterior diameter and organs that may be included within the field.
- Previous pelvic surgery gives higher risk, although there are contradictory studies.
- Co-morbid disease such as diabetes and hypertension give higher risk.
- Hypersensitivity syndromes, e.g. ataxia, telangectasia, give higher risk.
- Pre-existing vascular changes, e.g. haemorrhoids, can lead to higher incidence.

Co-existing disease or other characteristics may add to the chance of radiation enteritis occurring.[96] A history of pelvic inflammatory disease may increase the risk of radiotherapy symptoms by 15%.[97] Although pre-existing vascular changes may add to the risk attached to abdominal or pelvic radiotherapy, since these factors are present in older age groups it is difficult to distinguish their importance from age *per se* as a risk factor.

Treatment factors
- Extended field of radiation treatment is more likely to include small bowel within the field. Acute symptoms have been correlated with the volume of the field.[98]
- Dose of irradiation – it has been shown in laboratory studies that with a lower dose the cells along the villus more rapidly return to normal.
- Fractionation schedule – smaller individual doses given over an extended period are less likely to cause toxicity.

Attempts to minimise the risk may include reducing the volume of small bowel within the treatment field. In pelvic radiotherapy this is achieved with a full bladder, so that the small bowel is pushed out of the field, which reduces radiation enteritis.[99] The precision of planning and conformal techniques can also minimise toxicity.

What does it mean for the person having radiotherapy?

Few studies have explored how enteritis symptoms are experienced. Most have focused on the extent of symptoms rather than the distress or impact for the individual. Padilla, in a study of 101 patients from four radiation oncology clinics, tried to describe the impact of gastrointestinal side-effects on psychological and physical well-being.[100] Data were collected using a variety of quality-of-life and quantitative assessments. Few had problems with gastrointestinal symptoms. Psychological distress was linked with gastrointestinal symptoms in 21.5% of patients, whereas anxiety linked to distress was found in 11.8% and other side-effects in 5.5%. The most distressing of physical symptoms was fatigue. Padilla concluded that where side-effects were perceived to be a problem they also had an important impact on psychological and physical well-being. Although this study highlights some of the psychological issues related to radiation enteritis, the quantitative design precludes exploration of what impact the symptoms had on the individual, or exploration of what aspect of gastrointestinal symptoms was of greatest concern to those experiencing it.

Diarrhoea from acute radiation enteritis is often considered to be an inevitable consequence of radiation therapy, something that is to be suffered. This is described in one patient's account of his diarrhoea during pelvic radiotherapy (see Personal account 13.3).

These accounts have focused on the acute side of radiation enteritis and highlight that patients have numerous problems and feel that there is little that can be done. A low-residue diet and anti-diarrhoea medication have been reported as helpful in managing diarrhoea,[5] although the effectiveness of this approach is open to question since there remains a high incidence of enteritis, despite the use of medication.

Personal experience of symptoms is important in understanding how people interpret their symptoms. Padilla, in observing the impact of acute radiation enteritis,[100] may have found that this was not the most distressing of symptoms, but evidence suggests that if bowel problems persist and become chronic they impact greatly on quality of life.

Bowel symptoms, whether acute or chronic, can profoundly influence social and sexual life.[103] Although most people experience transient and minor symptoms, those who do have uncontrolled diarrhoea or enteritis can find that they become

Personal account 13.3

> Basically I had diarrhoea . . . it was bad news because no sooner had you put a clean pair of underpants on, then I would need to go again and, you know, unfortunately you missed and they were messed again. That was very difficult to take . . . The thing is because I was told, I knew it was going to be okay, if I hadn't been told that's the upsetting thing . . . I think if you know it's a limited time, it's a bit easier . . . needed to be near a toilet and to be perfectly honest some of the times that I would go would be quite unusual I mean it would be 2 am, 5am. I found that was difficult.[101]

Diarrhoea disrupts sleep, journeys, or social activities. Medication for diarrhoea can cause side-effects. One man described how he was left feeling remote and dizzy with codeine phosphate tablets:

> The diarrhoea hasn't really gone it's a little naughty but the tablets cause a stalling they certainly help. The tablets leave me with a funny feeling I don't know what it is erhm . . . a bit woozy it's a bit hard to explain I mean I can walk and get in or drive the car but at the same time they make you feel a bit woozy.

Others complained of getting constipated:

> The tablets they are giving me are blocking me up back-wise now and you know they've given me some other medicine to take for that and if I take too much of it I get terrible diarrhoea which I've got at the moment so you know you're doing one thing to stop one thing and you're taking something else and causing other problems.[101,102]

socially isolated, with the symptoms making them feel unclean and not sexually desirable. There is abundant information on the effects of radiation on morphology and intestinal tissue but little on the time-course of enteritis symptoms, or how individuals can cope with them.

Management

A number of management approaches to radiation enteritis have been reported. There is a distinction between acute and late enteritis and each is controlled differently. A key to the management of the problem is to assess accurately the extent of an individual's symptoms and possible causative mechanisms. Breath tests and faecal fat monitoring are not realistic in a clinical setting, but asking

Personal account 13.4

A man who had received pelvic radiotherapy for prostate cancer 6 months previously was well throughout treatment but had experienced proctitis at the end of it. Months went by with severe pain when opening his bowels. At clinic appointments he had been told he was constipated and he had received differing laxatives. During this time he had periods of diarrhoea and then constipation, the severe pain continued and he found that it was difficult to eat and was losing weight. After many months his cancer was 'cured' but he had despaired of all help; he described how desperate he felt, that 'life wasn't worth living like this'. Finally, with surgical investigations it was found that he had a stricture and required a colostomy to treat this late side-effect. Several months later he told how relieved he was to have someone take his symptoms seriously, and that if someone had listened before to how he was feeling things might not have been as bad.[101]

patients to complete a diary or log of their bowel habit can give valuable information as to the extent of the problem, and the pattern of symptoms. There are three approaches to management: diets, drugs that influence the aetiology, and anti-diarrhoeal agents.

Diet

A low-fat diet has been shown in studies to be beneficial in reducing diarrhoea. Experimental research has shown that specific and elemental diets are useful in protecting cell function during radiotherapy.[98] These alter the fat and lipid content of the diet, but are unpalatable and unlikely to be acceptable. Fat content in the diet has also been associated with bile acid malabsorption, and studies suggest that a 40 g low-fat diet can significantly reduce diarrhoea.[88,104] In practice, low-fat diets are rarely used and it is low fibre that patients are recommended, with the presumption that reducing bowel bulk will reduce symptoms. There is no clinical evidence that would suggest that this advice is of value, and indeed it may cause constipation. One problem with a low-fat diet is that some fat in the diet is inevitable, and therefore dietary control is unlikely to control all symptoms completely.

Drugs influencing aetiology

To combat bile acid malabsorption bile acid sequestrants (colestipol hydrochloride, cholestyramine) have been used in clinical trials. These drugs act to bind with bile acids in the intestine. Although successful in reducing diarrhoea, the side-effects outweigh benefits.[105] Further studies have used the bile acid sequestrant in combination with a 40 g low-fat diet, which resulted in significantly less diarrhoea compared to a low-fat diet without sequestrant.[106]

Anti-diarrhoeal agents

Anti-diarrhoeal agents such as codeine phosphate or Lomotil are often used for symptom management, but these are costly, may cause problems of constipation or dizziness, and may only produce short-term relief.

The management of chronic radiation enteritis is often difficult and is based on the cause of the problem. Strictures, fibrosis, haemorrhage, or ulceration require surgical investigations. Assessment is clearly very important and in the case of diarrhoea this may be a result of fat malabsorption or bacterial contamination. Studies suggest several strategies, that of a low-fat diet, bile acid sequestrants, antibiotics, or fermented milk, which may be useful in reducing diarrhoea symptoms, while non-steroidal anti-inflammatory agents, steroids and sulfasalazine have been suggested for proctitis (see Table 13.5). The use of a low-fat diet, bile acid sequestrants and antibiotics were found by Danielsson et al. to significantly reduce chronic diarrhoea.[88] Of the 20 (from a sample of 173) women who were investigated for chronic diarrhoea, 13 had bile acid malabsorption and 9 bacterial contaminations.

The use of bacterial cultures in fermented milk has been used clinically as a way of reducing over-

Table 13.5 Management of acute and late radiation enteritis

Acute	Late
Low-fat diet	Antibiotics
Anti-diarrhoea medication	Low-fat diet
Cholestyramine	Steroids
Sucralfate granules	

growth of pathogenic micro-organism in Sweden. There is little clinical evidence that this is effective. In a study by Henrikkson of 40 patients, the addition of a fermented milk (verum halsofil) did not significantly reduce bowel symptoms, and where this was administered to patients during treatment this increased the frequency of diarrhoea.[107]

Sucralfate, an agent used in inflammatory bowel disease, has been shown to have a protective 'coating' effect on the gastrointestinal mucosa.[108] Henriksson *et al.*, in a double blind trial of 70 people having radiotherapy for prostate or bladder cancer, found that sucralfate granules significantly improved diarrhoea symptoms and that they also reduced the late bowel disturbances up to 1 year following treatment.[109] An animal study exploring the efficacy of anti-inflammatory agents (aspirin, indometacin, piroxicam), misoprostol (prostaglandin analogue), and sucralfate found that these agents had no effect on proctitis signs.[110] Most often proctitis is treated symptomatically with low-dose topical steroids or local analgesic agents.

Many of the treatments mentioned in controlling symptoms of radiation enteritis have not been effectively tested and there is a need to improve the clinical assessment and diagnostic tests for radiation enteritis. The possible link between acute and chronic symptoms has been suggested; one study indicates that effective control of acute symptoms may reduce the incidence of chronic radiation enteritis. The question 'Does effective acute symptom management have an impact on later side-effects?' is an important issue for future research to address.[111]

Radiation skin reactions

Skin reactions from radiotherapy are considered a relatively infrequent complication to radiation therapy. Modern planning techniques and new methods of delivery such as conformal and intensity-modulated radiation therapy (IMRT), have resulted in smaller volumes of normal tissue being treated, and this has impacted on the number of radiation skin reactions observed. Although in theory a reduction in skin reactions should occur, the requirement for multiple beams tangential to the skin and high doses can result in increased skin reactions. Skin changes occur following treatment. Erythema and moist desquamation are often seen as bad signs and may induce fears of having had too much treatment – 'I've been burnt by the therapy'. Symptoms produce discomfort and may take many weeks or months to heal, with a subsequent impact on quality of life.

In the past, skin reactions were used as a way of monitoring radiotherapy dose. With improved technology some skin reactions have reduced, but have been replaced by wounds in difficult areas, such as skin folds or creases, that are troublesome to manage. The primary aim of modern management is to aid comfort and prevent infection until the skin has regrown. With the increasing prevalence of concomitant therapy, such as chemotherapy and surgery, and new techniques such as escalating radiotherapy dosage and accelerated regimes, it is clear that skin reactions will remain a problem.

Incidence of skin toxicity is unclear, with skin inflammation ranging from 66% to 83%.[112,113] Prevalence studies are rare and few cancer centres use assessments to monitor skin problems. What is known is that acute skin reactions are cumulative with radiotherapy treatment, and have a latent healing time after treatment has completed. This highlights the differing aetiology of radiation skin damage compared with conventional wounds.[114] Skin management varies considerably between cancer centres.[115,116] There is a need for studies to evaluate modern wound-care products in the context of radiotherapy skin reactions, and a need for innovation to improve this neglected area of radiotherapy side-effects.

Mechanisms
The underlying cause of skin reactions relates to the radiobiological damage to the dermis and epidermis. In normal tissue the epidermis has a renewing cell population in which cell production is balanced by cell loss. Superficial cells are shed and replaced by new cells formed by mitosis in the basal layer.[117,118] The average time for repopulation of cells is approximately 4 weeks. In radiation skin damage, this repopulation is impaired by radiobiological damage to the radiosensitive basal and suprabasal layer, and hence this affects

the integrity of the upper epidermis layer.[119] The associated erythema represents the secondary inflammation. Skin changes vary and are commonly classified as erythema, dry desquamation, moist desquamation, and necrosis.

These reactions may occur in isolation or in combination over a radiation field. Erythema is a dry, red, warm skin reaction that may feel sensitive and tight.[120] This often starts to occur 2–3 weeks into treatment and subsides 2–3 weeks after therapy. If repopulation of the cells does not keep pace with those being lost, then dry desquamation occurs. This is associated with dry peeling skin that itches. The discomfort of this reaction is compounded by the decreased ability of the sweat and sebaceous glands to produce sweat. This reaction can occur as early as 2–3 weeks into treatment. If new cell proliferation is inadequate and the epidermis layer becomes broken, then moist desquamation may occur. This has distinctive signs in that the skin blisters and sloughs, leaving the denuded areas of dermis exposed. These areas then exude serum, which is associated with pain and discomfort. Necrosis is an infrequent skin reaction caused by a combination of ischaemia and vascular occlusion, and is a result of cell death (see Table 13.6).

As in many radiation reactions, the link between acute and late effects is not known. The severity of an acute reaction may have a link to the cosmetic and functional impact on the area that was treated. Scarring from skin breakdown has an effect on body image, as well as on functional morbidity.

Table 13.6 Radiation-induced skin reactions

Early or acute radiation-induced effects	Late or chronic radiation-induced effects
Erythema	Atrophy
Dry desquamation	Thinning
Moist desquamation	Telangiectasia
Alopecia	Altered pigmentation
Reduced sweating	Fibrosis
Itching	Ulcerations
Changes in pigmentation	Necrosis
	Carcinogenesis

Incidence

The incidence of radiation-induced skin problems is relatively unknown. In a survey of radiotherapy units in the UK, Barkham found that skin reactions are relatively common: 83% of centres reported frequently seeing skin inflammation, dry desquamation was reported in 52% of centres, and moist desquamation in 12%.[113] Acute necrosis was rarely seen. King investigated the timing, onset, frequency, and duration of symptoms among a group of patients receiving radiotherapy.[5] Skin irritation was reported in the last week of radiotherapy in 87% of patients having treatment to the chest, and in the third week of treatment in 80% of patients receiving head and neck radiotherapy. Skin reactions continued to be troublesome in 9% of those treated with radiotherapy to the head and neck, 3 months post-treatment.

Like many of the radiation-induced side-effects, factors that influence the occurrence of toxicity are not certain. Clear treatment-related factors such as dose, volume, and fractionation are known to be influencing factors, but other skin variables are not clear.[121]

Treatment factors adversely affecting skin include:

- higher doses of radiation per fraction
- large treatment fields
- tangential fields
- raising the skin surface by wax or moulds
- electron beams – these have a shorter wavelength of radiotherapy and this may result in the skin receiving a larger dose compared to photon treatments.

Factors influencing skin vulnerability include:

- concurrent chemotherapy
- site of radiotherapy – skin folds are more susceptible to damage, e.g. axilla, groin, intramammary fold, perianal area, and head and neck
- skin areas susceptible to friction
- recent surgery to the skin area
- diabetes or vascular disease
- smoking[121,122]
- use of irritant skin-care products.[123]

As with many radiotherapy toxicities, it is difficult to predict those patients most at risk of developing radiation skin damage. Late toxicity is seen in less than 5% of patients and is considered a rare and unexpected complication of curative radiotherapy. Turesson and Thames measured early and late radiation skin damage following radiotherapy to the breast.[124] All patients had standard therapy; however, it was clear that the variation in tolerance to radiation was related to an individual's radiosensitivity. Neal *et al.* found that a significant factor in late toxicity was the dose variation within a field.[125]

The impact of skin reactions

The discomfort and distress of radiation-induced skin reactions is frequently under-represented as a toxicity, and often goes unnoticed as the physical appearance of the skin does not always correspond with the discomfort experienced by the patient. Pain is often associated with radiation-damaged skin, and can be exacerbated by incorrect wound management.[126] In a small study of women (n = 20) having radiotherapy for breast cancer, skin reactions were found to have an adverse affect on home life.[127] Some form of skin reaction occurred in every woman after radiotherapy, with moist desquamation occurring in 45%. The women complained of symptoms of itching and tenderness, a feeling of tightness, and throbbing of the skin. However, few complained of marked pain. The skin changes resulted in functional and body-image changes: skin damage limited household activities, the discomfort restricted what clothes could be worn, sleep disturbances were reported, and 10% said that the radiotherapy had affected sexual relationships. Few research studies have used qualitative accounts to explore the impact radiation skin reactions have on the individual. One patient with head and neck cancer in Wells' study reported being fearful of people observing him: 'I didn't want people looking surreptitiously at my burns'.[128] Skin was described as feeling 'raw' and as looking like 'crocodile skin', and was painful and itchy. The lack of qualitative research in this area shows how little we know about the impact of skin reactions. Patient accounts and subjective information are necessary to provide insights into how best to assess and support patients through these symptoms.

The management of radiation-induced skin reactions

Modern wound-care products are expensive, and therefore it is important that we utilise interventions based on evidence. Furthermore, although some interventions do not result in improved healing, outcomes such as reduced pain, improved comfort and self-care are still important outcomes. The latent healing period after therapy is completed means that wound healing is not the same as in conventional cases.[116] Assessment is fundamental in recognising the right approach for skin problems, but preventing skin damage and mediating skin problems is also an essential part of nursing care.

Assessment

The literature is full of descriptions of radiation-induced skin reactions, with scoring for toxicity based on observer reports. Most reflect only the observable reaction and not the subjective symptoms that patients experience. Conventional skin-assessment tools are often not applicable as the skin damage differs from conventional wounds. Digital photography has been shown to be an effective tool for recording skin erythema.[129]

The main aims for caring for impaired skin arising during the course of radiotherapy are to:

- prevent infection
- maximise patient comfort
- minimise trauma and prevent further skin damage.

Following completion of radiotherapy, healing is the priority.

One problem is that there are many assumptions made about how to care for the skin. Two randomised trials demonstrate that washing the skin with lukewarm water and a mild soap during radiotherapy is harmful.[130,131] The use of creams and ointments is considered to alleviate some of the discomfort of a dry skin.[121] Creams should not be allowed to build up on the skin, and therefore washing should be encouraged. Some creams are contraindicated (for example, petroleum jellies such as Vaseline) as these are poorly soluble and stay on the skin's surface. Lanolin-based creams such as E45 are also not recommended, as the lanolin content increases sensitivity. Topical steroid-based creams are often prescribed for the itching experienced with the dry desquamation; however, prolonged use of steroids is known to delay healing and has no beneficial effects if the skin is broken.[132] A recent randomised trial of calendula cream, which is derived from the marigold plant, against trolamine found statistically significant differences in reducing the incidence of grade 2 or higher skin reactions. While 84% of the women in this study used the cream successfully, 30% of these women reported the topical application difficult.[133] The routine use of moisturising creams may prevent the need for steroids. Talcum powder can also be soothing for dry desquamation, although there is little evidence of its efficacy. Clothes should be loose and made of cotton. Irradiated skin is more vulnerable to damage from sun exposure, therefore covering up irradiated skin and using sun blocks after completion of treatment is important.

The routine use of antiseptics such as proflavine in radiation wound management is not considered to confer any advantage over normal saline.[116] Morgan suggests that some products may also have toxic effects on healing tissue such as fibroblasts, and therefore normal saline is recommended for wound cleansing.[134] Dressings such as melonin and paraffin gauze were traditionally used for skin reactions; however, they stick to wounds and cause pain and trauma when removed. New dressings have since been developed, such as the alginates and hydrogels. Hydrogels are non-adhesive, absorb wound fluid slowly, have cooling properties and provide a moist environment to enhance re-epithelialisation.[135] Alginate sheets are recommended for wounds with moderate to high exudate during radiotherapy; for example, Sorbsan, which converts to a hydrophilic gel on contact with exudate or saline.[115,126] One of the benefits of alginates is their haemostatic properties, which are useful for areas of bleeding. During radiotherapy, treatment dressings within the radiation field usually need to be removed to prevent changes in dosimetry. In some palliative treatments, dressings may be left in place; it is therefore worth checking with the therapeutic radiographer. The use of adhesives such as tape or semi-permeable film dressings within the treatment field may add to skin damage. Occlusive dressings are ideal post-treatment; hydrocolloid sheets can be placed over an area of moist desquamation and left in place for up to 7 days. Several other dressings have been used in clinical practice or described in the literature, but there remains a paucity of evidence evaluating the effectiveness of interventions for the management of skin reactions.[136]

Case example 13.1 Managing skin reactions

After having a wide local excision for breast cancer and radiotherapy, Hannah started to develop a skin reaction. On assessment, the skin in the treatment field was covered in erythema with an area of moist desquamation in her intramammary fold. The overall skin reaction appeared minimal yet she was experiencing sharp burning pain in her breast, and pruritis around her nipple. Sleep was difficult and the pain caused her to worry about tumour progression. Hannah was anxious about her treatment, and the skin reaction very visibly reinforced the nature of her disease.

Nursing intervention not only addressed her anxiety but focused on the physical symptoms. Aqueous cream was applied to the erythema and a hydrocortisone cream applied to her nipple area. The moist desquamation was covered with a hydrogel sheet (Geliperm), which Hannah found soothing and which reduced the pain. Over the next 5 days, the area of moist desquamation enlarged; this was expected, as there is latent healing following radiotherapy. Subsequent to the deterioration the moist desquamation healed within 2 days.

Another example of the use of occlusive dressings can be shown by the case of Joe, who was 8 years old and having radiotherapy to his spine. Near the completion of his treatment he developed an area of moist desquamation on the anterior of his neck. He found it hard not to scratch and peel the dry skin. To prevent him damaging the skin further, Granuflex was applied to his neck. The thin wafer was used as it is more pliable and easier to mould onto the skin folds. A large border was left to enclose any exudates, and within 4 days Joe's skin had successfully healed.

The management of skin reactions is a neglected area of practice. There are few research studies to guide practitioners on how best to manage skin problems, and research is needed to evaluate modern skin-care products. Innovations such as the use of aloe vera creams, and evening primrose and lavender oils have positive anecdotal reports but clinical trials need to be established to evaluate these formally.[114] Skin reactions, not only those that are acute but also longer term ones, potentially cause pain and anxiety and should be taken seriously.

Sexual issues and radiotherapy

Sexuality and fertility are an important component of management in radiotherapy practice that is often overlooked by clinicians. Symptoms and side-effects during and following radiotherapy (for example, fatigue, pain, or diarrhoea) may have implications for sexual desire but can also affect sexual function. Talking about sexual issues prior to treatment is difficult, with the consequence that they are often ignored, avoided, or dismissed by staff, despite numerous reports that, for many, concerns over fertility or sexuality are common and affect physical and psychological well-being. Symptom management and support should include information on how radiotherapy impacts on fertility, libido, and sexual functioning.

Radiotherapy may affect sexual functioning both physically and psychologically, and these effects may be difficult to distinguish from cancer-related ones. Vaginal fibrosis, post-coital bleeding, sterility, and early menopause occur as a result of radiotherapy treatment.[137] Much of the literature focuses on the effects of radiotherapy on women with gynaecological malignancies, but men also have problems with radiotherapy treatment affecting libido and potency. The incidence of sexual problems varies considerably in studies. For example, in one study 50% of women treated for cervical cancer reported reduced sexual activity.[138] In genito-urinary cancer, impotence has been reported in about 35–40% of men following radiotherapy.[104] One problem is that the physical effects of the radiotherapy for genito-urinary and gynaecological cancer are often difficult to distinguish from the sexual dysfunction and impotence

that results from the initial disease or adjuvant therapies.

Abbitol and Davenport suggest that it is the physical effects of treatment that result in poor sexual function.[139] This has been disputed following studies where no positive correlation between patients with severe physical changes and those with the greatest decrease in sexual functioning were found.[140,141] Many studies highlight that the physical changes following radiotherapy do not necessarily inhibit sexual desire, but that changes in body image, misconceptions or fears about spreading cancer, or hastening recurrence may all have an impact on sexual function.[142] As with many symptoms, the cause of the problem may be multifactorial, with social, cultural, and other symptoms affecting the complexity of sexual desire and function.[143]

Physiological changes

In women treated with radiotherapy for gynaecological cancer, the vaginal canal and ovaries are the areas most sensitive to radiation therapy, and combined-modality treatments have a more profound effect.[144,145] If the radiation field includes vaginal tissue, a decrease in vaginal lubrication and sensation may result. The cells in the vagina have rapid cell renewal, which makes the epithelium very sensitive to radiation damage. Depletion of cell supply, slow occlusion of blood vessels, and gradual laying down of fibrosis result in narrowing and lack of elasticity in the vaginal canal.[142] Stenosis and/or shortening of the vagina are late effects that occur progressively over time, with a consequent reduction in size and diameter. In women, radiation to the ovaries causes premature menopause with loss of germinal epithelium and follicles. Very low doses of radiation (4–10 Gy) are required to stop ovulation, and permanent loss of menses is inevitable in women over the age of 40 years.[146] Younger women are more likely to remain functional, but with larger therapeutic doses, cessation of ovulation occurs in any age group (see Table 13.7).

In men, radiation to the genital regions as in treatment for prostate or bladder cancer, seminoma, or testicular cancer, can have consequences for sexual functioning. Impotence following external beam radiation therapy for prostate cancer can

Table 13.7 Possible effects of radiotherapy on the sexual organs

Women	Men
Pelvic fibrosis	Pelvic fibrosis
Atrophy of the vaginal wall	Decreased testosterone
Inelasticity of tissue	Pudendal or sympathetic nerve injury
Scarring	Decreased semen levels
Obliteration of small blood vessels	Aspermia
	Fibrosis of arteries
Thinning of epithelium	Reduction in penile blood pressure
Loss of lubrication	
Ulceration	

Table 13.8 Sexual dysfunction following radiotherapy

Women	Men
Pain on intercourse	Impotence
Post-coital bleeding	Pain on ejaculation
Early menopause	Decrease in semen volume
Decreased libido	Male menopause
Feelings of burning with semen	Decreased libido
Pelvic pain	

have physiological effects, causing fibrosis of the pelvic vasculature and damage to the pudendal or sympathetic pelvic nerves.[147,148] Vascular changes result in reduced penile blood pressures, which can contribute to arteriosclerotic changes in the pelvic arteries.[149] Radiotherapy may therefore accelerate changes that were already taking place through other diseases such as diabetes or hypertension. Decreased levels of testosterone may produce a reduction in libido. The testes are also highly radiosensitive. Radiotherapy to the retroperitoneum and pelvis (for example, for seminoma) may compromise gonadal function even at low doses, and erectile dysfunction is seen in 10% of cases.[150] Cessation of sperm production (aspermia) may be temporary in those men having lower doses of radiation, but can take 3–5 years to recover.

The common problem from these physiological changes is that they lead to pain on intercourse (dypareunia). Researchers report that 30–50% of women interviewed said that pain on intercourse was the main reason for their decreased enjoyment of sexual activity.[115] Women were also frightened that sex would be painful and this reduced sexual pleasure. Post-coital bleeding has also been found to be a problem.[137,139,151]

In men, the result of physical changes may be absolute as in the physical inability to have an erection, but they may also complain of symptoms of pain on ejaculation and a permanent decrease in semen volume (see Table 13.8).

Loss of reproductive function

The ovaries are very sensitive to radiation therapy, and if included within a treatment field will suffer ovarian failure. Shielding can sometimes maintain function, but despite this 30–50% of women lose ovarian function after irradiation.[152] The effect of this is that reproductive function is lost and women lose their childbearing ability. It may also induce early menopause, with premature ageing and feelings of diminished femininity.[153] Men treated with pelvic radiotherapy rarely report having discussed the possibility of infertility as a result of radiotherapy. Often they are considered by medical and nursing staff as too old for this to matter, but Schover found that this was a significant source of distress.[148] The focus with men undergoing radiotherapy is on the subsequent ability to have an erection, but this is not the only significant aspect of sexuality. As Burke suggests, many individuals 'may find it difficult to separate the pleasurable, from the reproductive aspects of sexual intercourse; consequently, once the reproductive function has gone, the reason for having intercourse has disappeared as well'.[154]

Gonadal shielding is available, and moving the ovaries outside the radiation field is sometimes possible. Sperm banking is often not considered prior to radiotherapy, as it has demonstrated little value to viable fertility. Many patients have reduced sperm counts before receiving therapy, but research is limited and for some individuals the opportunity to discuss the options is important and should not be dismissed.

Diminished interest in sex

In many studies, one of the most frequent reasons cited for reduction in sexual activity is loss of desire or interest in sex. Loss of libido may have physical causes, such as a reduction in the production of sexual hormones following ablative doses of radiotherapy, or adjuvant hormone treatment. Siebel and Graves, however, have found that loss of libido was not directly associated with the biological and physical changes resulting from radiotherapy.[140] In women, body image changes and worries concerning early menopause may add to the anxiety and distress, resulting in decreased libido. Sexual interest has been found to be at its lowest at completion of treatment, which suggests that it is a side-effect of treatment.[145] Symptoms such as fatigue, diarrhoea, dysuria, cystitis, nocturia, and rectal bleeding contribute to a decrease in desire for sexual intimacy. Concerns after treatment can vary greatly. Some people are fearful that they may spread the cancer or radiation through intercourse.

Fears and responses

It is often difficult to separate fears from the physical symptoms. Anderson reported that 60% of patients studied reported sexual dysfunction prior to a cancer diagnosis.[143] A combination of physical effects of disease and anxiety were found to lead to a decline in sexual activity. Fear of the disease still being present and of it being caused by sexual intercourse are common beliefs. Women with cervical cancer may see a link between sexual activity and the cancer, viewing the disease as a punishment.[155] Radiotherapy is sometimes perceived as not curative and used as a last resort. Anderson found that 17% of patients gave fear of recurrence as a reason for decline in sexual activity, believing cancer to be still in the body and that it would spread or damage their partner.[143] For example, a patient with bladder cancer undergoing pelvic radiotherapy believed that the epithelial debris he saw in his urine was the cancer seeding. He refrained from sex as he believed that these cancer cells would infect his partner and subsequently put her at risk of cancer. Understanding of how radiation affects such private and personal matters is often left unexplored by clinicians, and these fears may contribute to sexual dysfunction. Sexual issues may cause strain to marriage and personal relationships.

Management

Sexual dysfunction following radiotherapy is clearly a multifaceted problem, with both physical changes and psychological components influencing desire and function. There are many misconceptions in radiotherapy centres about the problem, and doubt about whether management of physical sexual dysfunction is appropriate or part of active symptom management. Information is often lacking about potential sexual problems, and this area is rarely monitored. Information about sexual issues in radiotherapy is neglected. In one study, only 30% of patients were given any information about potential sexual problems.[156] When asked whether they would have liked information, 40% of informants indicated that they would. Why is it then that clinicians are reluctant to address this issue? Possibly it is because it is presumed that older women will be offended, or assumptions are made that sex is no longer of interest to older women, particularly if they do not have a partner. Studies, however, have shown that a majority of older people may be sexually active.[157]

Lack of adequate information regarding sexual issues may also relate in part to the fact that information is often given prior to the start of treatment when worries and concerns surround side-effects and anxieties are about coping with the radiotherapy. Sexual issues may not be a concern until after therapy, when professional support is limited. In an interview study of men who were having or had had pelvic radiotherapy for prostate or bladder cancer, sexual concerns such as lack of libido or impotence were often ranked as a lower priority than urinary problems during and immediately after treatment. At 6 months post-treatment, however, loss of interest in sex was third in priority.[101] Sexual functioning and desire for sex may not be seen as important, when other side-effects are at their peak. Not uncommonly, the question of fertility or sexual function arises after side-effects of treatment have diminished. All too often, no pre-treatment counselling is offered and loss of fertility or potency comes as a bitter disappointment. The difficulty also arises when action has been delayed, fibrosis or strictures have developed, and intervention is often too late. The focus of health professionals is often on provision of information, but practical strategies as well as psychological insight need to be considered as integral to any intervention.

One of the most effective ways of preventing vaginal stenosis and adhesions is to use a vaginal dilator and douche as part of sexual rehabilitation after gynaecological radiotherapy.[158] Dilators need to be used over a long time period unless the patient has regular sexual intercourse,[142] although their use can be difficult and painful. The use of lubrication for a dry vagina reduces irritation and pain.

Decreased vaginal elasticity and scarring may make particular sexual positions uncomfortable, so suggesting different positions may help to increase comfort and satisfaction. For men, careful assessment of the cause of erectile dysfunction may help in providing solutions to the cause of diminished sexual potency; Doppler ultrasound studies can show whether the cause of erectile dysfunction is due to arterial changes. Penile implants, drug therapy, pumps, or prostheses may be used if dysfunction is permanent.[137]

Many individuals find discussing sexual issues embarrassing, although the opportunity to discuss sexual issues is reported to be helpful.[156] Women who are well informed during gynaecological treatment have been found to be more motivated towards recovery.[159] Although practical suggestions for women and men are available, it is clear that nurses and clinicians find difficulty with discussing sexual issues and that this impedes sexual rehabilitation. Counselling patients and partners has been shown to have beneficial effects. A crisis counselling service and intervention programme for women with genital malignancies has been demonstrated to be extremely effective in promoting sexual functioning when counselling was initiated shortly after diagnosis.[142]

Support following radiotherapy is important; however, sexual problems for many are all too frequently ignored. Providing information about potential sexual problems that may be experienced during and after radiotherapy legitimises this as an area of care that it is possible to discuss. Assessment and appropriate referral for sexual counselling is an essential element of the role of the nurse in the radiotherapy department.

Mucositis and radiation therapy

Mucositis resulting from radiation to the head and neck area is considered an inevitable consequence of radiation cancer treatment.[160] Terms such as stomatitis and mucositis are often used interchangeably; both mean mucosal damage in the oropharyngeal cavity. The degree of mucositis depends on many factors, such as the extent and dosage of radiotherapy treatment, and also the individual's pretreatment health, age, general oral hygiene, and smoking behaviour.[161] Although it is a symptom that occurs during radiation treatment and heals rapidly after therapy is finished, it can be distressing and is often identified by radiotherapy nurses as being difficult to manage. Mucositis is exacerbated by changes in saliva and taste, and affects eating and nutrition. Mucositis causes pain and sometimes sensations of coughing and choking, which can be frightening.

Physiological changes

Changes in the mucosal membranes occur early in radiotherapy treatment, as fast-growing cells such as those in the mouth are vulnerable to damage. They tend to appear in the beginning of the second week of treatment and persist for 2–3 weeks after completion of radiotherapy.[162] The homeostatic balance between new and old cells is lost. As cells are lost they are not replaced, causing denudation of the mucosal layers, with epithelial and vascular changes.[163] The direct damage caused by radiotherapy may also exacerbate infection or previous mouth problems.[164]

Different areas of the oral cavity are more sensitive than others to radiation treatment, and therefore the distribution of radiation side-effects may occur only in specific areas. The pharyngeal walls, tonsils, and buccal membranes are most vulnerable. The extent of mucosal reaction depends on several factors: those related to the treatment and those that relate to the patient's pre-existing problems. Acute radiation mucositis, including soreness and epithelial changes, often quickly recovers once therapy is finished. Longer-term effects such as saliva changes and dental problems or radionecrosis may never heal.[165] Although these longer-term problems occur in less than 5% of patients, radiotherapy to the head or neck carries a small risk of side-effects persisting long after treatment has finished.[162]

The extent of mucosal reactions depends on:

* radiation regimen
* dose
* fractionation
* area and volume
* anatomic location.

How treatment is delivered has important implications for how quickly side-effects are manifested. The shorter the time between doses the greater the severity of the reactions. For example, in hyperfractionated schedules, individuals develop mucositis that is severe, and often require a planned break in therapy to allow for some recovery before continuing treatment. Although treatment factors determine the extent of radiation mucositis, indirect factors such as the general health of the individual impact on the healing and treatment of mucositis.

Individual factors that increase vulnerability to mucositis include:

* age
* oral hygiene
* smoking/alcohol
* poor dental hygiene
* traumatising agents, i.e. dentures
* large amalgam fillings
* chemotherapy
* fungal infections.

Constant use of the mouth through talking, breathing, eating, and drinking makes any changes more noticeable. Distinct changes in taste and saliva flow are noticed within a few weeks of starting therapy.[166,167]

Mucositis begins with changes in feeling in the mouth. These may be subtle changes in saliva flow or consistency. As radiobiological damage occurs, more visible changes are seen with a whitish discoloration in areas of the mucosal membrane. Mild erythema occurs with epithelial cells diminishing, as well as inflammatory changes due to cell damage.[168] This causes redness and pain when eating or cleaning the mouth.

Erythema is less obvious with a reddish appearance; red patches occur with small white patches, sometimes in conjunction with ulceration. Often a fibrous exudate covers areas of mucositis, and ulcers underneath cause pain and bleeding. The first signs occur frequently in the second week of radiotherapy, but this may be more rapid in hyperfractionated treatment regimes. Patients complain of pain, burning and discomfort in the mouth, which is exacerbated by swallowing, eating, and breathing. Thickening of saliva is also a consequence of treatment as a result of damage to the salivary glands. Saliva helps in moistening the mouth, digesting food, and preventing infection. Loss of saliva (xerostomia) is one of the key problems and exacerbates other symptoms.[128]

The distress of mucositis is sometimes underestimated. Changes in saliva, taste, and soreness and pain have an important effect on quality of life. The focus of studies is often on healing and agents used in dealing with mucosal ulceration; however, it can be the additional symptoms that are particularly hard for people to deal with.[168] Wells,[128] in a study of how patients felt while undergoing head and neck radiotherapy, describes the trauma that these additional symptoms can cause:

> One lady having head and neck radiotherapy found that her saliva had changed during treatment: she was coughing up copious nasty tasting and sticky saliva: 'If I had known that something like that was going to happen I would have been prepared for it . . . I mean I could fill a carrier bag with this stuff in the night . . . when I was going on the tube . . . I used to get quite err, agitated, because you know this coughing used to sound so dreadful.

Wells found that these enduring unpleasant symptoms were a vicious circle for patients.[128] She describes the effects that radiation symptoms have on the people she interviewed:

> Mucositis changes affected one man's throat early in the radiotherapy. He wrote in his diary, 'Woke up at 4 am and had a fit of coughing, made my throat bleed' [day 3].

Others describe having a 'choked up feeling' that affected sleep. One man at interview described 'the biggest trouble was at night I couldn't sleep because of my throat'. Taste changes were also a distressing symptom. One man said:

> everything bland like mashed potato . . . you cannot describe what it's like losing your taste, that was the worse thing . . . you don't feel like eating and that makes you worse because you are not getting enough nourishment so you get tired, it's a sort of vicious circle . . .

Taste changes not only affect appetite but reduce the pleasure of eating and can result in a poor diet. One man said:

> I thought I was going to fade away, that's the only thing that worried me, I would have hated it for people to say to me, you do look ill, you're losing weight.

The combination of symptoms can result in feeling depressed and in social isolation. Thus patients undergoing head and neck irradiation need considerable support to cope with oral symptoms.

The management of radiation-induced mucositis

Oral care has been well addressed in the literature but knowledge about this radiation side-effect is still limited. It is difficult to manage, and healing will not occur while an individual is having radiotherapy treatment. Often the issues are different from mucositis due to chemotherapy. The aims are primarily to provide support, to give symptomatic relief, and to prevent secondary infection.

Much of the focus of research has been on which agents or chemicals are best used to rinse the mouth and provide oral care. However, it is often routine assessment and simple preventive strategies that are most effective in mediating patient symptoms. There are no clear answers in the research literature but it would appear that the distress from symptoms can be reduced by providing information, early assessment and support to help patients with pain, and saliva, and nutrition, and taste changes (see Box 13.2).[169]

Radiation mucositis cannot be avoided but its impact can be reduced and prevented by assessment of the oral cavity prior to treatment and

---

Box 13.2   Helpful and unhelpful strategies for managing decreased saliva[170]

Unhelpful strategies
- Smoking
- Alcohol
- Spicy foods
- Very hot or cold foods
- Citrus juices
- Commercial mouthwashes
- Coarse or hard foods

Helpful strategies
- Keeping your mouth clean after eating
- Taking frequent sips of water
- Use synthetic saliva when mouth feels dry
- Sucking on hard sugarless sweets or gum
- Using a cool mist vaporiser

---

elimination of sources of infection and chronic irritation. It is important that mouth care is performed frequently and consistently, and this is now considered more important than the specific oral care agents used.[171] Many of the mouth rinses that are anti-plaque or antibacterial (such as chlorehexidine) are ineffective, as the active ingredients require saliva to be effective. It is also important to brush teeth regularly, as reduction in saliva can cause plaque and dental problems. Encouraging fluids and regular sipping of water can help in reducing the unpleasantness of reductions in saliva. Studies have shown that artificial saliva is of minimal benefit for those with acute symptoms.[172] In a cross-over randomised trial, 12 out of 17 patients thought pilocarpine was more helpful.[173] Problems with managing associated drug symptoms such as nausea and sweating have diminished the likely value of pilocarpine. Assessing an individual's associated medications can also have substantial benefits on saliva flow.[174] Managing symptoms such as pain from the mucositis with either systemic analgesics or local analgesics such as sprays (e.g. Difflam) is important. Pain also affects swallowing and reduces nutritional intake. Preventing secondary infection is essential, and studies suggest that the use of nystatin pastilles is useful in reducing the development of fungal infections.[175]

Research to date has focused on cleansing agents, timing of mouth care and protective coatings. Sucralfate shows promise as a protective coating to prevent damage; it also improves comfort and reduces pain, and early studies have shown better healing.[173] Studies exploring pain relief have found anti-inflammatory (benzydamine) and steroid preparations of benefit in reducing inflammatory changes and delaying the onset of symptoms.[173,174] New agents such as human keratinocyte growth factors are in phase II studies are being evaluated to target cell growth and reduce inflammatory effects, and have been shown to reduce the length of time that mucositis occurs in initial small-scale studies.[175] Several interventions are helpful in preventing or reducing the severity of mucositis associated with radiotherapy but these are often of variable quality and there is still a need to evaluate newer agents and approaches to oral care.[176]

It is clear that there are no easy answers to the problems of radiation-induced mucositis; like many side-effects of therapy, their intense nature can cause great distress. What is important is to provide information and education for the patient in providing oral care. Unrealistic expectations of what mouth rinses and medications can provide do not help patients to cope with these distressing symptoms. It is vital to start preventive strategies at the onset of treatment, rather than waiting for problems to occur. Symptom management should encompass not only the mucosal reactions but also the decrease and changes in saliva.

The role of supportive care: can this make a difference to radiation side-effects?

Supportive care has been a key element in the discussion of the management of the radiation side-effects in cancer care. Supportive care is defined as the provision of information, counselling, social support, and side-effect management, with the aim of reducing radiotherapy morbidity. It is clear from the literature that few studies have been conducted to contribute to the knowledge that is required to provide evidence-based radiotherapy practice, and reflect the value or benefits of different approaches. The lack of consistency across the country and internationally in radiotherapy treatment strategies is also reflected in how adverse effects of therapy are managed.[177] As cancer treatments become more complex and chemotherapy regimes are increasingly combined with radiotherapy, nurses need to have the knowledge and skills to accurately assess and intervene.

Questions as to the best and most appropriate symptom management, follow-up services and surveillance during radiotherapy treatment are not adequately studied. The interface between follow-up care, physical and psychological needs, and community services has been a neglected area. Supportive care is a Cinderella area in radiotherapy and the literature attests to this, with less than 1% reflecting quality-of-life assessments or the impact that treatment can have on the individual, but it is clear that radiotherapy treatment can have a substantial impact on the person with cancer. The evidence about whether supportive and nursing care can make a difference to the individual, not only in terms of physical symptoms but also in terms of psychological distress, is as yet not clear, but it is likely to be of considerable benefit to well-being, recovery, and the experience of symptoms associated with radiotherapy treatment.

References

1. Munro A., Biruls R., Griffin A., Thomas H. and Vallis K. (1994). Distress associated with radiotherapy for malignant disease: a quantitative anlysis based on patients perceptions. *British Journal of Cancer* **60**, 370–374.
2. Wells M. and Faithfull S. (2003). The future of supportive care in radiotherapy. In Faithfull S. and Wells M. (eds.) *Supportive Care in Radiotherapy*. Edinburgh: Churchill Livingstone, pp. 372–381.
3. Forester B.M., Kornfield D. and Fleiss J. (1985). Psychiatric aspects of radiotherapy. *American Journal of Psychiatry* **142**, 22–27.
4. Christman N. (1990). Uncertainty and adjustment during radiotherapy. *Nursing Research* **39**, 17–20.
5. King K., Nail L., Kreamer K., Strohl R. and Johnson J. (1985). Patients' descriptions of the experience of receiving radiation therapy. *Oncology Nursing Forum* **12**, 55–61.
6. Peck A. and Boland J. (1977). Emotional reactions to radiation treatment. *Cancer* **40**, 180–184.

7. Fritzsche K., Liptai C. and Henke M. (2004). Psychosocial distress and need for psychotherapeutic treatment in cancer patients undergoing radiotherapy. *Radiotherapy and Oncology* **72**, 183–189.

8. Maraste R., Brandt L., Olsson H. and Ryde-Brandt B. (1992). Anxiety and depression in breast cancer patients at start of adjuvant radiotherapy. *Acta Oncologica* **31**, 641–643.

9. Hammick M., Tutt A. and Tait D. (1998). Knowledge and perception regarding radiotherapy and radiation in patients receiving radiotherapy: a qualitative study. *European Journal of Cancer Care* **7**, 103–112.

10. Young J. and Maher E. (1992). The role of a radiographer counsellor in a large centre for cancer treatment: a discussion paper based on an audit of the work of a radiographer counsellor. *Clinical Oncology* **4**, 232–235.

11. Gordils-Perez J., Rawlins-Duell R. and Kelvin J.F. (2003). Advances in radiation treatment of patients with breast cancer. *Clinical Journal of Oncology Nursing* **7**, 629–636.

12. Rotman M., Rogow L., DeLeon G. and Heskel N. (1977). Supportive therapy in radiation oncology. *Cancer* **39**, 744–750.

13. Hall E. (1988). Time, dose and fractionation in radiotherapy. In Hall E. (ed.) *Radiobiology for the Radiologist*. Philadelphia, PA: Lippincott, pp. 239–259.

14. Adamson D. (2003). The radiobiological basis of radiation side effects. In Faithfull S. and Wells M. (eds.) *Supportive Care in Radiotherapy*. Edinburgh: Churchill Livingstone, pp. 71–95.

15. Bomford C.K., Kinkler I.H. and Sheriff S.B. (1993). *Walter and Millers Textbook of Radiotherapy: Radiation Physics, Therapy and Oncology*, 5th edition. Edinburgh: Churchill Livingstone.

16. Fieler V. (1997). Side-effects and quality of life in patients receiving high-dose rate brachytherapy. *Oncology Nursing Forum* **24**, 545–553.

17. Faithfull S. (2005). FACET Developments in radiotherapy: treatment for cancer implications for practice. *European Journal of Cancer Care* **14**, 91–100.

18. Anscher M.S., Chen L., Rabbani Z. *et al.* (2005). Recent progress in defining mechanisms and potential targets for prevention of normal tissue injury after radiation therapy. *International Journal of Radiation Oncology Biology Physics* **62**, 255–259.

19. Powell S. and McMillan T. (1990). DNA damage and repair following treatment with ionizing radiation. *Radiotherapy and Oncology* **19**, 95–108.

20. Withers R. (1992). Biological basis of radiation therapy for cancer. *Lancet* **339**, 156–159.

21. Hopewell J., Calvo W. and Reinhold H. (1989). Radiation effects on blood vessels: role in late normal tissue damage. In Steel C., Adams G. and Horwich A. (eds.) *The Biological Basis of Radiotherapy*. Amsterdam: Elsevier, pp. 101–112.

22. Burnet N., Nyman J. and Turesson I. (1992). Prediction of normal-tissue tolerance to radiotherapy from in-vitro cellular radiation sensitivity. *Lancet* **399**, 1570–1571.

23. Bentzen S., Overgaard M. and Overgaard J. (1993). Clinical correlations between late normal tissue end-points after radiotherapy: implications for predictive assays of radiosensitivity. *European Journal of Cancer* **29A**, 1373–1376.

24. Hill R., Rodemann H., Hendry J., Roberts S. and Anscher M. (2001). Normal tissue radiobiology: from the laboratory to the clinic. *International Journal of Radiation Oncology Biology Physics* **49**, 353–365.

25. Munro A. (2003). Challenges to radiotherapy today. In Faithfull S. and Wells M. (eds.) *Supportive Care in Radiotherapy*. Edinburgh: Churchill Livingstone, pp. 17–30.

26. Dische S. (1995). Clinical radiobiology. In Price P. and Sikora K. (eds.) *Treatment of Cancer*. London: Chapman and Hall.

27. Sikora K. and Bosanquet N. (2003). Cancer care in the United Kingdom: new solutions are needed. *British Medical Journal* **327**, 1044–1046.

28. Trott K. and Kummermehr J. (1985). What is known about tumour proliferation rates to choose between accelerated fractionation or hyperfractionation? *Radiotherapy and Oncology* **3**, 1–9.

29. Saunders M. and Dische S. (1990). Continuous hyperfractionated accelerated radiotherapy (CHART) in non-small-cell carcinoma of the bronchus. *International Journal of Radiation Oncology Biology Physics* **19**, 1211–1215.

30. Price P. and McMillan T. (1994). Radiotherapy in the 21st century: a look forward. In Tobias J. and Thomas P. (eds.) *Current Radiation Oncology*. London: Edward Arnold, pp. 382–400.

31. Dodd J., Barrett A. and Ash D. (1992). *Practical Radiotherapy Planning*, 2nd edition. London: Edward Arnold.

32. Webb S. (1993). *The Physics of 3-Dimensional Radiation Therapy, Conformal Radiotherapy, Radiosurgery and Treatment Planning*. Medical Science Series. London: IOP Publications.

33. Colyer H. (2003). The context of radiotherapy care. In Faithfull S. and Wells M. (eds.) *Supportive Care in Radiotherapy*. Edinburgh: Churchill Livingstone, pp. 1–16.

34. Wells M. (2003). The treatment trajectory. In Faithfull S. and Wells M. (eds.) *Supportive Care in Radiotherapy*. Edinburgh: Churchill Livingstone, pp. 372–382.

35. Eardley A. (1986). Radiotherapy. *Nursing Times* **April 16**, 24–26.
36. Ward S., Viergutz G., Tormey D., DeMuth J. and Paulen A. (1992). Patients' reactions to completion of adjuvant breast cancer therapy. *Nursing Research* **41**, 362–366.
37. Timmermans L.M., Van Der Maazen R.W.M., Leer J.M. and Kraaimaat F.W. (2006). Palliative or curative treatment intent affects communication in radiation therapy consultations. *Psycho-oncology* **15**, 713–725.
38. Eardley A. (1986). Expectations of recovery. *Nursing Times* **23 April**, 53–54.
39. Kagan A., Levitt P., Arnold T. and Hatten J. (1984). Honesty is the best policy: a radiation therapist's perspective on caring for terminal cancer patients. *Clinical Oncology* **17**, 381–383.
40. Mitchell G. and Glicksman A. (1977). Cancer patients' knowledge and attitudes. *Cancer* **40**, 61–66.
41. Jahraus D., Sokolosky S., Thurston N. and Guo D. (2002). Evaluation of an educational program for patients with breast cancer receiving radiation therapy. *Cancer Nursing* **25**, 266–275.
42. Holland J. and Tross S. (1989). Psychological sequelae in cancer survivors. In Holland J. and Rowland J. (eds.) *Handbook of Psychooncology*. Oxford: Oxford University Press.
43. Porock D. (1995). The effect of preparatory patient education on the anxiety and satisfaction of cancer patients receiving radiotherapy. *Cancer Nursing* **18**, 206–214.
44. Strohl R. (1988). The nursing role in radiation oncology symptom management of acute and chronic reactions. *Oncology Nursing Forum* **15**, 429–434.
45. Kim Y., Rosecoe J.A. and Morrow G.R. (2002). The effects of information and negative affect on severity of side-effects from radiation therapy for prostate cancer. *Supportive Care in Cancer* **10**, 416–421.
46. Fitch M.I., Gray R.E., McGowan T. *et al.* (2003). Travelling for radiation cancer treatment: patient perspectives. *Psycho-oncology* **12**, 664–674.
47. Anderson B. and Tewfik H. (1985). Psychological reactions to radiation therapy: reconsideration of the adaptive aspects of anxiety. *Journal of Personality and Social Psychology* **48**, 1024–1032.
48. Holland J., Rowland A., Lebovitz A. and Rusalem R. (1979). Reactions to cancer treatment: assessment of emotional response to adjuvant radiotherapy as a guide to planned intervention. *Psychiatric Clinics of North America* **2**, 347–358.
49. Graydon J. (1988). Factors that predict patients' functioning following treatment for cancer. *International Journal of Nursing Studies* **25**, 117–124.
50. Eardley A. (1986). After the treatment's over. *Nursing Times* **April 30**, 40–41.
51. Stone H.B., Coleman C.N., Anscher M.S. and McBride W.H. (2003). Effects of radiation on normal tissue: consequence and mechanisms. *The Lancet Oncology* **4**, 529–536.
52. Stone H.B., Coleman C.N., Ansher M.S. and McBride W.H. (2003). Effects of radiation on normal tissue: consequences and mechanisms. *The Lancet Oncology* **4**, 529–536.
53. Khoo V. (2003). Other late effects. In Faithfull S. and Wells M. (eds.) *Supportive Care in Radiotherapy*. Edinburgh: Churchill Livingstone, pp. 348–371.
54. Maher E. (2000). Late radiation damage-whose point of view? *Radiotherapy and Oncology* **57**, S1–S2.
55. Truong P.T., Berthelet E., Lee J.C. *et al.* (2006). Prospective evaluation of the prevalence and severity of fatigue in patients with prostate cancer undergoing radical external beam radiotherapy and neoadjuvant hormone therapy. *Canadian Journal of Urology* **13**, 3139–3146.
56. Barsevick A., Dudley M., Beck S. *et al.* (2004). A randomized clinical trial of energy conservation for cancer-related fatigue. *Cancer* **100**, 1302–1310.
57. Dauz Williams P., Ducey K.A., Sears A.M. *et al.* (2001). Treatment type and symptom severity among oncology patients by self-report. *International Journal of Nursing Studies* **28**, 359–367.
58. Barsevick A.M., Dudley W.N. and Beck S.L. (2006). Cancer-related fatigue, depressive symptoms, and functional status. *Nursing Research* **55**, 366–372.
59. Dagneleie P., Pijls-Johannesma M., Lambin P. *et al.* (2007). Impact of fatigue on overall quality of life in lung and breast cancer patients selected for high-dose radiotherapy. *Annals of Oncology* **18**, 940–944.
60. Faithfull S. (2003). Fatigue and radiotherapy. In Faithfull S. and Wells M. (eds.) *Supportive Care in Radiotherapy*. Edinburgh: Churchill Livingstone, pp. 118–134.
61. Wells M. (2003). Pain and breathing problems. In Faithfull S. and Wells M. (eds.) *Supportive Care in Radiotherapy*. Edinburgh: Churchill Livingstone, pp. 160–181.
62. Haylock P. and Hart L. (1979). Fatigue in patients receiving localised radiation. *Cancer Nursing* **2**, 461–467.
63. Greenberg D., Sawicka J., Eisenthal S. And Ross D. (1992). Fatigue syndrome due to localised radiotherapy. *Journal of Pain and Symptom Management* **7**, 38–45.
64. Piper B. and Dodd M. (1991). Self-initiated fatigue interventions and their perceived effectiveness. *Oncology Nursing Forum* **18**, 39.

65. Nail L. (1993). Coping with intracavity radiation treatment for gynaecological cancer. *Cancer Practice* **1**, 218–224.

66. Faithfull S. (1991). Patients' experiences following cranial radiotherapy: a study of the somnolence syndrome. *Journal of Advanced Nursing* **16**, 939–946.

67. Faithfull S. and Brada M. (1998). Somnolence syndrome in adults following cranial irradiation for primary brain tumours. *Clinical Oncology* **10**, 250–254.

68. Goldstein D., Bennett B., Friedlander M. *et al.* (2006). Fatigue states after cancer treatment occur both in association with, and independent of, mood disorder: a longitudinal study. *Biomedical Chromatography* **9**, 240–243.

69. Fobair P., Hoppe R., Bloom J. *et al.* (1986). Psychosocial problems among survivors of Hodgkin's disease. *Journal of Clinical Oncology* **14**, 908–914.

70. Kobashi-Schoot J. (1985). Assessment of malaise in cancer patients treated with radiotherapy. *Cancer Nursing* **8**, 306–313.

71. Miaskowski C., Dodd M. and Lee K. (2004). Symptom clusters: the new frontier in symptom management research. *Journal of the National Cancer Institute Monographs* **32**, 139–143.

72. Oberst M., Hughes S., Chang A. and McCubbin M. (1991). Self-care burden, stress appraisal and mood among persons receiving radiotherapy. *Cancer Nursing* **14**, 71–78.

73. Richardson A. and Ream E. (1998). Recent progress in understanding cancer-related fatigue. *International Journal of Palliative Nursing* **4**, 192–198.

74. Richardson A. (1995). Fatigue in cancer patients: a review of the literature. *European Journal of Cancer Care* **4**, 20–32.

75. Winningham M. (1991). Walking program for people with cancer: getting strated. *Cancer Nursing* **14**, 270–276.

76. Pearce S. and Richardson A. (1994). Fatigue and cancer: a phenomenological study. *Journal of Cancer Nursing* **3**, 381–382.

77. Richardson A. and Ream E. (1997). Self-care behaviours initiated by chemotherapy patients in response to fatigue. *International Journal of Nursing Studies* **34**, 35–43.

78. Graydon J., Bubela N., Irvine D. and Vincent L. (1995). Fatigue-reducing strategies used by patients receiving treatment for cancer. *Cancer Nursing* **18**, 23–28.

79. Mock V. (2003). Clinical excellence through evidence-based practice: fatigue as a model. *Oncology Nursing Forum* **30**, 790–795.

80. Miaskowski C. and Lee K. (1999). Pain, fatigue and sleep disturbances in oncology outpatients receiving radiation therapy for bone metastasis: a pilot study. *Journal of Pain and Symptom Management* **17**, 320–332.

81. Winningham ML., Nail L., Barton Burke M. *et al.* (1994). Fatigue and the cancer experience: the state of the knowledge. *Oncology Nursing Forum* **21**, 23–36.

82. Mitchell S.A., Beck S.L., Hood L.E., Moore K. and Tanner E.R. (2007). Putting evidence into practice: evidence based interventions for fatigue during and following cancer and its treatment. *Clinical Journal of Oncology Nursing* **11**, 99–113.

83. Churnratanakul S., Wirzba B., Lam T. *et al.* (1990). Radiation and the small intestine: future perspectives for preventive therapy. *Digestive Disease* **8**, 45–60.

84. Gami B., Harrington K., Blake P. *et al.* (2003) How patients manage gastrointestinal symptoms after pelvic radiotherapy. *Alimentary Pharmacology and Therapeutics* **18**, 987–994.

85. Flickinger J., Bloomer W. and Kinsella J. (1990). Intestinal intolerance of radiation injury. In Galland R. and Spencer J. (eds.) *Radiation Enteritis*. London: Edward Arnold, pp. 51–65.

86. Yeoh E. and Horowitz M. (1988). Radiation enteritis. *British Journal of Hospital Medicine* **June**, 498–504.

87. Kinsella T. and Bloomer W. (1980). Bowel tolerance to radiation therapy. *Surgery Gynecology and Obstetrics* **151**, 273–284.

88. Danielsson A., Nyhlin H., Stendahl R., Stenling U. and Suhr O. (1991). Chronic diarrhoea after radiotherapy for gynaecological cancer: occurrence and aetiology. *Gut* **32**, 1180–1187.

89. Yeoh E., Lui D., and Lee N. (1984). The mechanism of diarrhoea resulting from pelvic and abdominal radiotherapy: a prospective study using selenium-75 labelled conjugated bile acid and cobalt-58 labelled cyanocobalamin. *British Journal of Radiology* **57**, 1131–1136.

90. Newman A. (1974). Breath – analysis tests in gastroenterology. *Gut* **15**, 308–323.

91. Stryker J., Hepner G. and Mortel R. (1977). The effect of pelvic irradiation on ileal function. *Radiology* **124**, 213–216.

92. Gray G. (1975). Carbohydrate digestion and absorption: role of the small intestine. *New England Journal of Medicine* **292**, 1225–1230.

93. Mennie A., Dalley V., Dinneen L. And Collier H. (1975). Treatment of radiation induced gastrointestinal distress with acetylsalicylate. *Lancet* **ii**, 942–943.

94. Martenson J., Hyland G., Moertl C. *et al.* (1996). Olsalazine is contraindicated during pelvic radiation therapy: results of a double blind, randomized clinical trial. *International Journal of Radiation Oncology Biology Physics* **35**, 299–303.

95. Keefe D.M., Gibson R.J. and Hauer-Jensen M. (2004). Gastrointestinal mucositis. *Seminars in Oncology and Nursing* **20**, 38–47.

96. Potish R., Jones T. and Levitt S. (1979). Factors predisposing to radiation-related small bowel damage. *Oncology* **132**, 479–482.

97. Perez C., Lee H., Georgia A. and Lockett M. (1994). Technical factors affecting morbidity in definitive irradiation for localized carcinoma of the prostate. *International Journal of Radiation Oncology Biology Physics* **4**, 811–819.

98. Levi S. and Hodgson H. (1990). Prevention of radiation enteritis. In Galland R. and Spencer J. (eds.) *Radiation Enteritis*. London: Edward Arnold, pp. 121–135.

99. Green N., Iba G. and Smith W. (1975). Measures to minimize small intestine injury in the irradiated pelvis. *Cancer* **35**, 1633–1640.

100. Padilla G. (1990). Gastrointestinal side-effects and quality of life in patients receiving radiation therapy. *Nutrition* **6**, 367–370.

101. Faithfull S. (1995). 'Just grin and bear it and hope that it will go away': coping with urinary symptoms from pelvic radiotherapy. *European Journal of Cancer Care* **4**, 58–165.

102. Faithfull S. (2000). *Supportive Care in Radiotherapy: evaluating the potential contribution of nursing*. PhD thesis, Institute of Cancer Research, London University, p. 294.

103. Hassey K. (1987). Radiation therapy for rectal cancer and the implications for nursing. *Cancer Nursing* **10**, 311–318.

104. Bosaeus I., Andersson H. and Nystrom C. (1979). Effect of low fat diet on bile salt excretion and diarrhoea in the gastrointestinal radiation syndrome. *Acta Radiologica Oncologica* **18**, 460–464.

105. Stryker J., Chung C. and Layser J. (1983). Colestipol hydrochloride prophlaxis of diarrhea during pelvic radiotherapy. *International Journal of Radiation Oncology Biology Physics* **9**, 185–190.

106. Chary S. and Thomson D. (1984). A clinical trial evaluating cholestyramine to prevent diarrhoea in patients maintained on low fat diets during pelvic radiation therapy. *International Journal of Radiation Oncology Biology Physics* **10**, 1885–1890.

107. Henriksson R., Franzen L., Sandstrom K. *et al.* (1995). Effects of active addition of bacterial cultures in fermented milk to patients with chronic bowel discomfort following irradiation. *Supportive Care in Cancer* **3**, 81–83.

108. Tarnawski A. (1984). Sucralfate: is it more than just a barrier. *Current Concepts in Gastroenterology* **June/July**, 5–12.

109. Henriksson R., Franzen L. and Littbrand B. (1992). Effects of sucralfate on acute and late bowel discomfort following radiotherapy of pelvic cancer. *Journal of Clinical Oncology* **10**, 969–975.

110. Northway M., Scobey M. and Geisinger K. (1988). Radiation proctitis in the rat: sequential changes and effects of anti-inflammatory agents. *Cancer* **162**, 1962–1969.

111. McGough C., Bladwin C., Frost G. and Andreyev H. (2004). Role of nutritional intervention in patients treated with radiotherapy for pelvic malignancy. *British Journal of Cancer* **90**, 2278–2287.

112. Dini D., Macchia R., Gozza A. *et al.* (1993). Management of acute radiodermatitis. *Cancer Nursing* **16**, 336–370.

113. Barkham A. (1993). Radiotherapy skin reactions and treatments. *Professional Nurse* **8**, 732–736.

114. Wells M. and Macbride S. (2003). Radiation skin reactions. In Faithfull S. and Wells M. (eds.) *Supportive Care in Radiotherapy*. Edinburgh: Churchill Livingstone, pp. 135–159.

115. Thomas S. (1992). *Current Practices in the Management of Fungating Lesions and Radiation Damaged Skin*. Bridgend Hospital: The Surgical Materials Testing Laboratory.

116. Lavery B. (1995). Skin care during radiotherapy: a survey of UK practice. *Clinical Oncology* **7**, 184–187.

117. Hilderley L. (1983). Skin care in radiation therapy: a review of the literature. *Oncology Nursing Forum* **10**, 144–162.

118. Sitton E. (1992). Early and late radiation-induced skin alterations: Part 1 Mechanisms of skin changes. *Oncology Nursing Forum* **19**, 801–807.

119. Hopewell J. (1990). The skin: its structure and response to ionizing radiation. *International Journal of Radiation Oncology Biology Physics* **57**, 751–773.

120. Dunne-Daly C. (1995). Skin and wound care in radiation oncology. *Cancer Nursing* **18**, 144–162.

121. Wells M., Macmillan M., Raab G. *et al.* (2004). Does aqueous or sucralfate cream affect the severity of erythematous radiation skin reactions? A randomised controlled trial. *Radiotherapy and Oncology* **73**, 53–162.

122. Porock D. and Kristjanson L. (1999). Skin reactions during radiotherapy for breast cancer: the use and impact of topical agents and dressings. *European Journal of Cancer Care* **8**, 143–153.

123. Porock D., Nikoletti S. and Cameron F. (2004). The relationship between factors that impair wound healing and the severity of acute radiation skin and mucosal toxicities in head and neck cancer. *Cancer Nursing* **27**, 71–78.

124. Turesson I. and Thames H. (1989). Repair capacity and kinetics of human skin during fractionated

radiotherapy: erythema, desquamation and telangiectasia after 3 and 5 years follow up. *Radiotherapy and Oncology* **15**, 169–188.

125. Neal A., Torr M., Helyer S. and Yarnold J. (1995). Correlation of breast dose inhomogeneity with breast size using three dimensional CT planning and dose volume histograms. *Radiotherapy and Oncology* **34**, 210–218.

126. Moody J.F. (1993). Radiation damaged skin: which treatment option and why? *Wound Management* **4(suppl.)**, 86–87.

127. Lawton J. and Twoomey M. (1991). Skin reactions to radiotherapy. *Nursing Standard* **6**, 53–54.

128. Wells M. (1995). *The Impact of Radiotherapy to the Head and Neck: a qualitative study of patients after completion of treatment*. MSc thesis, Institute of Cancer Research, Centre for Cancer and Palliative Care Studies, London, pp. 1–76.

129. Wengstrom Y., Forsberg C., Naslund I. and Bergh J. (2004). Quantitative assessment of skin erythema due to radiotherapy – evaluation of different measurements. *Radiotherapy and Oncology* **72**, 191–197.

130. Roy I., Fortin A. and Larochelle M. (2001). The impact of skin washing with water and soap during breast irradiation: a randomized study. *Radiotherapy and Oncology* **58**, 333–339.

131. Campbell I. and Illingworth M. (1992). Can patients wash during radiotherapy to the breast or chest wall? A randomized controlled trial. *Clinical Oncology* **4**, 78–82.

132. Bostrom A., Lindman H., Swartling C., Berne B. and Bergh J. (2001). Potent corticosteroid cream (mometasone furoate) significantly reduces acute radiation dermatitis: results from a double blind, randomized study. *Radiotherapy and Oncology* **59**, 257–265.

133. Pommier P., Gomez F., Sunyach M.P. *et al.* (2004). Phase III randomized trial of *Calendula officinalis* compared with Trolamine for the prevention of acute dermatitis during irradiation for breast cancer. *Journal of Clinical Oncology* **22**, 1447–1453.

134. Morgan D. (1993). Is there a role for antiseptics? *Journal of Tissue Viability* **3**, 80–84.

135. Crane J. (1993). Extending the role of a new hydrogel. *Journal of Tissue Viability* **3**, 98–99.

136. McQuestion M. (2006). Evidence-based skin care management in radiation therapy. *Seminars in Oncology Nursing* **22**, 163–173.

137. White I. and Faithfull S. (2003). Sexuality and fertility. In Faithfull S. and Wells M. (eds.) *Supportive Care in Radiotherapy*. Edinburgh: Churchill Livingstone, pp. 303–319.

138. Decker W. and Schwartzman C. (1962). Sexual functioning following treatment for carcinoma of the cervix. *American Journal of Obstetrics and Gynecology* **83**, 83.

139. Abbitol M. and Davenport J. (1974). The irradiated vagina. *Obstetrics and Gynecology* **44**, 249–256.

140. Siebel M. and Graves W. (1982). Sexual function after surgery and radiotherapy for cervical carcinoma. *The Southern Medical Journal* **75**, 11–15.

141. Hubbard J. and Singleton H. (1985). Sexual function of patients after carcinoma of the cervix treatment. *Clinics in Obstetrics and Gynaecology* **12**, 247–264.

142. Cartwright-Alcarese F. (1995). Addressing sexual dysfunction following radiation therapy for a gynaecologic malignancy. *Oncology Nursing Forum* **22**, 1227–1231.

143. Anderson B. (1987). Sexual function in women with gynaecological cancer. *Cancer* **60**, 317–323.

144. Lamb M. (1985). Sexual dysfunction in gynaecological oncology patients. *Seminars in Oncology Nursing* **1**, 9–17.

145. Flay L. and Matthews J.H. (1995). The effects of radiotherapy and surgery on the sexual function of women treated for cervical cancer. *International Journal of Radiation Oncology Biology Physics* **31**, 399–404.

146. Dembo A. and Thomas G. (1994). The ovary. In Cox J.D. (ed.) *Moss' Radiation Oncology*. St Louis, MO: Mosby, pp. 712–733.

147. Perez C., Fair W. and Ihde D. (1989). Carcinoma of the prostate. In DeVita V., Hellman S. and Rosenberg S. (eds.) *Cancer Principles and Practice of Oncology*. Boston: Jones & Bartlett, pp. 1023–1058.

148. Schover L. (1987). Sexuality and fertility in urologic cancer patients. *Cancer* **60**, 553–558.

149. Goldstein I., Feldman M., Deckers P., Babayan R. and Krane R. (1984). Radiation associated impotence: a clinical study of its mechanism. *Journal of the American Medical Association* **251**, 903–910.

150. Auchincloss S. (1989). Sexual dysfunction in cancer patients: issues in evaluation and treatment. In Holland J.C. and Rowland J.H. (eds.) *Handbook of Psychooncology: the Psychological Care of the Patient with Cancer*. New York: Oxford University Press.

151. Andelusi B. (1980). Coital function after radiotherapy for carcinoma of the cervix uteri. *British Journal of Obstetrics and Gynaecology* **87**, 821–823.

152. Schuster E., Unsain A. and Goodwin M. (1982). Nursing practice in human sexuality. *Nursing Clinics of North America* **17**, 345–349.

153. Shell J. (1990). Sexuality for patients with gynaecologic cancer. *Clinical Issues in Perinatal and Women's Health Nursing* **1**, 479–514.

154. Burke L. (1996). Sexual dysfunction following radiotherapy for cervical cancer. *British Journal of Nursing* **5**, 239–244.

155. Glasgow M., Haltin V. and Althausen A. (1986). *Sexual Response and Cancer*. New York: American Cancer Society.

156. Jenkins B. (1988). Patients' reports of sexual changes after treatment for gynaecological cancer. *Oncology Nursing Forum* **15**, 349–354.

157. Starr B. and Weiner M. (1981) The Starr–Weiner report on sex and sexuality in the mature years. New York: McGraw Hill.

158. Bransfield D., Herriot J. and Abbitol A. (1984). A medical chart for information about sexual functioning in cervical cancer. *Radiotherapy and Oncology* **1**, 317–323.

159. McMullin M. (1992). Holistic care of the patient with cervical cancer. *Nursing Clinics of North America* **27**, 847–858.

160. Wells M. (2003). Oropharyngeal effects of radiotherapy. In Faithfull S. and Wells M. (eds.) *Supportive Care in Radiotherapy*. Edinburgh: Churchill Livingstone, pp. 182–203.

161. Porock D., Nikoletti S. and Cameron F. (2004). The relationship between factors that impair wound healing and the severity of acute radiation skin mucosal toxicities in head and neck cancer. *Cancer Nursing* **27**, 7178.

162. Dreizen S. (1990). Description and incidence of oral complications. *NCI Monographs* **9**, 11–15.

163. Maciejewski B., Zajusz A., Pilecki B. *et al.* (1991). Acute mucositis in the stimulated oral mucosa of patients during radiotherapy for head and neck cancer. *Radiotherapy and Oncology* **22**, 7–11.

164. Squier C. (1990). Mucosal alterations. *NCI Monographs* **9**, 169–172.

165. Calman F. and Langdon J. (1991). Oral complications of cancer: preventative treatment is vital and many specialities are required. *British Medical Journal* **302**, 485–486.

166. Greenspan D. (1990). Management of salivary dysfunction. *NCI Monographs* **9**, 159–161.

167. Sonis S.T., Elting L.S., Keefe D. *et al.* (2004). Perspectives on cancer therapy-induced mucosal injury: pathogenesis, measurement, epidemiology and consequences for patients. *Cancer* **100(suppl.)**, 1995–2025.

168. Martin M. (1993). Irradiation mucositis: a reappraisal. Oral oncology. *European Journal of Cancer* **1 29**, 1–2.

169. Macmillan Practice Development Unit. (1995). *Managing Oral Care Problems throughout the Cancer Illness Trajectory*. London: Cancer Relief Macmillan Fund, The Institute of Cancer Research, The Royal Marsden NHS Trust.

170. Trinque J. and Meers K. (1992). Oral care of patients receiving radiation therapy to head and neck: practice corner. *Oncology Nursing Forum* **19**, 940–941.

171. Rubenstein E., Peterson D., Schubert M. *et al.* (2004). Clinical practice guidelines for the prevention and treatment of cancer therapy-induced oral and gastrointestinal mucositis. *Cancer* **100(suppl.)**, 2026–2046.

172. Davies A. and Singer J. (1994). A comparison of artificial saliva and pilocarpine in radiation induced xerostomia. *Journal of Laryngology and Oncology* **108**, 663–665.

173. Leslie M. and Glaser M. (1993). Impaired salivary gland function after radiotherapy compounded by commonly prescibed medications. *Clinical Oncology* **5**, 290–292.

174. McIlroy P. (1996). Radiation mucositis: a new approach to prevention and treatment. *European Journal of Cancer Care* **5**, 153–158.

175. Rubenstein E.B., Peterson D.E., Schubert M. *et al.* (2004). Clinical practice guidelines for the prevention and treatment of cancer therapy-induced oral and gastrointestinal mucositis. *Cancer* **100(suppl.)**, 2026–2046

176. Clarkson J.E., Worthington H.V. and Eden O.B. (2003). Interventions for preventing oral mucositis for patients with cancer receiving treatment. (Cochrane Review). *The Cochrane Library*, Issue 4. Oxford: Update Software.

177. Burnet N., Benson R. and Williams M. (2000). Improving cancer outcomes through radiotherapy. *British Medical Journal* **320**, 198–199.

CHAPTER FOURTEEN

Endocrine therapies

Deborah Fenlon

Introduction

The development of some cancers, notably breast and prostate cancers, is influenced by the normal body hormones. Changing the levels of these hormones can help in the treatment of the cancer. This manipulation of the hormones is known as endocrine therapy. Although endocrine therapy is not considered to be a primary, curative therapy it is frequently used for both adjuvant and neo-adjuvant treatment in the primary setting and for the control of metastatic disease. In recent years there has been a rapidly increasing understanding of the biology of cancer and the role of hormones in stimulating cancer growth. These advances are constantly leading to new treatments and may ultimately help to prevent some cancers.

While many of the drugs used for hormonal manipulation have few side-effects and are well tolerated, they are not without consequences that need to be considered when offering these treatments. In the past it has been shown that side-effects are under-reported by physicians,[1] so there is a risk that people may not be adequately prepared for the side-effects of endocrine therapies. The experience of endocrine therapy will depend on the context in which it takes place. For some, hormone treatment has little or no impact on life; others will achieve remission from their disease and so find that their quality of life is greatly improved. Others will find that the benefit they gain from treatment of the disease is countered by significant side-effects that are of such magnitude that treatment may be considered unacceptable.

Hormones are most commonly associated with sex hormones and with gender. An individual's identity is inextricably linked to being male or female, and sex hormones confer physiological femininity or masculinity on individuals. Within a culture that values and rewards attributes associated with gender, anxiety that one's femininity or masculinity may be altered as a result of treatment is common. A man may not be able to think of himself as a man unless he is fully virile, able to have intercourse and to engender children. Individuals may be concerned that masculine attributes such as courage, power, fighting spirit, justice, and technical achievement may be jeopardised or threatened as a result of hormonal treatment. Worse still, hormone therapy may even confer female attributes, such as enlarged breasts and hot flushes. Femininity is associated with the ability to conceive children. Identity as a woman may be tied up with the roles of wife and mother, and femininity is expressed through the way one looks. When a woman's hormones are altered as a result of cancer treatment, she risks losing all of this. Youth, beauty, sexual attractiveness and mothering may be threatened. Hormone treatment may result in the loss of the capacity to conceive and the onset of premature symptoms of menopause. While cancer inspires fear, the very treatments that are offered may strike at the root of an individual's being and cause questions about his or her identity and place in society.

How endocrine therapy works

As long ago as 1616, William Harvey noted that prostatic atrophy occurred after castration, and in 1896 it was observed that surgical removal of the ovaries of pre-menopausal women caused regression of breast cancer.[2] Tumours that arise in organs that are normally under endocrine control may be influenced by manipulating hormonal status. This premise is the basis for treatment of cancers of the breast, prostate, thyroid, and uterus. Other tumours, such as renal cell carcinoma and malignant melanoma, have shown responses to hormone therapies but they are not widely used in this context. Endocrine therapy is not normally regarded as a curative treatment. It causes disease regression, but does not eliminate disease altogether. This is probably due to tumours being made up of mixed cell populations, where some of the cells are sensitive to hormone deprivation and therefore die, while others are not sensitive and grow and spread. However, where a cancer becomes resistant to one hormone treatment, treatment with a different hormone may still cause a response, by affecting a different cell population.

Normal physiology

Hormones are chemicals produced by endocrine glands, which circulate in the body to affect other tissues and are used to control many different functions in the body. The hormones of most importance in cancer treatment are those produced in the hypothalamus, anterior pituitary, adrenals, and gonads. The hypothalamus governs the activity of the anterior pituitary gland via small polypeptide hormones such as thyrotrophin-releasing hormone (TRH) and luteinising hormone-releasing hormone (LHRH). In response, the anterior pituitary gland produces more complex hormones, such as thyroid-stimulating hormone (TSH), adrenocorticotrophic hormone (ACTH), follicle-stimulating hormones (FSH) and luteinising hormone (LH). These hormones then stimulate the target gland to produce its own hormones. The thyroid gland releases thyroxine, the adrenal gland produces corticosteroids, and the gonads produce oestrogens or androgens. High levels of end hormones, such as oestrogen, will provide negative feedback and inhibit the activity of the hypothalamus. As a result, the stimulatory system is switched off so that a constant balance of hormones in the bloodstream can be maintained. The purpose of these hormones is to control the growth and maturation of organs such as the breast, uterus, and prostate gland, as well as more general effects, on development and metabolism in the whole body. Growth hormone, which affects all cells, is controlled by a dual system of growth hormone-releasing factor (GHRF) and an inhibitory factor, known as somatostatin. Somatostatin affects many other physiological systems in the body, including glucagon, insulin and the pancreas.

Steroid hormones

Steroid hormones include hydrocortisone and the sex hormones, such as androgen and oestrogen. Hydrocortisone (cortisol) is produced by the adrenal glands and has an effect on the metabolism of all tissues in the body. Artificial replacements include cortisone, which is converted to hydrocortisone by the liver, prednisolone, dexamethasone, and betamethasone. Androgens are largely made by the testes; oestrogen and progesterone are produced by the ovaries. However, the testes do produce small amounts of oestrogen, the ovaries produce small amounts of androgens, and some sex hormones are produced in subcutaneous fat under the control of the adrenal gland. Male hormones are involved in the development of male genitalia and body hair (androgenic effect) and the development of muscle and skeletal tissues (anabolic effect). Oestrogens and progesterone are responsible for the development of the breasts and the endometrium, and are involved in the control of the processes of menstruation, pregnancy, and lactation.

Hormone receptors

Hormones exert their effect by acting on individual cells in the target gland. Protein hormones do not enter the cell but bind to receptors on the surface of the cell, which mediates the effect of the hormone. Steroid hormones do enter the cell but need to combine with cytoplasmic receptors in order to enter the nucleus and exert their effect. Each hormone has its own receptor, which cannot be activated by another hormone, and only the tissues that have specific hormone receptors will be affected by that particular hormone. Tumours that have hormone receptors are more likely to be responsive to hormone manipulation.

In breast cancer, the important hormone receptors are for oestrogen and progesterone. There is another receptor that is important when treating breast cancer, which is known as HER2. This receptor binds with human epidermal growth factor and stimulates the growth of breast cancer. Herceptin is a drug that has been designed to block the HER2 receptor and stop it working. Herceptin is a monoclonal antibody, not a hormone, although it works in a similar way. Herceptin only works in tumours that have high levels of HER2, which are found in about 20% women with breast cancer. Tumours that have neither oestrogen or progesterone receptors nor HER2 are known as triple negative tumours.

The overall response rate to hormone therapies in breast cancer is 30%, while in those that are oestrogen receptor positive (ER +ve) the response rate is 60%.[3] ER +ve tumours are more common in post-menopausal women and are associated with better prognosis, a longer disease-free interval and longer survival. Oestrogen receptor-negative tumours are unlikely to respond to hormone treatment. Prostate tissue contains androgen, oestrogen, and progesterone receptors and, as with breast cancer, those with high levels of hormone receptors are more likely to respond to hormonal therapy. It is not always possible to predict which tumours will respond to hormone therapy as the cell population may vary greatly, with some cells resembling the original tissue from which they arose and some that are different. Tumours that contain cells more similar to the original tissue are more likely to contain hormone receptors and to respond to hormone treatments. Although there is a growing understanding of the way that hormones work on the body it is not always possible to predict what effect they will have. This is because there are complex interactions between hormones and how they influence each other. As a result, it is important to test out any theory about the efficacy and safety of new drugs or herbal medicines before they are used in clinical practice.

The use of endocrine therapy

Endocrine therapy was largely developed in the treatment of metastatic disease and it is still most widely used in this area. It needs to be borne in mind that cure of metastatic cancer is not possible, so that the best quality of life is being sought. For many, endocrine therapy can bring about disease regression and relief of symptoms. However, for some, the side-effects experienced from treatment are great, therefore an accurate assessment of the unwanted effects is important when considering whether to continue or to change therapy. The chance of achieving a response with endocrine therapy varies according to the type of cancer and whether the tumours contain hormone receptors. In breast cancer, the overall response rate to endocrine therapy is 30–40%, although with prostate cancer it may be as high as 80%.[4] Where a response is seen to one endocrine treatment, it is more likely that a second-line hormone will also achieve a response, although this decreases with each subsequent treatment.[5] The disease is often slow to respond, so a rapidly progressing illness is treated with chemotherapy. In prostate cancer combining different hormone therapies gives a more complete reduction in androgen levels, which appears to translate into a greater clinical effect.[6] In breast cancer there does not appear to be an increased benefit when combining a variety of hormonal treatments.[5] Treatment for metastatic disease should continue until there is evidence of disease progression.

Endocrine therapy can also be used in the adjuvant, neo-adjuvant and preventive setting. The synthetic anti-oestrogen, tamoxifen, has been given for many years as an adjuvant treatment alongside primary surgery for breast cancer, as it has been demonstrated to delay relapse and prolong survival time in women with ER +ve tumours.[7] There is now a wealth of new hormone therapies being developed, which may prove to be of greater efficacy and less toxicity than tamoxifen. Current research is being conducted to establish the optimal use of these therapies to reduce breast cancer recurrence.

Tamoxifen has now been approved for the reduction of breast cancer risk.[8] However, its use also increases the risk of uterine cancer and thromboembolic events, such as stroke. It has now been demonstrated that raloxifene also reduces the risk of primary breast cancer and appears to have a lower side-effect profile than tamoxifen.[8]

Adjuvant and neo-adjuvant hormones are also used extensively in the treatment of prostate cancer. The use of adjuvant therapy has been demonstrated to reduce recurrence and improve survival rates in men with high-grade or locally advanced prostate cancer.[9] Neo-adjuvant hormone therapy reduces the volume of the prostate by up to 25%, thus reducing the amount of normal

tissues that is included in the radiation field. This results in lower rates of side-effects in the surrounding tissues, including the bowel and bladder, and erectile dysfunction may be minimised. It is possible that survival may also be improved.[9]

Endocrine treatments for different cancer sites

Breast cancer

Clinical and laboratory evidence now supports the theory that oestrogens play a primary role in the maintenance of growth of at least some breast carcinomas.[10] Many endocrine treatments in breast cancer are therefore aimed at either reducing the synthesis of oestrogen or opposing its action (see Tables 14.1 and 14.2). Surgical or radiation oophorectomy reduces oestrogen production by 90%. Ovary function can now be 'switched off' by the use of highly potent synthetic LHRH analogues, which initially stimulate the pituitary gland to produce LH, causing a rise in oestrogen levels. In women with metastatic disease

Table 14.1 Endocrine treatment for pre-menopausal women with breast cancer

Treatment	Drug name and dose	Mechanism of action	Unwanted effects
Oophorectomy		Decreases oestrogen production by 90% by surgical removal of ovaries.	Menopause, including hot flushes, infertility, dry vagina.
LHRH analogues		Decrease oestrogen production by preventing release of LH.	As above.
Leuprorelin	Prostap (3.75 mg s.c. once per month)		
Goserelin	Zoladex (3.6 mg s.c. once per month)		
Chemotherapy		Suppresses ovarian function.	As above.
Oestrogen antagonists		Oestrogen receptor antagonist.	Hot flushes, weight gain, changes in menstrual flow, thrombosis, endometrial hyperplasia, endometrial cancer,[18] retinopathy, tumour flare.
Tamoxifen	Nolvadex, tamofen (20 mg daily)		
Raloxifene			

Table 14.2 Endocrine treatment for post-menopausal women with breast cancer

Treatment	Drug name and dose	Mechanism of action	Unwanted effects	Notes
Oestrogen antagonists – tamoxifen	Nolvadex Tamofen (20 mg daily)	Competitive inhibitor of oestrogen, with some oestrogenic activity.[12]	Hot flushes, weight gain, thrombosis, endometrial hyperplasia, endometrial cancer,[13] retinopathy, tumour flare.	
– toremifene	Fareston (60 mg daily)			
– raloxifene	Evista			
Aromatase inhibitors – aminoglutethimide	Orimeten (250 mg daily)	Enzyme inhibition, preventing post-menopausal production of oestrogen.	Lethargy, nausea and vomiting, skin rash and fever, ataxia.[14]	Cortisone production also affected; need to give hydrocortisone replacement.
– trilostane	Modrenal (960 mg daily)		Diarrhoea, abdominal discomfort.	
Aromatase inhibitors – formestane	Lentaron (250 mg i.m. every 2 weeks)	As above.	Pain at injection site, rarely dizziness, lethargy, hot flushes.[15]	
– letrozole	Femara (2.5 mg p.o. daily)		Very mild side-effects, possibly arthralgia, fatigue, headache, nausea.[16]	
– anastrozole	Arimidex (1 mg p.o. daily)			
Progestins – medroxyprogesterone acetate – megestrol acetate	Farlutal, Provera (500 mg daily) Megace (160 mg daily)	Activation of the progesterone receptor affects oestrogen activity.	Stimulate appetite, weight gain, fluid retention, thromboembolic disorders, vaginal bleeding, tremors, sweating, Cushing-like features, muscular cramps, nausea and vomiting.[17]	

Table 14.2 Continued

Treatment	Drug name and dose	Mechanism of action	Unwanted effects	Notes
Oestrogens – stilboestrol	Stilboestrol (10–20 mg daily)	?Blocking oestrogen receptors or negative feedback on pituitary gland.	Nausea, fluid retention, thrombosis, withdrawal bleeding, tumour flare.	
Androgens – testosterone	Virormone (100 mg i.m. 2–3 times per week) Primotestan Depo (250 mg i.m. every 2–3 weeks)	Synthetic hormone with androgenic activity.	Oedema, nausea, dizziness, rash, facial hair, male pattern hair loss, headache, depression, deepening of the voice, increase sebum, increase in libido.	

this may cause a 'flare', or worsening of disease-related symptoms. However, after the initial stimulation of the pituitary, the high potency of these analogues causes over-stimulation of the pituitary and no further LH is released so that the ovaries are effectively 'switched off'. This process is reversible, so that if treatment is discontinued ovarian function will return. Drugs in this category include goserelin (Zoladex), leuprorelin, buserilin and triptorelin, and they may be used in either the adjuvant or metastatic setting in pre-menopausal women.[11]

Adjuvant chemotherapy often causes inhibition of menstruation and the nearer the woman is to her natural menopause, the less likely it is that her periods will return.[18] Adjuvant chemotherapy has been shown to confer a greater survival benefit on pre-menopausal women than on post-menopausal women,[19] and it has been suggested that this added benefit may be due to the suppression of ovarian function caused by chemotherapy.

Anti-oestrogens act by binding to oestrogen receptors, making them unavailable to endogenous oestrogens, without stimulating cell division.

Although originally thought of as anti-oestrogens, most of this group of drugs has mixed oestrogenic and anti-oestrogenic activity and so they are known as selective oestrogen receptor modifiers (SERMs). Tamoxifen is the major SERM, while newer ones, such as raloxifene and idoxifene are being developed and their role in the treatment of breast cancer and osteoporosis is still being investigated.[20] Most women with breast cancer will be treated with tamoxifen as it has been shown to substantially reduce the risk of cancer recurrence and subsequent death.[21] It appears that tamoxifen does have some oestrogenic activity,[12] continuing to cause proliferation of the lining of the womb, which results in an increased risk of endometrial cancer.[22] Most pre-menopausal women continue to ovulate and menstruate while on tamoxifen, although women who are near the natural menopause may be 'tipped into it' by tamoxifen. Both tamoxifen and raloxifene increase the risk for venous thromboembolic disease and hot flushes, while tamoxifen increases the risk for endometrial cancer and stroke.[13,23] It has also been suggested that tamoxifen and raloxifene might protect against coronary heart disease, due to an improvement in lipid profile, and osteoporosis, due to increased bone density.[24] Some herbal and food preparations, such as soy, contain molecules similar to animal oestrogens, which are known as phytoestrogens. These appear to have mild oestrogenic activity and some may be SERMs. Various claims are made about their use in reducing osteoporosis, and menopausal symptoms and even to prevent breast cancer. However, this is a very mixed group of substances and as yet there is little evidence to support their use or safety. To date, none of the SERMs have been proved to be superior to tamoxifen in treating breast cancer.[25] A new group of compounds, called SERDs (selective oestrogen receptor downregulators) is now being investigated and may be useful following the use of aromatase inhibitors.[25]

About 10% of oestrogen is made in subcutaneous fat under the control of the adrenal gland, by the conversion of androgens by aromatase enzymes. This oestrogen continues to be produced after menopause, and so hormonal treatments of breast cancer are effective both before and after menopause. A group of drugs called aromatase inhibitors can prevent these enzymes from working and inhibit the production of post-menopausal oestrogens. The first of this group was aminoglutethimide. Aminoglutethimide interfered with enzyme action in the adrenal gland and so corticosteroid replacement was necessary. More specific aromatase inhibitors, such as anastrozole and exemestane, have now been developed, which are associated with much lower toxicity. Side-effects of aromatase inhibitors include hot flushes, arthritis, arthralgia, myalgia, osteoporosis, diarrhoea, and visual disturbances.[26,27] These third-generation aromatase inhibitors are currently approved as first-line therapy for the treatment of post-menopausal women with metastatic estrogen-dependent breast cancer.[28] The use of an aromatase inhibitor as initial therapy, or after treatment with tamoxifen, is now recommended as adjuvant hormonal therapy for post-menopausal women with hormone-dependent breast cancer. Anastrozole, exemestane and letrozole have all been shown to confer longer disease-free survival than tamoxifen.[26,27,29] However, there is a concern that aromatase inhibitors increase the rate of bone loss in post-menopausal women and potentially increase the rate of fracture. Monitoring and treatment-management strategies to reduce bone loss risk are warranted in women receiving aromatase inhibitors for breast cancer.[30] Studies are ongoing to determine the optimal sequence and use of aromatase inhibitors and tamoxifen.

Research work on tumour biology is leading to an increased understanding of the role of hormones in tumour development and progression and, as a consequence, new treatments and improved methods of delivery are constantly being developed. Fulvestrant (Faslodex) is a molecule which resembles oestrogen but has the effect of destroying oestrogen receptors.[31] Fulvestrant has now been licensed for use in metastatic disease in the US, and studies are under way to determine whether it should be used in sequence or in combination with other hormonal therapies. Biological agents, such as lapatinib and gefitinib, inhibit cell receptor sites for growth factors involved in tumour growth. The combination of these agents with hormone therapies has been shown in laboratory studies to give increased inhibition to cancer cell growth.[32] These studies have yet to be translated into clinical use, but show promise for future benefits. Other hormones that are effective in breast cancer, such as progestogens and androgens, appear to oppose the action of oestrogen, although the mechanisms are not well understood. Progesterones cause increased appetite and weight gain. In the longer term, Cushingoid changes, including fat redistribution and diabetes, may occur. Androgens are now rarely used because of the severity of their side-effects. Aromatase inhibitors are now generally preferred to progestogens.

Male breast cancer

Breast cancer is much more rare in men than in women, accounting for less than 1% of all breast cancer cases,[33] and in 2002 the incidence, unlike in women, was not rising but stable.[34] In 2004 there were 324 cases in the UK, resulting in 92 deaths.[35] In some African countries the proportion of men with breast cancer is higher, although the reason for this is unclear.[34] Male breast cancer also occurs later in life and generally does not occur before the age of 55 years, with a median age of diagnosis at 68 years.[34] Breast cancer that occurs in men is more frequently hormone receptor positive and may therefore be more sensitive to hormone therapy.[34]

Due to the rarity of male breast cancer, the use of endocrine therapy has been based on evidence gathered from experience in women, despite the fact that the hormonal environment is clearly very different in men.[36] Nevertheless it appears that adjuvant tamoxifen can improve survival for men with breast cancer, and current advice is to give five years of adjuvant treatment.[37] Endocrine therapy has also been seen to be effective in men with metastatic breast cancer. About 85% of male breast cancers are ER +ve,[37] and approximately 79% of patients will respond to orchidectomy for an average duration of 30 months.[38] LHRH agonists are usually used in preference to surgery. Tamoxifen and the aromatase inhibitors may also be useful second-line therapies.[39]

Prostate cancer

Prostate cancer is the second most common cancer in men, accounting for 90% of cancer cases in men over the age of 65 years. There were 34 986 new cases of prostate cancer in the UK in the year 2004, with 10 000 deaths.[40] The number of cases doubled between 1990 and 2001, largely as a result of increased diagnosis due to the use of prostate-specific antigen as a diagnostic tool.[41] Endocrine therapy in prostate cancer is now being widely used for both neo-adjuvant, adjuvant, and metastatic disease. Currently 50–60% of men present with metastatic disease where hormone therapy is the mainstay of treatment. Endocrine treatments can achieve a response in 40–80% of men treated.[42] This high response rate makes it the treatment of choice for metastatic prostate cancer. However, as with breast cancer, this does not represent a cure, and most men will subsequently relapse after treatment with endocrine therapy (see Table 14.3).

Over 60 years ago, Huggins and Hodges observed that the prostate gland is dependent on androgens, and demonstrated a response to orchidectomy in patients with advanced prostatic cancer.[43] Androgen deprivation can produce symptomatic relief in 80–85% of patients, with a mean duration of response of about 18 months.[44]

The use of LHRH analogues suppresses the function of the testes in the same way as ovarian function is suppressed in women, resulting in a medical orchidectomy and depriving the tumour of androgens. After either of these treatments, men will usually lose their sex drive and ability to develop erections. Many will also suffer hot flushes. A smaller number (one study reported an incidence of 4.8%) will experience breast swelling and breast pain.[42] These side-effects can cause major changes to body image, which are rarely addressed in men with cancer. LHRH analogues used are buserilin, goserelin, leuprorelin, or triptorelin. Because of the initial stimulation of the pituitary, up to 5% of patients may suffer an increase in symptoms or 'flare' in the first 1–2 weeks of treatment.[42] This worsening of symptoms can result in increased bone pain or raised calcium levels in the blood. The effect of this 'flare' can be blocked by giving an anti-androgen, such as flutamide, for several days before and for 2 weeks after commencing treatment with LHRH analogues.[45]

Following treatment with either LHRH analogues or orchidectomy, circulating androgens are reduced by 90–95%, while the remaining 5% continue to be produced by the adrenal glands.[46] These androgens appear to be particularly active in the prostate gland and the levels of the potent androgen, dihydrotestosterone (DHT), are only reduced by 50–70% in the prostate gland following medical or surgical castration.[47] Thus, it is necessary to use anti-androgens to oppose the action of DHT. Anti-androgens compete with androgens for binding sites at the androgen receptor in the nucleus of prostate cancer cells. The combined use of medical or surgical castration and the administration of anti-androgens is known as combined androgen blockade (CAB).

There are two classes of anti-androgens: the steroidal, such as cyproterone acetate (Cyprostat), and the non-steroidal, such as flutamide (Drogenil), nilutamide, or bicalutamide (Casodex). It is unclear whether the non-steroidal anti-androgens are as effective as castration when used as single agents, but they may be used because the effect on sexual functioning appears to be less. Side-effects include gynaecomastia, breast tenderness, and bodily hair loss.[45] Hot flushes may also occur. The steroidal anti-androgens not only

Table 14.3 Endocrine treatment for prostate cancer

Treatment	Drug name and dose	Mechanism of action	Unwanted effects
Bilateral orchidectomy		Prevents androgen production.	Loss of sexual drive.
LHRH agonists			
Goserilin	Zoladex (3.6 mg s.c. once per month)	Decrease androgen production by preventing release of LH.	Tumour flare, hot flushes, decreased libido, impotence, depression.
Leuprorelin	Prostap (3.75 mg s.c. once per month)		
Buserilin	Suprefact (500 µg s.c. three times daily for 1 week, then intranasal six times daily)		
Triptorelin	De-capeptyl (3 mg i.m. every 4 weeks)		
Anti-androgens Steroidal:			
Cyproterone	Cyprostat (300 mg daily)	Block androgen receptors and inhibit release of LH.	Hepatotoxicity in long-term use.
Non-steroidal: Flutamide	Drogenil (250 mg daily)		Hot flushes, gynaecomastia, and breast tenderness, pruritus and nausea and vomiting.
Bicalutamide	Casodex (50 mg daily)		
Oestrogens Stilboestrol	Stilboestrol (1–3 mg daily)	Reduction in testosterone by negative feedback on the pituitary.	Gynaecomastia, weight gain, fluid retention, nausea and vomiting, impotence, cardiovascular disease, tumour flare.
Fosfestrol	Honvan (100–200 mg daily)		

block androgen receptors, but also inhibit the release of LH, causing a reduction in testosterone production. They may be used as a first-line treatment instead of orchidectomy or LHRH analogues. Sexual potency may also be retained. Side-effects include results of androgen deprivation, and liver dysfunction and fatigue have also been reported.[46]

In the past oestrogens, such as stilboestrol and fosfestrol tetrasodium (Honvan), were used. These cause a reduction in testosterone levels due to negative feedback on the pituitary. These are now rarely used due to side-effects, which include feminisation (such as gynaecomastia), erectile dysfunction, penile and testicular atrophy, weight gain, fluid retention, nausea, vomiting, and impotence. Cardiovascular disease is a major problem with oestrogen therapy and anticoagulation

therapy may be given to reduce cardiovascular complications.

Corticosteroids may have a use in those who have relapsed after first-line hormonal treatment as they reduce concentrations of ACTH and so interfere with the production of adrenal androgens. Second-line treatments have the much lower response rate of 30% at best.[46]

Endometrial cancer

The primary treatment for cancer of the womb is surgery and radiotherapy. Hormone therapy may be given as an adjuvant treatment, but the evidence to support this is poor and hormone therapy is usually reserved for treatment of metastatic disease. However, some endometrial cancers are hormone dependent and there is an overall response rate of 11–25% to progestogens such as medroxyprogesterone acetate (100–500 mg daily) or megestrol acetate (40–320 mg daily).[48] There are few data currently available on the use of aromatase inhibitors or SERMs in the treatment of endometrial cancer, and the epidermal growth factor receptor inhibitors (such as gefitinib and lapatinib) and monoclonal antibodies (such as trastuzumab) are currently being investigated.

Endocrine tumours and paraneoplastic syndromes

Tumours arising in endocrine glands may cause disturbances to normal hormonal levels, including tumours of the pituitary, thyroid, and adrenal gland (such as phaeochromocytoma), and carcinoid tumours. Treatment is usually by surgery and subsequent replacement and monitoring of hormone levels. Some tumours also produce inappropriate hormones and cause endocrine abnormalities not directly associated with the tumour. This is most common with lung cancer, where 12% produce endocrine abnormalities.[49] The hormones secreted include ACTH, ADH (antidiuretic hormone) and PTH (parathyroid hormone). These can cause effects such as Cushing's syndrome, hyponatraemia, and hypercalcaemia. Gynaecomastia, hyperthyroidism, and acromegaly may also be seen.

Pituitary adenomas

Tumours arising in the pituitary gland may cause disturbances in normal hormone levels. The pituitary may underfunction, resulting in a lack of growth hormone and gonadotrophins. Pressure on the hypothalamus may result in a lack of regulation of hormones, characterised by an increase in prolactin levels. The tumour cells may secrete excess amounts of hormones, such as growth hormone, prolactin, or ACTH. Treatment is primarily surgical, and will result in lifelong endocrine regulation and hormone replacement therapy (HRT).

Carcinoid tumours

Carcinoid tumours arise from enterochromaffin cells, which may be scattered throughout the body, but mostly occur in the intestine and the main bronchi. They are often multihormonal and secrete hormones such as ACTH, 5-HT (sero-

tonin) and 5-HTP (hydroxytryptophan). Excess levels of these hormones may result in carcinoid syndrome, which is characterised by cutaneous flushing (especially in the face and neck), diarrhoea, wheezing, and valvular heart disease. Where possible the tumour is treated by surgery. Carcinoid syndrome can be treated by the somatostatin analogue octreotide (Sandostatin).

Thyroid cancer

The treatment of thyroid cancer is thyroid ablation, usually by surgery or radiotherapy, followed by physiological HRT. This prevents hypothyroidism and maintains TSH at low levels, to minimise the chance of recurrence of a TSH-dependent tumour. Elderly patients who are unfit for surgery and have small, well-differentiated tumours that are dependent on TSH for growth may be treated by supraphysiological doses of thyroxine (levothyroxine) alone, which inhibits the secretion of TSH by negative feedback control. One study found that this interferes with quality of life by affecting sleep and energy levels, with emotional and social consequences.[50]

Renal cancer

Progestogens can be used in metastatic renal cancer with some effect, e.g. medroxyprogesterone acetate in a dose of 100–500 mg daily, but the chance of response is very low and may be less than 10%. Toremifene has also been used with effect in metastatic disease.[51]

Corticosteroid hormones

Corticosteroid hormones have an anti-tumour effect and may cause regression of breast cancer. They have a marked effect in acute lymphoblastic leukaemia, Hodgkin's disease, and non-Hodgkin's lymphomas, and are sometimes used in conjunction with chemotherapy regimens in order to boost their effectiveness. A more common use in oncology is for acute symptomatic relief or palliative care, due to their suppression of inflammatory and allergic disorders. The use of chemotherapy may result in patients requiring support in the form of multiple platelet and blood transfusions and, as a consequence, they are more vulnerable to reactions from transfusion and so hydrocortisone is routinely used to prevent allergic reactions in these patients.

Large doses or prolonged use may exaggerate some of the normal actions of corticosteroids. The mineralocorticoid effects are fluid retention, potassium loss, and hypertension. Glucocorticoid effects include diabetes, osteoporosis, myopathy, transient euphoria followed by depression, muscle wasting, and peptic ulceration. High doses may result in Cushing's syndrome, with moon face, redistribution of body fat, skin striae, and acne. Corticosteroids predispose to infection and they may mask signs and symptoms of infection.

Hydrocortisone is topically active and has a relatively low incidence of side-effects as it is the least active of this group, and is therefore used for inflammatory skin conditions, such as radiation inflammation. Prednisolone is most commonly used by mouth for long-term administration and has few mineralocorticoid effects. Dexamethasone is a very potent anti-inflammatory with virtually no mineralocorticoid effects, making it very useful where fluid retention would cause a problem, such as with cerebral oedema. Symptoms from brain tumours can be rapidly relieved by high doses of dexamethasone. Brain irradiation will initially cause an increase in inflammation, and so dexamethasone cover will normally be continued throughout a course of treatment.

Palliative care

Corticosteroids act as co-analgesics. That is, they are not true analgesics in the pharmacological sense, but contribute to pain relief by inhibiting production of prostaglandins and thereby reducing inflammation and oedema associated with tumour deposits. They are particularly useful in the treatment of neurological disturbances, such as raised intracranial pressure and brachial plexus damage, and are also effective in treating pain due to bone metastases or where capsular stretching occurs, as with liver disease. Commonly used drugs are prednisolone (30 mg), dexamethasone (4 mg), and hydrocortisone (120 mg).[52] They may also be used to combat difficult pain problems, such as bladder or rectal pain, particularly where there is thought to be a neuropathic component.[53] However, side-effects from long-term use are gen-

erally unacceptable, so corticosteroids will usually only be used for short-term pain relief.

Because of their anti-inflammatory action, corticosteroids also have a useful role to play in relieving the distress caused by breathlessness. They can reduce problems such as airways obstruction, tracheal tumour that causes stridor, lymphangitis carcinomatosis, pneumonitis, and superior vena cava (SVC) obstruction.[54]

The anti-emetic activity of steroids is unexplained, but may have a direct effect on the vomiting centre in the brainstem. It is particularly useful for chemotherapy-related nausea or where nausea is associated with hepatic involvement. It is best used in conjunction with other anti-emetic agents as it enhances their effects.[55]

Other uses include the treatment of hypercalcaemia, stimulating the appetite, and a general improvement in mood and malaise.[56] The wide application of corticosteroids makes them very useful agents in the control of advanced disease; however, their toxicity can be severe in the long term, so they are used with caution. Many of the beneficial effects are also short lived, so steroids should only be used for short periods. Patients taking high doses of steroids for acute episodes may also suffer a number of changes, which may be distressing. The typical round cheeks of the Cushingoid syndrome are a marked feature, which can be very noticeable and, in the eyes of the patient, a significant indicator of severe disease.

PROBLEMS FACED BY WOMEN HAVING ENDOCRINE TREATMENT

Many women are very aware of hormonal changes in their body as they have been accustomed to marking the changes caused by the menstrual cycle. They are familiar with the 'bloating' effect of progesterone due to fluid retention prior to menstruation, and the nausea and increased appetite during pregnancy. They are aware that significant body changes take place as a result of hormone changes, such as changes in the skin and hair, fluctuations in weight, and changes in the distribution of body fat. These changes are often unwelcome in the normal course of life and many women may, therefore, anticipate difficulties in adjusting to hormone therapies and will be looking for familiar signs.

Within current Western society, images of what is thought to be beautiful are conveyed powerfully and constantly by the media. Fashion magazines give an endless flow of advice to women about how to maintain their hair, skin, and 'youthful looks'. The 'body beautiful' is young, sexy, and thin. Hormone therapies affect every part of this image. Those that induce the menopause bring signs of ageing; many will reduce libido, and induce vaginal discharge, bleeding or dryness, and a frequent side-effect is weight gain. Some therapies may even induce masculinising changes, such as increased facial hair and hair loss from the head. At the same time as affecting a woman's self-image and self-esteem, her role as wife, lover, or mother is also affected. The experience of cancer itself may make a woman less fit and less physically able to undertake her normal activities in life. In addition to this, hormone therapy may render her infertile, interfere with her body image or sexuality, or affect her relationship with her partner.

For many women, the relief from symptoms caused by the disease may make hormone therapy well accepted. For others, especially those having hormone therapy as adjuvant treatment, the side-effects may be much more unacceptable and problems may easily be underestimated by health professionals.

Menopause

Menopause and menopausal problems may be induced in women having treatment for cancer. This may be a direct effect of hormonal manipulation with respect to hormonally dependent tumours, such as breast cancer, or it may be an indirect effect as a consequence of chemotherapy or oophorectomy for many other cancers.

Canney and Hatton have shown that 70% of women under the age of 65 years having adjuvant treatment for breast cancer will experience menopausal symptoms.[57] This may be as a consequence of discontinuing treatment with HRT, natural menopause, or the use of adjuvant drugs. In pre-menopausal women, chemotherapy, the use of

LHRH agonists, or oophorectomy will bring about cessation of ovarian function which may be permanent.[18] Even for post-menopausal women there is the chance of suffering menopausal symptoms. Those that have been taking HRT will be advised to stop, with the consequence that menopausal problems may return. Tamoxifen is widely used as an adjuvant treatment in this group owing to its efficacy in reducing mortality,[7] and its principal side-effect is hot flushes.[58] It is thought that a suddenly precipitated menopause may be associated with more symptoms than a normal one.[59] For women who are having a combination of chemotherapy and tamoxifen, it is even more likely that they will experience menopausal symptoms.[60]

Women who have had endometrial, cervical, or ovarian cancer may be told that they should not take HRT; however, there appear to be no data that suggest that HRT increases the risk of recurrence in these women.[61,62]

Experience of menopause

The experience of menopause is a very different transition for each woman. For some it is a time of major role change, when children are leaving home, and the menopause is a reminder of ageing, which may make them feel less attractive as a sexual partner. For others, it is dominated by physical effects such as hot flushes and night sweats, which interfere with their lives and can make them feel unwell. The medical response has been to regard the change as abnormal, a cessation of normal function, and therefore a condition to be treated with medication. Many women find that there is a dearth of information to help them to adjust or even to know what they should expect as normal.[63] However, it has been suggested that the menopause should, more constructively, be considered as a complex event, with physical, psychological, and social components, and that perimenopausal distress has many causes.[64]

As part of the 'beauty myth', old age can be dreaded by women in Western society. As Simone de Beauvoir said, 'old age looms ahead of us like a calamity'.[65] Menopause may be regarded as the start of old age. Women may find it difficult to accept treatment that induces menopause. Endocrine therapies, such oophorectomy and the use of LHRH analogues, are designed to bring about menopause, and as a consequnce cause infertility. Chemotherapy may also bring about an early menopause. Some of these changes are reversible and others are not. Initially it is not possible to know whether a woman is infertile and so it is important to advise the continued use of contraception. Barrier methods are more advisable as the contraceptive pill may interfere with the action of the endocrine treatments. It is important to consider whether the loss of fertility is an issue for the woman and is an important consideration when commencing treatment. In interviews with premenopausal women Singer and Hunter found that premature menopause resulted in negative repercussions on self-esteem and body image.[66] Women experienced feelings of bereavement due to lost fertility, and the level of distress was frequently underestimated by health professionals.

Hot flushes/night sweats

In a normal menopause it is likely that around 50% of women will suffer from hot flushes,[67] while the prevalence of flushes in women with breast cancer is 65%.[68] A study of 150 women with breast cancer showed the number of flushes to range from one to 25 per day, with a median of five, and that the problem was longlasting, with 23% of the sample still experiencing flushes more than 5 years after both menopause and cancer diagnosis.[69]

One woman described her hot flushes following treatment for breast cancer in this way:

> It's as though somebody has built a furnace inside of you and it's your whole body. It starts almost at your feet and works up and you just feel as though you are literally on fire inside . . .[70]

Some women find that the daytime flushes are quite bearable, but that waking many times during the night soaked in sweat is more distressing. Fenlon's study showed that women were more distressed about night sweats than they were about daytime hot flushes; 72% of women in her study reported having disturbed nights.[69]

> To me it felt like . . . probably like a child wetting the bed . . . very distressing, and, and in the morning I would really feel terribly upset, and, and that something when you are so out, so out of control.[70]

Bond *et al.* describe in one study how the basic problem for women experiencing menopause after breast cancer was one of vulnerability.[71] Women needed to find ways of coping with menopausal changes, but these were measured up against the risk that they may cause cancer recurrence, which left them emotionally vulnerable. While initially they minimised problems associated with the menopause as this was regarded as secondary to the cancer diagnosis, at a later stage they started to reflect on their experience and were confused about any menopausal problems they still faced. Health care professionals tended to focus on treatment and related side-effects, and women felt that they were unprepared for the changes of menopause, so that when they came to focus on 'becoming menopausal' they did not feel they had support from their health care providers and they had to find their own way to cope.

Fenlon found that a recurring problem for women with hot flushes was a need to regain control over their bodies.

> . . . it is frightening because you can't control your body; suddenly your body is out of control.[70]

Women tried to find ways to control their menopausal symptoms; this involved many adaptations to daily life and some things, such as coffee and alcohol, were now associated with something bad. Many of the women put a lot of time and effort into trying to regain control by searching their lives for causative factors for the flushes and attempting to avoid these factors (see Box 14.1). This included looking at all aspects of their life, what they did, where they went, what they ate and how they behaved. Numerous strategies were engaged to try to regain control of their lives, but in turn these had the consequence of limiting what they could do or where they could go. Control was regained, but at a price. Some reduced participation in public activities, meeting new people, or creating new relationships.

> . . . I could no sooner have a man sleeping in my bed than fly to the moon . . . there's no way I could enter into a new relationship now.[69]

The attempts to regain control included controlling the environment and the ambient

Box 14.1   Factors that make hot flushes worse, as described by women[69]

Drink
- Hot drinks (12)
- Coffee (5)
- Alcohol (1)
- Spirits (1)
- Wine (10)
- Red wine (2)

Time of day
- When waking (9):
  - woken by flush (4)
  - flush soon after waking (4)
- After breakfast (1)

Food
- Hot food (7)
- Eating late (1)
- Chocolate (1)
- Spicy food (1)
- Too much sugar (1)

Environment
- Hot weather (7)
- The wind (1)
- No control at work (3) or in public places (3)
- Hot (3) or stuffy (3) rooms
- Closed windows (2)

Stress
- Being stressed (13), including such stressors as:
  - work (5)

  - social events (1)
  - late nights (2)
  - making decisions(1)
  - making mistakes(1)
  - being rushed (2) or busy (1)
  - travelling (1)
  - not able to rest (1)
  - being anxious (5)
  - crowds (1)
  - too many dreams (1)

Clothing
- At night: duvets (1)
- In the day: wearing polyester (1) or man-made fibres (1)

Behavioural
- Sleeping on front
- Activity (2) or exercise (2)
- Exertion (1) or over-exertion (2)
- Cooking (1), hoovering (1) ironing (1)
- Standing all day at work (1)
- Holiday (1)
- Being overtired (1)
- Meetings at work (1)
- Walking in cold (1)
- Opening bowels (1)
- Driving (1)
- Taking a bath or shower (3)

temperature. Not only did they have to think about each environment as they entered it and how they would cope, but they also had to anticipate at the beginning of the day what they might face and what would be the most suitable clothing for the day. The factors mentioned included wearing layers, choosing breathable fabrics, such as silk and cotton rather than wool or manmade fibres, and avoiding clothes that were tight around the neck such as jumpers or polo necks. For some women this meant a change in the style of clothes that they wore, so that they had to change their outward image. Once they assessed the environment they could then adjust their clothing appropriately and, if possible, take other measures to control the environment, such as keeping the house cool or opening windows. A similar process

would occur at night, which is clearly disruptive to sleep, as the women frequently needed to get out of bed in order to seek cooling or to change wet clothes.

Other strategies included the use of fans, changing from taking baths to taking showers, or taking a cold bath, moving to a cooler area, going outside, and drinking plenty of water. Diet was examined for elements that might precipitate flushes. Women wrote about avoiding caffeine, spicy foods and alcohol in particular. Some tried to avoid dairy products. The most commonly quoted way of improving flushes was to have a cold drink ($n = 40$) or to drink water ($n = 24$). Another frequently mentioned method of regaining control was to take measures to reduce stress, which might just be about learning to become calmer, or might be about adopting strategies to reduce stress, such as relaxation, increasing rest time, or decreasing work demands.

In order to address the problems brought about by menopausal changes it is important to consider the context of a person's life and how these changes may impact upon them. An approach advocated by Kleinman for people suffering chronic conditions is to construct a mini-ethnography of the person's life and then work with them to address those areas that have significance or cause disruption to daily living.[72] Once an individual has been able to discuss their personal issues they then can begin to construct a way to deal with these. The role of the professional is to facilitate an understanding of the processes that are occurring and thus to help the individual to construct personal meaning and significance in the process.

In the context of cancer, women focus on maintaining long-term health and are concerned by the possibility of cancer recurrence, while the impact of short-term symptoms is minimised.[73] Both after the menopause,[74] and after breast cancer,[73] women look to re-evaluate their lives, and adjust to a new persona. This often includes taking up healthy lifestyle changes and adopting complementary and alternative medicines, including health foods, herbal medicines, and stress-reducing techniques.[75] This may be important by helping to increase feelings of control after menopause; and an enhanced sense of control can help to reduce the impact of menopausal symptoms.[76] Although evidence suggests that after breast cancer women are more likely to use complementary therapies for menopause,[77] they are also more vulnerable and feel the need for additional reassurance from health professionals.[73]

The approach to the management of menopause suggested here is based on allowing the women to take control by focusing on the problem as she views it and providing her with the information to make choices appropriate to her own needs. This strategy is outlined in Table 14.4. Assessment focuses on the problems as defined by the woman herself. The response of the health professional is to help the woman understand the physical changes in her body, to explore her response to these and to examine the options

available to help manage her difficulties. A targeted package of strategies, including pharmacological and non-pharmacological methods, is then developed to help the woman deal with her physical symptoms and help her cope. Herbal remedies need to be considered, as pharmacological treatments and an appropriate level of education must be provided in order for women to make informed decisions about their use. Although HRT is generally contraindicated, some women will be experiencing sufficiently severe difficulties to consider its use, and the risks and benefits will need to be carefully considered for each individual.

Non-pharmacological strategies for dealing with hot flushes

Women use many strategies in order to deal with hot flushes. Many of these are described above in the way that women respond to their experience of hot flushes. In diaries gathered from 150 women experiencing flushes, five categories of behaviours were described by Fenlon.[69] The most common was to have a drink, either water or a cold drink. The other categories related to controlling the environment, adjusting clothing, altering diet and reducing stress. See Box 14.2.

Ultimately many women find that the flushes are not changed by anything they do, but they learn to cope by adjusting the way that they feel about their flushes:

> . . . just accepting that those hot flushes are there, and just trying to um, just trying to stay calm when they happen, not try to fight them. Because I think they get worse if you try and fight them.[69]

Relaxation training

There is some evidence to suggest that the practice of relaxation can reduce hot flushes. Women have long reported that stressful incidents can initiate hot flushes.[78,79] It has been shown in laboratory conditions by Swartzman *et al.* that stress increases the number of flushes experienced over a 24-hour period.[80] This would suggest that reducing stress may reduce flushing. This was first demonstrated in 1984 by Germaine and Freedman who showed a 50% reduction in flushing using behavioural relaxation techniques compared with control.[81] Further small studies supported this finding.[82–85]

Table 14.4 Self-management approaches to menopausal difficulties after breast cancer

Self-management strategies used in menopause	Professional role
• Exploration of the meaning of menopause, for example the heralding of old age or change in social status	• To listen to the individual's narrative and facilitate exploration of meaning
• To identify priorities in symptom management	• To facilitate assessment of menopausal difficulties experienced, such as hot flushes, vaginal dryness
• To find out the causes of symptoms, either due to menopause or as a consequence of treatment for breast cancer	• To inform as to the different causes of symptoms due to cancer, its treatments and menopause
• To learn about the natural changes in the body associated with menopause	• To offer education about the physiology of menopause
• To learn and practise behavioural techniques to cope with hot flushes	• To teach about the role of behavioural techniques, such as distraction or paced respiration for hot flushes
• To learn and practise behavioural techniques to improve stress management	• To teach behavioural techniques, such as relaxation to aid stress management
• To discover and utilise specific strategies for managing vaginal dryness and painful intercourse	• To offer advice on the use of vaginal gels, vaginal oestrogen, or to offer sexual health counselling
• To learn about the risks and benefits of pharmacological interventions and to utilise those that are most appropriate	• To discuss the risks and benefits of HRT, progesterones, clonidine, SSRIs, bisphosphonates
• To learn about the risks and benefits of complementary interventions and to utilise those that are most appropriate	• To discuss the risks and benefits of soy, herbal medicines, acupuncture, vitamins
• To adopt healthy lifestyle measures, such as giving up smoking, increasing exercise, and adapting diet to maintain health	• To provide education as to the benefits of lifestyle measures which can improve health, specifically cardiac and bone health

A large, randomised controlled trial of 150 women with breast cancer has recently confirmed that hot flushes can be reduced by the use of relaxation techniques.[69]

Acupuncture
Several authors have discussed the positive benefits of acupuncture,[86,87] but there is a lack of appropriate studies to support these claims. Wyon *et al.* studied 24 healthy women with flushes and compared the use of superficial needle position and electrostimulated acupuncture.[88] Women kept log books and showed a significant reduction of flushes by 50% over 8 weeks. However, this study had no control group to allow for changes over time or for placebo response. Similarly, Cohen *et al.* claim a benefit for targeted acupuncture over generalised acupuncture, but their study size of 24 was too small to give a reliable result.[89]

Magnetic therapy
Carpenter *et al.* conducted a pilot study of 11 women to evaluate the use of magnetic therapy for hot flushes, which found that placebo was significantly more effective than magnetic therapy in reducing the frequency of hot flushes.[90]

Homeopathy
There are some studies to support the use of homeopathy for the relief of hot flushes, but they do not have control groups or use formal evaluative methods.[91,92] It is therefore difficult to know whether the benefit was gained due to the treatment itself or to some other factor.

Pharmacological agents for use in menopause
Hormone replacement therapy
It is not known whether it is safe to give HRT to women who have had breast cancer, and every

Box 14.2 Factors that relieve hot flushes as described by women[69]

Drink
- Having a cold drink (39) or plenty of cold drink (1)
- Drinking water (23) or fizzy water (1)
- Tea (1) or iced tea (1)
- Wine to help sleep (2)

Food
- Eating (4)

Environment
- Cold weather (1), cold day (3), cold night (1)
- Go outside (5), working outside (1), get fresh air (6)
- Go for a walk (2)
- Control atmosphere (4) by:
  - adjusting heating or clothing (1)
  - anticipating heat
  - keeping house (2) or room cool (1)
  - opening doors (1) and windows (5)
  - cool breeze (1), fan (2), cool floor (2)
  - cool wash (1)

Reducing stress
- Relaxing (2) or keeping calm (1)
- Resting (4)
- Not 'pushed for time' (1) or less stressed (2)
- Ways of reducing stress:
  - taking life easy (1)
  - having a holiday (1)
  - not working (1)
  - having an early night (1)
  - breathing exercises (5)
  - relaxation techniques (9) or to help sleep (3)

Clothing
- At night:
  - cotton sheets (3)
  - light blankets (2)
  - light or easily adjustable bed linen (3)
  - removing bed covers (6)
- Daytime:
  - wearing cotton (1)
  - man-made fibres (1)
  - wear removable layers (1)

Behavioural
- Cooling activities:
  - fanning (1)
  - taking a shower (1)
  - holding cold glass to face (1)
  - splashing face with cold water.
- Other strategies were:
  - getting out of bed (3),
  - getting up (1),
  - sitting down for a minute (1)
  - walking (2)
  - sleeping on back
- Distraction:
  - reading (2)
  - gardening (2)
  - keeping busy at work (1)

woman needs to consider the risks and benefits when making a decision as to whether to take HRT in any form. Some authors, such as Shoham and Kopernik, point out that the reduction in oestrogen levels at the time of the menopause has detrimental effects in almost every organ in the body, and that oestrogen should be given routinely to post-menopausal women in order to prevent these effects.[93] It has been shown that oestrogen protects against osteoporosis, reducing the number of hip fractures that occur;[94] reduces the incidence of colon cancer;[94] reduces urinary incontinence,[95] vaginal dryness and dyspareunia,[96] and hot flushes;[97] and may improve cognition.[98] Detrimental effects of oestrogen include an increase in pulmonary embolism, stroke, and cardiovascular disease,[94] although the evidence regarding coronary heart disease is not completely clear as the risk of cardiac disease increases in the first year of oestrogen use and then declines.[99] It may therefore be that oestrogen triggers disease in those who have pre-existing problems, but is protective in those without.

There appear to be differences between the use of oestrogen alone and oestrogen and progesterone combined. Oestrogen used alone is associated with a much higher rate of endometrial hyperplasia, while combined oestrogen and progesterone is similar to placebo for hyperplasia.[100] This suggests that combined HRT is safe with respect to uterine cancer, although Weiderpass *et al.* showed an increased risk of endometrial cancer with oestrogen used alone.[101]

With respect to breast cancer, it is known that oestrogen given to breast cancer cells *in vitro* stimulate cancer to grow,[49] and a number of studies have now shown that not only oestrogen, but also oestrogen and progesterone combined, as well as the synthetic hormone tibilone all increase the primary incidence of breast cancer.[94,102] What is not clear is whether this risk translates into an increased risk of recurrence in women who have already had breast cancer. Some authors point out that the biological appearance of tumours that occur during HRT use is less aggressive,[103] and that women have a better prognosis, lower incidence of metastasis, and improved life expectancy when breast cancer is diagnosed during HRT use.[93] Furthermore, the one study published on the incidence of recurrence in 2755 women taking HRT who had a diagnosis of breast cancer, showed that there was a lower risk of recurrence and mortality in women who used HRT than in women who did not.[104] The authors do not claim that HRT is protective against recurrence, but suggest that HRT after breast cancer may not have an adverse impact on recurrence and mortality.[104] Despite this finding, there is still concern about the use of HRT after breast cancer. A systematic review conducted by Pritchard *et al.* concluded that there was sufficient evidence to accept that the risk of breast cancer was increased with the use of HRT in women without a diagnosis of breast cancer.[105] From this the authors extrapolated that it is possible that there is an increased risk of recurrence and contralateral breast cancer associated with HRT in women with breast cancer.[105,106] While HRT is still generally regarded as contraindicated after breast cancer, there remains little evidence to support this concern.[62]

Alternatives to HRT

There are a variety of alternatives to HRT, but few address all the problems associated with low oestrogen levels. The physical changes of hot flushes, urogenital changes, osteoporosis, and cardiovascular disease may need to be treated separately. Hormones other than oestrogen, such as progesterone, synthetic oestrogens and phyto-

estrogens, may be helpful and these will be discussed first. Other measures to manage menopause include a variety of drugs, but also lifestyle measures, such as diet and exercise.

Progestogens.   Progestogens, such as medroxyprogesterone acetate, are used as a treatment for breast cancer and so there is an assumption that their use for the alleviation of menopausal symptoms is safe. They have proven to be effective in treating hot flushes in both men and women after cancer treatment, with reductions in flushes of up to 90%,[107,108] and having lasting benefit.[109] There are also herbal medicines, such as wild yam cream, which have progesterone-like activity, and which are used by some women.[110] The benefit of these has not yet been adequately demonstrated. There is also a multiplicity of active agents in such medicines and doubtful absorption through the skin.[111] It is possible that they may even be harmful.[112] Work by Komesaroff *et al.* measuring active hormones in the blood showed that the amount of the yam cream, Progest, absorbed through the skin was minimal, but this does not mean that it has no effect.[111] If it is accepted that combined HRT of oestrogen and progesterone together give a greater risk of primary breast cancer than oestrogen only,[102] it cannot be assumed that the use of progesterone is safe after breast cancer.

Selective   oestrogen   receptor   modulators (SERMs).   The selective oestrogen receptor modulators may have a role to play in the control of menopausal problems. An optimal SERM would act to provide the benefits of oestrogen in the central nervous system to reduce hot flushes, to prevent osteoporosis, to improve urogenital symptoms, and to decrease cardiovascular disease, while at the same time not have oestrogenic effects on the breast and the endometrium with the consequence of endometrial proliferation and increased cancer risk. The two major SERMs are tamoxifen and raloxifene. While these are antioestrogenic in the breast, they do have oestrogenic activity in the bones and reduce circulating cholesterol levels,[22] so there may be a role for these drugs in preventing some of the changes due to oestrogen withdrawal after menopause. The risks for tamoxifen are an increase in endometrial cancer and thromboembolic events.[22] With respect to bone density, it appears that tamoxifen decreases bone mineral density in pre-menopausal women, but prevents bone loss in post-menopausal women.[113] Tamoxifen also causes hot flushes,[58] and so while it is a useful drug for treating breast cancer, it is not effective for menopausal problems. In post-menopausal women raloxifene decreases bone turnover and increases bone mineral density, thereby reducing the incidence of vertebral fractures.[114] Unlike tamoxifen, raloxifene does not cause endometrial hyperplasia or cancer,[22] and may even reduce the risk of breast cancer.[115] However, raloxifene does not alleviate early menopausal symptoms, such as hot flushes and urogenital atrophy, and may even exacerbate some of them. Raloxifene may be an alternative for the prevention of osteoporosis and heart diseases in women with previous breast cancer, but it is not suitable for those with hot flushes.[114]

Phytoestrogens. Phytoestrogens are plant substances that mimic animal oestrogens and have been shown to have some oestrogenic effect in animals and humans.[116] They can be part of the diet or found in herbal remedies. They include many substances classified as lignans, isoflavones and coumestans.[117] Isoflavones are the most oestrogenically potent, and the major dietary isoflavones are genistein and daidzein.[117] Intestinal flora convert inactive plant precursors into compounds active in the human.[118] Phytoestrogens are found in plant sources such as soy beans and soy foods, linseed, sunflower and flax seeds, bean sprouts, whole grains, fruit and vegetables. They are also provided in herbal remedies such as red clover (*Trifolium pratense*), black cohosh (*Cimicifuga racemosa*), chaste berry (*Vitex agnus-castus*), dong quai (*Angelica sinensis*), hops (*Humulus lupulus*) and liquorice (*Glycyrrhiza glabra*).[116] In countries where the intake of these foods is high, it has been noted that both breast cancer and menopausal difficulties are lower in incidence than in the West.[119] It is thought that a high intake of phytoestrogens in the diet may be able to reduce the development of breast cancer,[119–121] to reduce hot flushes after menopause, and to protect against osteoporosis. However, Guthrie *et al.* point out that women who take high levels of phytoestrogens are also more likely to indulge in many other healthy lifestyle activities and that it is not possible to assign particular health benefits to one dietary component.[122] As the phytoestrogens have mixed oestrogenic effects in humans, it has been proposed that they may behave like SERMs. Further evidence is required to test the phytoestrogens as individual agents, as each have different actions.

Soy. Soy beans are one of the major dietary sources of phytoestrogens and contain high levels of isoflavones. The use of soy in the diet has been recommended to reduce hot flushes. A study on Japanese women has shown that the higher the intake of soy the lower the number of flushes experienced.[123] The promotion of soy as a safe alternative to HRT has resulted in a surge in uptake in women with breast cancer, who are six times as likely as women without breast cancer to be taking soy for menopausal symptoms.[124] However, the data to support the use of soy are still conflicting. Trials that support the use of soy include the work of Albertazzi *et al.* showing a 45% reduction in flushing versus 30% in placebo,[125] and that of Murkies *et al.* who showed a 40% reduction in a soy group compared with 25% in placebo.[126] Quella *et al.*[127] and van Patten *et al.*[128] did not demonstrate any benefit due to soy. Studies of isoflavone extract have also been unable to show an improvement in flushing using either 80 mg or 114 mg isoflavone.[129,130] Recent literature reviews continue to present conflicting studies, with Huntley and Ernst showing four studies that found soy to be effective and six finding it non-effective.[131] A review by Kronenberg and Fugh-Berman of 29 randomised trials supported the use of soy for hot flushes, but pointed out that isoflavone extracts are less effective than natural soy,[132] and a meta-analysis of placebo-controlled trials by Messina and Hughes suggested that soy is more effective in reducing flushes when there are a greater number of flushes initially.[133] Wuttke *et al.* could find no overall benefit using soy for hot flushes, but have suggested that soy may have a mild osteoprotective effect.[134]

The difficulties with achieving standardisation of results may be due to types and amount of product used. Many of the soy products available in the west are alcohol washed, and this may reduce the isoflavone content.[135] If soy products are effective, it is not clear whether supplements should be used or whether the effect will be greater by incorporating soy into the diet. Apart from mild gastrointestinal disturbances, soy appears to be safe to use.[125,128]

A consensus opinion by the North American Menopause Society concluded that although there are studies that support the use of isoflavones to reduce hot flushes, there are others that do not, and the balance of evidence is insufficient to support the use of isoflavones for menopause.[136] There are also inadequate data to evaluate the effect of isoflavones, such as soy, on breast and other female-related cancers, bone mass and vaginal dryness.

*Black cohosh (*Cimicifuga racemosa*).* There are many authors who discuss the use of the black cohosh for the relief of hot flushes,[110,132,137,138] but few randomised controlled studies to assess safety and efficacy. Black cohosh has been assumed to be a phytoestrogen due to the presence of the isoflavone formononetin, but recent laboratory analysis by Mahady *et al.* showed no evidence of the presence of formononetin.[139] The mechanism of the action of black cohosh has not been explained, and it may not be mediated by oestrogen receptors. Some authors have shown it has no oestrogenic effects on vaginal proliferation or blood hormone levels,[116,140] although conversely Wuttke *et al.* found some evidence of oestrogenic activity in the brain, bone, vagina, and bladder.[141] In relation to breast cancer risk, Amato *et al.* have shown that black cohosh does not stimulate the growth of human breast cancer cells in mice.[142] Several reviews of the literature suggest that there may be a mild effect on menopausal symptoms, especially hot flushes, and with mild, if any, side-effects.[143–146] Three studies have shown a reduction in flushes with the use of black cohosh. Liske *et al.* showed that 40 mg was as effective as 127 mg and reduced flushes by 70% in 149 women, but there was no control group in this study.[140] In a small study of 62 women Wuttke *et al.* showed that black cohosh was as effective as oestrogen when compared to placebo.[141] In breast cancer Hernandez Munoz and Pluchino found flushes to be less in women treated

with tamoxifen and black cohosh than in women taking tamoxifen only.[147] However, in a study of 85 women with breast cancer Jacobson *et al.* found that black cohosh was not more effective than placebo, and raised the concern about possible interactions with tamoxifen.[148] Despite the uncertainty about its mechanism of action, there is a growing use of black cohosh sold as Remifemin for alleviation of hot flushes.[144] Due to its limited oestrogenic effect, some authors have suggested that black cohosh is safe to use after breast cancer,[135] although it has not been tested for interactions with tamoxifen or the aromatase inhibitors. More recently, Wuttke *et al.* have raised a concern about the possibility that another component of black cohosh, genistein, might have a detrimental effect on the uterus, similar to oestrogen.[149]

*Dong quai (*Angelica sinensis*).* The amount of evidence available for other phytoestrogens is very limited. Dong quai has been shown to have weak oestrogen receptor binding,[116] and may not be safe to use as it has been shown to induce the activity of cultured breast cancer cells.[142] A study of 71 women treated for 6 months showed that dong quai was no better than placebo for the treatment of hot flushes.[150]

*Red clover (*Trifolium pratense*).* There is also a trend towards the use of red clover for hot flushes and other menopausal symptoms, and it has a clear oestrogenic effect. Liu *et al.* demonstrated oestrogen binding and oestrogenic activity in endometrial cells.[116] Tice *et al.* showed a reduction of flushes using two different formulations of red clover (Promensil and Rimostil), but suggested this was too small to be clinically significant.[151] van der Weijer and Barentsen showed a 44% reduction in flushes which was significant when compared to placebo,[152] although two previous placebo trials showed no reduction of flushing.[153] Red clover may have benefits to the heart and bone,[154] but has been shown to cause infertility in animals,[155] and contains coumarins, which may affect clotting.[153] There are no studies available to show any possible interactions with tamoxifen.

Overall, it appears that some phytoestrogens have oestrogenic effects in the body, but there is very little definitive data about either their safety or efficacy. Soy isoflavones have been the most extensively researched, appear to be safe and may have a variety of beneficial effects after menopause. Other herbal remedies have mixed oestrogenic effects, some of which may be harmful. Black cohosh may have a different mechanism of action not yet understood.

Selective serotonin reuptake inhibitors. Selective serotonin reuptake inhibitors (SSRIs) are agents which inhibit the reuptake of serotonin, which is involved in temperature regulation and thought to be implicated in the flush mechanism.[156] They include fluoxetine (Prozac), venlafaxine (Effexor), paroxetine (Seroxat) and sertraline (Lustral), which have all been shown to be effective in reducing flushing in women with breast cancer.[157,158] Venlafaxine 75 mg has been demonstrated to reduce flushes by up to 61%,[159] and paroxetine by 67%.[160] Venlafaxine is claimed to be currently the most effective non-hormonal option to reduce hot flushes in breast cancer patients.[161] Although it is claimed that SSRIs are well tolerated, mouth dryness, decreased appetite, nausea, and constipation are reported. Clayton et al. found that sexual problems due to SSRIs were consistently under-reported by physicians.[162] Somnolence and anxiety have also been reported,[160] and personal observation has shown a significant proportion of women reporting these symptoms as highly unpleasant. It is also possible that there may be interactions between SSRIs and tamoxifen. While the SSRIs may be highly effective for some women, they must be used with caution due to the level of side-effects.

Clonidine. Although the SSRIs mainly inhibit serotonin uptake, they also influence the reabsorption of norepinephrine (noradrenaline).[163] Clonidine is an anti-hypertensive which appears to be active through its effect on reducing central noradrenergic activation, and decreases the amount of norepinephrine in the brain. This effect raises the sweating threshold and ameliorates hot flushes.[164] Laufer et al. demonstrated that clonidine could suppress the occurrence of hot flushes by 46% at a dose of 0.4 mg per day.[165] The effectiveness of clonidine has since been supported by a number of studies, including in healthy women,[164] men with prostate cancer,[166] and women with breast cancer taking tamoxifen.[167,168] The largest of these studies ($n = 194$) found that 0.1 mg clonidine reduced hot flushes by 38% compared to 24% with placebo, although it also found that patients receiving clonidine were more likely to report difficulty sleeping (41% compared with 21%; $P = 0.02$).[167] Side-effects reported by Goldberg et al. included mouth dryness, constipation and drowsiness.[167] Although clonidine may be useful for some women it is accompanied by unpleasant side-effects, which may cause up to 40% of patients to discontinue treatment.[165]

Other agents. A variety of other agents have been used in the past with varying success. These include belladonna alkaloids,[169] and methyldopa. None of these agents has been demonstrated to be particularly useful.[170] The use of gabapentin was suggested in 2002 by Reidenbach,[171] and Loprinzi et al.,[172] and Pandya et al. have successfully utilised gabapentin to reduce hot flushes by up to 70% in women with breast cancer taking tamoxifen, although these studies were small and had no control group.[173] Side-effects included lightheadedness, dizziness, sleepiness, nausea, and rash.

Treating vaginal dryness
The symptoms of vaginal atrophy can be improved by the use of locally applied oestrogen or topical gels. A Cochrane review of vaginal oestrogen showed that creams, pessaries, tablets, and the estradiol vaginal ring were equally effective.[96] A possible concern with the use of vaginal oestrogen is that oestrogen is absorbed into the bloodstream to have systemic as well as local effects. However, there is minimal absorption of oestrogen through the vagina, and blood levels remain within normal menopausal limits.[96] As so little oestrogen is absorbed, the systemic adverse effects such as bleeding, breast tenderness, and endometrial stimulation are reduced with the use of local oestrogens. This Cochrane review states that the avoidance of systemic effects can be of advantage to women who have previously been treated for cancer.[96] As a treatment choice women appeared to find creams and pessaries to be messy and

application times difficult to remember. Overall, women favoured the estradiol-releasing vaginal ring for ease of use, comfort of product, and overall satisfaction.[96]

A more recent study showed that in post-menopausal women with breast cancer taking aromatase inhibitors, serum estradiol was raised after the use of a vaginal estradiol tablet from ≤5 pmol/l to 72 pmol/l at 2 weeks, and then reduced to a median of 16 pmol/l after 4 weeks.[174] The beneficial effect of aromatase inhibitors is achieved through the suppression of oestrogen to very low levels in this group of women. The vaginal estradiol tablet significantly raises systemic estradiol levels, at least in the short term. This reverses the estradiol suppression achieved by aromatase inhibitors in women with breast cancer, and is therefore contraindicated in these women.

Vaginal dryness can also be improved by the use of local topical gels. There is a range of gels available which range from simple moisturisers to polycarbophil gels which claim to improve vaginal moisture and elasticity. Gelfand and Wendman found one of these (Replens) to be effective in 80% of women.[175] A study by Bygdeman and Swahn showed that Replens significantly improved vaginal dryness, although dienoestrol cream was significantly better than Replens.[176] There was no information given as to patient preference or satisfaction between these two options.

Strategies for maintaining bone density
Until recently, HRT has been recommended for maintaining bone density after the menopause.[177] This is seen as a high-risk strategy for women who have had breast cancer and is unlikely to be recommended for this group. Other options include alterations to lifestyle – mainly diet and exercise. These are discussed in detail below. Raloxifene increases bone mineral density, although its role in women who have had breast cancer is unclear.[24] Bisphosphonates are a group of drugs (including clodronate, alendronate and pamidronate) which have no hormonal action, but are effective in reducing post-menopausal osteoporosis because they have a high affinity for bone mineral and inhibit bone resorption. They are effective in treating bone loss and reducing fractures that are induced by aromatase inhibitors.[178]

Lifestyle factors in dealing with symptoms of menopause
Diet
Alterations in diet can be useful for managing some menopausal changes and can affect long-term health. Diet is a well-established risk factor for cardiovascular disease and extensive work has been conducted to discover which food components provide protection or increased risk. A summary of the evidence has been provided by a review by Reddy and Katan.[179] Risk factors include being overweight and a high alcohol intake (more than one or two units per day). The main foods to avoid are saturated fatty acids and cholesterol, with unsaturated fats, fish, whole grains, soy, and fruit and vegetables being protective.[179]

The evidence for preventing osteoporosis through diet is more problematic. A recent overview of the latest evidence by Prentice suggested that where calcium intake is low (less than 400 mg/day) or in the elderly, there is a benefit in taking calcium supplementation along with vitamin D.[180] The evidence supports the use of calcium and vitamin D together, as either supplement given alone is less beneficial.[180] Other recommendations were to increase physical activity, reduce sodium intake, increase consumption of fruit and vegetables, avoid smoking, and maintain a healthy body weight, as low body weight is a risk factor for osteoporosis.[180] There is evidence that maintenance of calcium intake is important for bone health, and higher consumption of milk and cheese is associated with a lower risk of fracture. However, there is no evidence that calcium supplementation for women within 5 years of the menopause has any effect on the bone mineral density of trabecular regions of the skeleton, where the greatest loss of bone occurs.[180]

Many menopausal women search their diet for triggers for flushes and it is frequently suggested that avoidance of caffeine, alcohol, and spicy foods can reduce flushing.[181] Herbal supplements are frequently taken and these have been discussed above. No studies examining the effect of caffeine on flushing were found in the literature. Vitamin E was first suggested by Blatt *et al.* in 1953 to help relieve flushing.[182] This has been demonstrated to be effective by Barton *et al.* in a prospective randomised control using a daily dose of 800 IU of vitamin E, where flushes reduced by 25% over placebo.[183]

Evening primrose oil has been widely promoted for women's health and specifically to reduce hot flushes. Only one research paper was found examining the effect of evening primrose oil on hot flushes. This study of only 35 women showed placebo to be better than 2 g evening primrose oil taken over 6 months.[184] The study is too small to draw any conclusions.

Physical exercise

Physical exercise is an effective management strategy for many of the problems in menopause. General aerobic exercise improves cardiovascular health and reduces mortality from cardiac disease.[185] Weight-bearing exercise will prevent bone loss, although it does not appear to increase bone density.[186] It can also help to improve fitness and muscle strength, which will contribute to the prevention of falls and a lower risk of fracture.[187] Exercises focused specifically on the muscles of the pelvic floor can help to reduce urinary incontinence.[188] Swedish cohort studies have suggested that women who have undertaken regular aerobic exercise experience fewer menopausal symptoms, and especially fewer hot flushes, than other women.[189–191] The suggested rationale for the way in which flushes might be reduced is that it is due to the improvement in beta-endorphin production found after regular exercise.[190] However, similar Australian and American studies have not confirmed these reports.[192,193] A recent study by Lindh-Åstrand *et al.* showed that exercise reduced flushing by 50% in women who exercised for 36 weeks.[194] This study can be criticised as the data were only gathered on five women and there was no control group. Furthermore, there may be confounding factors when studying physical exercise. Guthrie *et al.* showed an association between physical exercise and lower body mass index and lower alcohol intake,[192] and Sternfeld *et al.* showed that lower body mass index is associated with reduced flushing.[193] Although Ivarsson *et al.* controlled for body mass index,[190] this association and others, such as alcohol intake, may need to be explored further.

Other problems for women on hormonal therapies

Changes in mood state

Alterations in hormones can have a profound effect on mood state. An increase in progesterone or testosterone will cause an initial feeling of well-being. This can be useful in the terminal stages of disease, but is not generally useful otherwise, as it is short-lived. Other changes, particularly a reduction in testosterone, may cause depression. This has also been noted with the use of some of the aromatase inhibitors. There is a general belief that menopause can cause depression, although it is unclear whether this is due to biological changes or whether it is largely the result of concurrent changes in lifestyle. This time of life is often associated with children gaining independence and this can be a blow to a mother's self-esteem. Individuals who perceive that their bodies are changing and becoming less attractive due to hormonal therapies may also suffer from lowered self-esteem, and this too can result in depression. For both men and women these difficulties may be secondary to concerns about cancer and their mortality, but they may all contribute to a depressive state. It is important to carefully assess an individual who suffers from depression, and to note whether this coincides with commencing hormone therapy, as for some it may be a major contributory factor.

Weight gain

Weight gain is common after treatment for cancer, although it is not completely clear what the role of hormone therapy is in this problem. Progestins and steroids can cause weight gain,[17] which may be difficult to control as they are associated with an increased appetite as well as fluid retention. The increased gain in weight is often seen in a Cushingoid distribution, with the typical 'moon face'. This may be distressing in the way it alters appearance. Tamoxifen has also been connected with weight gain.[195] It has been demonstrated that a high percentage of women treated for breast cancer with chemotherapy, with or without tamoxifen, gain weight, while those on tamoxifen gain more weight.[196,197] Pre-menopausal women put on more weight (3–4 kg) than post-menopausal women (1–2 kg). Part of the explanation for the findings in women with breast cancer may be a change in lifestyle. During treatment for cancer women may take less exercise and be less rigorous about dieting. The consequence for women may be further disruption to their self-image and feelings of femininity. Many women search for ways in which they can regain control over their lives after breast cancer, and advice about diet can help in this area. When giving advice, it is important to consider what they eat, but also to look at what else is happening in their lives and what physical activity they are able to undertake. However, it is also possible for women to feel guilty if they are unable to keep their weight at their accepted norm. If it is not acknowledged that tamoxifen contributes to this gain, then this may be perceived as another burden to bear.

Vaginal bleeding

Vaginal bleeding has been reported as the most distressing side-effect of hormonal therapy, followed by weight gain and hot flushes.[198] It is not known whether this distress is found only when women are not warned that bleeding is a possibility, as they will then be concerned about the cause. Tamoxifen can cause irregular periods in pre-menopausal women – either heavier or lighter – and can induce a discharge or bleeding in post-menopausal women. Progestins and oestrogens can also cause bleeding. Some hormones are associated with a withdrawal bleed, so that women should be warned about the possibility of bleeding as they discontinue the drug. Abnormal bleeding may be a sign of gynaecological cancers, and tamoxifen can cause a slight increase in the incidence of endometrial cancer.[13,199] For this reason, women need to be warned about the possibility of unusual bleeding and to report this to their doctor.

Sexuality

Combined with a loss of confidence and self-esteem following cancer diagnosis and treatment, physical changes that affect sexuality may also occur. Women with treatment-induced menopause have been shown to have reduced sexual functioning.[200] Reduction in oestrogen may cause a decreased libido, although this is gradual. This may exacerbate the effects of treatments such as chemotherapy or surgery. Loss of oestrogen also results in more fragile, less-well-lubricated vaginal mucosa and may be accompanied by irritation or itching. For some women the change in the acid balance of the vagina can lead to an increase in infections, such as thrush (*Candida albicans*). Over a period of time the vagina becomes shorter and narrower.

One woman's comments on her experience of sex after hormonal treatments were as follows:

> I know all the way through he was absolutely wonderful, but when it came to any sexual activity I don't think he fancied me very much. I really don't and I've put on a lot of weight. He's not a man to push himself forward any way too much so err . . . it affected me, I mean it still does, I still have no libido . . .[69]

> If one or other partner finds it a problem then it is a problem, but if you've both adjusted then it's not. The vagina is drier. It takes longer to be comfortable. One is getting older.[69]

Joint pains and stiffness

Joint pain was the major symptom found in a study of 114 post-menopausal women after treatment for breast cancer,[201] although McPhail and Smith found that joint pains were no more common in women with breast cancer than in an age-matched control population.[202] It is not clear how much joint pains are a consequence of breast cancer treatment, menopause, or normal ageing. However, it does appear that joint pains and stiffness can be a major problem when using aromatase-inhibiting drugs, such as arimidex.

Tumour flare

Some drugs may cause an initial worsening of symptoms, known as a 'tumour flare'. This is particularly important for those with bone disease. Initially bone pain may become more severe, but bone destruction can result in hypercalcaemia or spinal cord compression. Individuals at risk should be warned of relevant symptoms and watched carefully for these problems.

Much of the nursing care required for women facing these problems is rooted in helping to give realistic information about what they should expect, what is 'normal', and what practical measures they might be able to implement to help. However, listening and talking through difficulties may provide a positive focus for improving very difficult problems.

Problems faced by men having endocrine treatment

Many of the problems for men are similar to those faced by women. For those with breast cancer there may also be the added stigmatisation of suffering from a 'female' disease, as well as the feminising effects that can occur with some of the treatments.

Alterations in sexuality
Lion has defined sexuality as:

> . . . all those aspects of the human being that relate to being woman or man, and is an entity subject to lifelong dynamic change. Sexuality reflects our human character, not solely our genital nature.[203]

Therefore, in caring for a man having treatment that will affect his sexuality, it is important to consider both his ability to perform the sexual act and his feelings about sexuality, which are closely aligned to masculinity. Hormonal treatments or surgical interventions such as orchidectomy and prostatectomy not only directly affect the ability to function sexually (for example, the ability to have an erection), but are also profoundly threatening to masculinity, self-image, and esteem.

Hormonal treatments can have feminising effects. Loss of androgens, or treatment by oestrogen, can cause development of the breasts (gynaecomastia) and reduction in body and facial hair. These body-image changes can have a major impact on men causing reduced self-esteem and feelings of emasculation.[204] Colbourne also found that men may not be prepared for gynaecomastia, which may be associated with breast pain or tenderness, and appeared to be a long-term problem.[204] Furthermore, there is a lack of treatment to deal with gynaecomastia, which does not necessarily resolve after hormone treatment. Problems associated with gynaecomastia were reduced intimacy with partners, due to discomfort, and embarrass-

ment in social situations where it would be normal to reveal the chest, such as when taking exercise. Loss of fitness and weight gain may also be associated with detrimental changes to body image, where being masculine is associated with being fit and healthy.

The research that has been conducted on men's sexuality after cancer has largely been carried out in men who have had orchidectomy for testicular cancer. In this case only the affected testis is removed and therefore sexual functioning is less likely to be affected. Jones and Webb found that for these men the priority was shown to be one of having their cancer treated, while issues of fertility and sexuality were secondary, although some did express concern about losing their manhood.[205] More recently, Gascoigne et al. found that there was a greater effect on masculinity than had previously been suggested, and that merely the discovery of testicular symptoms produced embarrassment, fear of castration, and concern about masculinity.[206] It has also been shown that even among testicular cancer survivors a significant proportion suffer treatable sexual problems long after treatment has been discontinued.[207]

Where men have undergone radical prostatectomy for prostate cancer, health professionals may make the assumption that they have already lost sexual function. This is not always the case as nerve-sparing techniques have reduced the incidence of impotence from nearly 100% to about 32%,[207] and the issue may need to be addressed when giving hormone therapies. By offering information about sexuality and fertility, without waiting for the subject to be raised, nurses can help men to talk over problems that may be worrying. They can also help to redefine sexuality in broader terms, such as sharing, communication, and intimacy. Nurses may also be able to help consider choices about treatment that may affect sexuality. For example, given the choice, most men would prefer castration through drug treatment rather than surgical removal of the testes, although many who are suffering symptoms choose the surgery, since relief of symptoms may be achieved more quickly.[208] If symptoms are severe, such as spinal cord compression due to bone metastases, it may be considered necessary for surgical intervention to obtain a speedy response. In the absence of severe disease, one approach could be to use medical treatment to ascertain whether a hormonal response is likely, and follow up with surgical treatment if it proves to be effective. For those where there is no response, surgery would be spared and the effects of hormonal treatment could be reversed.

Many people with prostate cancer are elderly, and in the past health professionals may have assumed that sexuality is not an issue for them. This assumption is erroneous; older people often enjoy continued sexual interest, function, and satisfaction until the end of life,[209] and hormonal therapies have a profound effect on sexual function, which should not be dismissed. Furthermore, with the advent of screening, the age profile of men diagnosed with prostate cancer is reducing, yet Colbourne found that health professionals still behave as though prostate cancer was a disease of the elderly where issues of sexuality and fertility were not relevant.[204]

Loss of or reduction in sexuality may cause a fundamental alteration in the way a man feels about himself. Even when sexuality is not lost the enjoyment may be reduced, which may have an impact on a man and his relationship with any partner. Participants in Colbourne's study suggested that the trade-off for cure was the loss of an enjoyable sexual relationship.[204]

Hot flushes

Hot flushes have been reported to occur in over 75% of men who have undergone orchidectomy,[210] and during treatment with LHRH analogues, which have been shown to reduce quality of life. Colbourne found that men were not prepared for the intensity or frequency of flushing and that it restricted activity and caused disrupted sleep, with consequent daytime tiredness.[204] One informant described his flushes in this way:

> The big problem I had was sweats, which I can't tell you were minor things cos they weren't, they were really dramatic things, I'd sit in the office at work and I'd go blood red all over, and the sweat would just pump out of me and I'd end up with a shirt that was literally soaking, wringing wet . . .[204]

Hot flushes were an outward sign to others not only of illness or abnormality but also of a symptom normally associated with women and

the menopause. One man described flushing as 'having a granny'.

Treatments for flushes that are effective in women are likely to also be effective in men. It has also been shown that megestrol acetate can reduce the incidence of hot flushes by 50% or more in 74% of sufferers.[106]

Infertility

The assumption may often be made that as prostate cancer occurs in the older age group, most men with prostate cancer will not wish to father children. However, it is not uncommon for older men to marry women considerably younger than themselves, and so the possibility of preservation of sperm should not be dismissed. The threat of loss of fertility is also an issue for men whenever this occurs, even when they have had children, just as it is for women. Since men do not usually completely lose their fertility even into old age, this loss may be difficult. Furthermore the age profile of prostate cancer is shifting towards younger men, and health professionals may have to alter their assumptions about the needs of this group.

Conclusion

Endocrine therapies are becoming a valuable approach for the treatment of some cancers, most notably breast and prostate cancer. When given selectively, impressive responses may be achieved, often with minimal side-effects. Endocrine therapies are now increasingly used to reduce both mortality and morbidity from cancer. Future developments in tumour biology are pointing to a rapidly increasing role for hormones in the control of these cancers and an understanding of the complex interactions between hormones, diet and lifestyle in the development of cancer is leading to new approaches to both treatment and prevention of the disease.

References

1. Fellowes D., Fallowfield L.J., Saunders C.M. and Houghton J. (2001). Tolerability of hormone therapies for breast cancer: how informative are documented symptom profiles in medical notes for 'well-tolerated'

treatments? *Breast Cancer Research and Treatment* **66**, 73–81.

2. Beatson G.T. (1896). On the treatment of inoperable cases of carcinoma of the mamma: suggestions for a new method of treatment with illustrative cases. *Lancet* **2**, 104–107; 62–65.

3. Powles T. (1993). Progestins II: Megestrol acetate. In Powles T. and Smith I. (eds.) *Medical Management of Breast Cancer*. Cambridge: Dunitz.

4. Hardy J. (1995). Endocrine therapy in advanced malignancy. *European Journal of Palliative Care* **2**, 151–154.

5. Buzdar A. and Hortobagyi G. (1998). Update on endocrine therapy for breast cancer. *Clinical Cancer Research* **4**, 527–534.

6. Schellhammer P., Sharifi R., Block N. *et al.* (1997). Clinical benefits of bicalutamide compared with fluta-mide in combined androgen blockade for patients with advanced prostatic carcinoma: final report of a double-blind, randomized, multicenter trial. *Urology* **50**, 330–336.

7. Early Breast Cancer Trialists Collaborative Group. (1988). Effects of adjuvant tamoxifen and cytotoxic therapy on mortality in early breast cancer. An over-view of 61 randomized trials among 28 896 women. *New England Journal of Medicine* **319**, 1681–1692.

8. Vogel V.G., Costantino J.P., Wickerham D.L. *et al.* (2006). Effects of tamoxifen vs raloxifene on the risk of developing invasive breast cancer and other disease outcomes: the NSABP Study of Tamoxifen and Raloxifene (STAR) P-2 trial. [see comment] *Journal of the American Medical Association* **295**, 2727–2741.

9. Morton G.C. (2000). Early prostate cancer. *Current Problems in Cancer* **24**, 3–55.

10. Dowsett M. (1991). Reproductive endocrinology and endocrine effects of therapy. In Powles T.J. and Smith I.E. (eds.) *Medical Management of Breast Cancer*. London: Martin Dunitz.

11. Prowell T.M. and Davidson N.E. (2004). What is the role of ovarian ablation in the management of primary and metastatic breast cancer today? *Oncologist* **9**, 507–517, 2004.

12. Jackson I.M., Litherland S. and Wakeling A.E. (1991). Tamoxifen and other antioestrogens. In Powles T.J. and Smith I.E. (eds.) *Medical Management of Breast Cancer*. London: Martin Dunitz.

13. Fornander T., Rutqvist L.E. and Cedermark B. (1989). Adjuvant tamoxifen in early breast cancer: occurrence of new primary cancers. *Lancet* **I**, 117–120.

14. Coombes R.C., Powles T.J. and Easton D. (1987). Adjuvant aminoglutethimide therapy for postmeno-pausal patients with primary breast cancer. *Cancer Research* **47**, 2496–2499.

15. Coombes R.C. (1991). Clinical studies with 4-hydroxy-androstenedione in advanced breast cancer. In Coombes R.C. and Dowser M. (eds.) *4-Hydroxyandrostenedione – A New Approach to Hormone Dependent Cancer*. London: Royal Society of Medicine Services.

16. Dombernowsky P., Smith I., Falkson G. *et al.* (1998). Letrozole, a new oral inhibitor for advanced breast cancer: double-blind randomized trial showing a dose effect and improved efficacy and tolerability compared with megestrol acetate. *Journal of Clinical Oncology* **16**, 453–461.

17. Pannuti F., Martoni A., Zamagni C. and Melotti B. (1991). Progestins I: medroxyprogesterone acetate. In. Powles T. and Smith I. (eds.) *Medical Management of Breast Cancer*. Cambridge: Dunitz.

18. Goodwin P.J., Ennis M., Pritchard K.I., Trudeau M. and Hood N. (1999). Risk of menopause during the first year after breast cancer diagnosis. *Journal of Clini-cal Oncology* **17**, 2365–2370.

19. Padmanabhan N., Howell A. and Rubens R.D. (1986). Mechanisms of action of adjuvant chemotherapy in early breast cancer. *Lancet* **ii**, 411–414.

20. Wickerham D.L. (2003). Tamoxifen's impact as a pre-ventive agent in clinical practice and an update on the STAR trial. *Recent Results in Cancer Research* **163**, 87–95; discussion 264–266.

21. Baum M. (1998). Tamoxifen – the treatment of choice. Why look for alternatives? *British Journal of Cancer* **78**, 1–4.

22. Jordan V.C., Gapstur S. and Morrow M. (2001). Selective estrogen receptor modulation and reduction in risk of breast cancer, osteoporosis, and coronary heart disease. *Journal of the National Cancer Institute* **93**, 1449–1457.

23. Kinsinger L.S., Harris R., Woolf S.H., Sox H.C. and Lohr K.N. (2002). Chemoprevention of breast cancer: a summary of the evidence for the US Preventive Serv-ices Task Force. *Annals of Internal Medicine* **137**, 59–69.

24. Vogelvang T.E., van der Mooren M.J. and Mijatovic V. (2004). Hormone replacement therapy, selective estrogen receptor modulators, and tissue-specific com-pounds: cardiovascular effects and clinical implica-tions. *Treatments in Endocrinology* **3**, 105–115.

25. Johnston S.R. (2005). Endocrinology and hormone therapy in breast cancer: selective oestrogen receptor modulators and downregulators for breast cancer – have they lost their way? *Breast Cancer Research* **7**, 119–130.

26. Coombes R.C., Hall E., Gibson L.J. *et al.* (2004). A randomized trial of exemestane after two to three years of tamoxifen therapy in postmenopausal women with primary breast cancer. *New England Journal of Medicine* **350**, 1081–1092.

27. Goss P.E., Ingle J.N., Martino S. *et al.* (2003). A randomized trial of letrozole in postmenopausal women after five years of tamoxifen therapy for early-stage breast cancer. *New England Journal of Medicine* **349**, 1793–1802.

28. Brueggemeier R.W. (2006). Update on the use of aromatase inhibitors in breast cancer. *Expert Opinion on Pharmacotherapy* **7**, 1919–1930.

29. Baum M., Buzdar A.U., Cuzick J. *et al.* (2002). Anastrozole alone or in combination with tamoxifen versus tamoxifen alone for adjuvant treatment of postmenopausal women with early breast cancer: first results of the ATAC randomised trial. *Lancet* **359**, 2131–2139.

30. Mincey B.A., Duh M.S., Thomas S.K. *et al.* (2006). Risk of cancer treatment-associated bone loss and fractures among women with breast cancer receiving aromatase inhibitors. *Clinical Breast Cancer* **7**, 127–132.

31. Robertson J.F., Come S.E., Jones S.E. *et al.* (2005). Endocrine treatment options for advanced breast cancer – the role of fulvestrant. *European Journal of Cancer* **41**, 346–356.

32. Chu I., Blackwell K., Chen S. and Slingerland J. (2005). The dual ErbB1/ErbB2 inhibitor, lapatinib (GW572016), cooperates with tamoxifen to inhibit both cell proliferation- and estrogen-dependent gene expression in antiestrogen-resistant breast cancer. *Cancer Research* **65**, 18–25.

33. Borgen P.I., Wong G.Y., Vlamis V. *et al.* (1992). Current management of male breast cancer. A review of 104 cases. *Annals of Surgery* **215**, 451–457.

34. Giordano S.H., Buzdar A.U. and Hortobagyi G.N. (2002). Breast cancer in men. *Annals of Internal Medicine* **137**, 678–687.

35. Cancer Research UK. (2007). *UK Breast Cancer Incidence Statistics*. http://info.cancerresearchuk.org/cancerstats/types/breast/incidence/ (accessed 20 September 2007).
Cancer Research UK. (2007). *UK Cancer Incidence Statistics for Common Cancers*. http://info.cancerresearchuk.org/cancerstats/incidence/common-cancers/ (accessed 20 September 2007).

36. Nahleh Z.A. (2006). Hormonal therapy for male breast cancer: a different approach for a different disease. *Cancer Treatment Reviews* **32**, 101–105.

37. Gennari R., Curigliano G., Jereczek-Fossa B.A. *et al.* (2004). Male breast cancer: a special therapeutic problem. Anything new? *International Journal of Oncology* **24**, 663–670.

38. Judson I. and Powles T.J. (1988). Endocrine therapy. In Tiffany R. (ed.) *Oncology for Nurses and Health Care Professionals*, 2nd edition. Beaconsfield: Harper and Row.

39. Zabolotny B.P., Zalai C.V. and Meterissian S.H. (2005). Successful use of letrozole in male breast cancer: a case report and review of hormonal therapy for male breast cancer. *Journal of Surgical Oncology* **90**, 26–30.

40. Cancer Research UK. (2005). *UK Prostate Cancer Incidence Statistics*. http://info.cancerresearchuk.org/cancerstats/types/prostate/incidence/ (accessed 20 September 2007).

41. Quinn M., Wood H., Cooper N. and Rowan S. (2005). *Prostate Cancer Atlas of the United Kingdom and Ireland 1991–2000*. http://www.statistics.gov.uk/StatBase/Product.asp?vlnk=14059&Pos=&ColRank=1&Rank=272 (accessed 20 September 2007).

42. Denis L. (1993). Prostate cancer. Primary hormonal treatment. *Cancer* **71(suppl.)**, 1050–1058.

43. Huggins C. and Hodges C.V. (1941). Studies on prostatic cancer. I. The effects of castration, or of oestrogen and of androgen injection on serum phosphatases in metastatic carcinoma of the prostate gland. *Cancer Research* **1**, 293–297.

44. Shearer R. and Davies J.H. (1991). Studies in prostatic cancer with 4-hydroxyandrostenedione. In Coombes R.C. and Dowsett M. (eds.) *4-Hydroxyandrostenedione – A New Approach to Hormone Dependent Cancer*. London: Royal Society of Medicine Services.

45. McLeod D.G., Benson R.C. Jr., Eisenberger M.A. *et al.* (1993). The use of flutamide in hormone-refractory metastatic prostate cancer. *Cancer* **72(12 suppl.)**, 3870–3873.

46. Dearnaley D.P. (1994). Cancer of the prostate. *British Medical Journal* **308**, 780–784.

47. Labrie F. (1998). Combined androgen blockade and treatment of localized prostate cancer: a real hope when approaching the year 2000. *Endocrine Related Cancer* **5**, 341–351.

48. Gadducci A., Cosio S. and Genazzani A.R. (2006). Old and new perspectives in the pharmacological treatment of advanced or recurrent endometrial cancer: hormonal therapy, chemotherapy and molecularly targeted therapies. *Critical Reviews in Oncology/Hematology* **58**, 242–256.

49. Bunn P. and Ridgeway E.C. (1989). Paraneoplastic syndromes. In DeVita V., Hellman S. and Rosenberg S. (eds.) *Principles and Practice of Oncology*, 3rd edition. Philadelphia, PA: Lippincott.

50. Botella-Carretero J.I., Galan J.M., Caballero C., Sancho J. and Escobar-Morreale H.F. (2003). Quality of life and psychometric functionality in patients with differentiated thyroid carcinoma. *Endocrine-Related Cancer* **10**, 601–610.

51. Gershanovich M.L., Moiseenko V.M., Vorob'ev A.V. and Kiapiulia K. (1996). [Hormone therapy of

advanced renal cancer with high-dose toremifene (Fareston).] *Voprosy Onkologii* **42**, 105–109.

52. DeConno F. and Foley K. (1995). *Cancer Pain Relief: A Practical Manual.* Dordrecht: Kluwer.

53. Hanks G., Portenoy R., MacDonald N. and O'Neill R. (1993). Difficult pain problems. In Doyle D., Hanks G. and MacDonald N. (eds.) *The Oxford Textbook of Palliative Medicine.* Oxford: Oxford University Press.

54. Ahmedzai S. (1993). Palliation of respiratory symptoms. In Doyle D., Hanks G. and MacDonald N. (eds.) *The Oxford Textbook of Palliative Medicine.* Oxford: Oxford University Press.

55. Allen S. (1993). Nausea and vomiting. In Doyle D., Hanks G. and MacDonald N. (eds.) *The Oxford Textbook of Palliative Medicine.* Oxford: Oxford University Press.

56. Portenoy R. (1993). Adjuvant analgesics in pain management. In Doyle D., Hanks G. and MacDonald N. (eds.) *The Oxford Textbook of Palliative Medicine.* Oxford: Oxford University Press.

57. Canney P.A. and Hatton M.Q. (1994). The prevalence of menopausal symptoms in patients treated for breast cancer. *Clinical Oncology* **6**, 297–299.

58. Powles T.J., Jones A.L., Ashley S.E. *et al.* (1994). The Royal Marsden Hospital pilot tamoxifen chemoprevention trial. *Breast Cancer Research and Treatment* **31**, 73–82.

59. Chakravarti S., Collins W.P., Newton J.R., Oram D.H. and Studd J.W. (1977). Endocrine changes and symptomatology after oophorectomy in pre-menopausal women. *British Journal of Obstetric Gynaecology* **84**, 769–775.

60. Biglia N., Cozzarella M., Cacciari F. *et al.* (2003). Menopause after breast cancer: a survey on breast cancer survivors. *Maturitas* **45**, 29–38.

61. Mueck A.O. and Seeger H. (2003). Hormone therapy after endometrial cancer. *Journal of the British Menopause Society* **9**, 161–164.

62. Creasman W.T. (2005). Hormone replacement therapy after cancers. *Current Opinion in Oncology* **17**, 493–499.

63. Dickson G.L. (1990). A feminist poststructuralist analysis of the knowledge of menopause. *Advances in Nursing Science* **12**, 15–31.

64. Fugate-Woods N. (1970). Menopausal distress: a model for epidemiologic investigation. In Voda A., Dinnerstein M. and O'Donnell S. (eds.) *Changing Perspectives on Menopause.* Austin, TX: University of Texas Press.

65. De Beauvoir S. (1970). *Old Age.* London: Penguin Books.

66. Singer D. and Hunter M. (1999). The experience of premature menopause: a thematic discourse analysis. *Journal of Reproductive and Infant Psychology* **17**, 63–81.

67. Dennerstein L., Dudley E.C., Hopper J.L., Guthrie J.R. and Burger H.G. (2000). A prospective population-based study of menopausal symptoms. *Obstetrics and Gynecology* **96**, 351–358.

68. Carpenter J.S., Johnson D., Wagner L. and Andrykowski M. (2002). Hot flashes and related outcomes in breast cancer survivors and matched comparison women. *Oncology Nursing Forum* **29**, E16–E25.

69. Fenlon D. (2005). *Menopause after Breast Cancer: A Randomised, Controlled Trial of Relaxation Training to Reduce Hot Flushes.* PhD thesis, University of Southampton.

70. Fenlon D. and Rogers A. (2007). The experience of hot flushes after breast cancer. *Cancer Nursing* **30**, E19–E26.

71. Bond B., Hirota L., Fortin J. and Col N. (2002). Women like me: reflections on health and hormones from women treated for breast cancer. *Journal of Psychosocial Oncology* **20**, 39–56.

72. Kleinman A. (1988). *The Illness Narratives: Suffering, Healing and the Human Condition.* New York: Basic Books.

73. Knobf M.T. (2002). Carrying on: the experience of premature menopause in women with early stage breast cancer. *Nursing Research* **51**, 9–17.

74. Masse R. and Legare F. (2001). The limitations of a negotiation model for perimenopausal women. *Sociology of Health and Illness* **23**, 44–64.

75. Shen J., Andersen R., Albert P.S. *et al.* (2002). Use of complementary/alternative therapies by women with advanced-stage breast cancer. *BMC Complementary and Alternative Medicine* **2**, 8.

76. Reynolds F. (2000). Relationships between catastrophic thoughts, perceived control and distress during menopausal hot flushes: exploring the correlates of a questionnaire measure [In Process Citation]. *Maturitas* **36**, 113–122.

77. Harris P.F., Remington P.L., Trentham-Dietz A., Allen C.I. and Newcomb P.A. (2002). Prevalence and treatment of menopausal symptoms among breast cancer survivors. *Journal of Pain and Symptom Management* **23**, 501–509.

78. Reitz R. (1985). *Menopause – A Positive Approach.* London: Unwin.

79. Hunter M. and Liao K. (1995). Problem-solving groups for mid-aged women in general practice: a pilot study. *Journal of Reproductive and Infant Psychology* **13**, 147–151.

80. Swartzman L., Edelberg R. and Kemmann E. (1990). Impact of stress on objectively recorded menopausal hot flushes and on flush report bias. *Health Psychology* **9**, 529–545.

81. Germaine L.M. and Freedman R.R. (1984). Behavioral treatment of menopausal hot flashes: evaluation by objective methods. *Journal of Consulting and Clinical Psychology* **52**, 1072–1079.

82. Stevenson D.W. and Delprato D.J. (1983). Multiple component self-control program for menopausal hot flashes. *Journal of Behaviour Therapy and Experimental Psychiatry* **14**, 137–140.

83. Wijma K., Melin A., Nedstrand E. and Hammar M. (1997). Treatment of menopausal symptoms with applied relaxation: a pilot study. *Journal of Behaviour Therapy and Experimental Psychiatry* **28**, 251–261.

84. Freedman R.R. and Woodward S. (1992). Behavioral treatment of menopausal hot flushes: evaluation by ambulatory monitoring. *American Journal of Obstetrics and Gynecology* **167**, 436–439.

85. Fenlon D. (1999). Relaxation therapy as an intervention for hot flushes in women with breast cancer. *European Journal of Oncology Nursing* **3**, 223–231.

86. Towlerton G., Filshie J., O'Brien M. and Duncan A. (1999). Acupuncture in the control of vasomotor symptoms caused by tamoxifen. *Palliative Medicine* **13**, 445.

87. Tukmachi E. (2000). Treatment of hot flushes in breast cancer patients with acupuncture. *Acupuncture in Medicine* **18**, 22–27.

88. Wyon Y., Lindgren R., Hammar M. and Lundeberg T. (1994). [Acupuncture against climacteric disorders? Lower number of symptoms after menopause.] *Lakartidningen* **91**, 2318–2322.

89. Cohen S., Rousseau M. and Carey B. (2003). Can acupuncture ease the symptoms of menopause? *Holistic Nursing Practice* **17**, 295–299.

90. Carpenter J.S., Wells N., Lambert B. *et al.* (2002). A pilot study of magnetic therapy for hot flashes after breast cancer. *Cancer Nursing* **25**, 104–109.

91. Clover A. and Ratsey D. (2002). Homeopathic treatment of hot flushes: a pilot study. *Journal of the Faculty of Homeopathy* **91**, 75–79.

92. Thompson E.A. and Reilly D. (2002). The homeopathic approach to symptom control in the cancer patient: a prospective observational study. *Palliative Medicine* **16**, 227–233.

93. Shoham Z. and Kopernik G. (2004). Tools for making correct decisions regarding hormone therapy. Part I: background and drugs. *Fertility and Sterility* **81**, 1447–1457.

94. Beral V., Banks E. and Reeves G. (2002). Evidence from randomised trials on the long term effects of hormone replacement therapy. *Lancet* **360**, 942–944.

95. Moehrer B., Hextall A. and Jackson S. (2004) Oestrogens for urinary incontinence in women (Cochrane Review). *The Cochrane Library*, Issue 3. Oxford: Update Software.

96. Suckling J., Lethaby A. and Kennedy R. (2004). Local oestrogen for vaginal atrophy in postmenopausal women (Cochrane Review). *The Cochrane Library*, Issue 4. Oxford: Update Software.

97. MacLennan A., Lester S. and Moore V. (2004). Oral oestrogen replacement therapy versus placebo for hot flushes (Cochrane Review). *The Cochrane Library*, Issue 3. Oxford: Update Software.

98. Hogervorst E., Yaffe K., Richards M. and Huppert F. Hormone replacement therapy for cognitive function in postmenopausal women (Cochrane Review). *The Cochrane Library*, Issue 3. Oxford: Update Software.

99. Hulley S., Grady D., Bush T. *et al.* (1998). Randomized trial of estrogen plus progestin for secondary prevention of coronary heart disease in postmenopausal women. Heart and Estrogen/progestin Replacement Study (HERS) Research Group. *Journal of the American Medical Association* **280**, 605–613.

100. Lethaby A., Suckling J., Barlow D. *et al.* (2004). Hormone replacement therapy in postmenopuasal women: endometrial hyperplasia and irregular bleeding (Cochrane Review). *The Cochrane Library*, Issue 3. Oxford: Update Software.

101. Weiderpass E., Baron J.A., Adami H.O. *et al.* (1999). Low-potency oestrogen and risk of endometrial cancer: a case-control study. *Lancet.* **353**, 1824–1828.

102. Million Women Study Collaborators. (2003). Breast cancer and hormone replacement therapy in the Million Women Study. *Lancet* **362**, 419–427.

103. Holli K., Isola J. and Cuzick J. (1998). Low biologic aggressiveness in breast cancer in women using hormone replacement therapy. *Journal of Clinical Oncology* **16**, 3115–3120.

104. O'Meara E.S., Rossing M.A., Daling J.R. *et al.* (2001). Hormone replacement therapy after a diagnosis of breast cancer in relation to recurrence and mortality. *Journal of the National Cancer Institute* **93**, 754–762.

105. Pritchard K.I., Khan H. and Levine M. (2002). Clinical practice guidelines for the care and treatment of breast cancer: 14. The role of hormone replacement therapy in women with a previous diagnosis of breast cancer. *Canadian Medical Association Journal* **166**, 1017–1022.

106. Holmberg L. and Anderson H. (2004). HABITS (hormonal replacement therapy after breast cancer – is it safe?), a randomised comparison: trial stopped. *Lancet* **363**, 453–455.

107. Loprinzi C.L., Goldberg R.M., O'Fallon J.R. *et al.* (1994). Transdermal clonidine for ameliorating post-orchiectomy hot flashes. *Journal of Urology* **151**, 634–636.

108. Barton D., Loprinzi C., Quella S. *et al.* (2002). Depomedroxyprogesterone acetate for hot flashes. *Journal of Pain and Symptom Management* **24**, 603–607.

109. Quella S.K., Loprinzi C.L., Sloan J.A. *et al.* (1998). Long term use of megestrol acetate by cancer survivors for the treatment of hot flashes. *Cancer* **82**, 1784–1788.

110. Pick M. (2000). Herbal treatments for menopause. Black cohosh, soy and micronized progesterone. *Advances in Nursing Practice* **8**, 29–30.

111. Komesaroff P.A., Black C.V., Cable V. and Sudhir K. (2001). Effects of wild yam extract on menopausal symptoms, lipids and sex hormones in healthy menopausal women. *Climacteric* **4**, 144–150.

112. Gorski T. (2000). 'Wild Yam Cream' threatens women's health. *Quackwatchcom* www.quackwatch.com/01QuackeryRelatedTopics/wildyam.html (accessed 21 September 2007).

113. Powles T.J., Hickish T., Kanis J.A., Tidy A. and Ashley S. (1996). Effect of tamoxifen on bone mineral density measured by dual-energy X-ray absorptiometry in healthy premenopausal and postmenopausal women. *Journal of Clinical Oncology* **14**, 78–84.

114. Sismondi P., Biglia N., Roagna R. *et al.* (2000). How to manage the menopause following therapy for breast cancer. Is raloxifene a safe alternative? *European Journal of Cancer* **36(suppl.)**, S74–S76.

115. Jordan V.C. (2000). Tamoxifen: a personal retrospective. *The Lancet Oncology* **1**, 43–49.

116. Liu J., Burdette J.E., Xu H. *et al.* (2001). Evaluation of estrogenic activity of plant extracts for the potential treatment of menopausal symptoms. *Journal of Agricultural and Food Chemistry* **49**, 2472–2479.

117. Lethaby A.E., Kronenberg F., Roberts H. and Eden J. (2002). Phytoestrogens for menopausal symptoms (Protocol for a Cochrane Review). *The Cochrane Library*, Issue 1. Oxford: Update Software.

118. Adlercreutz H. and Mazur W. (1997). Phyto-oestrogens and Western diseases. *Annals of Medicine* **29**, 95–120.

119. Stephens F. (1997). Breast cancer: aetiological factors and associations (a possible protective role of phytoestrogens). *Australia and New Zealand Journal of Surgery* **67**, 755–760.

120. Ingram D., Sanders K., Kolybaba M. and Lopez D. (1997). Case–control study of phyto-oestrogens and breast cancer. *Lancet* **350**, 990–994.

121. Adlercreutz H. (2002). Phyto-oestrogens and cancer. *The Lancet Oncology* **3**, 364–373.

122. Guthrie J.R., Ball M., Murkies A. and Dennerstein L. (2000). Dietary phytoestrogen intake in mid-life Australian-born women: relationship to health variables. *Climacteric* **3**, 254–261.

123. Nagata C., Takatsuka N., Kawakami N. and Shimizu H. (2001). Soy product intake and hot flashes in Japanese women: results from a community-based prospec-tive study. *American Journal of Epidemiology* **153**, 790–793.

124. Newton K.M., Buist D.S., Keenan N.L., Anderson L.A. and LaCroix A.Z. (2002). Use of alternative therapies for menopause symptoms: results of a population-based survey. *Obstetrics and Gynecology* **100**, 18–25.

125. Albertazzi P., Pansini F., Bonaccorsi G. *et al.* (1998). The effect of dietary soy supplementation on hot flushes. *Obstetrics and Gynecology* **91**, 6–11.

126. Murkies A.L., Lombard C., Strauss B.J. *et al.* (1995). Dietary flour supplementation decreases post-menopausal hot flushes: effect of soy and wheat. *Maturitas* **21**, 189–195.

127. Quella S.K., Loprinzi C.L., Barton D.L. *et al.* (2000). Evaluation of soy phytoestrogens for the treatment of hot flashes in breast cancer survivors: a North Central Cancer Treatment Group Trial. *Journal of Clinical Oncology* **18**, 1068–1074.

128. Van Patten C.L., Olivotto I.A., Chambers G.K *et al.* (2002). Effect of soy phytoestrogens on hot flashes in postmenopausal women with breast cancer: a rand-omized, controlled clinical trial. *Journal of Clinical Oncology* **20**, 1449–1455.

129. St Germain A., Peterson C.T., Robinson J.G. and Lee Alekel D. (2001). Isoflavone-rich or isoflavone-poor soy protein does not reduce menopausal symptoms during 24 weeks of treatment. *Menopause* **8**, 17–26.

130. Nikander E., Kilkkinen A., Metsa-Heikkila M. *et al.* (2003). A randomized placebo-controlled cross-over trial with phytoestrogens in treatment of menopause in breast cancer patients. *Obstetrics and Gynecology* **101**, 1213–1220.

131. Huntley A. and Ernst E. (2004). Soy for the treatment of perimenopausal symptoms – a systemic review. *Maturitas* **47**, 1–9.

132. Kronenberg F. and Fugh-Berman A. (2002). Complementary and alternative medicine for menopausal symptoms: a review of randomized, controlled trials. *Annals of Internal Medicine* **137**, 805–813.

133. Messina M. and Hughes C. (2003). Efficacy of soy-foods and soybean isoflavone supplements for alleviating menopausal symptoms is positively related to initial hot flush frequency. *Journal of Medicinal Food* **6**, 1–11.

134. Wuttke W., Jarry H., Becker T. *et al.* (2003). Phyto-estrogens: endocrine disrupters or replacement for hormone replacement therapy? *Maturitas* **44(suppl.)**, S9–S20.

135. Gass M.L. and Taylor M.B. (2001). Alternatives for women through menopause. *American Journal of Obstetrics and Gynecology* **185(2 suppl.)**, S47–S56.

136. North American Menopause Society. (2000). The role of isoflavones in menopausal health: consensus opinion

of The North American Menopause Society. *Menopause* 7, 215–229.

137. Pepping J. (1999). Black cohosh: *Cimicifuga racemosa*. *American Journal of Health System Pharmacy* **56**, 1400–1402.

138. Kang H J., Ansbacher R. and Hammoud M.M. (2002). Use of alternative and complementary medicine in menopause. *International Journal of Gynaecological Obstetrics* **79**, 195–207.

139. Mahady G.B., Fabricant D., Chadwick L.R. and Dietz B. (2002). Black cohosh: an alternative therapy for menopause? *Nutrition in Clinical Care* **5**, 283–289.

140. Liske E., Hanggi W., Henneicke-von Zepelin H.H. *et al.* (2002). Physiological investigation of a unique extract of black cohosh (*Cimicifugae racemosae rhizoma*): a 6-month clinical study demonstrates no systemic estrogenic effect. *Journal of Womens Health and Gender Based Medicine* **11**, 163–174.

141. Wuttke W., Seidlova-Wuttke D. and Gorkow C. (2003). The Cimicifuga preparation BNO 1055 vs. conjugated estrogens in a double-blind placebo-controlled study: effects on menopause symptoms and bone markers. *Maturitas* **44(suppl. 1)**, S67–S77.

142. Amato P., Christophe S. and Mellon P. (2002). Estrogenic activity of herbs commonly used as remedies for menopausal symptoms. *Menopause* **9**, 145–150.

143. Lieberman S. (1998). A review of the effectiveness of *Cimicifuga racemosa* (black cohosh) for the symptoms of menopause. *Journal of Womens Health* **7**, 525–529.

144. McKenna D.J., Jones K., Humphrey S. and Hughes K. (2001). Black cohosh: efficacy, safety, and use in clinical and preclinical applications. *Alternative Therapies in Health and Medicine* **7**, 93–100.

145. Ernst E. (2002). Herbalism and the menopause. *Journal of the British Menopause Society* **June**, 72–74.

146. Borrelli F. and Ernst E. (2002). *Cimicifuga racemosa*: a systematic review of its clinical efficacy. *European Journal of Clinical Pharmacology* **58**, 235–241.

147. Hernandez Munoz G. and Pluchino S. (2003). *Cimicifuga racemosa* for the treatment of hot flushes in women surviving breast cancer. *Maturitas* **44(suppl. 1)**, S59–S65.

148. Jacobson J.S., Troxel A.B., Evans J. *et al.* (2001). Randomized trial of black cohosh for the treatment of hot flashes among women with a history of breast cancer. *Journal of Clinical Oncology* **19**, 2739–2745.

149. Wuttke W., Rimoldi G., Christoffel J. and Seidlova-Wuttke D. (2006). Plant extracts for the treatment of menopausal women: Safe? *Maturitas* **55(suppl. 1)**, S92–S100.

150. Hirata J.D., Swiersz L.M., Zell B., Small R. and Ettinger B. (1997). Does dong quai have estrogenic effects in postmenopausal women? A double-blind, placebo-controlled trial. *Fertility and Sterility* **68**, 981–986.

151. Tice J.A., Ettinger B., Ensrud K. *et al.* (2003). Phytoestrogen supplements for the treatment of hot flashes: The Isoflavone Clover Extract (ICE) Study; a randomized controlled trial. *Journal of the American Medical Society* **290**, 207–214.

152. van de Weijer P. and Barentsen R. (2002). Isoflavones from red clover (Promensil®) significantly reduce menopausal hot flush symptoms compared with placebo. *Maturitas* **42**, 187.

153. Fugh-Berman A. and Kronenberg F. (2001). Red clover (*Trifolium pratense*) for menopausal women: current state of knowledge. *Menopause* **8**, 333–337.

154. Clifton-Bligh P.B., Baber R.J., Fulcher G.R., Nery M.L. and Moreton T. (2001). The effect of isoflavones extracted from red clover (Rimostil) on lipid and bone metabolism. *Menopause* **8**, 259–265.

155. Vincent A. and Fitzpatrick L.A. (2000). Soy isoflavones: are they useful in menopause? *Mayo Clinic Proceedings* **75**, 1174–1184.

156. Berendsen H.H.G. (2002). Hot flushes and serotonin. *Journal of the British Menopause Society* **March**, 30–34.

157. Barton D., La Vasseur B., Loprinzi C. *et al.* (2002). Venlafaxine for the control of hot flashes: results of a longitudinal continuation study. *Oncology Nursing Forum* **29**, 33–40.

158. Loprinzi C.L., Sloan J.A., Perez E.A. *et al.* (2002). Phase III evaluation of fluoxetine for treatment of hot flashes. *Journal of Clinical Oncology* **20**, 1578–1583.

159. Loprinzi C.L., Kugler J.W., Sloan J.A. *et al.* (2000). Venlafaxine in management of hot flashes in survivors of breast cancer: a randomised controlled trial. *Lancet* **356**, 2059–2063.

160. Stearns V., Isaacs C., Rowland J. *et al.* (2000). A pilot trial assessing the efficacy of paroxetine hydrochloride (Paxil) in controlling hot flashes in breast cancer survivors. *Annals of Oncology* **11**, 17–22.

161. Mom C.H., Buijs C., Willemse P.H.B., Mourits M.J.E. and de Vries E.G.E. (2006). Hot flushes in breast cancer patients. *Critical Reviews in Oncology/Hematology* **57**, 63–77.

162. Clayton A.H., Pradko J.F., Croft H.A. *et al.* (2002). Prevalence of sexual dysfunction among newer antidepressants. *Journal of Clinical Psychiatry* **63**, 357–366.

163. Kent J. (2000). SnaRIs, NaSSAs and NaRIs: new agents for the treatment of depression. *Lancet* **335**, 911–918.

164. Freedman R.R. and Dinsay R. (2000). Clonidine raises the sweating threshold in symptomatic but not in asymptomatic postmenopausal women. *Fertility and Sterility* **74**, 20–23.

165. Laufer L.R., Erlik Y., Meldrum D.R. and Judd H.L. (1982). Effect of clonidine on hot flashes in postmenopausal women. *Obstetrics and Gynecology* **60**, 583–586.

166. Bressler L.R., Murphy C.M., Shevrin D.H. and Warren R.F. (1993). Use of clonidine to treat hot flashes secondary to leuprolide or goserelin. *Annals of Pharmacotherapy* **27**, 182–185.

167. Goldberg R.M., Loprinzi C.L., O'Fallon J.R. *et al.* (1994). Transdermal clonidine for ameliorating tamoxifen-induced hot flashes. *Journal of Clinical Oncology* **12**, 155–158 [Published erratum appears in *Journal of Clinical Oncology* **14**, 2411 (1996).]

168. Pandya K.J., Raubertas R.F., Flynn P.J. *et al.* (2000). Oral clonidine in postmenopausal patients with breast cancer experiencing tamoxifen-induced hot flashes: a University of Rochester Cancer Center Community Clinical Oncology Program study. *Annals of Internal Medicine* **132**, 788–793.

169. Loprinzi C.L., Barton D.L. and Rhodes D. (2001). Management of hot flashes in breast-cancer survivors. *The Lancet Oncology* **2**, 199–204.

170. Shanafelt T.D., Barton D.L., Adjei A.A. and Loprinzi C.L. (2002). Pathophysiology and treatment of hot flashes. *Mayo Clinic Proceedings* **77**, 1207–1218.

171. Reidenbach F. (2002). Gabapentin may relieve tamoxifen-related hot flushes. *The Lancet Oncology* **3**, 393.

172. Loprinzi L., Barton D.L., Sloan J.A. *et al.* (2002). Pilot evaluation of gabapentin for treating hot flashes. *Mayo Clinic Proceedings* **77**, 1159–1163.

173. Pandya K., Thummala A., Griggs J. *et al.* (2004). Pilot study using gabapentin for tamoxifen-induced hot flashes in women with breast cancer. *Breast Cancer Research and Treatment* **83**, 87–89.

174. Kendall A., Dowsett M., Folkerd E. and Smith I. (2006). Caution: vaginal estradiol appears to be contraindicated in postmenopausal women on adjuvant aromatase inhibitors. *Annals of Oncology* **17**, 584–587.

175. Gelfand M.M. and Wendman E. (1994). Treating vaginal dryness in breast cancer patients: results of applying a polycarbophil moisturizing gel. *Journal of Women's Health* **3**, 427–434.

176. Bygdeman M. and Swahn M.L. (1996). Replens versus dienoestrol cream in the symptomatic treatment of vaginal atrophy in postmenopausal women. *Maturitas* **23**, 259–263.

177. US Preventive Services Task Force. (2002). Postmenopausal hormone replacement therapy for primary prevention of chronic conditions: recommendations and rationale. *Annals of Internal Medicine* **137**, 834–839.

178. Gnant M. (2006). Management of bone loss induced by aromatase inhibitors. *Cancer Investigation* **24**, 328–330.

179. Reddy K. and Katan M. (2004). Diet, nutrition and the prevention of hypertension and cardiovascular diseases. *Public Health Nutrition* **7**, 167–186.

180. Prentice A. (2004). Diet, nutrition and the prevention of osteoporosis. *Public Health Nutrition* **7**, 227–243.

181. Shaw C.R. (1997). The perimenopausal hot flash: epidemiology, physiology, and treatment. *Nurse Practitioner: American Journal of Primary Health Care* **22**, 55–56.

182. Blatt M., Weisbader H. and Kuppperman H.S. (1953). Vitamin E and climacteric syndrome. *Archives of Internal Medicine* **91**, 792–799.

183. Barton D.L., Loprinzi C.L., Quella S.K. *et al.* (1998). Prospective evaluation of vitamin E for hot flashes in breast cancer survivors. *Journal of Clinical Oncology* **16**, 495–500.

184. Chenoy R., Hussain S., Tayob Y. *et al.* (1994). The effect of oral gamolenic acid from evening primrose oil on menopausal flushing. *British Medical Journal* **308**, 501–503.

185. Fang J., Wylie-Rosett J., Cohen H.W., Kaplan R.C. and Alderman M.H. (2003). Exercise, body mass index, caloric intake, and cardiovascular mortality. *American Journal of Preventive Medicine* **25**, 283–289.

186. Sharkey N.A., Williams N.I. and Guerin J.B. (2000). The role of exercise in the prevention and treatment of osteoporosis and osteoarthritis. *Nursing Clinics of North America* **35**, 209–221.

187. Forwood M.R. and Larsen J.A. (2000). Exercise recommendations for osteoporosis. A position statement of the Australian and New Zealand Bone and Mineral Society. *Australian Family Physician* **29**, 761–764.

188. Teunissen T.A., de Jonge A., van Weel C. and Lagro-Janssen A.L. (2004). Treating urinary incontinence in the elderly – conservative therapies that work: a systematic review. *Journal of Family Practice* **53**, 25–30.

189. Hammar M., Berg G. and Lindgren R. (1990). Does physical exercise influence the frequency of postmenopausal hot flushes? *Acta Obstetrica Gynecologica Scandinavica* **69**, 409–412.

190. Ivarsson T., Spetz A.C. and Hammar M. (1998). Physical exercise and vasomotor symptoms in postmenopausal women. *Maturitas* **29**, 139–146.

191. Hammar M.L., Hammar-Henriksson M.B., Frisk J., Rickenlund A. and Wyon Y.A. (2004). Few oligo-amenorrheic athletes have vasomotor symptoms. *Maturitas* **34**, 219–225.

192. Guthrie J.R., Smith A.M., Dennerstein L. and Morse C. (1994). Physical activity and the menopause experience: a cross-sectional study. *Maturitas* **20**, 71–80.

193. Sternfeld B., Quesenberry C.P.J. and Husson G. (1999). Habitual physical activity and menopausal symptoms: a case–control study. *Journal of Women's Health* **8**, 115–123.

194. Lindh-Åstrand L., Nedstrand E., Wyon Y. and Hammar M. (2004). Vasomotor symptoms and quality of life in previously sedentary postmenopausal women randomised to physical activity or estrogen therapy. *Maturitas* **48**, 97–105.

195. Rohatgi N., Blau R. and Lower E.E. (2002). Raloxifene is associated with less side effects than tamoxifen in women with early breast cancer: a questionnaire study from one physician's practice. *Journal of Women's Health and Gender Based Medicine* **11**, 291–301.

196. Demark-Wahnefried W., Winer E. and Rimer B. (1993). Why women gain weight with adjuvant chemotherapy for breast cancer. *Journal of Clinical Oncology* **11**, 1418–1429.

197. Hoskin P.J., Ashley S. and Yarnold J.R. (1992). Weight gain after primary surgery for breast cancer – effect of tamoxifen. *Breast Cancer Research and Treatment* **22**, 129–132.

198. Leonard R.C.F. and Lee L. (1995). *Choice of Endocrine Treatment for Advanced Breast Cancer: Clinicians' and Patients' Perspectives*. Fourth Nottingham International Breast Cancer Conference. Nottingham: Zeneca.

199. Stearns V. and Gelmann E. (1998). Does tamoxifen cause cancer in humans? *Journal of Clinical Oncology* **16**, 779–792.

200. Ganz P.A., Rowland J.H., Meyerowitz B.E. and Desmond K.A. (1998). Impact of different adjuvant therapy strategies on quality of life in breast cancer survivors. *Recent Results in Cancer Research* **152**, 396–411.

201. Carpenter J.S. and Andrykowski M.A. (1999). Menopausal symptoms in breast cancer survivors. *Oncology Nursing Forum* **26**, 1311–1317.

202. McPhail G. and Smith L.N. (2000). Acute menopause symptoms during adjuvant systemic treatment for breast cancer: a case-control study. *Cancer Nursing* **23**, 430–443.

203. Lion E.M. (1982). *Human Sexuality in Nursing Process*. New York: John Wiley.

204. Colbourne L.C. (2005). *Testicular and Prostate Cancer: Explaining the Treatment and Post Treatment Experience of Couples*. PhD thesis, Southampton University.

205. Jones L. and Webb C. (1994). Young men's experiences of testicular cancer. In Webb C. (ed.) *Living Sexuality: Issues for Nursing and Health*. London: Scutari Press.

206. Gascoigne P., Mason M.D. and Roberts E. (1999). Factors affecting presentation and delay in patients with testicular cancer: results of a qualitative study. *Psycho-oncology* **8**, 144–154.

207. Ofman U. (1993). Psychosocial and sexual implications of genitourinary cancers. *Seminars in Oncology Nursing* **9**, 286–292.

208. Chadwick D., Gillatt D. and Gingell J. (1991). Medical or surgical orchidectomy: the patients' choice. *British Medical Journal* **302**, 572.

209. Butler R.N. and Lewis M.I. (1987). Myths and realities of sex in the later years. *Providers* **13**, 11–13.

210. Charig C.R. and Rundle J.S. (1989). Flushing: long term side effect of orchiectomy in treatment of prostatic carcinoma. *Urology* **33**, 175–178.

CHAPTER FIFTEEN

Complementary and alternative therapies in cancer care

Caroline Hoffman

Introduction

The purpose of this chapter is to give cancer nurses a level of knowledge and understanding about complementary and alternative therapies for people affected by cancer. In this chapter there will be opportunities to understand more about what these therapies are, who is using them and why, to take a look at the evidence base for these therapies and to hear a little from both practitioners and people with cancer who have experienced the therapies for themselves. It is also hoped that the reader will be better informed when people with cancer come along who are either using or thinking of using some of these therapies. What this chapter will not do is make the reader an expert in the field, but rather it offers signposts for both nurses and those they care for to obtain accurate and helpful information in this area.

Defining complementary and alternative therapies

Complementary therapies may be defined as those therapies that are used alongside conventional medical treatments, whereas alternative therapies are those that are used in place of conventional medical treatments for any health condition. The term 'complementary and alternative medicine' is usually referred to as CAM. The group of therapies that form part of CAM may vary according

to the definition that is adopted. Defining which therapies may be included as complementary is not an exact science as experts may disagree as to which therapies should be included or excluded. The British House of Lords (2000) Science and Technology Select Committee published a special report on complementary and alternative medicine classifying therapies into different systems and classifying therapies into three groups, professionally organised alternative therapies, complementary therapies, and alternative disciplines (see Box 15.1).[1] This classification was done for

Box 15.1 Categories of CAM disciplines from House of Lords Report[1]

Group 1: Professionally organised therapies
Acupuncture, chiropractic, herbal medicine, homeopathy, osteopathy.

Group 2: Complementary therapies
Alexander technique, aromatherapy, Bach and other flower remedies, bodywork therapies including massage, counselling stress therapy, hypnotherapy, meditation, reflexology, shiatsu, healing, Maharishi Ayurvedic medicine, nutritional medicine, yoga.

Group 3: Alternative disciplines
- *3a: long-established and traditional systems of healthcare* – anthroposophical medicine, Ayurvedic medicine, Chinese herbal medicine, Eastern medicine (Tibb), naturopathy, traditional Chinese medicine
- *3b: other alternative disciplines* – crystal therapy, dowsing, iridology, kinesiology, and radionics.

operational purposes. The Cochrane Collaboration[2] defines CAM as a broad domain of healing resources that encompasses all health systems, modalities, and practices and their accompanying theories and beliefs, other than those intrinsic to the politically dominant health systems of a particular society or culture in a given historical period.[2]

Possibly the most clear definition to date is that from the USA National Center for Complementary and Alternative Medicine which classifies CAM therapies into five categories, or domains,[3] which in summary is as follows:

1. *Alternative medical systems* built upon complete systems of theory and practice. Examples of alternative medical systems include homeopathic medicine and naturopathic medicine, traditional Chinese medicine and Ayurveda.
2. *Mind–body interventions* use a variety of techniques designed to enhance the mind's capacity to affect bodily function and symptoms. Other mind–body techniques include meditation, prayer, mental healing, and therapies that use creative outlets such as art, music, or dance.
3. *Biologically based therapies* use substances found in nature, such as herbs, foods, and vitamins. Some examples include dietary supplements,[3] herbal products, and the use of other so-called natural but as yet scientifically unproven therapies (for example, using shark cartilage to treat cancer).
4. *Manipulative and body-based methods* are based on manipulation and/or movement of one or more parts of the body. Some examples include chiropractic or osteopathic manipulation and massage.
5. *Energy therapies* involve the use of energy fields and include therapies intended to affect energy fields that purportedly surround and penetrate the human body. Examples include qi gong, Reiki, and therapeutic touch.

An integrated approach to cancer care includes the best of the orthodox medical treatments and the best evidence-based, supportive complementary modalities that relieve many of the physical and emotional symptoms that people with cancer may experience.[4] The Prince's Foundation for Integrated Health in the UK has adopted the term 'integrated' (or 'integrative' as it is referred to in the USA),[5] with reference to this combined approach to healthcare. This term 'integrated' is often used in preference to 'complementary', as it better acknowledges a collaborative working between conventional and complementary health care practitioners to best support the ongoing needs of the people with cancer or other illnesses.

This chapter will focus mostly on complementary therapies for cancer, those that can be used alongside, and in combination with, orthodox medical treatments.[6] In cancer care, complementary therapies may be used before, during and after medical treatments. Some of the therapies discussed in this chapter, if used to the exclusion of conventional medical treatments, would be regarded as alternative. The chapter will not focus on alternative cancer therapies, but does discuss them briefly so that nurses can help guide people with cancer appropriately regarding these alternative approaches to cancer. Broadly speaking, there is a lack of rigorous scientific evidence to support these alternative approaches, but more detail will be found on this towards the end of this chapter.

The use of CAM in cancer

The use of CAM by people with cancer has been surveyed extensively throughout the Western world. In a review of 26 surveys looking at complementary and alternative therapies in cancer care from 13 countries, Ernst and Cassileth found that 7–64% of patients with cancer used these therapies, with an average of 31% across all studies.[7] In a European survey of 14 countries, Molassiotis *et al.* found that an average of 35.9% of people (a range of 14.8–73.1%) with cancer ($n = 956$) used some form of complementary or alternative medicine.[8] In a study looking at the prevalence of complementary therapy use by women with breast cancer in the South Thames region of London, Rees *et al.* found that 22.4% of women diagnosed with breast cancer ($n = 1023$) over the last 7 years had consulted a complementary practitioner in the previous 12 months; 31.5% of these women had done so since diagnosis.[9] In as Israeli study performed by Paltiel *et al.*

($n = 526$), 51% of participants had used complementary therapies since their diagnosis,[10] compared with the findings of Boon *et al.*, where 66.7% ($n = 557$) of a Canadian sample of breast cancer survivors were using these therapies.[11] In an Australian study looking at the use of complementary and alternative therapy use amongst people with advanced cancer ($n = 111$), 48% of participants used these therapies.[12] They found that overall, CAM users reported higher levels of anxiety and pain, less satisfaction with conventional medicine, and lower need for control over treatment decisions compared to non-users. However, it is interesting that the researchers found many of these findings were reversed between users and non-users who were getting towards the end of life.

Virtually all studies conducted internationally report that, where detailed, people who seek complementary therapies are better educated, of higher socio-economic status, and more likely to be female and also younger than those who do not.[8,13,14] On the financial side, some of the reason for this may be that, with the exception of a few voluntary organisations and hospitals providing complementary therapies, most people need to pay for these therapies out of their own pockets.

Care strategy 15.1

The surveys regarding CAM in cancer use performed to date found that there is anything between a 7% and 66% chance that people with cancer will be using some form or another of CAM, so it is an important question for nurses to enquire about when speaking with people with cancer who come to them for support. It is also worth bearing in mind the kind of people who are more likely to use CAM: younger women, with a better education or a higher socio-economic status.

CAM therapies used by people with cancer

The provision of complementary therapies for people affected by cancer has been growing worldwide. There is no set range of complementary therapies that people with cancer are using, and it has been found through a systematic review[7] that

the range is as wide as from diets and relaxation to Iscador (mistletoe therapy) and traditional Chinese medicine.[7] The most commonly noted complementary and alternative therapies across all studies include mind–body approaches (meditation, relaxation, hypnotherapy, visualisation, and other imagery techniques), reflexology, dietary approaches and food supplements, Chinese medications, botanical preparations, homeopathy and spiritual healing.[7]

Herbal medicines and remedies were most commonly used by Europeans with cancer,[8] with herbal medicines and remedies being the most commonly used, together with homeopathy, vitamins/minerals, medicinal teas, spiritual therapies, and relaxation techniques. Herbal medicine use was found to triple from before to after a cancer diagnosis.

In a guide of UK complementary therapy services produced by Macmillan Cancer Support in 2002, the available services were as follows: hospices provide 36%, hospitals 31%, and up to 20% is based in the voluntary sector.[6] Over 90% of services offer touch therapies such as massage, aromatherapy and reflexology. Relaxation and visualisation is offered in over 80% of services, healing and energy work including Reiki, spiritual healing and therapeutic touch are also widely available in 45% of services.

Reasons for using CAM in cancer

Complementary therapies may be used alongside conventional medical treatments for a variety of reasons, including the belief on the part of users that they:

- may help cure cancer, prevent it recurring
- boost the immune system
- reduce the symptoms of cancer or the side-effects of cancer treatment
- assist their body to heal
- are perceived as non-toxic
- are holistic by nature
- enhance well-being
- give a feeling of control with respect to their treatment, or allow more patient participation in treatment

- help with the emotional or mood disturbance that may occur as a result of diagnosis, treatment, and prognosis.[8,14–16]

Downer et al.[14] and Paltiel et al.[10] suggested that people who use complementary and alternative therapies in cancer care may do so because they are suffering from more emotional or social distress or despair, and Boon et al. suggest that people using these therapies may have a lesser belief than non-users in the power of conventional medicine to cure their condition than non-users.[11] Downer et al. reported that those using complementary therapies were shown to be more anxious, had concern over the side-effects of conventional treatment, or concern about being left in a 'no hope' situation from conventional medicine.[14] Complementary therapy users also believed that conventional therapies have side-effects and weaken the body's natural defences, while also wanting more control over treatment decisions.[10]

In order to better understand how people with cancer use complementary therapies, a longitudinal study using a biographic narrative approach is currently being performed by Corner and Harewood of people with cancer who have declared themselves to be users or non-users of these therapies.[17] These authors also acknowledge that the use of both complementary and alternative therapies amongst people with cancer represents a naturally occurring system of consumer-led and self-managed health care from which conventional health care systems may be able to learn.

Disclosure of CAM usage

One of the most concerning aspects of this turn to complementary therapies is the fact that many people with cancer who are using them do not feel that they can tell their doctors. This is from fear of ridicule or being told 'well it won't do you any harm', both of which are equally disempowering for people wishing to help themselves or manage symptoms that are poorly controlled with conventional medicines. This is an area where nurses looking after these people can help when taking a nursing history or enquiring about how people are supporting themselves through the experience of

cancer and its treatments. While some authors report that this unhelpful attitude amongst some members of the medical profession is improving,[17] from recent conversations that the author has had with women with breast cancer at the time of writing this chapter, there is still a long way to go in order to allow people with cancer to feel that they can safely and fully disclose the nature and extent of CAM usage. The danger inherent with this lack of disclosure is the risk of interactions between conventional medicines and some complementary therapies, particularly herbal medicines or dietary supplements, and the possibility that these might affect the therapeutic impact of conventional cancer treatments. This will be discussed in more detail later in this chapter.

It is interesting to note that Molassiotis et al. found that the main reasons that people with cancer gave for not using CAM were that they were happy with the conventional treatment they received ($n = 236$; 43.4%), some had never thought of CAM ($n = 82$; 15.1%), and others said that they did not believe in it.[8]

How do complementary therapies work?

Trained in a conventional Western medical model, many nurses find it easy to compartmentalise symptoms that people suffer from. It is easy to think of physical, mental or emotional symptoms experienced by people when they are ill. Increasingly the link between mind and body is being understood better by science, and over the last 20 years there has been groundbreaking work done revealing the complex link between the mind and the body and how each influences the other, not as previously thought simply 'one-way traffic' from the brain to the body.[18]

Using complementary therapies can have the effect of inducing a response which brings the mind and body back into a better state of balance or homeostasis. Another way of putting this is that it helps achieve a balance in the autonomic nervous system, where sympathetic and parasympathetic drives are in better balance. When in this state, the body's own natural healing mechanisms can work more effectively. There is a natural mechanism in the body to heal and repair itself, which on the simplest level is seen in the repair of damaged tissue. In the same sense, the mind has a natural longing or desire to be in a state of balance and to have 'some peace of mind'. This can be particularly helpful when a person's world has been turned upside down through the experience of a cancer diagnosis and its treatments and possible consequences. Using complementary therapies can help facilitate this process and also, as a result, can be found to help reduce the severity of symptoms in many situations. While this idea may seem oversimplified, through using different complementary therapies, people can help come to know and understand themselves better, raise their levels of self-awareness, and find more appropriate ways of coping with cancer and the stressors of everyday life.

An integrated approach to cancer care

Complementary therapies are best used in a fully integrated way for people with cancer. This means that both the doctor and the therapists should be fully informed of the current medical and complementary treatments that the person is having, to ensure their safety and to optimise effectiveness on all sides. Breast Cancer Haven, a registered charity which has day centres offering free support, information and complementary therapies to people affected by breast cancer, has developed a model of integrated health care showing how this can work (see Figure 15.1). In this model it can be seen that there is regular correspondence between the hospital/general practitioner (GP) and complementary therapy teams to communicate the medical condition of the patient and their treatment, any complementary therapies being undertaken, and the outcome of such therapies.

Research into CAM and cancer

In recent years, there have been a number of projects, particularly in the UK and US, reviewing the current evidence base for complementary therapies, including the area of cancer care.

In the UK there is an ongoing project funded by the Department of Health which provided funds for the Research Council for Complementary Medicine (RCCM) to systematically review the clinical evidence for complementary therapies in three health care areas including cancer. The NHS Priorities Project is a 3-year project which is being conducted by the Research Council for Complementary Medicine in collaboration with the School of Integrated Health, University of Westminster, London, UK.

The aims are to:

- carry out a detailed review and critical appraisal of the published research in specific complementary therapies, focusing on key areas of NHS priority
- make this information available to health care professionals, researchers and the public via the internet
- maintain an evidence-based information resource that reflects current research evidence, and to establish an ongoing process for updating this information.

The main outcome of the project is the Complementary and Alternative Medicine Evidence Online (CAMEOL) database,[19] providing a review of the evidence available aimed at health care professionals where, to date, 13 different reviews have been performed giving the current state of evidence for a number of different complementary and alternative therapies in cancer care, or looking at common cancer symptoms and reviewing the state of the evidence for complementary therapies to assist with these.

In 2006 in Great Britain, the National Library for Health (NLH)[20] launched its own CAM specialist library which is looking at the following topics at the first stage of the library's development: acupuncture, aromatherapy, chiropractic, herbal medicine, homeopathy, hypnosis, massage, meditation, osteopathy, reflexology, and yoga. In the future other therapies will be included in the systematic search for resources, and the library eventually will provide information on a broader range of CAM therapies, including dietary and nutritional therapies.

The Cochrane Library has on its database an increasing number of systematic reviews and meta-analyses of complementary therapies research,[21] and this is a useful source of research-based information when searching for evidence.

In order to develop and promote research into complementary therapies in the UK, in 2004, the National Cancer Research Institute (NCRI) developed a Complementary Therapies Clinical Studies Development Group (CTCSDG),[22] one of 23 groups covering major cancer sites and other generic issues. The group is composed of oncologists, complementary therapists, academic researchers, complementary therapy users, health economists, statisticians, and representatives from research networks. The group was created to build a portfolio of high-quality research into complementary (not alternative) therapies in cancer. It has identified three priority areas:

1 physical and psychological effects of specific complementary therapies in cancer patients
2. safety of complementary interventions when used with conventional cancer treatments
3. use of complementary therapies to control adverse physical and psychological effects of conventional cancer treatments.

To achieve these aims the group offers support, advice, and guidance to individuals and groups wishing to develop studies on complementary therapies in cancer care; it does not actually fund the studies itself, but helps to create studies that would be more likely to get funding as they are well designed.

In the US, the National Institutes of Health (NIH) have a dedicated centre for the study of complementary therapies, entitled the National Center for Complementary and Alternative Medicine (NCCAM),[3] which is one of the 27 institutes and centres that make up the NIH. The NIH is one of eight agencies under the public health service (PHS) in the Department of Health and Human Services (DHHS). NCCAM is dedicated to exploring complementary and alternative healing practices in the context of rigorous science, training CAM researchers, and disseminating authoritative information to the public and professionals.

Their four primary areas of focus for NCCAM are:[3]

1. *research* – they support clinical and basic science research projects in CAM by awarding grants

across the country and around the world; they also design, study, and analyse clinical and laboratory-based studies on the NIH campus in Bethesda, Maryland
2. *research training and career development* – they award grants that provide training and career-development opportunities for predoctoral, postdoctoral, and career researchers
3. *outreach* – they sponsor conferences, educational programmes, and exhibits, operate an information clearinghouse to answer inquiries and requests for information, provide a website and printed publications, and hold town meetings at selected locations in the US
4. *integration* – to integrate scientifically proven CAM practices into conventional medicine, they announce published research results, study ways to integrate evidence-based CAM practices into conventional medical practice, and support programmes to develop models for incorporating CAM into the curriculum of medical, dental, and nursing schools.

From this work there are many valuable research projects being performed that are adding to the evidence for the different complementary therapies in cancer care.

Education in CAM for cancer

There is no global standard of training and practice in complementary therapies. At present, a number of complementary therapies may be studied at degree, masters or PhD level with academic institutions, examples of which in the UK include the University of Westminster's Department of Complementary Therapies in the School of Integrated Health.[23] This kind of education would be regarded as a 'gold standard' for the training of therapists in the current health climate. There are still many complementary therapy courses offered by therapy schools not associated with any formal educational system run throughout the UK and in other parts of the world, the standards of training from which may vary. Little exists to date for the training of complementary therapists in the area of cancer. This is a developing area and one where cancer nurses will be able to support and collaborate with academic institutions in the training and development of complementary therapists to ensure that they can work at a safe level with people affected by cancer.

Regulation in CAM

The process of regulation of CAM in the UK is a slow, ongoing process. Most complementary therapy bodies in the UK are self-regulated, with only osteopathy and chiropractic being statutorily regulated in the same way as nurses, doctors, and other allied health professionals. While there are some therapies organised by very well-established and regarded professional bodies, such as the British Acupuncture Council, other professional complementary therapy self-regulatory bodies are not so well developed. It is the aim of most self-regulating CAM professional bodies to head towards statutory regulation. This is a slow and difficult process which may take several more years to achieve in some of the most popular and well-regarded CAM therapies such as homeopathy, acupuncture, and herbal medicine. This may cause a potential difficulty for people with cancer, who may wish to access the services of a well-qualified CAM therapist, to be able to know which therapists are best trained and most regulated. In the UK, The Prince's Foundation for Integrated Health has created a booklet that is available on its website to help guide people looking for CAM practitioners.[5] The foundation is supporting the process of regulation for complementary therapies, and similar processes examining the standards of education and practice are happening in countries as far as the US and Australia where different healthcare systems are in place. The hope for this in the future is that they ensure, as far as possible, safety and quality of standards of care for any person seeking a CAM practitioner.

Provision and availability of complementary therapy services

An increasing number of complementary therapies for people with cancer are being offered in the hospital and hospice settings.[6] These environments can offer a safe and appropriate service for people with cancer when used in an integrated way. The Prince's Foundation for Integrated Health and the National Council for Hospice and Specialist Palliative Care Service have produced *National Guidelines for the Use of Complementary Therapies in Supportive and Palliative Care* which is a valuable guide to any health care organisation wishing to develop a service of complementary therapies, as well as being a useful guide for cancer nurses to understand more about the issues of service development and delivery including policy development.[24] While many complementary therapy services are developing, each person with cancer generally receives a quota of treatments, sometimes as little as four hours during their cancer treatments. This restriction is generally due to a high demand and lack of resources for any service that is free of charge.

There are a number of charities and other voluntary or not-for-profit organisations offering complementary therapies to people with cancer. In the UK, one of the best known and established of these is the Bristol Cancer Help Centre,[25] which has been running for over 25 years. A pioneer in its field offering high standards of care, it is a residential centre offering information and complementary therapies to people affected by cancer, and many other centres have been inspired by the work of this centre. A possible drawback of this centre is that it generally relies on payment for its services.

Breast Cancer Haven (BCH) is an example of a registered charity which provides day centres offering support, counselling, information and complementary therapies free of charge to people affected by breast cancer.[26] Staffed by cancer nurses, counsellors, and complementary therapists, Havens offer help before, during and after medical treatment for breast cancer. Each person with breast cancer attending the centre is offered a minimum of 30 hours' individual and group therapy time free of charge. Carers are also offered counselling and the opportunity to join a support group. BCH has two Havens in England, London and Hereford, with an additional centre planned for Yorkshire and plans for further centres around the country. Working in a fully integrated way with hospital cancer teams and community cancer

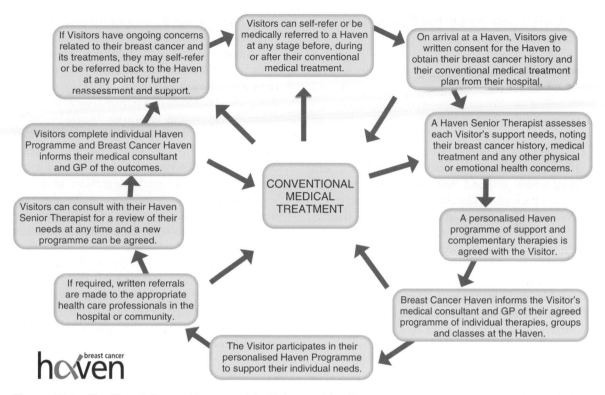

Figure 15.1 The Breast Cancer Haven model of integrated health care.

nurses, BCH ensures that all its treatments are safe and appropriate, working from the best available evidence for each therapy. The Breast Cancer Haven model of integrated health care is included in Figure 15.1.

In other countries, the US and Australia for example, most of the therapy provision for cancer comes either through hospitals or designated centres such as Commomweal located on the coast north of San Fransisco, USA,[27] or The Gawler Foundation, in the countryside near Melbourne, Australia.[28] Centres like these offer wonderful programmes and retreats for people affected by cancer, but there is generally a charge for the programmes.

Guiding people with cancer seeking complementary therapies

In order to be able to guide people to safe and appropriate complementary therapies, cancer nurses need to be familiar themselves with what is available in terms of complementary therapy services and also with the appropriate guidance to give people looking for CAM practitioners. Documents produced by the Prince's Foundation for Integrated Health *Complementary Healthcare: A Guide for Patients* or NCCAM's document *Selecting a Complementary and Alternative Medicine (CAM) Practitioner*[3] are very helpful. The implications of this for people with cancer is that complementary therapists may have limited knowledge of working with people with cancer and little understanding of their needs. Nurses should have some basic knowledge themselves to guide people with cancer appropriately when seeking out complementary therapy practitioners. It is important for nurses to ensure that the person wants to be engaged in the particular complementary therapy on offer and that it is safe and appropriate for that person. A particular therapy should never be forced on any person simply because this is the only complementary therapy on offer or available at that time.

The evidence base for CAM in cancer

As with many fields of nursing, the evidence base for the use of CAM therapies in cancer care and with other health conditions is under development and growing fast, with an increase in interest in their area. Many universities are now setting up departments of complementary therapies, and within these there is rigorous research being performed. This is good news for complementary therapies as more rigorous trials are now being performed which can add to the evidence base in this field. As with any area of research, there is tough competition for funding from the small number of sources that may choose to fund CAM therapies in cancer.

In this chapter, there will be a review of the evidence for the use of complementary therapies in cancer care on a the basis of the hierarchy of evidence. Where they exist, meta-analyses and systematic reviews will be looked at first, then randomised controlled trials (RCTs) and other studies including any qualitative studies that may have been performed. In addition to this, there is a more practical clinical dimension added to the information presented here, from asking both complementary therapists and people with cancer alike how they have found the various therapies useful. There is also a section on safety. Unfortunately this review, while being systematic, is not complete, as much of the systematic review work of CAM in cancer is still in progress.

There are a couple of areas that have not been included in the CAM review for reasons explained below.

1. Manipulative therapies such as osteopathy and chiropractic are not included in this review and should be used cautiously by people with cancer. While these therapists are amongst the most highly skilled and well-established and regulated of complementary therapists in the UK, unless working with the most recent X-rays and scan results, there may be risks that these therapies could exacerbate problems for people with bony metastases or reduced bone density. If people with cancer wish to use manipulative therapies, they should discuss this with their oncologist and the manipulative therapist concerned.

2. Nutritional and dietary therapies for cancer. This is a large topic and one that can arguably be regarded as good basic health care rather than complementary therapies. No one would argue that everyone, ill or well should be eating a healthy diet, balanced between the food groups with plenty of fresh fruit and vegetables. However, in cancer care there are debates about the value of excluding meat as a preventative for colon cancer, or dairy products in the case of women with oestrogen-positive breast cancers; however, the current evidence does not help us to know which is the best way to advise patients. So often, as with many other things in life, moderation is the key and eating as good a quality food as is available. However, in the table on alternative therapies, a couple of alternative diets are discussed for information.

The following tables give information from systematic review in relation to the following symptoms for cancer:

Table 15.1: Acupuncture for pain
Table 15.2: Acupuncture-point stimulation for nausea and vomiting
Table 15.3: Acupuncture for hot flushes
Table 15.4: Hypnosis in cancer care
Table 15.5: Hypnosis for nausea and vomiting
Table 15.6: Aromatherapy and massage in cancer care
Table 15.7: Homeopathy in cancer care
Table 15.8: Reflexology in cancer care
Table 15.9: Yoga in cancer care
Table 15.10: Meditation in cancer care
Table 15.11: Mindfulness-based stress reduction (MBSR) in cancer care
Table 15.12: Chinese herbal medicine for side-effects of chemotherapy
Table 15.13: Western herbal medicine
Table 15.14: Black cohosh for hot flushes
Table 15.15: Mistletoe (*Viscum album*) in cancer care
Table 15.16: Essiac in cancer care
Table 15.17: Bach flower remedies in cancer care
Table 15.18: Alternative therapies for cancer

Table 15.1 Acupuncture for pain

Therapy	Evidence for use	What practitioners say	What users say	Safety/precautions
Acupuncture: the insertion of fine sterile disposable needles into certain points on the body. Its mode of action is thought to stimulate the release of endorphins and enkephalins as well as the distribution of many neurotransmitters and neuromodalities.	A recent systematic review suggests that more appropriately powered studies should be performed.[29] It is worth noting that the most recent and rigorous studies showed positive results. One high-quality study showed significant results with ear acupuncture and cancer pain.[30]	Acupuncture has been used for centuries in the management of pain for all types. It often takes a regular course of acupuncture treatments to significantly reduce more chronic pain (6 treatments), whereas acute pain can often be treated more quickly.	With the pain from secondary bone cancer, I found that the acupuncture treatments were useful in addition to the pain medication I was receiving. I also found the sessions relaxing and I slept better as a result.	• Acupuncture is generally a safe therapy when administered by well-trained and qualified acupuncturists. • Acupuncture-point stimulation by any method is safe with minimal, transient and rare side-effects.[31] • For people with lymphoedema, needling into the affected area should be avoided.

Table 15.2 Acupuncture-point stimulation for nausea and vomiting

Therapy	Evidence for use	What practitioners say	What users say	Safety/precautions
Acupuncture-point stimulation on acupuncture point P6.	A Cochrane review of acupuncture point stimulation for chemotherapy-induced nausea and vomiting from 11 trials ($n = 1247$) suggested a biological effect.[32] They found electroacupuncture to be effective for acute first-day vomiting after chemotherapy. Self-administered acupressure appears to have reduced chemotherapy-induced nausea severity and can readily be taught to patients. Neither acupressure nor electrostimulation offered significant relief for delayed symptoms.	When the P6 point is located accurately on the lower inner forearm, stimulation to this point is found to help with nausea and vomiting of all kinds, including that induced by chemotherapy.	I found it helpful to use the commercial products for travel sickness which I found at the chemist to help with nausea during my chemotherapy. These are like a round button on a piece of elastic that can be worn on the inner forearm to stimulate the acupuncture point. If I forget these, I find that pressing the point with my thumb can also be helpful.	• Acupuncture-point stimulation by any method is safe with minimal, transient and rare side-effects.[31] • For people with lymphoedema, needling into the affected area should be avoided.

Table 15.3 Acupuncture for hot flushes

Therapy	Evidence for use	What practitioners say	What users say	Safety/precautions
Acupuncture for hot flushes.	A systematic review of the research evidence for the effectiveness of acupuncture for the treatment of hot flushes in cancer patients was performed, revealing three RCTs, nine uncontrolled studies and one qualitative study.[33] The uncontrolled studies suggested that acupuncture may show benefits for the alleviation of hot flush symptoms resulting from tamoxifen use in women, or from castration therapy in men.	Acupuncture given as an individual prescription or in the more general form or auricular (ear) acupuncture seems to help the women with breast cancer who are suffering from hot flushes, in terms of their frequency and severity.	I find that the acupuncture always gives me a good night's sleep when normally I would wake up several times in the night from hot flushes. Following my course of acupuncture I found that my frequency of hot flushes reduced. I was no longer getting them at night, and in the day they were down to a quarter of what they were before and not so intense. In addition I was less moody.	• Acupuncture-point stimulation by any method is safe with minimal, transient and rare side-effects.[31] • For people with lymphoedema, needling into the affected area should be avoided.

Table 15.4 Hypnosis in cancer care

Therapy	Evidence for use	What practitioners say	What users say	Safety/precautions
Hypnosis	One review[34] of studies to date has explored the usefulness of hypnosis for the management of pain, hot flushes, nausea and vomiting, immune function, and general quality of life which has shown proven efficacy in actual symptom management.[34] Another review of hypnotherapy for cancer procedures and distress in children found seven RCTs and one controlled trial.[35] Studies here reported positive results including statistically significant reductions in pain and anxiety for children undergoing bone marrow aspirations or lumbar punctures.	Patients enjoy the hypnotic experience. They obtain relief without destructive or unpleasant effects. It is a skill that individuals can easily learn, that provides a personal sense of mastery and control over their problems and that counters feelings of helplessness and powerlessness.	I found that I could apply the hypnotherapy I learned to manage post-operative pain and anxiety to the nausea and vomiting I experienced during chemotherapy. From this point of view I have found learning hypnosis very useful indeed.	• It is safe and does not produce adverse effects or drug interactions.[34,35] • There is no reduction of normal function or mental capacity and no development of tolerance to the hypnotic effect.

Table 15.5 Hypnosis for nausea and vomiting

Therapy	Evidence for use	What practitioners say	What users say	Safety/precautions
Hypnosis is a procedure in which a therapist suggests that the client experiences changes in sensation, perception, thought and behaviour.	A systematic review of the evidence on the effectiveness of hypnosis for chemotherapy-induced nausea and vomiting involving six RCTs, five of which involved children.[32] Studies were small but included comparison against other therapies and no treatment. Studies reported positive results including statistically significant reductions in anticipatory and chemotherapy-induced nausea and vomiting.	Hypnosis works on the principle that the recipient can learn to achieve a deeply relaxed state whereby they can be desensitised to stressful situations. Usually done through a series of half to one hour appointments, the person can be given a post-hypnotic suggestion which enables them to induce the hypnotic state after the treatment course is completed, including when going for chemotherapy, anticipatory nausea prior to treatment, as well as for a range of other fears and anxieties related to cancer, its treatments and possible outcomes.	I thought I would be stuck feeling ill throughout all my chemotherapy treatments, so I decided to get some help to learn how I could do something for myself to ease the distress. I was surprised that it helped me so much, as I really didn't expect it to. I was also able to apply what I learned to other aspects of my treatment and recovery from cancer.	• Hypnosis can sometimes exacerbate psychological problems in people who are vulnerable psychologically. • Hypnosis should be avoided in people suffering from established psychosis, borderline psychosis, and those with personality disorders.

Table 15.6 Aromatherapy and massage in cancer care

Therapy	Evidence for use	What practitioners say	What users say	Safety/precautions
Aromatherapy and massage	A Cochrane review looked at the evidence for aromatherapy and massage for symptom relief in patients with cancer.[36] Eight randomised controlled trials met the inclusion criteria ($n = 357$). The most consistently found effect of massage or aromatherapy massage was on anxiety, with four trials ($n = 207$) showing a reduction of between 19% and 32%. Contradictory evidence exists as to any additional benefit conferred by the addition of aromatherapy. The impact of massage/aromatherapy on depression was variable. Of three trials ($n = 120$), only one found a significant difference in this symptom. Three studies found a reduction in pain ($n = 117$) following intervention, and two ($n = 71$) found a reduction in nausea.	Many people affected by cancer find great comfort from the feeling of touch as well as the well-being experienced from the odour of the aromas which have a direct effect on the limbic system of the brain and so can affect mood state and well-being. The chemical contents of the different essential oils lend themselves to being used to help with symptomatic relief.	Until I had cancer and had a massage, my body had not been touched for 13 years. I found great comfort from this experience as well as a deep sense of relaxation. I could not sleep well during my treatment, but found that putting a few drops of lavender oil on a tissue near my pillow did help me sleep better at night.	• Essential oils used in topical aromatherapy massage are plant products and, in general, should be used under the guidance of a trained aromatherapist. • While there are some oils containing substances that are contraindicated for people with cancer,[37] these oils are generally not available over the counter in pharmacies or via reliable essential oil suppliers. • Gentle therapeutic massage is safe for people at any stage of the cancer journey. • Massage does not stimulate the circulation or lymphatic system any more than gentle exercise, so is not regarded as a risk to spreading cancer around the body.[38]

Table 15.7 Homeopathy in cancer care

Therapy	Evidence for use	What practitioners say	What users say	Safety/precautions
Homeopathy: homeopathic remedies are thought to trigger the body's own defence and self-regulatory response; however, their mode of action is unclear. Using minute doses of substances, they act as a stimulus to the body. The idea that the effects of homeopathy are completely due to placebo have not been sustained.[39]	From a review of the efficacy of homeopathic therapy in cancer care, six out of a potential 55 studies met the inclusion criteria for the review.[40] Five out of the six studies yielded positive results, which suggest the effectiveness of homeopathy in cancer care in the areas of chemotherapy-induced stomatitis,[41] radiodermatitis,[42,43] and general adverse events from radiotherapy. Breast cancer survivors suffering from menopausal symptoms experienced a general improvement in their quality of life. There is currently a Cochrane review in progress of homeopathy for adverse events in cancer management.[44]	People with cancer can be helped greatly in terms of symptomatic relief with homeopathy. This has happened when dealing with pain, including pain from metastatic spread, hot flushes, grief and low mood as well as the side-effects of radiotherapy and chemotherapy. Two homeopathic remedies that can be useful when undergoing radiotherapy are called X Ray and Rad Brom. These can be taken in a 30C potency each day that radiotherapy is given, to ease the local skin and general side-effects from radiotherapy.	I was feeling extremely low and tearful, grieving, I think, for the loss of my health and very afraid of the treatment for my cancer. The homeopath gave me a remedy called Ignatia and within days I was feeling a lot better within myself. Starting radiotherapy brought me to my knees, I felt exhausted and lightheaded, unable to think as well as getting sore skin over the area. I was recommended some homeopathic remedies which enabled me to cope and not feel so tired.	• Homeopathic substances, being highly diluted and given in a minimal dose, do not hold risk of chemical interactions with other pharmaceutical agents and are therefore safe for people undergoing cancer treatments. NB: This is in contrast to herbal medicines (which are different from homeopathic remedies), which are made from raw plant materials and for which there is a known list of interactions with pharmacological agents.

Table 15.8 Reflexology in cancer care

Therapy	Evidence for use	What practitioners say	What users say	Safety/precautions
Reflexology stimulates areas on the feet which are thought to have a relationship to the rest of the body. The practitioner works on the feet according to the look and feel of the particular areas, to rebalance the body and reduce symptoms.	A Cochrane review of reflexology for symptom relief in patients with cancer has been performed, but, at the time of writing this chapter, it has been withdrawn from publication.[45] In a small randomised study ($n = 30$), state anxiety was evaluated amongst patients receiving second- and third-cycle chemotherapy, finding significant decrease in state anxiety following reflexology compared to controls ($P < 0.0001$).[46] In another study[47] evaluating the effect of foot reflexology in patients with lung or breast cancer ($n = 23$), there was found to be an immediate positive effect of foot reflexology with a reduction in pain and anxiety.[47] A further study found that patients with metastatic disease who reported pain ($n = 36$) also found it to be beneficial in the short term.[48]	Reflexology can be helpful as it is a gentle non-invasive technique that can be given to most people affected by cancer as it works on the area of the feet.

The powerful ability of this therapy to help to reduce the severity of symptoms related to cancer and its treatments is one that makes it so popular. | When I was having chemotherapy I was constantly feeling tired. I found that a regular reflexology treatment really picked me up and I left the treatment feeling light and energised.

I have had significant pain in by back due to cancer but find that weekly reflexology helps to ease the pain a lot. I always get a good night's sleep after my treatment. | • Reflexology is a safe therapy for people with cancer as it uses only touch, usually to the soles of the feet.
• The amount of pressure used depends on the tolerance of the recipient and can be done with more or less pressure accordingly. For patients with very sensitive feet, a pair of thick socks may be worn. |

Table 15.9 Yoga in cancer care

Therapy	Evidence for use	What practitioners say	What users say	Safety/precautions
Yoga is the integration or harmonisation of the mind, body and breath. Yoga uses stretches, postures and breathing exercises to achieve this.	In a systematic review of the literature evaluating the effectiveness of yoga as a supportive therapy in cancer, only four RCTs and three uncontrolled studies were found.[49] There is some limited evidence to suggest that yoga can reduce sleep disturbance,[50] and increase emotional well-being and spiritual integration.[51]	Yoga can be a useful tool at all stages of cancer and yoga practice can be adapted to suit even the most ill, e.g. breathing exercises can be performed. Yoga is excellent to help with mobility following cancer surgery and for example, with breast cancer; these exercises can also help in the prevention of the development of lymphoedema. The calming and energising effects of regular yoga practice cannot be overemphasised.	Following my cancer surgery, I was given a few post-operative exercises by the physio, but other than that, I was pretty scared of moving too much in case I made matters worse. When I had finally recovered from my surgery and could exercise again, I was frightened to go to an exercise class given by someone who did not understand what I had been through. I found an experienced yoga teacher especially trained to look after people who have had cancer and other illnesses, so was guided by her to a point that I was then able to join a more general yoga class nearer my home.	• People with cancer should seek out a suitably qualified yoga teacher who is experienced in working with people with a cancer diagnosis. They can be found in the Iyengar Yoga Institute and with teachers trained in yoga therapy.

Table 15.10 Meditation in cancer care

Therapy	Evidence for use	What practitioners say	What users say	Safety/precautions
Meditation includes techniques such as awareness of the breath, repeating a mantra or witnessing of thoughts to focus the attention and to bring about a state of self-awareness and inner calm.[52]	A systematic review of meditation in cancer has been performed, which included four RCTs and three uncontrolled studies.[53] The review found that meditation may have the potential to provide benefit to patients as a supportive therapy. There is some limited evidence that meditation can increase positive coping and optimism, and reduce the severity of chemotherapy and nausea.	The practice of meditation gives people with cancer and their carers a self-management tool to help cope with the stresses of diagnosis and treatments, as well as a tool to help people gain a sense of peace and calm in everyday life.	I used my meditation technique when I went in for a scan. This not only gave my mind something to do so it helped me manage my fear of the outcome, but also helped me to be less anxious about being in the scanner. Since learning meditation, I find I am coping better with my life in general, I learned it originally to help with the cancer but find that it has helped me cope with my family relationships and coping at work as well. My meditation practice is my lifeline, I find it helps keep me centred and calm despite the uncertain future I have since cancer.	• Meditation is a safe practice which can be taught to anyone with cancer. • If active psychosis or severe depression are present, then it is advised to wait until these states have passed before beginning meditation practice.

Table 15.11 Mindfulness-based stress reduction (MBSR) in cancer care

Therapy	Evidence for use	What practitioners say	What users say	Safety/precautions
Mindfulness-based stress reduction (MBSR) is an eight-week participatory programme to help cultivate mindfulness, our ability to be present and aware in each moment. It is taught using mindfulness techniques including a mindful body scan, meditation and yoga stretches.	A systematic review of MBSR for people affected by cancer was performed where three RCTs and six uncontrolled trials were found.[54] The studies reported positive results, including improvements in mood state, sleep quality and reductions in stress. A dose-response effect has been observed between practice of MBSR and improved outcomes.	I am currently teaching MBSR to women who have had breast cancer. Some of these women are finding that this course is enabling them to take time for themselves, to do life-enhancing practices such as mindfulness meditation and mindful yoga stretches. These women are seeing for themselves what impact that has on their managing their lives and coping with 'living with cancer'.	In moments of panic and stress, I get a hot flush reaction so now I return to the breath. By using this calming method to help with stress, I don't get so many hot flushes. When I came to the MBSR programme I could not allow myself to accept that there was the possibility that I didn't have MS, (in addition to my cancer), despite medical proof that I didn't. Physical symptoms which to me indicated that I must have the illness (MS) are now beginning to dramatically subside. I believe I now have a tool to enable me to maximise my life opportunities – to enjoy whatever life throws at me from here on – even the bad bits.	• Patients with cancer are able to participate fully in the programme. If any of the mindful yoga stretches seem inappropriate for that person, then they are invited to 'do them in their imagination', or just do the bits they can. • MBSR training is not suitable for people with acute episodes of psychosis, borderline personality disorder or severe depression.

Table 15.12 Chinese herbal medicine for side-effects of chemotherapy

Therapy	Evidence for use	What practitioners say	What users say	Safety/precautions
Chinese medical herbs for side-effects of chemotherapy.	A Cochrane review of the use of Chinese medical herbs for chemotherapy side-effects in colorectal cancer patients reviewed four relevant trials ($n = 342$), all of which were of low quality.[55] Findings suggested that decoctions of Huangqi compounds (which contains the herb Astralgus spp.) may result in a decrease in the rate of leucopenia and an increase in the proportions of T lymphocyte subsets, stimulate immunocompetent cells, and decrease side-effects of nausea and vomiting in patients treated with chemotherapy. Huangqi did not affect levels of antibodies in the blood.	Chinese herbal medicines have been used for centuries in China and the East, so while the clinical trials may be limited there is much evidence from case studies for their effectiveness.	I have found Chinese herbs a great support following my cancer treatment. I was feeling very tired having had surgery, chemotherapy and radiotherapy. The herbal pills were a great support to me in helping to regain my energy and my zest for life after all the treatment I had gone through.	• No evidence of harm arising from the use of Huangqi decoctions was found.[55] • As Chinese herbal medicines in general are not free from potential harm, (allergic reactions and nephropathy have been noted from their use[55]), patients should ensure they are going to a well-qualified practitioner who uses a high quality of herbal medicines.

Table 15.13 Western herbal medicine

Therapy	Evidence for use	What practitioners say	What users say	Safety/precautions
Herbal Medicine (Western) herbalists utilise a range of herbs traditionally used for their medicinal properties.	There is one systematic review of the prevalence of complementary/ alternative medicine in cancer, which identified nine studies involving the use of herbal medicines.[7] A systematic review of RCTs for the efficacy of ginger for nausea and vomiting evaluated six studies, three of which evaluated post-operative nausea and vomiting, two of which found ginger equal in effect to metoclopromide (anti-emetic).[56] The one study evaluating chemotherapy-induced nausea favoured ginger over placebo.[57]	In cancer care, herbal medicines can be used in the following way: • *pre- and post-surgery* to support cardiovascular, immune and liver function in preparation for, through, and after surgery • *chemotherapy* alongside and after chemotherapy to minimise damage to healthy tissue and support/restore key functions, and help treat side-effects such as oral and digestive, sleeping, immune, and vein/circulation problems, anxiety • *radiotherapy* supporting liver function, protecting lung and heart function and preventing inflammation, using safe topical creams or gels	I have been taking herbs from the herbalist to help with my hot flushes which have improved out of sight. When I had chemotherapy, I took slippery elm powder to help soothe my insides, which really helped me to cope with the treatment and I was able to eat without discomfort. I found it difficult to sleep as I was so worried about my cancer treatment and coping with my kids. I found the herbal preparation I was given from the herbalist helped me to feel calmer so I slept better and was not so short-tempered with the children.	• Herbal medicine in the hands of an expert herbal practitioner (in the UK a member of the National Institute of Medical Herbalists, MNIMH, or the College of Practitioners of Phytotherapy, CPP), who uses a reputable supplier and only dispenses a herbal prescription tailored to the individual following a detailed medical consultation is considered safe herbal medicine. • Reported adverse reactions to herbs are almost exclusively based on self-administered herbal medicines bought over the counter (OTC), in concentrated forms and usually in doses far exceeding those stated. Due to lack of quality control, OTC herbal products are frequently found not to contain the correct herb or may be contaminated.

- *menopausal or hormone drug-induced symptoms* treatment for hot flushes, mood changes, vaginal dryness, and other menopausal symptoms
- *recovery and to regain and maintain health and immunity* restorative tonics, energy and immune-supporting foods.

In a consultation with a qualified and experienced medical herbalist, a full medical history is taken including any medications that the person may be on or be going to have in the near future. Herbs are prescribed according to the person as a whole and their particular symptoms.
People receiving herbs are reviewed regularly and a new prescription of herbs is made up according to their changing condition.

I took slippery elm powder to soothe my digestive tract during chemotherapy, which has helped the acid feeling in my stomach. I noticed my bowel movements were easier too.

- Some research has identified possible areas where herbs may interfere with the metabolism of chemotherapy,[59] or by the anti-oxidant-related protection of tumour cells from oxidative damage.[60,61] Advice which has followed this in an American cancer centre,[13] is that herbs and supplements beyond the recommended daily doses should not be taken for a week before chemotherapy and radiotherapy. It is recommended that people should discuss this with their oncologist and herbalist.

Table 15.13. continued

Table 15.13 Continued

Therapy	Evidence for use	What practitioners say	What users say	Safety/precautions
		It is safe for people with cancer to drink herbal teas to help, such as peppermint, ginger, chamomile etc, but they are never recommended to self-medicate with over-the-counter herbs. In terms of enhancing cancer treatment, there is evidence that herbs and supplements can: • decrease or protect against specific toxicities of conventional treatments • increase the sensitivity of cancer cells to chemo- and radiosensitisation by a variety of mechanisms • protect against myelosuppressive effects of chemotherapy and radiotherapy • act synergistically on the same targets as certain chemotherapies.[58]		

Table 15.18 Alternative therapies for cancer

Therapy	Definition	Evidence for use	Safety/precautions
Di Bella regimen	This regimen consists of melatonin, bromocriptine, retinoids, and either somatostatin or octreotide.	Two research studies have not shown any benefit for this treatment.[82,83]	This therapy is not recommended.
Gerson therapy	This is a dietary regimen that aims to detoxify and re-energise the body and support the liver through a low-salt, high-potassium diet achieved by juicing of a gallon of fruit and vegetables per day in addition to coffee enemas.	There are no well-conducted clinical trials to support the use of this regime as a cancer cure; one review was flawed with non-randomised comparisons and subgroup analysis.[84]	This regime is very time consuming and almost impossible for a person with cancer to do alone due to the constant need for enemas and juicing.
Laetrile	This consists of a single compound 'Vitamin B17' isolated from a natural substance – apricot kernels.	Phase II trials have shown no benefit and some toxicity with laetrile.[85]	Risk of toxicity from large doses of laetrile.
Macrobiotic diet	Devised by a Japanese, George Ohsawa in the 1930s, it is a mostly vegetarian high-fibre, low-fat diet, with an emphasis on whole grains, legumes, fresh vegetables and occasional fish.	On the basis of available evidence and the similarity of dietary recommendations for chronic disease prevention, the macrobiotic diet may carry a reduced cancer risk; however, further research into this is needed.[86]	This diet can be bulky and difficult to digest for some people with cancer. The foods in this diet are so limited there may be a risk of nutritional deficiency.
Metabolic therapy	These therapies are based on the idea that cancer and other illnesses result from an accumulation of toxins in the colon which lead to liver failure and death. Diets include low salt, high potassium, high doses of vitamins, minerals, and enzymes, several litres of fruit and vegetable juice daily, and detoxification by means of high colonic irrigation with herbs, coffee or enzymes.	A case series of 11 patients with adenocarcinoma of the pancreas receiving a metabolic regime reported encouraging findings, which is serving as the basis of a RCT.[87]	As there is so much variation in the different metabolic regimes, it is hard to know which if any or all of the aspects are an essential part of their process. It does make sense to eat a very healthy diet if diagnosed with cancer, but it raises the issue about the necessity to go to extremes.

Table 15.18 Continued

Therapy	Definition	Evidence for use	Safety/precautions
Mushrooms (Coriolus versicolor)	Medicinal mushrooms are commonly prescribed in Japan to help people with cancer. They contain the substance PSK, regarded as an anti-tumour polysaccharide–protein complex.	Data collected from controlled clinical trials are suggesting that these mushrooms may well be beneficial. In one study, those with colorectal cancer taking the PSK extracts, disease-free survival was higher than in those on chemotherapy alone.[88]	This appears to be a safe therapy with no adverse side-effects found in trials to date.[88]
Pau d'arco tea	This tea comes from the bark of a South American tree which has been used as a remedy since Inca times for many ailments including cancer. The active ingredient of lapachol has been isolated.	Lapachol has been shown to have anti-tumour effects in animal studies, but does not seem to affect human cancers.[89]	May induce nausea and vomiting.
Shark cartilage	The basis of taking shark cartilage for cancer is through the erroneous idea that sharks do not get cancer, but animal researchers have found they do.	The shark cartilage is thought to have some anti-angiogenesis properties, but none of this is proven in phase I/II clinical trial.[90]	This preparation is expensive and has no proven value for cancer.
Vitamin C (high dose)	Nobel Laureate, Dr Linus Pauling, coined the term 'orthomolecular' to describe the treatment of disease with large quantities of nutrients. Megavitamin and orthomolecular therapy, adding minerals and other nutrients remain popular despite being unproven.	Pauling's claims that vitamin C could cure cancer were not confirmed by clinical trials.[91,92]	Toxicity does not normally occur as vitamin C is water-soluble and readily excreted by the body. Excess ascorbic acid in the urine can give a false-positive test for sugar. High doses of vitamin C may interfere with copper absorption and there is some question as to the risk of developing renal stones.[93]

Summary of use of complementary therapies in cancer care

As can be seen from these tables, there are a wide variety of therapies that can be used to help people before, during and after cancer treatments, some of which offer support, for example massage and reflexology, and others which give the person help to learn a new form of self-management, for example meditation and yoga. At different stages, different therapies may be appropriate. For example, if people are in the middle of treatment and are feeling tired, a relaxing hands-on therapy might be just what is needed. For others where treatment is completed or nearing completion, the person may wish to develop further strategies to help support themselves and to develop new and better habits for a healthier lifestyle in the future. It is often the case that the developing of cancer can highlight difficulties in relationships or the desire to change jobs or to reduce levels of stress in daily life. Many people can find complementary therapies helpful in spending some time with themselves, gaining a clearer perspective on their lives and what they need or want.

Alternative therapies for cancer

Some alternative therapies have been added for information in Table 15.18, so that cancer nurses might be able to know a little about each therapy, but these therapies on their own without medical input are not recommended. Cancer is an illness that is difficult to treat with conventional medicine, and alternative therapies certainly do not offer any guarantees of cure. Having said this, there are a few patients, who, having been told that nothing more can be done with conventional medicine, have taken an alternative therapies route and healed themselves. One example of this healing from cancer is the experience of Dr Ian Gawler, a former vet from Australia who then went on to set up a foundation and residential centre called The Gawler Foundation, near Melbourne, Australia to support people with cancer. The reason that this is mentioned is that some people with cancer, usually against the advice of their medical staff, take this stance to follow an alternative route, and if this does occur, they should be encouraged to have regular medical checks and monitoring from the oncology team so that appropriate care may be offered to them if needed.

References

1. House of Lords. (2000). *6th Report of the House of Lords Science and Technology Committee.* www.publications.parliament.uk/pa/ld/ldselect.htm (accessed 2 August 2007).
2. The Cochrane Collaboration. www.cochrane.co.uk/en/thecochranecollaboration.htm (accessed 9 August 2007).
3. National Center for Complementary and Alternative Medicine. http://nccam.nih.gov/health/whatiscam/ (accessed 2 August 2007).
4. Cassileth B.R., Deng G., Vickers A.J. *et al.* (2005). *Integrative Oncology: Complementary Therapies in Cancer Care.* Hamilton Ontario, Canada: BC Decker.
5. The Prince's Foundation for Integrated Health. www.fih.org.uk (accessed 2 August 2007).
6. Macmillan Cancer Relief. (2002). *Directory of Complementary Therapy Services in UK Cancer Care: Public and Voluntary Sectors.* London: Macmillan Cancer Relief.
7. Ernst E. and Cassileth B. (1998). The prevalence of complementary/alternative medicine in cancer: a systematic review. *Cancer* **83**, 777–782.
8. Molassiotis A., Fernandez-Ortega P., Pud D. *et al.* (2005). Use of complementary and alternative medicine in cancer patients: a European survey. *Annals of Oncology* **16**, 655–663.
9. Rees R.W., Feigel I., Vickers A. *et al.* Prevalence of complementary therapy use by women with breast cancer: a population-based survey. *European Journal of Cancer* **36**, 1359–1364.
10. Paltiel O., Avitzour M., Peretz T. *et al.* Determinants of the use of complementary therapies by people with cancer. *Journal of Clinical Oncology* **19**, 2439–2448.
11. Boon H., Stewart M.A.K., Gray R. *et al.* (2000). Use of complementary/alternative medicine by breast cancer survivors in Ontario: prevalence and perceptions. *Jounal of Clinical Oncology* **18**, 2515–2521.
12. Correa-Velez I., Clavarino A., Barnett A. and Eastwood H. (2003). Use of complementary and alternative medicine and quality of life: changes at the end of life. *Palliative Medicine* **17**, 695–703.
13. Cassileth B.R. and Vickers A.J. (2005). High prevalence of complementary and alternative medicine use amongst cancer patients: implications for research and clinical care. *Journal of Clinical Oncology* **23**, 2590–2592.

14. Downer S.M., Cody M.M., McCluskey P. *et al.* (1994). Pursuit and practice of complementary therapies by cancer patients receiving conventional treatment. *British Medical Journal* **309**, 86–89.

15. Polley M., Hoffman C., Brydon N. *et al.* (2006). The benefits of individualised complementary therapy programmes for women with breast cancer at Breast Cancer Haven (Poster) 5th European Breast Cancer Conference, Nice, France, 2006 March 21–25. *European Journal of Cancer* **4**, 89.

16. Helyer L.K., Chin S., Chui B.K. *et al.* (2006). The use of complementary and alternative medicines among patients with locally advanced breast cancer – a descriptive study. *BMC Cancer* **6**, 1–8. www.biomedcentral.com/1471-2407/6/39 (accessed 2 August 2007).

17. Corner J. and Harewood J. (2004). Exploring the use of complementary and alternative medicine by people with cancer. *NT Research* **9**, 101–109.

18. Sapolsky R.M. (1998) *Why Zebras don't get Ulcers*. New York: WH Freeman and Company.

19. Research Council for Complementary Medicine: Complementary and Alternative Medicine Evidence On Line (CAMEOL). www.rccm.org.uk/cameol/Default.aspx (accessed 2 August 2007).

20. The National Library for Health CAM Specialist Library. www.library.nhs.uk/cam (accessed 2 August 2007).

21. The Cochrane Library. www.cochrane.co.uk/en/thecochranecollaboration.htm (accessed 9 August 2007).

22. National Cancer Research Institute Complementary Therapies Clinical Studies Development Group (CTCSDG). www.ncrn.org.uk/csg/groups.asp?groupID=22 (accessed 2 August 2007).

23. University of Westminster's School of Integrated Health. www.wmin.ac.uk (accessed 2 August 2007).

24. The Prince's Foundation for Integrated Health and the National Council for Hospice and Specialist Palliative Care Service. (2003). *National Guidelines for the Use of Complementary Therapies in Supportive and Palliative Care*. London: The Prince's Foundation for Integrated Health.

25. Bristol Cancer Help Centre. www.bristolcancerhelp.org (accessed 2 August 2007).

26. Breast Cancer Haven. www.breastcancerhaven.org.uk (accessed 2 August 2007).

27. Commonweal Cancer Help Programme. www.commonweal.org/programs/cancer-help.html (accessed 2 August 2007).

28. The Gawler Foundation. www.gawler.org (accessed 2 August 2007).

29. Lee H., Schmidt K. and Ernst E. (2005). Acupuncture for cancer-related pain – a systematic review. *European Journal of Pain* **9**, 437–444.

30. Alimi D., Rubino C., Pichard-Léandri E. *et al.* (2003). Analgesic effects of auricular acupuncture for cancer pain. *Journal of Clinical Oncology* **21**, 4120–4126.

31. Ezzo J.M., Richardson M.A., Vickers A. *et al.* (2006). Acupuncture-point stimulation for chemotherapy-induced nausea or vomiting (Cochrane Review). *The Cochrane Library,* Issue 2. Oxford: Update Software.

32. Richardson J., Smith J., McCall G. *et al.* (2005). Hypnosis for chemotherapy-induced nausea and vomiting. A systematic review. *Complementary and Alternative Medicine Evidence On Line (CAMEOL)* www.rccm.org.uk/cameol/Default.aspx (accessed 2 August 2007).

33. Smith J., Richardson J., Filshie J. *et al.* (2005). Acupuncture for hot flushes as a result of cancer treatment: a systematic review. *Complementary and Alternative Medicine Evidence On Line (CAMEOL)* www.rccm.org.uk/cameol/Default.aspx (accessed 2 August 2007).

34. Liossi C. (2006). Hypnosis in cancer care. *Contemporary Hypnosis* **23**, 47–57.

35. Richardson J., Smith J.E. and Pilkington K. (2001). Hypnosis for procedure-related pain and distress in paediatric cancer patients: a systematic review of effectiveness and methodology related to hypnosis interventions. *Journal of Pain and Symptom Management* **31**, 70–84.

36. Fellowes D., Barnes, K. and Wilkinson, S. (2004). Aromatherapy and massage for symptom relief in patients with cancer (Cochrane Review). *The Cochrane Library*, Issue 3. Oxford: Update Software.

37. Tisserand R. and Balacs T. (1995). *Essential Oil Safety: A Guide for Health Care Professionals*. Edinburgh: Churchill Livingstone.

38. Kassab S. and Stevensen C. (1996). Common misunderstandings about complementary therapies for patients with cancer. *Complementary Therapies in Nursing and Midwifery* **2**, 62–65.

39. Linde K., Clausius N., Ramirez G. *et al.* (1997). Are the clinical effects of homeopathy placebo effects? A meta-analysis of placebo-controlled trials. *Lancet* **350**, 834–843.

40. Milazzo S., Russell N. and Ernst E. (2006). Review: efficacy of homeopathic therapy in cancer treatment. *European Journal of Cancer* **42**, 282–289.

41. Oberbaum M., Yaniv I., Ben-Gal Y. *et al.* (2001). A randomised controlled clinical trial of the homeopathic medication Traumeel S® in the treatment of chemotherapy-induced stomatitis in children undergoing stem cell transplantation. *Cancer* **92**, 684–690.

42. Balzarini A., Felisi E., Martini A. *et al.* (2000). Efficacy of homeopathic treatment of skin reactions during radiotherapy for breast cancer: a randomised double-blind clinical trial. *British Homeopathic Journal* **89**, 8–12.

43. Kulkarni A., Nagarkar B.M. and Burde G.S. (1988). Radiation protection by use of homeopathic medicines. *Hahnemann Homeopathic Standard* **12**, 20–23.

44. Kassab S., van Haselen R., Fisher P. and McCarney R. (2004). Homeopathy for adverse events of cancer

management. (Protocol). *The Cochrane Library*, Issue 3. Oxford: Update Software.

45. Fellowes D., Gambles M., Lockhart-Wood K. *et al.* (2000). Reflexology for symptom relief in patients with cancer. (Protocol). *The Cochrane Library*, Issue 1. Oxford: Update Software.

46. Quattrin R., Zanini A., Buchini S. *et al.* (2006). The use of reflexology foot massage to reduce anxiety in hospitalised cancer patients in chemotherapy treatment: methodology and outcomes. *Journal of Nursing Management* **14**, 96–105.

47. Stephenson N.L.N., Weinrich S.P. and Tavakoli A. (2001). The effects of foot reflexology on anxiety and pain in patients with breast and lung cancer. *Oncology Nursing Forum* **27**, 67–72.

48. Stephenson N., Dalton J.A. and Carlson J. (2003). The effect of foot reflexology on pain in patients with metastatic cancer. *Applied Nursing Research* **16**, 284–286.

49. Richardson J., Smith J., Hoffman C. *et al.* (2005). Yoga as a supportive therapy in cancer: a systematic review. 2005. (Online) (access August 2006) Available from URL. *Complementary and Alternative Medicine Evidence On Line (CAMEOL)* www.rccm.org.uk/cameol/Default. aspx (accessed 2 August 2007).

50. Cohen L., Warneke C., Fouladi R.T. *et al.* (2004). Psychological adjustment and sleep quality in a randomised trial of the effects of Tibetan yoga intervention in patients with lymphoma. *Cancer* **100**, 2253–2260.

51. Targ E.F. and Levine E.G. (2002). The efficacy of a mind–body-spirit group for women with breast cancer: a randomised controlled trial. *General Hospital Psychiatry* **24**, 238–248.

52. Canter P.H. (2003). The therapeutic effects of meditation. Editorial. *British Medical Journal* **326**, 1049–1050.

53. Richardson J., Smith J., Hoffman C. and Pilkington K. (2005). Meditation as a supportive therapy in cancer: a systematic review. *Complementary and Alternative Medicine Evidence On Line (CAMEOL)* www.rccm.org.uk/cameol/Default.aspx (accessed 2 August 2007).

54. Smith J.E., Richardson J., Hoffman C. *et al.* (2005). Mindfulness-based stress reduction as supportive therapy in cancer care: systematic review. *Journal of Advanced Nursing* **52**, 315–327.

55. Taixiang W., Munro A.J. and Guanjian L. (2005). Chinese medical herbs for chemotherapy side effects in colorectal cancer patients (Cochrane Review). *The Cochrane Library*, Issue 1. Oxford: Update Software.

56. Ernst E. and Pittler M.H. (2000). Efficacy of nausea and vomiting: a systematic review of randomised clinical trials. *British Journal of Anaesthesia* **84**, 367–371.

57. Pace J.C. (1987). Oral ingestion of encapsulated ginger and reported self-care actions for the relief of chemother-apy associated nausea and vomiting. *Dissertations Abstracts International* **47**, 3297-B.

58. Yance D. (2005). A novel approach to cancer treatment: Botanicals that inhibit angiogenesis and/or enhance non-specific biological immune response. www.centrehealing.com/Resources/A%20Novel%20Approach%20to%20Cancer.pdf (accessed 2 August 2007).

59. Mathijssen R.H., Verweij J., de Bruijn P. *et al.* (2002). Effects of St John's Wort on irinotecan metabolism. *Journal of the National Cancer Institute* **94**, 1247–1249.

60. Labriola D. and Livingston R. (1999). Possible interactions between dietary antioxidants and chemotherapy. *Oncology* **13**, 1003–1008.

61. Memorial Sloan-Kettering Cancer Center. (2004). *Information Resource: About Herbs, Botanicals and other Products.* www.mskcc.org/aboutherbs (accessed 2 August 2007).

62. Borrelli F. and Ernst E. (2002). *Cimicifuga racemosa*: a systematic review of its clinical efficacy. *European Journal of Clinical Pharmacology* **58**, 235–241.

63. Uebelhack M.D., Blohmer M.D., Graubaum H.-J. *et al.* (2006). Black cohosh and St John's wort in climacteric complaints. *Obstetrics and Gynaecology* **107**, 247–255.

64. Mckenna D.J., Jones, K., Humphrey S. *et al.* (2001). Black cohosh: efficacy, safety, and use in clinical and preclinical applications. *Alternative Therapy, Health and Medicine* **7**, 93–100.

65. Blumenthal M. (1998). *German Federal Institute for Drugs and Medical Devices. Commission E. The Complete German Commission E Monographs: Therapeutic Guide to Herbal Medicines.* Austin, TX: American Botanical Council.

66. European Medicines Agency Press Office. (2006). *EMEA Public Statement on Herbal Medicinal Products Containing Cimicifuga racemosa rhizome (Black Cohosh, Root) – Serious Hepatic Reactions.* London: European Medicines Agency Press Office. www.emea.eu.int/pdfs/human/hmpc/26925906en.pdf (accessed 2 August 2007).

67. Richardson J., Smith J. and Pilkington K. (2005). European mistletoe extract (*Viscum album*), as an adjunctive (survival and supportive) cancer therapy. A systematic review. *Complementary and Alternative Medicine Evidence On Line (CAMEOL).* www.rccm.org.uk/cameol/include/login.aspx?ReturnUrl=%2fcameol%2fDefault.aspx (accessed 9 August 2007).

68. Ernst E., Schmidt K. and Steuer-Vogt M.K. (2003). Mistletoe for cancer? A systematic review of randomised clinical trials. *International Journal of Cancer* **107**, 262–267.

69. Kienle G.S., Berrino F., Bussing A. *et al.* (2003). Mistletoe in cancer: a systematic review on controlled clinical trials. *European Journal of Medical Research* **8**, 109–119.

70. Kleijnen J. and Knipschild P. (1994). Mistletoe treatment for cancer: review of controlled trials in humans. *Phytomedicine* **1**, 255–260.

71. Hajto T., Hostanska K., Frei K. *et al.* (1990). Increased secretion of tumour necrosis factor α, interleukin-1 and interleukin-6 by human mononuclear cells exposed to galactoside-specific lectin from clinically applied mistletoe extract. *Cancer Research* **50**, 3322–3326.

72. Horneber M.A., Bueschel G., Huber R. *et al.* (2001). Mistletoe therapy in oncology (Protocol). *The Cochrane Library*, Issue 1. Oxford: Update Software.

73. Loewe-Mesch A. (2002). Die Mistletherapie in der biologischen Tumorbegleitbehandlung. *Erfahrungsheilkunde* **4**, 256–258.

74. Pilkington K. and Richardson J. (2005). Essiac in cancer: a review of the systematic reviews. *Complementary and Alternative Medicine Evidence On Line (CAMEOL)* www.rccm.org.uk/cameol/Default.aspx (accessed 2 August 2007).

75. Kaegi E. (1998). Unconventional therapies for cancer: 1. Essiac. *Canadian Medical Association Journal* **158**, 897–902.

76. Barnard J. and Bach E. (1931). The twelve healers. Republished in Barnard J. (ed.) (1998). *The Collected Writings of Edward Bach*. Bath: Ashgrove Press.

77. Anon. (1995). *The Work of Edward Bach. An Introduction and Guide to the 38 Remedies*. London: Wigmore Publishing Ltd.

78. Ernst E. (2002). Flower remedies': a systematic review of the clinical evidence. *Wiener Klinische Wochenschrift* **114**, 963–966.

79. Von Ruhle G. (1995). Pilotstudie zur Anwendung von Bach Blütentherapie bei Ernstgebärenden mit verlängerter Tragzeit. *Erfahrungsheilkunde*, **44**, 854–860.

80. Cram J.R. (2002). Flower essence in the treatment of major depression. *Complementary and Alternative Medicine* **January**, 8–15.

81. Walach H., Rilling C. and Engelke U. (2001). Efficacy of Bach flower remedies in test anxiety: a double blind, placebo controlled, randomised trial with partial crossover. *Anxiety Disorders* **15**, 359–366.

82. Italian Study Group for the Di Bella Multitherapy Trials. (1999). Evaluation of an unconventional cancer treatment (Di Bella multitherapy): results of phase II trials in Italy. *British Medical Journal* **318**, 224–228.

83. Buiatti E., Arniani S., Verdechhia A. *et al.* (1999). Results from a historical survey of the survival of cancer patients given Di Bella multitherapy. *Cancer* **86**, 2143–2149.

84. Hildenbrand G.L., Hildenbrand L.C., Bradford K. *et al.* (1995). Five year survival rates of melanoma patients treated by diet therapy after the manner of Gerson: a retrospective review. *Alternative Therapy Health and Medicine* **1**, 29–37.

85. Moertel C.G., Fleming T.R., Rubin J. *et al.* (1982). A clinical trial of Amygdalin (Laetrile) in the treatment of human cancer. *New England Journal of Medicine* **306**, 201–206.

86. Kushi L.H., Cunningham J.E., Hebert J.R. *et al.* (2001). The macrobiotic diet in cancer. *Journal of Nutrition* **131**, 3056S–3064S.

87. Gonzalez N.J. and Isaacs L. (1999). Evaluation of pancreatic proteolytic enzyme treatment of adenocarcinoma of the pancreas with nutrition and detoxification support. *Nutrition and Cancer* **33**, 117–124.

88. Mitomi T., Tsuchiya S., Iijima N. *et al.* (1992). Randomised controlled study on adjuvant immunochemotherapy with PSK® in curatively resected colorectal cancer. *Diseases of the Colon and Rectum* **35**, 123–130.

89. Block J.B., Serpick A.A., Miller W. *et al.* (1974). Early clinical studies with lapachol (NSC-11905). *Cancer Chemotherapy Reports* **4**, 27–28.

90. Miller D.R., Anderson J.J., Stark J.L. *et al.* (1998). Phase I/II trial of the safety and efficacy of shark cartilage in the treatment of advanced cancer. *Journal of Clinical Oncology* **16**, 3649–3655.

91. Moertel C.G., Fleming T.R., Creagan, E.T. *et al.* (1985). High dose vitamin C versus placebo in the treatment of patients with advanced cancer who have had no prior chemotherapy. *New England Journal of Medicine* **312**, 137–141.

92. Creagan E.T., Moertel C.G. and O'Fallon J.R. (1979). Failure of high-dose vitamin C (absorbic acid) therapy to benefit patients with advanced cancer. *New England Journal of Medicine* **301**, 687–690.

93. Iqbal K., Kahn A. and Kattak M. (2002). Biological significance of absorbic acid (vitamin C) in human health: a review. *Pakistan Journal of Nutrition* **3**, 5–13.

CHAPTER SIXTEEN

Hereditary cancer

Audrey Ardern-Jones, Sarah Thomas, Rebecca Doherty and Rosalind Eeles

Cancer genetics is an important specialty in cancer care, for both patients with cancer and their families. Although at the cellular level cancer is always a genetic condition, it is not always an inherited genetic disorder. Indeed, only 5–10% of cancers are thought to be inherited due to alterations in high-risk genes. However, for families with an inherited cancer susceptibility, the risk of developing cancer is high compared with the normal population cancer risk. The importance of genetics in cancer care is to accurately quantify the cancer risk, and advise on its application to cancer management and its implications for individuals seeking advice regarding prevention strategies. Families who carry an identified alteration in a cancer predisposition gene need specialist care and understanding. The implications of living with a known cancer gene mutation are far-reaching, and although not all individuals who carry cancer predisposition genes develop cancer, the concern for the whole family is paramount. This chapter does not describe in detail the syndromes associated with hereditary cancers but highlights important issues surrounding testing and genetic counselling. Further information about the rare inherited conditions that affect children or adults with cancer can be found in other textbooks.[1,2]

The genetic material

Humans are composed of cells. Each nucleated cell contains the entire human genome, which has been estimated to contain approximately 20 000 to 25 000 genes.[3] The human genome is composed of DNA (deoxyribose nucleic acid), a long, complex molecule in the form of a double helix. The basic element of DNA is a nucleotide, which is a carbon sugar (deoxyribose) with an attached phosphate group and a base, which may be a purine (adenine, A, or guanine, G) or pyrimidine (cytosine, C, or thymine, T). The nucleotides are joined together by phosphodiester bonds between the sugar molecules to form a linear strand. The double helix is formed by two DNA strands linked together with the sugar phosphate backbones on the outside of the molecule and the bases on the inside, orientated such that hydrogen bonds form between opposing purine and pyrimidine bases. The base pairing is strict, with A always pairing with T, and C always pairing with G. This strict base pairing results in two DNA strands, which are termed 'complementary' to each other. The linear sequence of bases is important as it codes for specific amino acids. Each group of three adjacent bases (codon) is a code for a single amino acid or a stop or start signal; hence, the linear DNA sequence forms the genetic code for the formation of specific proteins, which are composed of these amino acids. Proteins direct the function of cells and therefore the entire organism; hence the DNA structure stores all the necessary information for the correct functioning of an individual.[4]

A gene is a sequence of DNA, which can code for a specific protein or have a specific function, such as regulating the expression of other genes. The gene sequence may contain both coding areas for amino acids (exons) and non-coding areas (introns). It is interesting to note that only 3–5% of the DNA in the human genome is used to code for proteins. The function of the remaining 95% of the genome is not well understood, but is likely to be involved with the structure and maintenance of the genome.

The sequence of adjacent base pairs in a gene may vary between individuals. This may be a normal variation (which results in the differences observed between two individuals and is termed 'genetic polymorphism'), or an abnormal alteration in the sequence of adjacent base pairs in a gene (termed a 'mutation').

Different types of mutations exist in genes; for example, a change that alters only one single base to another is known as a point mutation. Alternatively, other mutations include the deletion of an existing base and insertions or deletions of multiple bases, or even the rearrangement of the correct bases into an incorrect order. All types of mutations can result in the incorrect amino acid(s) being incorporated into a protein, thereby changing the structure and/or function of the protein. Alternatively, a mutation may result in the formation of a stop codon, which terminates the coding sequence and results in production of a shortened or truncated protein. These changes may result in an abnormal protein that does not function correctly. Fortunately, not all genes are functional, so mutational changes in the genetic code do not always result in abnormal proteins.

Mutations in the DNA sequence of a gene are copied and transferred from parent to progeny cells through the process of mitosis. If this mutation occurs in a somatic cell (that is, all the cells of the body other than the ova and sperm, or germ cells), then only the progeny cells from the original cell will contain this abnormality and all the other cells of the organism will have a normal genetic code. This is termed a 'somatic mutation' and is the likely mechanism of formation of sporadic (non-inherited) cancers. As the germ cells are unaffected by mutation, then the somatic mutation will not be passed to subsequent genera-

tions of the organism. If a mutation affects a germ cell (a germline mutation) then the abnormal gene may be passed to the next generation, and this forms the mechanism of familial predisposition to specific cancer syndromes.[5]

Genetic inheritance

Humans are diploid organisms; that is, they contain two copies of the entire genetic code in each cell, one copy from each parent. The genetic code is arranged in the form of chromosomes, which are long lengths of DNA condensed into a compact structure. Each copy of the genetic code consists of 22 pairs of autosomal chromosomes and two sex chromosomes, hence the full genetic complement consists of 44 autosomal chromosomes and two sex chromosomes. The term 'homologous chromosomes' refers to a pair of matching chromosomes, one from each parent. These matching chromosomes are not exact copies of each other, but are similar in that the specific genes (loci) are aligned in the same position on each homologous chromosome. The actual genes can be of different sequences due to genetic polymorphism. The term 'allele' refers to a version of a gene; hence, each nucleated cell contains two alleles (versions) of each gene. The genetic code inherited by an individual is termed the 'genotype', whereas the appearance of an individual (for example, hair colour) is termed the 'phenotype'.[6]

The major contributor to the understanding of the role of inheritance was Gregor Mendel in 1865. Indeed, it was through his novel experiments on plant breeding that he discovered statistical ratios that made sense in calculating the outcomes of cross-breeding in plants. These ratios were an important advance and led to the classification of inheritance patterns as dominant, recessive, or sex-linked. Dominant inheritance refers to the expression of a phenotype determined by the inheritance of a single allele; Huntingdon's disease is an example of this type of inheritance. Recessive inheritance refers to the expression of a phenotype determined by the inheritance of two alleles containing mutations; if only one is inherited then that phenotype is not expressed, as the recessive allele is dominated by the homologous normal allele. Cystic fibrosis is the most common recessive inherited genetic disease in UK Caucasians; both parents must be carriers of the recessive gene in order to produce a child with cystic fibrosis. Sex-linked inheritance is the inheritance of genes located on the sex chromosomes; haemophilia is a well-described X-linked disease that is passed down through unaffected female carriers to affected sons on the X chromosome.

It must be remembered that, except for sex-linked inheritance, the inheritance of a germline mutation in a gene is not dependent on the sex of an individual; male and females may equally be carriers. However, the phenotypic expression of the gene may depend on the sex of the individual. For example, men and women can inherit breast and ovarian cancer predisposition genes, but men rarely develop breast cancer and cannot develop ovarian cancer, while still being able to pass on the gene to the next generation.

The phenotypic expression of an inherited gene depends on the penetrance of the gene. A highly penetrant gene is one that is usually expressed if inherited. For example, a carrier of either of the cancer predisposition genes known as *BRCA1* or *BRCA2* has a 40–85% lifetime expectancy of development of breast cancer, depending on ethnicity, and a risk of ovarian cancer that varies with the gene inherited.[7] The penetrance of a gene will depend on many factors, including the sex of the individual (for example, a male carrying a mutation in the *BRCA1* gene rarely develops breast cancer), the presence of carcinogens, or the effect of other genes. The penetrance of germline cancer predisposition genes has been estimated, but the estimations are continually refined as further knowledge of cancer genetics is gained.[8]

Cancer predisposition genes

Cancer predisposition genes are genes that, when disrupted by germline mutations, can predispose to the development of cancer. The understanding of these genes and the developments in the field of cancer molecular biology have been extraordinarily rapid in the last decade. Three types of cancer predisposition genes have been identified.

Oncogenes

Oncogenes are genes that may cause cancer when activated by a mutation. They are commonly forms of normal genes (proto-oncogenes) with important cell-regulatory functions; mutations will therefore tend either to increase gene expression or lead to uncontrolled activity of the proteins encoded by the oncogene. Germline oncogenes tend to show a dominant pattern of inheritance and the only examples currently identified in the human are the *Ret* and *Met* oncogenes in multiple endocrine neoplasia (MEN),[9] and familial papillary renal cell cancer syndromes, respectively. Current opinion is that somatic oncogene activation is an important step in sporadic tumour carcinogenesis.

Tumour suppressor genes

In contrast to oncogenes, tumour suppressor genes lead to cancer predisposition when inactivated. The normal function of tumour suppressor genes is to inhibit cell proliferation and growth; hence loss of function will result in uncontrolled cell division. Germline mutations in tumour suppressor genes tend to show recessive inheritance at the cellular level, as both copies of the gene must be inactivated before cancer can develop, otherwise the remaining normal copy of the gene will still produce adequate quantities of the relevant protein for the normal functioning of a cell.

Despite the recessive molecular mechanism, the inheritance of phenotype is said to be dominant. An individual inheriting a single mutation is said to have inherited a dominant cancer predisposition, as the remaining allele may be affected by mutation during the course of a lifetime. Knudson's hypothesis describes this as the 'second hit', where the second allele of the tumour suppressor gene undergoes a somatic mutation (see Figure 16.1).[10] That single cell is therefore rendered null for the normal tumour suppressor gene. This cell may now go on to divide in an uncontrolled manner and develop into a cancer, as normal tumour suppressor gene function is lost.

Recessive genetic inheritance by phenotypically dominant inheritance is a difficult concept to introduce in genetic counselling; the inherited mutation on its own is not sufficient to cause cancer and often it is unknown which factors

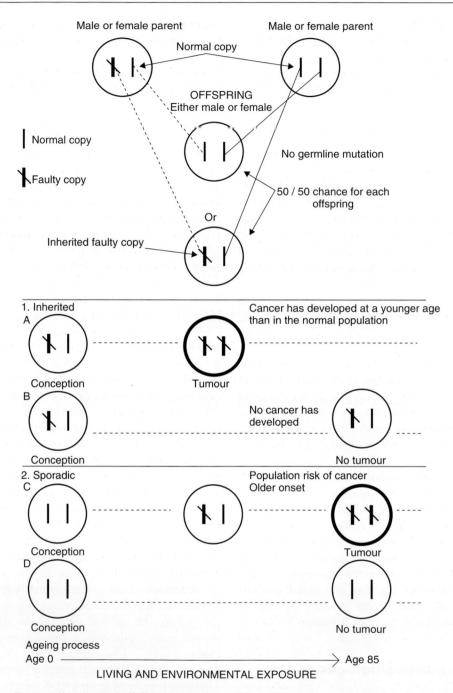

Figure 16.1   Dominantly inherited adult-onset cancer predisposition gene, e.g. breast/ovarian syndrome.

result in the mutation of the remaining normal allele. These factors may include diet, chemicals, viruses, replication error, and occupational exposure to carcinogens. Many identified inherited germline cancer predisposition genes appear to show this type of inheritance, the most well-characterised being the breast and colon cancer predisposition genes.

DNA repair genes

These are involved in correcting DNA replication errors, which are common events during the natural process of DNA replication. Similar to tumour suppressor genes, repair gene mutations tend to show a recessive genotypic inheritance, but a phenotypically dominant expression, as a somatic mutation of the remaining normal copy of the gene commonly occurs during the lifetime of the individual in at least one somatic cell. The main example in humans is the syndrome HNPCC (hereditary non-polyposis colorectal cancer), where germline alteration in any of the six genes that have so far been identified can cause this syndrome, characterised by colon carcinomas and other tumours.[11]

Cancer development

The origin of cancer may be an inherited susceptibility, environmental influences, or a combination of both. The main common inherited cancer syndromes are summarised in Table 16.1. The global incidence of cancer is increasing, mainly due to increased longevity: by the year 2020 there may be 20 million new patients diagnosed with cancer each year.[12]

As with sporadic cancer, hereditary cancer varies considerably; for example, in terms of the ages at which people develop the disease, differences in tumour grading and clinical staging, and length of survival. A cancer predisposition may be inherited from the maternal or paternal side of the family or, in rare instances, from both sides of the family. Intermarriage (consanguinity) can complicate this further. Certain types of tumour may be more commonly linked with a hereditary cancer diagnosis. Several authors suggest that women with breast cancer who have germline *BRCA1* mutations are more likely to have high-grade tumours that are negative for oestrogen and progesterone receptors, do not express *HER2*, and are more likely to be positive for p53 protein, compared to non-carriers.[13–15] Women of unknown genetic status with these tumour characteristics have between a 10% and 27% chance of carrying a mutation in the *BRCA1* gene.[13] More recently, Foulkes *et al.* discovered an association between germline *BRCA1* mutation and the expression of stratified epithelial cytokeratin 5 and/or 6.[16]

Understanding a cancer family history and detecting who is at risk

It is estimated that one in three people will develop cancer in their lifetime;[17] most families therefore have some history of cancer. However, as stated earlier, only a small proportion of these cancers have a hereditary cause. More than 200 types of hereditary cancer syndromes are known, and these account for 5–10% of all cancers diagnosed.[18] Individuals who have a hereditary predisposition have a high risk of developing cancer, and if they have already developed one cancer, they have a higher than average risk of developing a second one.

Oncology nurses are in a position to identify appropriate patients for referral to a cancer genetics clinic as they have direct contact with the patient and their family and can be sensitive to their fears. However, it can be difficult to collect an accurate family history. There are many sensitive issues that may need to broached. Family life today is complex, and many people may not be in touch with their relatives, or may know little information about the family. Furthermore, there are such issues as non-paternity, partnership splits, and death in the family that can make it difficult for the patient when talking about the past.

Analysing a family history is a complex process. Family history information is collected in the form of a family tree, or pedigree. Guidelines about how to draw a Family tree can be found at www.clingensoc.org.

Information that it is particularly important to record is:

- cancer type
- age of diagnosis (as a general rule cancers under the age of 50 years are considered young)
- whether affected family members have died
- multiple or bilateral cases of cancer in one individual
- intermarriage between family members
- ethnicity.

- *First-degree relatives* are those that are one step away on the family tree, for example your mother, father, brothers, sisters and children.

Table 16.1 Summary of main common inherited cancer syndromes. Adapted from Firth H. and Hurst J. (2005). *Oxford Desk Reference Clinical Genetics.* Oxford: Oxford University Press.[19]

Syndrome	Main gene(s)	Cancer types/features	Risks	Inheritance
FAP (familial adenomatous polyposis)	*APC*	Classical FAP is defined when >100 adenomatous polyps are found in the colon. Attenuated FAP may lead to less (2–100 polyps); extracolonic features include osteomas, epidermoid cysts, CHRPEs (congenital hypertrophy of the retinal pigment epithelium), upper gastrointestinal polyposis and malignancy, desmoid tumors, and an increased risk of peri-ampullary carcinoma, papillary thyroid, brain tumours, hepatoblastoma and sarcomas	Up to 100% risk of colonic cancer by age 50 years if untreated	Autosomal dominant
Hereditary non-polyposis colorectal cancer (HNPCC or Lynch syndrome)	*MLH1, MSH2, MSH6, PMS2*	Mainly colon cancer and endometrial cancer, but also increased risk of cancers of the ovary, urothelium, stomach, brain, and small bowel. Hepatobiliary and pancreatic cancers have also been reported	60–80% risk of colorectal cancer over lifetime; 40–60% risk of endometrial cancer over lifetime	Autosomal dominant
Breast and ovarian cancer	*BRCA1, BRCA2*	Mainly breast and ovary, but also increased risk of fallopian tubes, peritoneum, prostate, and pancreas, and melanoma	40–80% risk of breast cancer over lifetime; 10–60% risk of ovarian cancer over a lifetime	Autosomal dominant
von Hippel–Lindau disease (VHL)	*VHL*	Haemangioblastomas of the cerebellum and spinal cord, retinal angiomas, renal cell carcinoma, phaeochromocytomas, and renal, pancreatic, and epidymal cysts	By age 60 years, 84% for cerebellar haemangioblastoma, 70% for retinal angioma, and 69% for renal cell carcinoma	Autosomal dominant
Li–Fraumeni syndrome	*TP53*	Breast cancer, soft tissue sarcomas, osteosarcoma, brain tumours, adrenocortical cancer, Wilms' tumour, and phyllodes tumour	Estimated to be 73% in males and nearly 100% in females	Autosomal dominant
Cowden's syndrome	*PTEN*	Breast cancer, thyroid cancer, endometrial cancer, facial trichelemmomas, acral keratoses, papillomatous papules, mucosal lesions	Mucocutaneous lesions are found in >90% of mutation carriers; 66% have breast or thyroid disease or both	Autosomal dominant

- *Second-degree relatives* are two steps away on the family tree, for example aunts, uncles, grandparents, nephews and nieces
- *Third-degree relatives* are those that are three steps away on the family tree, for example great

aunts and great uncles, great grandparents, cousins.

It may not always be possible for the oncology nurse to gather an accurate and extended family history, however on referral to a genetics centre, specialist nurses and genetic counsellors can help the patient to explore their family history more fully.

Box 16.1 lists factors in a family history that may lead to referral to a cancer genetics unit:

Box 16.1 Factors in a family history that may lead to a referral to a cancer genetics unit. Adapted from Bancroft E., Ardern-Jones A. and Lynch E. (2006). Cancer genetics: the importance of obtaining a family history. *Nursing Times* 102, 28–29.[20]

1. Young age of onset, e.g. breast cancer under 40 years, bowel cancer under 50 years
2. Autosomal dominant pattern of inheritance (e.g. successive generations affected)
3. Multiple cases of cancer in one individual
4. The occurrence of more than one rare tumour in a family, e.g. sarcomas, brain tumours
5. The occurrence of the same cancer multiple times in an individual or cancers known to be related, e.g. breast and ovarian, bowel and uterine
6. Ashkenazi Jewish ancestry in a family with multiple cases of breast and/or ovarian cancer.

In the cancer genetics clinic, there are certain features that a counsellor will recognise as typical of an inherited cancer syndrome. For example, if several family members on either the maternal or paternal side have developed the same or related cancers, particularly involving two or three first-degree relatives, then this pattern is highly suggestive of the presence of a cancer predisposition gene. Another important factor to consider when analysing a family pedigree is the age of onset; on average, the age of onset of inherited cancers is lower than that of sporadic cancers. It is important to remember that even in a family with an inherited predisposition, it is possible for some family members to develop cancer by chance alone (these are referred to as sporadic cases, or phenocopies).

Verification of family history is important for accurate genetic counselling, Commonly, the histories that people report initially are inaccurate, and further research and collection of histological reports are necessary. If family members have died, it is wise to collect copies of death certificates or medical records to establish the cause of death. The ages of family members and dates when the cancer was diagnosed in the family are essential. The collection of this family history information must be sensitively handled as family members have often experienced bereavement, and simply talking about past experiences may be profoundly distressing.

The phenotypic appearance of the individual attending the clinic is also of great importance. It is therefore necessary to take note of any significant features that may suggest a known hereditary condition; for example, skin trichilemmomas and large head circumference, which can occur in Cowden's syndrome. This rare syndrome may also predispose to the development of both breast and thyroid cancers.[21]

Through the counselling process it may be necessary to make estimates of environmental exposures such as sun exposure and smoking, as well as to clarify the ethnic background of the family members seeking counselling, as this may have an impact on cancer risk. For example, women of Ashkenazi Jewish origin who have developed breast cancer younger than 40 years of age have a higher chance of carrying an alteration in one of the breast cancer susceptibility genes, *BRCA1* or *BRCA2*, than a woman from another ethnic group.[22]

What happens at an appointment at a cancer genetics clinic?

It is normal for most genetic centres to send out a questionnaire before patients are seen in a genetics centre. This gives the centre the opportunity to verify the information where possible, and then for the families to be assessed before attending the clinic. In some clinics patients are telephoned by a genetic/nurse counsellor before attending a clinic, as they may be requested to get a relative's death certificate or approach living relatives with cancer for consent so that the genetics team can access their medical records. However, it is not always possible to gather complete information about a family, especially in the UK which has a diverse range of cultures and changing family structures. In some families, previous generations may have been lost as a result of war or disease or through immigration and loss of contact. The staff at the cancer genetics clinic will take this into account and will advise on information available.[20]

Once the appointment is made, the family may be discussed in a multidisciplinary meeting and then seen by one of the genetics team. It may be one of several appointments that the individual will have with the genetics team or simply a one-off appointment, depending on the particular situation of the family. The family history is reviewed with the patient, and the risk of there being a genetic susceptibility to developing cancer is discussed. Issues around genetic testing may be raised if appropriate, and screening for the patient themselves and other at-risk family members is discussed. It is important for the genetic/nurse counsellor to explore psychological issues, as often individuals require support for bereavement and cancer anxiety. Further referral for ongoing counselling may be needed.[5]

If there are medical issues, such as the patient wishing to discuss prophylactic surgery, the patient should ideally be seen in a clinic where there are appropriate clinicians available to discuss medical management. For these people it is also important that there are nurse specialists or counsellors available to support patients.

Genetic counselling

The term 'genetic counselling' has evolved over the years to include psychosocial issues that are paramount as part of the process of counselling. The complex process of genetic counselling addresses problems associated with diagnosis, risk assessment, and the explanation of all the possible options available to help with the burden associated with genetic risk. The essence of genetic counselling is to make known to the counsellee(s) the information about an inherited disorder that is of concern, and to help to evaluate the alternative options stemming from the many concerns that may be raised by the counsellee during the session. This may include advising the person seeking genetic counselling about the different

services (i.e. screening or support) that are available to both the patient and the family.[5]

The meaning and presentation of risk and screening issues

Epidemiological studies of many human cancers have demonstrated a modest (two- or threefold) increase in risk of cancer amongst first-degree relatives of individuals with a similar cancer.[23] Family members may well be advised to seek screening for these cancers; however, genetic cancer risk is multidimensional and hard to define. As well as the probability and consequence of a cancer developing, it is important for an individual to consider the possible implications of knowing about cancer risk and how that may impact on behaviour (for example, the decision to take preventive action or no action at all).[24]

McAllister suggests that for some individuals, beliefs about risk perception can form part of a process of coping and coming to terms with living with being 'at risk'.[25] This study, looking at families with hereditary non-polyposis colorectal cancer, found 28% of respondents said that they expressed fear and anxiety about their risk and appeared to be mixing up their experience of cancer in their family and their own risk of developing cancer. There is evidence that suggests that being identified as 'at risk', because of either genetic testing or pedigree analysis, may also have a negative effect upon psychological well-being, and individuals may be fearful and anxious about their risks of developing cancer.[26,27]

One of the most important reasons for identifying hereditary cancer is to enable family members who are not affected by cancer to seek preventive strategies for the future; that is, to seek screening, surveillance, or surgery. There is evidence to show that early detection may prevent the onset of metastatic cancer. In addition, by providing cancer-risk information it may be possible to facilitate informed choices of anti-cancer treatments or surveillance programmes.

Referral patterns
Members of families with a high risk of cancer are referred to the regional genetics services that serve

the UK. Within these units there are multidisciplinary teams including specialists in cancer genetics. Referrals are made by the general practitioner (GP), hospital doctors, or other health professionals. A government white paper has highlighted best practice for referral patterns,[28] and the Human Genetics Commission also outlines best practice for genetic testing services.[29] Thus the government has invested considerable sums of money into education and information to be made available for the public interest regarding genetics. Cancer genetics is becoming an increasingly important part of genetics services and has now become the largest single reason for referral to the regional genetics centres in the UK.

Screening issues

Cancer-risk notification is fraught with ethical dilemmas. There is sometimes little more to offer the majority of 'at-risk' family members other than surveillance or lifestyle advice. Given the climate of present-day health care and rationing, the implications of cancer screening are controversial.[30] Members of families with a known genetic condition are potentially engaged in everyday bioethical decision making,[31] and there can be problems with disclosing information following a cancer genetics consultation to family members, particularly in relation to screening recommendations for their relatives. Individuals are recommended to share information, but it can be argued that is it unethical to recommend, for example, breast and ovarian screening, in the knowledge that the uptake of screening in certain countries where some of their kin live is not feasible due to limiting advances in health technology.

Screening

As well as the psychological and social costs, screening is expensive and benefits are not proven for all the screening programmes. Genetic counsellors are involved in planning screening programmes for family members at risk of hereditary cancer, and a referral to a clinic for this purpose can be seen by some members of the medical profession to have little benefit to the patient. This may cause disruption and anxiety for people

Personal account 16.1

The following is a personal account explaining how, in Iran, screening is only available privately, so if someone cannot afford to pay for it they do not have it arranged. Nancy who is from Iran illustrates this. She compares the health care system in Iran with that in England:

> They have it in Iran as well, but obviously it depends if somebody can afford it, they go and have it done. If they cannot afford it, they cannot have it done; it's as simple as that. It's not available for everybody. I am grateful that [screening in England] it's available free for everybody. So no matter where you come from or what's your material situation, you can afford to go and get screened.[32]

who believe that a prevention programme is important.

There is a need for evidence-based advice to be given to families seeking guidance with regard to screening programmes. Thus families with a high risk of developing cancer are guided by criteria derived from protocols advised by the National Institute for Health and Clinical Excellence (NICE).[33] These guidelines are drawn from research projects that have been published in scientific journals.

Personal account 16.2

The following is the personal account of a family member seeking screening for hereditary colon cancer:

> I think that, as a lot of people feel, that if you have somebody close to you . . . [that has developed cancer] you immediately start to worry . . . but it didn't worry me unduly . . . until my mother's sister died and I thought 'no, all three sisters in the family, that is a bit too much' . . . I thought I might be in line for it. . . . the thought of cancer frightens me . . . I had to press [my GP] very hard . . . and I had to go to another doctor . . . he had never written to the hospital. . . . I don't think that he particularly wanted me to go to the hospital . . . I don't have much confidence in that doctor.[34]

In fact, the patient referred to in this letter came from a high-risk hereditary non-polyposis colorectal cancer (HNPCC) family and colonoscopy screening is clearly recommended as a beneficial procedure with proven benefits.[35]

Recently, people have been divided into three different catogories with regard to cancer risk – high, moderate and low (or population) risk.[33] This can be confusing for some people who feel that they have fallen into the wrong category.

Most cancer genetic risk-prevention programmes include screening as a tool to detect early signs of cancer so that it may then be cured. Screening is planned in accordance with age and may need to be followed for long periods of time.

There are concerns that the advances in genetic technology may result in more widespread knowledge of susceptibility, and that screening services will be offered to those at risk, without consideration of the consequences. The possible harm (for example, anxiety) that may arise from a screening test for any person may be very small in comparison with the potential harm from not offering screening, and screening may be life-saving by enabling treatment of a potentially fatal cancer. However, despite the wide publicity and optimism amongst the lay public regarding the benefits of screening, some families may have problems with their family doctors arranging a referral for appropriate screening. At this point in time, ovarian screening, prostate cancer screening, and mammography in the under 40–50-year age group are being evaluated by various research studies, which hope to provide an evidence base for future screening guidelines.

Diagnostic genetic testing

Cancer genetic testing aims to identify an alteration in a known cancer predisposition gene. In the public health system, this commonly involves offering testing to an affected family member in order to maximise the chance of an alteration being found.

Testing for a cancer-causing mutation may not find an alteration in the gene – the individual must be aware of this. This may be for several reasons, including the fact that modern technology is limited, the patient having the test may have developed cancer by chance, there is a mutation present in the gene that is being looked at but it has been missed, or that there is a mutation present in a gene/genes yet to be identified. Testing families with HNPCC needs to start with microsatellite testing on the tumour sample as a first stage before testing the DNA. It may take a few months to complete the search for the gene alteration. Testing in the UK has improved as a result of NICE guidelines improving both genetic testing times and the quality of the genetic test. These improvements have only emerged in the last year or so, since 2006.

If a mutation is found, this means that this is likely to be the reason for the development of the particular cancer in the individual concerned. This may have predictive implications for other cancers. This is hard for some families as the quote from Fiona below shows; she was unaffected and had had prophylactic mastectomies despite not knowing her genetic status, while her sister had an uninformative genetic test result:[36]

> I think when your mother dies young we were quite young so you don't think too much about it um and then when your father dies and cancer is becoming part of your life and then your sister gets it, even then I think I still put it down to it's just a coincidence, we're just extremely unlucky people, but for a third sister to get it you just think the odds are against us now, there's obviously something genetic there.

The counselling process with the affected person informs the individual about the further cancer risks both to the person having the test and for their relatives. For example, the breast/ovarian cancer gene *BRCA1* confers a high risk for contralateral breast cancer, as well as the development of both breast and ovarian cancer, and a small increased risk of other cancers.

In a dominantly inherited condition there is always a 50/50 chance that all first-degree family members have a chance of inheriting the same mutation in the family. This may or may not cause concerns and worries for other family members.

Counselling sessions for genetic testing may include several consultations with the individual, who may need to take time before undergoing such a test. Talking through all the implications with the multidisciplinary team members is important. The preparation time is described in Box 16.2.

Box 16.2 Predictive genetic testing

In this case, a known mutation in the family has been identified and a person who has not developed cancer is seeking a test to know whether or not they carry this same mutation.

Informed consent
Full understanding of the implications of finding out whether or not the individual seeking testing carries the mutation in the family is required.

Session 1
Here, the risks and benefits of the test and the current risk factors associated with becoming a known carrier of the disease are explained. This is important, as statistical evidence associated with gene penetrance does change. Informing the person about implications of undergoing genetic testing and explaining all the options that are available for them should they find that they are a carrier is important. Assessing that they have not been coerced into undergoing such a test, and exploring psychological risk factors are also aims of this first session. If they have a history of depression or suicidal ideation then it is essential that they have the opportunity to meet with a clinical psychologist for further support and assessment before undergoing testing. Leaflets are available via the Association of British Insurers (ABI) for patients considering testing (www.abi.org.uk). It is important to get to know the individual in this session, to listen to and understand their fears, and assess their support networks whether these are through their family or friends.

Session 2
This involves further discussion regarding all the emotional implications surrounding such a test. Are there any anxieties about taking this test? This session should include time to establish a good relationship with the genetic counsellor, who will be there when they have their results. Part of the process is preparing for both a positive result and a negative result. Plans for either result may be mapped out on paper.

This plan includes all the screening options and surgical options. When the person seeking the testing is confident and comfortable with all his or her information, a blood sample can be taken. If there is a known mutation in the family, the predictive test does not take very long (about 4 weeks). It is also important to discuss the fact if they do not carry the gene then there may be no need to continue with the screening that has been recommended unless there is a significant history on the other side of the family. Some people are distressed at the thought of not having screening in the future especially if they have been attending a screening clinic for many years. Also, there is evidence of survivor guilt if they are negative for the mutation in the family. This should all be explained, along with the fact that it is quite normal for individuals who are found to be positive for the gene to be upset for some days following the news. Studies have shown that over time the psychological impact of a positive result for some predictive tests is not detrimental to a person's psychological state.[37]

The individual is encouraged to bring a friend or partner with them for their results.

Session 3
Test results are given, and partners or a friend may or may not be present with them for their results. At this session arrangements are made for follow-up support, and the planned programme is arranged for screening or preventive surgery options. Patients who are found to be positive for the gene need careful follow-up over a period of time. Many people are very emotional and upset when told the news that they are a gene carrier, despite careful preparation. Research has shown that distress and anxiety reduce after a month.[38] Carrier clinics for gene mutation carriers are offered in some areas, as well as support groups and education days.

Ethical issues surrounding genetic testing

Many of the ethical issues surrounding genetic testing concern confidentiality and the duties of the individuals sharing information with their family. For example, who should take the responsibility for informing other family members about a possible genetic risk or a 'positive' genetic test, and is there a duty to do so? For some, the effect of informing others can be devastating.[39] If the patient does not wish to warn relatives about cancer risk, does the problem then become one for the professional? In general, this important consideration related to the professional ethics of genetics is difficult if one assumes that genetic testing is always a 'family affair'. Arguably, although it is assumed to be a family affair, the individual rights of the person seeking genetic counselling for him or herself need to be considered. After all, one brother or sister may wish to know and another may not wish to know, because of the fear of discrimination. The rights of an individual to decide to know or not are paramount.[40]

The Human Genetic Commission has been asked to advise ministers on the complex issues surrounding the rapid advances in genetics and genetic testing.[29] This commission has a facilitative and advisory role, and aims to improve the level of informed debate about the implications of the development of human genetics. It incorporates a Genetic Discrimination Monitoring Group whose aim is to minimise discrimination for those people with genetic disorders. Family communication may differ between ethnic groups or those with different cultural backgrounds. Indeed, the culture of a given group may be very different from that of another culture. For example, in African-American culture, family sharing and a sense of spirituality are often highly valued, and decisions may be made collectively.[41] This may differ from the ethic of many Europeans whose values are based on the notions of the individual and his right to choose for himself.[42]

Genetic testing is centred around helping individuals to decide whether or not the genetic test that they are considering is worth taking. The genetic counsellor aims to work with that individual to explore all the pros and cons of each decision as part of the pre-test informed consent process. On the one hand, establishing the test itself is a scientific process, and on the other hand, the level of predictive power that justifies the test is a professional ethical question.[43] Assessing the test and its value includes a professional judgement about the clinical significance of any of the results that may affect not only the individual, but also the family.

There is a probability component in estimating whether or not an individual who chooses to have a predictive cancer genetic test will develop cancer or not. Certainly, the knowledge that an individual may have inherited a cancer susceptibility gene provides important information. This information is of clinical significance as preventive procedures may reduce morbidity and mortality in a known gene carrier. It is as well to note that there is an element of probability and uncertainty in clinical advice given concerning many cancer genes. The main considerations attributable to predictive cancer genetic testing are the knowledge that probability does not equate with certainty, and that individuals who are otherwise healthy are faced with the knowledge of carrying a genetic mutation that they may or may not pass to their offspring with associated risk of developing cancer. This knowledge is linked in with modifying factors, which are not only genetic but also have environmental influences. For example, if a woman carries either of the two known breast cancer genes (*BRCA1* or *BRCA2*), it is not certain that she will develop breast or ovarian cancer but merely that she has a cancer risk estimated from the latest gene penetrance studies.[7]

The examples below illustrates the fear and concern associated with a genetic test.

Anna said:

> When I was asked if I would like to find out if I had the gene . . . I discussed it with my sisters . . . and I said my reaction is that I don't want to know, and they said 'I'd agree with you . . . I wouldn't want to know either, because like what are you going to do . . . if you find out you've got the gene . . .?'.[34]

Penny felt:

> I am not sure [about genetic testing] . . . it is one of those things that I am trying not to think much about because I am not sure what my answer would be . . . I would be quite happy to have the test, if there is a fair chance that it was going to be negative . . .[34]

Prophylactic surgery

Prophylactic surgery is an option for the treatment of individuals at a high risk of developing cancer. In certain areas of cancer risk management, surgery has an established preventive role. For example, in the treatment of patients with multiple endocrine neoplasia type-2 syndrome, prophylactic total thyroidectomy is advocated to prevent the development of medullary thyroid cancer. Prophylactic colectomy is normally advised for individuals who have familial adenomatous polyposis, as surgery aims to prevent the inevitable progression of colonic adenomas to invasive cancers.[11]

In conditions where the cancer risk is lower, such as inherited breast and ovarian cancer, surgery is offered as a management option rather than being recommended. As well as reducing ovarian cancer risk by as much as 96%,[44] prophylactic oophorectomy has been demonstrated to reduce the risk of breast cancer by approximately half, depending on the woman's age at surgery.[45,46] There is also evidence that the reduction in risk of breast cancer from prophylactic breast surgery may be as high as 90%,[47-49] although there is some concern that current information regarding residual breast and ovarian cancer risk may contain bias inherent to the way the studies are currently performed.[49]

The sensitivity and specificity of surveillance techniques can also play a role in decisions about surgery. While the risk of ovarian cancer in a woman with a *BRCA*1 or *BRCA*2 mutation may not be as high as the risk of breast cancer, there is not as much evidence to show that ovarian cancer surveillance is as effective at detecting early-stage ovarian cancer as mammography is with early-stage breast cancer. There may be women who therefore choose to pursue prophylactic oophorectomy for ovarian cancer risk reduction, while managing their breast cancer risk through regular surveillance.

Although surgery offers high preventive rates for some of these inherited cancer syndromes, it is never without trauma, fear, and an impact on an individual's life when they opt for what may be considered a 'life-saving option'. The long-term follow-up of family members who have opted for surgery should continue, and the family history remains along with the continued concern for others in the family who may have already developed cancer.

The cost of prophylactic surgery in psychological terms has yet to be fully studied and understood. A very recent quantitative study surveyed women who had had prophylactic surgery as well as women who were at risk and had not undergone surgery. The majority of women reported satisfaction with bilateral prophylactic mastectomy and experienced psychosocial outcomes similar to women with similarly elevated breast cancer risk who did not undergo prophylactic mastectomy. This study suggests bilateral prophylactic mastectomy appears to neither positively nor negatively impact long-term psychosocial outcomes.[50]

Personal account 16.3

Susan (whose sister died at the age of 29 years, as did her mother and three sisters) said:

> Now that I am thirty-two . . . I am thinking . . . 'oh well there is hope because I am going to have this mastectomy' . . . so I pin all my hopes on that mastectomy . . . and if it means that I do not have two lumps around my body that didn't work for me . . . [she could not breast feed her child], as far as I am concerned [they are] two big bombs waiting to go off . . . I can't see another way . . . I wanted to have a baby before I died . . . I wanted to have that emotion . . . I could not face death without having a child . . . which is selfish because I was going to leave that child behind . . . I wasn't going to wait for the cancer to get me . . . I was going to get the cancer before it got me . . .[34]

Cultural issues in genetic counselling

The process of communication is at the core of genetic counselling. Genetic counselling encompasses issues including plans for continuing medical management, genetic testing, and how to communicate with other family members about genetics and risk. In all cases, such issues require sensitive handling; it is also important, however, to have an awareness of the individual's ethnicity and culture and how it might influence reactions to these issues. Ethnicity and culture can affect virtually all aspects of genetic counselling, and from an ethical and moral perspective, the goal of providing equal access and quality of services for all individuals requires that health care professionals are sensitive, knowledgeable, and skilled in working with individuals from diverse cultures and ethnic communities.[51]

Beliefs and expectations concerning medical treatment and practitioners can influence how the patient perceives genetic counselling.[52] Rapp[53] and Weil[54] have identified how religious and spiritual beliefs may affect how patients understand and respond and how they may have a major influence on the use of genetic tests and interventions. It is important that these beliefs are acknowledged and respected.[55] If they are ignored, it may lead to the patient withdrawing, withholding information, feelings of anger or shame, or even failing to attend appointments and non-compliance.[51]

Family dynamics can play an important role in genetic counselling and decision making. Cultural experiences and expectations may influence decision making. Decisions relating to reproduction or screening may be perceived to include other family members. This involves a broad spectrum of cultural issues relating to family authority, cohesion and support, and/or the relationship of the individual and family to the social or religious community.[56,57]

Communication barriers extend beyond those involving non-fluency in English. Although the person's first language may be English, they may be unfamiliar with the terms and concepts used in cancer genetics, Western medicine, and genetic counselling. Weil[51] and Mittman et al.[57] have also identified cultural differences in the degree of emotion expressed and self-revelation involved in communication with health care professionals.

The 'culture of cancer' and influence of the media

The media's influence on the culture of cancer is documented in the literature. Its depiction as 'the killer disease' provides a negative response. The language of warfare is regularly used in newspaper journals and on television programmes, fuelling anxiety for many people, especially those with a cancer risk. Cancer becomes a disease that personifies death itself. In this context, time is particularly needed in the complex process of cancer genetic counselling. The language of warfare is very often reflected in the language used by families discussing their cancer risk. The meta-phoric personification of cancer as the 'enemy' is profound, and linked with images from the media and film world. For example:

> Cancer is such an awful illness and it still keeps evading every doctor, research scientist as to a cure, as to why it happens . . . it must be one hell of a disease . . . it reminds me of Dr Hannibal in *The Silence of the Lambs*, he was a psychopathic killer, who used his victims through their brains, he got to them through the way he spoke . . . I thought he was a very clever, very, very, clever guy . . . and that is how I feel about cancer, it is clever, it is a smart cookie . . .[34]

The cancer nurse is well suited to deconstructing and understanding stories and myths long believed by the devastated families with inherited cancers. Telling the story, listening to the story, and empathising and understanding that cancer is a complicated illness is important. Lay people very often misinterpret the metastatic cancer process and confuse metastatic tumours with new primary tumours. In this way, individuals fear for themselves, believing that they are in line for many different types of cancer. Explanation of this process may decrease anxiety for some family members. Understanding the disease, the treatments, and the illness process is important. Some family members have never had the chance to do this and therefore feel a sense of confusion: they 'haven't liked to ask Dad' about the real truth about a family member's illness.

The following in an extract from Lisa's view of her genetic risk:

> I think [my grandmother's death] never really was explained to me . . . I just knew she was very ill and it was a cancer . . . but exactly what and why I didn't know . . . I didn't really register anything, that there might be a genetic link . . . so what can you do about it . . .?[34]

This example highlights the fact that some people are unaware of the cancer development in another family member. Lisa lives in a family with a dominantly inherited colon cancer gene. Her mother is terrified of developing the disease that killed her own mother and her two sisters. Cancer remains confusing to her and the genetic link has been her mother's prime concern. Screening for colon cancer is recognised as a positive management strategy for hereditary colon cancer risk.[11]

Family dynamics are very important, and one should establish with the family involved in the genetic counselling process the social relationships within the family. This is helpful to both the counsellor and the family member, as other members of the family may seek genetic counselling. Social relationships can be drawn in the format of a genogram (a family tree that shows the social relationship patterns in the family). It is essential to provide a confidential place of knowledge giving. All family members visiting the cancer genetics clinic are assured of their privacy with regard to the genetic counselling process. Any information about a cancer diagnosis or medical matter concerning a person who is alive should be given with written consent from the individual to whom the information pertains.

Psychological morbidity

It is important to be aware of any psychopathology that may occur as part of the experience of belonging to a family with a high cancer risk. The many bereavements in the family, and in particular the loss of a parent, may make it difficult for people to accept their own personal cancer risks. Unresolved bereavement, cancerphobia, or excessive anxiety states all need expert assessment by a clinical psychologist.

Discrimination and insurance

Fear of discrimination may exist for people known to be at high risk of developing cancer. The ABI Code of Practice on Genetic Testing regulates the behaviour of insurance companies who belong to the ABI when dealing with any genetic test information disclosed to them by an individual applying for insurance. Insurers are also bound by the Moratorium, agreed with the government in 1999, and the Concordat and Moratorium of 2005. This moratorium has been extended until 2011 and sets down that no predictive genetic test results be requested by ABI insurance companies unless the patient is requesting insurance cover

over a certain financial limit.[58] However, if a person who has a positive result following a Huntingdon's predictive genetic test seeks insurance over a certain threshold, they are bound to inform the insurance company about their results.

New developments

Preimplantation genetic diagnosis (PGD) involves *in vitro* fertilisation (IVF) and embryo biopsy to prevent pregnancies affected with serious life-threatening diseases. This technique has been used in the past mainly for hereditary disorders causing lifelong disability or death in early life, or for cases where there is no possible option of treatment. It has been used for cancer conditions such as familial adenomatous polyposis coli (FAP) and multiple endocrine neoplasia. More recently there has been much debate over the licence granted by the Human Fertilisation and Embryology Authority (HFEA) to use PGD in the UK for 'lower penetrance' mutations in adult-onset hereditary breast cancer (BRCA) and hereditary non-polyposis colorectal cancer (HNPCC) adult-onset families where individuals do not always develop the disease even if the mutation is inherited. A recent qualitative study debated the ethical and social issues with BRCA patients,[59] and, as a *BRCA1* carrier and past medical doctor involved in PGD, the author Bryan recommends in her chapter on PGD that families carefully weigh the wide range of views and the options available.[60]

Conclusions

Cancer genetics is a developing specialty, and oncology nurses may well be involved with caring for patients who have developed hereditary cancer. They may need to refer patients on to the cancer genetic services if needed. Nurses who choose to work in cancer genetic clinics need to understand the state of flux of knowledge, along with the many psychosocial implications that affect not only the person seeking the counselling but also other family members. This knowledge is both predictive and prognostic, and has many implications for families.

The language of cancer genetics needs to be explained to family members seeking counselling. The changing and cutting-edge nature of this specialty is both exciting and symbolic of the complexities associated with a rapidly developing technological age. These developments are interlinked with cost cutting budgets and constraints in practice as well. Scientific discoveries leading to improving cancer care need careful consideration and understanding from a holistic perspective. The scientific discoveries are moving at a great pace, and by understanding the molecular basis of the mechanics of the genetic changes, there is hope for further discoveries leading to new treatments, useful screening, and perhaps a cure for inherited cancer. Already certain patients are being offered chemotherapy regimes in the research setting to help manage their condition, after suggestion that cells carrying mutations in cancer predisposition genes might be sensitive to inhibition of an enzyme called Poly (ADP-ribose) polymerase.[61] As this is a fast-moving field, the absolute risk figures can change with time as more knowledge becomes available. Also, it may not be long before pathology diagnostics make it clear at the moment of diagnosis whether or not a cancer patient is likely to be a gene mutation carrier. This new knowledge will greatly impact on the clinicians who are informing patients about their cancer diagnosis.[62]

If, however, predictions for improved diagnosis are borne out, then it is essential to process the knowledge in human terms. Understanding cancer risk is complex, and each individual has their way of believing the facts and relating to them in meaningful ways according to experience. Cancer nurses need to have the education to both support and provide information for those patients and their families who have developed cancer as the result of an inherited condition.

References

1. Eeles R.A., Ponder B.A.J., Easton D.F. and Horwich A. (eds.) *Genetic Predisposition to Cancer*, 2nd edition. London: Chapman and Hall.
2. Hodgson S.V., Foulkes W., Eng C. and Maher E. (eds.) (2006). *A Practical Guide to Human Cancer Genetics*, 3rd edition. Cambridge: Cambridge University Press.
3. Stein L.D. (2004). Human genome: end of the beginning. *Nature* **431**, 915–916.
4. Suzuki D.T., Griffiths A.J.F., Miller J.H. and Lewontin R.C. (1986). *An Introduction to Genetic Analysis*, 3rd edition. New York: W.H. Freeman.
5. Schneider K. (2002). *Counseling about Cancer: Strategies for Genetic Counseling*, 2nd edition. New York: John Wiley and Sons.
6. Jones S. and van Loon B. (1993). *Genetics for Beginners*. Cambridge: Icon Books.
7. Ford D., Easton D.F., Stratton M.R. *et al.* (1998). Genetic heterogeneity and penetrance analysis of the *BRCA1* and *BRCA2* genes in breast cancer families. *American Journal of Human Genetics* **62**, 676–689.
8. Easton D. (2004). From families to chromosomes: genetic linkage, and other methods for finding cancer predisposition genes. In Eeles R.A., Ponder B.A.J., Easton D.F. and Horwich A. (eds.) *Genetic Predisposition to Cancer*, 2nd edition. London: Chapman and Hall, pp. 21–40.
9. Eng C. and Ponder B. (2004). Multiple endocrine neoplasia type 2. In Eeles R.A., Ponder B.A.J., Easton D.F. and Horwich A. (eds.) *Genetic Predisposition to Cancer*, 2nd edition. London: Chapman and Hall, pp. 105–118.
10. Knudson A.G. (1985). Hereditary cancer, oncogenes and antioncogenes. *Cancer Research* **45**, 1437–1443.
11. Hodgson S. and Murday V. (2004). Screening and management of familial colon cancer. In Eeles R.A., Ponder B.A.J., Easton D.F. and Horwich A. (eds.) *Genetic Predisposition to Cancer*, 2nd edition. London: Chapman and Hall, pp. 331–338.
12. Anonymous (2001). News. *European Journal of Cancer Care* **10**, 228–233.
13. Lakhani S.R., van de Vijver M.J., Jacquemier J. *et al.* (2002). The pathology of familial breast cancer: predictive value of immunohistochemical markers estrogen receptor, progesterone receptor, HER-2, and p53 in patients with mutations in *BRCA1* and *BRCA2*. *Journal of Clinical Oncology* **20**, 3752–3753.
14. Armes J.E. and Venter D.J. (2002). The pathology of inherited breast cancer. *Pathology* **34**, 309–314.
15. Møller P., Borg A., Evans D.G. *et al.* (2002) Survival in prospectively ascertained familial breast cancer: analysis of a series stratified by tumour characteristics, BRCA mutations and oophorectomy. *International Journal of Cancer* **20**, 555–559.
16. Foulkes W.D., Stefansson I.M., Chappuis P.O. *et al.* (2003). Germline *BRCA1* mutations and a basal epithelial phenotype in breast cancer. *Journal of the National Cancer Institute* **95**, 1482–1485.
17. Office for National Statistics. www.statistics.gov.uk/CCI/nugget.asp?ID=915&Pos=1&ColRank=1&Rank=294 (accessed 6 September 2007).

18. McKusick V. (1998). *Mendelian Inheritance in Man.* Baltimore, MA: Johns Hopkins University Press.

19. Firth H. and Hurst J. (2005). *Oxford Desk Reference Clinical Genetics.* Oxford: Oxford University Press.

20. Bancroft E., Ardern-Jones A. and Lynch E. (2006). Cancer genetics: the importance of obtaining a family history. *Nursing Times* **102**, 28–29.

21. Eng C. (1998). Genetics of Cowden syndrome: through the looking glass of oncology. *International Journal of Oncology* **12,** 701–710.

22. Abeliovich D., Kadouri L., Lerer I. *et al.* (1997). The founder mutations in 185delAG and 5382insC in *BRCA*1 and 617delT in *BRCA*2 appear in 60% of ovarian cancer and 30% of early-onset breast cancer patients among Ashkenazi women. *American Journal of Human Genetics* **60**, 505–514.

23. Easton D.E. and Peto J. (1990). The contribution of inherited predisposition to cancer incidence. *Cancer Surveys* **9**, 395–416.

24. Evers-Kiebooms G., Cassiman J.-J., van den Berghe H. and d'Ydewalle G. (eds.) (1987). *Genetic Risk, Risk Perception and Decision Making.* New York: Liss.

25. McAllister M. (2003). Personal theories of inheritance, coping strategies, risk perception and engagement in hereditary non-polyposis colon cancer families offered genetic testing. *Clinical Genetics* **64**, 179–189.

26. Watson M., Lloyd S., Davidson J. *et al.* (1999). The impact of genetic counselling on risk perception and mental health in women with a family history of breast cancer. *British Journal of Cancer* **79**, 868–874.

27. Appleton S., Fry A., Rees G., Rush R. and Cull A. (2000). Psychological effects of living with an increased risk of breast cancer: An exploratory study using telephone focus groups. *Psycho-oncology* **9**, 511–521.

28. Department of Health. (2003). *Our Inheritance, Our Future.* London: Department of Health.

29. Human Genetics Commission. (2003). *Genes Direct. Ensuring the Effective Oversight of Genetic Tests Directly to the Public.* London: Human Genetics Commission.

30. Stewart-Brown S. and Farmer A. (1997). Screening could seriously damage your health. *British Medical Journal* **314**, 533–534.

31. Featherstone K., Atkinson P., Bharadwaj A. and Clarke A.J. (2006). *Risky Relations: Family and Kinship in the Era of New Genetics.* Oxford: Berg.

32. Thomas S.G. (2005). *Women's Experiences of Living with an Inherited Breast/Ovarian Cancer Family History: Stories from Different Ethnic Groups.* MSc thesis, Kings College, London.

33. National Institute for Health and Clinical Excellence. (2006). *Clinical Guidance: Familial Breast Cancer: The Classification and Care of Women at Risk of Familial Breast Cancer in Primary, Secondary and Tertiary Care (partial update of CG14).* London: National Institute for Health and Clinical Excellence.

34. Ardern-Jones A.T. (1997). *Living with a Cancer Legacy – The Experience of Hereditary Cancer in the Family.* MSc thesis, University of London, Institute of Cancer Research.

35. Vasen H.F.A., Mecklin J.-P., Meera-Khan P. *et al.* (1991). The International Collaborative Group on Hereditary Non-Polyposis Colorectal Cancer (ICG-HNPCC). *Diseases of the Colon and Rectum* **34**, 424–425.

36. Ardern-Jones A.T., Kenen R., Lynch E., Doherty R. and Eeles R. (2007). Is no news good news. *European Journal of Cancer Care* (in the press).

37. Kash K., Dabney M. and Boolbol S. (2004). Psychological issues in cancer genetics. In Eeles R.A., Ponder B.A.J., Easton D.F. and Horwich A. (eds.) *Genetic Predisposition to Cancer*, 2nd edition. London: Chapman and Hall, pp. 404–413.

38. Reichelt J.G., Heimdal K., Møller P. and Dahl A.A. (2004). BRCA1 testing with definitive results: a prospective study of psychological distress in a large clinic-based sample. *Familial Cancer* **3**, 21–28.

38. Foster C., Evans D.G., Eeles R. *et al.* (2002). Predictive testing for *BRCA1/2*: attributes, risk perception and management in a multi-centre cohort. *British Journal of Cancer* **86**, 1209–1216.

39. Hallowell N., Foster C., Eeles R., Ardern-Jones A. and Watson M. (2004). Accommodating risk: responses to *BRCA1/2* genetic testing of women who have had cancer. *Social Science and Medicine* **59**, 553–565.

40. Clarke A., Richards M., Kerzin-Storrar *et al.* (2005). Genetic professioinals' reports of nondisclosure of genetic risk information within families. *European Journal of Human Genetics* **13**, 556–562.

41. Martin J.N., Hecht M.L. and Larkey L.K. (1994). Conversational improvement strategies for interethnic communication: African American and European American perspectives. *61 Communication Monographs* **236**, 353–372.

42. Lerman C., Peshkin M.S., Hughes C. and Isaacs M.D. (1998). Family disclosure in genetic testing for cancer susceptibility: determinants and consequences. *Journal of Health Care, Law and Policy* **1**, 353–372.

43. Geller L.N., Alper J.S., Billings P.R., Barash C.L., Becwith J. and Natowicz M. (1996). Individual family and societal dimensions of genetic discrimination: a case study analysis. *Science and Engineering Ethics* **2**, 71–88.

44. Olopade O. and Artioli G. (2004). Efficacy of risk-reducing salpingo-oophorectomy in women with BRCA-1 and BRCA-2 mutations. *The Breast Journal* **10(suppl. 1)**, S5–S9.

45. Rebbeck T.R., Lynch H.T., Neuhausen S.L. *et al.* (2002). The Prevention and Observation of Surgical End Points

Study Group: prophylactic oophorectomy in carriers of *BRCA1* or *BRCA2* mutations. *New England Journal of Medicine* **346**, 1616–1622.

46. Hartmann L.C., Schaid D.J., Woods J.E. *et al.* (1999). Efficacy of bilateral prophylactic mastectomy in women with a family history of breast cancer. *New England Journal of Medicine* **340**, 77–84.

47. Rebbeck T.R., Friebel T., Lynch H.T. *et al.* (2004). Bilateral prophylactic mastectomy reduces breast cancer risk in *BRCA1* and *BRCA2* mutation carriers: The PROSE study group. *Journal of Clinical Oncology* **22**, 1055–1062.

48. Meijers-Heijboer H., van Geel B., van Putten W.L.J. *et al.* (2001). Breast cancer after prophylactic bilateral mastectomy in women with a BRCA1 or BRCA2 mutation. *New England Journal of Medicine* **345**, 159–164.

49. Klaren H.M., van't Veer L.J., van Leeuwen M.A. *et al.* (2003). Commentary: Potential for bias in studies on efficacy of prophylactic surgery for BRCA1 and BRCA2 mutation. *Journal of the National Cancer Institute* **95**, 941–947.

50. Geiger A.M., Nekhlyudov L., Herrington L.J. *et al.* (2007). Quality of life after bilateral prophylactic mastectomy. *Annals of Surgical Oncology* **14**, 686–694.

51. Weil J. (2001). Multicultural education and genetic counseling. *Clinical Genetics* **59**, 143–149.

52. Greb A. (1998). Multiculturalism and the practice of genetic counseling. In Baker D.L., Schuette J.L., Uhlmann W.R. (eds.) *A Guide to Genetic Counseling*. New York: Wiley-Liss, pp. 171–198.

53. Rapp R. (1999) *Testing Women, Testing the Fetus: The Social Impact of Amniocentesis in America*. New York: Routledge.

54. Weil J. (1991). Mothers' postcounseling beliefs about the causes of their children's genetic disorders. *American Journal of Human Genetics* **48**, 145–153.

55. Cohen L.H., Fine B.A. and Pergament E. (1998). An assessment of ethnocultural beliefs regarding the causes of birth defects and genetic disorders. *Journal of Genetic Counseling* **7**, 15–29.

56. Wang V.O. (2001). Multicultural genetic counselling: then, now, and in the 21st century. *American Journal of Medical Genetics* **106**, 208–215.

57. Mittman I., Crombleholme W.R., Green J.R. and Golbus M.S. (1998). Reproductive genetic counseling to Asian-Pacific and Latin American immigrants. *Journal of Genetic Counseling* **7**, 49–70.

58. Department of Health (2005). *Genetics and Insurance Committee, Fourth Report from January 2005 to December 2005*. London: Stationery Office.

59. Menon U., Harper J., Sharma A. *et al.* (2007). Views of BRCA gene mutation carriers on preimplantation genetic diagnosis as a reproductive option for hereditary breast and ovarian cancer. *Human Reproduction* **22**, 1573–1577.

60. Bryan E. (2007). Afterward. In Bryan E. *Singing the Life*. London: Vermillion, pp. 278–296.

61. McCabe N., Lord C.J., Tutt A.N. *et al.* (2005). BRCA2-deficient CAPAN-1 cells are extremely sensitive to the inhibition of Poly (ADP-Ribose) polymerase: an issue of potency. *Cancer Biology and Therapy* **4**, 934–936.

62. Scott R. (2006). Future Implications for Genetic Testing. Oral presentation at IMPACT and AIDIT conference, Szczecin, Poland, 28–30 November, 2006.

Part 4

The Management of Cancer-related Problems

Introduction

Cancer causes a large range of difficult and distressing problems, as a result of either the disease process itself, or its treatment. In the preceding section on 'The Experience of Treatment', problems associated with treatment are identified and nursing strategies for managing these examined. This section focuses more directly on those problems, which are primarily (although not exclusively) the result of the disease process. The problems and difficulties that often accompany cancer cannot be neatly divided into those resulting from treatment and those arising from the disease itself. These are not mutually exclusive; therefore a rather arbitrary distinction is made here. Several common cancer-related problems have been identified, however, and are explored with particular reference to the contribution that nursing could make to their control or management. A departure from the traditional notion of symptom management is made, and a more radical and person-centred approach is proposed.

Symptom management has been dominated by the successes achieved in cancer pain control using powerful drugs. This perhaps unintentionally set a path for the construction of care, which has placed heavy emphasis on a biomedical model of management, and the search for new and better drugs first for pain, and then for other symptoms common in cancer. This has led to the orientation of care around the 'relief' of the symptom experienced, and the neglect of other equally important aspects, such as suffering, distress, and ability to function independently.

The limitations of this model of 'symptom control' are well rehearsed in the literature, and surround the biomedical relationship to 'the body' since this:

- regards the body as an external object to the enquiries that yield knowledge of it
- assumes that the practitioner is in control of the body of the 'patient', and diagnosis and treatment therefore requires them to be subordinate to the practitioner
- deals with malfunctioning organs and related symptoms and not the 'body', which constitutes the actual person.[1,2]

The assumption that symptoms are reflections of disordered bodily processes, where the physician's task is to decode patients' descriptions of these in order to diagnose disease, is inadequate. Instead, a meaning-centred approach has been proposed,[3,4] which seeks to access an individual's interpretation of their illness and to assist them to construct new understanding of their illness. In this context, therefore, the term 'symptom' is highly problematic because of the assumption that this is universally defined and can be managed beyond the person by the health carer, with little reference to social or cultural influences. It also inherently excludes the person's own narrative and personal meanings from the therapeutic process. The terms 'problem' and 'need' are preferable, since these suggest something that is difficult to deal with or understand. The power for action and ownership of these, however, remains with the person experiencing the problem. Looked at in this way, it is possible to see that as health carers we have no right to 'manage' these problems, only to assist in their containment, and both the sufferer and health carer have a mutual need to understand them:[5]

> There is more to what people experience and know than they are able to express and we are able to hear.[6]

Problems associated with cancer and its treatment may be viewed both positively and negatively. Where a problem provides legitimisation to rest or temporarily to cease demanding activities, it may be interpreted as beneficial. More commonly it is interpreted as a sign of disease progression, failure of treatment, or imminent death. The meanings attributed to cancer-related symptoms and how people respond to and cope with problems are unique. These are influenced by an individual's life history and the wider culture in which understanding of illness develops.[7,8] Gender, personality traits, health beliefs, socio-economic status, environmental factors, and health carers themselves are all potent in either exacerbating or containing the problems that result from cancer.[9] This implies that health carers must disentangle what is 'really going on' from a person's account of their problem and any distress or difficulty associated with it. Their experience is of only secondary importance within the biomedical process of naming a symptom. Practitioners who use such a reductionist approach may respond to complex situations by applying a diagnosis based upon professional knowledge, discarding the subjective expressions of the person experiencing it since they do not 'fit' the diagnostic picture.[10]

Nurses have a tremendous contribution to make in helping people to articulate and interpret their problems and through this become better at managing them for themselves. Nurses' expertise lies not in telling people what ails them, but in working alongside them to clarify the totality of their experience. Even when cure is not possible, understanding the meaning problems hold for an individual can be a powerful source of support and comfort.

In this section, expert nurses have set out to articulate a way of working with people who have cancer in order to assist them in managing their problems. Many common problems are discussed. Some, such as pain, compromised nutrition, wounds, and the risk of infection, have been widely documented and researched. Others, such as breathlessness, ascites, confusion, and lymphoedema, have received less attention.

The section begins its consideration of the clinical management of cancer-related problems by focusing on nursing's contribution to the management of cancer pain. As one of the most commonly associated symptoms of cancer, it is not surprising that pain is often one of the most feared, and perhaps the most catastrophised, of all cancer symptoms. Despite the considerable attention paid by health care professionals to this phenomenon, pain continues to be inadequately controlled.

References

1. Lynon M.L. and Barbalet J.M. (1994). Society's body: emotion and the 'somatization' of social theory. In Csordas T.J. (ed.) *Embodiment and Experience.* Cambridge: Cambridge University Press.
2. Corner J. and Dunlop R. (1997). New approaches to care. In Clark D., Ahmedzai S. and Hockley J. (eds.) *New Themes in Palliative Care.* Milton Keynes: Open University Press.
3. Cassel E.J. (1982). The nature of suffering and the goals of medicine. *New England Journal of Medicine* **306**, 639–645.
4. Good B.J. and DelVecchio Good M.J. (1980). The meaning of symptoms – a cultural hermeneutic model for clinical practice. In Eisenberg I. and Kleinman A. (eds.) *The Relevance of Social Science for Medicine.* Dordrecht: Reidel.
5. Corner J. (2004). Working with difficult symptoms. In Payne S., Seymour J. and Ingleton C. (eds.) *Palliative Care Nursing.* Maidenhead, Berkshire: Open University Press.
6. Halldorsdottir S. and Hamrin E. (1995). Experiencing existential changes: the lived experience of having cancer. *Cancer Nursing* **19**, 29–36.
7. Kleinman A. (1988). *The Illness Narratives: Suffering, Healing and the Human Condition.* New York: Basic Books.
8. Benner P. and Wrubel J. (1989). *The Primacy of Caring. Stress and Coping in Health and Illness.* Menlo Park, CA: Addison-Wesley.
9. Vessey J. and Richardson B. (1993). A holistic approach to symptom assessment and intervention. *Holistic Nursing Practice* **7**, 13–21.
10. Schön D. (1983). *The Reflective Practitioner.* London: Maurice Temple Smith.

CHAPTER SEVENTEEN

Pain

Meinir Krishnasamy

Evidence indicates that half of all patients who experience cancer pain receive inadequate relief, even though research suggests that it is possible to relieve 80–90% of cancer pain.[1-3] Pain is often the primary reason for seeking medical attention. For the individual subsequently diagnosed with cancer, it becomes a potent symptom, signifying the presence of disease or intimating its progression. Cancer, pain, and death may consequently become fused in the mind of the individual. Because of this, pain management will only be effective if a patient-centred approach to care is embraced by health professionals.[4] Unfortunately, there is little evidence to suggest that cancer pain management is either patient centred or holistic.[5]

The World Health Organization promotes the concept of 'total pain',[6] which acknowledges that it has physical, emotional, social, and spiritual components.[7] Without attention to each of these facets of the pain experience, patient-centred care will continue to be an anomaly, and the statistics for unrelieved pain are unlikely to improve. As long ago as 1979, McCaffrey stated that 'everything written or said about pain is worthless in the hands of a practitioner who doubts that a patient has pain'.[7] The patient, she asserts, is 'the only authority about the pain he experiences'. An acceptance of pain, when reported by individuals, irrespective of whether or not there is verifiable tissue damage, is therefore fundamental to effective pain management.[8]

Pain is deeply personal – neither solely shaped nor confined by a biological reality.[5] It is a complex biocultural event and, as such, one of nursing's greatest potential contributions to pain management is to facilitate the expression of each individual's experience of pain.[9]

Managing cancer pain

Evidence-based clinical guidelines set out essential aspects of effective pain management,[10] and yet in reality these recommendations are only partly adopted in practice.[11] Some of the key recommendations emphasised in the guidelines include: pain intensity must be quantified, pain must be adopted as an organisational priority, pain assessment must be standardised across the organisation, selected pharmacological and non-pharmacological interventions should be used, and minimum standards for clinicians' pain assessment skills should be established.[10,12]

The aims and principles of cancer pain management are to:

- recognise and promptly assess pain in patients with cancer
- identify psychological and spiritual influences on pain perception and management
- alleviate pain at night, at rest, and on movement

- maximise independence and possible quality of life
- address and thus relieve current and future fears about pain
- provide support and encouragement for family members and friends and professional caregivers
- invite participation of the patient, family, and/ or friends
- adopt a collaborative, multidisciplinary approach
- design unique analgesic regimes tailored to each patient's needs and tolerance
- regularly follow up the outcome
- refer early to specialist services if pain control is not achieved.[13]

Without comprehensive assessment taking account of the many interdependent facets of pain it is unlikely that the principles outlined above will be met.

Several pain-assessment instruments are now widely available, and evidence indicates that no one approach consistently shows greater sensitivity than others in their ability to detect changes in pain.[14] The core elements of cancer pain assessment include questions around:

- *intensity* – how severe is the pain?
- *character* – how would you describe your pain?
- *location* – where is your pain? Does your pain go anywhere else?
- *timing* – when does your pain occur?
- *associated factors* – what makes your pain worse or better?
- *implications of pain* – how does this pain affect your daily living?

An awareness of misconceptions that may hamper the process of assessment will facilitate effective nursing management.

Some common misperceptions about pain management are that:

- real pain has an identifiable, physical cause
- psychogenic pain (i.e. one better understood through the language of psychology rather than physiology) does not really hurt and may even be comparable to malingering
- members of the health care team are capable of making accurate inferences about the nature, severity, and existence of an individual's pain, based on professional knowledge and the patient's behavioural and physiological expressions of the pain
- the severity and duration of pain can be predicted by the nature of the cancer and the cause and location of the pain
- patients should be encouraged to have a high tolerance for pain
- patients in severe pain always look distressed
- pain can be understood in isolation solely as a facet of the cancer diagnosis.[8,15–17]

Box 17.1   Some factors affecting an individual's perception of pain[5,7,15,17]

• Fatigue	• Cultural norms and
• Insomnia	expectations of pain
• Discomfort	expression and behaviour
• Anxiety	• Religious or spiritual
• Depression	beliefs
• Anger	• Familial support
• Fear	• Social support network
• Sadness	• Perceptions of self
• Boredom	• Altered self-image and
• Isolation	self-esteem
• Withdrawal	• Loss of income
• Loneliness	• Professional expectations
• Perceptions of the	of causes of pain behaviour
significance of the	• Professional expectations
pain and its meaning	of pain behaviour
• Cultural identity	• Fear of being on 'a
	collision course with death'

Traditionally, medical management had involved identification of a relationship between pain and a noxious stimulus or abnormal neurophysiological activity.[7] When a cause for the pain is found, the doctor explains to the patient why he experiences pain, and prescribes 'appropriate' analgesia. However, in the light of the factors affecting perception of pain, administering analgesia in isolation is clearly insufficient if pain relief is to be effective.

What happens when no cause for an individual's pain can be found? For many in this situation, their experience is left unverified and may ultimately result in stigmatisation or rejection by professionals, family, and friends. Exploring what pain means to the person experiencing it, and attempting to understand it within the context of social and cultural characteristics, is a means of overcoming the difficulty of identifying a cause. Unfortunately, there is currently little evidence of nurses' ability to enter into such profoundly therapeutic relationships with people in pain.

An appreciation of pain pathways and analgesic regimes (described later in this chapter) is central to effective nursing care. This may be especially important when complex pain syndromes such as bone and neuropathic pain impact on an individual's quality of life. However, nursing's critical contribution to cancer pain management will only be realised as we begin to nurture the therapeutic skills necessary to help others to articulate the experience of illness, as we begin to understand and work with what we are told about pain. Nevertheless, this is notoriously difficult as pain, like so many other symptoms discussed in this chapter, is deeply resistant to simple expression in everyday language or speech.[3] How many times have you been told, 'I just can't explain what it feels like' or 'I know it sounds stupid but I just can't point to where it is'?

As health care professionals, we may compound the unspeakable nature of pain, demanding acquiescence in an objective rhetoric so that symptoms may be validated, and the 'right' to help for them is justified.[18] Nurses are ideally placed to redress this bias. By directing assessment at the person and not the pain, we are likely to be effective in a way that has previously been unattainable (see Care strategy 17.1).

An overview of analgesic drugs

The World Health Organisation has developed a guide for the selection of analgesic drugs to manage cancer pain.[6] These steps, commonly referred to as the 'three-step analgesic ladder', have become the mainstay of pharmacological management of mild, moderate, and severe cancer pain (see Box 17.2).[19]

Care strategy 17.1   Working with an individual – 'I'm much more than just a cancer patient'

Valuable questions to ask to try and evaluate a patient's pain include:

- When did you first notice you were ill?
- How have things been since you were told about the cancer?
- How have things been with and for your family or friends?
- What was happening in your life when the cancer was diagnosed?
- What plans or life events has it disrupted or destroyed?
- Did you experience any pain when you were first ill?
- When did you first experience any pain?
- Is the pain the same now or has it changed?
- What makes it worse and what makes it better?
- What are your expectations, fears, and hopes for the future?
- What does the pain mean to you?

Unfortunately, there are many unwanted side-effects of these medications. The most prevalent are nausea, vomiting, and constipation. For those who are eating well or who have previously been taking opioids, an anti-emetic is less likely to be necessary. For some, nausea is only a problem for the first few days following initial prescription or while doses are being increased incrementally until pain control is achieved, while others may require indefinite anti-emetic cover. Nursing approaches to managing nausea and vomiting are discussed later in this chapter. Aperients should always be prescribed with opioids unless specific complications such as bowel obstruction contraindicate this. Combining a softening laxative (e.g. lactulose) with a stimulant (e.g. senna) may often be more effective.[23]

Drowsiness, urinary retention, confusion, hallucinations, itching, and bronchospasm have also been documented as side-effects of opioid medication.[13] Respiratory depression is not a problem when using strong opioids regularly by mouth to relieve pain. Indeed, circumstantial evidence suggests that the competent use of morphine to relieve pain facilitates better rest, dietary intake, and mobility, thus prolonging lives.[17] Addiction

Box 17.2 The three-step analgesic ladder

Mild pain
Drugs of choice – non-narcotics:

- paracetamol, aspirin, or non-steroidal anti-inflammatory drugs (NSAIDs)
- combining paracetamol and NSAIDs is more effective than using either alone.

Moderate pain
Drugs of choice – weak opioids:

- dextropropoxyphene (Distalgesic), codeine, or dihydrocodeine.

Severe pain
Drugs of choice – strong opioids:

- morphine, hydromorphone, oxycodone methadone, fentanyl (transdermal patch - long acting, subcutaneous injections (very short action time; fentanyl lozenges)
- combining two strong opioids or mixing a weak and strong opioid is not advisable. Remember that most patients with cancer require strong opioids.

Adjuvant drugs/co-analgesics:

- corticosteroids for nerve and bone pain and for painful hepatomegaly and headache from raised intracranial pressure
- antidepressants, anti-arrhythmic, and anticonvulsant drugs can all be used to alleviate nerve pain
- antispasmodics for reduction of muscle spasm
- biphosphonates for relief of bone pain
- antibiotics or antirheumatic drugs for alleviation of co-existing pathologies.[6,19–22]

opioids over a short period of time, or have rapidly increasing pain over a short period of time.[26] The cause of pain wind-up is usually inadequate treatment of pain or misdiagnosis of neuropathic pain. It can usually be prevented by comprehensive pain assessment and complex analgesic regimens, but it will not be relieved by opioid prescription.[26]

Surgery, radiotherapy, nerve blocks, transcutaneous nerve stimulation (TENS), heat, cold, and cordotomy (although only occasionally used) are also effective methods of pain relief.[17] Increasing attention is being given to interventions that rely more on psychological and cultural influences on pain.[27] Expert opinion and patient self-report attest to their benefit, but there is limited level I (systematic review) or II (randomised controlled trial) evidence to support their safety or efficacy. Data from descriptive studies and expert opinion suggest that complementary interventions can reduce the level of analgesics required by some patients, and for patients sensitive to opioids these approaches may offer considerable benefit.[28–31]

Care strategy 17.2 Examples of non-pharmacological interventions

• Relaxation	• Imagery
• Hypnosis	• Distraction
• Acupuncture	• Music therapy
• Visualisation	• Reflexology
• Art therapy	• Massage
• Biofeedback	

is not a problem when morphine is used to treat opioid-responsive pain,[17] and this should not be used as a reason to withhold opioids from patients with cancer.[24]

Physical dependence, manifested as irritability, chills, sweating, abdominal pain, diarrhoea, and anxiety, if opioids are stopped suddenly, should not be confused with psychological addiction.[19]

For some patients, cancer pain increases with time and seems resistant to increasing doses of analgesia. This may be due to progression of the disease or to a phenomenon called 'pain wind-up', where patients require increasing doses of

Providing nursing care for a person experiencing cancer pain is a considerable nursing challenge. Its complexity demands that nurses open their minds to different ideas of ways in which to interact with people in pain.[5] This also involves relying on a process of individualising established components of pain relief.

- Don't wait until pain becomes severe before intervening.
- Use a variety of pain relief measures, but above all, include what the patient says works.

Box 17.3   Guidelines for use of morphine for cancer pain in adults[17,19,25,26]

- *Administration*:
  - The optimal route of administration of opioids is by mouth, but if patients are unable to swallow drugs, rectal and subcutaneous routes can be used, as the bio-availability and duration of action are the same. Morphine suppositories are widely available in several doses, but if you do have trouble accessing them, they can be prepared easily in hospital pharmacies.
  - Morphine can be given *subcutaneously* every 4 hours or by continuous infusion. When converting from oral to subcutaneous morphine for chronic pain the dose should be divided by two (the precise ratio probably lies between 1:2 and 1:3). Other opioids such as *diamorphine* and *hydromorphone* may be preferred to morphine for parenteral use. However, neither drug is more effective than morphine, but both are more potent. The relative potency ratio of oral morphine to subcutaneous diamorphine is 1:3.
  - *Morphine should not be given intramuscularly for chronic cancer pain* as subcutaneous administration is easier and less painful for the patient.
  - If patients have generalised oedema, tend to develop erythema, soreness, or sterile abscesses with subcutaneous administration, have coagulation disorders, or poor venous circulation, subcutaneous administration is contraindicated and intravenous (IV) administration should be considered instead. IV administration should also be considered if patients have indwelling central catheters or peripheral IV access. *The relative potency of oral to intravenous morphine is about 1:3.* Bolus IV doses of morphine will be higher in potency because of greater peak effects.
  - *Controlled-release morphine tablets should not be crushed* as this alters their dissolution and absorption characteristics. *Vaginal or rectal administration is also contraindicated*, as reduced bio-availability and haphazard absorption are likely. Sublingual and nebulised routes of morphine administration for pain management are not recommended as there is little evidence of predictability of absorption rates.
- Dose titration should involve the prescription of immediate-release morphine (oral morphine in solution or immediate release tablets) every 4 hours. The same dose should be used for breakthrough pain and can be given as frequently as required, e.g. every hour. There is no evidence to suggest that patients experience any significant adverse effects when the full dose is administered for breakthrough pain. If immediate-release morphine is not available, the total daily dose requirement should be based on an individual's previous analgesic intake. Breakthrough pain should be managed with non-steroidal anti-inflammatory drugs or with another short-acting opioid. If available, morphine sulphate injection solution can be administered orally or rectally for breakthrough pain.
- *Controlled-release morphine*, which provides cover over a 12-hour period, should not be used when attempting to titrate the analgesic dose, as its delayed peak plasma concentration makes it more difficult to assess the adequacy of the dose given, and to respond quickly to patients' needs. Several formulations are available but there is no evidence that they differ in their duration of effect or relative analgesic properties. However, care needs to be taken if changing between preparations, as there may be possible variations in release profiles and bio-availability.
- *Once stabilised*, patients using a 4-hourly regimen based on immediate-release morphine can continue to use the same dose for breakthrough pain. However, if a patient's pain is controlled using a 12-hourly regimen, the immediate-release morphine dose used to counteract breakthrough pain should be *one-third of the regular 12-hourly dose*.
- If a patient's pain returns consistently before the next dose of regular analgesia is due, the 4- to 12-hourly prescription should be increased. Relying solely on breakthrough analgesia to 'top up' the analgesic requirement will not only result in greater inconvenience for the patient, but may also lead to increased adverse side-effects. For some patients, however, a 12-hourly regime is inadequate to control their pain, and controlled-release morphine may be required with an 8-hourly regime if their pain is to be effectively managed.
- Fentanyl, methadone and buprenorphine are well absorbed sublingually and may be used as alternatives to subcutaneous morphine. Buprenorphine is commonly used sublingually and may be a useful alternative for low-dose oral morphine where patients have difficulty swallowing. Evidence of efficacy in long-term use is limited. Early indications suggest that fentanyl provides continuous, controlled systemic delivery of analgesia for 72 hours via transdermal patches. It appears to be well tolerated and effective, but further evidence of its place in the routine management of cancer pain is required.
- Advising a patient to take a double dose of their immediate-release morphine at bedtime, to prevent night-time waking and disturbed sleep, is a widely accepted practice, which appears to have no adverse effects. However, no formal research evidence is available to support this practice.

- How active does the patient want to be in managing his or her care and what means of patient education and information provision best suits his or her needs?
- How active can the patient be in managing his or her care and who else in the patient's support network should be involved?
- What are the individual's subjective perceptions of the severity of pain and the distress caused by it?
- What is the best way of assessing efficacy of pharmacological and non-pharmacological interventions? Are pain charts and/or patient diaries practicable?

Pain mechanisms

Of the many kinds of nerve, only a few are concerned with nociception and the transmission of impulses associated with pain. Some nerves carry nociceptive impulses, while others carry impulses that directly affect the perception of pain. Three types of neurone seem to be involved with pain transmission:

- *large, heavily myelinated A-beta fibres* – these respond to light pressure, and their stimulation leads to the sensation of tenderness
- *smaller, thinly myelinated A-delta fibres and fine, unmyelinated C fibres* – A-delta and C fibres are the principal transmitters of pain impulses, although other fibres may also be involved. Damage to these fibres results in intense pain. The A-delta fibres give rise to sharp pain, while the C fibres give rise to dull, persistent pain.

One of the earliest theories of pain was the specificity theory. It was postulated that there were special receptors for each type or modality of pain, e.g. Meissner's corpuscles responded exclusively to touch, Pacinian corpuscles to pressure, Ruffini and Krayse end-organs to heat and cold, and free nerve endings to pain. Melzack and Wall went on to show that these assumptions were over-simplified, assuming a 'rigid, fixed relationship between a neural structure and a psychological experience'.[32]

The pattern theory of pain followed the specificity theory. Criticised for discounting psychological aspects of the pain experience, the pattern theory was based on the belief that excessive stimulation of the skin receptors created particular patterns of nerve impulses that were summated in the dorsal horn of the spinal cord and consequently caused pain.

However, the most widely recognised pain theory is the gate control theory (GCT), first espoused by Melzack and Wall in 1965.[32] The theory proposes that:

- the transmission of nerve impulses is modulated by a spinal gating mechanism in the dorsal horn (substantia gelatinosa)
- larger fibres tend to close the gate (inhibit transmission), while smaller fibres tend to open the gate (facilitate transmission)
- descending impulses from the cerebral cortex influence the gate mechanism
- a system of specialised conducting fibres activates selective cognitive processes that influence the gating mechanism via descending fibres.

Pain occurs when spinal cord transmission exceeds a critical level. Despite its advantages over earlier pain theories, the GCT has been criticised for lacking detail about the interactions it proposes. Nevertheless, it is still the most important working model for pain researchers.[27,32–34]

Bone pain[35–40]

Bone metastases are the most common cause of cancer pain. Any part of the skeleton may be involved, but the axial skeleton and the proximal limb bones are particularly susceptible to metastatic disease. Approximately 50% of all bone metastases, usually resulting from bloodborne spread, arise from breast, lung, and prostate tumours.

Once inside the bone, pressure on the periosteum, nerves, and muscles surrounding the bone may lead to pain. Pain-sensitive nerve endings located in the periosteum or joints may be activated by mechanical stimuli, i.e. expansion of the tumour within the bone and/or chemical stimuli, e.g. prostaglandins. Prostaglandin production by bone metastases causes osteolysis and lowers the peripheral pain threshold.

Characteristics of bone pain

- *Base of skull metastases* – metastatic spread to the head and neck (including orbital, parasagittal, middle fossa, jugular foramen, and clivus metastases, sphenoid sinus metastases and odontoid fracture) may result in aching facial pain, as well as severe headache, sometimes exacerbated by neck flexion (depending on the sites involved). Diplopia, papilloedema, nasal stuffiness, a sense of fullness in the head, hoarseness, dysphagia, dysarthia, trapezius muscle weakness and ptosis, paralysis of the tongue, weakness of the sternomastoid, and stiff neck may also accompany bony metastatic spread to the head and neck region.
- *Bone metastases to C7–T1* may result in constant aching along the paraspinal areas radiating to both shoulders. One or other arm may also be affected where the patient experiences radiating pain to the ulnar region. The patient may also describe tenderness or pain when the spine is touched, parasthesia and numbness in the ulnar aspect of an arm, and progressive weakness of the triceps or hand.
- *L1 metastases* may be accompanied by aching in the mid-back and sacroiliac joints and a radiating pain in the groins. Pain may be exacerbated when the patient lies down.
- Aching pain in the sacral or coccygeal region characteristic of *sacral metastases* may be relieved by sitting or walking. Perianal sensory loss, bowel and bladder dysfunction, and impotence may also accompany sacral metastases.

Management

Although some bone metastases cause no pain, small localised metastases can cause severe pain where there is associated nerve involvement or damage. Alternatively, for other patients, disseminated bone diseases may result in only minimal discomfort or no pain.

Bone pain is generally only partly opioid responsive. A combination of NSAIDs and morphine should therefore be used as first-line treatment. NSAIDs inhibit prostaglandin production stimulated by bone metastases. NSAIDs are classified under several different chemical classes, with marked variations reported in patients' analgesic response to the various drugs. Therefore, if bone pain is not controlled with one particular NSAID, there is merit in trying a different drug from a different class. However, there is never an indication to use two NSAIDs concurrently.

Corticosteroids (e.g. dexamethasone, with a starting dose of 8 mg) can be useful in the management of pain caused by bone metastases. However, their side-effect profiles make corticosteroids unacceptable as first-line or long-term therapy in the management of painful bone lesions.

Radiotherapy is the most effective single therapy for the treatment of local metastatic bone pain, with response rates as high as 80% consistently reported.[36] For some patients, radiotherapy can achieve complete pain relief, although the mechanisms by which pain control is achieved are poorly understood. Reduction of tumour bulk as cells are killed may result in a reduction in the pain experienced, but it may also be that pain-mediating agents released as a result of treatment, in conjunction with osteoclast/osteoblast interaction, contribute to pain relief. When used to manage pain caused by localised metastasis, pain relief may occur within 2–3 days, with a maximum benefit seen at around 2–3 weeks following treatment. Immediate pain relief after local irradiation is rare. Therefore, it is important to continue with, and where necessary increase, the patient's analgesic regime throughout radiotherapy and for the immediate period following treatment.

Studies comparing the benefits of a single fraction of 8 Gy with a course of 5–10 fractions of 20–30 Gy have demonstrated few advantages of multiple fractionation over a single dose,[36] although multiple fraction regimes continue to be the treatment of choice where there is concern over possible fracture or nerve involvement. Radiotherapy has been demonstrated to help prevent pathological fractures and promote healing following a pathological fracture.

For patients with more widespread disease, hemi-body irradiation may be required, with a single dose of 8 Gy to the lower body or 6 Gy to the upper body, as appropriate. However, side-effects from hemi-body irradiation may be particularly distressing and up to two-thirds of patients may experience nausea, vomiting, or diarrhoea. The majority of patients will experience bone marrow suppression, and in some instances patients may experience radiation pneumonitis. Despite this, for patients whose pain is resistant to other forms of management, hemi-body irradiation has been shown to achieve effective pain relief, which, for the majority of terminally ill patients, may be maintained until death. In addition, pain relief may be achieved within 24–48 hours. As with any treatment, the side-effects of therapy must be balanced against patients' subjective wishes and the potential benefits of treatment.

For patients whose pain does not respond to radiotherapy or who relapse after an initial response, there is little evidence that retreatment with radiotherapy is effective. Alternative approaches such as treatment with strontium-89 (SR-89),[39] or intravenous bisphosphonates[38] may be more appropriate.

Surgery may be useful in managing pain caused by a pathological fracture resulting from bone metastases, or where there is a high risk of pathological fracture. Internal fixation is the preferred management when long bones are affected, but is not feasible for rib fractures or vertebral collapse, when local radiation should be used. As with any therapy, the benefits of treatment must be weighed against any possible costs to the individual. For patients in the advanced stages of illness, attempts at internal fixation with the associated demands of analgesia and risks posed by post-operative complications of bed-rest may be inappropriate, and local irradiation should again be the treatment of choice.

Radioactive isotopes used in the management of multiple painful bone metastases have demonstrated some promising results. The most widely reported in the management of pain caused by bone metastases is strontium-89 (SR-89). SR-89 is a calcium analogue with a half-life of 50.5 days. It is taken up by bone tissue and has the capacity to deliver therapeutic levels of radiation to a bone site for several months. It has been demonstrated to bring about equally effective pain relief when compared with five daily fractions or a single fraction of local radiotherapy given to patients with metastatic prostate cancer, and has also been shown to be an effective adjunct to local radio-

therapy with the same cancer group.[39] Its potential to benefit terminally ill patients is limited, as a period of 7–20 days is required before pain relief is achieved. Despite its radioactive properties, SR-89 poses a minimal threat to patients or health care professionals. Careful handling of any excreta is required, and gloves should be worn when disposing of any urine or faeces, or when blood is taken. Ideally patients should be discouraged from using bedpans, and where a patient is incontinent of urine sensitive explanation should be given, prior to administration of the isotope, of the need to catheterise the patient for a period of 1 week after treatment.

Bisphosphonates, chemical analogues of pyrophosphate, are powerful inhibitors of osteoclastic function. They have become the treatment of choice when managing malignant hypercalcaemia, and have also demonstrated some potential as analgesic agents in patients with multiple myeloma, prostate, or breast cancer. The most widely used and evaluated to date is clodronate. Despite evidence to suggest that intravenous bisphosphonantes do relieve malignant bone pain, potential differences among them, the existence of dose-dependent effects, and lack of information relating to the long-term risks of their use have led to the conclusion that they should only be used at present with patients who have severe bone pain that is resistant to management with opioids, NSAIDs, and corticosteroids.[38]

Varying degrees of pain relief from bone metastases caused by breast and prostatic cancer have been reported as a result of chemotherapy. However, it is not clear whether symptom relief is brought by tumour regression or whether pain relief obtained as a result of chemotherapy administration occurs independently of tumour response.

Contradictory evidence of the efficacy of repeated doses of calcitonin in the management of bone pain characterises the current state of knowledge regarding its use as an adjuvant analgesic. As its benefits and long-term risks are unknown at this time, it should only be considered as an experimental treatment. Similarly, contradictory findings have been reported with L-dopa, and its use is currently not recommended for routine trials.

Neuropathic pain[41-45]

Neuropathic pain is non-nociceptive (i.e. visceral, somatic, or muscle spasm pain caused by stimulation of nerve endings), and may arise from disturbances of function or pathological change in peripheral and/or central nervous systems.

Neuropathic pain is therefore not a discrete entity. It may comprise:

- peripheral nerve injury (deafferentation pain), e.g. neuroma or nerve infiltration
- central nervous system injury, e.g. spinal cord compression
- mixed peripheral and central injury, e.g. post-herpetic neuralgia.

Distinguishing characteristics include the following:

- abnormalities in pain quality – generally referred to as allodynia, hyperalgesia, and hyperpathia. Allodynia, hyperalgesia, and hyperpathia are commonly referred to as dysesthesia, and associated sensations include tingling, prickling, electricity-like effects, burning, and lancinating pain. Allodynia is pain caused by a stimulus that does not normally lead to pain, e.g. temperature or pressure; hyperalgesia refers to an increased response to a stimulus that does not normally cause pain; hyperpathia refers to pain caused in a relatively anaesthetic area of the body by an exaggerated reaction to a stimulus
- pain distribution consistent with neural damage
- evidence of neural injury or disease.

Major causes of neuropathic pain in patients with cancer

Neuropathic pain can be caused by compression or infiltration of nerves by tumour, nerve trauma due to diagnostic or surgical procedures, nervous system injury including spinal cord compression, and following chemotherapy or radiotherapy.

Specific causes include the following:

- cranial nerve involvement due to base of skull metastases mainly from breast, lung or prostate cancers; leptomeningeal metastases; or infiltration from head and neck tumours

- post-herpetic neuralgia, frequently seen in association with malignancy
- intercostal nerve injury due to rib metastases
- tumour invasion of the sciatic notch
- epidermal tumour masses or leptomeningeal metastases, which may lead to dermatomal pain
- radiculopathy, which is exacerbated by coughing, and sneezing. Painful radiculopathy may be an indication of spinal cord compression and therefore requires urgent magnetic resonance imaging (MRI) scanning. Complaints of central back pain occurring in a rapid crescendo pattern may be an especially significant sign of probable cord compression
- brachial plexus infiltration, most commonly as a result of lymph node metastases from breast cancer or lymphoma, or direct infiltration from a pancoast tumour
- direct extension of colorectal or cervical carcinomas, sarcoma, lymphoma, or breast metastases, which may cause lumbosacral plexopathy
- neuronopathy or ganglionopathy, which may present with dysesthesias, parasthesias, and sensory loss in extremities, resulting in paraneoplastic peripheral neuropathy
- high-dose intrathecal and epidural injections of opioids, which may result in neuropathic pains; approximately 20% of patients who receive anaesthetic epidural injections experience neuropathic pain
- chronic neuropathic pain, characterised by a burning or constricting sensation in the chest wall, axilla, or medial arm; this has been reported to affect as many as 20% of women post-mastectomy. Patients undergoing surgery for head and neck tumours or thoracotomy for lung tumours may also experience considerable neuropathic pain, which varies in onset and duration. Thoracotomy and post-mastectomy pain usually develops shortly after surgery, while pain associated with neck block dissection may not occur for weeks or months after treatment
- radiotherapy, which may lead to myelopathy, plexopathy, and neuropathy. Radiation myelopathy most commonly occurs after radiotherapy for extraspinal tumours, while brachial plexopathy may follow chest wall and axillary radiotherapy. Sacral plexus irradiation has

been reported to result in paresthesias, distal weakness, and pain in lower extremities

- vinca alkaloids (especially vincristine), and cis-platinum: these are known to cause painful neuropathy in some patients receiving chemotherapy. Paclitaxel and more rarely cytarabine have also been associated with the development of peripheral neuropathy. Withdrawal of the causative agent may result in resolution of the pain over some months; however, cisplatinum may cause persistent neuropathies even after withdrawal

- large doses of parenteral dexamethasone: these may be followed by a burning sensation in the perineum. This may be prevented by slow infusion.

Care strategy 17.3 Important factors to consider if neuropathic pain is suspected

1. Does the patient describe tingling or burning pain?
2. Do bed covers or underclothes cause severe pain?
3. Is the pain felt locally, does it radiate, cause an after-sensation, or is it a delayed sensation occurring some time after the stimulus?
4. Does the patient describe any associated weakness, vasomotor or dystrophic changes?
5. Does the patient have a primary tumour known to cause neuropathic pain as a consequence of metastatic spread or direct/primary infiltration/nerve damage?
6. Has the patient received cancer treatments with the potential to cause neuropathic pain?
7. Is the patient immunocompromised? Infection can cause peripheral neuropathy with intractable, escalating pain.
8. Does the patient have non-malignant degenerative disease of the spine, osteoporosis, aortic aneurysm, vasculitis, metabolic abnormalities, or nutritional deficiencies, all of which are known to cause central or peripheral neuropathies?

The use of opioids in the management of neuropathic pain remains controversial. Further evidence is required, which takes into account the plethora of aetiological and pathological mechanisms prevalent amongst heterogeneous groups of patients with cancer who present with neuropathic pain. Evidence available to date suggests a continuum of opioid responsiveness for patients, and best practice guidelines advocate that a com-

bination of opioid, non-opioid, and adjuvant analgesics be used judiciously, after a thorough examination of the patient, including computed tomographic and MRI scans where appropriate.

NSAIDs and adjuvant analgesics have been widely used in the management of neuropathic pain. Combinations of non-steroidals and an opioid are regularly used in clinical settings, and their efficacy is widely acknowledged.

First-line adjuvant analgesia in the management of neuropathic pain

Adjuvant analgesics, i.e. drugs with primary indications other than analgesia, particularly tricyclic antidepressants such as amitryptyline, are accepted agents in the management of neuropathic pain. Evidence suggests that neuropathic pain responds more quickly to antidepressant medication than does depression, and thus requires lower doses. However, full dosage may be necessary and should not be withheld. Other heterocyclic antidepressants, e.g. trazodone, may be less effective as they have different side-effect profiles to the tricyclics and should be used with caution (see Care strategy 17.4). Recent evidence attests to the benefits of gabapentin in the treatment of neuropathic pain.[44] Gabapentin is an anti-epileptic originally synthesised as a cyclic analogue of gamma aminobutyric acid (GABA), to be used to reduce seizure frequency when added to conventional anti-epileptic drugs. Data from large clinical trials indicate that it has similar efficacy to tricyclic antidepressants and carbemazepine, but may have fewer side-effects. The most notable are somnolence and dizziness. Evidence suggests that higher analgesic response rates may be observed when gabapentin is prescribed with opioids, because of a synergistic interaction.[42]

Second-line adjuvant analgesia

- Baclofen appears to be useful in trigeminal neuralgia. The usual dose is 20–120 mg.
- Oral local anaesthetics such as tocainide may be useful in either continuous or lancinating dysesthesias. They may be helpful alternatives when patients experiencing continuous dysesthsias have not responded to tricyclic antidepressants.
- Neuroleptic drugs such as fluphenazine and haloperidol can be used in low doses (2–8 mg

Care strategy 17.4   Recommended dose ranges of antidepressants/anticonvulsants

Tricyclic antidepressants
- Amitryptyline – start with 10–25 mg orally, increasing gradually to 150 mg
- Desipramine – start with 10–25 mg orally, increasing gradually to 150 mg
- Imipramine – start with 15.5 mg orally, increasing gradually to 150 mg
- Clomipramine – start with 10 mg orally, increasing gradually to 150 mg

Adjuvant anticonvulsants
- Carbamazepine – 200–400 mg three times a day (starting with 100 mg)
- Gabapentin – used in divided doses from 300 mg to a maximum of 3600g per day; but if patients have any brain damage the dose must be started lower (100 mg) and built up slowly
- Phenytoin – 300–400 mg (starting with 100 mg)

Anticonvulsant drugs such as carbamazepine have been found to be particularly effective in the management of lancinating pains. Phenytoin, valporic acid, and clonazepam may also be effective.

Care strategy 17.5   Relaxation – some recommendations for practice

Teaching a patient, family member or friend a relaxation technique is relatively quick and easy and the rewards can be significant. There are many forms of relaxation but progressive muscle relaxation (PMR) appears to be the most commonly used by nurses in their daily practice.[5] PMR involves tensing and then relaxing separate muscle groups throughout the body one after the other. Below are some basic phrases you may find helpful to use with patients and family members.

- Find yourself a quiet place. This may be your bedroom or a favourite spot in the garden.
- Make sure that you are sitting or lying comfortably and loosen any tight clothing.
- You may choose to have music playing or to sit in silence. Tell your family or friends that you are setting this time aside so that they do not disturb you. They may even choose to join you.
- You may choose to focus on a picture or a flower or just look at a distant point. You may prefer to close your eyes.

Most relaxation texts will emphasise the importance of deep breathing and of beginning the relaxation process by taking several deep breaths. For some patients with advanced disease, deep breathing may cause discomfort or even cause additional distress, e.g. patients with lung cancer who are breathless. Therefore, before beginning the relaxation process ask your patient about his or her breathing and find the most appropriate breathing pattern for him or her. If the patient is breathless try suggesting: 'Be aware of your breathing just for a moment and then just try to maintain a comfortable breathing pace throughout the relaxation period'.

   If the patient can breathe normally you may choose to say: 'As you breathe in count 1-2-3 slowly, hold your breath for 1-2-3 and breathe out 1-2-3-4-5-6'.

   The next few steps are part of the process of progressive muscle relaxation. They are directed at relaxing the shoulders but can be applied to any part of the body.

- Once you have found a comfortable, well-supported position, slowly and gently draw your shoulders up towards your ears. Hold them in that position for as long as is comfortable for you (about half a minute to a minute).
- After you have felt the tension in your shoulders slowly let them relax, lowering your shoulders gently back to their usual position. Be aware of a release in tension as you do this.
- Some people talk about thinking of feelings of warmth and peace as they relax their shoulders, letting go of pain, fear, and anxiety.
- If you feel able, repeat this action a second time.

Some people prefer to set aside 20–30 minutes during the day to carry out relaxation of all muscle groups within the body. Others find that repeating some form of relaxation for as little as 5–10 minutes, two or three times a day, helps prevent tension from building up.

per day) for neuropathic pain. However, the benefits of their prolonged use as adjuvant analgesics must be weighed against the risk of developing tardive dyskinesia.

- Anxiolytics such as alprazolam or clonazepam may also be useful in the management of neuropathic pain. Oral alprazolam (0.25–2 mg three times a day) has been shown to be helpful in some patients with phantom limb pain, while oral clonazepam (0.5–4 mg twice a day) may be useful in the management of lancinating pains.

Additional approaches to the management of neuropathic pain include:

- sympathetic blockade (e.g. nerve blocks)
- epidural injections (particularly bupivocaine, which has been shown to be effective with patients unresponsive to opioid treatment)
- neurosurgical interventions (although success rates are limited)
- and neurostimulation (e.g. TENS).

References

1. Hanks G.W. (1995). Problem areas in pain and symptom management in advanced cancer patients. *European Journal of Cancer Care* **31a**, 869–870.
2. Menzies K., Murray J. and Wilcock A. (2000). Audit of cancer pain management in a cancer centre. *International Journal of Palliative Nursing* **6**, 443–447.
3. Dahl J.L. (2004). Pain: impediments and suggestions for solutions *Journal of the National Cancer Institute Monographs* **32**, 124–126.
4. Hiscock M. (1993). Psychological aspects of acute pain. *Professional Nurse* **December**, 158–160.
5. Lanceley A. (1995). Wider issues in pain management. *European Journal of Cancer Care* **4**, 153–157.
6. World Health Organization. (1990). *Cancer Pain Relief and Palliative Care*. Geneva: World Health Organization.
7. McCaffrey M. (1979). *Nursing the Patient in Pain*. London: Harper and Row, pp. 13–14.
8. Merskey H. (1976). Psychiatric aspects of the control of pain. In Bonica J.J. and Albe-Fessard D. (eds.) *Advances in Pain Research and Therapy*, Vol. 1. New York: Raven Press, pp. 711–716.
9. Bates M.S. (1987). Ethnicity and pain: a biocultural model. *Social Science and Medicine* **24**, 47–50.
10. Oncology Nursing Society. (2004). *Cancer Pain Management ONS Positions.* www.ONS.org (accessed 3 August 2007).
11. Cohen M.Z., Easley M.K., Ellis C. *et al.* (2003). Cancer pain management and the JCAHO's pain standards: an institutional challenge. *Journal of Pain and Symptom Management* **25**, 519–527.
12. National Comprehensive Cancer Network. (2004). *Guidelines for Supportive Care – Cancer Pain.* Jenkintown: National Comprehensive Cancer Network.
13. Foley K.M. (1985). The treatment of cancer pain. *New England Journal of Medicine* **313**, 84–95.
14. Jensen M.P. (2003). The validity and reliability of pain measures in adults with cancer. *The Journal of Pain* **4**, 2–21.
15. Kleinman A. (1988). *The Illness Narratives: Suffering, Healing and the Human Condition.* New York: Basic Books.
16. Sternbach R.A. (1974). *Pain Patients: Traits and Treatment.* London: Academic Press, pp. 20–51.
17. Twycross R. (1988). The management of pain in cancer: a guide to drugs and dosages. *Oncology* **2**, 35–44.
18. Heath C. (1989). Pain talk: the expression of suffering in the medical consultation. *Social Psychology Quarterly* **52**, 113–125.
19. National Council for Hospices and Specialist Palliative Care Services (1994). *Guidelines for Managing Cancer Pain in Adults.* London: National Council for Hospices and Specialist Palliative Care Services.
20. Redmond K. (1996). Advances in supportive care. *European Journal of Cancer Care* **5(suppl. 2)**, 1–7.
21. Twycross R. (1984). Control of pain. *Journal of the Royal College of Physicians of London* **18**, 32–37.
22. Bruera E., Macmillan K., Hanson J. and MacDonald R. (1989). The cognitive effects of administration of narcotic analgesics in patients with cancer pain. *Pain* **39**, 13–16.
23. Sykes N.P. (1991). A clinical comparison of laxatives in a hospice. *Palliative Medicine* **5**, 307–314.
24. Schug S.A., Grond S., Zech D., Jung H., Meuser T. and Stobbe B. (1992). A long-term survey of morphine in cancer pain patients. *Journal of Pain and Symptom Management* **7**, 259–266.
25. Expert Working Group of the European Association for Palliative Care (1996). Morphine in cancer pain: modes of administration. *British Medical Journal* **312**, 823–826.
26. Virtual Medical Centre. *Cancer Pain.* www.virtualcancercentre.com (accessed 3 August 2007).
27. Wentworth Dolphin N. (1983). Neuroanatomy and neurophysiology of pain: nursing implications. *International Journal of Nursing Studies* **20**, 255–263.
28. Syrjala K.L., Cummings C. and Donaldson G.W. (1992). Hypnosis or cognitive behavioral training for the reduc-

tion of pain and nausea during cancer treatment: a controlled clinical trial. *Pain* **48**, 137–146.

29. Hammar M., Frisk J., Grimas O. *et al.* (1999). Acupuncture treatment of vasomotor symptoms in men with prostatic carcinoma: a pilot study. *Journal of Urology* **161**, 853–856.

30. Vickers A.J. and Cassileth B.R. (2001). Unconventional therapies for cancer and cancer-related symptoms. *The Lancet Oncology* **2**, 226–232.

31. Deng G. and Cassileth B.R. (2005).To what extent do cancer patients use complementary and alternative medicine? *Nature Clinical Practice Oncology* **2**, 496–497.

32. Melzack R. and Wall P. (1988). *The Challenge of Pain.* London: Penguin Books.

33. Astley A. (1990). A history of pain. *Nursing* **4**, 33–53.

34. Melzack R. and Wall P. (1965). Pain mechanisms: a new theory. *Science* **150**, 971–979.

35. McDonald N. (1995). Principles governing the use of cancer chemotherapy in palliative medicine. In Doyle D., Hanks G. and MacDonald N. (eds.) *The Oxford Textbook of Palliative Medicine.* Oxford: Oxford University Press, pp. 105–117.

36. Hoskin P. (1995). Radiotherapy in symptom management. In Doyle D., Hanks G. and McDonald N. (eds.) *The Oxford Textbook of Palliative Medicine.* Oxford: Oxford University Press, pp. 117–129.

37. Portenoy R. (1995). Adjuvant analgesics in pain management. In Doyle D., Hanks G. and McDonald N. (eds.) *The Oxford Textbook of Palliative Medicine.* Oxford: Oxford University Press, pp. 187–203.

38. Ernst S., Brasher P., Hagen N. *et al.* (1997). A randomized, controlled trial of intravenous clodronate in patients with metastatic bone disease and pain. *Journal of Pain and Symptom Management* **13**, 319–326.

39. Kan M. (1995). Palliation of bone pain in patients with metastatic cancer using strontium-89 (Metastron). *Cancer Nursing* **18**, 286–291.

40. O'Brien T. (1993). Pain. In Saunders C. and Sykes N. (eds.) *The Management of Terminal Malignant Disease.* London: Edward Arnold, pp. 33–62.

41. Breitbart W. (1998). Psychotropic adjuvant analgesics for pain in cancer and AIDS. *Psycho-oncology* **7**, 333–345.

42. Billings A. (1994). Neuropathic pain. *Journal of Palliative Care* **10**, 40–43.

43. Martin L.A. and Hagen N.A. (1997). Neuropathic pain in cancer patients: mechanisms, syndromes and clinical controversies. *Journal of Pain and Symptom Management* **14**, 99–117.

44. Bennett M.I and Simpson K.H. (2004). Gabapentin in the treatment of neuropathic pain. *Palliative Medicine* **18**, 5–11.

45. Caraceni A., Zecca E., Bonezzi C. *et al.* (2005). Gabapentin significantly improves analgesia in people receiving opioids for neuropathic cancer pain. *Cancer Treatment Reviews* **31**, 58–62.

CHAPTER EIGHTEEN

Nausea and vomiting

Meinir Krishnasamy

Cancer continues to be widely conceived of as an uncontrollable, capricious disease.[1] It may be suffused with feelings of fear, shame, and repulsion, feelings culturally and socially affiliated with physical manifestations such as vomit or malodorous wounds. Cancer and its treatment transpose many individuals to a world where previously private phenomena such as vomiting are moved into a public arena. It is unsurprising therefore that nausea, vomiting, and retching have repeatedly been identified by patients as being among the most disruptive, distressing, and feared side-effects of radiotherapy and chemotherapy.[2,3]

> While physicians are concerned with disease, clients are concerned with illness . . . This distinction defines a crucial domain for nursing. Nursing uses the model of illness and the model of disease and mediates the two.[4]

Disease refers to the way in which doctors and nurses frame illness within physiological and pathological theoretical models.[5] Illness refers to patients' perceptions, experiences, interpretations, and patterns of coping with symptoms or problems.[1] Inherent to any discussion of effective interventions for nausea and vomiting is the premise that the individual's experience of illness forms the cornerstone of nursing care. Regardless of the goal of treatment, whether it be prophylaxis or symptom control, the individual's beliefs and anxieties will strongly influence their ability to continue with any course of treatment, and to live with a life-threatening disease.[2] The importance of understanding the enormity of the impact of a symptom upon an individual's being is powerfully described by one young person:

> The severity of nausea and vomiting at times made the thought of death seem an almost welcome relief.[6]

For many, treatment becomes intolerable as a consequence of poorly controlled nausea and/or vomiting, while for some life itself may seem to be too high a price to pay for such anguish and suffering.[7] Persistent nausea and vomiting is known to be a factor in half of all missed appointments and delays in treatment, and for some leads to withdrawal from potentially curative treatment altogether.[6] Nausea and vomiting are among the most distressing side-effects of cancer therapy.[8–10]

Nausea, vomiting, and retching are discrete entities (see Box 18.1), and yet evidence suggests that patients are commonly invited to respond to questions, or to complete self-report measures, without prior clarification of the problem being explored.[2] Two-thirds of medical, surgical, gynaecological, and oncology patients are unfamiliar with the term nausea, using the term 'sick at stomach' instead, while the phrase 'throw up' is most frequently used to refer to vomiting.[10]

Assessment

Misunderstandings over terms such as 'nausea' and 'vomiting' may lead to confusion and subsequently to poor management. Careful exploration of the nature, duration, subjective feelings, and physical manifestations of the symptom being experienced is fundamental. Measures of nausea and vomiting exist; however, these may not be either reliable or valid when used in everyday practice.

Box 18.1   The concepts of nausea, vomiting, and retching

- *Nausea* – a subjective phenomenon; an unpleasant sensation experienced in the back of the throat and the epigastrium, which may or may not result in vomiting. It has been described as an autonomic response, a conscious recognition of a desire to vomit.
- *Vomiting* – the forceful expulsion of stomach, duodenum, or jejunum contents through the oral cavity. As the stomach contents become trapped between the forceful contractions of the muscles of the abdomen and diaphragm, intragastric pressure builds up, the oesophageal sphincters open, and vomiting follows.
- *Retching* – an attempt to vomit without bringing anything up. Retching is controlled by the respiratory centre in the brainstem. The respiratory centre lies near the vomiting centre. It shares the common neural pathway of the fifth, seventh, tenth, and twelfth cranial nerves, which are responsible for the changes in rate and depth of respiration that accompany nausea and vomiting.[2,11]

Objective observation tools used in studies measure the number of times emesis or retching occurs. They have several limitations. They fail to assess the perception of the distress caused by these symptoms and assume that nausea is an observable problem. The need for an observer to be present prevents measurement over time; observation is impractical in a busy ward or clinic setting. The advantages of using self-report questionnaires or diaries are clearly apparent. Visual analogue scales (VASs) offer a ready means of accessing subjective perceptions of symptoms, providing that the anchor statements at each end

of the scale are meaningful to the person completing the tool. Although well recognised as being reliable, valid, and sensitive, VASs can be confusing, and translating feelings into a quantifiable mark on a scale is difficult.[12] Guidance may need to be given on how to complete these. Where self-report measures such as VASs are to be used, it is important to ensure that they address both the occurrence of the symptom and the degree of distress caused by it.[10] For example, consider Figure 18.1.

From the first VAS shown in Figure 18.1, it could be assumed that this person vomits very little, and as such experiences minimal distress. However, each time he vomits, he might interpret it as a manifestation of worsening disease. Fearing that with greater disease activity vomiting might become persistent, the distress experienced may become so intense that it almost leads to a life perceived to be devoid of any pleasure. To date, we know little of the consequences of cumulative distress resulting from anticipatory and prolonged nausea and vomiting.[3] Without the added insight gained from the second VAS, or during skilled communication, management of the symptom and attempts at facilitating self-care may be ineffective.

Aspinall wrote in 1976:

> The many books and articles about nurse care planning and implementation generally start with the problem, which supposedly has already been identified in some way . . . they [the books] usually encourage the nurse to use another approach if her action is unsuccessful, rather than consider the possibility that the patient's disturbed or changed functioning may stem from a problem totally different from the one originally identified.[13]

If a nurse is to attach the correct diagnosis, facilitate subjective expression of the nature and meaning of the symptom, and plan effective care, then adequate theoretical knowledge and an ability to combine analytical and intuitive methods of thinking is needed. It is also important to draw upon what Benner and Wrubel[14] describe as 'perceptual awareness',[14] where *knowing how* (theoretical knowledge) and *knowing that* (practical knowledge[15]) work to complement each other. In Figure 18.2, the physiological mechanisms (the

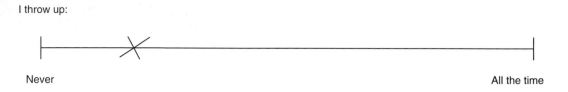

I throw up:

Never   All the time

This gives an idea of how often this person vomits but it doesn't tell us whether:

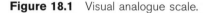

Throwing up:

Doesn't bother   Destroys all
me at all   pleasure I have

Figure 18.1 Visual analogue scale.

knowing how) of nausea and vomiting are outlined. Pharmacological interventions for cancer-induced nausea and vomiting are outlined in Box 18.2.

Patterns of nausea and vomiting

Nausea and vomiting can be compounded by the memories of previous treatment cycles; anticipatory, acute post-treatment or delayed onset nausea and vomiting can complicate effective control.[19]

The emetogenic potential of cancer chemotherapy varies greatly (see Table 18.1). Most drugs do not cross the blood–brain barrier and therefore appear to initiate vomiting through mechanisms other than direct stimulation of the CTZ, such as irritation of the CTZ via a peripheral pathway.[2,20] Chemotherapy regimes that use several drugs associated with moderate to severe emetogenic potential are associated with higher risk of nausea and vomiting.[21]

Anticipatory nausea and vomiting may occur moments before administration of the drug(s) or at any time when the individual thinks of aspects of the chemotherapy experience. For some people the smell of the hospital and the sight of the infusion pump may act as potent triggers. Other patients have described tastes and sounds, even the sight of nurses or doctors involved with their care, as potentiating factors.[9] Factors associated with an increased risk of anticipatory nausea and vomiting are listed in Box 18.3.

Anxiety and hostility may also contribute to the development of anticipatory nausea and vomiting, although the relationship between anxiety, nausea, and vomiting remains unclear.[22]

Nurses play a crucial role in the prevention and early detection of anticipatory nausea and vomiting.[2] Through sensitive questioning and an accepting and knowledgeable response, nurses can avoid considerable suffering and give enhanced meaningful support.

Radiation-induced nausea and vomiting is related to the dose and type of treatment. Radiotherapy to the upper gastrointestinal tract can result in vasculitis and direct irritation of the oesophageal mucosa, leading to nausea and

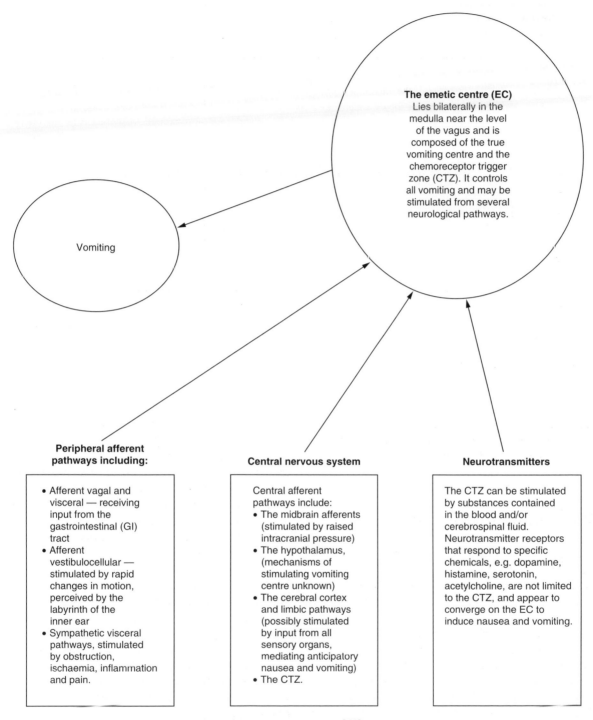

Figure 18.2   Physiological mechanisms of nausea and vomiting.[2,4,16]

Box 18.2   Pharmacological interventions for cancer-induced nausea and vomiting

- *Aprepitant* is a neurokinin type 1 (NK-1) receptor antagonist.[17] It exerts anti-emetic activity by blocking the NK-1 receptor. The endogenous neurotransmitter that usually binds to the NK-1 receptor is the 11-amino acid techykinin called substance P that is involved in many inflammatory and noxious reactions such as emesis. This new class of drug seems to be providing hope for the continued improved pharmacological management of chemotherapy-induced nausea and vomiting.
- *Phenothiazines, e.g. prochlorperazine, chlorpromazine* exert their primary effect as dopamine antagonists, inhibiting transmission in the chemoreceptor trigger zone (CTZ). Associated with extrapyramidal reactions, acute dystonic reactions, autonomic and hypersensitivity reactions, they must be used with caution. Akathesia, described as feeling jittery and sleepy at the same time, is a common side-effect of phenothiazines, and its occurrence warrants discontinuation of the drug.[2,10]
- *Serotonin antagonists, e.g. ondansetron, granistron, tropistron* act by blocking serotonin-type receptors and have two possible sites of action: the vagal afferent peripheral nerve terminals, and the central terminals of the same afferent nerves.[10] Although serotonin receptor antagonists have become first-line treatment in preventing acute post-chemotherapy nausea and vomiting, and have minimal side-effects, their ability to prevent delayed nausea and vomiting is less apparent.
- *Palonosetron* is a new serotonin antagonist. It shares many of the characteristics of the existing available drugs in its class, however it has a much stronger affinity for the $5HT_3$ receptor as well as a markedly longer half life (37 hours versus 3–9 hours).
- *Substituted benzamide, e.g. metoclopramide* – metoclopramide has been proven to be an effective anti-emetic against strongly emetogenic chemotherapy, including cisplatinum-based regimes.[2] It appears to have two modes of action, including dopamine antagonist activity and promotion of gastric emptying, limiting reflux and retching.[10] It has several potential distressing side-effects, including extrapyramidal reactions, diarrhoea, fatigue, and sleepiness.
- *Corticosteroids* – dexamethasone is commonly used in conjunction with other anti-emetics, especially ondansetron and metoclopramide, when aggressive treatment regimes are administered. The exact mechanism of action of corticosteroids is unknown but it is postulated that they manifest antiprostaglandin activity.[18]
- *Benzodiazepines, e.g. lorazepam, diazepam* – benzodiazepines appear to act at thalamic, limbic, and hypothalamic levels of the central nervous system, although their exact mechanism is not known. They produce anxiolytic, sedative, hypnotic, skeletal muscle relaxant and anticonvulsant effects.[10] As they are capable of producing all levels of central nervous system depression, they should be used with caution with elderly patients and with patients with poor respiratory function.
- *Antihistamines, e.g. diphenhydramine (Piriton)* – their primary site of action is in the CTZ, although they are ineffective as single-agent anti-emetics. They are most commonly used alongside phenothiazines or metoclopramide, incorporated into aggressive anti-emetic regimens to help prevent extrapyramidal reactions.[18]
- *Butyrophenones, e.g. droperidol, haloperidol* act as dopamine antagonists in the CTZ and also have a sedating and anxiolytic effect. Hypotension and extrapyramidal reactions are significant side-effects.[18]
- *Cannabinoids, e.g. marijuana* – their mode of action is unknown but the anti-emetic effect may be related to the 'high' achieved by adequate blood concentration. Memory loss, mood changes, inco-ordination, euphoria, and hallucinations have all been documented as side-effects.[10]

Table 18.1   Emetic potential of commonly used cancer chemotherapy agents[21]

Highly emetogenic	Moderately emetogenic	Low emetogenic potential
Cisplatin	Doxorubicin	Etoposide (dose and route dependent)
Dacarbazine	Procarbazine	Hydroxyurea
Cychlophosphamide	Carboplatin	5-Fluorouracil (5-FU)
BCNU	Mitomycin-C	Bleomycin
	Ifosfamide and mesna	Vinblastin
	Mitoxantrone	Vincristine
	Cytosine arabinoside	Methotrexate (dose related)
	Daunorubicin	Busulfan
	Carmustine	Taxol
	CCNU	Taxotere

Box 18.3 Factors associated with increased risk of anticipatory nausea and vomiting[16]

- Being under 50 years of age
- Previously poorly controlled nausea and vomiting
- Subjective perceptions of the severity of the symptoms
- A sense of increased warmth and weakness following therapy
- A history of motion sickness.

vomiting.[2] Symptoms may occur early in the course of treatment and as quickly as within 2 hours of completing each radiotherapy fraction. Consequently, an individual's predisposition to anticipatory nausea and vomiting is great. Stomatitis, xerostomia, dysguesia, and abdominal cramping may all contribute to radiotherapy-induced nausea and vomiting,[23] and for some individuals, anorexia and persistent retching rapidly result in a sore, dry mouth and abdominal cramping. Meticulous mouth care is therefore necessary, alongside prompt initiation of an effective antiemetic regime.

Symptoms that persist or develop 24 hours or more after chemotherapy are defined as delayed nausea and vomiting. Its aetiology is unclear but may be due to the ongoing effect that the antimetabolites of cancer-related treatments continue to have on either the central nervous system or the gastrointestinal tract.[18] As the blood levels of chemotherapeutic agents fall, the neurotransmitters that mediate nausea and vomiting are no longer 'blocked'.[2] Nurses need to develop tools to evaluate symptom-management strategies for use at home. As increasing numbers of patients attend hospital on a day-care basis, and political influences encourage the shift towards more home-based therapies and skilled care planning, and meaningful nursing outcome measures are paramount.

Non-pharmacological interventions

Non-pharmacological interventions that may help with nausea and vomiting are shown in Box 18.4. The benefits of many of these measures rely on anecdotal evidence. These present nurses with many challenging and important areas for future research. Richardson suggests several key areas for future research, which are outlined below.[3]

Considerable research efforts over the past decade have significantly improved the management of cancer-induced nausea and vomiting. However, the application of these findings within a holistic model of care continues to present cancer and palliative practitioners with a substantial therapeutic challenge.

Box 18.4 Non-pharmacological interventions for nausea and vomiting

- *Self-care facilitation* – Orem defines self-care as 'the personal care that individuals require each day to regulate their own functioning and development'.[24] It has been suggested as a means of promoting enhanced symptom control and as a means of encouraging individuals with cancer to avoid the regression sometimes associated with the disease.[3,24] Nausea and vomiting may demand of an individual a new set of self-care actions. Where possible, the person will respond to these challenges, but when, as with a major life-event such as a diagnosis of cancer, self-care agency is overwhelmed, help is needed. Nurses have a key role to play in planning, designing, and evaluating new modes of self-care management.
- *Progressive muscle relaxation, humour, music, exercise, hypnosis, and systematic desensitisation* – these activities redirect an individual's attention away from nausea and vomiting.[10] Whether their success is due to cessation of the symptoms or to perceptual exchange is unclear, but currently available evidence supports their effectiveness and continued use.
- *Patient education and written information* – patient education is an integral part of symptom management, and written instructions are often indispensable for a group of people bombarded by disease-related information and psychological trauma.[2]

Areas for future nursing research

Potential areas for research include:[3]

- studies to explore the interface between pharmacological, behavioural, and self-care interventions in seeking to control chemotherapy-induced nausea and vomiting

- investigation of the potential relationships between intervening variables such as age, gender, diagnosis, cancer treatment, self-concept, self-care agency, locus of control, and the cancer patient's performance of self-care behaviour
- development and testing of valid and reliable measures of self-care behaviours performed, and their effectiveness
- descriptive studies to assess how individuals monitor and react to symptoms over the course of chemotherapy, and relate such symptoms to self-care behaviour.

References

1. Donnelly E. (1995). Culture and meanings of cancer. *Seminars in Nursing Oncology* **11**, 3–8.
2. Hogan C.M. (1990). Advances in the management of nausea and vomiting. *Nursing Clinics of North America* **25**, 475–497.
3. Richardson A. (1991). Theories of self-care: their relevance to chemotherapy-induced nausea and vomiting. *Journal of Advanced Nursing* **16**, 671–676.
4. Dougherty M. and Tripp-Reimer T. (1990). Nursing and anthropology. In Johnson T.M. and Sargent C.F. (eds.) *Medical Anthropology: A Handbook of Theory and Method.* New York: Greenwood, pp. 174–186.
5. Kleinman A. (1988). *The Illness Narratives: Suffering, Healing and the Human Condition.* New York: Basic Books.
6. Stroudermire A., Contanch P. and Laszlo J. (1984). Recent advances in the pharmacologic and behavioural management of chemotherapy induced emesis. *Archives of Internal Medicine* **144**, 1029–1033.
7. Khan D.L. and Steeves R. (1995). The significance of suffering in cancer care. *Seminars in Oncology Nursing* **11**, 9–16.
8. Coates A., Abraham S., Kay S., Sowerbutts T., Frewin C. and Fox R. (1983). On the receiving end: patient perceptions of the side-effects of cancer chemotherapy. *European Journal of Cancer and Clinical Oncology* **14**, 203–208.
9. Nerenz D., Leventhal H. and Love R. (1982). Factors contributing to emotional distress during cancer chemotherapy. *Cancer* **50**, 1020–1027.
10. Rhodes V., Johnson M. and McDaniel R. (1995). Nausea, vomiting and retching: the management of the symptom experience. *Seminars in Oncology Nursing* **11**, 256–265.
11. Norris (1982). *Concept Clarification in Nursing.* London: Aspen.
12. Gift A.G., Plaut S.M. and Jacox A.K. (1986). Psychological and physiologic factors related to dyspnoea in subjects with chronic obstructive pulmonary disease. *Heart and Lung* **15**, 595–601.
13. Aspinall M.J. (1976). Nursing diagnosis – the weak link. *Nursing Outlook* **24**, 433–437.
14. Benner P. and Wrubel J. (1982). Skilled clinical knowledge: the value of perceptual awareness. *Nurse Educator* **May–June**, 11–17.
15. Polyani M. (1962). *Personal Knowledge.* London: Routledge and Kegan Paul.
16. Morrow G.R. (1984). Clinical characteristics associated with the development of anticipatory nausea and vomiting in cancer patients undergoing chemotherapy treatment. *Journal of Clinical Oncology* **2**, 1170–1179.
17. Aapro M. and Johnson. J. (2005). Chemotherapy-induced emesis in elderly cancer patients: the role of 5-HT3 receptor antagonists in the first 24 hours. *Gerontology* **51**, 287–296.
18. Gralla R.J. (1993). Antiemetic therapy. In DeVita V., Hellman S. and Rosenberg S. (eds.) *Principles and Practice of Oncology*, 4th edition. Philadelphia, PA: Lippincott, pp. 2238–2347.
19. Eick-Swigart J. (1995). What cancer means to me. *Seminars in Oncology Nursing* **11**, 41–42.
20. Fiore J.J. and Gralla R.J. (1984). Pharmacologic treatment of chemotherapy-induced nausea vomiting. *Cancer Investigations* **2**, 351–361.
21. Chabner B.A. (1993). Anticancer drugs. In DeVita V., Hellman S. and Rosenberg S. (eds.) *Principles and Practice of Oncology*, 4th edition. Philadelphia, PA: Lippincott, pp. 328–339.
22. Ingle R.J., Burish T.G. and Wallston K.A. (1984). Conditionability of cancer chemotherapy patients. *Oncology Nursing Forum* **11**, 97–102.
23. Holmes S. (1991). The oral complications of specific anticancer therapy. *International Journal of Nursing Studies* **28**, 343–360.
24. Orem D. (1991). *Nursing: Concepts of Practice*, 4th edition. St Louis, MO: Mosby Yearbook.

CHAPTER NINETEEN

Fatigue

Meinir Krishnasamy

Fatigue is one of the most common symptoms experienced by people with cancer.[1] It is a nebulous concept, difficult to define, and intensely personal. The North American Nursing Diagnosis Association defines fatigue as 'an unremitting and overwhelming lack of energy and an inability to maintain usual routines'.[2] Carpenito describes fatigue as 'an overwhelming, sustained sense of exhaustion and decreased capacity for physical and mental work'.[3] People who experience fatigue describe it in many different ways, including, tiredness, lack of energy, lethargy, weakness, depression, anxiety, exhaustion, impaired mobility and functional capacity, motivation and concentration span, sleepiness, drowsiness, heaviness, an inability to carry on, as well as many other sensations.[4–9] Evidence indicates that fatigue limits social activities, results in loss of valued activities, impacts family life and relationships, and results in feelings of social isolation and lowered self-esteem.[10–14] Guilt, anger, and boredom have all been reported as accompanying cancer-related fatigue.[10,11]

The manifestations of fatigue identified in studies of cancer-related fatigue are outlined in Figure 19.1.

Models of fatigue have focused on its six distinct dimensions:[2]

- *temporal* – refers to the timing of fatigue, its onset and duration, and its pattern[2]
- *sensory* – refers to subjective experiences of fatigue, factors that exacerbate and alleviate it, and the presence of any concurrent problems, for example pain, nausea, or breathlessness[17]
- *cognitive/mental* – focuses on the ability to concentrate, changes in attention span, memory recall, and degree of alertness[2,17,18]
- *affective/emotional* – refers to changes in mood, distress, and anxiety caused by the fatigue[2,17,18]
- *behavioural* – refers to functional status, ability to undertake work, social and recreational activities, changes in sleep pattern, and nutritional intake[17,18]
- *physiological* – refers to findings from the medical history, including stage of disease and its symptoms, side-effects of malignancy and treatment, concurrent diseases, past coping mechanisms, and family history.[2,17,18]

A definitive classification system by which to diagnose and grade cancer-related fatigue is now available through the International Classification of Diseases (ICD-10).[19–21] This clinically useful classification system defines cancer-related fatigue as:

- the presence of six or more out of 11 possible fatigue symptoms including for example, 'diminished energy', 'increased need to rest', 'significant fatigue', present every day or nearly every day during the same 2-week period in the past month
- the symptoms cause clinically significant distress or impairment in important aspects of functioning

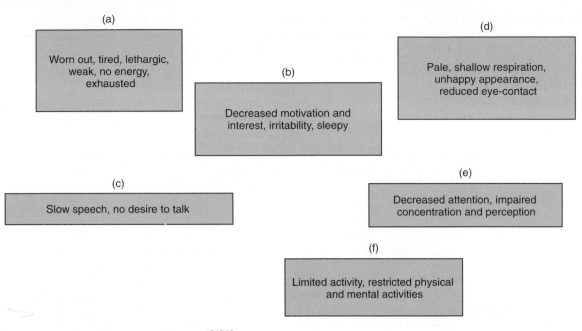

Figure 19.1 Manifestations of fatigue.[1,9,15,16]

- the symptoms result from cancer or cancer treatment
- the symptoms are not primarily a consequence of co-morbid psychiatric disorders.

In addition to objective screening and assessment, nurses must also recognise that effective management of cancer-related fatigue relies on exploring the meaning of the problem with individuals. For the person with cancer, fatigue may be the first sign of ill-health, leading him or her to seek medical advice. It may therefore become a potent symbol of the presence of disease, possessing great significance for the patient and family. Thorough assessment of the problem in all its complexity is therefore essential to effective person-centred care. Asking about duration, recuperative purpose, predictability, response to self-care measures, its nature, and the distress associated with it contribute to the developemnt of an individualised plan of care. Despite the development of numerous fatigue-assessment scales over the past decade, psychometrically sound, clinically applicable instruments continue to need further refinement.[22] Single-item instuments such as visual analogue fatigue scales provide easy

approaches to standardised screening of fatigue intensity,[22,23] while more complex instruments such as the Cancer Fatigue Scale,[24] or Multidimensional Fatige Symptom Inventory[25] provide opportunity for in-depth assessment of fatigue across all its dimensions. As fatigue is a subjective sensation, one of the most clinically useful ways to measure it is through the use of symptom diaries, which have been shown to be an efficient way to recognise the severity, pattern, and impact of cancer-related fatigue experienced and reported by individuals.[26]

Despite a recognition of the prevalence of fatigue as a consequence of cancer and its treatment, little is known of the meanings inherent for the individuals experiencing it and the families and professionals witnessing it. With a few exceptions, little has been documented of the experience of living with cancer-related fatigue.[9,27–30]

In a phenomenological study undertaken to describe the experiences of six individuals with chemotherapy-induced fatigue, Pearce and Richardson found that psychological and emotional distress were more commonly reported consequences of fatigue than were physical manifestations.[9] They report one patient's experience of

Table 19.1   Some descriptions of the fatigue of advanced cancer by patients, family members, and friends

Patient	Patient subjective descriptors	Relative or friend descriptors
David	*I just feel exhausted, no energy to do anything, you can sleep anytime.*	Just more and more tired, and losing weight, and not doing anything (Jennie, David's wife).
Michael	*It's like you're so heavy, drained of energy.*	it's just cut him off from everybody because it's too much of an effort, he's got no energy to spare (Judith, Michael's wife).
Ruth	*Some days I don't think I can physically get myself up out of bed, and I've got no energy.*	I fell for her so much because she wants to be busy, to see friends, but she's exhausted, just exhausted (Francis, Ruth's friend).
Beth	*I feel so tired but I want to be able to get up but I feel I physically can't*	Some days you can almost feel the tiredness, it's so draining (Howard, Beth's husband).
Allan	*It's so heavy, like a weight coming down on you.*	He's just not the same person, always busy, but he tells me it's like a weight on him, and I think I can understand, like after I had an operation once, but I think it's very different too (Sandra, Allan's wife).
Enid	*It's a terrible tiredness, it makes you feel exhausted.*	She's got half, well not a quarter, of the energy she used to have, no get up and go (Frank, Enid's friend).

feeling extremely depressed and of having almost suicidal thoughts during her chemotherapy. She made sense of these extremely distressing emotions by stating: 'I think it may have been the realisation of my illness for the first time'. Other studies have found that physical limitations imposed by the fatigue are more commonly referred to.[30] Similarly, relatives and friends tend to describe the impact of fatigue in physical terms. Krishnasamy undertook a detailed case study of 15 patients with advanced cancer who were experiencing fatigue.[12] The study also involved interviews with nominated friends or relatives and health professionals, and a case note analysis. Table 19.1 shows examples of these patients' and family members' descriptions of the fatigue accompanying advanced cancer.

The meanings inherent in these descriptions suggest that fatigue is much more than simply a physical problem; there are clear emotional, psychological, and social consequences of fatigue. This presents nurses with a considerable challenge, where the language used to describe the fatigue experience, especially within the last months of life, may convey little of its psychological distress. This remains hidden, and therefore nurses' ability to support patients experiencing distress will be limited.

Fatigue continues to be for the greater part a 'socially invisible' consequence of cancer,[31] the experience of which is far more complex than simply a lack of visibility.[32] It contributes to a complex world in which illness is a product of personal idealisation and social construction. It has a profound effect on an individual's ability to live a 'normal life', and their perception of self. All aspects of life may be affected, forcing withdrawal from family, work, social, and recreational activities, all of which may previously have been powerful in reinforcing feelings of self-worth and self-esteem. As a consequence of this forced withdrawal from daily life, intense feelings of isolation and lack of motivation to continue to try to undertake normal functions have been described as a result of fatigue following chemotherapy.[9] Similarly, fatigue resulting from breathlessness has been found to cause withdrawal and isolation.[33] This may be especially true with tumours associated with extreme fatigue such as mesothelioma.

Krishnasamy[12] commented as follows in her research field notes after an interview with a gentleman with small-cell lung cancer:

It seems to me that he felt the illness didn't show tiredness to begin with, he talked about things getting worse, of wanting to do things but not being able, I could feel his sense of dismay, knowing that there was more to come.

The consequences of social definition, interpretation, and judgement of obscure or 'invisible' phenomena such as fatigue[34] are powerfully demonstrated in this description of the impact of chronic disability:[35]

It was not just that people acted differently towards me, but rather I felt differently towards myself . . . it [illness] left me feeling alone and isolated despite strong support from family and friends . . . a diminution of everything I used to be [pp.71–76].

Evidence from the cancer literature suggests that fatigue has been hidden from the consciousness of well-meaning professionals and researchers, with little appreciation of the consequences of its obscurity for patients and relatives, or for the development of true patient-centred care:

One cannot separate life experience from a person's unique interpretation of his or her illness and the ability and desire to get well. Expressions of hope, love, anger, fear, and loss provide the nurse with a lived dialogue, and offer the opportunity for interpretation of events in a way that has particular meaning for the patient.[36]

Further exacerbating nurses' inability to help patients and their families to manage cancer-induced fatigue is a lack of understanding of helpful behaviours identified by patients themselves. Although some work is now emerging within the field of chemotherapy- and radiotherapy-induced fatigue, much remains to be explored.[37–39] Box 19.1 lists activities reported as being helpful in alleviating fatigue. Few of these interventions have been evaluated through empirical research studies. Nevertheless, these accounts provide invaluable insight and information for planning future nursing intervention studies.

A comprehensive understanding of the possible causes and contributing factors of fatigue will lead to a precise nursing diagnosis.[17] At present, this is unlikely, as much research has yet to be undertaken before the nature of the relationship between factors contributing to fatigue and the resultant subjective experiences can be understood.

Box 19.1   Strategies in alleviating fatigue

Helpful strategies identified by patients receiving chemotherapy and radiotherapy[2,40,41]
- Resting or sleeping during the day
- Prioritise activities
- Reading/listening to the radio/watch television
- Walking/gentle exercise
- Relaxation/massage
- Learning coping skills, e.g. goal planning, activity pacing
- Maintaining a diary or journal to map patterns of fatigue
- Information seeking
- Boosting nutritional intake
- Quiet or stimulating environment
- Social support, being with family or friends
- Effective management of physical symptoms, e.g. pain, nausea.

Helpful strategies identified by patients experiencing the fatigue of advanced cancer, and their relatives, friends, and professional carers
- Talk to someone about it – tell them how awful it is
- Help to give it a language you can work with
- Help family and friends understand it
- Help patients describe the fears and meanings associated with the fatigue of dying.

Figure 19.2 shows the complexity of the variety of factors thought to influence fatigue in cancer.

Patients treated with radiotherapy and chemotherapy often describe feelings of general malaise, incorporating feelings of lack of energy and tiredness. Between 65% and 100% of patients receiving radiotherapy as a treatment for cancer experience fatigue, with the most severe side-effects occurring during the last week of treatment.[4,17,42] For many, it may continue to be a problem for several months after treatment has ended.[17] Studies involving patients receiving chemotherapy for a variety of different types of cancer report incidences of fatigue ranging from 59% to 82%.[43] There is considerable evidence documenting the occurrence of fatigue after surgery;[44] this may be especially problematic where adjuvant chemotherapy or radiotherapy may have to be administered prior to, or immediately following surgery. Surgical procedures performed as pallia-

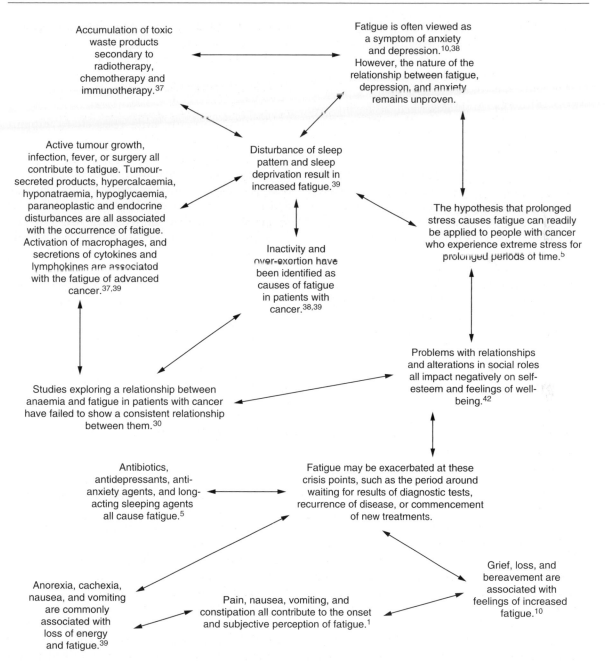

Figure 19.2 The complexity of fatigue in cancer.

tive interventions for patients who may have already undergone months, even years, of anti-cancer treatment may confer considerable relief of acute symptoms, but at the expense of exacerbating profoundly debilitating fatigue.

Successive reports of the symptoms of advanced cancer suggest that fatigue is experienced by between 50% and 75% of patients.[45] Despite its prevalence, the impact of the fatigue of advanced cancer continues to be poorly understood as papers referring to it focus on a physiological consideration of asthenia. Asthenia is a medical term used to describe pathological fatigue associated with various diseases, and in particular with acute and chronic infections, as well as the fatigue of advanced cancer. It is described as having two predominant symptoms – fatigue and generalised weakness – but no recognised body of knowledge about its aetiology or treatment currently exists.[45,46] Research to date has failed to differentiate between fatigue or tiredness as a component of cancer treatment, and fatigue or tiredness as a facet of advanced, terminal illness.

The ways in which fatigue is expressed and experienced are only just beginning to be explored. Fatigue as a feature of depression is one such area.[47] The perceptions of distress caused by fatigue and the intensely personal meanings attached to the phenomenon may play a significant part in altered mood state. Cimprich concluded that subjects who report a depressed mood state tend to have lower self-ratings of attentional functioning than those with a more positive mood state.[48] A relationship between perceptions of distress caused by unrelieved symptoms, and alterations in mood state is thought to exist.[49] The importance of working with patients to explore the meanings conferred by them onto their fatigue is therefore further supported. An in-depth interview study of 20 patients receiving a variety of ongoing treatments for cancer suggested that affective expressions of fatigue appeared to be strongly interwoven with its physical dimensions, leading us to question whether a factor such as sadness leads to tiredness (or vice versa), which then leads to decreased motivation and inactivity (or vice versa), with the inactivity then leading to sadness (or vice versa).[30] As nurses, we are ideally placed to begin to explore some of these fundamental problems with our patients.

The purpose of interventions targeted at cancer-related fatigue has been defined as facilitating patients adaptation to and understanding of it by:

- reducing the actual level of patients' fatigue by treating factors known to increase it, such as poor control of other symptoms

- reducing the impact of fatigue on patients' lives so that individuals can engage in activities they value
- reducing the distress associated with fatigue in order to enhance patients' quality of life.[40]

There is currently little research to support specific interventions for managing fatigue induced by cancer treatments, and some of the most common interventions, such as the suggestion of rest, are based on little or no scientific evidence and may in fact prove to be detrimental.[50] Winningham warns that 'unnecessary bed rest and prolonged sedentarism can contribute significantly to the development of fatigue and may result in rapid and potentially irreversible losses in energy and functioning'.[50] Improved psychological status, decrease in fatigue, and increased feelings of vigour have been reported in groups of women with breast cancer following initiation of exercise.[51,52] By far the most convincing evidence to support a clinical intervention for fatigue includes data from a series of robust studies of exercise across differing cancer populations and with people of varying disease stages. The benefits of participation in exercise programmes have been demonstrated to be:

- enhanced quality of life
- increased exercise and activity tolerance without compounding fatigue
- increased functional capacity and physical performance
- greater feelings of control
- decreased perceptions of fatigue
- enhanced psychosocial well-being.[41,52–54]

Energy conservation, enhancing energy sources, and preventing energy waste are three potential strategies for managing fatigue identified in the literature. Vincent suggests that a multimethod fatigue therapy programme, including energy-conservation activities, a planned exercise programme, stress reduction instruction, and nutritional counselling, may prove to be especially helpful for people with chronic fatigue.[55] Stress management and energy conservation appear to be the two most widely reported facets of care currently employed. Stress management has been defined as incorporating 'counselling' (facilitating a trusting relationship with the person with cancer), patient education, meditation, exercise, muscle relaxation, biofeedback, time management, and diversional activities, e.g. games, music, or reading.[6] Energy conservation focuses attention on the value of rest, setting priorities in valued activities and roles, and delegating tasks.[6,54] There is some evidence of the potential benefits of exercise and energy-conserving strategies to patients with advanced cancer,[54] but these interventions may prove to be of little relevance to this group of patients unless provided alongside in-depth emotional support:

> She told me it's no good all the things that used to help don't now. She listed lots of things like activity pacing and goal planning, although she didn't call them that, but they just didn't work for her anymore.[12]

Activity pacing, goal setting, and identification of priority activities have repeatedly been identified as potentially helpful interventions to manage fatigue.[2] However, the unpredictability and severity of the fatigue experienced by patients with advanced cancer may mean these interventions may prove to be less effective with this group. Further research is needed. For those experiencing chemotherapy- and radiotherapy-related fatigue, anticipating when fatigue is most likely to occur may allow forward planning. Activities can then be planned to avoid high fatigue times; routine rest periods can be set and requests for help with daily activities targeted effectively for patients and their families. Fatigue following radiotherapy has been found to occur most often in the afternoon, and planning for a nap or rest periods at that time can be helpful.[10] Work by Bredin *et al.*, evaluating a nursing approach to managing breathlessness for patients with advanced lung cancer, presents as one of its therapeutic interventions the need to be able to help patients to plan and organise their days around prioritised activities.[56] The notion of balancing daily activities in relation to a 'breathing cost' may have an important contribution to make to the development of a nursing strategy for helping patients to live with the fatigue of advanced cancer, where each activity incurs an 'energy cost'. One of the key therapeutic aspects of their intervention is

a commitment to explore the existential meaning of the cancer and its many ramifications.

If we accept that caring is attending to a person's wholeness,[57] we must develop the skills to work with individuals in such a way that phenomena such as fatigue cannot be reduced to specific component parts. For individuals who experience cancer-related fatigue, it mediates between the 'I' of pre-cancer person and the 'me' as cancer patient. It becomes a representation of self:[35]

> ... there is another aspect of my fatigue that cannot be eased by rest. This is a sense of tiredness and *ennui* with practically everything and everybody, a desire to withdraw from the world, to crawl into a hole and pull the lid over my head [p. 77].

References

1. Nail L.M. (2002). Fatigue in patients with cancer. *Oncology Nursing Forum* **29**, 537.
2. Piper B., Lindsay D. and Dodd M. (1987). Fatigue mechanisms in cancer patients: developing a nursing theory. *Oncology Nursing Forum* **14**, 17–23.
3. Carpenito L. (1995). Fatigue. In Carpenito L. (ed.) *Handbook of Nursing Diagnosis*, 5th edition. Philadelphia, PA: Lippincott.
4. Haylock P. and Hart L. (1979). Fatigue in patients receiving localised radiation. *Cancer Nursing* **2**, 461–467.
5. Varricchio C. (1985). Selecting a tool for measuring fatigue. *Oncology Nursing Forum* **12**, 122–127.
6. Aistars J. (1987). Fatigue in the cancer patient: conceptual approach to a clinical problem. *Oncology Nursing Forum* **14**, 25–30.
7. Pickard-Holley S. (1991). Fatigue in cancer patients. A descriptive study. *Cancer Nursing* **14**, 13–19.
8. Armes J. (1995). *Cancer Patients' Experiences of Fatigue in Cancer*. BSc dissertation, University of Hull.
9. Pearce S. and Richardson A. (1996). Fatigue in cancer: a phenomenological perspective. *European Journal of Cancer Care* **5**, 111–115.
10. Ferrell B., Grant M., Dean G., Funk, B. and Ly J. (1996). 'Bone tired': the experience of fatigue and its impact on quality of life. *Oncology Nursing Forum* **23**, 1539–1547.
11. Ream E. and Richardson A. (1996). The role of information in patients' adaptation to chemotherapy and radiotherapy: a review of the literature. *European Journal of Cancer Care* **5**, 132–138.
12. Krishnasamy M. (1997). Exploring the nature and impact of fatigue in advanced cancer. *International Journal of Palliative Nursing* **3**, 126–131.

13. Magnusson K., Moller A., Ekman, T. and Wallgren A. (1999). A qualitative study to explore the experience of fatigue in cancer patients. *European Journal of Cancer Care* **8**, 224–232.

14. Holley S. (2000). Cancer-related fatigue. Suffering a different fatigue. *Cancer Practice* **8**, 87–95

15. Grandjean A. (1968). Fatigue. Its physiological and psychological significance. *The Ergonomics Research Society* **11**, 427–436.

16. Cimprich B. (1992). Attentional fatigue following breast cancer surgery. *Research in Nursing and Health* **15**, 199–207.

17. Gall H. (1996). The basis of cancer fatigue: where does it come from? *European Journal of Cancer Care* **5(suppl. 2)**, 31–34.

18. Nail L. and King K. (1987). Fatigue. *Seminars in Nursing Oncology* **3**, 257–262.

19. Portenoy R. and Itri L.M. (1999). Cancer-related fatigue: guidelines for evaluation and management. *Oncologist* **4**, 1–10.

20. Cella D., Davis K., Breitbart W., Curt G. and The Fatigue Coalition. (2001). Cancer-related fatigue: prevalence of proposed diagnostic criteria in a United States sample of cancer survivors. *Journal of Clinical Oncology* **19**, 3385–91.

21. Sadler I.J., Jacobsen P., Booth-Jones M., Belanger H., Weitzner M.A. and Fields K.K. (2002). Preliminary evaluation of a clinical syndrome approach to assessing cancer-related fatigue. *Journal of Pain and Symptom Management* **23**, 406–16.

22. Wu H.S. and McSweeney M. (2001). Measurement of fatigue in people with cancer. *Oncology Nursing Forum* **28**, 1371–84.

23. Glaus A. (1998). Fatigue in patients with cancer. Analysis and assessment. *Recent Results in Cancer Research* **145**, 1–172.

24. Okuyama T., Akechi T., Kugaya A., Okamura H., Shima Y., Maruguchi M., Hosaka T. and Uchitomi Y. (2000). Development and validation of the cancer fatigue scale: a brief, three-dimensional, self-rating scale for assessment of fatigue in cancer patients. *Journal of Pain and Symptom Management* **19**, 5–14.

25. Stein K.D., Martin S.C., Hann D.M. and Jacobsen P.B. (1998). A multidimensional measure of fatigue for use with cancer patients. *Cancer Practice* **6**, 143–152.

26. Richardson A. (1995). Fatigue in cancer patients: a review of the literature. *European Journal of Cancer Care* **4**, 20–32

27. Rhodes V., Watson P. and Hanson B. (1988). Patients' descriptions of the influence of tiredness and weakness on self-care abilities. *Cancer Nursing* **11**, 186–194.

28. Ream E. and Richardson A. (1997). Fatigue in patients with cancer and chronic obstructive airways disease: a phenomenological enquiry. *International Journal of Nursing Studies* **34**, 44–53.

29. Jamar S. (1989). Fatigue in women receiving chemotherapy for ovarian cancer. In Funk S., Tornquist E., Champagne M. *et al.* (eds.) *Key Aspects of Comfort: Management of Pain, Fatigue and Nausea.* New York: Springer, pp. 224–228.

30. Glaus A., Crow R. and Hammond S. (1996). A qualitative study to explore the concept of fatigue/tiredness in cancer patients and in healthy individuals. *European Journal of Cancer Care* **5(suppl. 2)**, 8–23.

31. Alonzo A. (1985). An analytical typology of disclaimers, excuses and justifications surrounding illness. A situational approach to health and illness. *Social Science and Medicine* **21**, 153–162.

32. Thorne S. (1993). *Negotiating Health Care. The Social Context of Chronic Illness.* London: Sage.

33. Brown M., Carrierri V., Janson-Bjerklie S. and Dodd M. (1986). Lung cancer and dyspnoea: the patient's perception. *Oncology Nursing Forum* **13**, 19–24.

34. Czechmeister C. (1994). Metaphor in illness and nursing: a two-edged sword. A discussion of the social use of metaphor in everyday language, and implications of nursing and nursing education. *Journal of Advanced Nursing* **19**, 1226–1233.

35. Murphy R.F. (1987). *The Body Silent.* London: W.W. Norton.

36. Ryder R. and Ridley M. (1990). The place from which the patient comes. *Journal of Professional Nursing* **6**, 255.

37. Richardson A. and Ream E. (1997). Self-care activities initiated by chemotherapy patients in response to fatigue. *International Journal of Nursing Studies* **34**, 35–43.

38. Nail L., Jones S., Greene D., Schipper D. and Jensen R. (1991). Use and perceived efficacy of self-care activities in patients receiving chemotherapy. *Oncology Nursing Forum* **18**, 883–887.

39. Graydon J., Bubela N., Irvine D. and Vincent L. (1995). Fatigue reducing strategies used by patients receiving treatment for cancer. *Cancer Nursing* **18**, 23–28.

40. Ream E. and Stone P. (2004). Clinical interventions for fatigue. In Armes J.P., Krishnasamy M. and Higginson I. (eds.) *Fatigue in Cancer.* Oxford: Oxford University Press, pp. 255–271.

41. Ream E., Richardson A. and Alexander-Dann C. (2002). Facilitating patients' coping with fatigue during chemotherapy-pilot outcomes. *Cancer Nursing* **25**, 300–308.

42. Kobashi-Schoot J., Hanewald G., VanDam F. and Bruning P. (1985). Assessment of malaise in cancer patients treated with radiotherapy. *Cancer Nursing* **8**, 306–313.

43. Nerenz D., Leventhal H. and Love R. (1982). Factors contributing to emotional distress during cancer chemotherapy. *Cancer* **50**, 1020–1027.

44. Rhoten D. (1982). Fatigue and the postsurgical patient. In Norris C. (ed.) *Concept Clarification in Nursing*. Rockville, MD: Aspen, pp. 277–300.

45. Bruera E. and MacDonald N. (1988). Overwhelming fatigue in advanced cancer. *American Journal of Nursing* **January**, 99–100.

46. Morant R. (1991) Asthenia in cancer patients: a double-edged inflammatory response against the tumour? *Journal of Palliative Care* 7, 22–24.

47. Visser M. and Smets E.M.A. (1998). Fatigue, depression and quality of life in cancer patients: how are they related? *Journal of Supportive Care in Cancer* 6, 101–108.

48. Cimprich B. (1993). Development of an intervention to restore attention in cancer patients. *Cancer Nursing* 16, 83–92.

49. Love R., Leventhal H., Easterling D. and Nerenz D. (1989). Side effects and emotional distress during cancer chemotherapy. *Cancer* **63**, 604–612.

50. Winningham M. (1991). Walking programme for people with cancer. Getting started. *Cancer Nursing* **14**, 270–274.

51. Kirshbaum M.N. (2007). A review of the benefits of whole body exercise during and after treatment for breast cancer. *Journal of Clinical Nursing* 16, 104–121.

52. Mock V., Dow K.H., Mears C.J. *et al.* (1997). Effects of exercise on fatigue, physical functioning, and emotional distress during radiation therapy for breast cancer. *Oncology Nursing Forum* **24**, 991–1000.

53. Dimeo F., Tilmann M., Bertz H., Kanz L. and Mertelsmann J. (1997). Aerobic exercise in the rehabilitation of cancer patients after high dose chemotherapy and autologous peripheral stem cell transplantation. *Cancer*, **79**, 1718–1722.

54. Porock D., Kristjanson L., Tinnelly K., Duke T. and Blight J. (2000). An exercise intervention for advanced cancer patients experiencing fatigue: a pilot study. *Journal of Palliative Care* **16**, 30–36.

55. Vincent L. (1992). Management of fatigue in cancer patients. In Bailey C. (ed.) *Cancer Nursing – Changing Frontiers – 7th International Conference on Cancer Nursing*, 16–21 August, Vienna, Austria. Oxford: Rapid Communications, pp. 91–94.

56. Bredin M., Corner J., Krishnasamy M. *et al.* (1999). Multicentre randomised controlled trial of nursing intervention for breathlessness in patients with lung cancer. *British Medical Journal* **318**, 901–904.

57. Picard C. (1991). Caring and the story: the compelling nature of what must be told and understood in the human dimension of suffering. In Gaut D. and Leininger M. (eds.) *Caring: The Compassionate Healer*. New York: National League for Nursing Press, pp. 89–98.

CHAPTER TWENTY

Breathlessness

Christopher Bailey

Common definitions of breathlessness suggest that it is 'the sensation of difficult breathing', 'the sensation of difficult, uncomfortable breathing',[1] 'an uncomfortable awareness of breathing'.[2] Ripamonti and Fusco wisely point out, however, that:[2]

> ... although everybody has experienced the sensation and has an intuitive understanding of this symptom, there is no universal agreement as to its definition [p.204].

Even more importantly, perhaps, they suggest that breathlessness:

> ... is frequently described by patients in terms such as fatigue upon breathing, air hunger, suffocation, choking or heavy breathing that incorporates suffering, and fear and anguish ... when speaking about 'their' dyspnea [p.204].

Ahmedzai, writing in the first edition of the *Oxford Textbook of Palliative Medicine*, commented that:[3]

> ... it is helpful to think of dyspnoea as the major part of 'total respiratory distress' which would encompass the physical, psychological, and social manifestations [p.352].

In a later edition of the same book, the authors write that:[4]

A breath is a vital sign of a living creature. When one dies, one expires. A breath, however, serves more than physiological purposes. A sigh often carries unspeakable messages from the inner being. Hence the essence of a breath is filled with physiological, psychological, and spiritual signals [p.587].

Breathlessness accounts for a high proportion of the disability, impaired life quality, and human suffering experienced by people with respiratory disease. It is more than a sensation, and more than unpleasant; because it affects so many aspects of a person's day-to-day life and experience, it is difficult to think of it as just a symptom.

Booth acknowledges that breathlessness is a 'devastating' symptom of advanced cancer, and can present such a challenge to those trying to manage or alleviate it that:[5]

> ... it is not uncommon for even palliative care physicians to feel uncertain about how to manage it and to become pessimistic about the outcome of their therapies [p.304].

Breathlessness causes a great deal of suffering, and though much of the literature on managing it derives from studies of patients with non-malignant disease, it is a major issue for people with cancer.

Data on the prevalence of breathlessness in cancer are complex, however. Twycross and Lack, for example, indicate that some 30% of people terminally ill with cancer and 65% of people with lung cancer will experience breathlessness.[6] Ripamonti and Fusco found that in advanced cancer patients the prevalence of dyspnoea increases from referral to palliative care services (15–55 5%) to the last week of life (18–79%), with severity reported to be moderate to severe in 10–63% of cases.[2] A study by Reuben and Mor in the US showed that 70% of terminally ill cancer patients were breathless at some time in the last 6 weeks of life,[7] and in a study of 135 patients with advanced cancer, Bruera *et al.* found that 55% had a symptom score of ≥30/100 for dyspnoea, arguing that this represents major impairment in function and quality of life.[8] Dudgeon *et al.* found that of a sample of 923 outpatients with cancer, 46% had some degree of shortness of breath, although only 4% had been diagnosed with lung cancer, and only 5.4% had lung metastases.[9]

People with cancer are often breathless as a result of a specific pathophysiological cause (including obstruction of the superior vena cava or bronchus, lymphangitis, pleural effusion, or cardiovascular complications).[10] Treatment should focus on reversible causes where possible, alongside appropriate management of symptoms.[11,12] Surgery, radiotherapy, chemotherapy, and administration of steroids, are important treatments for obstruction of the upper airways by primary or secondary tumours.[13] Mediastinal obstruction, or obstruction of the bronchus, can be treated with radiotherapy, chemotherapy, and again, steroids. It may be possible to treat obstruction locally with laser therapy, cryotherapy, or stenting.[11] Pleural effusions, most common in tumours of the lung or breast, can be drained (although fluid frequently reaccumulates), or pleuradesis performed.

If it is not possible to reverse the cause of breathlessness, drug treatment is often seen as the principal means of alleviating the symptom. Lymphangitis, in which the lymphatic system of the lungs is affected by tumour, is unlikely to respond to treatment, but palliation may be achieved by a combination of dexamethasone and oral morphine.[13] Thomas and von Gunten suggest that glucocorticoids may be useful for bronchospasm, superior vena cava syndrome, carcinomatous lymphangitis, or radiation pneumonitis; they also point out that antibiotics may be used if appropriate for infections, and anticoagulants for the prevention and treatment of pulmonary emboli.[11] Ripamonti adds that pulmonary infections are in fact responsible for the death of almost half of all patients with advanced cancer.[10]

Bronchodilators may be useful for patients whose breathlessness is exacerbated by reversible airways disease. Reversibility can be assessed by measuring the patient's peak expiratory flow rate (PEFR) before and half an hour after a standard dose of a drug such as salbutamol. An improvement of more than 15% suggests that the patient will benefit from the appropriate bronchodilator.[13]

Respiratory sedatives are often recommended for alleviating breathlessness:[3]

> In the palliation of dyspnoeic patients with advanced cancer, neurological disease, or cardiorespiratory disease, the main benefit comes from the suppression of respiratory awareness [p.361].

Morphine has been the drug most commonly referred to in this respect. While the mode of action of morphine in breathlessness is not well understood, oral morphine has been shown to improve exercise tolerance in patients with chronic obstructive pulmonary disease (COPD).[14] Ripamonti suggests, in fact, that most studies of systemically administered morphine show that it has potential benefits in the alleviation of breathlessness.[10,15]

Nearly 20 years ago, Higginson and McCarthy conducted a study evaluating the work of domiciliary terminal care support teams in Bloomsbury Health Authority in London.[16] Fourteen items, agreed by support teams to be independent objectives of care and measures of the condition and further needs of dying patients and their families, were graded on a seven-point scale.[16] In all, the symptoms of 86 patients were rated throughout the period that patients were under the care of the support teams. While pain was found to be the most common symptom at referral (41% of patients), assessment scores improved after the first week of care, and in the last week of life. By contrast, the 13 patients with breathlessness at referral all had breathlessness at death. In addition, five patients developed breathlessness after referral. Symptom control scores suggested that 'pain was controlled very early in care, while dyspnoea was not controlled at all' (p.266). The authors point out that a full range of treatments, including opioids, bronchodilators, anxiolytics, and corticosteroids, was used by the support teams, and acknowledge that:[16]

> . . . results suggest that treatment may not be sufficiently effective. The existing measures may have poor efficacy, or they may be applied too late [p.267].

Ten years later, Edmonds *et al.* used a similar approach to assess the effect of palliative care teams in controlling symptoms in inpatients at a large London hospital, and in this case found that improvements were achieved in, for example, pain, mouth discomfort, anorexia, nausea, vomiting, constipation, breathlessness, and psychological distress.[17]

Studies such as that of Higginson and McCarthy have been particularly influential in the development of innovative (especially non-pharmacological) approaches to the management of breathlessness in lung and other cancers.[16]

Chest physiotherapy is usually seen as alleviating breathlessness by removing excess secretions, but techniques of breathing control have also been developed within physiotherapy to avoid breathlessness at rest or on exertion. Breathing control involves relaxing the upper chest and shoulders, and breathing at the normal rate using the lower chest (this is sometimes referred to as 'diaphragmatic breathing').[18] Gallo-Silver and Pollack provide helpful guidelines on how to practise using the diaphragm during breathing, which can be summarised as:[19]

- recline in a comfortable position
- breathe in a natural way (possibly in through nose, out through mouth)
- place a small object (e.g. book) on your tummy
- place hands at sides
- while breathing, focus on the object on your tummy
- see if it rises as you breathe in, and falls as you breath out

- practise making it rise and fall as you breathe in and out (see p.269).

The aims of breathing retraining are to:

- promote a relaxed and gentle breathing pattern
- minimise the work of breathing
- establish a sense of control
- improve ventilation at the base of the lungs
- increase the strength, co-ordination, and efficiency of the respiratory muscles
- maintain mobility of the thoracic cage
- promote a sense of well-being.

Breathing control can be used to climb stairs, breathing in as one step is climbed, and out as the next is climbed, and walking at a slightly slower pace, reducing the degree of breathlessness. The technique can also be applied on hills or slopes, on level ground if necessary, or to recover the breath when stationary. Lower-chest breathing is often grouped together in interventions for breathlessness with pursed lip breathing (PLB).[19,20] While PLB is thought to be a more effective pattern of respiration, it probably does not decrease the work of breathing. The source of symptom benefit from PLB may be due to decreased airway collapse, enlarged tidal volume, and slowed respiration.[21]

Often, breathlessness can lead a person to breathe with the upper chest and shoulders in a rapid, shallow manner.[22] Gasping for air increases the resistance to flow, which increases energy expenditure. Using accessory respiratory muscles, which are not as efficient as primary respiratory muscles, leads more quickly to fatigue, and to greater oxygen consumption. As the rate of breathing increases, the depth often decreases, creating a larger dead space in the lungs and reducing the amount of oxygen available to the body. In effect, this response to inadequate ventilation actually places even greater demands on the respiratory system.

Breathing retraining is intended to encourage as efficient a breathing pattern as possible, and to reverse as far as possible the ineffective response that has developed.

Research study 20.1

Roberts D.K., Thorne S.E. and Pearson C. (1993). The experience of dyspnoea in late-stage cancer: patients' and nurses' perspectives. *Cancer Nursing* **16**, 310–320.[23]

Arguing that there were gaps in our knowledge of the management of breathlessness in cancer, and that to understand breathlessness we must appreciate it from the point of view of those who are experiencing it, Roberts and colleagues set out in this study to answer the question, *What is the meaning of dyspnoea in late-stage cancer?*

In order to do this, they employed a wide range of data-collection methods, including self-report patient surveys of the frequency and nature of breathlessness, chart audits, interviews with patients and nurses, participant observation, questionnaires (e.g. about the nature, extent and context of breathlessness, and related symptoms), and specially adapted visual analogue scales (e.g. to measure usual severity and peak severity). The intention in using this extensive range of methods was to provide 'a richer and more accurate description and interpretation of the phenomenon than would any one data source alone' (p.312).

A sub-sample of 10 patients with a range of different cancers (lung, breast, throat, stomach, prostate and kidney) were interviewed, together with 12 nurses. Roberts and her colleagues identified three key themes from the interview data: *barriers in daily life*, *coping in isolation*, and *inconsistent understanding* (i.e. shown by health care professionals of experience of breathlessness). Breathlessness was a barrier to activity 'invading' daily lives (p.315); there were few if any recognised strategies for coping with breathlessness – patients 'figured it out for themselves' (p.315); discrepancies in nurses' interpretations of the frequency, effects, and implications of breathlessness, and differing views of the effectiveness of various management strategies, were common. They conclude that the study shows patients coping 'in isolation' with 'an extremely troublesome symptom' (p.318) and that:

> understanding the meaning of the symptom for the patient is a foundation for effective management [p.319].

All in all, this study provides a wealth of insight and information into the nature and impact of breathlessness in cancer, and has had strong influence upon subsequent work to develop non-pharmacological interventions for this distressing experience.

Breathlessness can be a frightening experience: anyone who has experienced, say, asthmatic attacks, or altitude sickness, or, indeed, anyone whose children have experienced breathlessness can testify to that. The experience of people whose breathlessness occurs in the context of a potentially life-limiting disease such as cancer can be extraordinarily vivid and powerful. As Roberts *et al.* pointed out:[23]

> . . . patients' interpretations of what the signal of shortness of breath meant in relation to their disease seemed . . . the predominant influencing factor in shaping their experience with dyspnoea [p.315].

> The sensation aroused by dyspnoea created a barrier to comfort and peace of mind . . . patients lived with the life-threatening potential of breathlessness [p.311].

She describes one woman who avoided any activity that made her aware of her breathing, despite being able to bath, walk, and dress independently, because she believed that being breathless would make her cancer spread. Breathlessness can represent a threat to life itself:

> It starts to feel like you're choking. Someone's taking the breath away from me [p.314]

and:

> I panic a bit sometimes, because deep down I know that [this breath] could be my last one . . . It's an awful feeling [p.314].

Steele and Shaver also identify that breathlessness constitutes a serious threat:[24]

> . . . the experience of dyspnoea incorporates cognitive interpretation of the event as threatening

and suggest that this is why activity is circumscribed:

> . . . motivation to alleviate threat through behaviours such as slowing or cessation of activities that evoke dyspnoea would be expected [p.67].

While it is understandable that both patients and carers respond to breathlessness in this way,

Box 20.1   A programme of research into managing breathlessness in lung cancer

Corner J., Plant H. and Warner L. (1995). Developing a nursing approach to managing dyspnoea in lung cancer. *International Journal of Palliative Nursing* **1**, 5–11.[25]

• Outlined approach and model for working with breathlessness in lung cancer

Bailey C. (1995). Nursing as therapy in the management of breathlessness in lung cancer. *European Journal of Cancer Care* **4**, 184–190.[26]

• Focused on broader rehabilitative goals of therapy, including managing function and psychosocial burden

Corner J., Plant H., A'Hern R. and Bailey C. (1996). Non-pharmacological intervention for breathlessness in lung cancer. *Palliative Medicine* **10**, 299–305.[27]

• Reported findings of first randomised control trial into non-pharmacological intervention (*n* = 34)

Corner J. and O'Driscoll M. (1999). Development of a breathlessness assessment guide for use in palliative care. *Palliative Medicine* **13**, 375–384.[28]

• Development of breathlessness assessment guide

O'Driscoll M., Corner J. and Bailey C. (1999). The experience of breathlessness in lung cancer. *European Journal of Cancer Care* **8**, 37–43.[29]

• The experience of breathlessness in lung cancer – study of 52 patient records

Bredin M., Corner J., Krishnasamy M. *et al.* (1999). Multicentre randomised controlled trial of nursing intervention for breathlessness in patients with lung cancer. *British Medical Journal* **318**, 901–904.[30]

• Multicentre randomised controlled trial (RCT) of nursing intervention for breathlessness in lung cancer (*n* = 119)

Plant H., Bredin M., Krishnasamy M. and Corner J. (2000). Working with resistance, tension and objectivity: conducting a randomised controlled trial of a nursing intervention for breathlessness. *NT Research* **5**, 426–436.[31]

• Interview study with specialist nurses participating in RCT

Froggatt K., Corner J. and Bredin M. (2002). Dissemination and utilisation of an intervention to manage breathlessness: letting go or letting down? *NT Research* **7**, 223–232.[32]

• Critical analysis of methods of disseminating findings from studies of intervention for breathlessness

the objective of therapy remains to roll back inactivity, or loss of function, and to work with the heavy psychological burden that is so influential in restricting freedom.

Our own work has focused on developing and evaluating an intervention that addresses both the functional and the psychosocial aspects of breathlessness (see Box 20.1). This work had its early origins in a recognition of the importance of an 'ecologic' model of dyspnoea, 'a framework for guiding nursing science', which:

> . . . unlike the linear, reductionist biomedical model with notions of cause, disease, and cure . . . acknowledge[s] the interactive effects of multivariate individual and environmental influences upon individual adaptations and health outcomes.[24]

Corner *et al.* proposed an 'integrative model', in which the emotional experience of breathlessness is considered as inseparable from the sensory experience and the biological mechanisms.[25] This model was used as the basis for a non-pharmacological intervention for breathlessness, developed for the outpatient setting, which draws on breathing retraining, relaxation, and biofeedback techniques. The intervention, which was the subject of a randomised controlled trial (RCT),[27] consisted of the following strategies:

• detailed assessment of breathlessness
• exploration of meaning of breathlessness
• advice and support on ways of managing breathlessness
• breathing retraining

- goal setting
- meditative and progressive muscle relaxation
- early recognition of need for other interventions.

This study showed that using the intervention led to important improvements in participants' experience of breathlessness, including:

- breathlessness at worst: improved by 35%
- distress caused by breathlessness: improved by 53%
- functional capacity: improved by 17%
- difficulty in performing activities of daily living: reduced by 21%.[27]

From the beginning, it was anticipated that the meaning of breathlessness in the context of severe, life-threatening illness would be an important factor in patients' experiences, and that managing breathlessness would involve working with its meaning.

A small study, conducted in parallel with the main evaluation study, was developed to record and assess nurse-researchers' perceptions of the intervention.[26] Using an exploratory single case design, interviews were conducted with the three nurse-researchers working in the outpatients' clinic at that time.[33]

Evidence from interviews with the nurse-researchers suggested that the deep emotional consequences of breathlessness in lung cancer have a profound influence on how the intervention is realised in practice. The value of attention paid to psychosocial issues was at least as great as the value of breathing retraining. As one nurse-researcher said:

> ... the [practical] framework that we give people, actually helps them cope, and that has to ... go alongside talking about emotional issues, and the difficulties ...

Referring to a man she was seeing in the clinic, she gave an example of how this worked in practice:

> ... last week he was talking about ... walking up the car park ... it goes up a bank ... it sort of steps up. Well, for all the people who attend it's a problem, because they have to park their cars on the third level,

and having talked about the difficulties of any kind of incline they then have to climb up to get back to their car. So I walked back to his car with him, slowly, to see how it was for him ... we had this little conversation while I went up to the car with him   the fact that I walked to the car with him obviously means something enormous ... he actually lives with his son, who he feels a tremendous burden on ... I always got a feeling ... that they feel no one really cares about them ... I think this was like he did matter to me ... almost a confirmation of it, 'cos I bothered to walk up to his car with him ...

The opportunity to accompany this man to the car park was a means of rehearsing an aspect of breathing retraining in a practical situation. It was also a means of working socially with a client whose sense was that his illness had made him a burden and that he was therefore not entitled to make claims upon people's time and care. Being a burden, and being beyond the reach of care, are part of illness and breathlessness, and are approached, with the physical experience of breathlessness, as a single, integrated phenomenon.

The same nurse-researcher refers to her clients' feelings of loss of worth again in another interview:

> ... there is ... this need to give something back ... it's almost self-respect ... to say that they are still wanted and needed ... I had a really long conversation with him telling me the most economical way to use my washing machine ... and another time he told me about cooking nectarines, well I thought it was just so important to listen to that.

Breathlessness can restrict our ability to carry out our customary daily personal and work-related activities, and can leave us feeling disconnected from the social world, which in other circumstances would be a vital source of pride and self-esteem.

As Charmaz points out:[34]

> Chronically ill persons frequently experience a crumbling away of their former self-images without simultaneous development of equally valued new ones. The experiences and meanings upon which these ill persons had built former positive self-images are no longer available to them [p.168].

The nurse-researcher referred to above is addressing some of the overall effect of breathlessness when she responds to her client's wish to pass on his domestic skills. The physical losses caused by breathlessness, evident in the man's difficulty in walking to his car, go hand in hand with the social ones, played out at home and in his relationship with his son; together, they constitute lost elements of a 'positive self-image', and it is towards this that the nurse is directing her attention and support by reciprocating her client's offer of insight into domestic and culinary skills.

Night-time panic attacks exemplify the way in which breathlessness is not a sensation, not an emotion, and not a physical process, but all three of these, at least, and also a dynamic, fluctuating state. Responding therapeutically to panic attacks makes great demands on both the client, and the nurse, and organisations working with people with cancer have developed a number of strategies for managing panic, including the 'panic hand'.[35] Panic in breathlessness is an escalating predicament in which normal breathing patterns collapse, awareness is acute, and fear takes hold. Sleep becomes impossible and panic rises. The essence of panic is that catastrophe appears imminent and inescapable; with breathlessness, panic can frequently revolve around the idea that suffocation and death are close. One nurse-researcher working with people in one of our early studies of nurse-led clinics described her client's experience in this way:

> . . . his breathing was bad, he used to come in at night with these panic attacks, he couldn't sleep . . . because he was so frightened, and a lot of the work I did with him was with strategies for coping with the night, and getting to sleep, and ways of calming himself down at night . . . he used to get breathless at night . . . it was just because he would go to bed and think about his breathing and think he wouldn't be able to breathe and then get in a panic about it . . .

It is, then, appropriate to apply the practical discipline of breathing retraining to a highly charged emotional situation such as this (and it is true to say that part of what the nurse is doing is responding to a pathological process). The nurse, however, is aware and involved in the predicament as a whole, and is called upon to work with a high level of distress.

Fabricius suggests that being 'with' and 'for' the patient is a therapeutic response to distress:[36]

> . . . by 'being for the patient' . . . I mean allowing the patient, to some extent, to use the nurse, psychically, as the sort of object he needs. Often this will be, to use Bion's term, as a container for whatever of his anxieties are at the moment intolerable to him, and of course this . . . is a maternal function [p.101].

Fabricius points out that nurses are often unable to meet the demands made on them by patients:[36]

> . . . the sheer quantity, as well as force, of the projections that are thrust on them are too much for any human unless she herself is held in a supportive, containing structure [p.103].

She suggests that facilitated small-group meetings for nurses to discuss anything to do with their relationships with patients and the feelings aroused by them represent progress towards such a structure. Franks *et al.* add that the effectiveness of this type of group work appears to depend on there being a balance between the *structure* the group provides and *space* for personal reflection it gives: when we are trying to deal with the anxiety caused by working closely with patients, we need some kind of 'defence' against it, and stable, well-facilitated small-group discussion may be able to provide this.[37] In our own work with lung cancer patients with breathlessness, we held structured one-to-one sessions for members of the team to reflect on their experiences of working with patients, which in fact provided a lot of insight into the realities of our work.

Johnson and Moore have written insightfully about some of the challenges of working with people with cancer-related breathlessness.[38] They point out that in the light of positive findings from studies of a non-pharmacological intervention for breathlessness (see Box 20.1), nurses and others have been encouraged to adopt a similar approach in their own work. Putting this kind of intervention into practice, they believe, is challenging not only because of the kind of organisational change that is required, but also because confidence has to be gained in using the techniques involved, and because existing professional roles impose a series of limitations. They rightly stress that:

> In the research studies . . . psychological demands on the nurses using the intervention were acknowledged and access to supervision and support was considered an essential part of the intervention. Nurses worked in pairs and had support from the research team [p.36]

and emphasise that while it may be difficult to arrange, it is nevertheless:

> . . . imperative . . . that nurses working within clinical practice ensure they have access to a similar level of support and supervision to maintain their own psychological well-being [pp.36–37].

The benefits for people with cancer related breathlessness offered by the type of non-pharmacological intervention outlined here, and the potential rewards for health care professionals in terms of achieving genuinely therapeutic goals, are, however, substantial, if the challenges of implementing change can be successfully met.[39] And in recent years, this has been recognised in the recommendation of such approaches by the National Institute of Health and Clinical Excellence:[40]

> . . . non-drug interventions for breathlessness should be delivered by a multidisciplinary group, coordinated by a professional with an interest in breathlessness and expertise in the techniques (for example a nurse, physiotherapist or occupational therapist). Although support may be provided in a breathlessness clinic, patients should have access to it in all care settings [p.7]

and the Scottish Intercollegiate Guidelines Network:[41]

> Breathlessness clinics led by nurses or physiotherapists should be made available to all lung cancer patients [p.38].

The conceptualisation put forward by Corner *et al.*, which treats the emotional experience of breathlessness as inseparable from the sensory experience and the biological mechanisms,[25] challenges us to look outside the neat but limited and impersonal categories represented by conventional symptomatology. We have to develop therapeutic responses that genuinely address the broad range of needs flowing from the embodied experience of various forms of distress, including consequential social losses and their implications for self-concept and suffering. The nociceptive model described by Steele and Shaver might suggest that one dimension of a phenomenon (*distress*, for example) can be addressed independently of another (*sensation*, for example).[24] Corner *et al.*, however, suggest that breathlessness should be:[25]

> . . . understood holistically in the context of an individual's life, illness experience and its meaning [p.6].

Embodied experience is not neatly packaged, and individual 'items' of need are not always clearly linked to a discrete and well-defined intervention. Addressing needs as if they were discrete, separate entities, without listening to and working with the whole story, as it were, can leave fundamental fears, distress and suffering relatively untouched. As one nurse-researcher involved in an early study of nurse-led intervention for breathlessness commented:

> People don't even know that they're anxious . . . it's so much part of your physiological activity that you don't know what's doing what . . . it's impossible to start saying there are components of it, to even talk about components seems to be wrong . . . you have to treat it as a whole experience, and it must have intense meaning to people.

A key part of the response demanded by Corner's conceptualisation is the 'containing, supportive structure' referred to by Fabricius,[36] extended by nurse to client and, as importantly, by co-workers and institution to nurse.

The questions raised about the practical arrangements required by such a response (raised in one form by Johnson and Moore[38]) are raised in a slightly different way by Allan in her study of nursing on a fertility unit.[42] Nursing care on the unit was 'good enough' (a mixture of emotional awareness and emotional distance) Allan suggests, partly because 'nurses in this setting were not encouraged to recognise feelings arising from their interactions with patients' and 'had not been offered clinical supervision' (p.58), and partly because nurses' 'emotional distance or non-caring . . . was a defence against the anxiety caused by the pain of infertility' (p.55). In these circumstances it is, one feels, inevitable that at times 'patients were left alone in their distress and their feelings denied' (p.59). Allan's study leaves us pondering the question of whether 'good enough' is, given the constraints and demands upon us, good enough; or whether, given the moral imperatives of caring, a way must be found to establish supportive structures for staff and clients alike so that in health care institutions patients are not 'left alone in their distress'.

Breathlessness is not just a symptom, it is lived experience. For some patients with lung cancer, it is fear of dying, and care in these circumstances might include the kind of supporting structure that allows this to be articulated safely, to become more a part of an unfolding and progressing 'story':

> . . . one lady . . . I turned to put the pulse oximeter, turned it on, and to put it on her, and as I turned my back to her, she said, 'Am I going to die of this?' And, I mean the fact that I'd done something, moved away to do something technical and turned my back, allowed her to say the thing that she really wanted to say, and it was about allowing that person to be in a totally private place with someone who appeared to be very comfortable and safe to ask that question of.

For some, breathlessness is panic, and things that cannot be accomplished, and care is tackling panic, and accomplishing some of those things:

> . . . teaching a few simple strategies to manage those attacks, and techniques and new ways of breathing . . . by the next session . . . he'd only had minor attacks of breathlessness at night, so he was beginning to master these awful panics . . . then . . . teaching a bit more, like how do you use these breathing techniques to manage stairs . . . he could recover quicker at the top by using diaphragmatic breathing . . . timing your breathing while you're walking . . . talking about sleeping and those sorts of things, and getting a bit further with them about what they both felt about it and the future . . .

Fabricius asks how nurses can be psychotherapeutic, and what hinders them from being so.[36] The priorities and ordering of nursing situations, the routine; the way in which 'symptoms' are dealt with at a high level of abstraction and distance from the individual; the prevalence of models or algorithms which 'stand for' human experiences without making them real; the splitting of human experience into disembodied parts, setting aside the undisciplined, disorderly whole; all of this stands in the way, provides a means to become detached and to leave potentially painful things untouched.

Acknowledgement

This chapter is adapted and expanded from 'Nursing as therapy in the management of breathlessness in lung cancer', first published in the *European Journal of Cancer Care* 1995 **4**, 184–190, with the permission of Blackwell Science Ltd.

References

1. Renfroe K.L. (1988). Effect of progressive muscle relaxation on dyspnoea and state anxiety in patients with chronic obstructive pulmonary disease. *Heart and Lung* **17**, 408–413.
2. Ripamonti C. and Fusco F. (2001). Respiratory problems in advanced cancer. *Supportive Care in Cancer* **10**, 204–216.
3. Ahmedzai S. (1995). Palliation of respiratory symptoms. In Doyle D., Hanks G. and McDonald N. (eds.) *The Oxford Textbook of Palliative Medicine*. Oxford: Oxford University Press.
4. Chan K-S., Sham M.M.K., Tse D.M.W. and Thorsen A.B. (2004). Palliative medicine in malignant respiratory diseases. In: Doyle D., Hanks G., Cherny N. and Calman K. (eds.) *The Oxford Textbook of Palliative Medicine*, 2nd edition. Oxford: Oxford University Press.
5. Booth S. (2006). Palliative care for intractable breathlessness in cancer. *European Journal of Cancer Care* **15**, 303–314.
6. Twycross R.G. and Lack S.A. (1986). *Therapeutics in Terminal Cancer*. London: Churchill Livingstone.
7. Reuben D.B. and Mor V. (1986). Dyspnoea in terminally ill cancer patients. *Chest* **89**, 234–236.
8. Bruera E., Schmitz B., Pither J., Neumann C.M. and Hanson J. (2006). The frequency and correlates of dyspnea in patients with advanced cancer. *Journal of Pain and Symptom Management* **19**, 357–362.
9. Dudgeon D.J., Kristjanson L., Sloan J.A., Lertzman M. and Clement K. (2001). Dyspnea in cancer patients: prevalence and associated factors. *Journal of Pain and Symptom Management* **21**, 95–102.
10. Ripamonti C. (1999). Management of dyspnea in advanced cancer patients. *Supportive Care in Cancer* **7**, 233–243.
11. Thomas J.R. and von Gunten C.F. (2002). Clinical management of dyspnoea. *The Lancet Oncology* **3**, 223–228.

12. Jennings A.L., Davies A.N., Higgins J.P.T. and Broadly K. (2003). Opioids for the palliation of breathlessness in terminal illness (Cochrane Review). *The Cochrane Library*, Issue 1. Oxford: Update Software.

13. Cowcher K. and Hanks G.W. (1990). Long-term management of respiratory symptoms in advanced cancer. *Journal of Pain and Symptom Management* **5**, 320–330.

14. Light R.W., Muro J.R., Sato R.I. *et al.* (1989). Effects of oral morphine on breathlessness and exercise tolerance in patients with chronic obstructive pulmonary disease. *American Review of Respiratory Diseases* **139**, 126–133.

15. Abernethy A.P., Currow D.C., Frith P. *et al.* (2003). Randomised, double blind, placebo controlled crossover trial of sustained release morphine for the management of refractory dyspnoea. *British Medical Journal* **327**, 523–528.

16. Higginson I. and McCarthy M. (1989). Measuring symptoms in terminal cancer: are pain and dyspnoea controlled? *Journal of the Royal Society of Medicine* **82**, 264–267.

17. Edmonds P.M., Stuttaford J.M. and Penny J. (1998). Do hospital palliative care teams improve symptom control? Use of a modified STAS as an evaluation tool. *Palliative Medicine* **12**, 345–351.

18. Gallo-Silver L. and Pollack B. (2000). Behavioural interventions for lung cancer-related breathlessness. *Cancer Practice* **8**, 268–273.

19. Webber B. (1991). The role of the physiotherapist in medical chest problems. *Respiratory Disease in Practice* **February/March**, 12–15.

20. Kersten L. (1989). *Comprehensive Respiratory Nursing*. Philadelphia, PA: WB Saunders.

21. Mueller R.E., Petty T.L. and Filley G.F. (1970). Ventilation and arterial blood gas changes induced by pursed lips breathing. *Journal of Applied Physiology* **28**, 784–789.

22. Gift A.G., Moore T. and Soeken K. (1992). Relaxation to reduce dyspnoea and anxiety in COPD patients. *Nursing Research* **41**, 242–246.

23. Roberts D., Thorne S.E. and Pearson C. (1993). The experience of dyspnoea in late-stage cancer: patients' and nurses' perspectives. *Cancer Nursing* **16**, 310–320.

24. Steele B. and Shaver J. (1992). The dyspnoea experience: nociceptive properties and a model for research and practice. *Advances in Nursing Science* **15**, 64–76.

25. Corner J., Plant H. and Warner L. (1995). Developing a nursing approach to managing dyspnoea in lung cancer. *International Journal of Palliative Nursing* **1**, 5–11.

26. Bailey C. (1995). Nursing as therapy in the management of breathlessness in lung cancer. *European Journal of Cancer Care* **4**, 184–190.

27. Corner J., Plant H., A'Hern R. and Bailey C. (1996). Non-pharmacological intervention for breathlessness in lung cancer. *Palliative Medicine* **10**, 299–305.

28. Corner J. and O'Driscoll M. (1999). Development of a breathlessness assessment guide for use in palliative care. *Palliative Medicine* **13**, 375–384.

29. O'Driscoll M., Corner J. and Bailey C. (1999). The experience of breathlessness in lung cancer. *European Journal of Cancer Care* **8**, 37–43.

30. Bredin M., Corner J., Krishnasamy M. *et al.* (1999). Multicentre randomised controlled trial of nursing intervention for breathlessness in patients with lung cancer. *British Medical Journal* **318**, 901–904.

31. Plant H., Bredin M., Krishnasamy M. and Corner J. (2000). Working with resistance, tension and objectivity: conducting a randomised controlled trial of a nursing intervention for breathlessness. *NT Research* **5**, 426–436.

32. Froggatt K., Corner J. and Bredin M. (2002). Dissemination and utilisation of an intervention to manage breathlessness: letting go or letting down? *NT Research* **7**, 223–232.

33. Yin R. (1994). *Case Study Research. Design and Methods*, 2nd edition. London: Sage.

34. Charmaz K. (1983). Loss of self: a fundamental form of suffering in the chronically ill. *Sociology of Health and Illness* **5**, 168–195.

35. Wessex Cancer Trust. (2002). *Coping with Breathlessness due to Cancer*. Southampton: Wessex Cancer Trust, Southampton. www.wessexcancer.org (accessed 7 August 2007).

36. Fabricius J. (1991). Running on the spot or can nursing really change? *Psychoanalytic Psychotherapy* **5**, 97–108.

37. Franks V., Watts M. and Fabricius J. (1994). Interpersonal learning in groups: an investigation. *Journal of Advanced Nursing* **20**, 1162–1169.

38. Johnson M. and Moore S. (2003). Research into practice: the reality of implementing a non-pharmacological breathlessness intervention into clinical practice. *European Journal of Oncology Nursing* **7**, 33–38.

39. Hately J., Scott A., Laurence V., Baker R. and Thomas P. (2001). *A Palliative Care Approach for Breathlessness in Cancer: a Clinical Evaluation*. London: Help the Hospices.

40. National Institute for Clinical Excellence. (2005). *Lung Cancer: the Diagnosis and Treatment of Lung Cancer* (Clinical Guideline 24). London: National Institute for Clinical Excellence. www.nice.org.uk/guidance/CG24/niceguidance/pdf/English (accessed 7 August 2007).

41. Scottish Intercollegiate Guidelines Network. (2005). *Management of Patients with Lung Cancer: a National Clinical Guideline*. Edinburgh: Scottish Intercollegiate Guidelines Network. www.sign.ac.uk/guidelines/published/index.html (accessed 7 August 2007).

42. Allan H. (2001). A 'good enough' nurse: supporting patients in a fertility unit. *Nursing Inquiry* **8**, 51–60.

CHAPTER TWENTY-ONE

Wound management

Meinir Krishnasamy

In his book *The Body Silent*, Murphy reminds us that illness is 'not simply a physical affair . . . it is our ontology, a condition of our being in the world' (p. 77).[1] Illness, especially when it is associated with disfigurement or alterations in body image, confers on people a loss of self-esteem, a stigma, resulting in a 'spoiled identity'.[2] When the disfigurement is associated with the disease of cancer, the potential for negative self-perception through acceptance of a subjectively created or objectively projected spoiled identity is enormous.[3] Where self-perception is altered by the presence of a physical wound, whether visible or otherwise, profoundly negative associations may occur. In extreme cases, a person may identify him- or herself with the malignant wound, believing himself to be foul, odorous, or repulsive. The consequences for an individual's quality of life, self-esteem and well-being are enormous.

Skilled technical and physiological knowledge is necessary if avoidable wounds are to be prevented, wounds caused by any number of invasive procedures and treatments are to be managed effectively, uncomplicated wound healing is to be facilitated, or when complete healing is not feasible, if discomfort and distress are to be minimised. Alongside technical proficiency, nurses must also convey compassion (as illustrated in Personal account 21.1).[4–6]

Personal account 21.1[6]

I was so shocked when I saw the wound, it was leaking and black, and the smell was very strong. As soon as I began to unpack the items on the dressing trolley he fixed his eyes on me, waiting for me to show signs of repulsion, I think. I stopped and asked him if he minded me seeing the wound and him like this.

The wound had broken through, out onto his lower abdomen, but the area to be cleaned and dressed spread down to his genital area. He was very thin. He started to tell me how disgusting he found the wound and how he was ashamed of having it on his stomach. His wife sat quietly trying very hard to be absorbed in a book. He talked about it as though it were something alien that had taken over his body.

By the time he had finished talking, the technical dressing was over, but the effects of the interaction, of asking him what this wound meant to him were far-reaching. This time became an opportunity for intense personal interaction and over the course of the next ten days, the three of us began to talk about their sadness and fears about the future.

Wound healing

Irrespective of the nature or type of wound, the same basic processes are required to bring about wound healing, and yet wound care has altered so dramatically over the past 20 years that nurses often feel overwhelmed by the array of dressings and treatments available.[5,7] Most products on the market provide passive support for wound healing by creating an environment favorable to repair (that is, clean, moist, insulated, and protected). There are also emerging therapies designed to actively manipulate the repair process. Nevertheless, despite the plethora of dressings and agents available there is very little robust evidence to indicate the most effective ways of managing cancer-related wounds. Nurses therefore must make product and management decisions based on wound characteristics and response to treatment.

The most widely available wound dressings continue to be:[8,9]

- *absorbent dressings* – e.g. gauze, gamgee, and lint, are highly absorbent, but have a tendency to adhere to wound surfaces, causing trauma and pain on removal
- *low-adherence dressings* – those that have one non-adherent surface intended for direct contact with the wound. They are for use on minor wounds with minimal exudate
- *tulle dressings* – sheets of gauze impregnated with various amounts of paraffin, antiseptics, or other agents. They too are best used with low-exudate wounds
- *semi-permeable dressings* – clear polyurethane film coated with adhesive. When used with low-exuding wounds, they conform well and allow unimpeded observation of the wound site
- *polysaccharide dressings* – work by exerting osmotic action at the wound surface. They are available as pastes, beads, and ointments and are intended to be used during the inflammatory phase of sloughy or infected wounds
- *hydrogels* – especially suited for use in cavities and are effective débriding/desloughing agents. They provide a cooling action and may reduce pain on contact with the wound surface
- *hydrocolloids* – form a gel, which creates an ideal, moist, wound healing environment and protect fragile skin and areas of the body affected by urinary or faecal incontinence or frictional forces
- *silver dressings* – release a steady amount of silver to a wound and provide antimicrobial or anti-

bacterial action. They can manage minimal, moderate or heavy exudates depending on which type of dressing is used
- *alginates* – intended for use on moderately or heavily exudating wounds. On absorbing secretions they form a gel, creating optimum humidity and temperature for wound healing
- *collagens* – used for partial- and full-thickness wounds, infected and non-infected wounds, tunnelling wounds and wounds with minimal to heavy exudate. They encourage the deposition and organisation of newly formed collagen fibres and granulation tissue in the wound bed
- *foam dressings* – highly absorbent materials suitable for a wide range of granulating wounds. They provide thermal insulation to the wound, creating a moist healing environment. They may be used in conjunction with topical antibiotics for infected wounds. They may be used as primary or secondary dressings.

There are many types of wounds and several methods exist to classify them. However, there is to date no universally accepted classification system and wounds may be described as:

- mechanical injuries, incorporating abrasions, lacerations, penetrating wounds, bites, and surgical wounds
- burns and chemical injuries, incorporating superficial, deep dermal, and full-thickness thermal, chemical, electrical, and radiation burns
- chronic ulcerative wounds, which can be divided into decubitus ulcers (pressures sores), leg ulcers (venous, ischaemic, or traumatic), and ulcers arising from systemic infections, radiotherapy, or malignant disease[8]
- acute wounds, which include surgical and traumatic wounds
- chronic wounds, which include the ulcers, malignant and fungating wounds.[5]

Patients with cancer are at risk of developing any one of these many types of wounds.

Principles of wound healing

Damaged tissue passes through a number of phases of repair following injury. Inflammatory, destructive, proliferative, and maturation phases are characterised by numerous overlapping processes involving cell regeneration and proliferation, and collagen production.[9] In the surgical management of wound healing, four types of repair are recognised and a brief overview of the types of wound healing and phases involved is outlined below.[8]

Primary closure

Clean surgical wounds or newly inflicted traumatic injuries are managed by primary closure. When wounds heal by primary closure, granulation tissue and scar formation are visible. An acute inflammatory phase begins within a few minutes of injury, resulting in constriction of smooth muscle, reduced blood flow, and aggregation of collagen and platelets at the wound site.[10] Activation of the clotting mechanism occurs and results in the production of a clot or plug, which brings about haemostasis, while supporting and strengthening the injured tissue.[8] As the capillary walls at the damaged site become permeable, serum, leucocytes, erythrocytes, and antibodies pass into the wound. During the destructive phase of wound healing, and within hours of clot formation, polymorphonuclear leucocytes and macrophages begin the process of removing debris and bacteria from the wound site.[8,9,11] After a period of about 24 hours, epidermal cells begin to grow across the surface of the wound underneath the now dried scab, and depending on the nature and size of the wound, this process will continue for 2–3 days.

Open granulation

When drawing the edges of a wound together immediately is inadvisable, for example following major surgery, or when there is a considerable risk of infection, open granulation becomes the healing method of choice.[8] Open granulation is by necessity a slower process than primary closure, involving the progressive filling of the wound with granulation tissue. Granulation tissue is composed of collagen, a complex mixture of proteins and polysaccharides, salts, and other colloid materials.[8] When the wound cavity is almost filled with granulation tissue, the epithelium around the wound margin becomes active and strands of collagen are drawn across the surface of the wound.[11] This early collagen is very delicate and the wound needs to be stabilised to prevent damaging its delicate

structure. Collagen growth is dependent upon a good supply of oxygen and an adequate supply of vitamin C.[12]

Delayed or secondary closure

Delayed primary closure occurs following infection, breakdown of the healing process, or when there is a poor blood supply.[8] Delayed primary closure involves leaving the wound open for 3–4 days before closure is undertaken, or involves resuturing of a previously closed wound.

During the maturation phase of healing, fibroblasts begin to leave the wound, and as a result of dehydration and reorganisation of collagen fibres, the edges of the wound are drawn together through a process of contraction.[9,12] However, open granulation and contraction may be unacceptable where the scar left by the injury is to be visible, as contraction, especially of a facial wound, may result in distortion of surrounding features.

Grafting or flap formation

Grafting involves the removal of a portion of skin from one anatomical site, usually the thigh or buttock, to be placed onto a wound elsewhere. Despite offering rapid potential for healing, grafting results in the patient having two wounds instead of one. There is also considerable anecdotal evidence that donor sites cause greater pain than the original wound.

Skin flaps involve raising a portion of skin and subcutaneous tissue and rotating it to cover an area of skin loss.[8] Adequate blood supply, and prevention of infection and stress at the graft or flap site are essential factors in the success of these procedures.

Assessment

Nursing management of wounds will only be effective if based on informed decisions following a thorough assessment of objective and subjective information.[5] Recent developments in the availability of digital technology, along with emerging evidence of improved patient outcomes and cost-effectiveness of using digital wound-imaging software, offers a new and exiting avenue for nurses to pursue within oncological

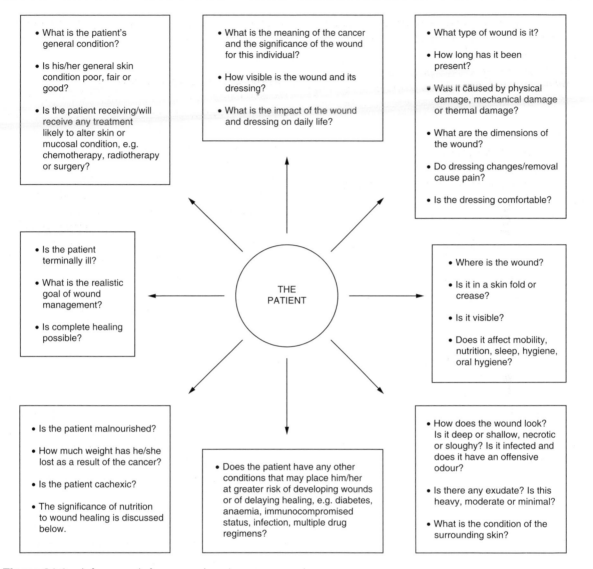

- What is the patient's general condition?

- Is his/her general skin condition poor, fair or good?

- Is the patient receiving/will receive any treatment likely to alter skin or mucosal condition, e.g. chemotherapy, radiotherapy or surgery?

- What is the meaning of the cancer and the significance of the wound for this individual?

- How visible is the wound and its dressing?

- What is the impact of the wound and dressing on daily life?

- What type of wound is it?

- How long has it been present?

- Was it caused by physical damage, mechanical damage or thermal damage?

- What are the dimensions of the wound?

- Do dressing changes/removal cause pain?

- Is the dressing comfortable?

- Is the patient terminally ill?

- What is the realistic goal of wound management?

- Is complete healing possible?

THE PATIENT

- Where is the wound?

- Is it in a skin fold or crease?

- Is it visible?

- Does it affect mobility, nutrition, sleep, hygiene, oral hygiene?

- Is the patient malnourished?

- How much weight has he/she lost as a result of the cancer?

- Is the patient cachexic?

- The significance of nutrition to wound healing is discussed below.

- Does the patient have any other conditions that may place him/her at greater risk of developing wounds or of delaying healing, e.g. diabetes, anaemia, immunocompromised status, infection, multiple drug regimens?

- How does the wound look? Is it deep or shallow, necrotic or sloughy? Is it infected and does it have an offensive odour?

- Is there any exudate? Is this heavy, moderate or minimal?

- What is the condition of the surrounding skin?

Figure 21.1   A framework for comprehensive assessment.

wound management.[13] Along with skilled, technical knowledge, nurses must also be prepared to enter into a relationship with the patient, which engenders trust and a mutual respect (see Figure 21.1):

> Nursing is a metaphor for intimacy . . . Nurses do for others publicly what healthy persons do for themselves behind closed doors . . . [they] are there to hear secrets especially those born of vulnerability . . . and nurses

are indelibly identified with those terribly personal times.[14]

A detailed assessment of a person's wound status includes, but may not be limited to, its location, size, colour, type of wound tissue, exudate, odour, wound margins, pain, dressing management, adjunctive therapies, the person's interpretation of the cancer, the wound and associated disease stage.[9] The rationale for wound dressing is shown in Figure 21.2.

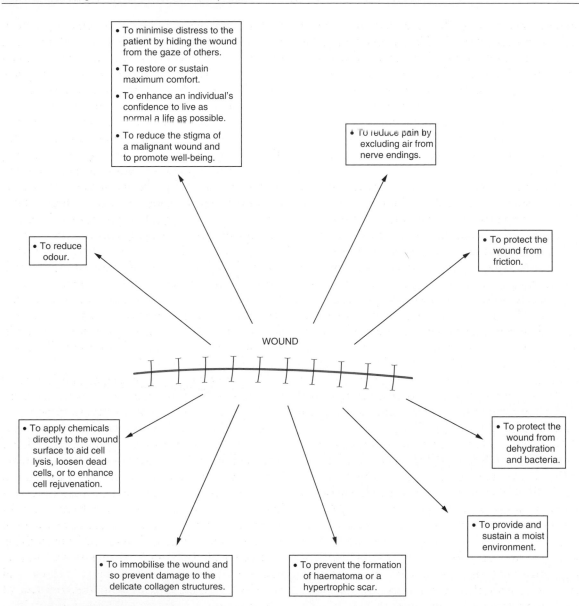

Figure 21.2 Rationale for dressing a wound.[8,10,11]

Factors interfering with normal processes of wound healing in cancer

Over the past few years, researchers have begun to define a multi-step process necessary to address complex or chronic wounds. The concept of *wound bed preparation* is gaining increasing momentum amongst nurses as its offers a systematic approach (the TIME approach) to removing barriers to healing, including **T**issue (non-viable), **I**nfection or inflammation, **M**oisture imbalance and non-advancing or undermining **E**dges (TIME).[9,15,16] The emerging view is that chronic or delayed-healing wounds are characterised by resident cells that have undergone phenotypic changes that need to be corrected for optimal healing to occur.[17] With this understanding, the potential to revolutionise chronic wound management through the use of gene and stem cell therapies is being evaluated. In recent years, the use of maggots (larval therapy) appears to offer a safe and effective method of debriding tissue for wound bed preparation. Further research is needed to establish clinical utility and patient acceptability of their use.[18,19]

The ageing process is associated with reduced tissue elasticity, increased likelihood of systemic diseases, impaired immune and inflammatory responses, and generally impaired vascularity. Since cancer is recognised as being primarily a disease of old age, these factors are all likely to complicate wound healing. Impaired oxygen supply further compounds the healing process. Phagocytes cannot function effectively when oxygen availability is reduced, and as this deficit may arise as a consequence of inadequate lung and cardiovascular function, patients with primary lung cancer or secondary metastatic spread to the lungs may be highly susceptible to delayed wound healing. Chemotherapy commonly results in anaemia, further compromising oxygen availability.

Nutritional status influences wound healing. Efficient wound healing is dependent on the availability of adequate energy, and yet cancer causes metabolic demands that greatly exceed energy of injury or stress, and the greater the impact on nutritional intake as a result of the demands of the tumour upon nutritional requirements and extent of catabolism.[20] Any form of trauma, and particularly nutritional consequences for those who may have a diagnosis of cancer, results in a triggering of a hypothalamic chain of events that culminates in a physiological state known as catabolism, where plasma proteins are utilised to satisfy increased energy demands at a time when carbohydrate stores are depleted.[21]

Nutritional requirements for the wound-healing process include copper, iron, zinc, magnesium, the fat-soluble vitamins A and K, and the water-soluble vitamins B_1, B_5, and C.[21] In cancer, the risk of malnutrition as a result of anorexia, nausea and vomiting, malabsorption, cachexia, anxiety, and depression, leading to increased metabolic rate or reduced intake, as well as

tumour-induced metabolic requirements, is great. Undernourishment delays wound healing owing to a reduction in collagen synthesis, while plasma proteins essential for effective wound healing may be utilised elsewhere to satisfy increased energy requirements.[22] The protein demands for tissue repair are consequently unmet. The role of assessing patients' nutritional status and needs for dietary supplements in promoting wound healing is of central importance. Most chemotherapeutic agents adversely affect dietary intake, often resulting in prolonged periods of reduced food intake. This can lead to weight loss, progressive disability, and malnutrition. Nausea and vomiting, diarrhoea, food aversion, and taste changes are but a few of the consequences of chemotherapy, which indirectly impact on wound healing. Similarly, radiotherapy directed at the gastrointestinal tract can result in severe nutritional deficiencies. Malabsorption and malnutrition may arise as a result, as well as severe nausea and vomiting, diarrhoea, and abdominal cramps.[20]

Early detection of potential wound infections is important. Signs of inflammation and discharge are commonly relied upon to alert us to potential problems. However, for the individual with cancer, such indicators may be of limited value if treatment has induced neutropenia, if steroids are being taken, or if tumour-related complications result in inadequate inflammatory response. Swelling, redness, and discharge may all be absent.[17] An effective defence system is a critical component of effective wound healing, but for patients receiving a plethora of drugs and treatments that impact significantly upon immunological status and capacity for inflammatory response, the risk of infection and delayed wound healing is considerable. Steroids are especially potent inhibitors of inflammatory response to injury.[17] Anticoagulants may cause haemorrhage and interfere with clot and scar formation. Chemotherapeutic agents and immunotherapies have the capacity to suppress immune response and to enhance vulnerability to viral and bacterial infection, as well as impairing clotting and healing.[9] Varying degrees of tissue injury arising from radiotherapy can result in the development of an actual wound, which may become the focus for a local infection, or the site of a systemic infection.

Fungating wounds

Of all the lesions experienced by individuals with cancer, perhaps the most distressing for patients, relatives, and health professionals alike are fungating wounds. When malignant tumour cells infiltrate and erode through the skin a wound is said to be 'fungating'.[5] Breast cancer, melanoma, bladder, colon, kidney, ovary, uterus, stomach, head and neck, and lung cancers all have this potential. Fungating wounds often occur in locally advanced, metastatic, or recurrent disease, but this is not always the case. They are often characterised by malodorous exudate, whether serous or blood, which may seep out onto clothing, causing extreme distress.[4] Fungating wounds may cause withdrawal from social activities, or daily life, as the persistent odour or heavily exudating wound necessitates frequent dressing changes.[4,5]

Addressing the psychological impact of a fungating wound, alongside highly skilled physical wound management, is of paramount importance.

The aims of managing fungating wounds are to:

- control tumour growth
- prevent and halt surface bleeding
- where possible, restore skin integrity.[5]

Treatment may include major therapeutic modalities such as chemotherapy, radiotherapy, surgery, hormone manipulation, or a combination of these. Local treatment includes haemostatic agents and topical metronidazole, along with systemic analgesics, antibiotics, or clotting factors as necessary.[4,5] Currently available wound dressings are frequently inadequate for fungating wounds, and work is under way between nurse-researchers and industry to develop and evaluate dressings developed specifically to manage exudating, fungating wounds.[5] Until such time as there are proven data to support the use of a dressing designed specifically for fungating wounds, dressings should be chosen following a consideration of problems identified during a thorough assessment.

Irrespective of the nature of the wound being managed, the rationale for dressing it, the requirements of the wound, and the individual's wishes and expectations form the basis of the decision-making process. Meaningful assessment of outcomes of care, and evaluation of interventions employed can only be undertaken successfully following consideration of the processes described above. Once appropriate dressings are identified, planning how the wound can best be managed, in partnership with the person and their immediate carers, will offer a greater chance of mutual achievement of an agreed outcome. Together a plan can be drawn up of care where wound management is far more than simply a physical affair, reflecting an attempt to respect individuality and circumstance.

References

1. Murphy R.F. (1987). *The Body Silent.* London: WW Norton.
2. Goffman E. (1963). *Stigma. Notes on the Management of Spoiled Identity.* New York: Simon and Schuster.
3. Kleinman A. (1988). *The Illness Narratives: Suffering, Healing and the Human Condition.* New York: Basic Books.
4. Wilson V. (2005). Assessment and management of fungating wounds: a review. *British Journal of Community Nursing*, **10**, S28–S34.
5. Grocott P. (2000). The palliative management of fungating malignant wounds. *Journal of Wound Care* **9**, 4–9.
6. Gaut D. and Leininger M. (eds.) (1991). *Caring: The Compassionate Healer.* New York: National League for Nursing Press.
7. Wilkes L., White K., Smeal T. and Beale B. (2001). Malignant wound management: what dressings do nurse use? *Journal of Wound Care* **19**, 65–69.
8. Thomas S. (1990). *Wound Management and Dressings.* London: Pharmaceutical Press.
9. Hess C.T. and Kirsner R. (2003). Uncover the latest techniques in wound bed preparation. Specific strategies, innovative products advance the healing process. *Nursing Management* **34**, 54–56.
10. Miller M. (1994). Wound care. The ideal healing environment. *Nursing Times* **90**, 62, 64, 66.
11. Quick A. (1994). Dressing choices. *Nursing Times* **90**, 68.
12. Brunner L. and Suddarth D. (eds.) (1992). *The Textbook of Adult Nursing.* London: Chapman and Hall.
13. Santamaria N. and Clayton L. (2000). Cleaning up. The development of the Alfred/Medseed Wound Imaging System. *Collegian* 7, 14–15, 17–18.

14. Fagin C. and Diers D. (1983). Nursing as metaphor. Occasional notes. *New England Journal of Medicine* **309**, 116.

15. Dowsett C. and Ayello E. (2004). TIME principles of chronic wound bed preparation and treatment. *British Journal of Nursing* **13**, S16–S23.

16. Fletcher J. (2003). The benefits of applying wound-bed preparation into practice. *Journal of Wound Care* **12**, 347–349.

17. Falanga V. (2004). The chronic wound: impaired healing and solutions in the context of wound bed preparation. *Blood Cells Molecular Diseases* **32**, 88–94.

18. MacDougall K.M. and Rodgers F.R. (2004). A case study using larval therapy in the community setting. *British Journal of Nursing* **13**, 255–260.

19. Fear M. (2004). The use of maggots as a new treatment in the community. *Nursing Times* **100**, 48–50.

20. Holmes S. (1987). Malignant disease: nutritional implications of disease and treatment. *Cancer and Metastasis Reviews* **6**, 357–381.

21. Hallett A. (1994). Vital ingredients. *Nursing Times* **90**, 64, 66, 68.

22. Senter H. and Pringle A. (1985). *How Wounds Heal: A Practical Guide for Nurses.* Cheshire: Wellcome Foundation.

CHAPTER TWENTY-TWO

Lymphoedema

Anne Williams

Introduction

Lymphoedema is a chronic and often progressive condition, usually presenting as limb swelling but sometimes involving the trunk, genitalia, or head and neck. Insufficiency of the lymphatic system leads to an accumulation of fluid and proteins in the tissues and a subsequent chronic inflammatory condition, often complicated by skin changes and infection.[1] Lymphoedema has a wide range of causes that may be cancer or non-cancer related. This chapter will focus on lymphoedema following cancer and will explore relevant pathophysiology, discuss lymphoedema incidence, and highlight the impact of lymphoedema on individuals. It will then outline treatment approaches, drawing on the developing evidence base within this relatively new speciality.

The lymphatic system

The lymphatic system is a one-way drainage system that removes excess interstitial fluid, plasma proteins, cells, and debris from the tissues, returning it to the blood vascular system (see Figure 22.1). It plays an important role in maintaining fluid balance, has an immune function, and also transports fats and proteins.[2]

Box 22.1   The lymphatic system

A dense network of initial lymphatics (sometimes called lymph capillaries) is present in the superficial dermis of the skin and mucous membranes. These are blind-ended, with a single cell wall and are supported by elastic fibres and anchoring filaments which enable the vessels to open and close in response to changing tissue pressures. This allows fluid to enter the lymphatic system from the interstitial tissues. The initial lymphatics drain into pre-collector and larger collector vessels, consisting of contractile muscular segments, separated by valves. Lymph is propelled towards the deeper lymphatics by peristaltic-like movements of the collectors, passing through a series of lymph nodes before moving into increasingly larger lymphatic trunks that eventually drain into the venous system at the base of the neck. Around 700 lymph nodes are present in the body and act as filter stations, regulating the protein content of lymph and producing lymphocytes.

Each collector drains a specific area of skin and the larger vessels also drain lymph from muscles, joints and deeper organs. Groups of collector lymphatics drain into specific regional lymph nodes. Where lymph nodes and/or vessels have been damaged, collateral pathways in the initial lymphatics and pre-collectors provide opportunity for lymph to be redirected towards alternative regional nodes. The movement of lymph through the system depends on the intrinsic contractibility of lymphatics but is influenced by the muscle pump, the pulsation of blood vessels, gut motility and changes in intrathoracic and intra-abdominal pressures brought about by respiratory movements.[3]

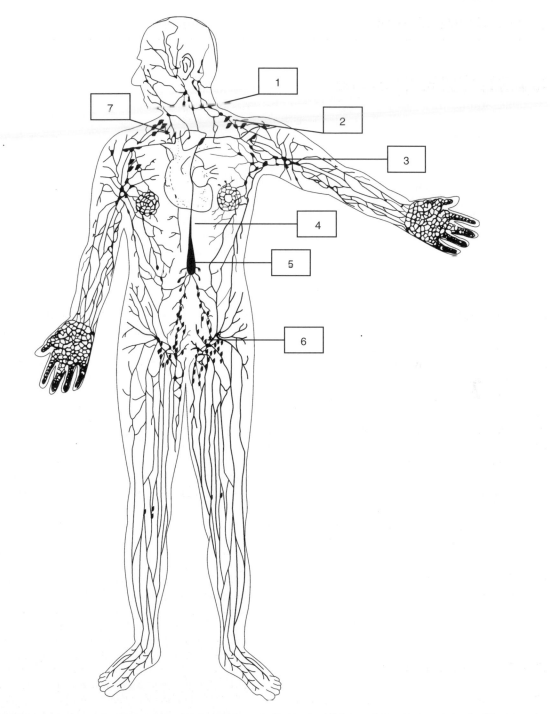

Figure 22.1   Main lymph trunks and lymph node groups in the body. (1) Internal jugular lymph trunk; (2) supracla-vicular lymph nodes; (3) axillary lymph nodes; (4) thoracic duct; (5) cisterna chyli; (6) inguinal lymph nodes; (7) right lymphatic duct.

Lymphoedema and cancer

Lymphoedema is associated with a variety of different cancers including breast, malignant melanoma, genitourinary malignancies, and sarcoma. Studies of breast cancer-related lymphoedema predominate in the literature (see Box 22.2). Clark et al.[4] have reported a 21% incidence of breast cancer-related lymphoedema, with significant risk factors identified as mastectomy, hospital skin puncture and body mass index (BMI) >26.[4] In this study, 80% of those with lymphoedema developed the problem in the first year following treatment. Previous research has highlighted the increased risk of lymphoedema following surgery and radiotherapy to the axilla.[5] Approaches to managing the axilla have now changed, and more recently there is evidence that sentinel node biopsy reduces arm morbidity.[6,7] The literature is limited, however, by the lack of standardisation in methods used for identifying and quantifying lymphoedema.[8,9] It is clear, however, that as survival rates improve and many women also undergo long-term chemotherapy for invasive or metastatic disease, breast cancer-related lymphoedema continues to be a significant problem.

Serpell et al. described a 29% incidence of lymphoedema following inguinal node dissection in the management of invasive malignant melanoma.[10] A 48% risk of temporary oedema in the 12 months post-treatment has also been reported in this group.[11] Gynaecological cancers are also associated with lower limb lymphoedema.[12,13] and Robinson et al. reported a 30% incidence of lymphoedema after treatment for soft tissue sarcoma of the lower limb or pelvis.[14]

Lymphoedema may develop many years after cancer treatment, and the International Society of Lymphologists recognises a latent, subclinical stage of lymphoedema.[15] It is significant that a new-onset lymphoedema or worsening swelling may be indicative of recurrent cancer in patients who have been disease free. In patients with advanced cancer, problems such as tumour obstruction, immobility, cardiac, renal or hepatic failure will also exacerbate lymphoedema, with some drugs also producing additional fluid retention.

Lymphoedema prevention

To date there is no good evidence to suggest that lymphoedema can be prevented, although there is specific advice that should be given to people at risk of lymphoedema, including:

- avoid skin injury, scratches, insect bites and burns on or near the affected limb
- avoid venepuncture, injections and having blood pressure taken on the affected limb
- minimise any activities that exacerbate the lymphoedema such as standing for long periods if the leg is swollen or using the swollen arm to carry heavy bags.[16]

Further work is required to fully understand the factors that increase lymphoedema risk and evaluate the role of interventions that aim to prevent or reduce swelling, including the prophylactic use of compression hosiery and exercise.[17] Todd and Topping have shown that there is a lack of consensus on written information on shoulder mobilisation provided for women following breast cancer, despite the fact that this may impact on rates of seroma formation and lymphoedema incidence.[18] The need for health care professionals to communicate accurate information about lymphoedema to all patients at risk of lymphoedema has been clearly identified.[19]

Box 22.2 Recent studies of the pathogenesis of breast cancer-related lymphoedema

The traditional view that lymphoedema is a direct result of lymph drainage failure due to lymph node removal is now being questioned. Pain et al. have shown that the risk of developing lymphoedema after breast cancer may be partly predetermined as a result of pre-operative differences in lymphatic function.[20] Variations in lymphatic function have been identified in some groups,[21] and may account for the uneven distribution of swelling in women with arm lymphoedema, where the arm is swollen but the hand is spared, for example. It is not clear how these findings relate to other types of cancer-related lymphoedema.

Diagnosis of lymphoedema

Prompt diagnosis and treatment are important. Many breast cancer centres provide care for people with lymphoedema but there is evidence that lymphoedema services are often inadequate and unstructured, with significant numbers not receiving appropriate treatment.[22]

Lymphoedema is usually defined as swelling of >3 months' duration that initially may be soft, pitting, and reduce on elevation.[15,22] There are often characteristic changes in limb size and shape, with skin folds developing, particularly near joints. Eventually, the swelling may become fibrotic (hard) and will no longer 'pit' to finger pressure. Fibrosclerotic changes lead to a positive Stemmer's sign, the inability to pinch up the thickened skin at the base of the second toe. This is a differential diagnostic sign for lower limb lymphoedema. Skin and tissue changes can also occur including dry skin, hyperkeratosis (scaly skin), increased fat deposition, and papillomatosis, a bulging cobblestone effect usually seen in lower limb swelling. Increased vulnerability to fungal and bacterial infections is common, and cellulitis has been identified in 29% of patients with lymphoedema.[22]

Diagnosis is usually made from the patient's history, clinical examination and measurement. Investigations are not usually indicated in cancer-related lymphoedema although magnetic resonance imaging, vascular studies, ultrasound or *in vivo* visualisation of lymphatic vessels using lymphoscintigraphy may be used to confirm diagnosis, assess cancer status, or exclude other pathology such as venous disease.

The impact of lymphoedema

Lymphoedema is associated with a variety of problems that impact on quality of life including shock, fear, frustration, and negative body image.[23] Franks *et al.* have highlighted the difficulties experienced by people with lower limb lymphoedema in terms of physical and social functioning and pain.[24] A study of women with lower limb lymphoedema after treatment for gynaecological cancers identified the paucity of research in this area and described particular problems with clothing and difficulties with daily activities such as housework, driving, and walking.[25]

Studies of women with breast cancer-related lymphoedema have clearly shown the psychological morbidity and altered sensations that can result in significant distress.[26,27] Several authors have described the evaluation of quality-of-life tools in this group, highlighting the need for appropriate and clinically meaningful outcome measures to adequately assess the impact of lymphoedema.[28,29]

Additionally, issues relating to information seeking and coping with lymphoedema and, more specifically, the attitudes and comments of others, have been described.[30,31] The psychological and psychiatric morbidity associated with lymphoedema should not be underestimated and health professionals have an important role in providing the long-term support and resources required by individuals with this chronic condition.

Treating lymphoedema

Historically, the current approach to lymphoedema treatment originated in Austria and Germany in the 1970s and was introduced to the UK in the 1980s.[32] Most of the early lymphoedema clinics were sited in cancer or palliative care units but, increasingly, primary care-based services are developing to address the wider need.[33] Lymphoedema management combines meticulous skin care, isotonic exercises, manual lymphatic drainage massage, and compression therapy.[32] Principally, this approach aims to optimise the function of the lymphatic system, reverse the changes taking place in the tissues, and prevent further deterioration. Treatment interventions are summarised in Table 22.1.

Accurate diagnosis is crucial to identify the cause of swelling and a comprehensive assessment is necessary including medical history, clinical examination and measurement. Skill and flexibility are required to develop a treatment programme based on individual need, and practitioners need to work in partnership with patients to achieve realistic outcomes.

Table 22.1   Treatment interventions

Intervention	Rationale	Comments
Skin care	To maintain skin integrity and minimise the risk of infection.	• Daily washing and moisturising with a suitable emollient • Checking for signs of skin changes or damage
Compression therapy:[39] • hosiery garments • multilayer bandaging • intermittent compression pumps (used with caution)	To prevent accumulation of fluid by raising interstitial pressure, reducing capillary filtration and encouraging fluid to move towards the root of the limb.	• A wide range of standard and custom-made hosiery is available • Garments should be fitted by experienced practitioners • Multilayer bandaging consists of stockinette layer, padding and layers of short stretch bandages, with a digit bandage • This provides a variation in pressure peaks of sub-bandage pressures to enable oedema reduction
Exercise	To enhance lymph flow without increasing capillary filtration, improve the muscle pump action and reduce musculoskeletal problems.	• Exercise is individualised depending on ability and lifestyle • Activities such as walking and swimming are encouraged • Breathing techniques are also used • The effect may be improved by wearing hosiery or bandages
Manual lymphatic drainage or simple lymphatic drainage[32]	To redirect the lymph along the superficial and deeper lymphatics, from the swollen, congested areas towards healthy lymphatics (often through collateral pathways).	• Manual lymphatic drainage (MLD) is a gentle but very specific massage • Treatment includes the neck, trunk and limb • The movements enhance the contraction of lymphatics • Practitioners should be qualified in the Vodder, Földi, Casley Smith or Leduc methods of MLD in order to treat lymphoedema • Simple lymphatic drainage (SLD) is a simplified version of MLD designed for use by patients • Appropriate teaching in SLD is required for this to be successful

Many patients with cancer-related lymphoedema present with mild, relatively uncomplicated swelling, requiring support with self-management practices. This is referred to as *maintenance treatment* and may include daily skin care, exercises, simple lymphatic drainage (a type of self-massage), and wearing of compression hosiery garments. Those with more severe lymphoedema require *intensive treatment* to reduce limb volume and improve shape and skin condition.[32] This usually consists of a 2–4-week course of daily manual lymphatic drainage massage and multilayer bandaging, and is sometimes referred to as decongestive lymphatic therapy (DLT) or complex decongestive therapy (CDT).

Self-management of lymphoedema within the maintenance phase requires motivation and perseverance and patients often have to make a number of lifestyle adjustments. A telephone survey of patients with stable lymphoedema explored long-term compliance with treatment and highlighted their experiences of adaptation and self-management,[34] reflected in the following comments:

I have to get up nearly an hour earlier in the morning to allow time to put my stockings on after doing the massage and exercises.

I can't be spontaneous as I have to fit in my self-management routine every day, even on holiday.

I miss walking in bare feet.

I no longer go on holiday to hot climates for fear of getting an infection again.

Surgery, once the mainstay of treatment for lymphoedema in the UK, is rarely used now and the use of diuretics is discouraged as these do not address the functional changes within the lymphatic system and are only indicated if there are concurrent problems such as cardiac failure. Intermittent compression pumps are also used with extreme caution, particularly in cancer-related lymphoedema following lymphadenectomy. While these may push fluid to the root of the limb, leading to fibrosis in this area, they also increase the risk of genital oedema.[35]

Evidence base

A Cochrane review of physical therapies for lymphoedema has highlighted the limited evidence base for lymphoedema treatment.[36] Studies of DLT provide some insight into expected treatment outcome,[37,38] although methods used to measure limb volume are not consistent and results are often not comparable, providing little scope for meta-analysis at present. Improvements in quality of life following treatment have been reported by several authors particularly in terms of physical mobility, function, and reduction in pain.[24,28]

Several studies have examined the efficacy of specific interventions. Badger *et al.* demonstrated that a period of multilayer bandaging followed by elastic compression hosiery was more effective at reducing excess limb volume and providing long-term control of lymphoedema, than hosiery alone.[39] Manual lymphatic drainage for breast cancer-related lymphoedema has also been evaluated.[40,41] and although results are not fully conclusive,[42] and patient samples are small, there is evidence to support its use, particularly at an early stage when lymphoedema is relatively mild.[43]

One study that examined the effects of self-management techniques including gentle arm exercise and deep breathing, reported a statistically significant reduction in limb volume and symptoms such as arm heaviness and tightness.[11] There is also a growing body of literature encouraging the use of active exercise programmes in women with breast cancer-related lymphoedema and challenging previous beliefs that people with lymphoedema should avoid all strenuous activities.[17,45]

There is substantial scope for further research into lymphoedema. Currently there is much expertise amongst practitioners and patients, however, and this is reflected in the development of a number of consensus documents. The British Lymphology Society and Lymphoedema Support Network, a patient-run organisation, have produced guidelines on the management of cellulitis in lymphoedema.[46] Substantial work is also being undertaken by the Lymphoedema Framework Project in the development of best practice guidelines for lymphoedema.[33]

Summary

Cancer-related lymphoedema is a significant problem for some patients and may lead to long-term difficulties in patients who are otherwise disease-free. Appropriate and comprehensive treatments can do much to improve quality of life. Health care professionals need to be able to identify lymphoedema in its early stages, provide information for those at risk of the problem, and be aware of local services for treatment and referral. Substantial expertise exists relating to lymphoedema and its management and the evidence base is gradually developing. The future development of multi-centre trials will address important clinical questions and provide exciting challenges for lymphoedema practitioners, patients and researchers.

References

1. Stanton A. (2000). How does tissue swelling occur? The physiology and pathophysiology of interstitial fluid formation. In Twycross R., Jenns K. and Todd J. (eds.).

Lymphoedema. Oxford: Radcliffe Medical Press, pp. 11–21.

2. Földi M. and Földi E. (2003). Physiology and pathophysiology of the lymphatic system. In Földi M., Földi E. and Kubik S. (eds.) *Textbook of Lymphology for Physicians and Lymphedema Therapists.* Munich and Jena: Urban and Fischer, Elsevier.

3. Vaqas B. and Ryan T.J. (2003). Lymphoedema: pathophysiology and management in resource-poor settings-relevance for lymphatic filariasis control programmes. *Filaria Journal* **2**, 4. www.filariajournal.com/content/2/1/4 (accessed 7 August 2007).

4. Clark B., Sitzia J. and Harlow W. (2005). Incidence and risk of arm oedema following treatment for breast cancer: a three year follow-up study. *Quarterly Journal of Medicine* **98**, 343–348.

5. Kissin M.W., Querci della Rovera G., Easton D. and Westbury G. (1986). Risk of lymphoedema following the treatment of breast cancer. *British Journal of Surgery* **73**, 580–584.

6. Golshan M., Martin W.J. and Dowlatshahi K. (2003). Sentinel lymph node biopsy lowers the rate of lymphedema when compared with standard axillary lymph node dissection. *American Surgeon* **69**, 209–211.

7. Mansel R.E., Fallowfield L., Kissin M. *et al.* (2006) Randomized multicentre trial of sentinel node biopsy versus standard axillary treatment in operable breast cancer: the ALMANAC Trial. *Journal of the National Cancer Institute* **98**, 599–609.

8. Williams A.F., Franks P.J. and Moffatt C.J. (2005). Lymphoedema: estimating the size of the problem. *Palliative Medicine* **1**, 300–313.

9. Armer J.M. and Stewart B.R. (2005). A comparison of four diagnostic criteria for lymphedema in a post-breast cancer population. *Lymphatic Research and Biology* **3**, 208–217.

10. Serpell J.W., Carne P.W. and Bailey M. (2003). Radical lymph node dissection for melanoma. *Australian and New Zealand Journal of Obstetrics and Gynaecology* **73**, 294–299.

11. Wrone D.A., Tanabe K.K., Cosimi A.B. *et al.* (2000). Lymphedema after sentinel lymph node biopsy for cutaneous melanoma: a report of 5 cases. *Archives of Dermatology* **136**, 511–514.

12. Nesvold I.L. and Fossa S.D. (2002). Lymphedema after surgical treatment of cervical and vulvar cancer: routines and needs before discharge. *Tidsskrift for den Norske Loegeforen* **122**, 2531–2533.

13. Ryan M., Stainton M.C., Slaytor E.K. *et al.* (2003). Aetiology and prevalence of lower limb lymphoedema following treatment for gynaecological cancer. *Australian and New Zealand Journal of Obstetrics and Gynaecology* **43**, 148–151.

14. Robinson M.H., Spruce L., Eeles R. *et al.* (1991. Limb function following conservation treatment of adult soft tissue sarcoma. *European Journal of Cancer* **27**, 1567–1574.

15. International Society of Lymphology. (2003). *The Diagnosis and Treatment of Peripheral Lymphedema.* Consensus Document of the International Society of Lymphology. *Lymphology* **36**, 84–91.

16. Lymphoedema Support Network. (2006). *Preventative Advice for Patients at Risk of Developing Lymphoedema of the Leg(s).* LSN Factsheet, London: Lymphoedema Support Network.

17. Lane K., Worsley D. and McKenzie D. (2005). Exercise and the lymphatic system: implications for breast-cancer survivors. *Sports Medicine* **35**, 461–471.

18. Todd J. and Topping A. (2005). A survey of written information on the use of post-operative exercises after breast cancer surgery. *Physiotherapy* **91**, 87–93.

19. Ridner S.H. (2006). Pretreatment lymphedema education and identified educational resources in breast cancer patients. *Patient Education and Counselling* **61**, 72–79.

20. Pain S.J., Purushotham A.D., Barber R.W. *et al.* (2004). Variation in lymphatic function may predispose to development of breast cancer-related lymphoedema. *European Journal of Surgical Oncology* **30**, 508–514.

21. Stanton A.W., Modi S., Mellor R.H. *et al.* (2006). A quantitative lymphoscintigraphic evaluation of lymphatic function in the swollen hands of women with lymphoedema following breast cancer treatment. *Clinical Science* **110**, 553–561.

22. Moffatt C.J., Franks P.J., Doherty D.C. *et al.* (2003). Lymphoedema: an underestimated health problem. *Quarterly Journal of Medicine* **96**, 731–738.

23. Morgan P.A., Franks P.J. and Moffatt C.J. (2005). Health-related quality of life with lymphoedema: a review of the literature. *International Wound Journal* **2**, 47–62.

24. Franks P.J., Moffatt C.J., Doherty D.C. *et al.* (2006). Assessment of health-related quality of life in patients with lymphedema of the lower limb. *Wound Repair and Regeneration* **14**, 110–118.

25. Ryan M., Stainton M.C., Jaconelli C. *et al.* (2003). The experience of lower limb lymphoedema for women after treatment for gynaecologic cancer. *Oncology Nursing Forum* **30**, 417–423.

26. Tobin M.B., Lacey H.J., Meyer L. and Mortimer P.S. (1993). The psychological morbidity of breast-cancer-related swelling. *Cancer* **72**, 3248–3252.

27. Woods M. (1993). Patients' perceptions of breast cancer-related lymphoedema. *European Journal of Cancer Care* **2**, 125–128.

28. Sitzia J. and Sobrido L. (1997). Measurement of health-related quality of life patients receiving conservative

treatment for limb lymphoedema using the Nottingham Health Profile. *Quality of Life Research* **6**, 373–384.

29. Coster S., Poole K. and Fallowfield L.J. (2001). The validation of a quality of life scale to assess the impact of arm morbidity in breast cancer patients post-operatively. *Breast Cancer Research and Treatment* **68**, 273–282.

30. Johansson K., Homstrom H., Nilsson I. *et al.* (2003). Breast cancer patients' experiences of lymphoedema. *Scandinavian Journal of Caring Sciences* **17**, 35–42.

31. Williams A.F., Moffatt C.J. and Franks P.J. (2004). A phenomenological study of the lived experiences of people with lymphoedema. *International Journal of Palliative Nursing* **10**, 279–286.

32. Foldi E., Foldi M. and Weissleder H. (1985). Conservative treatment of lymphoedema of the limbs. *Angiology* **36**, 171–180.

33. Morgan P. and Moffatt C. (2006). The National Lymphoedema Framework Project. *British Journal of Community Nursing, The Lymphoedema Supplement* **11(suppl. 4)**, S19–S22.

34. Rose K.E., Taylor H.M. and Twycross R.G. (1991). Long-term compliance with treatment in obstructive arm lymphoedema in cancer. *Palliative Medicine* **5**, 52–55.

35. Boris M., Weindorf S. and Lasinski B.B. (1998). The risk of genital edema after external pump compression for lower limb lymphedema. *Lymphology* **31**, 15–20.

36. Badger C., Preston N., Seers K. and Mortimer P. (2004). Physical therapies for reducing and controlling lymphoedema of the limbs (Cochrane Review). *The Cochrane Library*, Issue 3. Oxford: Update Software.

37. Ko D.S., Lerner R., Klose G. *et al.* (1998). Effective treatment of lymphoedema of the extremities. *Archives of Surgery* **133**, 452–458.

38. Szuba A., Strauss W., Sirsikar S.P. *et al.* (2002) Quantitative radionuclide lymphoscintigraphy predicts outcome of manual lymphatic therapy in breast cancer-related lymphedema of the upper extremity. *Nuclear Medicine Communications* **23**, 1171–1175.

39. Badger C.M.A., Peacock J.L. and Mortimer P.S. (2000). A randomised, controlled, parallel-group clinical trial comparing multilayer bandaging followed by hosiery versus hosiery alone in the treatment of patients with lymphoedema of the limb. *Cancer* **88**, 2832–2837.

40. Williams A.F., Vadgama A., Franks P.J. and Mortimer P.S. (2002). A randomized controlled crossover study of manual lymphatic drainage therapy in women with breast cancer-related lymphoedema. *European Journal of Cancer Care* **11**, 254–261.

41. Johansson K., Albertsson M., Ingvar C. *et al.* (1999). Effects of compression bandaging with or without manual lymph drainage treatment in patients with post-operative arm lymphedema. *Lymphology* **32**, 103–110.

42. Andersen L., Højris I., Erlandsen M. *et al.* (2000). Treatment of breast-cancer-related lymphedema with or without manual lymphatic drainage. A randomised study. *Acta Oncologica* **39**, 399–405.

43. McNeely M.L., Magee D.J., Lees A.W. *et al.* (2004). The addition of manual lymph drainage to compression therapy for breast cancer related lymphedema: a randomized controlled trial. *Breast Cancer Research and Treatment* **86**, 95–106.

44. Moseley A.L., Piller N.B. and Carati C.J. (2005). The effect of gentle arm exercise and deep breathing on secondary arm lymphedema. *Lymphology* **38**, 136–145.

45. Ahmed R.L., Thomas W., Yee D. and Schmitz K.H. (2006). Randomized controlled trial of weight training and lymphedema in breast cancer survivors. *Journal of Clinical Oncology* **24**, 2765–2772.

46. British Lymphology Society. (2006). *Consensus Document on the Management of Cellulitis in Lymphoedema*. Sevenoaks: British Lymphology Society.

CHAPTER TWENTY-THREE

Malignant ascites

Nancy Preston

Management of malignant ascites results in 6% of hospice admissions and can affect up to 40% of patients with metastatic peritoneal deposits.[1] Ascites is a collection of fluid in the peritoneal space which may develop as a result of malignancy. The primary cancer sites where malignant ascites is most common are the ovary, breast, colon, stomach, and pancreas. Any tumour with metastatic peritoneal deposits may result in the development of ascites.

Common symptoms

As fluid accumulates the abdomen becomes distended, giving rise to a range of symptoms including:

- indigestion
- loss of appetite
- altered bowel habit
- abdominal discomfort
- abdominal distension
- changes in body image
- disruption in daily activities and lifestyle
- nausea and vomiting
- ankle oedema
- fatigue
- shortness of breath.

Individually, each symptom can be managed. Indigestion can be treated with regular antacids or even systemic H_2 antagonists. If this is controlled, appetite might be improved but the ascites squashes the stomach, hence satiety is easily reached. Laxatives can help to maintain soft stool, and mild pain killers might be needed for abdominal discomfort. A new wardrobe of clothes may be required as the waistline can increase considerably with ascites. With the change in size, patients' body image may alter. For some, this is not seen as a problem as their lives are predominantly based within the home, but for others this may have far-reaching effects upon femininity and sexuality. As the ascites increases so do the symptoms and this can mean becoming increasingly limited in what is manageable at home. Fatigue and breathlessness are an increasing consequence of the ascites, and the only way to resolve these problems is to remove the fluid.

Pathophysiology

Ascites is a type of oedema. Malignant ascites is an umbrella term, which denotes ascites arising from a malignancy. The causes of malignant ascites are quite distinct from the causes of non-malignant ascites that may result, for example, from cirrhosis of the liver or heart failure. Malignant ascites has been classified into four types: central, peripheral, mixed and other (see Table 23.1).[2] A central ascites results from pressure from liver metastases forcing fluid out of the general

Table 23.1 Types of malignant ascites

Classification	Proportion (%)	Definitions
Central ascites	15	Massive hepatic metastases causing fluid to be forced out of the venous system – transudate (low in protein)
Peripheral ascites	50	Lymphatic obstruction coupled with increased permeability of the peritoneal capillaries – exudates (high in protein)
Mixed ascites	15	Mixture of the above causes
Remaining ascites	20	Chylous ascites, or unknown cause

circulation. There may also be some disruption in the rennin–angiotension–aldosterone system. This ascites is usually a transudate with a low protein content. Peripheral ascites is the most common form and is usually an exudate, with a high protein content. This arises due to two main causes: increased permeability of the peritoneal capillaries, and lymphatic obstruction. Increased permeability of the peritoneal capillaries results in excess fluid production. This has limited exit routes due to the obstruction of lymphatic vessels draining the peritoneal cavity by tumour cells.[3] Flow rates from the peritoneal cavity are about a quarter the rate of people without a malignancy.[4]

It is important to know which type of ascites is being managed, to choose the appropriate treatment.

Managing ascites

Treatment for ascites can either be palliative or anti-cancer. There are few well-conducted studies to base treatment upon. Decisions need to be made from the best evidence available, clinical opinion, and being guided by pathophysiology.

Anti-cancer treatments

The aim of anti-cancer treatment is to remove the tumour, thereby reducing the ascites. A number of experimental drugs have been used against ascites. Most of these are biological therapies which are expensive and involve frequent hospital stays. Only tumour necrosis factor has been evaluated in a randomised controlled trial (RCT).[5] Although in early studies it had looked hopeful, in the RCT it was shown to have no effect.

Palliative treatments

Systematic reviews have identified few trials of the main palliative treatments, namely drainage and diuretic therapy.[6] Two surveys in the UK[6] and Canada[7] found that drainage or paracentesis is used in 98% of centres. However, in Canada paracentesis was seen as effective by 78% of physicians; in the UK only 44% felt this. Diuretic therapy was seen as preferable by 62% of physicians in the UK.

Paracentesis

Anyone with cancer presenting with abdominal distension thought to be due to malignant ascites needs to have this diagnosis confirmed. This is done through cytology, where fluid removed at drainage is examined for malignant cells. Ascites can result from other medical conditions, hence it is imperative to demonstrate that the ascites has occurred due to malignancy. Any drainage of the peritoneal cavity has the risk of bowel perforation. As fluid builds up, so the bowel can float upwards. Insertion of any drainage tube should be carried out with ultrasound guidance, so that the largest area of fluid can be identified and marked for drainage.[8]

Drainage is carried out under local anaesthetic and can be uncomfortable. Further, paracentesis, although offering relief from symptoms, is only temporary and the fluid will re-accumulate. Repeated drainage may result in protein depletion, hypotension, and infection.[9] Many people who have intractable ascites spend their preterminal and terminal days requiring frequent hospital admissions for drainage.[10] Interviews with women with ascites undergoing drainage of their ascites with a suprapubic catheter showed that they welcomed drainage due to the relief it brought, and minimal discomfort.[6] The experience of discomfort changed when a peritoneal drainage catheter was used, with some women refusing the procedure due to pain during the procedure but particularly afterwards. However, there are no well-conducted studies evaluating paracentesis.

In an attempt to reduce hospital admissions, a protocol has been evaluated in which a catheter is left in the abdomen to allow continuous drainage. The catheter is tunnelled under the skin and sutured into place. The exit site is cared for as a stoma, with the fluid collected in a catheter bag. A number of studies have been carried out following people with indwelling drains, but none were RCTs. In a number of cases there were problems with peritonitis and the need to resite the catheter. Without a comparison it is unclear how much more beneficial this approach is. In one trial, 16 out of 40 people approached declined the continuous drainage catheter saying they would prefer weekly drainage.[11] Overall repeated paracentesis seems to be acceptable to most people.

Diuretic therapy
Consensus as to the use of diuretic therapy has yet to be achieved. Discrepancies may be due to differences in prescribed diuretic dosages and/or the type of ascites being treated – central or peripheral ascites.

There have been no published randomised studies to evaluate the role of diuretics in managing malignant ascites. Diuretics such as spironolactone compete with aldosterone for receptors on the proximal tubule of the kidney, inhibiting the effect of aldosterone. In one study success was measured by a weight loss of 0.5 kg per day.[12] This was achieved in 13 out of 16 cases. However, a similar study, which also measured weight loss, assessed whether fluid had moved out of the peritoneal cavity.[13] In this study they found weight loss was associated with fluid movement in central ascites but not peripheral ascites. They felt that the weight loss was due to dehydration in peripheral ascites, and was thus dangerous and not recommended.

Peritoneovenous shunts
Peritoneovenous shunts were developed for use with intractable ascites as a result of cirrhosis of the liver. This method involves implanting a catheter under the skin running from the peritoneal cavity back into the general circulation, usually via the superior vena cava or right atrium. The two sections are connected by a one-way valve allowing fluid to move in one direction only. Fluid moves upwards owing to changes in intrathoracic and intraperitoneal pressure achieved through normal breathing. A pressure of 3 cm of water is required to open the valve.[14] Patients are asked to wear abdominal binders and to carry out breathing regimes, where they breathe against a pressure for 15 minutes, four times a day, in order to maximise the pressure changes. Peritoneovenous shunts are physiologically based in that they avoid problems of protein depletion. There are two main types of shunt: LeVeen and Denver. Both have been involved in clinical studies with patients with malignant ascites but neither has proved superior. They differ in that the Denver shunt has a valve that can be massaged each day to increase the flow and to push through debris in the catheter that may otherwise occlude it.

Both are usually inserted under local anaesthetic and a review of the literature of studies using shunts shows variable success rates.[6] However, these studies are poorly conducted and rarely define what they mean by successful. Further, they are associated with a number of deaths. Other complications include overload, thrombosis, infection, bleeding, and respiratory distress. Fewer studies seem to be conducted, perhaps showing it is becoming less well used and less appropriate for palliative care.

Summary of treatments
Many strategies have been tested for controlling malignant ascites. Unfortunately, there has been little formal assessment undertaken to examine what individuals with ascites themselves feel about these various treatments. Only the good acceptance of women undergoing paracentesis using a suprapubic catheter has been demonstrated. Personal accounts 23.1 and 23.2 of two women with ascites demonstrate that the way in which individuals interpret the problem is crucial to how they choose to have their symptom managed. For the majority, malignant ascites occurs at a time when emphasis should be upon

minimal intervention and enabling patients to remain as free of hospital admissions and invasive procedures as possible. Evaluation of all methods currently employed, incorporating the perception of outcome from patients, doctors, and nurses, is required. A novel nursing approach to ascites management through breathing exercises and abdominal binding has been conducted to increase the time between drainage.[6] However, too few people were entered and the approach needs further evaluation, although early results were promising.

The experience of ascites

A great deal has been written about the various treatments for malignant ascites, although there is no consensus of opinion as to the optimal treatment. Few studies have formally asked people about their experience of ascites, or their views on the treatments offered to them. What is apparent from talking to women with ascites is that they have very different experiences. They interpret their ascites according to the meanings they attach to it and its relationship to their prognosis.

Meaning will be dependent upon an individual's own perceptions, which in turn will be influenced by culture, society, and environment. It is possible that ascites was wrongly construed as pregnancy in the past, as implied by Jane Rogers in *Mr Wroe's Virgins*,[15] a story set in the early part of the 19th century. The story describes a religious group built up around the teachings and prophecy of Mother Southcote. At the age of 60 she appeared to be pregnant and died during childbirth:

> For she was sixty years of age, unmarried, and had never known a man. Yet she was with child . . . When the time for the child's birth came and passed with no sign of deliverance, her suffering heart broke, letting the captive spirit escape from earthly trials . . . The child born of Mother Southcote was a spirit.

The explanation for her pregnancy may have been malignant ascites as a result of cancer. The pains she suffered could have been those associated with bowel obstruction. When an individual is left without adequate explanation for her ascites, she may believe that the distended abdomen is caused by the presence of tumour. She may fear that the pressure is damaging her organs and it will undoubtedly serve as a daily reminder of the disease. This is illustrated by Jenny's experience in Personal account 23.1. A contrasting experience is offered in Personal account 23.2.

Personal account 23.1

Jenny is 43. Having been diagnosed for a year with ovarian cancer, Jenny's disease relapsed after first-line therapy. She was prescribed a taxane but continued to be troubled with recurrent ascites. Her appearance was very important to her: Jenny liked to look glamorous. Her husband also dressed well, and they enjoyed an active social life.

Jenny would come into hospital for drainage, when she felt her ascites was gross, when clothes looked awful, and she could no longer cope with the distress caused by her condition. She also associated her ascites with the fear that her chemotherapy was not working. Her ascites was an outward manifestation of the danger her disease posed. Jenny found it very hard to accept that the fluid was not causing her any physical harm, because the feelings she experienced were so great. She would frequently request the fluid to be drained, often when there was insufficient fluid to remove. Her self-image was crucial to maintaining her sense of normality. Her appearance was paramount; it represented the woman she was before becoming a cancer patient. The ascites disrupted this self-image, forcing an unwelcome and painful redefinition of self.

Results from the interview study with women with ascites found the experience to be very difficult.[6] Few women understood what ascites was and most did not know it was connected to their cancer. Some believed it was urine, chemotherapy build-up, and a side-effect of trial drugs. The impact of the ascites was negative, with about a quarter saying it was the worst part of their cancer journey. All symptoms improved after drainage, except emotional discomfort. Perhaps this related to women's realisation that their cancer was not going to be cured and the ascites was an outward manifestation of their cancer's ongoing growth. As the ascites made the cancer visible it was harder to ignore. Some spoke of the associations with pregnancy, with one woman being asked by a work colleague when her baby was due.

Personal account 23.2

Elizabeth had a different experience of ascites. She was 73, and thought of herself as a survivor, having lived through the war and had seven children. When diagnosed with cancer she thought 'that was it' and was amazed that the hospital could offer any treatment. Everything from then on was a bonus: 'living on borrowed time'. Friends constantly visited her at home; although she rarely left home, she didn't feel embarrassed about her appearance. She thought it funny that people might think 'How can that old girl be pregnant?'. She rarely complained of side-effects even though she was often unwell from her treatment.

Her ascites accumulated every 2 weeks, but this did not appear to be a problem for her. She would telephone the ward after 2 weeks telling staff she felt 'a bit uncomfortable'. She would have 10–13 litres of fluid drained. Elizabeth's expectations were markedly different from Jenny's as she saw the ascites as simply an inevitable consequence of her cancer.

References

1. Reynard C. and Mannix K. (1989). Management of ascites in advanced cancer – a flow diagram. *Palliative Medicine* **4**, 45–47.
2. Runyon B.A., Hoefs, J.C. and Morgan, T.R. (1988). Ascitic fluid analysis in malignancy-related ascites. *Hepatology* **8**, 1104–1109.
3. Feldman G.B. (1975). Lymphatic obstruction in carcinomatous ascites. *Cancer Research* **35**, 325–332.
4. Bronskill M.J., Bush R.S. and Ege G.N. (1977). A quantitative measurement of peritoneal drainage in malignant ascites. *Cancer* **40**, 2375–2380.
5. Hirte H.W., Miller D., Tonkin K. *et al.* (1997). A randomized trial of paracentesis plus intraperitoneal tumor necrosis factor-alpha versus paracentesis alone in patients with symptomatic ascites from recurrent ovarian carcinoma. *Gynecology Oncology* **64**, 80–87.
6. Preston N. (2004). *The Development of a Nursing Therapy for the Management of Malignant Ascites.* PhD thesis, University of London.
7. Johnson I.S., Rogers C., Biswas B. and Ahmedzai S. (1990). What do hospices do? A survey of hospices in the United Kingdom and Republic of Ireland. *British Medical Journal* **300**, 791–793.
8. Ross G.J., Kessler H.B., Clai M.R. *et al.* (1989). Sonographically guided paracentesis for palliation of symptomatic malignant ascites. *American Journal of Roentgenology* **153**, 1309–1311.
9. Kehoe K.C. (1991). Malignant ascites: etiology, diagnosis and treatment. *Oncology Nursing Forum* **18**, 523–530.
10. Belfort M.A., Stevens P.J., DeHaek K., Soeters R. and Krige J.E. (1990). A new approach to the management of malignant ascites; a permanently implanted abdominal drain. *European Journal of Surgical Oncology* **16**, 47–53.
11. Young D.S., Lentz S.S., Barrett R.J., Homesley H.D. and Moore J.S. (1992). Outpatient management of malignant ascites using ultrasound, a trocar, and a Tenckhoff catheter. *International Journal Gynecological Cancer* **2**, 175–178.
12. Greenway B., Johnson P.J. and Williams R. (1982). Control of malignant ascites with spironolactone. *British Journal of Surgery* **69**, 441–442.
13. Pockros P.J., Esrason K.T., Nguyen C., Duque J. and Woods S. (1992). Mobilization of malignant ascites with diuretics is dependent on ascitic fluid characteristics. *Gastroenterology* **103**, 1302–1306.
14. LeVeen H.H., Christoudias G., Ip M. *et al.* (1974). Peritoneovenous shunting for ascites. *Annals of Surgery* **180**, 580–591.
15. Rogers J. (1991). *Mr Wroe's Virgins.* London: Faber and Faber.

CHAPTER TWENTY-FOUR

Bone marrow suppression: neutropenia and thrombocytopenia

Ruth Dunleavey

Introduction

Bone marrow suppression (BMS) is a reduction in the formation of red and white blood cells and platelets in the bone marrow. In cancer, BMS may be secondary to the disease process or may result from the therapy used to treat it. It is a particular problem amongst people undergoing chemotherapy. Cytotoxic drugs arrest the multiplication of malignant cells by interfering with the process of cell division. Because most chemotherapy lacks the specificity to target cancer cells alone, cytotoxic drugs also interfere with cell division amongst healthy groups of cells. Cells that are rapidly dividing, such as blood cells, are particularly vulnerable.

Blood cells are made in the bone marrow which is found inside the long bones of the body and in the sternum, pelvis, and skull. They originate from a 'great, great-grandfather' cell known as the pluripotent stem cell (see Figure 24.1).[1] Pluripotent stem cells have the unique capacity to produce daughter cells that either mature into further stem cells or differentiate into specific types of blood cell.

A normal white blood count is $4\text{--}10 \times 10^9/l$. Neutrophils make up approximately 40–60% of this. Neutrophils have a very short life span, living for only 7–8 hours in peripheral blood.[2] Neutropenia is usually graded by the National Cancer Institute (NCI) system (see Table 24.1).[3] The depth and duration of neutropenia has been demonstrated to bear a very close correlation with the acquisition of infection, the majority of severe infections occurring when the neutrophil count falls below $0.1 \times 10^9/l$.[4] People receiving chemotherapy are considered to be at greatest risk of becoming neutropenic following their first cycle of treatment.[5,6]

The normal range for platelets is $150\text{--}400 \times 10^9/l$ and thrombocytopenia occurs when the level falls below this. Thrombocytopenia is also graded by the NCI system (see Table 24.1).[3]

The rest of this chapter examines some of the key clinical issues in the care of neutropenic and thrombocytopenic patients, with particular emphasis on the care of patients with haematological malignancies. It begins with a discussion of febrile neutropenia followed by an evaluation of two strategies aimed at the prevention of infection amongst the neutropenic patient – namely the neutropenic diet and protective isolation. Care of the neutropenic patient is then discussed in the context of current health care trends such as early discharge from hospital and outpatient care of oncology patients. Finally there is an exploration of some of the issues involved in caring for the patient with thrombocytopenia.

Neutropenia and the cancer patient

. . . considering neutropenia exclusively as the numerical value of the absolute neutrophil count limits its conceptualizations to physiologically related aspects, minimizes its complexities and neglects dimensions of human response and the patient experience.[7]

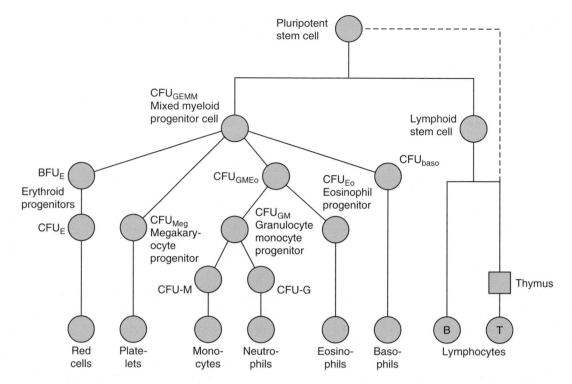

Figure 24.1 Blood cell formation (haemopoiesis). Diagrammatic representation of the bone marrow pluripotent stem cell and the cell lines that arise from it. Various progenitor cells can now be identified by culture in a semi-solid medium by the type of colony they form. Baso, basophil; BFU$_E$, burst-forming unit; CFU, colony-forming unit; E, erythroid; Eo, eosinophil; GEMM, mixed granulocyte, erythroid, monocyte, megakaryocyte; G, granulocyte; M, monocyte; Meg, megakaryocyte. Reproduced with the permission of Blackwell Scientific Publications from Hoftbrand A.V. and Pettit J.E. (1993). *Essential Haematology*, 3rd edition.[1]

Table 24.1 National Cancer Institute neutropenia grading[4]

Grade	Neutrophils (×10⁹/l)	Platelets (×10⁹/l)
1	≥1.5 to < 2.0	<LLN to 75
2	≥1.0 to <1.5	>50 to ≤75
3	≥0.5 to <1.0	>10 to ≤50
4	<0.5	<10

LLN, lower limit of normal.

Infection has now superseded bleeding as the primary cause of death amongst people having chemotherapy.[8,9] Infection in a neutropenic patient usually – although not always – becomes manifest through a febrile episode. Differing definitions of febrile neutropenia can be found. In DeVita's *Cancer: Principles and Practice of Oncology* it is classified as:

1. a single temperature of greater than 38.3°C or greater than or equal to 38°C over at least one hour
2. an absolute neutrophil count (ANC) of less than 0.5×10^9/l or less than 1.0×10^9/l with predicted rapid decline to 0.5×10^9/l.[10]

Neutropenia is a problem amongst the oncology population for a number of reasons. First, there is the obvious risk of infection and life-threatening sepsis which results from having an inadequate neutrophil count. Second, it may lead to chemotherapy delays and dose reductions which threaten the overall efficacy of treatment regimens.[11] Finally the very experience of neutropenia in itself can be discomforting and debilitating.

Although not historically considered to be a symptomatic condition, neutropenia has been associated with fatigue, malaise and decreased functioning with activities of daily living [7,12,13] It is not uncommon to hear people describe feelings of weakness at certain stages in their treatment cycle, which they consider to correspond with periods of reduced white blood count. The development of tools such as the FACT-N quality-of-life scale, specifically designed for this patient population, are helping us to gain a greater understanding of neutropenia from the patient's perspective. [12]

Nursing management of a person with neutropenia cannot be examined in isolation from medical management. Over the last three decades there have been enormous changes in this. Not only have there been significant improvements in infection prophylaxis and treatment – particularly of fungal infections [14] – but there has also been the development of colony-stimulating factors (CSFs – see Box 24.1). This has led to a decreased duration of neutropenia in certain populations and has facilitated new treatment modalities such as peripheral blood stem cell transplantation (PBSCT) requiring shorter periods of hospitalisation and allowing outpatient transplantation programmes (see Box 24.2). [15]

Neutropenia – managing acute infection

While neutropenia is a potential complication for any cancer patient receiving bone marrow-suppressing chemotherapy, it is a particular issue among patients with haematological malignancies because of the immunosuppressive nature of both their disease and treatment. This immunosuppression may be compounded by a number of factors which have been well described in the literature (see Box 24.3). The combination of general immunosuppression combined with a reduced neutrophil count means that even a small infection can very quickly escalate into life-threatening septic shock.

Neutropenic people are at risk of infection from a variety of organisms, although improvement in the management of early bacterial infections coupled with changes in the medical management of some malignancies has meant that infections from organisms such as viruses (e.g. cytomegalovirus (CMV)), protozoa (e.g. *Pneumocystis carinii*) and fungi (e.g. *Aspergillus*), which usually arise later in the period of neutropenia, have assumed much greater significance, particularly in the haematology population. Nevertheless, bacterial infections are still the most common cause of infection among neutropenic patients, with a trend towards more gram-negative

Box 24.1 Colony-stimulating factors (CSFs)

One important factor which has facilitated current trends towards reduced hospitalisation and techniques such as PBSCT is the development of colony-stimulating factors. Granulocyte-colony stimulating factor (G-CSF) and granulocyte-macrophage stimulating factor (GM-CSF) were introduced in the 1980s. These are cytokines, substances which are endogenous to the body and can be produced commercially using recombinant techniques. Parenteral administration of these cytokines stimulates neutrophil production.

CSFs bring about a reduction in the length of neutropenia. The benefit of this is not only to reduce the incidence of febrile neutropenia. It also facilitates the delivery of chemotherapy on time and reduces the need for dose delays and reductions because of neutropenia. These compromises in dose intensity of chemotherapy have been found in studies of breast cancer and lymphoma to be detrimental to the extent that they reduce disease-free survival. [16,17]

More recently a new CSF has entered the market which is a pegylated version of G-CSF. The advantage of this is that it only needs to be administered weekly rather than daily. Whereas G-CSF is a small molecule which is rapidly excreted by the kidneys, the addition of a polyethylene glycol (PEG) molecule onto this creates a much larger molecule. Pegylated G-CSF is non-toxic, pH neutral, water soluble, and capable of lasting for much longer periods *in vivo*. Elimination is via the kidneys, and pegylated G-CSF levels will remain elevated until sufficient numbers of normal neutrophils have developed to eradicate it from the bloodstream.

Box 24.2 Peripheral blood stem cell transplantation

Peripheral blood stem cell transplantation (PBSCT) has now largely replaced bone marrow transplantation. It is a procedure where 'bone marrow' cells are collected either from a patient while they are in remission or from a matched donor.

PBSCT mobilisation requires the administration of intermediate doses of chemotherapy in conjunction with growth factors. It has been found that when the bone marrow begins to recover there is a short period of time during which progenitor cells (stem cells) are mobilised from their normal environment in the bone marrow into the peripheral circulation. These cells can be harvested with the use of a cell separator in a process know as leukopheresis. The products can then be preserved and frozen in preparation for transplantation. During a peripheral blood stem cell transplant the patient receives a high, myeloablative dose of chemotherapy in the same way that they would with a conventional bone marrow transplant, and their marrow is rescued by re-infusion of the stem cells.

The advantages of this technique over using bone marrow are threefold:

- the cells engraft more quickly, leading to a rapid recovery of blood count and speedy discharge home from hospital
- it is available to people unable to undergo a general anaesthetic
- it is cheaper than bone marrow transplantation.

For these reasons, high-dose therapy with stem cell rescue is being offered to a wide range of people who would previously not have been eligible for transplantation such as the elderly, or people with poor performance status. The role of stem cell transplantation for the management of solid tumours did not fulfil its earlier promise, although the technique is being investigated in solid tumours because of its immunotherapeutic effects.[18] To date it remains principally a therapy for haematological malignancies.

---

infections in recent years.[23,24] The increasing prevalence of resistant strains of micro-organisms such as vancomycin-resistant enterococci (VRE) is of concern. VRE bacteraemia may be associated with a mortality rate of greater than 70%.[24]

The key to good management of infection lies with prompt recognition of the early signs followed by immediate action, and this requires the highest level of nursing skill. With the exception of fever, signs and symptoms of the infective process are usually very mild or absent in neutropenic populations.[25] Furthermore, even fever may not always be present as it may be masked, for example, by medications such as steroids or paracetamol. Other early symptoms include irritability, confusion, or drowsiness accompanied by haemodynamic changes – usually tachycardia and blood pressure alterations.[26,27] If severely immunosuppressed, the patient may be unable to mount an adequate immune response, resulting in general vascular collapse.

In the past, the literature classified septic shock into stages beginning with a hyperdynamic state (warm shock) which progresses to cold shock when the body's compensatory mechanisms fail and the patient begins to experience multisystem failure.[28] While of some use in clarifying a complex phenomenon, the pattern of changes associated with infection is extremely varied and may not follow any real chronology. Today the terms 'warm' and 'cold' shock have largely been superseded by 'the septic syndrome'. The septic syndrome describes a continuum which begins with a localised infection and progresses to a systemic one (septicaemia).[29]

Statistics regarding the incidence of sepsis are varied and difficult to interpret, but the consensus of opinion suggests that the death rate from septic shock ranges between 25% and 50%, rising to 75% amongst the cancer population, and is greater than 90% if more that one infecting organism is involved.[25,26,29]

Amongst the neutropenic, pyrexia should always be treated as indicative of an infection until proven otherwise. Febrile neutropenia is an oncological emergency requiring immediate action. Different institutions have different policies regarding the specific management of febrile

Box 24.3   Factors predisposing the person with cancer to infection

Although neutrophil count is probably the single most important factor when considering infection amongst people with cancer, there are also a number of other issues that should be considered, which relate to the general level of immucompetence of that individual.

The human immune system can be divided into two components: the non-specific and the specific. Non-specific immunity refers to the first line of defence against infection and it includes surface membrane barriers and non-specific cellular and chemical defences such as neutrophils, macrophages, and a range of cytokines. The second 'specific' line of defence refers to the white blood cells, particularly the lymphocytes, which have the ability to recognise foreign antigens and immobilise, incapacitate, or destroy them. Both systems operate in conjunction with one another.

Lines of defence may be compromised in people with cancer for a variety of reasons (see below). Chemotherapy and sometimes radiotherapy can disrupt the mucosal surfaces and deplete the neutrophil and lymphocyte count. The potential for infection is further exacerbated by factors such as age,[19] concomitant medical problems (e.g. diabetes, rheumatoid arthritis), and poor nutritional status, as well as the general stress of being diagnosed as a cancer patient.[20] Furthermore the hospital environment provides a major source of pathogenic organisms.[21,22]

Disease-related factors
- Defective T-cells found in people with lymphoma, multiple myeloma, and the leukaemias are associated with humoral defence deficits
- Bone marrow infiltration, tumour obstruction, and erosion
- Cachexia
- Stress
- Extremes of age and poor nutritional status
- Concomitant disease (renal failure, liver disease, diabetes, cardiac disease)
- Splenectomy
- Advanced disease stage
- Graft-versus-host disease.

Treatment-related factors
- Chemotherapy or radiotherapy to the bone marrow cause bone marrow suppression
- Steroids cause depression of neutrophil chemotaxis, decreased leucocyte adherence, depressed monocyte bactericidal activity, decreased endocytosis, and decreased lymphocyte function
- Surgery leads to a fall in lymphocytes and is immunosuppressive
- Invasive procedures such as insertion of an intravascular device provide a route for micro-organisms
- Some regimens are damaging to mucosal surfaces and can potentiate bacterial translocation
- Prolonged antibiotic therapy
- Prior chemotherapy or bone marrow transplant, particularly in association with immunosuppressive therapy.

Environmental factors
- The hospital environment is potentially hostile because of the large number of micro-organisms it harbours, particularly in inhalational equipment, nebulisers, food sources, contaminated air/water, and through hand-to-hand transmission.

neutropenia, but most will implement measures when the temperature rises above 38°C or 38.5°C.

The first step is to take the relevant specimens for microbiology. In the haematology setting a septic work-up generally involves drawing blood for culture, taking sputum and urine specimens, and possibly taking central line exit site swabs. Once again, institutional procedures vary regard-

ing not only the specimens taken but also the frequency with which a septic work-up is performed in patients who have protracted spells of febrile neutropenia.

One area in which there is overall agreement is in the timing of initiating antibiotics. Intravenous antibiotics must be given immediately. More than 70% of people will respond if antibiotics are given within the first 24 hours, compared with only

22% if they are delayed to the third day following the development of symptoms.[30]

Neutropenia – prevention of infection

There is a considerable body of nursing and medical literature largely dating from the 1970s, which explores the optimal environment in which to place the neutropenic patient. An environment has been sought which protects the patient from organisms that might cause febrile neutropenia and sepsis.

While the logic of providing a clean environment for the immunocompromised patient seems irrefutable, for some time it has been widely conceded that for the majority of people with neutropenia the primary source of bacterial infection is their own body. Schimpff *et al.* analysed the organisms leading to infective episodes among a population of people with neutropenia.[21] It was discovered that the vast majority of these were caused by the person's own commensal organisms – that is that *most infections were caused by bacteria that already inhabited the affected patient*. In 47% of cases these were organisms that were acquired during hospitalisation.

Nevertheless, the management of the neutropenic patient in many institutions still incorporates strategies aimed at minimising contact with pathogens. Such measures range from sophisticated endeavours to decolonise the gastrointestinal tract with antibiotics, to expensive air filtration and strict isolation policies. The enormous variation in institutional practices regarding management of a person who is neutropenic can be confusing to both the patient and nurse alike. Although there are many areas of disparity within the topic of neutropenic care, just two have been selected for discussion here, namely the neutropenic diet and protective isolation.

Neutropenic diet

A number of common foodstuffs have been found to contain potentially pathogenic bacteria such as *Escheria coli*, *Pseudomonas aeruginosa* and Klebsiella.[31,32] Such organisms are frequently associated with sepsis in the neutropenic individual.

For this reason dietary recommendations have traditionally been made to neutropenic patients – particularly those undergoing bone marrow transplant – resulting in 'clean', 'sterile' or 'low bacterial' diets.[33] Box 24.4 lists some of these recommendations.

Box 24.4 Dietary recommendations and restrictions during neutropenic periods[6,13,34–37]

Restrictions
- Raw or unpasteurised milk or milk products including cheese or yoghurt
- Raw or undercooked meats, fish, poultry, eggs, tofu, cold smoked fish
- Aged cheese (brie, camembert)
- Salad-based dressings with cheese base
- Unwashed raw fruit and vegetables
- Delicatessen meats, processed luncheon meat, rare and medium cooked meat, raw eggs, seafood, lasagne, pizza
- Any foodstuff containing nuts or raisins
- Unsterilised water, unpasteurised beer.

Recommendations
- Food to be served on sterile plates and trays covered during transport
- Cooked foods from multiserve containers be served to neutropenic people first.

While clean diets vary between institutions, the basic philosphy of diet modification is the same in that it aims to expose the patient to the minimum possible number of pathogens by including only cooked or highly processed foods. Foodstuffs associated with high microbial loads (salad, raw fruit, certain diary products) are thus eliminated. Despite the presence of potential pathogens, the link between bacteria-laden foodstuff and infection has not been definitively proven.

> There is lack of empirical evidence substantiating the ability of reduced microbial diets to diminish rates of infection, morbidity or mortality.[34]

Nevertheless, dietary restrictions are still imposed in many centres. Hartkopf Smith and

Galford Besser surveyed 156 oncology centres to establish their dietary recommendations for neutropenic inpatients.[37] This survey excluded people undergoing bone marrow transplant but extended to all other categories of neutropenic patient. Seventy-eight per cent of centres imposed some dietary restrictions. Peeled fruits, raw potatoes, raw eggs, and rare and medium-cooked meats were restricted at more than 60% of institutions. Raisins and dried fruit, potato salad, and beer were restricted at 40% of institutions. The evidence for specific restrictions was not always clear.

Not only have the infective implications of dietary modification never been fully evaluated, but neither have the nutritional consequences. A feature of clean diets is that they are potentially unappetising and restrictive at a time when the patient's nutritional requirements are high.[34] This raises another important point regarding dietary practices, and that is the issue of patient acceptability.

DeMille et al. looked at the role of a neutropenic diet amongst a population of outpatients receiving chemotherapy and at high risk of developing neutropenia, in a small pilot study which excluded bone marrow transplant and haematology patients.[33] Although the population was only small (23 patients), the observations were interesting. Approximately one-third of patients were found to be non-compliant with their diet. Despite this there were no significant differences in the rates of febrile admissions or positive blood cultures between compliant and non-compliant patients.

There appears to be a trend in many centres towards reducing restrictive dietary practices.[35]

In the absence of data from large, randomised, controlled trials it is possible that such initiatives are partly driven by clinical observations and patient compliance issues as noted above.[33]

Protective isolation

Following the same rationale as the neutropenic diet, there has been a longstanding policy of isolation for the neutropenic patient – especially the neutropenic haematology and bone marrow transplant patient. Protective isolation aims to minimise the number of organisms with which an individual will have contact. Various types of

isolation exist, ranging from highly sophisticated protective isolation units incorporating air filtration devices to simple isolation (basically a single room).

Air filtration may incorporate laminar air flow (LAF), usually in conjunction with high standards of sterility. This is the most rigorous level of air filtration. High-efficiency particulate air (HEPA) filtration is a less-intensive approach allowing a slightly larger number of particles into the clinical area. While air filtration is undoubtedly effective in removing highly pathogenic Aspergillus spores, there is controversy about the overall benefit it confers.[38–40]

The use of air-filtration devices is generally restricted to the highest-risk neutropenic individuals such as those undergoing bone marrow transplant. It is more common for patients who are less immunocompromised to be confined to a single room on an ordinary ward during periods of neutropenia. The usefulness of this strategy has been disputed. Nauseef and Maki[41] studied a large group of people who were neutropenic after chemotherapy and found there was no advantage to nursing them in a single room compared with the general ward (see Research study 24.1). They also noted that such isolation strategies can be psychologically discomforting to people, and hence questioned their utility.

A number of studies have endeavoured to explore the psychological effects of isolation.[42] This has been a difficult task, in part because of the number of other psychological factors confronting the neutropenic patient – and specifically the febrile neutropenic patient. Physically they are likely to be feeling unwell, possibly deprived of sleep, perhaps in pain, and generally vulnerable. Psychologically, people in isolation have to contend with being away from their loved ones, facing a serious illness and possibly confronting death for the first time. Some of the literature describes the loneliness and stressfulness of isolation:[43,44]

> . . . it makes you feel like . . . like you're in an institution, where people are just wandering in and out and you really don't matter as an individual.[45]

Mank reviewed the isolation literature with a view to revising the practice at his institution.[46]

Research study 24.1

Nauseef W.M. and Maki D.G. (1981). A study of the value of simple protective isolation in patients with panuocytopenia. *New England Journal of Medicine* **304**, 448–453.[41]

This piece of research was carried out in Wisconsin between 1977 and 1978. It was conducted by two clinicians hoping to identify whether expensive isolation and disinfection procedures were necessary to prevent neutropenic sepsis. Furthermore, they had observed that extreme forms of isolation can have adverse psychological effects on people and were concerned about the rationale behind such practices.

The study sample consisted of people either with acute lymphocytic leukaemia or aplastic anaemia, who had been admitted to hospital for longer than a week. They were undergoing remission-induction therapy or treatment for a relapse. People were randomised into either protective isolation or standard hospital care. Protective isolation was defined by the Centres for Disease Control. Their recommendations were for a single room with private toilet and use of clean gown, gloves, and mask for anyone entering. Standard care consisted of an ordinary two-bedded room with a sign on the door reminding people coming in to wash their hands. Neither group was given gut decontamination or sterile food.

In total 37 people were enrolled on to the study, experiencing 43 episodes of neutropenia in all. Both groups were comparable in terms of age, blood count, therapy and admission time. The study found no statistically significant differences in infection rate between the two groups. Unfortunately, no formal analysis was made of quality of life. However, although the majority of people tolerated the conditions, even amongst this small sample, two individuals had to break isolation because of psychological distress. Nauseef and Maki state:

> On the basis of our data, we concluded that simple protective isolation alone, as practiced in most hospitals, offers no appreciable benefits to people with granulocytopenia in reducing infections or improving the rate of leukaemic remission, and that it does not prolong survival. In view of the added costs and the emotional deprivation that patient and family must endure, its use should be re-evaluated.[41]

This study can be criticised for its small sample size and lack of statistical significance. However, despite being performed almost 30 years ago there have been few further attempts at confirmatory studies since.

For his search he utilised key words; 'protective isolation', 'protective environment', 'patient isolators', 'neutropenia', 'bone marrow transplantation' and 'peripheral blood stem cell transplantation'. One-hundred and sixty publications on protective isolation for people with neutropenia were found, but only six were prospective, randomised studies – and even these provided conflicting reports on the efficacy of isolation. Mank concluded that although there was 'a plethora of opinion from respected authorities or expert committees', this was largely based on clinical experience or descriptive studies rather than randomised controlled trials. In conclusion he felt he had failed to locate enough evidence to support maintaining protective isolation.

Similarly Russell *et al.* chose to abandon the strict isolation practices in their bone marrow transplant unit, partly as a result of a nursing strike that depleted staff and rendered such labour-intensive measures inoperable.[47] They failed to demonstrate any increase in infections or mortality as a result. The option to go home during the transplant period even when profoundly neutropenic is now offered routinely in this institution.

Neutropenia – research and practice

Neutropenic diet and protective isolation are only two of many nursing issues that arise in the care of people with neutropenia. Other topics which also provoke discussion are the management of central lines, optimal mouth care regimens, the use of masks, gowns and overshoes, and personal hygiene measures. Indeed, with perhaps the exception of hand-washing, which is now universally accepted as being the principal measure in the prevention of infection, most other nursing strategies for the management of people with neutropenia are still the subject of debate.[48,49]

Although the nursing literature often provides prescriptive advice in these areas, it is not always supported by research. Where research is cited, studies are often small, not statistically significant, and involve divergent patient populations. There have been few new research studies in this area in recent years.

Over the last two decades there has been considerable discussion of 'evidence-based care' – indeed, 'evidence' may well be one of the most fashionable words in health care at the moment.[50] As a result of this there have been a number of attempts at assessing the clinical relevance of the literature on neutropenia. Several nursing reviews have attempted to identify the level of evidence supporting the various interventions which have been put forward for the care of the neutropenic person.[6,13,36]

Larson and Nirenberg examined the evidence on low-microbial diets, protective clothing/environment, personal hygiene, and oral care.[36] They omitted discussion of the management of intravascular devices and hand hygiene, as these topics are not specific to people with neutropenia and have a broad literature already. They also omitted studies on people receiving bone marrow transplants alone because transplants are not used in many common cancers.

Their findings are illustrated in Table 24.2. Level 1 refers to the highest level of evidence – that is a randomised controlled trial. Only one level 1 study was identified and this was for the sucking of ice chips to prevent mucositis. Most of the other common nursing interventions for neutropenic populations were supported by low levels of evidence. Clean diets were supported by level 4 evidence (well-conducted qualitative studies) and protective isolation measures by level 5 or 6 evidence (well-conducted case studies or poorly controlled/uncontrolled studies).

West and Mitchell reviewed the data relating to the care of a person with neutropenia following outpatient stem cell transplantation.[13] They looked at antimicrobial prophylaxis, dietary restrictions, oral care, hand-washing and hygiene practices, central line care, and the use of CSFs. A similar review by Shelton examined the research on infection control measures with reference to

Table 24.2 Evidence base for various clinical practices to reduce the risk of infection in neutropenic patients with cancer. Reproduced with permission, from Larsen E. and Nirenberg A. (2004). Evidence-based nursing practice in hospitalized neutropenic patients with cancer. *Oncology Nursing Forum* **31**, 717–723[36]

Level[a]	Source of evidence	Clinical practice
1	Integrative reviews, meta-analysis of multiple, well-designed, randomised controlled trials of adequate quality	Ice chips to prevent mucositis
2	At least one properly designed, randomised, clinical trial of appropriate size	None found
3	Well-designed trial without randomisation	Influenza immunisation for staff
4	Well-conducted qualitative systematic review of non-experimental design studies	Low-microbial diets (no evidence of benefit)
5	Well-conducted case–control study	None found
6	Poorly controlled or uncontrolled study	Patients wear high-efficiency masks outside the room, have private room isolation, are treated with oral care regimens (e.g. chlorhexidine, honey, calcium phosphate)
7	Conflicting evidence with weight of evidence supporting the recommendation or meta-analysis showing a trend, National Institutes of Health consensus reports, and published practice guidelines	Patients are under protective isolation, do not wear cover gowns, and have antiseptic bathing. Visitors and pets are restricted and screened. Plants and flowers are restricted
8	Qualitative designs, case studies and opinions from experts	None found

[a]Levels of evidence as designated by Ropka and Spencer-Cisek.[51] The lower the number the stronger the evidence.

the neutropenic person with leukaemia.[6] Shelton utilised the Oncology Nursing Society's evidence-based guidelines, which have four levels of evidence base ranging from weak to strong.

In both papers, although a thorough overview of the literature was provided, it was not always clear which research study was being proposed to support the specific guidelines that were made, or the level of this evidence behind each guideline. Their recommendations regarding diet and environmental factors are summarised in Table 24.3.

The lack of clinical trials on which to build practice in this field is largely a reflection of the technical difficulty of such studies – principally in controlling the large number of variables that can impact infection rates. For example, institutions vary significantly in their prophylactic antibiotic regimens, mouth care and central line-dressing policies. Any endeavour at assessing one variable of neutropenic care must take into account all of these and a multitude of other related factors. Furthermore the extent to which findings can be applied to different cancer populations is unknown. For example, to what degree can a study conducted with people undergoing allogeneic bone marrow transplant for leukaemia be applied to a population of patients with lymphoma – let alone to a population of outpatients receiving chemotherapy for breast cancer?

Table 24.3 Guidelines for the nursing care of neutropenic populations[6,13]

Practice	Shelton[6]	Level of evidence cited	West and Mitchell[13]	Level of evidence cited
Population	Neutropenic patient with leukaemia		Outpatient haemopoietic stem cell transplant patient	
Environment	HEPA for stem cell transplant patients/ patients with prolonged neutropenia. Otherwise no routine barrier precautions/protective isolation	Moderate	Outpatient population. Limit exposure to bacterial, viral, and fungal infections. Patients to wear mask to and from clinic and when out in public	Recommendation based on Centres for Disease Control (CDC) guidelines
	No fresh flowers or plants	High	Avoid fresh flowers and plants	Expert opinion
Patient care practices	Good hand hygiene	High	Meticulous hand hygiene	Unspecified
Diet	No special dietary considerations	Moderate	Quote CDC guidelines – 'all foods should be well cooked, and all raw foods, including seafood, mayonnaise and raw eggs should be avoided during the neutropenic period'	Level of evidence unspecified
Oral care	Frequent oral care including toothbrushing and gentle flossing as tolerated. Rinse mouth with any palatable solution, but use antimicrobial mouth rinses when poor oral hygiene or gingivitis is present	High	Oral care four to six times daily and as needed including dental care and mouthwashes 'best suited to the patients needs and preferences'	Level of evidence unspecified

Neutropenia – care in context

The nursing management of the neutropenic person is constantly evolving in parallel with their medical management. Recent medical innovations include the aforementioned CSFs, which have brought about a reduction in neutropenia in certain populations and have rendered the condition altogether more 'manageable'. Concurrent with the development of CSFs there has been a shift in ethos from inpatient to outpatient care – a change that has been largely driven by economic motives. Much of the literature on this subject arises from the US where hospitalisation is the single largest component of direct medical costs, accounting for 40–50% of total cancer care costs.[52] Hospitalisation for febrile neutropenia constitutes a large proportion of this.[5,25] Both these trends are accompanied by a change in attitude in the current literature in which the neutropenic population is no longer treated as a homogenous group to whom 'blanket' policies can be applied.

A number of recent initiatives have involved the identification of 'risk groups' of neutropenic patients in order to implement management strategies that are more appropriate to their needs. For example, risk-assessment strategies have been employed to identify populations that might benefit from the early introduction of CSFs. Current recommendations are that CSFs should not be applied routinely to all populations of patients undergoing cytotoxic therapy, but only in situations in which there is a high risk of febrile neutropenia.[53] Checklists such as the Risk Assessment for Neutropenic Complications Tool[54] have been developed by chemotherapy nurses to identify high-risk groups for febrile neutropenia in whom CSFs could be introduced early in order to prevent treatment delays and life-threatening sepsis (see Box 24.5).

Other institutions have introduced policies for outpatient management of people with neutropenic sepsis. The febrile neutropenic person is assessed in the emergency department, and if they fulfil the necessary criteria they are discharged home with the appropriate medication, advice and support. They are usually given an initial dose of intravenous antibiotics followed by oral antibiotics to take at home, or in some cases

Box 24.5   Risk factors for neutropenic complications[54]

- Treatment with a chemotherapy regimen with at least a 40% risk of febrile neutropenia
- Patient older than 70 years
- Bone marrow involvement or compromise
- Open wounds
- Occurrence of febrile neuropenia in a previous course of therapy
- Serum albumin level of less than 3.5 g/dl
- First-cycle absolute neutrophil count (ANC) less than 500/mm³.

oral antibiotics may be administered from the beginning.

Once again, such a strategy is not appropriate for all but only for those at low risk of complications. The Multinational Association for Supportive Care in Cancer (MASCC) conducted a multicentre study in order to identify low-risk persons with neutropenia for whom outpatient management was an option.[55] Characteristics which were considered predictive of favourable outcome were:

- burden of illness with no, mild, or moderate symptoms
- absence of hypotension
- absence of chronic obstructive pulmonary disease
- solid tumour or no prior fungal infection in haematological tumours
- absence of dehydration
- good performance status
- age less than 60 years.[55]

At this point it should be added that effective outpatient care of the neutropenic patient is also dependent on an optimal social environment and a supportive carer. Caring for a person with chemotherapy-induced neutropenia is stressful for families, and the role of the nurse in educating and supporting them is pivotal.[56]

In conclusion, after many years of discussing the optimal management of the neutropenic person, there would still appear to be no simple answers. However, recent changes in the management of neutropenic patients facilitated by the development of CSFs, and coupled with a general shift towards outpatient management, has altered the complexion of neutropenia. In the future it may be that an extensive risk assessment of people at risk of neutropenia will be performed in order to guide their management, and subsequent research projects will concentrate on subgroups of patients in order to obtain more meaningful data about specific populations.

Bone marrow suppression – thrombocytopenia

Normal clotting occurs at the culmination of a complex series of events known as the coagulation cascade. Alteration of any single component in this pathway results in aberrant clotting, which may manifest itself as either thrombosis or haemorrhage. Clinically significant haemostatic abnormalities are thought to affect as many as 15% of cancer patients, with the incidence rising to up to 90% following chemotherapy.[57] These disorders may be the result of either the primary malignancy or the therapy employed to treat it.[58]

Clotting defects are multifactorial in their aetiology and may result from secretions from the tumour cell itself, or damage to the liver, spleen, or bone marrow. However, the most usual single cause of serious haemorrhage, particularly amongst people with leukaemia, is thrombocytopenia.[16]

Thrombocytopenia may be the result of chemotherapy administration or due to disease factors as in the case of the haematological malignancies. Cancer-related bone marrow suppression can cause thrombocytopenia in people with acute leukaemia. Some people with lymphoma or chronic lymphoblastic leukaemia experience increased peripheral platelet destruction due to hypersplenism. People with solid tumours may also experience disease-related thrombocytopenia as a result of marrow infiltration by the tumour. Bone marrow secondaries are commonly observed in breast cancer and prostate cancer. Less commonly, they can be seen in a variety of other tumour types including lung cancer and melanoma.[58]

The availability of platelet concentrates has made thrombocytopenia treatable. This has facili-

tated intensive chemotherapy regimens and also allowed supportive care for disease-related thrombocytopenia. The use of platelet transfusions continues to increase. There was a 2.3% increase in the demand for platelet concentrates in hospitals in England in 2001–2002 compared with the previous year (i.e. 215 050 adult doses in total).[59]

Management of thrombocytopenia

Education is extremely important in the management of thrombocytopenia. People undergoing chemotherapy need to understand what thrombocytopenia is and when their counts are low. It is important for the nurse to be able to recognise the signs and symptoms of a low platelet count (bruising, bleeding, purpurae, and epistaxis), and to offer counselling about how to modify lifestyle to minimise risk of bleeding. For example, it might be suggested to avoid heavy manual labour and contact sports or to use a soft toothbrush and an electric razor to minimise trauma to the gums and face.[60] Steroids and non-steroidal anti-inflammatory drugs prolong clotting times. Where possible, these should be avoided, although in reality this may sometimes lead to clinical dilemmas in which the potential risk of bleeding needs to be weighed against important symptom control measures such as pain relief.

Although there have been considerable advances in platelet transfusion over the last 40 years, some areas continue to provoke debate. The use of prophylactic platelets is one such area.

Prophylactic platelet transfusions have become common practice for people with marrow failure, and studies have indicated that platelet transfusion decreases morbidity (but not mortality) in people with thrombocytopenia through marrow failure.[61] However, transfusion is not without risk.

The first risk is that of refractoriness. It is suggested that following as few as one or two platelet transfusions, it is possible to become refractory to their beneficial effects;[62] between 15 and 20% of those who are frequently transfused become seriously refractory.[63]

Second, there is the risk of a transfusion reaction. This is relatively common, occurring in 30%

of transfusions, and is the result of leucocyte contamination or cytokine release from the transfused product.[62] It is manifested as chills, rigors, and rashes. Not only can this be extremely frightening, but it also negates any benefit from the transfusion, as the platelets are consumed in the ensuing immune activity. Some units routinely administer steroid and antihistamine 'cover' pretransfusion, although there are concerns about the risk of avascular necrosis and also increased risk of fungal infection from the excessive use of steroids.[60,64–66] In recent years there has been a movement towards employment of leucocyte filters. Not only do these minimise reactions but they are also thought to prevent or delay refractoriness and prevent the transmission of some blood-borne infections.[67]

Infection is the third potential complication of transfusion. Although platelets can be screened for known infections such as CMV and human immunodeficiency virus (HIV), there is a theoretical concern of transmission of organisms not yet known. Other platelet-associated risks include transfusion-related acute lung injury.[59]

Traditionally, prophylactic transfusions have been administered when the platelet count falls below $20 \times 10^9/l$, although this practice has been questioned in recent years.[60] A randomised study of women with gynaecological cancer compared prophylactic platelet infusions at counts of $20 \times 10^9/l$ and counts of $5 \times 10^9/l$. Transfusion at a count of $5 \times 10^9/l$ was found to be just as safe as $20 \times 10^9/l$.[68] Other studies have demonstrated a safe threshold at $10 \times 10^9/l$.[69]

On the basis of such research the British Committee for Standards in Haematology have made a number of recommendations.[59] Their advice also concurs with that of the American Society of Clinical Oncology.[70] These are:

- a threshold of $10 \times 10^9/l$ is as safe as higher levels for people without additional risk factors. Risk factors include sepsis, concurrent use of antibiotics or other abnormalities of haemostasis
- for people without any risk factors, a threshold of $5 \times 10^9/l$ may be appropriate if there are concerns that alloimmunisation could lead to platelet refractoriness. However, accurate counting of low platelet numbers may create difficulties when trying to reduce the threshold below $10 \times 10^9/l$
- a specific threshold for transfusion may not be appropriate for people with chronic stable thrombocytopenia who are best managed on an individual basis depending on the degree of haemorrhage.

The issue of quality of life and thrombocytopenia has not been clearly addressed in the literature but, as in the case of neutropenia, this is a consideration for people receiving platelet transfusions – particularly in the palliative setting. The benefits of transfusion need to be weighed against the fact that people may find themselves spending periods of time in hospital awaiting treatment, may be subjected to repeated painful and often difficult cannulations, and are at risk of unpleasant transfusion reactions.

Conclusion

Much nursing time and energy is spent in the management of the person with neutropenia and thrombocytopenia. Care of this population has changed in recent decades in line with medical changes and new approaches to management.

The observation that there has been little new research in the field of neutropenic care in recent years is disappointing, but perhaps not surprising, reflecting both the technical difficulties behind such research as well as current trends within oncology. The nurse still plays a key role in caring for the neutropenic and thrombocytopenic patient. She is responsible not only for managing active infection and bleeding, but also for promoting a safe environment through instituting appropriate, research-based policies, and by educating and supporting people through the neutropenic and thrombocytopenic period.

References

1. Hoffbrand A.V. and Pettit J.E. (1993). *Essential Haematology*. Oxford: Blackwell Scientific.
2. Cappozzo C. (2004). Optimal use of granulocyte-colony stimulating factor in patients with cancer who are at risk

for chemotherapy-induced neutropenia. *Oncology Nursing Forum* **31**, 569–574.

3. National Cancer Institute Therapy Evaluation Team (1999). *Common Toxicity Criteria Manual version 2.* http://ctep.cancer.gov/forms/CTCManual_v4_10-4-99.pdf (accessed 7 August 2007).

4. Bodey G. (1982). Infections in patients with cancer. In Holland J.F. and Frei E. (eds.) *Cancer Medicine.* Philadelphia, PA: Lea and Febinger, pp. 1339–1372.

5. Lyman G.H. and Kuderer N.M. (2004). The economics of the colony-stimulating factors in the prevention and treatment of febrile neutropenia. *Critical Reviews in Oncology/Haematology* **50**, 129–146.

6. Shelton B.K. (2003). Evidence-based care for the neutropenic patient with leukaemia. *Seminars in Oncology Nursing* **19**, 133–141.

7. Crighton M.H. (2004). Dimensions of neutropenia in adult cancer patients. *Cancer Nursing* **27**, 275–284.

8. Bick R.L. (1992). Coagulation abnormalities in malignancy. *Seminars in Thrombosis and Haemostasis* **18**, 353–372.

9. Carlson A.C. (1985). Infection prophylaxis in the patient with cancer. *Oncology Nursing Forum* **12**, 56–64.

10. Segal B.H., Walsh T.J. and Holland S.M. (2001). Infections in the cancer patient. In DeVita V.T., Hellman S. and Rosenberg S.A. (eds.) (2001). *Cancer: Principles and Practice of Oncology.* Philadelphia, PA: Lippincott Williams and Wilkins, p. 2804.

11. Lyman G.H., Dale D.C. and Crawford J. (2003). Incidence and predictors of low dose-intensity in adjuvant breast cancer chemotherapy: a nationwide study of community practices. *Journal of Clinical Oncology* **21**, 4524–4531.

12. Calhoun E.A. (2002). A neutropenia specific quality of life instrument: rationale for the development of FACT-N. *Proceedings of the American Society of Clinical Oncology* **21**, 375a.

13. West F. and Mitchell S.A. (2004). Evidence-based guidelines for the management of neutropenia following outpatient haematopoietic stem cell transplantation. *Clinical Journal of Oncology Nursing* **8**, 601–613.

14. Marr K.A. (2003). New approaches to invasive fungal infections. *Current Opinion in Hematology* **10**, 445–450.

15. Ringden O. and Le Blanc K. (2005). Allogeneic hematopoietic stem cell transplantation: state of the art and new perspectives. *Acta Pathologica Microbiologica et Immunologica Scandinavica* **113**, 813–830.

16. Budman D.R., Berry D.A., Cirrincione C.T. *et al.* (1998). Dose and dose intensity as determinants of outcome in the adjuvant treatment of breast cancer. *British Journal of the National Cancer Institute* **90**, 1205–1211.

17. Kwak L.W., Halpern J., Olshen R.A. *et al.* (1990). Prognostic significance of actual dose intensity in diffuse large cell lymphoma; results of a tree-structured survival analysis. *Journal of Clinical Oncology* **8**, 963–977.

18. Lundqvist A. and Childs R. (2005). Allogeneic hematopoietic cell transplantation as immunotherapy for solid tumors: current status and future directions. *Journal of Immunotherapy* **28**, 281–288.

19. Hood L.E. (2002). Chemotherapy in the elderly; supportive measures for chemotherapy-induced myelotoxicity. *Clinical Journal of Oncology Nursing* **7**, 185–190.

20. Ames B.N. (1995). Understanding the causes of aging and cancer. *Microbiologica* **11**, 305–308.

21. Schimpff S.C., Young V.M., Greene W.H. *et al.* (1972). Origin of infection in acute nonlymphocytic leukaemia. Significance of hospital acquisition of potential pathogens. *Annals of Internal Medicine* **77**, 707–714.

22. Schimpff S.C., Scott D.A. and Wade J.C. (1994). Infections in cancer patients: some controversial issues. *Supportive Care in Cancer* **2**, 94–104.

23. Pizzo P.A. (1989). Combating infections in neutropenic patients. *Hospital Practice* **22**, 93–110.

24. Vento S. and Cainelli F. (2003). Infections in patients with cancer undergoing chemotherapy: aetiology, prevention and treatment. *The Lancet Oncology* **4**, 595–604.

25. deLalla F. (2003). Outpatient therapy for febrile neutropenia. *Pharmacoeconomics* **21**, 397–413.

26. Hartnett S. (1989). Septic shock in the oncology patient. *Cancer Nursing* **12**, 191–201.

27. Cunneen J. (2004). The puzzle of sepsis: fitting the pieces of the inflammatory response with treatment. *Advanced Practice in Acute Clinical Care* **15**, 18–44.

28. Barry S.A. (1989). Septic shock: special needs for patients with cancer. *Oncology Nursing Forum* **16**, 31–35.

29. Truett L. (1991). The septic syndrome. *Cancer Nursing* **14**, 175–181.

30. Bodey G., Jadeja L. and Elting L. (1985). *Pseudomonas* bacteremia: retrospective analysis of 140 episodes. *Annals of Internal Medicine* **145**, 1621–1629.

31. Carter L.W. (1993). Bacterial translocation: nursing implications in the care of patients with neutropenia. *Oncology Nursing Forum* **21**, 1241–1250.

32. Remington J.S. and Schimpff S.C. (1981). Please don't eat the salads. *New England Journal of Medicine* **304**, 433–435.

33. DeMille D., Deming P., Lupinacci P. and Jacobs L.A. (2006). The effect of the neutropenic diet in the outpatient setting: a pilot study. *Oncology Nursing Forum* **33**, 337–343.

34. Rust D.M., Simpson J.K. and Lister J. (2000). Nutritional issues in patients with severe neutropenia. *Seminars in Oncology Nursing* **16**, 152–162.

35. Wilson B.J. (2002). Dietary recommendations for neutropenic patients. *Seminars in Oncology Nursing* **18**, 44–49.

36. Larson E. and Nirenberg A. (2004). Evidence-based nursing practice in hospitalized neutropenic patients with cancer. *Oncology Nursing Forum* **31**, 717–723.

37. Hartkopf Smith L. and Galford Besser S. (2000). Dietary restrictions for patients with neutropenia: a survey of institutional practices. *Oncology Nursing Forum* **27**, 515–576.

38. Pizzo P.A. (1989). Considerations for the prevention of infectious complications in patients with cancer. *Reviews of Infectious Disease* **II(suppl. 7)**, 1551–1563.

39. Armstrong T.S. (1994). Protected environments are discomforting and expensive and do not offer meaningful protection. *American Journal of Medicine* **76**, 685–689.

40. Meyers J.D. (1990). Fungal infections in bone marrow transplant patients. *Seminars in Oncology Nursing* **17**, 10–13.

41. Nauseef W.M. and Maki D.G. (1981). A study of the value of simple protective isolation in patients with pancytopenia. *New England Journal of Medicine* **304**, 448–453.

42. Holland J., Plumb M., Yates J. *et al.* (1977). Psychological response of patient with acute leukaemia to germ-free environments. *Cancer* **40**, 871–879.

43. Collins C., Upright C. and Aleksich J. (1989). Reverse isolation: what patients perceive. *Oncology Nursing Forum* **16**, 675–679.

44. Hjermstad M.J., Loge J.H., Evensen S.A. *et al.* (1999). The course of anxiety and depression during the first year after allogeneic or autologous stem cell transplantation. *Bone Marrow Transplantation* **24**, 1219–1228.

45. Krishnasamy M. (1994). *What Do Cancer Patients Identify as Supportive and Unsupportive Behaviours of Nurses?* MSc dissertation, University of Surrey.

46. Mank A. and van der Lelie H. (2003). Is there still an indication for nursing patients with supportive care in cancer risk index: a multinational scoring system for identifying low-risk febrile neutropenic cancer patients. *Journal of Clinical Oncology* **18**, 3038–3051.

47. Russell J.A., Poon M., Jones A.R., Woodman R.C. and Reuther B.A. (1992). Allogeneic bone marrow transplantation without protective isolation in adults with malignant disease. *Lancet* **339**, 38–40.

48. Steere A.C. and Mallison G.F. (1978). Handwashing practices for the prevention of nosocomial infections. *Annals of Internal Medicine* **83**, 683–690.

49. Gould D. (1994). Nurses' hand decontamination practice: results of a local study. *Journal of Hospital Infection* **28**, 15–29.

50. Rycroft-Malone J., Seers K., Titchen A. *et al.* (2004). What counts as evidence in evidence based practice? *Journal of Advanced Nursing* **47**, 81–90.

51. Ropka M.E. and Spencer-Cisek P. (2001). PRISM: priority symptom management project phase I: assessment. *Oncology Nursing Forum* **28**, 1585–1594.

52. Schuette H.L., Tucker T.C., Brown M.L., Potosky A.C. and Samuel T. (1995). The costs of cancer care in the United States: implications for action. *Oncology* **11**, 19–22.

53. National Comprehensive Cancer Network. (2005). *NCCN Clinical Practice Guidelines in Oncology: Myeloid Growth Factors in Cancer Treatment*. www.nccn.org/professionals/physician_gls/PDF/myeloid_growth.pdf (accessed 7 August 2007).

54. Donohue R. (2006). Development and implementation of a risk assessment tool for chemotherapy-induced neutropenia. *Oncology Nursing Forum* **33**, 347–352.

55. Klastersky J., Paesmans M., Rubenstein E.B. *et al.* (2000). The multinational association for supportive care in cancer risk index: a multinational scoring system for identifying low-risk febrile neutropenic cancer patients. *Journal of Clinical Oncology* **18**, 3038–3051.

56. Eggenberger S.K., Krumwiede N., Meiers S.J., Bliesmer M. and Earle P. (2004). Family caring strategies in neutropenia. *Clinical Journal of Oncology Nursing* **8**, 617–621.

57. Goad K.E. and Gralnick H.R. (1996). Coagulation disorders in cancer. *Haematology/Oncology Clinics of North America* **10**, 457–484.

58. Rosen P.J. (1992). Bleeding problems in the cancer patient. *Haematology/Oncology Clinics of North America* **6**, 1315–1329.

59. Kelsley P. (Chairman) (2003). Guidelines for the use of platelet transfusions; British Committee for Standards in Haematology, Blood Transfusion Task Force. *British Journal of Haematology* **122**, 10–23.

60. Tauchmanova L., De Rosa G., Serio B. *et al.* (2003). Avascular necrosis in long-term survivors after allogeneic or autologous stem cell transplantation: a single center experience and a review. *Cancer* **97**, 2453–2461.

61. Roy A.J., Jaffe N. and Djerassi I. (1973). Prophylactic platelet transfusions in children with acute leukaemia. *Transfusion* **13**, 283–290.

62. Kaushansky K. (1996). The thrombocytopenia of cancer. *Haematology/Oncology Clinics of North America* **10**, 431–455.

63. Bayer W.L., Bodensteiner D.C., Tilzer L.L. and Adams M.E. (1992). Use of platelets and other transfusion products in patients with malignancy. *Seminars in Thrombosis and Haemostasis* **18**, 308–391.

64. Socie G., Cahn J.Y., Carmelo J. *et al.* (1997). Avascular necrosis of bone after allogeneic bone marrow transplantation: analysis of risk factors for 4388 patients by the Société Française de Greffe de Moelle (SFGM). *British Journal of Haematology* **97**, 865–870.

65. Hamblin T.J. (1997). Clinician's overview of platelet support. *Transfusion Science* **18**, 351–353.

66. Mollison P.L., Engelfreit C.P. and Contreras M. (1993). *Blood Transfusion in Clinical Medicine.* Oxford: Blackwell Scientific, p. 684.

67. Higgins V.L. (1996). Leucocyte-reduced blood components: patient benefits and practical applications. *Oncology Nursing Forum* **23**, 659–667.

68. Fanning J., Hilgers R.D., Murray K.P., Bolt K. and Aughenbaugh D.M. (1995). Conservative management of chemotherapy-induced thrombocytopenia in women with gynaecologic cancers. *Gynaecologic Oncology* **59**, 191–193.

69. Callow C.R., Swindell R., Randall W. and Choprah R. (2002). The frequency of bleeding complications in patients with haematological malignancy following the introduction of a stringent prophylactic transfusion policy. *British Journal of Haematology* **118**, 677–682.

70. Schiffer C.A., Anderson K.C., Bennett C.L. *et al.* for the American Society of Clinical Oncology. (2001). Platelet transfusion for patients with cancer: clinical practice guidelines for the American Society of Clinical Oncology. *Journal of Clinical Oncology* **19**, 1519–1538.

CHAPTER TWENTY-FIVE

Change in eating habits

Jane Hopkinson

Introduction

We eat to live; but eating contributes far more to our experience of living than merely sustaining bodily functions.

> Food and eating habits and preferences are not simply matters of 'fuelling' ourselves, alleviating hunger pangs, or taking enjoyment in gustatory sensations. Food and eating are central to our subjectivity, or our sense of self, and our experience of embodiment, or the ways in which we live in and through our bodies.[1]

Nutritional science is concerned with the study of what we should take into our bodies to promote, maintain or restore our health. Yet our diet often deviates from one that is appropriate for optimal health. Our eating habits do not only have the purpose of keeping our bodies stoked with the nutrients necessary for survival; they are also shaped by the meaning of foods for ourselves and others. These meanings evolve over time through our interactions with others. We learn that certain foods are good or bad and come to associate them with emotions and moral values.[2] Sweets and cakes are enjoyable, but bad foods over which we should exercise control. So eating becomes intertwined with our identity, as certain foods and patterns of dietary intake come to represent desirable and undesirable personal characteristics. Eating is therefore far more than a practical and functional activity necessary to exist; it is part of being, where being is what it means to live.

This chapter examines how nurses can help people live with changes in eating habits when they have cancer. It looks beyond the possibilities of help offered by biomedicine in the form of pharmacological and nutritional interventions. Non-invasive intervention for changing eating habits may be able to complement biomedical approaches to the problem and offer a unique nursing contribution to the support of people living with eating difficulties associated with cancer.

The nature of change in eating habits

People with cancer may perceive changes in dietary intake and patterns of taking food across their cancer journey, including prior to diagnosis. The prevalence of the symptom varies according to diagnosis and stage of disease. Between 30% and 80% of people with advanced cancer are reported to have anorexia.[3] However, the proportion of people with cancer who experience the symptom as being troublesome is unknown. It seems likely that the degree to which eating habits are experienced as problematic varies across time in response to treatments, other symptoms, social circumstances, and disease status. A survey of 199 people with advanced cancer found 76% to have experienced a decline in their food intake since first becoming unwell. Of these people, 43% were concerned about their eating habits.[4]

What is known about changing eating habits across the cancer journey?

Research into the eating habits of people with cancer has taken one of three approaches. One approach has been to examine the potential for food to be used as treatment for the disease. The goal is to make people better. A second approach has been to search for ways in which food might help manage disease by arresting or reversing symptoms. The goal here is better function in spite of disease. The third approach is a newly emergent line of study that seeks to alleviate eating-related distress. The goal is to help people feel better.

Making people better

There is much interest in the ability of food to promote health. It is known that a diet high in fibre, fruit, and vegetables lowers the risk of contracting cancer.[5] It seems logical that certain foods or dietary supplements might therefore be able to arrest tumour growth once cancer is diagnosed. The popularity of alternative therapies is increasing, with 'designer diets' seen as having the potential for treating cancer, although none as yet have been proven effective.[6] Work is ongoing, such as that looking at the effects of n-3 polyunsaturated fatty acids found in fish oil on both chemotherapy treatments and cancer cachexia.[7] The benefits of fruit, vegetables, and vitamin supplements that contain polyphenols and antioxidants that may slow tumour growth, need to be tested in clinical trials.[8] So, research has yet to demonstrate the efficacy of dietary change in contributing to the management of disease progression. Indeed, the use of dietary supplements, such as minerals and vitamins, during cancer treatment can attenuate its effectiveness. It is for this reason that the American Institute for Cancer Research cautions the use of multivitamins during treatments, recommending intake of no more than the level of dietary reference intakes.[9]

Helping people function better

While it is yet to be proven that diet has a part to play in the treatment of cancer, optimising nutritional status may, nevertheless, be important. Diet may be important to enhancing outcomes from treatments by improving survival time and/or limiting treatment-related morbidity. Tolerance of potentially curable treatment and subsequent morbidity and mortality has been found to be related to pretherapy nutritional status and weight. Those with weight loss prior to treatment have been shown to have poorer survival and be less able to tolerate treatments.[10] Nutritional counselling has been demonstrated to improve protein and energy intake.[11,12] The provision of nutritional support during radiotherapy and chemotherapy has been found to limit weight loss compared with controls receiving no support.[13–15] But, reduction in food intake alone cannot explain the weight loss and nutritional deficits that can accompany cancer.[16] Brown conducted a systematic review of randomised controlled trials where nutritional counselling was offered.[11] The findings across studies were consistent. Intake was enhanced but this was not reflected in measures of survival, quality of life, weight, improved nutritional status, or tumour response to treatment. However, either there may be benefits that have still to be recognised, or perhaps it is yet to be demonstrated that certain groups of patients benefit where others do not.

Optimising nutritional status may also be important to the management of cancer cachexia. Cachexia is a syndrome resulting from primary metabolic response to a tumour and secondary contributory factors, such as reduced dietary intake. Artificial nutritional support, either parental or enteral, has been found to be of no benefit in terms of the survival of people with advanced cancer and cachexia. The outcomes of oral nutritional support in people with advanced cancer are, as yet, unknown.[17]

One way of understanding cachexia is as weight change caused by an imbalance between energy intake and energy expenditure. Personal characteristics (leading to secondary cachexia) and disease-related factors (leading to primary cachexia) influence energy balance. Hence, interventions that correct energy imbalance can be: increasing food intake, decreasing energy expenditure, minimising factors that affect food intake and energy expenditure, and suppressing inflammatory response to the tumour.[11,18] From this perspective the future of managing cancer cachexia lies in combination treatments, such as nutraceuticals (foods with pharmacological properties), offered alongside interventions that conserve energy and consider individual response to symptoms. Many authors urge routine assessment/screening to identify problems with weight and eating in people with involuntary wasting, that might be ameliorated by such an approach.[11,19,20]

Drug trials with patients who have cachexia have demonstrated a placebo effect where controls gain weight.[21] While the reasons for weight gain are poorly understood, they imply that there is potential for non-pharmacological intervention having beneficial outcomes.

Helping people feel better

Little work has been done that examines the experience of living with changing eating habits and cancer. This seems surprising in light of the prevalence of the symptoms and growing interest in the potential for diet to complement pharmacological approaches to illness management. By better understanding the meaning of changing eating habits it might be possible to both enhance the well-being of people living with the symptom, and also enhance the compliance, and hence effectiveness, of any nutritional or pharmacological intervention.

The implications of changing eating habits: sources of distress

In a study of people with advanced cancer,[4,22,23] patients were found to believe that little could be done to help with changing eating habits. In consequence, concerns had not been raised with nurse specialists or other health care professionals. However, more than half the sample was found to be manipulating their diet with the intention of enhancing their well-being, managing other symptoms of their disease, or arresting the progression of cancer.

The study was an exploratory study of the experience of changing eating habits of 30 people with advanced cancer under the care of two community palliative care teams working in the South of England. The participants were invited to talk about their eating habits and weight, describing any changes they had noticed since first considering themselves unwell. Any expressed concerns relating to eating and weight were explored in detail during the interviews.

The self-perceived difficulties experienced in consequence of changing eating habits were wide ranging, and spanned all four of the widely accepted domains of health-related quality of life: physical, psychological, social, and spiritual. Physical changes, including declining desire and ability to eat, were believed to lead to other symptoms that compromised quality of life, such as weakness and changed physical appearance. The inability to continue to participate in established patterns of taking food within one's social network and manage weight through eating led to feelings of isolation and loss of control that compromised quality of life in the psychological domain. The social domain was compromised because social occasions often involved the accepting and sharing of food. Relationships could change where food refusal was interpreted as rebuffing a caring act. Finally, declining appetite and loss of weight symbolised illness and approach of death, prompting concerns of a spiritual nature. Figure 25.1 gives examples of some of the concerns expressed by the study participants (all names have been changed to protect the anonymity of the participants).

The concerns about changing eating habits expressed by the 30 people with advanced cancer studied may be shared by people earlier in their cancer journey. This is yet to be demonstrated empirically.

Strategies to help people live with changing eating habits

The nurse specialists who were supporting the people who participated in the study above, detailed the help that they were offering in response to the eating-related concerns of which they were aware. In addition to nutritional supplements and medications, they recommended:

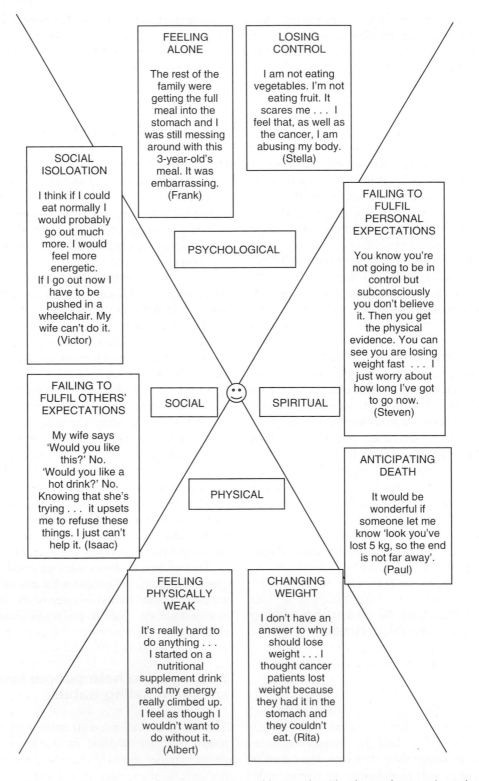

Figure 25.1 Examples of eating-related concerns expressed by people with advanced cancer in each of the four health-related quality-of-life domains.

the routine assessment of physical problems, offering tips for physical problems, and providing information. Information was seen as important to help people understand the cause of eating change. It was also seen as important to give insights into other people's experience of changing eating habits to lessen feelings of isolation. Table 25.1 details all the nurse participants' recommendations for helping people with concerns, alongside recommendations found in the literature (presented in italic). It is interesting that both the nurse participants in the study and the literature focus on identifying helpful interventions for physical changes that can cause concern to people with cancer.

At the more general level of principles for palliative care, the literature emphasises a shift in the purpose of interventions when cancer becomes advanced. This shift is from the goal of optimising nutrition and survival to that of improving quality of life.[31–33] It has been recommended that in order to enhance quality of life, overall distress for patients and families, including physical, psychosocial, and existential issues, should be addressed through the facilitation of disclosure and acknowledgement of individual concerns.[19,24,34] Psychological and behavioural interventions, such as attention to ambience at meal times and relaxation techniques have been suggested to have the potential to help with distress.[35] Written information and nutritional counselling have also been recommended as being helpful.[34]

Of note is the lack of attention paid, both in the literature and by health care professionals involved in the study described above, to the potential for eating changes to impact on relationships. While there is acknowledgement that changing eating habits are a source of conflict between the person with cancer and those involved in their care,[36,37] little is offered in the way of suggestions of how to help with a difficulty such as:

> Because I can't be persuaded to eat anything else, there's an atmosphere in this house . . . Always hassle. I used to like being here. I hate it now.
>
> Ron

It may be that many concerns that arise in consequence of changing eating habits can not be addressed by working with the person with cancer

in isolation from their social network. The rhetoric of palliative care supports family-centred care. However, there is still much work to be done in establishing appropriate and effective interventions for carers.[38]

Implications for practice

Helping people to live with eating changes across their cancer journey may involve more than consideration of nutritional intake and treatment of disease. It may be possible to complement these very important interventions with strategies that can enhance well-being for those who live with the symptom, and their families.

Routine and recurrent assessment of change in eating habits is important if difficulties with eating that are amenable to intervention are to be identified and acted upon. Assessment is key to establishing if other symptoms, such as pain, depression, nausea, constipation, or breathlessness are impacting on dietary intake.

Assessment also facilitates communication and the opportunity to explore the meaning of eating changes and how they are shaping life for the person with cancer. By asking about past and present eating habits, the nurse can begin to build a picture of the changes that have taken place. This approach affords the opportunity to acknowledge the symptom as potentially troublesome and, through assessment and dialogue, find out about the concerns these changes have raised. Understanding the patient's particular beliefs about eating and emotions evoked by food can help tailor interventions so that they are appropriate to the problems that are particular to the individual. Information and tips on commonly experienced problems can be offered in response to need and preference. Urging increased dietary intake with suggestions such as 'eat whatever you want' without specific recommendations may be unhelpful.[26] Similarly, offering general advice, such as 'little and often' may be equally unhelpful if offered without consideration of context to the person who can 'eat little but not often'. Consideration can be given to the appropriateness of further screening and/or referral for specialist advice from other professionals, such as dieticians,

Table 25.1 Interventions/advice offered by nurse specialists in response to patients' concerns about eating habits (interventions/advice in italics are additional recommendations found in published papers)

Quality-of-life domain	Problem causing concern	Intervention/advice
Physical	Decline in food intake	Eat at time in the day when most hungry
		Eat at a time which is easiest, e.g. least pain/fatigue
		Eat energy- and protein-rich foods
		Try nutritional supplements in different ways e.g. ice cubes
		Take a diet that is easy to eat, e.g. soft diet, soups and puddings
		Try eating what you fancy
		Try experimenting with different foods and flavours
		Try eating little and often
		Try to avoid drinking prior to or during meals
		Try avoiding fatty/greasy foods that delay stomach emptying
		Try gentle exercise before eating
		Consider if environment is conducive to eating, e.g. appearance of food
		Offer information booklets on optimising nutritional intake e.g. Cancerbackup
		Assess bowel habits
		Assess fit of dentures
	Nausea	Assess for a pattern to the experience of nausea
		Assess compliance with medications
		Take anti-emetic pre-meal
		Take medications routinely
		Try cold foods with no odour
		Try avoiding fatty/greasy foods that delay stomach emptying
		Try ginger flavours
	Dry mouth	Routinely assess mouth
		Sip fluids when eating
		Try sucking pineapple chunks or ice chips
		Try moist food
		Try sucking sweets
		Vaseline for dry lips
	Weakness	Assess need for help with shopping and meal preparation
		Try buying pre-prepared meals
		Offer aids e.g. straws/easy grip cutlery
	Taste change	*Regular oral hygiene*
		Prepare foods in ways that do not create odour e.g. microwave
		Try non-metallic utensils
		Try cold foods
		Try experimenting by adding flavouring, e.g. salt, sugar, spices, herbs
	Food aversions	*Advise of potential of developing food aversion*
		Avoid favourite foods at time of treatment
Psychological	Feeling isolated by eating habits	Seek concerns
		Listen to concerns
		Information about changes in eating/weight that can accompany cancer
		Explain declining food intake is a common problem
Social	Eating habits perceived as antisocial (dribbling)	Referral to dietician and speech therapist
	Ill-fitting clothes	Help apply for a grant for new clothes
Spiritual	Weight loss symbolising decline	Discussion of prognosis

Source of suggestions in italics: references 24–30.

speech therapists, occupational therapists and physiotherapists.

Seeking information about the experience of eating and exploring feelings and attitudes about food is challenging. This is because it is likely to lead to discussions of relationships, death, and dying, which reveal the limitations of personal autonomy and medical science in eradicating disease and its consequences. However, if eating changes can bring about rupture between body, self, and society,[39] then it is an approach that can support the renegotiation of identity through encouraging story telling.[40] It is an approach where the skill of listening can become therapy, not only through the facilitation of story telling, but through opening up the opportunity for personal knowledge of illness to come together with nursing knowledge, revealing possibilities and choices that can enhance well-being.[41]

Encouraging people to express concerns and problems has the potential to open up opportunities for further professional interventions. In addition, for some it will facilitate personal decision making and action in self-managing eating-related concerns. People may be empowered through support to help themselves.

Implications for research

Decline in food intake and weight loss have implications for morbidity and prognosis. It is unsurprising and desirable that biomedical science seeks to arrest or reverse these symptoms through drug and nutritional interventions. Making people better by eradicating disease or improving function by arresting symptoms is to be championed. However, there is also a little explored potential for helping people live with the symptoms. This is an approach that through understanding the meaning of the symptoms, aims to complement conventional treatments. Non-invasive interventions across the cancer journey may lead to enhanced nutritional status, delayed weight loss, mitigation of distress, and enhancement of quality of life. Much empirical work is still to be done seeking and evaluating supportive interventions for troublesome eating changes that can accompany cancer.

Conclusion

Nurses can help people live with changing eating habits across the cancer journey. To help someone manage the everyday activity of eating when it becomes a troublesome symptom of illness challenges nurses to look beyond the practical problem of compromised nutrition. The challenge is to seek the meaning of the change for the individual and other members of their social network. Acknowledging and responding to concerns about eating habits may be one of the most effective caring activities that the nurse can offer to someone with cancer.

References

1. Lupton D. (1996). *Food, the Body and the Self*. London: Sage.
2. Lupton D. (1994). Food, memory and meaning: the symbolic and social nature of food events. *Sociological Review* **42**, 664–685.
3. Poole K. and Froggatt K. (2002). Loss of weight and loss of appetite in advanced cancer: a problem for the patient, the carer, or the health professional? *Palliative Medicine* **16**, 499–506.
4. Hopkinson J.B., MacDonald J., Wright D.N.M. and Corner J.L. (2006). The prevalence of concern about weight loss and change in eating habits in people with advanced cancer. *Journal of Pain and Symptom Management* **32**, 322–331.
5. Shaw C. and Lewis S. (2005). *Cancer: Food, Facts & Recipes*. London: Hamlyn.
6. Cohen J. and Lefor A.T. (2001). Nutritional support and cancer. *Nutrition* **17**, 698–699.
7. Baracos V.E., Mazurak V.C. and Ma D.W.L. (2004). n-3 Polyunsaturated fatty acids throughout the cancer trajectory: influence on disease incidence, progression, response to therapy and cancer-associated cachexia. *Nutritional Research Reviews* **17**, 177–192.
8. McCarthy D.O. (2003). Rethinking nutritional support for persons with cancer cachexia. *Biological Research for Nursing* **5**, 3–17.
9. Norman H.A., Butrum R.R., Feldman E. *et al.* (2003). The role of dietary supplements during cancer therapy. *The American Society for Nutritional Sciences Journal of Nutrition* **133**, 3794S–3799S.
10. Andreyev H.J.N., Norma A.R., Oates J. and Cunningham D. (1998). Why do patients with weight loss have a worse outcome when undergoing chemotherapy for gastrointestinal malignancies? *European Journal of Cancer* **34**, 503–509.

11. Brown J.K. (2002). A systematic review of the evidence on symptom management of cancer-related anorexia and cachexia. *Oncology Nursing Forum* **29**, 517–532.

12. Ovesen L., Allingstrup L., Hannibal J., Mortensen E.L. and Hansen O.P. (1993). Effect of dietary counseling on food intake, body weight, response rate, survival, and quality of life in cancer patients undergoing chemotherapy: a prospective, randomized study. *Journal of Clinical Oncology* **11**, 2043–2049.

13. Persson C., Johansson B.K., Sjoden P.O. and Glimelius L.G. (2002). A randomised study of nutritional support in patients with colorectal and gastric cancer. *Nutrition and Cancer* **42**, 48–58.

14. Cella D., Paul D., Yount S. *et al.* (2003). What are the most important symptom targets when treating advanced cancer? A survey of providers in the National Comprehensive Cancer Network (NCCN). *Cancer Investigation* **21**, 526–535.

15. Ravasco P., Monteiro-Grillo I. and Camilo M.E. (2003). Does nutrition influence quality of life in cancer patients undergoing radiotherapy? *Radiotherapy Oncology* **67**, 213–220.

16. Tisdale M.J. (2002). Cachexia in cancer patients. *Nature Reviews* **2**, 862–871.

17. Strasser F. (2003) Eating-related disorders in patients with advanced cancer. *Supportive Care in Cancer* **11**, 11–20.

18. Brown J.K, Byers T., Doyle C. *et al.* (2003). Nutrition and physical activity during and after cancer treatment: an American Cancer Society guide for informed choices. *Cancer Journal for Clinicians* **53**, 268–291.

19. Strasser F. and Bruera E. (2002). Update on anorexia and cachexia. *Hematology/Oncology Clinics of North America* **16**, 589–617.

20. Thoresen L., Fjeldstad I., Krogstad K., Kaasa S. and Falkmer U.G. (2002). Nutritional status of patients with advanced cancer: the value of using the subjective global assessement of nutritional status as a screening tool. *Palliative Medicine* **16**, 33–42.

21. Dahele M. and Fearon K.C.H. (2004). Research methodology: cancer cachexia syndrome. *Palliative Medicine* **18**, 409–417.

22. Hopkinson J.B. and Corner J.L. (2006). Helping patients with advanced cancer live with concerns about eating: a challenge for palliative care physicians. *Journal of Pain and Symptom Management* **31**, 293–305.

23. Hopkinson J.B., Wright D.N.M. and Corner J.L. (2006). The experience of weight loss in people with advanced cancer. *Journal of Advanced Nursing* **54**, 304–312.

24. Hill D. (2001). A practical approach to nutritional support for patients with advanced cancer. *International Journal of Palliative Nursing* **7**, 317–321.

25. Berteretche M.V., Dalix A.M., d'Ornano A.M. *et al.* (2004). Decreased taste sensitivity in cancer patients under chemotherapy. *Supportive Care in Cancer* **12**, 571–576.

26. Whitman M.M. (2000). The starving patient: supportive care for people with cancer. *Clinical Journal of Oncology Nursing* **4**, 121–125.

27. Shaw C. (1997). Nutrition and cancer. *Nursing Times* **93**, 1–6.

28. Wilkes G. (2000). Nutrition: the forgotten ingredient in cancer care. *American Journal of Nursing* **100**, 46–51.

29. Eberhardie C. (2002). Nutrition support in palliative care. *Nursing Standard* **17**, 47–52.

30. Grant M. and Kravits K. (2000). Symptoms and their impact on nutrition. *Seminars in Oncology Nursing* **16**, 113–121.

31. Arbolino L. and Sacchet D. (2000). Advanced cancer patient. *Topics in Clinical Nutrition* **15**, 12–19.

32. Bachmann P., Marti-Massoud C., Blanc-Vincent M.P. *et al.* (2003). Summary version of the Standards, Options and Recommendations for palliative or terminal nutrition in adults with progressive cancer. *British Journal of Cancer* **89(suppl. 1)**, S107–S110.

33. Holder H. (2003). Nursing management of nutrition in cancer and palliative care. *British Journal of Nursing* **12**, 667–668, 670, 672–674.

34. Strasser F. (2003). Eating-related disorders in patients with advanced cancer. *Supportive Care in Cancer* **11**, 11–20.

35. Higginson I. and Winget C. (1996). Psychological impact of cancer cachexia on the patient and family. In Bruera E. and Higginson I. (eds.) *Cachexia-anorexia in Cancer Patients*. Oxford: Oxford University Press, pp. 172–184.

36. Holden C.M. (1991). Anorexia in the terminally ill cancer patient: the emotional impact on the patient and the family. *Hospice Journal: Physical, Psychological and Pastoral Care of the Dying* **7**, 73–84.

37. Meares C.J. (1997). Primary caregiver perceptions of intake cessation in patients who are terminally ill. *Oncology Nursing Forum* **24**, 1751–1757.

38. Harding J. and Higginson I.J. (2003). What is the best way to help caregivers in cancer and palliative care? A systematic literature review of interventions and their effectiveness. *Palliative Medicine* **17**, 63–74.

39. Williams S.J. (2000). Chronic illness as biographical disruption or biographical disruption as chronic illness? Reflections on a core concept. *Sociology of Health and Illness* **22**, 40–67.

40. Mathieson C.M. and Stam H.J. (1995). Renegotiating identity: cancer narratives. *Sociology of Health and Illness* **17**, 283–306.

41. Paterson J. and Zderad L. (1976). *Humanistic Nursing*. New York: John Wiley.

CHAPTER TWENTY-SIX

Sexuality and cancer

Isabel White

Michel Foucault, a philosopher and sociologist, remains one of the most influential writers on sexuality, exploring this complex concept within its socio-cultural and historical contexts.[1] He asserted that in contrast to being stable and pre-ordained by hormonal influences and anatomical structures, sexuality and its expression is multi-faceted, diverse and, most importantly, socially constructed by men, women and thus society. Foucault rejected the popular hypothesis that sexuality is repressed at both an individual and societal level. Instead, his critique illuminates the extensive and never-ending discourse on sexuality that has developed in Western cultures from the beginning of the 19th century to the present day. Hence, in exploring sexuality within cancer care it is imperative that nurses and other health care professionals acknowledge the paradox created by their personal and collective values, beliefs, and assumptions with regard to the importance of sexuality and its expression for those coping with the rigors of modern cancer treatment. For it is those beliefs and attitudes that frequently dictate the comfort or discomfort we experience in addressing sexuality through the development and delivery of contemporary cancer services.[2,3]

With improvements in the treatment of many types of cancer, there is increasing emphasis on the quality of life for *survivors*. Cancer is increasingly experienced as a chronic as opposed to acutely fatal illness, and so greater emphasis needs to be placed on understanding the challenges of living with the physical, psychological, and relationship consequences of both illness and treatment. While there is acknowledgement that the impact of cancer and its treatment on a person's sexuality is an important topic for research within cancer care, published literature tends to limit its exploration to a narrow biomedical view of sexual dysfunction and its medical or pharmacological management. While biomedical perspectives are clearly relevant, it is also important to understand the psychological response of the individual with cancer and the subsequent impact on the couple relationship as a key source of both difficulty and support.[4]

Sexuality embraces the internalised image we hold of ourselves (self-concept); the feelings we have about ourselves (self-esteem); and how we would like other people to see us. Sexuality incorporates more than sexual desires, expression, and orientation, and includes touching, intimacy, and the physical closeness of others. Sexuality is also influenced by our personality and roles held within our families, relationships, work, and society.[5]

For some, sexuality also encompasses their identity as someone who is, or has the potential to be, fertile. Fertility concerns are often addressed as an integral component of sexuality and may be used by some health professionals as an indirect and perhaps less-embarrassing way of discussing the sexual consequences of therapy.[6]

This can be an appropriate strategy to adopt where the person with cancer is of reproductive age and still has the capacity to be fertile. It may be unhelpful where the person has lost their reproductive potential through ageing, as a direct result of cancer treatment or is someone who values their sexual expression as a distinct and separate aspect of their life and relationships.

While the importance of sexuality to a person's quality of life is recognised, many health professionals remain reluctant to address the sexual consequences of cancer therapy as part of their professional practice.[6–8] Lawler explored the social and psychological difficulties nurses face in dealing with body parts and functions considered taboo and normally only encountered within the context of close personal or intimate relationships.[9] She suggested the cultural (sexual) meanings embedded in body parts such as the breasts and genitalia often create embarrassment in care delivery. Her research discovered that while nurses were taught how to perform various body care procedures, they did not know 'how to manage socially what those procedures entailed, nor how they might respond emotionally to what they had to do' (p.122).

Serious illness and disability remove a person from their accustomed personal, social, and sexual relations, threatening self-esteem and attractiveness at a time when the need for intimacy and belonging may be greatest.[10] Even before confirmation of a diagnosis of cancer, psychological and physical effects of the illness can impinge upon a person's sexuality. The development of symptoms such as abnormal bleeding, lethargy, weight loss, and pain have the potential to cause a negative change in one's self-concept and body image. This ultimately affects a person's self-esteem and self-confidence, and in turn impacts on sexual expression.

During the period of diagnosis and treatment, not only may anxieties and fears lessen the desire for sex, but sexual expression may be considered a low priority while the person comes to terms with the threat of the diagnosis and copes with the demands of treatment side-effects.[10–12] There may be uncertainties about the future, perceived or actual threat to fertility and body image, and the experience of pain and disfigurement. Shame and guilt about the perceived causes of the cancer, and feelings of helplessness and isolation may lead

to an increase in anxiety and depression, which in turn will adversely affect sexual interest and the ability to respond sexually to a partner.[13,14]

A woman following creation of a stoma describes the interplay between the psychological, physical and functional elements of sexual expression eloquently:

> I mean internally, by losing your rectum, are you the same person internally? What effect will it have to have a penis pressing against the walls of your vagina when there is no rectum? And if you have got that vigilance there as well, and this affects sexual response . . . you are lying on the bed and half of you is on auto-pilot and the other half of you is thinking, hang on, is the bag still safe, or, oh yuk, I can hear it go gurgle, gurgle or squish, squish? [p.409][15]

The interrelationship of this woman's physical and psychological experiences of external disfigurement and changed internal anatomy resulted in a loss of spontaneity and increased self-consciousness during periods of intimacy. As Manderson illustrates, 'Pleasurable sex, idealized, is about being able to lose control, but people can only lose control when they are confident their bodies are in control in the first place' (p. 409).[15]

It is important to recognise that the diverse manifestations of altered sexuality more frequently result from the complex interplay of physical symptoms, psychological reactions, and partner or couple responses to both cancer and its treatment, as opposed to a more obvious causal relationship such as the erectile failure associated with radical prostatectomy. Hence, it is imperative that nurses in cancer care adopt a broad definition of altered sexuality and develop an inclusive frame of reference for sexual health assessment in cancer care.

Table 26.1 lists some possible effects of cancer treatment on sexual functioning.

Cancer can cause a loss of sexual desire throughout the illness experience. Feeling sexually unattractive due to alopecia, nausea, vomiting, altered bowel habit, and disfiguring surgery is common. Women may experience intense symptoms from treatment-induced menopause such as irritability, hot flushes, loss of sexual interest, and vaginal dryness.[16,17]

Effects of pelvic or breast radiotherapy such as vaginal stenosis and fibrosis, or changes in breast

Table 26.1 Possible effects of cancer treatment on sexual function

Site of cancer	Cancer treatment	Functional changes	Potential impact on sexuality
Head and neck	Removal of all or parts of the facial and oral structures, laryngectomy, head and neck radiotherapy	Dysphagia, dysphasia, trismus, changes in salivary texture and volume, taste changes, skin alterations, loss of voice and normal breathing mechanisms (tracheostomy)	Altered appearance and communication difficulties leading to social anxiety and avoidance, difficulty in kissing, decreased sensory perception
Breast	Mastectomy, breast-conservation treatment (local excision and radiotherapy), prosthesis, reconstruction, adjuvant hormone therapy and/or chemotherapy	Scarring, changes in colour, texture, and sensation in the breast tissues, temporary or permanent infertility, nausea, vomiting, alopecia, hot flushes, atrophic vaginitis, weight gain, fatigue	Reduced or loss of sexual interest, difficulty in sexual arousal, dyspareunia secondary to vaginal dryness/vaginitis, reduced sexual enjoyment
Cervical, endometrial, and ovarian	Wertheim's hysterectomy, oophorectomy, external beam pelvic radiotherapy and brachytherapy, adjuvant or concurrent chemotherapy	Removal of top third of vagina, infertility and menopausal changes, vaginal dryness, stenosis and fibrosis, bowel changes, cystitis, radiation skin reactions, fatigue, nausea, vomiting, alopecia, weight gain	Reduced or lost sexual desire, dyspareunia secondary to vaginal dryness and stenosis, reduced depth of vaginal penetration, potential for altered orgasmic sensation associated with loss of uterine contractions during orgasm
Vulva	Partial or radical vulvectomy, vulval radiotherapy	Scarring and altered appearance of external genitalia, loss of clitoris, sensory changes (numbness), narrowing of vaginal introitus, moist desquamation	Dyspareunia due to narrowed vaginal introitus, reduced or absent orgasmic capacity, difficulty in becoming sexually aroused due to reduced sensitivity
Testicular	Orchidectomy, retroperitoneal lymph node dissection, pelvic/ abdominal radiotherapy, systemic chemotherapy	Altered scrotal appearance (prosthesis), inability to ejaculate or retrograde ejaculation, infertility (temporary or permanent), fatigue, alopecia, nausea and vomiting	Reduced sexual interest due to fatigue and altered body image, erectile difficulties due to fatigue, altered orgasmic sensation due to ejaculatory changes
Prostate	Radical prostatectomy, pelvic radiotherapy, hormone therapy (adjuvant or sole therapy)	Erectile dysfunction (temporary or permanent), transient painful ejaculation, permanent reduction in semen volume, infertility, urinary incontinence, bowel changes, hot flushes, loss of muscle tone, changes in hair distribution, fatigue	Loss of sexual desire due to reduced testosterone levels and fatigue, erectile dysfunction due to hormonal, nerve and/or vascular changes, altered orgasmic sensation due to ejaculatory changes

Table 26.1 Continued

Site of cancer	Cancer treatment	Functional changes	Potential impact on sexuality
Colorectal	Abdominoperineal resection, sphincter-sparing surgery, pelvic radiotherapy and/or adjuvant or chemoradiation	Scarring, loss of rectum, stoma formation, altered bowel habit, radiation-induced skin reactions, fatigue, infertility, alopecia, nausea and vomiting	Loss of sexual desire due to altered body image and fatigue, erectile dysfunction due to nerve and vascular changes, dyspareunia

sensation may also be experienced. Studies of the psychosocial and sexual effects of radiotherapy and surgery on women with cervical cancer suggest that symptoms and anxieties experienced by the women negatively affect their feelings of attractiveness and self-confidence; as a result sexual difficulties may persist long after completion of treatment.[18,19]

Men may experience loss of desire, ejaculation and erectile difficulties as unwanted effects of surgery, radiotherapy, or hormone therapy.[20]

Psychosexual adjustment following treatment for cancer is dependent on numerous factors: the meaning of the loss (for example, a breast or limb), pre-illness psychosexual functioning, the specific treatment and site of the cancer, and interpersonal relationships.[6,10,14] The roles of the partner and family are important in enabling psychosexual adjustment and reducing feelings of isolation and abandonment.[5,6] Without communication and understanding, even the strongest of relationships can be destroyed. One man in Schover's book[6] had lost interest in sex due to the fatigue associated with his treatment for chronic leukaemia and spoke of the importance of support from his partner:

> Going through this illness really has reminded me how much I love you and value your support. I think our marriage has always been good, but sometimes we've taken each other for granted. I think I often don't tell you how I feel, and I just wanted you to know how important you are to me [p.40].

The experience of cancer and its treatment can expose and challenge pre-illness sexual and relationship strengths and limitations. An insight into the experience of one female patient is described in Personal account 26.1.

A significant proportion of the patient education literature offering practical advice regarding sexual difficulties associated with cancer has tended to come from America.[6,21–23]

However an increasing number of UK-based cancer charities (Cancerbackup, Prostate Cancer Charity, Breast Cancer Care, Cancer Research UK) now produce high-quality, peer-reviewed web-based materials and information booklets that address a range of sexual concerns associated with cancer and its treatment. Patients should be encouraged to access these resources, particularly if there is a sense that they are finding it difficult to acknowledge their need for further information about this intimate and private aspect of their lives.

While there is an expanding awareness of sexuality across the lifespan within contemporary Western society, it remains difficult for many people to ask for information or help with sexual concerns. Research suggests that many health care professionals are too embarrassed to discuss sexual issues; some feel it is not relevant to their management of the effects of illness and treatment. Although an increasing number of education programmes offer information about sexual dysfunction and cancer, there is often inadequate focus on the communication and assessment skills necessary to place this knowledge at the patient's disposal.[7–10,24–26]

To be able to offer professional help, a knowledgeable and non-judgemental approach is needed, as well as being comfortable with sexual attitudes and behaviours that may be different from one's own. Skilled communication is also

Personal account 26.1

I met Diana when she was undergoing pelvic radiotherapy for the treatment of cervical cancer. She would come to the department with her husband; they seemed a close couple, spending lots of time together now they were both retired. In the last week of Diana's treatment, I had scheduled some time to talk to her and her husband about resuming sexual contact and to answer any questions or concerns she still had about the use of vaginal dilators. When it came to her turn to be seen, her husband had popped out of the department for a cigarette and she indicated she would prefer it if we just started, as she would pass on anything not already covered in our previous joint meetings. I began by reminding her of the information we had already discussed about the effects of radiation on the vaginal tissues and the need for use of intimate lubricants to assist in making intercourse more comfortable. I also touched on the myths some people hold with regard to pelvic cancer and radiotherapy, such as transmitting cancer or radiation to a partner through sexual contact. The discussion seemed to be going smoothly and I was just about to congratulate myself on a job well done when Diana smiled broadly at me and said:

Isabel, thanks for all that but to be honest I am just going to tell him I can't have sex any more because I'm radioactive! You see he is a lovely husband and has been a great dad to our two boys but he's never been very good in bed. Since I got this cancer I've been bleeding after, you know, and I'm tired all the time, so sex is just a weekly chore I have to go along with after *Antiques Road Show* every Sunday. If this is an excuse I can use to let him down gently and let me off the hook too then that's a good thing, isn't it?

While I was sad for Diana that sex had never been a particularly enjoyable part of her relationship with Jim, I could sense that she was reluctant to consider the steps necessary to alter that.

Identified problems
- Diana's pre-existing dissatisfaction with her sexual relationship
- Lack of communication with her husband regarding her sexual needs
- Impact of post-coital bleeding as a symptom of illness
- Further loss of sexual interest associated with recent surgery and fatigue resulting from pelvic radiotherapy
- Anxiety about resuming sexual relationship post-treatment.

Interventions and recommendations
- Active listening to Diana's story to identify and pick up cues to conduct a comprehensive assessment of her sexual concerns
- Provision of information with regard to the causes of loss of sexual interest and the contribution of anxiety in maintaining difficulties
- Discussion of fears and reluctance in talking to her husband, and the importance of couple communication
- Practical advice regarding resumption of sexual expression post-treatment, e.g. use of dilators, vibrators, personal lubricants, relaxation exercises, and alternative sexual positions to reduce any pain experienced
- Provision of information about sources of both general and specialist sexual and relationship counselling should Diana wish to pursue this.

While I had made Diana aware that there were services where she and Jim could get further help if they wanted to explore changes to their sexual relationship in the future, we both acknowledged that she was happy to let this aspect of her relationship come to what she saw as a natural conclusion.

required to educate and support the patient and their partner in a positive way.[3,5,27]

A guide to talking about sexual issues is provided in Care strategy 26.1.

Health professionals in cancer care are not expected to be experts in all aspects of sexual function or dysfunction, but patients and their partners should be able to expect practitioners who can explain the potential impact of cancer and treatment effects on the relevant stages of the human sexual response cycle.[30] This should include changes to sexual interest/desire levels,

Care strategy 26.1   A guide to talking about sexual issues

As in other aspects of sensitive communication, there is no definitive formula. Each patient, partner, practitoner and context is different, and the questions you ask will depend on the factors deemed relevant to that situation, the verbal and non-verbal cues identified, and the practitioner's '. . . humility to be able to listen without needing to "know", to take the risk of hearing without the certainty of answers'.[28] The following are examples of communication principles that can be used to create opportunity for patients, partners and practitoners to broach the subject of sexuality.

Do:
• create an atmosphere that is comfortable and private
• act in a professional and caring manner
• acknowledge the sensitivity of the topic and explore its relevance to planning care and rehabilitation
• spend some time establishing a rapport with the person before proceeding to issues that are more sensitive
• be alert to cues, giving them permission to discuss sexual issues
• include the partner whenever possible.

Don't:
• assume anything
• prejudge individuals or relationships
• presume you share and understand the same language and meaning about sex.

During nursing assessment, ask:
• do you currently have a partner?
• how does your partner feel about your illness?
• has this illness affected your relationship in any way?
• is the physical/sexual side of your relationship important to you/your partner?
• has your sexual relationship been affected by this illness or treatment?

or

• are you worried about the effects of this treatment or illness on your relationship (intimate or sexual)?
• have you coped with times like this before?
• what do you want most from your partner now?
• what would help you most? Is there any way I can help you with that?
• what do you think your partner's reaction would be?[29]

In providing information try to:
• find out the patient/couple's existing knowledge about the disease and treatment and what their doctor has told them. Correct any myths and misconceptions and build on previous knowledge. Offer manageable pieces of information and explore any anxieties they have about the illness and treatment:
  – what do you understand about your illness or treatment?
  – what worries you most about your illness or treatment?

Where sexual issues are already a priority for the patient/partner to discuss, then these initial open questions may prompt direct or indirect discussion of sexual concerns. If this appears not to be the case, the sexual impact of illness, treatment, or supportive care (e.g. drug side-effects) strategies may be best addressed along with other essential components of treatment effects. Sometimes sexuality can be raised through a general statement that gives the patient and their partner the opportunity to ask further specific questions should they wish, or simply to note the general information being given. For example:

• many patients lose their confidence in being sexual because of tiredness, worries, or symptoms associated with their illness or treatment. Do you have any concerns in this area?

Let them know that they can talk to someone in their treatment team about it and about any specialist sources of treatment and sexual counselling that are available. Let patients know that sexuality is a recognised and important part of their care, that it is OK to talk or ask about any concerns they have.

impact on female sexual arousal or male erections, likelihood of pain during sex, ability to achieve orgasm/ejaculation associated with surgery, radiotherapy, chemotherapy, endocrine therapy, and the sexual side-effects of medication.

Practitioners are likely to have differing levels of knowledge, experience and interpersonal skills in relation to addressing the sexual consequences of cancer and its treatment. What is important to recognise is that all practitioners can offer some level of sexual assessment and supportive care, even if the more specialist or complex aspects of sexual health care are managed through referral to other designated services. The *P LI SS IT* model is a guide to the different levels of intervention possible in the management of sexual difficulties.[31] It broadly mirrors the levels of generic psychological service provision recommended within the recent UK supportive and palliative care policy guidance for adults with cancer.[32]

Nurses will differ in their ability to meet the specialist knowledge and skills associated with each stage; however, what is most important is that every nurse can address the issue, listen, and then refer on when she feels she has reached the limit of what she can offer at an individual and service level.

P refers to *permission* This means allowing someone to feel at ease with their own sexuality and making it explicit that this topic is a legitimate aspect of supportive cancer care. In Personal account 26.1, Diana is given the opportunity to express concerns about her sexuality, her relationship with her husband, and what she wants in relation to her rehabilitation goals. Asking questions in a sensitive manner and listening carefully to the replies can be supportive in itself. Not everyone wants to discuss sexual problems, but they need to know they can should the occasion arise in the future. As discussed earlier, the threat of the illness may override issues of sexuality. A crisis such as new diagnosis, recurrence, or treatment setbacks may not be the most appropriate time.

There is no research to suggest the best time to broach sexual consequences of cancer and its treatment, although there is agreement that discussion should be an integral part of supportive care at diagnosis, treatment, and follow-up.[32] The admission period provides an ideal opportunity to get to know someone, to find out their story and any concerns they may have. The assessment is pivotal to meeting needs; however, lip service is often paid to assessing sexuality. One reason may be because assessment tools tend to divide the body and mind into separate entities, and to begin an intimate conversation relating to a person's sexuality or sexual functioning is often challenging. A more effective strategy might be to ask the person to tell their story: 'Tell me about your illness, how it all began'. Through this approach cues can be picked up, allowing the conversation to be fluid, moving gently from less-sensitive topics to issues that are more sensitive.

When giving information it is essential to allow patients and their partners to express their anxieties and fears. Talking generally about the effects of treatment on sexual functioning will provide an opportunity to individualise the discussion at a pace dictated by the couple and their specific circumstances.

LI refers to *limited information*. Providing information should be limited to immediate needs. In Diana's situation, these include explaining how cancer treatments and worry can exacerbate pre-existing problems, how to use vaginal dilators and lubricants, helping her to clarify her goals for recovery post-treatment, putting her sexual problems in perspective, and reducing anxiety. It can also incorporate correcting myths and misconceptions such as 'Is cancer contagious?' or 'Can radiation be sexually transmitted?'. Talking about treatment sequelae should include information about possible impairments directly resulting from treatment, e.g. vaginal dryness and fibrosis. Once treatment is over, getting on with life is a high priority. Resuming sexual relationships, returning to work, and socialising once again may be difficult.[18] Support and advice are essential to enable adjustment. Being more forthright but gentle, by asking 'How are things going sexually for you and your partner?' is possible, if done sensitively and in privacy.

SS refers to *specific suggestions*. This includes giving information about strategies to help overcome specific sexual problems related to the disease or treatment. This might be about the the need to try alternative forms of sexual expression following pelvic cancer treatment, the use of drugs for erectile dysfunction, or the management of a stoma during sexual activity. Following reconstruction of the penis, breast, vulva, or vagina, specific advice about what to expect after the operation, together with assessment and discussion of sexual expression and goals, are essential to aid adaptation. Although surgical reconstruction has the potential to improve body appearance and feelings of masculinity and femininity, function will be altered. Among the changes there will be different sensations and altered appearance. Specific advice may also include using alternative sexual positions for where the vagina or penis may have been shortened, or how to modify present sexual activities when there are symptoms such as pain or fatigue.

IT refers to *intensive therapy*. This is normally intervention by a specialist in psychosexual therapy, medicine, or related fields such as erectile dysfunction services and couple counselling. Practitioners need to recognise their limitations and refer on where appropriate. For instance, in Diana's situation if she wanted to address pre-existing sexual difficulties with her husband, a psychosexual therapist would probably be an appropriate referral. When a sexual difficulty is identified, the nurse needs to know what services are available locally and to be able to discuss the possible treatment interventions with the patient or couple prior to onward referral with the patient's consent.

Nurses need organisational support to discuss their difficulties and experiences, access specialist

Research study 26.1

Hedestig O., Sandman P., Tomic R. and Widmark A. (2005). Living after external beam radiotherapy of localized prostate cancer: a qualitative analysis of patient narratives. *Cancer Nursing* **28**, 310–317.[33]

This qualitative study provides a detailed description of the process of recovery and adjustment for 10 Swedish men following external beam radiotherapy for localised prostate cancer. The men (aged 61–69 years, all married) were interviewed (taped and transcribed verbatim) in their own homes between 15 and 36 months post-completion of radiotherapy, with 8 of the 10 being interviewed on a second occasion to expand on topics raised in the first interview.

A qualitative content analysis of the transcripts revealed four key themes:

To bear the emotional experience of the illness alone, A sense of being exposed, Striving for a sense of having control in a new life situation and Striving to become reconciled with a new life situation [p.312].

As the themes suggest, the dominant experience of these men was of managing their emotional reactions to illness and treatment without sharing concerns with their wives, although some of the participants found it helpful to speak to other men going through the same experience. The men expressed embarrassment in having to expose a private part of their body to female health professionals, and favoured male nurses and physicians with whom to discuss erectile difficulties. The men appeared to struggle to achieve a sense of control in the face of an illness and treatment that were exemplified by uncertainty and mystery. As a coping strategy, they sought to live in the present and to accept the changes associated with their lives after cancer treatment such as bowel, bladder, and sexual effects, and the self-monitoring of prostate-specific antigen (PSA) levels as a way of having control over disease progression.

Limitations
As a qualitative study, the findings favour depth of exploration over breadth and do not attempt to be representative of all men with prostate cancer after external beam radiotherapy. The findings are also a product of their cultural context. The study would have yielded even greater insight regarding the men's management of an altered sexual self if their partners had been interviewed, as it is difficult to fully appreciate sexual adjustment without knowledge of the couple context.

This research highlights the gendered experience of cancer and the need for health professionals to be more aware of and responsive to the different ways in which men disclose sexual concerns (e.g. the use of humour) and manage the emotional burden of illness and its treatment.

training and education as appropriate, and build confidence and competence in this complex aspect of care and rehabilitation.

Challenging the taboo of sexuality and overcoming the fear and embarrassment of talking about patient's sexual concerns can be satisfying and enlightening, both professionally and personally. Supporting patients to understand and cope with sexual concerns enables one to cross the boundaries of intimacy and view the 'person with cancer' as someone with specific sexual desires, needs, attitudes, and behaviours. Whenever the sexual consequences of cancer and its treatment are considered relevant by those personally affected, it is incumbent upon practitioners who claim to offer holistic care to ensure sexuality, in all its diversity and dimensions, is an integral element of contemporary cancer care and rehabilitation.

References

1. Foucault M. (1979). *The History of Sexuality Vol. 1, An Introduction.* Harmondsworth: Penguin Books Ltd, p. 35.
2. Savage J. (1988). Sexuality: expectations of nurses. *Radical Community Medicine* **Winter**, 19–22.
3. White I. (2002). Facilitating sexual expression: challenges for contemporary practice. In Heath H. and White I. (eds.) *The Challenge of Sexuality in Health Care.* Oxford: Blackwell Science Ltd, pp. 243–263.
4. White I. (2005). Evidence-based cancer care: sexuality. *European Journal of Cancer Care* **14**, 289–299.
5. Wells D. (ed.) (2000). *Caring for Sexuality in Health and Illness.* Edinburgh: Churchill Livingstone.
6. Schover L.R. (1997). *Sexuality and Fertility After Cancer.* New York: John Wiley and Sons Inc.
7. Stead M.L., Brown J.M., Fallowfield L. and Selby P. (2003). Lack of communication between healthcare professionals and women with ovarian cancer about sexual issues. *British Journal of Cancer* **88**, 666–671.
8. Weijts W., Houtkoop H. and Mullen P. (1993). Talking delicacy: speaking about sexuality during gynaecological consultations. *Sociology of Health and Illness* **15**, 295–314.
9. Lawler J. (1991). *Behind the Screens: Nursing Somology and the Problem of the Body.* London: Churchill Livingstone.
10. Heath H. and White I. (eds.) (2002). *The Challenge of Sexuality in Health Care.* Oxford: Blackwell Science Ltd.
11. Juraskova I., Butow P., Robertson R. *et al.* (2003). Post-treatment sexual adjustment following cervical and endo-metrial cancer: a qualitative insight. *Psycho-oncology* **12**, 267–279.
12. Faithfull S. (1995). 'Just grin and bear it and hope that it will go away'. Coping with urinary symptoms from pelvic radiotherapy. *European Journal of Cancer Care* **4**, 158–165.
13. Cartwright-Alcarese F. (1995). Addressing sexual dysfunction following radiation therapy for a gynecologic malignancy. *Oncology Nursing Forum* **22**, 1227–1231.
14. Bancroft J. (1989). *Human Sexuality and its Problems*, 2nd edition. Edinburgh: Churchill Livingstone.
15. Manderson L. (2005). Boundary breaches: the body, sex and sexuality after stoma surgery. *Social Science and Medicine* **61**, 405–415.
16. Kunkel E.J., Chen E.I. and Okunola T.B. (2002). Psychosocial concerns of women with breast cancer. *Primary Care Update in Obstetrics and Gynaecology* **9**, 129–134.
17. Berglund G., Nystedt M., Bolund C., Sjoden P. and Rutquist L. (2001). Effect of endocrine treatment on sexuality in premenopausal breast cancer patients: a prospective randomized study. *Journal of Clinical Oncology* **19**, 2788–2796.
18. Cull A., Cowie V.J., Farquharson D.I.M. *et al.* (1993). Early stage cervical cancer: psychosocial and sexual outcomes of treatment. *British Journal of Cancer* **68**, 1216–1220.
19. Juraskova I., Butow P., Robertson R. *et al.* (2003). Post-treatment sexual adjustment following cervical and endo-metrial cancer: a qualitative insight. *Psycho-oncology* **12**, 267–279.
20. Potosky A.L., Legler J., Albertsen P.C. *et al.* (2000). Health outcomes after prostatectomy or radiotherapy for prostate cancer: results from the Prostate Cancer Outcomes Study. *Journal of the National Cancer Institute* **92**, 1582–1591.
21. Schover L.R. (1988). *Sexuality and Cancer: For the Man Who Has Cancer, and His Partner.* New York: American Cancer Society.
22. Schover L.R. (1988). *Sexuality and Cancer: For the Woman Who Has Cancer, and Her Partner.* New York: American Cancer Society.
23. Fincannon J.L. and Bruss K.V. (2003). *Couples Confronting Cancer: Keeping your Relationship Strong.* New York: American Cancer Society.
24. Meerabeau L. (1999). The management of embarrassment and sexuality in health care. *Journal of Advanced Cancer* **29**, 1507–1513.
25. Matocha L.K. and Waterhouse J. (1993). Current nursing practice related to sexuality. *Research in Nursing and Health* **16**, 371–378.
26. Lewis S. and Bor R. (1994). Nurses' knowledge of and attitudes towards sexuality and the relationship of these

with nursing practice. *Journal of Advanced Nursing* **20**, 251–259.

27. Waterhouse J. (1996). Nursing practice related to sexuality: a review and recommendations. *Nursing Times Research* **1**, 412–418.

28. Clifford D. (1998). Psychosexual awareness in everyday nursing. *Nursing Standard* **12**, 42–45.

29. Monroe B. (1998). Gender and sexuality. In Oliviere D., Hargreaves R. and Munroe B. (eds.) *Good Practices in Palliative Care: A Psychosocial Perspective.* Aldershot: Ashgate Publishing Ltd, pp. 95–119.

30. Masters W. and Johnson V. (1966). *Human Sexual Response.* Boston, MA: Little Brown & Co.

31. Annon J.S. (1974). *The Behavioral Treatment of Sexual Problems.* Honolulu: Mercantile Printing.

32. National Institute for Clinical Excellence (NICE). (2004). *Improving Supportive and Palliative Care for Adults with Cancer: The Manual.* London: NICE.

33. Hedestig O., Sandman P., Tomic R. and Widmark A. (2005). Living after external beam radiotherapy of localized prostate cancer: a qualitative analysis of patient narratives. *Cancer Nursing* **28**, 310–317.

CHAPTER TWENTY-SEVEN

Anxiety and depression

Annabel Pollard and Meinir Krishnasamy

Psychosocial distress is a common consequence of cancer diagnosis and treatment. While many patients experience diagnosable psychiatric disorders, such as anxiety and depression, a significant minority experiences subclinical levels of severe distress. Both depression and anxiety of themselves can exacerbate distress, and both are associated with additional suffering. Understanding the aetiology of adjustment to cancer, anxiety, and depression is the focus of this chapter.

Theoretical assumptions

Anxiety and depression in the context of cancer are responses to sometimes overwhelming life events. Understanding how someone develops an anxiety or mood disorder is as important as understanding the specific signs and symptoms of these disorders, as treatment will need to take into account the unique response of each individual.

Brennan provides a useful conceptual model of how individuals adjust to cancer as a life-changing event.[1] The Social–Cognitive Transition Model of Adjustment integrates psychological theories from the cognitive, trauma, and adjustment literature, and Brennan suggests that life-threatening events such as cancer challenge core mental assumptions about the self and the world. Since these assumptions are essentially cognitive maps, or internal representations of the world, they help us to predict the future with some sense of certainty and to make meaning out of everyday experiences. Over time these 'maps' are built up, continually refined, and expanded. Many assumptions are unconscious but serve an organising function within which to assimilate new experiences, in essence adding to a person's existing 'map'. When an individual's perceptions of danger or threat are activated by a diagnosis of cancer, fundamental assumptions about the world may be significantly disturbed, and individuals may exhibit symptoms of stress, anxiety, and depression as they struggle to fit new experiences into their existing knowledge and assumptions about the world.[1]

Psychological disorders such as anxiety and depression develop when an individual's ability to incorporate new challenges to existing fundamental assumptions is overwhelmed. This chapter considers anxiety and depression within the context of Brennan's model.

While distress, anxiety, sadness, and grief may be a normal response to life-threatening events or prolonged illness, these emotional responses are often integral to adjusting to a changed situation. However, for a considerable minority who have cancer the severity of these responses may require expert psychological intervention.[2,3]

Anxiety

Moderate to severe anxiety has been reported in numerous studies of people with a range of cancer diagnoses.[4] Between 30% and 40% of people with cancer have been found to report moderate to high levels of anxiety,[4,5] and anxiety is one of the most frequently cited reasons for psychological referral.[6]

Symptoms of anxiety

While mediated psychologically, anxiety has evolved as an evolutionary biological response to perceived danger or threat. Irrespective of cause, anxiety disorders are characterised by an emotional state typified by a cluster of emotions including feelings of fear, dread, impending doom, apprehension, or a vague sensation or emotion that is experienced as unpleasant and is difficult to define.[7] People with cancer also experience more specific situationally bound anxiety or worry associated with treatment, for example when undergoing new procedures or awaiting test results.[8]

Typically people with anxiety will also experience physiological symptoms of heightened autonomic arousal, mediated by neuroendocrine responses.[9] Sympathetic responses include restlessness, insomnia and nightmares, shortness of breath, sweating, irritability, headaches, palpitations or pounding heart, and hyperventilation. Other symptoms include gastrointestinal symptoms such as dry mouth, nausea, anorexia, and diarrhoea. These physical symptoms and heightened state of arousal are frequently experienced as aversive in themselves.

People who are anxious may also describe feeling overwhelmed by persistent worrying thoughts that are intrusive (patients may say they cannot 'escape' from these thoughts) and which tend to focus on catastrophic or 'worst possible' outcomes; other symptoms of anxiety include disturbances to concentration and memory. Features of post-traumatic stress, especially intrusive symptoms, such as recurrent thoughts about the treatment or diagnosis have been reported in cancer populations.[10] People tend to use the term anxiety to cover a wide range of psychological and physiological reactions to cancer, they may have some symptoms of anxiety in the absence of a clinically diagnosable disorder. The 'emotional rollercoaster' often described by people with cancer can often refer to the frequent upsurges in anxiety symptoms that are experienced across the disease continuum. The degree to which the anxiety response is pathological and/or requires treatment depends on the number and severity of symptoms and degree of impairment in overall functioning.

Aetiology

In the cancer setting, anxiety responses tend to be acute and time limited; however, some people will experience a more chronic anxiety. For example, many people experience recurrent situational anxiety, related to a crisis or a transitional period in the cancer trajectory – for example, commencing new treatment, awaiting scan results, or on completion of treatment.[11] However, for a subset of individuals the symptoms will persist and will adversely affect quality of life, and ability to comply with treatment or make treatment-related decisions.[6]

Anxiety related to organic factors such as health status is the second most frequent source of anxiety for patients receiving treatment for cancer.[11] Poorly controlled symptoms (for example, pain), abnormal metabolic states (for example, hypoglycemia, hypocalcaemia), hormone-secreting tumours (for example, parathyroid or paraneoplastic syndromes), and anxiety-producing drugs (for example, steroids, anti-emetics, interferon) are the most common sources of anxiety of this type. Adjustment disorder, pain, adverse drug reactions, delirium, organic anxiety, and other organic mental disorders may also lead to anxiety in an individual with advanced or terminal cancer.[6,12]

For some individuals a diagnosis of cancer and its many associated complications may reactivate a pre-existing anxiety disorder. There is some evidence that some individuals are more physiologically susceptible to anxiety and may give a history of being generally more anxiety prone.

Psychological treatment for anxiety disorders

From a nursing perspective, a thorough assessment is essential to understanding the nature, severity and frequency of psycho-physiological symptoms. Effective communication is vital to elicit and respond to psychosocial cues from each person. Effective communication and gentle exploration of concerns may help to make sense of worrying thoughts and fears – for example what meanings a particular source of worry or anxiety has for the person.

People respond well to having their concerns heard and normalised. Gentle encouragement to talk with a professional, or family member about the illness and its impact on their life may help resolve 'normal' anxieties. At the same time, be watchful for individuals whose anxiety may require a referral for specialist intervention.[4]

Treatment for anxiety is based on the number, type, and severity of symptoms described by the individual and depending on these may require specific targeted interventions or a more general treatment approach.

Evidence-based, clinical practice guidelines for the psychosocial care of adults with cancer suggest that cognitive-behavioural therapy, supportive psychotherapy, and group therapy have been associated with improvements in anxiety.[4] A variety of specific psychologically based interventions have been shown to be effective in treating anxiety including:

- relaxation
- guided imagery
- systematic desensitisation
- problem solving
- crisis intervention
- supportive interventions
- psycho-educational strategies.

Attendance at support groups, use of relaxation, and meditation are all interventions shown to reduce anxiety and, more importantly, can be incorporated into healthy behaviours by the people with cancer themselves and their family members.

Pharmacological management of anxiety

Pharmacological intervention in the treatment of anxiety in cancer and palliative care involves the use of medications including:[12,13]

- benzodiazepines, e.g. midazolam, lorazepam, diazepam, clonazepam
- non-benzodiazepines, e.g. buspirone
- neuroleptics, e.g. methotrimeprazine, chlorpromazine, haloperidol

- antihistamines, e.g. hydroxyzine
- tricyclic antidepressants
- selective serotonin re-uptake inhibitors, e.g. mirtazapine.

Depression

Normal responses to cancer (diagnosis, treatment, recurrence, advanced disease, or terminal illness) include feelings of shock, disbelief, sadness, and often a period of mourning evidenced by withdrawal. People are perceived to be coping well when they demonstrate a sense of adjustment – that is managing the threat without significant psychological distress. In general, psychological adjustment occurs as the individual incorporates new information and understandings into their experience. While distress is common, people are not considered to be depressed unless their mood has an adverse effect on overall functioning. Depression may be considered a psychological response to circumstances perceived by the individual as overwhelming. Some people may be more prone to depression than others genetically, or through learnt behavioural responses. Like all mood disorders, symptoms of depression are experienced on a continuum of severity. The degree to which depression is pathological and/or requires treatment depends on the number and severity of symptoms and degree of impairment in overall functioning.

The incidence of depression has been found to range from 4.5% to 42% in populations of people with cancer, and is said to increase as pain, advanced disease, level of dependency, and disability increase.[14,15]

Aetiology

Depression in cancer is multifactorial. Psychologically people often present with depression after a chronically stressful period of time, for example when they feel exhausted and at the end of their reserves; this may often be at the end of treatment. However, many other factors contribute to depression including drugs given to combat the cancer itself, as well as drugs used to relieve the symptoms of the disease and its treatments.[12,16] Box 27.1 outlines some of the factors that may predispose someone with cancer to depression.

Box 27.1 Predisposing factors for depression

- A family history of depression or suicide
- A family or personal history of alcoholism
- A previous psychiatric illness, especially depression, also drug abuse or a previous suicide attempt
- Past coping strategies: does the individual employ acceptance–resignation, information-seeking or confrontational coping strategies?
- Patients with advanced disease have a higher incidence of depression than those individuals with newly diagnosed cancer
- Cancer treatments, e.g. some cytotoxic drugs
- Medications.

Types of depression

Depression is classified as one of the mood disorders. Mood disorders are categorised by alterations in mood listed in the *Diagnostic and Statistical Manual* (DSM-IV).[17] Unipolar depression is generally diagnosed when a person has experienced one or more episodes of depressive symptoms over a period of not less than two weeks. Bipolar disorder is characterised by both manic and depressive symptoms.

Depression is now recognised as a significant co-morbidity in the context of cancer.[18] However, health professionals (and individuals diagnosed with cancer) occasionally persist in the view that depression in the context of diagnosis of cancer, is not a 'real' depression, believing that there is an understandable reason to feel depressed.[19] Depression diagnosis is highly skewed towards somatic symptoms.[13] There is also significant co-morbidity between depression and anxiety.[4]

One of the main problems associated with detecting depression in cancer is disentangling symptoms of depression from symptoms of the disease itself or its treatment.[19] In the context of cancer diagnosis and treatment, greater reliance must be placed on the psychological symptoms including dysphoric mood, hopelessness, worthlessness, guilt, and suicidal ideation.[20]

In advanced cancer, the physical manifestations of depression such as fatigue, anorexia, or insomnia are all too likely to be present as a result of the impact of the tumour, making accurate assessment of depression especially difficult.[2,15] The importance of potentiating factors of depression, such as functional limitation or metastatic disease, chronic fatigue, or unresolved pain, has clear implications for thorough assessment of depression and the initiation of prompt intervention. Potentiating factors include:[12]

- people with relentless physical symptoms, especially uncontrolled pain
- medications: corticosteroids, e.g. prednisolone and dexamethasone, cimetidine, diazepam, indomethacin, levodopa, methyldopa, pentazocine, phenmetrazine, phenobarbital, propranolol, and oestrogens; chemotherapy, especially vincristine, vinblastine, procarbazine, L-asparaginase, interferon, amphoteracin-B are also linked to the onset of depressive symptomatology
- whole-brain irradiation
- metabolic disturbances, nutritional abnormalities, endocrine imbalance, and neurological imbalance.

Case study 27.1

Bridget, a 54-year-old woman diagnosed with advanced breast cancer presented with symptoms of psychological distress. She was referred by her breast nurse consultant to a clinical psychologist. On assessment with the psychologist she clearly described a variety of symptoms that had been present for several weeks including mildly lowered mood (dysphoria), tearfulness nearly every day, loss of pleasure (anhedonia), hopelessness, loss of concentration, and sleep disturbance. She was not suicidal and had not experienced any thoughts of suicide. On discussion she suggested that she had felt somewhat depressed since her diagnosis 5 years previously. One of the major recent changes was an increase in pain and other symptoms associated with side-effects of treatment and advanced disease. She described herself as a perfectionist and 'someone who suppresses my emotions'. She had no history of depression in herself or her family of origin, or other history of mental health problems. She had a supportive family and in particular a happy relationship with her husband. She was reluctant to take medication. She was diagnosed with a mild depression and agreed to pursue a course of psychotherapy.

Case study 27.2

Jane was a 50-year-old woman with advanced breast cancer. She was initially diagnosed in her early forties and had had two recurrences, each 7 years apart. Diagnosed with her second recurrence she presented for a routine pretreatment visit to plan some radiotherapy. She presented as both agitated and dysphoric (lowered mood every day for most of the day), she experienced worry and depressive rumination about a variety of issues. She had significant sleep disturbance and loss of appetite. There was distinct loss of pleasure in anything. She had difficulty concentrating. These symptoms had been present and escalating for several weeks. She was highly suicidal and described both means and plans. She had never been depressed in the past. The apparent trigger for her depression was a conflict with a close family member some 6 months previously. She was diagnosed with an agitated depression, admitted to a psychiatric unit and commenced on medication. After several weeks her mood improved. She then commenced psychotherapy and cognitive-behavioural therapy to assist her to disentangle the variety of medical and other stressors that had contributed to her depression.

Treatment of depression

The optimum management of depression has been described as being a combination of supportive psychotherapy, cognitive-behavioural techniques, and antidepressant medications.

Non-pharmacological approaches

Nurses are generally sensitive to alterations in patient mood and play a significant role in identifying psychological distress and in referring on to other health care professionals for more intensive support. Advanced communication skills are essential to identification of distress, and there is extensive evidence that nurses (and other health care professionals) benefit from additional training to assist them to identify emotional cues and communicate effectively in the context of cancer.[21]

Generally the goals of psychologically based treatments are to alleviate distress and enhance coping through a variety of techniques. Supportive psychotherapy aims to facilitate discussion and exploration of the existential issues inherent in cancer diagnosis and treatment, for example, fears,

mortality, loneliness, and loss. The process of supportive psychotherapy is a means to validate emotional distress, and frequently people need to hear that their distress is 'normal'. Enhancing coping through problem solving, information seeking, and identifying areas of control are vital steps in assisting individuals to work through psychological concerns.

Cognitive-behavioural therapy is a well-established treatment for depression in the non-cancer setting. There is increasing evidence that cognitive-behavioural techniques of managing specific psychological difficulties are helpful. Cognitive-behavioural techniques include a variety of techniques that encourage patients to adapt cognitions or thinking (e.g. cognitive restructuring) and behaviours (e.g. relaxation and imagery) to assist in coping with their changed situation. These techniques have been shown to be easy for people to learn and to use.[22] A recognition of the growth in use of these techniques has led to a demand for an increase in the research knowledge base of nursing in examining their effectiveness.

Cognitive and behavioural interventions

Cognitive interventions

The enhancement of well-being through maximising beneficial coping strategies is one means of reducing psychological distress. Coping strategies are those processes people use to try to manage real or perceived deficiencies between demands imposed by a crisis such as a diagnosis of cancer and the resources available to respond to it. The two forms of coping mechanisms most commonly referred to in the literature are problem solving and emotional-orientated strategies. Problem-solving strategies work in two ways. They help to reduce the demands placed on an individual by the stressor, whatever that may be. They increase the resources available to deal with a stressor by developing new skills or promoting existing beneficial coping mechanisms.

Behavioural interventions

One of the most commonly used behavioural techniques is progressive muscle relaxation (PMR). PMR involves tensing and then relaxing separate muscles groups throughout the body one after the other. Teaching a patient, family member, or friend a relaxation technique is relatively quick and easy and yet the rewards can be significant in both the short and longer term.

An in-depth exploration of the various forms of psychological therapies can be found in the *Handbook of Psycho-oncology*, edited by Holland and Rowland.[13]

Pharmacological management of depression
The main drugs used in the pharmacological management of depression in cancer and palliative care are:

- tricyclic antidepressants, e.g. amitriptyline, dothiepin
- second-generation antidepressants, e.g. trazodone, mianserin
- psychostimulants, e.g. dextroamfetamine
- monoamine oxidase inhibitors, e.g. phenelzine
- lithium carbonate
- benzodiazepines, e.g. alprazolam
- fluoxetine hydrochloride (Prozac).

All antidepressants have side-effects and these should be explained clearly.

Occasionally, electroconvulsive therapy may be warranted for depressed people with cancer with psychotic features or for whom pharmacological intervention carries too many side-effects.[12,13]

Suicide

Cancer is a chronic illness, and for many the dying process can become long and extremely burdensome. The attitude towards suicide for the majority of health care professionals is that it is something to be avoided at all costs, but for many individuals suicide may reflect an attempt to retain some degree of control or to secure a 'dignified death'.

Despite the fact that people with cancer are at increased risk of suicide relative to the general population, particularly in the terminal stages of illness, there is agreement that very few individuals with cancer actually do commit suicide.[23] Men more than women with cancer have been identified as being at increased risk of suicide relative to

the general population. Taking analgesic and sedative drugs is the most common way of committing suicide.[24]

There is growing evidence that people with particular kinds of cancers are at increased risk of suicide. Those diagnosed with lung, pharyngeal, and oral cancers are at particular risk.[23,25] Identifying reasons why particular individuals or groups may be prone to suicide may allow early, appropriate intervention and help to reduce the risk. The onset of oral, pharyngeal, and lung cancers is often associated with extensive tobacco and alcohol intake. Heavy smoking and drinking may signify a vulnerable group who tend to utilise maladaptive coping skills, and as such they may be more prone to suicide as a coping strategy.[25] The disfiguring surgery associated with head and neck tumours, loss of vocal communication for those with pharyngeal tumours, and the marked weight loss and cachexia associated with lung tumours may also contribute to the suicidal potential of these individuals.[23]

As with anxiety and depression there are well-recognised predisposing factors that can help to alert nursing staff to those individuals most at risk of suicide. Those with advanced disease and a poor prognosis are most at risk of suicide because of the likelihood of multiple symptoms such as pain, delirium, depression and hopelessness, and fatigue. Feelings of loss of control and helplessness, pre-existing psychopathology, for example, alcoholism, substance abuse, major mental illness, and prior suicide history, also contribute to heightened risk of suicide.[26–29]

Assessment of suicide risk and appropriate interventions based on skilled interaction may often help to prevent suicide.[25] Many of the guidelines for assessment and evaluation of suicide risk in an individual with cancer outlined below are well-suited for use by nurses who are in close day-to-day proximity to those who may be at risk. The principles of assessing risk of suicide are as follows:

- establish a rapport with the person based upon trust and a non-judgemental approach
- invite them to describe their understanding of, and response to, the cancer diagnosis, its treatment and symptoms experienced. It is

important that he or she is asked to talk about everything that is important or meaningful. An agenda set by the doctor or nurse may omit the most salient points

- be vigilant – is the individual displaying any evidence of depression or delirium?
- is there any evidence of uncontrolled pain? Does he or she talk of fatigue, exhaustion, feelings of loss of control, hopelessness or helplessness?
- what is the person's past history? Is there any evidence of pre-existing pathology, such as depression or previous suicide attempt? Is there any history of family suicide?

Although nurses are ideally placed to help to find meaning or reasons for suicidal thoughts, as well as an understanding of how serious the person's intention really is, multidisciplinary management is essential for the individual who displays serious suicidal intent.

The role of health care professionals

Health professionals must confront difficult and tragic situations daily. This may lead to a protective defensiveness that helps shut out the most confronting aspects of their daily work. For example, by not addressing distress the health professional manages to protect themself from exposure to that distress. Effective communication skills, a knowledge of one's skill set and limitations, and good assessment skills are all vital in ensuring that people with anxiety and depression are appropriately identified and referred for care by suitably qualified members of the health care team.

Once again, the contribution of nursing lies with substantiating an appreciation of each individual's needs. Supportive interventions designed to help people to identify and respond positively to sources of anxiety and depression where they are able should be offered, or prompt referral for pharmacological, psychiatric, or psychological assessment and care initiated when appropriate.

Some potential future nursing research questions include:

- how effective is progressive muscle relaxation as a means of helping patients to minimise the anxiety of a distressing symptom, e.g. breathlessness, fatigue, nausea, and vomiting?
- can family/friends benefit from psychotherapeutic interventions?

Nursing interventions known to be effective in helping to manage anxiety in the early stages of illness (for example, relaxation and massage) should be systematically evaluated with patients in the latter stages of their disease.

References

1. Brennan J. (2004). *Cancer in Context*. Oxford: Oxford University Press.
2. Bukberg J., Penman D. and Holland J. (1984). Depression in hospitalised cancer patients. *Psychosomatic Medicine* **46**, 199–212.
3. Lampic C., Wennberg A., Schill J. *et al.* (1994). Anxiety and cancer related worry of cancer patients at routine follow-up visits. *Acta Oncologica* **33**, 119–125.
4. National Breast Cancer Centre and National Cancer Control Initiative. (2003). *Clinical Practice Guidelines for the Psychosocial Care of Adults with Cancer*. Campersdown, New South Wales: National Breast Cancer Centre.
5. Derogatis L.R., Morrow G.R., Fetting J., Penman D. and Piasetsky S. (1983). The prevalence of psychiatric disorder among cancer patients. *Journal of the American Medical Association* **249**, 751–757.
6. Noyes R., Holt C. and Massie M.J. (1998). Anxiety disorders. In Holland J.C. (ed.) *Psycho-oncology*. Oxford: Oxford University Press, pp. 548–563.
7. Stefanek M., Shaw A., Degeorge D. and Tsottles N. (1989). Illness-related worry among cancer patients: prevalence, severity and content. *Cancer Investigation* **7**, 365–371.
8. Wright E.P., Selby P.J., Crawford M. *et al.* (2003). Feasibility and compliance of automated measurement of quality of life in oncology patients. *Journal of Clinical Oncology* **21**, 374–382.
9. Leigh H. and Reiser M.F. (1985). *The Patient: Biological, Psychological and Social Dimensions of Medical Practice*. New York: Plenum Press.
10. Widows M.R., Jacobsen P.B. and Fields K.K. (2000). Relation of psychological vulnerability factors to posttraumatic stress disorder symptomatology in bone marrow transplant recipients. *Psychomatic Medicine* **62**, 873–882.

11. Massie M. (1990). Anxiety, panic and phobias. In Holland J. and Rowland J. (eds.) *Handbook of Psycho-oncology. Psychological Care of the Patient with Cancer.* Oxford: Oxford University Press, pp. 300–309.

12. Breitbart W., Cochinov H.M. and Passik S. (1998). Psychiatric aspects of palliative care. In Doyle D., Hanks G. and Macdonald N, (eds.) *Oxford Textbook of Palliative Medicine*, 2nd edition. New York: Oxford University Press, pp. 933–956.

13. Holland J. and Rowland J. (eds.) (1990). *Handbook of Psycho-oncology. Psychological Care of the Patient with Cancer.* Oxford: Oxford University Press.

14. Golden R., McCartney C., Haggerty J., Raft D. and Nemeroff C.B. (1991). The detection of depression by patient self-report in women with gynaecologic cancer. *International Journal of Psychiatry in Medicine* **21**, 17–27.

15. Carroll B.T., Kathol R.G., Noyes R., Wald T.G. and Calmon G.H. (1993). Screening for depression and anxiety in cancer patients using the Hospital Anxiety and Depression Scale. *General Hospital Psychiatry* **15**, 69–74.

16. Miaskowski C. (2000). The need to assess multiple symptoms. *Management Nursing* **3**, 115.

17. Spitzer R.L., Gibbon M., Skodol A., Williams J. and First M. (2002). *Diagnostic and Statistical Manual for the DSM-IV-TR Casebook. A Learning Companion to the Diagnostic and Statistical Manual of Mental Disorders*, 4th edition. Arlington: American Psychiatric Publishers, Inc.

18. Ronson A. (2004). Psychiatric disorders in oncology: recent therapeutic advances and new conceptual frameworks. *Current Opinion in Oncology* **16**, 318–323.

19. Endicott J. (1983). Measurement of depression patients with cancer. *Cancer* **53**, 2243–2248.

20. Breitbart W. (1995). Identifying patients at risk for, and treatment of major psychiatric complications of cancer. *Supportive Care in Cancer* **3**, 45–60.

21. Pollard A. and Swift K. (2003). Communication skills in palliative care. In O'Connor M. and Aranda S. (eds.) *Palliative Care Nursing: A Guide to Practice*, 2nd edition. Melbourne: Ausmed Publications, pp. 23–40.

22. Holland J., Morrow G. and Schmale A. (1991). A randomised clinical trial of alprazolam versus patients with progressive muscle relaxation in cancer patients with anxiety and depressive symptoms. *Journal of Clinical Oncology* **9**, 1004–1011.

23. Holland J.C. and Gooen-Piels J. (2000). Principles of psycho-oncology. In Bast R.C., Kufe D.W., Pollock R.E. *et al.* (eds.) *Cancer Medicine*, 5th edition. Hamilton, Ontario: BC Decker Inc., section 9.

24. Bolund C. (1985). Suicide and cancer I. Demographic and social characteristics of cancer patients who committed suicide in Sweden, 1973–1976. *Journal of Psychosocial Oncology* **3**, 17–30.

25. Breitbart W. and Krivo S. (1998). Suicide. In Holland J.C. and Rowland J. (eds.) *Handbook of Psycho-oncology. Psychological Care of the Patient with Cancer.* Oxford: Oxford University Press, pp. 541–547.

26. Lynch M. (1995). The assessment and prevalence of affective disorders in advanced cancer. *Journal of Palliative Care* **11**, 10–18.

27. Levin R.B. and Gross A.M. (1985). The role of relaxation in systematic desensitisation. *Behavioural Research Therapy* **23**, 187–196.

28. Faberow N.L., Schneidman E.S. and Leonard C.V. (1963). Suicide among general medical and surgical hospital patients with malignant neoplasms. *Medical Bulletin* **9**, Washington, DC: US Veterans Administration

29. Beck A., Kovacs M. and Weisman A. (1975). Hopelessness and suicidal behaviour: an overview. *Journal of the American Medical Association* **234**, 1146–1149.

CHAPTER TWENTY-EIGHT

Delirium

Meinir Krishnasamy

Caring for someone who is delirious is enormously challenging. It is often painful for all involved as the confusion, like cancer itself, gives rise to feelings of conflict, shame, isolation, and disempowerment in those witnessing its effects:

> . . . cancer appears to have become the metaphor of the deepest fears held about the inevitable disintegration and decay of the body [p. 268].[1]

Despite being a common symptom of cancer and occurring with the same frequency as depression, confusion or delirium is poorly recognised by health care professionals.[2] Throughout this chapter the terms confusion and delirium are used interchangeably. It is estimated to occur in approximately 10% to 15% of medically hospitalised patients and in up to 80% of patients with terminal illness.[3] It is associated with significantly increased morbidity and mortality, and interferes with self-care activities such as taking medications, maintaining activities, eating, hygiene practices, and informing physicians and nurses of changes in symptoms – all of which can impact an individual's quality of life and that of the family around them. Early symptoms of delirium are often misdiagnosed as anxiety, anger, depression, or psychosis.[4,5] Subsequently, treatment is often delayed until symptoms are severe, causing undue distress to the individual experiencing the confusion and to family and friends witnessing the changes in their behaviour and personality. The necessity for an appreciation of early signs of confusion, and an ability to differentiate those signs from the manifestations of anxiety, depression, and dementia, are important if nurses are to contribute meaningfully to the management of this difficult symptom.

Delirium, anxiety, depression, and dementia share many common manifestations, compounding accurate assessment and prompt intervention. Manifestations of anxiety and depression have been described in the previous chapter and therefore will not be outlined again here. Delirium, however, may be accompanied by any number of concurrent symptoms, including alterations to:

- level of consciousness
- attention
- thinking
- perception
- emotion
- memory
- psychomotor behaviour
- sleep–wake cycle.[6,7]

Differentiating between dementia and delirium can be extremely difficult because they share common features.[8] A useful *précis* of the key differences between the two conditions is shown in Table 28.1.

Whatever the symptom, delirium, dementia, anxiety, or depression, the single most important factor in effective intervention is skilled assessment.

Table 28.1 Features of delirium and dementia. Reproduced with permission from the American Medical Association from Lipowski Z. (1987). Delirium (acute confusional states). *Journal of the American Medical Association* **258**, 1789–1792[6]

Features	Delirium	Dementia
Onset	Acute, often at night	Insidious
Course	Fluctuating, with lucid intervals during the day, worse at night	Stable over course of day
Duration	Hours to weeks	Months or years
Awareness	Reduced	Clear
Alertness	Abnormally high or low	Usually normal
Attention	Lacks direction and selectivity, distractibility, fluctuates over course of day	Relatively unaffected
Orientation	Usually impaired for time, tendency to mistake unfamiliar for familiar place and persons	Often impaired
Memory	Immediate and recent impaired	Recent and remote impaired
Thinking	Disorganised	Impoverished
Perception	Illusions and hallucinations, usually visual and common	Often absent
Speech	Incoherent, hesitant, slow or rapid	Difficulty in finding words
Sleep–wake cycle	Always disturbed	Fragmented sleep
Physical illness or drug toxicity	Either or both present	Often absent

Identifying those at risk

Assessment and management of delirium require thorough knowledge of its diagnostic criteria, aetiology, signs and symptoms, appropriate intervention strategies, and monitoring techniques. It is important to differentiate delirium from dementia. There are significant differences between the two conditions including:

- delirium is potentially reversible – dementia is not
- the onset of delirium is hours to days whereas the onset of dementia is longer (months to years)
- delirium has significant impact on the sleep–wake cycle whereas dementia does not
- both are disorders of cognition but delirium has a significant alteration in arousal and attention – a patient with dementia is alert with usually no disturbance of consciousness.[9]

For the purpose of this project delirium is defined according to The *Diagnostic and Statistical*

Manual of Mental Disorders (DSM-IV), fourth edition as:

- a disturbance in consciousness (reduced clarity of environment awareness) with impaired ability to focus or shift attention
- a change in cognition (memory impairment, disorientation, language disturbances) or the development of perceptual disturbance that is not better accounted for by a pre-existing, established, or evolving dementia
- a disturbance that has evolved over a short period of time (hours or days) and fluctuates during the course of the day
- there is evidence from the history, physical examination, or laboratory findings that the disturbance is caused by physiological consequence of a general medical condition.[10]

As a range of underlying conditions are commonly associated with delirium, almost anyone with a diagnosis of cancer is at risk of experiencing some degree of confusion. For example, central nervous system disorders, metabolic disorders, cardiopulmonary disorders, and systemic illnesses resulting from neoplasm, infection or substance intoxication, or withdrawal. Medications known to have an association with delirium include drugs commonly prescribed to patients with cancer, for example analgesics, particularly opiates, anticonvulsants, antimicrobials, corticosteroids, gastrointestinal medications, muscle relaxants, immunosuppressive agents, and psychotropic medications with anticholinergic properties.[11]

In addition:[12,13]

- older people with cancer may have an increased risk of developing delirium as they may be especially sensitive to the potential causes listed below
- individuals with a past history of depression may be more likely to experience an episode of delirium as a consequence of a cancer diagnosis
- decreased mobility, compromised functional status, poor quality of sleep, and decreased contact with family and friends have all been shown to increase an individual's predisposition to confusion.[14]

Assessment of an individual suspected of developing confusion therefore requires great care and must involve key members of his or her social support network. In Box 28.1 some of factors that might contribute to a confusional state are shown.

One of the most important aspects of caring for an individual who has begun to exhibit signs of confusion is to try to retain a sense of wholeness, of personhood, for as long as possible. As the confusion establishes itself, there may be periods of lucidity when the person will be aware of alterations in their behaviour. Appropriate reassurance at this time that they are experiencing reversible manifestations of the cancer or its treatment will be enormously comforting. Relatives and friends also need to be aware of this information. Explain to them that the confusion is not a sign of mental illness. Someone who is left to contemplate this frightening symptom is likely to become increasingly distressed and subsequently more confused.[15] Family and friends will become increasingly despondent and may even withdraw at a time

Box 28.1 Factors for consideration in the assessment of someone who is confused[3,4,12]

- Is there any reason to suspect hyponatraemia, uraemia or hypercalcaemia, or any other metabolic abnormality?
- Does the patient have any respiratory complications?
- Are there likely to be, or is there evidence of current changes in renal and hepatic function?
- Is the patient in pain?
- Is there any reason to suspect brain metastases?
- When did the patient last pass urine?
- Is the patient constipated?
- Is the patient currently receiving chemotherapy or immunotherapy? L Asparaginase, 5-fluorouracil (5-FU), intrathecal methotrexate, nitrogen mustard, procarbazine, and chlorambucil can all cause delirium. Interleukin 2, lymphokine-activated killer cells, and interferon also have a potential to cause confusion.
- Has he/she been started on a new drug within the last 48 hours and what combination of drugs is the patient receiving? Opiates, non-steroidal anti-inflammatory drugs, psychotropics, corticosteroids, histamine blockers, hyoscine, oral hypoglycaemic drugs, digoxin, and anti-parkinsonian drugs may all cause confusion.
- Alcohol and diazepam withdrawal can lead to confusional states.
- A chest or urine infection, heart failure, hepatic failure, or renal failure can lead to confusion.

when most reassurance that they are loved and valued is needed:

> We must work harder at being human all of us: those who are disabled, those who are normal, those who are professional helpers [p.227].[16]

A brief cognitive assessment, consistently performed, can be used to ensure that confusion is not missed.[12] Non-threatening questions such as 'How have you been feeling?' are a simple and safe way to start the assessment. Once set at ease, questions about address, telephone number, and family members' names can be asked without seeming too intrusive or judgemental. When confused, someone may be easily disadvantaged during an assessment, particularly in an unfamiliar environment. Do they wear glasses or use a hearing aid?

Are these available to him or her? Is the environment quiet, well-lit, and free of instruments that might appear threatening or frightening? Have they recently received their first dose of morphine, cyclizine, or any other sedating agents? If patients display any signs of delirium, an appropriately qualified clinician should then screen for delirium using a standardised instrument such as the Confusion Assessment Method.[17] Where the screen indicates further assessment, a clinician with the necessary expertise should use a detailed instrument such as the Memorial Delirium Assessment Scale[18] to confirm or reject a diagnosis of delirium.

Involving family and friends

Family members may often be the only ones aware of subtle differences in behaviour. Family and friends can offer a very important insight into the 'normal' cognitive function and any recent changes in memory or impaired thinking.[12] They may also offer an invaluable insight into the person's awareness and acceptance of their diagnosis and prognosis, highlighting causes for the confusional state that may otherwise remain hidden. For some, the diagnosis of cancer or a prognosis of terminal illness is unbearable, making them become paranoid, withdrawn, and detached. Unable to tolerate the sadness or fear of dying, they may feel that somebody is trying to kill or harm them.[15] Educating the family is very important to reduce their fear and distress. If the delirium is expected to resolve then a clear explanation of its cause should be given. If, however, it is a part of the final stages of illness then reassurance that the person will not suffer, and explanation of the use of sedation is crucial.

Managing delirium

The most appropriate approach for managing confusion is to identify underlying causes and associated symptoms. Pharmacological management is outlined in Care strategy 28.1. Very few studies have evaluated the effect of non-pharmacological interventions aimed at managing

confusion in the cancer population. Most of the psychological and supportive interventions described in the literature are based on anecdote and offer little in the way of research-based practice guidelines. Observation, the use of constraints, a structured daily routine, and minimal room changes have all been reported as being helpful in supporting the confused individual.[8] However, many of these recommendations are believed to arise from current practices, which nurses seem to find unacceptable, ineffective, or impractical.[19]

For the majority of cancer-related symptoms it is possible to offer involvement in decisions about care. Confusion precludes this collaboration. Sometimes the decision involves sedating someone who is quite frail and who it is known may develop a chest infection by virtue of the sleep induced by sedative agents and the resultant inactivity.[15] As a team, along with the family, one of the concepts that may be helpful is to consider whether the time spent awake is of any value. Are they continually muddled and distressed when awake or are there times when they are still able to enjoy being with family and friends? It may be apparent, especially in the last few days of life, that an individual is only settled when sleeping.

If someone who is confused refuses medication, concealing medication in food or drink is inadvisable, as this may serve only to heighten an individual's mistrust when this is discovered.[15]

Terminal restlessness

Cawley and Webber found that nurses repeatedly identify terminal restlessness as a poorly managed symptom that is extremely distressing for family and friends, and often leaves doctors and nurses feeling compromised by the need to sedate patients heavily during the last few days of life.[19] Delirium during the last 24–48 hours of life (commonly referred to as terminal restlessness) may not be reversible and is most probably due to the influence of irreversible processes such as multiple organ failure.[5]

Managing terminal restlessness is an extremely challenging process, compounded by:

- multifactorial aetiology: one study suggests that a cause is identified in less than 50% of terminally ill patients with cognitive failure[15]
- an often irreversible cause
- inappropriateness of invasive or complex diagnostic assessment.[5]

It appears to be one of the most difficult symptoms to control without also causing sedation in patients with advanced cancer.[20] Traditionally, the treatment of delirium for a terminally ill individual has focused on sedating the patient, which diminishes the possibility of managing any potentially treatable causes; at the same time, unnecessary invasive tests to clarify confusional states in terminally ill patients (i.e. 24–48 hours prior to death) should be avoided, since they may often be of limited value.[21–26] One study reported that researchers were able to identify the cause of delirium in 44% of a group of patients with advanced cancer, noting an improvement in 33% of patients following treatment aimed at identifiable causes.[27] Others suggest that many reversible causes of delirium, even those occurring during the terminal stages of cancer (for example, renal failure, dehydration, hypoxia, or hypercalcaemia), can be identified by a series of simple examinations, including:

- review of medications
- complete blood count
- electrolytes
- urea
- creatinine
- glucose and calcium levels
- pulse oximetry.[23]

Whether these apparently simple medical examinations are acceptable to seriously ill individuals is unknown. The need for sensitive nursing care to help to elicit patients' preferences for their last days and weeks of life is clear.

Choice of drug must therefore be based on each individual's unique needs. If the intention is to attempt to improve sensory capacity and cognitive functioning, neuroleptic drugs such as haloperidol should be used. When improvement in cognition cannot be achieved, ensuring comfort and minimising distress for the patient and family are paramount.

Care strategy 28.1 Pharmacological management of confusion and terminal restlessness[3,20,26]

- Haloperidol, a neuroleptic, is useful in treating agitation, fear and paranoia. Many patients with delirium can be managed with oral haloperidol, but if necessary the addition of parenteral lorazepam may be more effective in rapidly sedating agitated, delirious patients.
- If benzodiazepines are used in palliative care, oxazepam and lorazepam are the preferred drugs. Adding lorazepam to a regime of haloperidol has been described as a useful means of treating a patient with agitated delirium. However, lorazepam alone has been shown to be ineffective and in some cases was even found to worsen symptoms. Perhaps the only setting in which benzodiazepines in isolation have an established role is in the management of terminal restlessness. In palliative care the cornerstones of therapy are neuroleptic and benzodiazepine drugs.
- Phenothiazines (such as thioridazine, chlorpromazine, and methotrimeprazine) are recommended for severe symptoms when sedation is required. McIver et al. found that small doses of chlorpromazine rapidly relieved the distress of restlessness in terminal cancer and that rectal administration was as effective as intravenous administration, making it a useful drug for patients being cared for at home.[26] At times, however, it may be necessary to sedate patients deeply to control terminal restlessness. Sensitive nursing directed at supporting relatives and friends is paramount at this distressing and difficult time in the patient's illness. Wherever appropriate, patients' wishes for sedation or otherwise will have been gently explored, allowing an opportunity for autonomy of choice right up until the time of death.
- Methotrimeprazine is commonly used to control confusion and agitation in terminal restlessness. However, it causes excessive sedation at a time when patients and relatives have very little time left to spend together. Its potential for causing hypotension and excessive sedation are important limiting factors.
- Midazolam is also used to control agitation. Unlike haloperidol, but similar to methotrimeprazine, midazolam aims only to sedate and will not improve cognition. It should be used when the goal of treatment is quiet sedation only.

Sedation and ethics

During the last days and hours of life, up to 20% of patients will be suffering from 'terminal restlessness' or a delirium that may need to be treated with sedation to unconsciousness – terminal sedation.[23,25] There is, however, serious concern that this is a guise for euthanasia or physician-assisted suicide. Others believe that the intention and motivation of the practitioner is critical, where the intention is to induce and maintain deep sleep, but not deliberately cause death. The argument that terminal sedation is ethically and legally distinct from physician-assisted suicide was endorsed by the United States Supreme Court in 1997 when it pronounced that terminal sedation intended for symptom relief is not assisted suicide, but a licensed practice of palliative care.[28,29]

References

1. Parker J. (1981). Cancer passage: continuity and discourse in terminal care. In Benner P. and Wrubel J. (eds.) (1989). *The Primacy of Caring. Stress and Coping in Health and Illness.* Menlo Park, CA: Addison-Wesley, pp. 256–312.

2. Wein S. (1999). Cancer. In Robinson R.G. and Yates W.R. (eds.) *Psychiatric Management of the Medically Ill.* New York: Marcel Dekker, pp. 229–251.

3. Breitbart W. (1995). Identifying patients at risk for, and treatment of major psychiatric complications of cancer. *Supportive Care in Cancer* **3**, 45–60.

4. Zimberg M. and Berenson S. (1990). Delirium in patients with cancer: nursing assessment and intervention. *Oncology Nursing Forum* **17**, 529–537.

5. Breitbart W. (1994). Psycho-oncology: depression, anxiety, delirium. *Seminars in Oncology* **21**, 754–769.

6. Lipowski Z. (1987). Delirium (acute confusional states). *Journal of the American Medical Association* **258**, 1789–1792.

7. Macleod A.D. and Whitehead L.E. (1997). Dysgraphia and terminal delirium. *Palliative Medicine* **11**, 127–132.

8. Nicholas L.M. and Linsay B.A. (1995). Delirium presenting with symptoms of depression. *Psychosomatics* **36**, 471–479.

9. Fleishman S. and Lesko L. (1985). Delirium in cancer patients: spotting it early, finding the cause. *Primary Cancer Care* **5**, 23–27.

10. American Psychiatric Association. (1994). *Diagnostic and Statistical Manual of Mental Disorders, DSM-IV,* 4th edition. Washington: American Psychiatric Association.

11. Ingham J.M. and Caraceni A.T. (1998). In Berger E., Portenoy R. and Weissman D.E. (eds.) *Principles and Practice of Supportive Oncology.* Philadelphia, PA: Lippincott-Raven, pp. 477–495.

12. Weinrich S. and Sarna L. (1994). Delirium in the older person with cancer. *Cancer* **74**, 2079–2091.

13. Holland J. and Massie M. (1987). Psychosocial aspects of cancer in the elderly. *Clinical Geriatric Medicine* **3**, 533–539.

14. Fleishman S. and Lesko L. (1990). Delirium and dementia. In Holland J. and Rowland J. (eds.) *Handbook of Psycho-oncology. Psychological Care of the Patient with Cancer.* Oxford: Oxford University Press, pp. 342–355.

15. Murphy G.E. (1977). Suicide and attempted suicide. *Hospital Practice* **12**, 78–81.

16. Kleinman A. (1988). *The Illness Narratives: Suffering, Healing and the Human Condition.* New York: Basic Books.

17. Inouye S.K., Van Dyck C.H., Alessi C.A. *et al.* (1990). Clarifying confusion: The Confusion Assessment Method. A new method for the detection of delirium. *Annals of Internal Medicine* **113**, 941–948.

18. Breitbart W., Rosenfeld B., Roth A. *et al.* (1997). The Memorial Delirium Assessment Scale. *Journal of Pain and Symptom Management* **13**, 128–137.

19. Cawley N. and Webber J. (1995). Research priorities in palliative care. *International Journal of Palliative Nursing* **1**, 101–113.

20. Steifel F., Fainsinger R. and Bruera E. (1992). Acute confusional states in patients with advanced cancer. *Journal of Pain and Symptom Management* **7**, 94–98.

21. Lichter I. and Hunt E. (1990). The last 48 hours of life. *Journal of Palliative Care* **6**, 7–15.

22. Back I. (1992). Terminal restlessness in patients with advanced malignant disease. *Palliative Medicine* **6**, 293–298.

23. de Stoutz N., Tapper M. and Faisinger R. (1995). Reversible delirium in terminally ill patients. *Journal of Pain and Symptom Managemen,* **10**, 249–253.

24. Cody M. (1990). Depression and the use of antidepressants in patients with cancer. *Palliative Medicine* **4**, 271–278.

25. Power D., Kelly S., Gilsenan J. *et al.* (1993). Suitable screening tests for cognitive impairment and depression in the terminally ill—a prospective prevalence study. *Palliative Medicine* **7**, 213–218.

26. McIver B., Walsh D. and Nelson K. (1994). The use of chlorpromazine for symptom control in dying cancer

patients. *Journal of Pain and Symptom Management* **5**, 341–345.

27. Bruera E., Macmillan K., Hanson J. and MacDonald R. (1989). The cognitive effects of administration of narcotic analgesics in patients with cancer pain. *Pain* **39**, 13–16.

28. Chater S., Raymond V. and Paterson J. (1998). Sedation for intractable distress in the dying – a survey of experts. *Palliative Medicine* **12**, 255–269.

29. Burt R.A. (1997). The Supreme Court Speaks. *New England Journal of Medicine* **337**, 1234–1236

CHAPTER TWENTY-NINE

Acute events in cancer

Stephen O'Connor

Introduction

Considerable progress in treatment outcomes and overall cancer survivorship have been achieved in recent years as a result of improvements in cancer treatment modalities and developments in supportive therapies which have dramatically altered the experience of cancer for many.[1] Notwithstanding this, the individual's cancer journey may be marked by unanticipated and unpredictable events occurring either as a result of the disease process or its treatment,[2] which require rapid diagnosis and treatment if their impact and severity are to be minimised. Spinal cord compression, superior vena cava obstruction and hypercalcaemia are more common in advanced disease,[1,3] but are potentially reversible, and the nurse's role in recognising, assessing and acting upon the early signs of these events is paramount.[4–7]

Hypercalcaemia

Hypercalcaemia is the most common life-threatening metabolic complication of malignancy, affecting 10–20% of cancer patients,[8,9] although this figure is likely to be an underestimate.[10] The figure may be as high as 20–40% in head and neck, breast, lung and prostate cancers, multiple myeloma, and lymphoma where it is indicative of a poor prognosis,[11] most patients dying of refractory hypercalcaemia or the effects of their disease within a few months.[12] Minor elevations (up to 2.8 mmol/l) may remain asymptomatic in many patients, but higher plasma calcium levels can cause renal failure, coma and cardiac arrest,[1,12] so it should always be regarded as a medical emergency requiring immediate treatment if the patient's survival chances are to be improved.

Pathophysiology of hypercalcaemia

The pathophysiology of hypercalcaemia is multifactorial, several different mechanisms being responsible for its onset in malignant disease,[11] where it may occur slowly, remaining undiagnosed until symptoms manifest themselves, or swiftly, causing a rapid decline in cardiac, renal and neurological status.[8] Numerous non-malignant conditions such as thyrotoxicosis, renal failure, and primary hyperparathyroidism, or treatment with thiazide diuretics and various hormone therapies may themselves potentiate a raised serum calcium,[8,11] but the commonest form of hypercalcaemia in malignancy is humoral hypercalcaemia of malignancy (HHM), which results from the dysregulation of endogenous parathyroid hormone-related peptide (PTHrP) by malignant cells in such a way that it gains access to the circulation from which it is normally excluded.[13] Here, it interacts with transforming growth factors (TGFα, TGFβ), epidermal growth factor, and interleukins α and β to stimulate osteoclastic bone resorption and enhanced calcium reabsorption in the renal tubules giving rise to elevated serum calcium levels.[13] HHM is most commonly seen in squamous-cell carcinomas of the head and neck, lung, oesophagus, and skin, although it also occurs in renal, bladder, ovarian, and some endocrine cancers.[11,13]

Hypercalcaemia in breast and prostate cancer is more likely to occur as a result of osteoclastic activity directly mediated by bone metastases,[11,13] in which the same chemical and hormonal mediators stimulate osteolysis and the release of calcium into the plasma. Here it exerts the same effects upon smooth muscle and nerve tissue by altering cell membrane permeability to calcium, sodium, and potassium ions.[14,15] Myeloma proteins may also elevate serum calcium by impairing osteoblastic function in bone tissue, but these must be significantly elevated in order for this to occur,[16,17] while the over-production of calcitrol, derived from vitamin D in granulomatous tumours such as Hodgkin's and non-Hodgkin's lymphomas leads to changes in extracellular calcium and phosphate concentrations by stimulating absorption of dietary calcium in the gastrointestinal tract and its mineralisation in bone.[18] Calcitrol and PTH normally counteract the effects of each other, but the hepatic hydroxylation of calcitrol in lymphoma is not subject to this negative feedback mechanism and the hypercalcaemic effects of each are thus compounded.[18]

Diagnosis and initial interventions for hypercalcaemia

Eighty-five per cent of people with hypercalcaemia will have demonstrable changes on X-ray or bone scan,[1] although this will be due to bone metastases or primary osteolytic tumours in only 20–30% of cases.[8] The presence of clinical signs may provide sufficient justification for the immediate treatment of suspected hypercalcaemia and may prevent irreversible end-organ damage, although non-malignant causes such as diabetes mellitus, cerebral metastases, hepatic or renal failure, and neutropenic sepsis should also be investigated.[12] Differential diagnosis depends upon a raised corrected serum calcium, the normal range being 2.1–2.6 mmol/l,[11,12] and treatment may vary depending upon whether the patient is symptomatic or not. When assessing an individual's serum calcium level a 'corrected' serum calcium

may need to be calculated. This takes into account serum albumin levels and allows for an increase in ionised (biologically active) calcium in cachexic or malnourished individuals where serum protein will be low.[8] A corrected serum calcium is calculated thus:

$$\text{Corrected calcium} = \text{measured calcium} + (40 - \text{albumin}) \times 0.02 \text{ mmol/l}.$$

The therapeutic goal of therapy is a reduction in calcium resorption from bone tissue and an increase in renal calcium excretion,[3] although tumour control is the only effective measure in the long term.[9,11,17] In mild hypercalcaemia (<3.0 mmol/l), symptoms may be alleviated by encouraging the individual to increase their fluid intake to 4 l per day followed by oral biphosphonates if serum calcium continues to rise.[11] Severely cachexic individuals or those with advanced disease may struggle to take adequate fluids however, and intravenous infusions of 4–6 l/day of saline should increase calcium excretion from the kidneys, although fewer than 30% of patients will achieve normocalcaemia with hydration alone.[11] A potassium-sparing loop diuretic such as furosemide may be used to increase calcium excretion,[15] although the dosage needs to be moderate if further instability in fluid volume is to be avoided.[11] Thiazide diuretics, which increase tubular calcium absorption, are contraindicated however, and should not be used in hypercalcaemia.

Biphosphonate therapy

Biphosphates such as sodium clodronate, sodium etidronate and sodium pamidronate have become the mainstay of treatment for hypercalcaemia of malignancy in the last decade.[11,19] They are potent inhibitors of osteoclastic bone resorption and achieve normocalcaemia in 70–80% of patients within days of administration.[1,20] They are also effective against the actions of PTHrP in humoral hypercalcaemia of malignancy,[20] and some third-generation drugs such as zoledronic acid have been demonstrated to exert additional anti-tumour effects against some cancers.[20–23]

Normocalcaemia elicited by sodium pamidronate ranges from 1.8 to 46.6 days,[20] and has a longer time to relapse than either sodium clodronate or sodium etidronate, though zoledronate is more potent still and has a rapid onset of action.[11,24] Side-effects are generally few and limited to skin irritation at the infusion site and a flu-like reaction on first administration in about one-fifth of patients,[11] but the more powerful drugs zoledronate and ibandronate can cause transient hypocalcaemia and hypophosphataemia in addition to these.[11,20,25] Ross *et al.* advocate as short an administration time as possible,[20] although rapid administration may lead to the deposition of calcium complexes in the kidneys with consequent kidney failure,[26] and the nurse should not attempt to exceed the manufacturer's recommended infusion times which are currently 15 minutes for zoledronate and 2–24 hours for pamidronate.[27,28] The nurse should also check serum creatinine before each dose and ensure that the patient is adequately hydrated, discontinuing therapy if renal function deteriorates during the infusion.[29,30]

Biphosphonates are poorly absorbed by the gastrointestinal tract, although preparations such as oral clodronate are useful in the management of mild or asymptomatic hypercalcaemia and for those wishing to remain at home,[11,31] although there may be problems with adherence to oral regimes over time.[32,33] The only adverse effects of oral administration are epigastric pain and oesophagitis, but these can be overcome by advising the recipient to drink a large glass of water (180–240 ml) with each dose and remain upright for 30 minutes after ingestion.[31]

Other treatments for hypercalcaemia

Corticosteroids decrease absorption of calcium from the gut and inhibit osteoclast-mediated bone resorption.[11] They are effective in the treatment of hypercalcaemia caused by Hodgkin's and non-Hodgkin's lymphomas, myeloma, and metastatic breast cancer but require 3–5 days in which to work.[8,17,18] They may cause gastrointestinal disturbance, opportunistic infections, hyperglycaemia, and osteoporosis with prolonged use and should be used for as short a time as possible before titrating downwards.[11]

Calcitonin, an endogenous peptide hormone produced by the thyroid and parathyroid counteracts the actions of PTH in a negative feedback mechanism, by depressing osteoclastic activity and encouraging the growth of new bone.[34] It is particularly useful for granulomatous tumours such as multiple myeloma where abnormal vitamin D metabolism contributes towards increased calcium absorption.[34] It works rapidly but has a short duration (3–4 days), requiring repeated intramuscular or intravenous injections, and may cause nausea, facial flushing, tingling, and an unpleasant taste.[11,34] It may also elicit acute hypocalcaemic reactions when given in combination with biphosphonate therapy,[11] and resistance or the development of antibodies to the commonly used salmon calcitonin may make it unacceptable in the management of those with advanced disease, although it may be useful for severe symptomatic hypercalcaemia as an adjunct to biphosphonates.[35]

Gallium nitrate has also been used in the treatment of malignant hypercalcaemia and is thought to inhibit osteoclast-mediated bone resorption, stimulate bone formation, and alter the mineral composition of bone by enhancing calcium and phosphate re-uptake.[36,37] It may be useful for cancers associated with accelerated bone loss such as multiple myeloma,[37] and has been well tolerated in a number of randomised trials where it produced a higher rate and longer duration of normocalcaemia than calcitonin, etidronate, and pamidronate. It may also be useful for tumours associated with high levels of PTHrP which limits the effectiveness of some calcium-lowering biphosphonates,[36] but it is normally given as a 5-day continuous intravenous infusion requiring close monitoring of renal function and adequate hydration. Its clinical usefulness is limited therefore, as is the use of plicamycin (mithramycin), a potent inhibitor of RNA synthesis within osteoclasts which decreases bone resorption in up to 80% of tumour-mediated hypercalcaemias.[1,11] Repeated doses of this irritant drug may be required every 3–7 days and may cause rebound hypercalcaemia unless the underlying disease is successfully treated.[11] It may also cause thrombocytopenia, stomatitis, and nephrotoxicity, and is generally no longer used in the management of malignant hypercalcaemia, its toxicity profile and the advent of effective third-generation biphosphonates rendering it unacceptable as a first-line treatment for hypercalcaemia of malignancy (personal communication S. Armitage, Royal Marsden Hospital Medicines Information Service. 9 August 2005).[35]

Care issues in the management of an acute hypercalcaemic crisis

Hypercalcaemia can be an extremely distressing experience for both the individual and family members, who may find changes to the cognitive functioning, physical appearance and self-care ability of their family member disturbing. In the most severe or acute cases, the individual may suffer extreme thirst and become agitated in their quest for adequate hydration, while others may become weak, lethargic, and unresponsive to those around them. Cognitive dysfunction may lead to hallucinations and confusion, the individual having little personal insight and losing their orientation to time, place, and space. Personal carers may no longer be recognised and come under accusation or suspicion, necessitating the individual's admission to hospital as a crisis in care develops, whereupon the hospital ward may be seen as a threatening, hostile environment rather than place of care and safety. The need for immediate treatment is paramount therefore,[4-7] and requires early recognition of warning signs such as extreme thirst, constipation, nausea and vomiting, polyuria, and subtle changes in mentation. These should alert the nurse to the likelihood of its existence and the need to initiate appropriate biochemical tests.[38] Dignity and personal safety should be maintained at all times and it may be necessary to re-evaluate the required skills-mix or staffing levels on the unit since these patients may be more liable to falls, accidental injury, and very occasionally, inappropriate social behaviour. They may also require greater assistance with self-care activities and personal hygiene, and infusion sites may need to be resited or adequately splinted to prevent their accidental removal.

Hypercalcaemia is, unfortunately, an indicator of advanced disease, and it may be appropriate to withhold medical treatment where it frequently recurs.[11,12] It is important in such cases to elicit both the individual's and family members' understanding of the prognosis, as the advice and support of the hospice or palliative care team may

be warranted in this difficult time of transition.[39,40] Care interventions in such instances should be aimed at helping the individual to remain at home or their preferred place of death if possible, by empowering them to make informed decisions so that they can have a peaceful and dignified death.[40] This does not necessarily obviate the further use of biphosphonates however, as these can provide symptomatic benefit throughout the terminal phase of the individual's life and significantly improve their quality of life in the 'living–dying' interval.[39]

Spinal cord or cauda equina compression

Spinal cord compression is diagnosed in approximately 5–10% of cancer patients,[3-5,41-43] although its incidence is increasing as a result of improvements in screening, magnetic resonance imaging (MRI), and cancer therapies that have increased cancer patient longevity.[42,44] The spinal cord is the commonest destination for bone metastases,[45] the highest incidence being in breast, lung, prostate, melanoma, and renal cell tumours which share a common affinity for bone tissue,[5,46-50] although up to 40% of all cancer patients exhibit signs of spinal metastases on post mortem examination.[42,47] Spinal cord compression is also the second commonest cause of neurological complications after brain metastases, and a significant cause of morbidity and mortality.[42,46,51] although primary tumours of the central nervous system (see Table 29.1) are rarely responsible for spinal cord

Table 29.1 Primary central nervous tumours giving rise to spinal cord compression

Tumour type	Common location
Chordoma	Extradural
Meningioma, neurofibroma, schwannoma	Intradural extramedullary
Astrocytoma, epenymoma, haemangioblastoma, lipoma, glioma	Intramedullary

compression, the majority of cases arising from extradural, blood-borne metastases.[6,12,46] Cauda equina compression is diagnosed less frequently and is considered a rare complication of metastatic disease,[52,53] although its presence may be occluded by the presence of concomitant spinal cord compression which affects different regions of the spine in 10–38% of cases.[42,46,54–56]

Breast, lung and prostate cancers account for more than 50% of malignant spinal cord compression,[42,57] which is also commonly found in multiple myeloma, lymphoma, and melanoma,[6,58,59] but any cancer which has the propensity to metastasise to bone may cause this debilitating condition which can cause pain, permanent damage to the central nervous system, paraplegia, and deterioration in the patient's quality of life and functional status unless treated immediately,[4,5,60] necessitating immediate intervention irrespective of its cause or the disease status of the individual affected.[5,38,51,61]

Early warning signs of spinal cord compression

Back pain and tenderness are experienced by up to 94% of patients on presentation,[46,62] and may be localised or radicular in nature.[5,43,61,63] Its insidious onset may be attributed to other causes such as arthritis – especially in the elderly,[64] but it is essential to differentiate the pain associated with spinal cord compression from degenerative spinal problems or acute trauma such as a herniated disc.[65] Unlike non-malignant back pain, the pain arising from spinal cord compression is not alleviated by lying down and may be worse at nighttime, although standing, walking, coughing and sneezing can also exacerbate it.[5,43,46] Pain may be absent, however, in lymphoma, and lung and renal disease,[43] so it is vital that spinal or cauda equina compression are not summarily dismissed as possible causes of urinary hesitancy, a sluggish bowel, numbness, 'pins and needles', weakness or 'heaviness' in the lower limbs in the absence of pain.

Radicular pain, described as a tight, band-like constriction around the torso is less common than localised pain, but indicative of advancing neurological damage.[5,46,66] It is always bilateral when thoracic nerves are damaged, whereas cervical or lumbosacral involvement may manifest themselves bilaterally or unilaterally.[3,43] A positive Lhermitte's sign may provide early indication of spinal cord involvement. This may induce a tingling or 'electric shock' sensation in the back or lower limbs when asked to flex or extend the head and neck, whilst hyper-reflexivity of the extensor plantar response demonstrated by a positive Babinsky reflex is regarded as a positive indicator,[65] though its absence does not exclude the possibility that spinal cord compression has occurred.[67] The use of a body outline or a dermatome chart may prove useful in identifying the likely level of spinal cord compression,[68] and normal neurological functioning above this area will help to eliminate brain metastases as the likely cause of sensorimotor or neurological deficits. These may include a loss of proprioception or stiffness in the affected limbs, 'foot-drop' or unsteady gait, parasthesiae and loss of sensation to pain, cold, and heat, although their significance may go unrecognised or be attributed to non-malignant causes on occasions.[46]

Eighty per cent of those diagnosed whilst ambulatory have a chance of recovery, but this is reduced to only 5% in those diagnosed once paraplegia has occurred.[46,69] Education about the relative risk and early warning signs of spinal cord compression is crucial therefore,[3] but the nurse should place emphasis upon the positive outcomes associated with early diagnosis. A leaflet reiterating the information given and containing out-of-hours contact numbers will reinforce the need to contact the oncology team without delay,[5] and may limit the onset of progressive nerve damage, pain, incontinence, and paralysis, which could occur without additional warning in a matter of hours.[1,5,12]

Diagnostic techniques

X-rays are a useful first-line measure and will identify spinal metastases in up to 83–85% of spinal cord compressions,[38,46] although one study of 201 spinal cord compression patients by Husband *et al.* found that only one-third of paraspinal masses detected at the site of extradural spinal cord compression by MRI had previously been detected by plain radiographic examination,[55] and it has been estimated that approximately 50% of the bone must be damaged in order for these to be visible on a plain film. MRI is therefore regarded as the most accurate diagnostic tool for the diagnosis of spinal cord compression and often identifies previously unsuspected tumours in addition to establishing the extent and required treatment volume for known lesions.[70,71] Husband *et al.* regard an urgent MRI scan as mandatory in the aftermath of a negative plain X-ray wherever neurological deficits are observed,[55] although treatment may be commenced in the presence of positive neurological signs in circumstances where a full MRI scan may be contraindicated or is otherwise deemed unacceptable.[7] Interest is also growing in the use of positron emission tomography (PET) scans which can detect very small lesions within the spine in addition to providing clinically useful information about neuronal dysfunction and impaired metabolic activity within the spinal cord.[72–74]

Good communication is essential prior to diagnostic tests and is a fundamental component of the nurse's role when caring for those with suspected spinal cord compression.[5] The benefits of providing sensory and procedural information so that individuals can create a cognitive map or anticipatory schema are well known,[75] and will prepare them for the unfamiliar experience they are about to encounter. Similarly, many value the presence of a familiar face on the way to or throughout the procedure, and timely assessment of their analgesic, anxiolytic or premedication requirements will also help to lessen the discomfort of a lengthy or uncomfortable scan. In some cases, the administration of an opioid analgesic or muscle relaxant may be appropriate,[5] and catheterisation, fluid balance, or blood glucose monitoring may also be indicated, depending upon the procedure being undertaken.[76]

Interventions for spinal cord compression

Interventions for spinal cord compression are primarily palliative,[46,60] and are aimed at restoring optimal neurological function, controlling pain and maintaining the stability of the spine by debulking the tumour or controlling its growth,[4,38] before permanent neurological dysfunction occurs.[63] The choice of treatment depends upon the number and level of spinal lesions, the rate of neurological deterioration, the sensitivity of the tumour to radio- or chemotherapy, and any prior treatments given.[7] The most commonly used treatments are corticosteroids, primarily dexamethasone.[5,43] These have analgesic, oncolytic and anti-inflammatory properties, and successfully reduce oedema around the lesion,[5,46,77] maintaining ambulation in 81% of those diagnosed with progressive loss of function. Doses up to 100 mg may be followed by a daily divided dose of 96 mg for 3 days prior to dose reduction,[5,46,78] although high-dose regimens remain controversial and may be contraindicated in patients with diabetes, hypertension, peptic ulcer, and other steroid sensitivities where radiotherapy alone may prove effective as long as it is started prior to the onset of neurological damage,[79] or within 24 h of medullary compression.[69]

Radiotherapy is the treatment of choice for radiosensitive tumours such as lymphoma, myeloma, seminoma, Ewing's sarcoma and neuroblastoma.[43] It has a moderately good outcome for spinal cord compression in breast and prostate cancers, but others such as non-small-cell lung cancer, melanoma, renal cell carcinoma, and soft tissue sarcomas are relatively radioresistant and require surgical intervention.[43,52] Common treatment dosages range from 2–4 Gy in 10 daily fractions to the two vertebral bodies above and below the lesion,[38,46] although doses of 4–8 Gy per day may be required in order to elicit a favourable outcome depending upon the type of tumour and any prior exposure to radiotherapy.[69] There is also increasing interest in hypofractionated radiotherapy regimes. One large (n = 300) randomised controlled trial by Maranzano *et al.* comparing the efficacy of two consecutive daily doses of 8 Gy over split 3- and 5-day regimens delivering 15 Gy found no significant difference in duration, response, survival, or toxicity between the three,[80] thus shorter regimens may be preferable in respect of patient comfort, convenience, and the quality of life.[80–83]

Possible adverse reactions to radiotherapy include myelosuppression, skin problems, nausea and vomiting, gastrointestinal disturbance, or heartburn, depending upon the site irradiated,[38] so the role of the nurse in assessment, symptom management, and patient education is crucial throughout the course of treatment. Recent interest has been shown in the efficacy of bisphosphonates such as sodium pamidronate and sodium clodronate in the management of spinal cord compression, but while they are effective in the prevention of complications such as pain and pathological fractures related to bone metastases,[43,84–86] their efficacy in the management of spinal cord compression has not been proven.[85,87]

Surgery remains the treatment of choice where the stability of the spine is already compromised, the tumour is radioresistant, or has relapsed after unsuccessful irradiation, and in patients with an unknown primary or an uncertain diagnosis in which it may be used to establish the nature and extent of a suspected lesion prior to its removal.[45,69] Surgery is not generally indicated, however, for myeloma, lymphoma, breast or prostate metastases, which have a 70–88% chance of responding to radiotherapy alone,[78] and may be unnecessary for lymphoma, myeloma, neuroblastoma, or germ cell tumours, which respond well to cytotoxic chemotherapy and radiotherapy.[43] Surgical decompression and spinal fixation may be indicated when a spinal lesion causes compression of the spinal cord or other neural elements,[42,88] although subsequent radiotherapy may well be advantageous.[89] Surgery may be complicated by pre-operative radiotherapy, however, one retrospective study ($n = 85$) by Ghogawala *et al.* demonstrating a threefold increase in wound complications in those receiving radiotherapy before decompression.[54] Additional risks to surgery include a 6–10% chance of mortality, further deterioration in neurological status and post-operative complications such as infection, haemorrhage, and cerebrospinal fluid leakage,[5,38,46] so it is used primarily to treat progressive neurological deficits or spinal instability. Interventions such as decompression laminectomy and fusion with or without radiotherapy may elicit marked improvements in pain, neurological, and functional status as long as paraplegia is not present.[42,46]

Rehabilitation following spinal cord compression

An individual's potential for successful rehabilitation depends upon clinical status at diagnosis and their response to treatment, although intensive multiprofessional effort will significantly improve outcomes for all those affected by spinal cord compression.[90] However, while physical function may be restored by treatment, patients are likely to have impaired mobility for a period of time and the role of physiotherapists, occupational therapists and others is crucial. Many will require intensive physiotherapy, wheelchairs, braces, and other mechanical aids, and the nurse can greatly assist them in their recovery by promoting and assessing the individual's confidence in their use. Most will still require some level of protection from potential injury, and it may be necessary to remind them to place their feet appropriately when standing or transferring from bed to chair, assess skin integrity in those remaining immobile for long periods of time, and promote good body alignment when at rest.[5] Careful assessment of bowel and bladder function will promote continence and prevent infection which might prevent successful rehabilitation, while a practical, problem-solving approach to expressed concerns will promote patient confidence, autonomy and independence.[91] Patients should be encouraged to express their anxieties for the future, and short-term goals negotiated so that their outcomes are both measurable and attainable.[5] Assessment of the individual's coping strategies, psychological adjustment, and locus of control[92] will enable the nurse to amend these goals while continuing to promote personal autonomy and social engagement, although these may require additional time and planning.[93] Sexual dysfunction may give rise to role anxiety, altered self-concept, or feelings of inadequacy although empathy, understanding, and the promotion of sexuality through alternative means such as dress, personal grooming, and the promotion of privacy for the expression of intimacy with others will greatly assist them in coming to terms with permanent or temporary losses of this nature, though professional counselling may be required where this remains an issue.[93]

Superior vena cava obstruction

Pathophysiology of superior vena cava obstruction

Superior vena cava obstruction (SVCO) is a rare but distressing and potentially life-threatening circulatory condition which affects individuals with cancer and, in 3–5% of cases, non-malignant conditions such as thyroid goitre, aortic aneurism, mediastinal fibrosis, and histoplasmosis.[94] It is commonly associated with carcinomas of the lung and non-Hodgkin's lymphoma, which together account for 84 97% of cases, metastatic breast disease, which may be responsible for as many as 10% of cases, and, more rarely, mediastinal tumours such as mesothelioma, thymoma, thymic carcinoid, and germ cell tumours.[95–97] Iatrogenic causes include superior vena cava thrombosis following the insertion of a cardiac pacemaker or central venous catheter.[94] The incidence of SVCO in small-cell lung cancer is more than five times greater than in non-small-cell lung cancer, one Cochrane systematic review reporting an incidence of 10% and 1.7% respectively in newly diagnosed lung cancer patients where it may be a presenting symptom of their disease.[96]

The superior vena cava is especially vulnerable to obstruction because of its thin walls, low venous pressure,[7,94] and the fact that it occupies a non-distensible space surrounded by inflexible structures such as the trachea, bronchus, sternum and pulmonary artery.[94,95] Occlusion of the vessel by a primary tumour, metastatic disease, thrombus, or enlarged lymph node obstructs the venous return of blood to the heart causing venous stasis of the head, arms, and upper chest, decreased cardiac output, and orthopnoea,[15,95] the main danger to patients arising from airway obstruction or laryngeal, bronchial, and cerebral oedema. The rate of onset is usually insidious, most individuals experiencing symptoms 4–6 weeks prior to diagnosis,[98] although the onset is likely to be more acute when the vessel is obstructed above the entry of the azygos vein, which normally facilitates collateral drainage via the internal mammary, lateral thoracic, paraspinous, and oesophageal veins.[94]

Clinical manifestations and diagnosis of superior vena cava obstruction

In the majority of cases, a differential diagnosis can be made on the basis of the presenting clinical picture, individuals with SVCO usually presenting with pronounced oedema of the face and neck, upper trunk and an elevated venous pressure leading to non-pulsatile distension of the neck

Table 29.2 Frequency of signs and symptoms in superior vena cava obstruction[94]

Presenting symptom	Frequency (%)
Venous distension of the neck	66
Dyspnoea	60
Venous distension of chest wall	54
Facial swelling	50
Cough	24
Cyanosis	20
Arm swelling	18
Chest pain	15

veins, and periorbital oedema.[3,7,96] They may also present with shortness of breath and hoarseness, and suffer from cough or stridor (see Table 29.2), although it is necessary to eliminate other possible causes for these symptoms, especially in lung cancer, which may have alternative aetiologies. Acute or severe blockage may cause visual and cognitive changes, headaches, dizziness, and acute respiratory distress as an adequate collateral circulation via the azygos vein may not have developed.[94,96] These, together with cyanosis, syncope, and coma are less common but indicative of advanced disease and require urgent medical intervention.[95]

A plain chest X-ray reveals a widened mediastinum or a right-sided mass in approximately 60–80% of cases,[94,95] while a computed tomography (CT) or MRI scan may provide important information on the location and extent of the obstruction, the integrity of vital structures such as the vocal cord or bronchi, and enable the blockage and any collateral blood flow to be visualised. CT scans also enable mediastinoscopy, bronchoscopy or fine needle aspiration of any mass, which may prove useful in lymphoma and germ cell tumours which are potentially curable with appropriate treatment.[12,99] CT scans are also useful in defining the required size and location of the treatment field for radiotherapy, and providing a clinical baseline for the evaluation of an individual's response to cytotoxic chemotherapy, while a contrast venogram or, increasingly, a radionuclide study may be used to identify possible stenosis and the extent of any thrombus formation prior to stenting.[94,96] Invasive tests are generally minimised, however, because of the risk of haemorrhage,[12] or thrombus formation,[95] and may not be appropriate in those with a very poor prognosis when treatment decisions are unlikely to be affected by their outcome.[1]

Clinical management of superior vena cava obstruction

The successful management of SVCO depends upon the elimination of underlying disease and the alleviation of life-threatening symptoms associated with it.[95] Nursing measures such as reassurance, elevation of the head, assistance with activities of daily living, and the initiation of oxygen therapy may provide symptomatic relief and allow time for a definitive histology to be obtained.[95,100] Constrictive clothing and interventions such as blood pressure monitoring via the affected limbs should also be avoided. A high-dose corticosteroid such as dexamethasone will significantly reduce laryngeal or cerebral oedema,[94,95] although oedema may worsen temporarily if administered alongside radiotherapy, as a result of ionisation at the tumour site.[81,96] Advice about the likelihood and transience of this side-effect is crucial if further anxiety is to be minimised, and it may be appropriate to administer a diuretic such as furosemide, which can provide symptomatic relief.[94,95,101] The total daily dose of steroids should be given singly in the morning or twice daily at breakfast and lunchtime, as this will lessen the cognitive arousal and insomnia associated with their use later in the day without compromising the therapeutic outcomes of therapy.[102]

Radiotherapy is the mainstay of treatment for SVCO due to its therapeutic action across a broad range of cancers, loco-regional effect, and patient tolerance at small doses, and is particularly useful for chemotherapy resistant tumours or non-small-cell carcinomas of the bronchus.[1,69] However, the therapeutic benefits of radiotherapy are often offset by the discomfort and inconvenience of having to travel to regional radiotherapy centres, long waiting times, unanticipated delays in treatment and, with fractionated regimes, frequent separation from loved ones which may impact upon their real or perceived quality of life in the last stages of the disease process.[83] There is, moreover, evidence that some radiographers are reluctant to use single fractionated doses in spite of a growing evidence base supporting simpler treatment regimes for the palliation of symptoms in advanced disease,[1,96,103] and this may place individuals in a 'double jeopardy' situation where the impact of treatment may add to rather than ameliorate the effects of their cancer.[104] Notwithstanding this, SVCO is a debilitating condition and radiotherapy plays an invaluable role in its management,[1,12,94] particularly in radiotherapy naive patients where symptom responses in the region of 94% have been reported in a number of studies.[96] However, many may have unnecessary concerns about its side-effects,[82] or unrealistic expectations about its effectiveness, over half the respondents in one study anticipating that it would 'heal' or make them well again in spite of being informed that it was being given with palliative intent.[105] It can therefore be distressing if the relief of symptoms is not immediately apparent or they appear worse in the immediate aftermath of treatment.[81,106] so reassurance and explanation by the nurse of the actions, timescales, and anticipated side-effects of radiotherapy are important.

In holistic terms, cytotoxic chemotherapy has some advantages over radiotherapy for the management of SVCO in chemotherapy-responsive tumours as it can be administered in the individual's local hospital and may only require a single infusion or bolus. It also has systemic effect which may be useful in metastatic disease, allowing radiotherapy to be used for the treatment of recurrence should this occur.[1] Symptom response to palliative chemotherapy for SVCO in lung cancer ranges from 60% for non-small-cell lung cancer to 77% for small-cell lung cancer,[96] and intensive regimes such as MACOP-B (methotrexate with leucovirin, doxorubicin, cyclophosphamide, vincristine, prednisone, and bleomycin) may indeed prove curative in lymphoma and germ cell tumours,[99,107] making it an effective first-line treatment for SVCO in both acute and advanced disease. These results are significantly increased when radiotherapy and chemotherapy are given together however, with some chemoradiotherapy regimes eliciting response rates as high as 83.3%

in SVCO associated with some lymphomas,[99,107] though sample sizes in such studies tend to be small.[97] More recent studies have advocated the percutaneous placement of expandable metal stents as a primary treatment for SVCO.[108–110] These provide rapid and effective relief of SVCO with immediate correction of the circulatory problem in 95% of cases, although the size and statistical power of such studies is low, no doubt as a result of the high cost of stents and the relatively low numbers of routine insertions carried out. They do have considerable benefit in non-small-cell lung cancer as long as SVCO is identified early, so that the complications associated with the concomitant anti-thrombolytic therapy can be minimised.[96] For a summary of the treatments and treatment outcomes for SCVO see Table 29.3.

Table 29.3 Treatment and treatment outcomes in SVCO

Treatment	Use	Treatment outcomes
Radiotherapy[a]	Non-small-cell lung cancer	Single fraction may be adequate to elicit relief of symptoms,[95] although this may take up to 14 days to occur[96]
	Small-cell lung cancer	Radiotherapy not indicated
	Indeterminate diagnosis/others	Initial short course of radiotherapy while awaiting definitive diagnosis[95]
Cytotoxic chemotherapy[a]	Small-cell lung cancer	Relief of symptoms in 76.9% of cases. Objective tumour response in 68.4% of cases – similar to those for small-cell lung cancer in general[96]
	Non-small cell lung cancer	Objective response rates much lower than in small-cell lung cancer, in the region of 20–40% compared with 50–80%
	Lymphoma and germ cell tumours	Aggressive treatment warranted and may result in long-term recurrence particularly if aligned to radiotherapy.[99] Treatment with MACOP-B particularly effective for mediastinal large B-cell lymphomas[107]
Surgical stenting	All malignancies	Provides rapid relief of symptoms within 12–24 h,[108,110] and is useful for relapse after alternative treatment or those with persistent SVCO provided these are recognised swiftly. Survival period often shorter than those reported for radiotherapy, chemotherapy or chemoradiotherapy although symptomatic benefit makes this worthwhile and endovascular stenting is increasingly proposed as the primary treatment of choice for all SVCO[96,108,109]
Corticosteroids	All malignancies	Used routinely – especially with radiotherapy though evidence base to support their use in SVCO is lacking.[97] High doses should be used for minimum period possible[96]

[a]The effectiveness of treatment appears not to depend upon any particular radiotherapy fractionation schedule or chemotherapy regime though clinical responses to radiotherapy appear higher in radiotherapy naive patients (94% versus 70%). Relief from SVCO was higher in synchronous chemoradiotherapy regimes (83.3% of patients) than those receiving radiotherapy or chemotherapy in isolation, although the absolute numbers treated ($n = 18$) were small.[96]

Conclusion

Spinal cord compression, superior vena cava obstruction, and hypercalcaemia carry a high risk of morbidity and mortality in advanced cancer and can have a devastating impact upon the real or perceived quality of life of those affected by them. Morbidity and mortality need not be a defining feature of these acute events however, and the nurse's ability to recognise and act upon the signs associated with each makes a significant contribution to positive clinical outcomes in such cases. Considerable progress in the medical management of each has been made in recent years as older interventions have been superseded by newer and better therapies; but the nurse's role in respect of patient education, rehabilitation, psychological, social, and spiritual care remains unchanged. Nursing interventions have the potential to limit the physiological impact of the acute event or its treatment upon the individual, and make a significant contribution towards the optimisation of biopsychosocial, sexual and spiritual health in the aftermath of an acute event, which makes the care of individuals experiencing acute events in advanced cancer one of the most challenging but rewarding aspects of cancer care.

References

1. Souhami R.L. and Tobias J. (2005). *Cancer and its Management*. Oxford: Blackwell Scientific.
2. Johnston P. and Spence R. (2002). *Oncological Emergencies*. Oxford: Oxford University Press.
3. Yarbro C., Frogge M.H. and Goodman M. (2003). *Cancer Symptom Management*. Boston, MA: Jones and Bartlett.
4. Leon T.G. and Pase M. (2004). Essential oncology facts for the float nurse. *Medical Surgical Nursing* **13**, 165–171, 189.
5. Wilkes G.M. (2003). Spinal cord compression. In Yarbro C.H., Frogge M.H. and Goodman M. (eds.) *Cancer Symptom Management*. Boston, MA: Jones and Bartlett, pp. 359–373.
6. Tan S.J. (2002). Recognition and treatment of oncologic emergencies. *Journal of Infusion Nursing* **25**, 182–188.
7. King P.A. (1995). Oncologic emergencies: assessment, identification, and interventions in the emergency department. *Journal of Emergency Nursing* **21**, 213–218.
8. Moore J.M. (1998). Metabolic emergencies: hypercalcemia. In Gross J. and Johnson B. (eds.) *Handbook of Oncology Nursing*. Boston, MA: Jones and Bartlett, pp. 675–691.
9. Heys S.D., Smith I.C. and Eremin O. (1998). Hypercalcaemia in patients with cancer: aetiology and treatment. *European Journal of Surgical Oncology* **24**, 139–142.
10. Lamy O., Jenzer-Closuit A. and Burckhardt P. (2001). Hypercalcaemia of malignancy: an undiagnosed and undertreated disease. *Journal of Internal Medicine* **250**, 73.
11. Hussein M. and Cullen K. (2003). Metabolic emergencies. In Johnston P. and Spence R. (eds.) *Oncologic Emergencies*. Oxford: Oxford University Press, pp. 51–73.
12. Neal A.J. and Hoskin P.J. (2003). *Clinical Oncology: Basic Principles and Practice*. London: Arnold.
13. Yen Y., Chu P.G. and Feng W. (2004). Paraneoplastic syndromes in cancer: case 3, parathyroid hormone-related hypercalcemia in cholangiocarcinoma. *Journal of Clinical Oncology* **22**, 2244–2245.
14. Tortora G.J. (2005). *Principles of Anatomy and Physiology*. Chichester: John Wiley and Sons.
15. Ganong W.F. (2005). *Review of Medical Physiology*. New York: Lange Basic Science.
16. Bone H. (2000). Bone disease in malignancy. In Hosking D. and Ringe, J. (eds.) *Treatment of Metastatic Bone Disease*. London: Taylor and Francis, pp. 57–75.
17. Hosking D. and Ringe J. (2000). *Treatment of Metastatic Bone Disease*. London: Taylor and Francis.
18. Marshall W.J. and Bangert S.K. (2004). *Clinical Chemistry*. Philadelphia, PA: Elsevier Health Sciences.
19. Heatley S. (2004). Metastatic bone disease and tumour-induced hypercalcaemia: treatment options. *International Journal of Palliative Nursing* **10**, 41–46.
20. Ross J.R., Saunders Y., Edmonds P.M. *et al.* (2004). A systematic review of the role of biphosphonates in metastatic disease. *Health Technology Assessment* **8**, 1–192.
21. Wellington K. and Goa K.L. (2003). Zoledronic acid: a review of its use in the management of bone metastases and hypercalcaemia of malignancy. *Drugs* **63**, 417–437.
22. Neville-Webbe H.L. and Coleman R.E. (2003). The use of zoledronic acid in the management of metastatic bone disease and hypercalcaemia. *Palliative Medicine* **17**, 539–553.
23. Berenson J.R. (2001). Zoledronic acid in cancer patients with bone metastases: results of phase I and II trials. *Seminars in Oncology* **28**, 25–34.
24. Major P., Lortholay A., Hon J. *et al.* (2001). Zoledronic acid is superior to pamidronate in the treatment of hypercalcaemia of malignancy: a pooled analysis of two

randomised controlled trials. *Journal of Clinical Oncology* **19**, 558–567.

25. Peter R., Mishra V. and Fraser W.D. (2004). Lesson of the week: severe hypocalcaemia after being given intravenous bisphosphonate. *British Medical Journal* **328**, 335–336.

26. Chang J.T., Green L. and Beitz J. (2003) Renal failure with the use of zoledronic acid. *New England Journal of Medicine* **349**, 1676–1679.

27. Novartis (2004) *Zometa® (Zoledronic Acid) Injection Prescribing Information*. East Hanover, NJ: Novartis.

28. Novartis (2004) *Aredia® (Pamidronate Disodium) Injection Prescribing Information*. East Hanover, NJ: Novartis.

29. Wickersham R.M. and Novack K.K. (2004). *Drug Facts and Comparisons*. St Louis, MO: Facts and Comparisons Inc.

30. Beckwith M.C. and Tyler L.S. (2004) *Cancer Chemotherapy Manual*. St Louis, MO: Facts and Comparisons Inc.

31. Body J.J. (2001). Dosing regimens and main adverse effects of biphosphonates. *Seminars in Oncology* **28**, 49–53.

32. Body J.J. and Mancini I. (2002). Bisphosphonates for cancer patients: why, how, and when? *Supportive Care in Cancer* **10**, 399–407.

33. Body J.J. (2004). Hypercalcemia of malignancy. *Seminars in Nephrology* **24**, 48–54.

34. Glynne P., Allen A. and Pusey C. (2002). *Acute Renal Failure in Practice*. London: Imperial College Press.

35. Esbrit P. and Hurtado J. (2002). Treatment of malignant hypercalcaemia. *Expert Opinion on Pharmacotherapy* **3**, 521–527.

36. Leyland-Jones B. (2004). Treating cancer-related hypercalcemia with gallium nitrate. *Journal of Supportive Oncology* **2**, 509–516, 516–520.

37. Chitambar C.R., Bockman R., Leyland-Jones B. *et al.* (2003). Update on gallium nitrate in cancer and cancer-related hypercalcemia and skeletal complications. *Seminars in Oncology Nursing* **30(suppl. 5)**, 1–41.

38. Yarbro C. H., Frogge M.H. and Goodman M. (2002). *Clinical Guide to Cancer Nursing*. Boston, MA: Jones and Bartlett.

39. O'Connor M. (2004). Transitions in status from wellness to illness, illness to wellness. In Payne S., Seymour J. and Ingleton C. (eds.) *Palliative Care Nursing*. Maidenhead: Open University Press, pp. 126–141.

40. Aranda S. and Kelso J. (1997). The nurse as coach in care of the dying. *Contemporary Nurse* **6**, 117–122.

41. Pease N.J., Harris R.J. and Finlay I.G. (2004). Development and audit of a care pathway for the manage-

ment of patients with suspected malignant spinal cord compression. *Physiotherapy* **90**, 27–34.

42. Ryken T.C., Eichholz K.M., Gerszten P.C. *et al.* (2003). Evidence-based review of the surgical management of vertebral column metastatic disease. *Neurosurgical Focus* **15**, 1–10.

43. Gucalp R. and Dutcher J. (2005). Oncologic emergencies. In Kasper D.L., Fauci S., Longo D.L. *et al.* (eds.) *Harrison's Principles of Internal Medicine*. New York: McGraw Hill, pp. 575–582.

44. Gabriel K. and Schiff D. (2004). Metastatic spinal cord compression by solid tumors. *Seminars in Neurology* **24**, 375–383.

45. Preciado D.A., Sebring L.A. and Adams G.L. (2002). Treatment of patients with spinal metastases from head and neck neoplasms. *Archives of Otolaryngeal Head and Neck Surgery* **128**, 539–543.

46. Agrawal M. and Khleif S.N. (2003). Neurologic emergencies. In Johnston P. and Spence R. (eds.) *Oncologic Emergencies*. Oxford: Oxford University Press, pp. 27–49.

47. Bilsky M.H., Boland P.J., Panageas K.S. *et al.* (2001). Intralesional resection of primary and metastatic sarcoma involving the spine: outcome analysis of 59 patients. *Neurosurgery* **49**, 1277–1287.

48. Healey J.H. and Brown H.K. (2000). Complications of bone metastases: surgical management. *Cancer* **88**, 2940–2951.

49. Coleman R.E. (1997). Skeletal complications of malignancy. *Cancer* **80**, 1588–1594.

50. Arbit E. and Galicich J.H. (1995). Vertebral body reconstruction with a modified Harrington rod distraction system for stabilization of the spine affected with metastatic disease. *Journal of Neurosurgery* **83**, 617–620.

51. Rude M. (2000). Selected neurologic complications in the patient with cancer. Brain metastases and spinal cord compression. *Critical Care Nursing Clinics of North America* **12**, 269–279.

52. Ampil F.L., Burton G.V., Mills G.M. *et al.* (2001). Cauda equina compression in breast cancer–incidence and treatment outcome. *European Journal of Gynaecological Oncology* **22**, 257–259.

53. Gale J., Mead G.M. and Simmonds P.D. (2002). Management of spinal cord and cauda equina compression secondary to epidural metastatic disease in adults with malignant germ cell tumours. *Clinical Oncology* **14**, 481–490.

54. Ghogawala Z., Mansfield F.L. and Borges L.F. (2001). Spinal radiation before surgical decompression adversely affects outcomes of surgery for symptomatic metastatic spinal cord compression. *Spine* **26**, 818–824.

55. Husband D.J., Grant K.A. and Romaniuk C.S. (2001). MRI in the diagnosis and treatment of suspected malignant spinal cord compression. *British Journal of Radiology* **74**, 15–23.

56. Muhlbauer M., Pfisterer W., Eyb R. and Knosp E. (2000). Minimally invasive retroperitoneal approach for lumbar corpectomy and anterior reconstruction. *Journal of Neurosurgery* **93**, 161–167.

57. Heys S.D., Currie D. and Eremin O. (1997). The management of patients with advanced cancer (III). *European Journal of Surgical Oncology* **23**, 361–365.

58. Ruckdeschel J.C. (2005). Early detection and treatment of spinal cord compression. *Oncology* **19**, 81–86, 89–92.

59. Loblaw D.A., Laperriere N.J. and Mackillop W.J. (2003). A population-based study of malignant spinal cord compression in Ontario. *Clinical Oncology* **15**, 211–217.

60. Levack P., Graham J. and Kidd J. (2004). Listen to the patient: quality of life of patients with recently diagnosed malignant cord compression in relation to their disability. *Palliative Medicine* **18**, 594–601.

61. Schiff D. (2003). Spinal cord compression. *Neurologic Clinics* **21**, 67–86.

62. Quinn J. and De Angelis L.M. (2000). Neurologic emergencies in the cancer patient. *Seminars in Oncology* **322**, 544–545.

63. Manfredi P.L., Gonzales G.R., Sady R., Chandler S. and Payne R. (2003). Neuropathic pain in patients with cancer. *Journal of Palliative Care* **19**, 115–118.

64. Fitzsimmons D. (2004). What are we trying to measure? Rethinking approaches to health outcome assessment for the older person with cancer. *European Journal of Cancer Care* **13**, 416–423.

65. Arce D., Sass P. and Abdul-Khoudoud H. (2001). Recognizing spinal cord emergencies. *American Family Physician* **64**, 631–638.

66. Robinson J.R. (2003). Lower extremity pain of lumbar spine origin: differentiating somatic referred and radicular pain. *Journal of Manual and Manipulative Therapy* **11**, 223–234.

67. Glick T.H., Workman T.P. and Gaufberg S.V. (1998). Spinal cord emergencies: false reassurance from reflexes. *Academic Emergency Medicine* **5**, 1041–1043.

68. Bonica J.J. (1990). *The Management of Pain*. Philadelphia, PA: Lea and Febiger.

69. Centeno C. and Gonzalez C. (2003). Radiotherapy for palliation of symptoms. In Fisch M.J. and Bruero E.D. (eds.). *Handbook of Advanced Cancer Care*. Cambridge: Cambridge University Press, pp. 27–39.

70. Maranzano E., Trippa F., Chirico L., Basagni M.L. and Rossi R. (2003). Management of malignant spinal cord compression. *Tumori* **89**, 469–475.

71. Kim J.K., Learch T.J., Colletti P.M. *et al.* (2000). Diagnosis of vertebral metastasis, epidural metastasis, and malignant spinal cord compression: are T(1)-weighted sagittal images sufficient? *Magnetic Resonance Imaging* **18**, 819–824.

72. Francken A.B., Hong A.M., Fulham M.J. *et al.* (2005). Detection of unsuspected spinal cord compression in melanoma patients by 18F-fluorodeoxyglucose-positron emission tomography. *European Journal of Surgical Oncology* **31**, 197–204.

73. Poggi M.M., Patronas N., Buttman J. *et al.* (2001). Intramedullary spinal cord metastasis from renal cell carcinoma: detection by positron emission tomography. *Clinical Nuclear Medicine* **26**, 837–839.

74. Baba H., Uchida K., Sadato N. *et al.* (1999). Potential usefulness of 18F-2-fluoro-deoxy-D-glucose positron emission tomography in cervical compressive myelopathy. *Spine* **24**, 1449.

75. Laszlo E., Artigiani R., Combs A. and Csanyi V. (1996). *Changing Visions, Human Cognitive Maps: Past, Present and Future*. Westport CT: Praeger.

76. Hambleden S.M. and Lowe V.J. (2003). Clinical 18F-FDG oncology patient preparation techniques. *Journal of Nuclear Medicine Technology* **31**, 3–10.

77. Sorensen S., Helweg-Larsen S., Mouridsen, H. and Hansen H.H. (1994). Effect of high-dose dexamethasone in carcinomatous metastatic spinal cord compression treated with radiotherapy: a randomised trial. *European Journal of Cancer* **30**, 22–27.

78. Abrahm J.L. (1999). Management of pain and spinal cord compression in patients with advanced cancer. *Annals of Internal Medicine* **131**, 37–46.

79. Maranzano E., Latini P., Beneventi S. *et al.* (1996). Radiotherapy without steroids in selected metastatic spinal cord compression patients: a phase II trial. *American Journal of Clinical Oncology* **19**, 179–183.

80. Maranzano E., Bellavita R., Rossi R. *et al.* (2005). Short-course versus split-course radiotherapy in metastatic spinal cord compression: results of a phase III, randomized, multicenter trial. *Journal of Clinical Oncology* **23**, 3358–3365.

81. Wells M. (2003). Pain and breathing problems. In Faithfull S. and Wells M. (eds.). *Supportive Care in Radiotherapy*. Edinburgh: Churchill Livingstone, pp. 160–182.

82. Wells M. (2003). The treatment trajectory. In Faithfull S. and Wells M. (eds.). *Supportive Care in Radiotherapy*. Edinburgh: Churchill Livingstone, pp. 39–59.

83. Colyer H. (2003). The context of radiotherapy care. In Faithfull S. and Wells M. (eds.). *Supportive Care in Radiotherapy*. Philadelphia, PA: Elsevier, pp. 1–16.

84. Pavlakis N. and Stockler M. (2005). Bisphosphonates for breast cancer (Cochrane Review). *The Cochrane Library*, Issue 2. Oxford: Update Software.

85. Roque M., Martinez M.J., Alonso-Coello P. *et al.* (2005). Radioisotopes for metastatic bone pain (Cochrane Review). *The Cochrane Library*, Issue 4. Oxford: Update Software.

86. Shaughnessy A. (2003). Does biphosphonate therapy decrease fractures in patients with bone metastases? *Evidence-Based Practice* **6**, 6.

87. Small E.J., Smith M.R., Seaman J.J., Petrone S. and Kowalski M.O. (2003). Combined analysis of two multicenter, randomized, placebo-controlled studies of pamidronate disodium for the palliation of bone pain in men with metastatic prostate cancer. *Journal of Clinical Oncology* **21**, 4277–4284.

88. Papadopoulos S.M., Selden N.R., Quint D.J. *et al.* (2002). Immediate spinal cord decompression for cervical spinal cord injury: feasibility and outcome. *Journal of Trauma* **52**, 323–332.

89. Regine W.F., Tibbs P.A., Young A. *et al.* (2003). Metastatic spinal cord compression: a randomized trial of direct decompressive surgical resection plus radiotherapy vs radiotherapy alone. Proceedings of the American Society for Therapeutic Radiology and Oncology, 45th Annual Meeting. Salt Lake City, Utah. *International Journal of Radiation Oncology Biology Physics* **57**, S125.

90. Cox Martin S. and Curtin M. (2002). Spinal cord lesions. In Turner A., Foster M. and Johnston S.E. (eds.) *Occupational Therapy and Physical Dysfunction*. Edinburgh: Elsevier Health Sciences, pp. 417–440.

91. Baxter T. and McKenna H. (2002). Upper limb trauma. In Turner A., Foster M. and Johnson S.E. (eds.) *Occupational Therapy and Physical Dysfunction*. Edinburgh: Elsevier Health Sciences, pp. 441–454.

92. Livneh H. (2000). *Psychosocial Adaptation to Chronic Illness and Disability*. Gaithersburg, MD: Aspen.

93. Falvo D.R. (2005). *Medical and Psychosocial Aspects of Chronic Illness and Disability*. Boston, MA: Jones and Bartlett.

94. Read P.W. and Kelly M. (2003). Superior vena cava syndrome. In Fisch M.J. and Bruero E.D. (eds.) *Handbook of Advanced Cancer Care*. Cambridge: Cambridge University Press, pp. 488–490.

95. Shah A.R. and Kennedy M.J. (2003). Cardiovascular emergencies. In Johnston P. and Spence R. (eds.) *Oncologic Emergencies*. Oxford: Oxford University Press, pp. 1–25.

96. Rowell N.P. and Gleeson F.V. (2005). Steroids, radiotherapy, chemotherapy and stents for superior vena caval obstruction in carcinoma of the bronchus (Cochrane Review). *The Cochrane Library*, Issue 3. Oxford: Update Software.

97. Ostler P.J., Clarke D.P., Watkinson A.F. and Gaze M.N. (1997). Superior vena cava obstruction: a modern management strategy. *Clinical Oncology* **9**, 83–89.

98. Stewart I.E. (1996). Superior vena cava syndrome: an oncologic complication. *Seminars in Oncology Nursing* **12**, 312–317.

99. Savarese D.M., Zavarin M., Smyczynski M.S., Rohrer M.J. and Hutzler M.J. (2000). Superior vena cava syndrome secondary to an angiotropic large cell lymphoma. *Cancer* **89**, 2515–2521.

100. Aurora R., Milite F. and Vander E.N.J. (2000). Respiratory emergencies. *Seminars in Oncology* **27**, 256–269.

101. Myckatyn T.M., Kassen B.O. and Legiehn G.M. (2002). Volume dependent superior vena cava syndrome related to stenosis after central venous catheterisation. *Canadian Journal of Surgery* **45**, 385–387.

102. Bedor M., Alexander C. and Edelman M.J. (2005). Management of common symptoms in advanced lung cancer. *Current Treatment Options in Oncology* **6**, 61–68.

103. Bentzen S.M., Hoskin P., Roos D. and Nielsen O.S. (2000). Fractionated radiotherapy for metastatic bone pain: evidence-based medicine or . . . ? *International Journal of Radiation Oncology Biology Physics* **46**, 681–683.

104. Munro A.J. (2003). Challenges to radiotherapy today. In Faithfull S. and Wells M. (eds.) *Supportive Care in Radiotherapy*. Edinburgh: Churchill Livingstone, pp. 17–38.

105. Koller M., Lorenz W., Wagner K. *et al.* (2000). Expectations and quality of life of cancer patients undergoing radiotherapy. *Journal of the Royal Society of Medicine* **93**, 621–628.

106. Devereux S., Hatton M.Q. and Macbeth F.R. (1997). Immediate side effects of large fraction radiotherapy. *Clinical Oncology* **9**, 96–99.

107. Martelli M.P., Martelli M., Pescarmiona E. *et al.* (1998). MACOP-B and involved field radiation therapy is an effective therapy for primary mediastinal large B-cell lymphoma with sclerosis. *Annals of Oncology* **9**, 1027–1029.

108. Garcia M.R., Bertoni H., Pallota G. *et al.* (2003). Use of self-expanding vascular endoprostheses in superior vena cava syndrome. *European Journal of Cardiothoracic Surgery* **24**, 208–211.

109. Patel T.M., Shah S.C., Ranjan A. *et al.* (2003). Stenting through a portocath for totally occluded superior vena cava in a case of non-Hodgkin's lymphoma. *Journal of Invasive Cardiology* **15**, 86–88.

110. Marcy P.Y., Magne N., Bentolila F. *et al.* (2001). Superior vena cava obstruction; is stenting necessary? *Supportive Care in Cancer* **9**, 103–107.

Part 5

Needs and Priorities in Cancer Care

Introduction

This final section brings together the themes of health and its influences, the need to set priorities in caring, and the relationships between local, international, and global health policy. This is not presented as a coherent, seamless text, but rather as a series of chapters examining needs and priorities in a number of areas. Important to the subjects chosen is to identify needy groups where there are particular challenges to providing care. For this reason children and adolescents, older people, people from minority ethnic groups, people who live long term with cancer, and people who are dying have been selected as warranting review as priority groups in need of care. The issues for each are very different; they do, however, represent some of the core factors that are important as determinants of health: age, social and economic status, race, and gender.

The needs of children and adolescents have been singled out, since cancer in childhood, although fortunately rare, is a high-ranking cause of death after accidents. Cancer in childhood represents a rather unique case; it is not a story of disadvantage and neglect, rather one of success. The cancers that occur in childhood are different in character from those in adulthood; many, certainly in younger children, have a congenital origin. As a result of important developments in the treatment of cancer in children these have become curable for a significant proportion of children. These successes are among the most celebrated in the cancer science story, and have been made possible by the organisation of children's cancer services. Owing to the relative rarity of childhood cancers, children's cancer services have been developed as a collective endeavour, with centres collaborating in a national and international research effort; it has therefore been possible to evaluate advances in an efficient and co-ordinated manner. The benefits discovered through studies are now finding a place in practice earlier than would be the norm for adults.

The emotive nature of cancer in children attracts generous donations from the public, further supporting research, treatment, and care. Despite this positive message, cancer in children and adolescents is devastating for parents and demanding for health professionals and requires unique skills. Unusually, this area of care requires a different environment, since it is parents who are the front-line carers, not health professionals; care and often treatment must therefore be mediated through a family-centred model. Adolescents need to be delegated such authority in a controlled and supportive manner; health professionals here must negotiate a delicate and shifting balance between the adult–child, near-adult–parent dynamic that inevitably becomes part of illness. In managing the care for children and adolescents, an eye must also be kept on the future, since it is the very real prospect of cure from cancer that brings with it risks of long-term damage, secondary cancers, infertility, possible learning difficulties, and adult life potentially disrupted by a cancer history.

For older people (those over the age of 65 years) a different picture emerges. Here, genuine concerns over suboptimal treatment exist, due to older people being characterised as too frail for the demands of cancer treatment and therefore excluded from it or given 'gentle' treatment; or, more disturbingly, the question sometimes arises of whether they are considered not to warrant the same intensity of effort as is directed at younger people. A research literature around any aspect of cancer or its treatment in older people is virtually absent, calling into question whether cancer exists as a distinct experience at the extremes of age; we simply do not know.

Likewise, studies surrounding race and cancer are absent, and the issues for people from a whole range of cultural and racial groups within society are little understood. More worrying is the possibility that insensitivity to issues of race, by the majority groups represented by most health carers, could lead to a form of racism in cancer care and treatment, at best because of a crude awareness of the complexity of agendas and influences in a racially diverse society. At worst, there may exist an overt neglect of the needs of people from minority groups.

In this new edition we have added chapters concerning the issues around long-term survival for cancer, the important agenda of user involvement in the development of cancer services and the concept of promoting self-management as a dynamic within care systems. As cancer detection and treatment increasingly deliver longer survival for people with cancer, the importance of the community of individuals who have experienced cancer, its treatment and its after-effects, comes to the fore. The voice of service users and consumers is now recognised as an important dynamic in learning about how care and treatment should be delivered and that consumers are a powerful influencing body. Nurses and other health professionals need to be better equipped to work in partnership with service users in delivering health care and developing future services.

For people whose disease management may be encompassed by palliative care (that is, they have advanced cancer or are dying), the issues are different. A specific system of care with relatively ample resources exists, founded in the hospice movement, and has now developed into a myriad of services with similar ideals. The issues here are to re-examine the ideals and achievements of this field of care; to explore whether, in adopting a different approach to care, it has resisted the problems explored in Part 1, and whether palliative care too falls prey to the conflicts and anxieties imposed by the sheer difficulty of caring for people facing death. The section ends with an exploration of research into cancer care; the potential contribution of nursing to cancer through a nursing research agenda is advocated.

CHAPTER THIRTY

The needs of children and adolescents

Fay Scullion and Jenny Thompson

Cancer is a very rare disease in childhood and is still seen universally as a disease affecting the ageing population, so when children, adolescents, and their parents and carers are faced with a cancer diagnosis their first experiences are of shock, disbelief and extreme threat.

The entire family is affected in an alien way, as they face traumatic experiences way beyond their control, that they have never experienced previously. The cancer diagnosis imposes considerable stress upon the whole family as they face interactions with clinicians and embark upon a journey that faces the usage of equipment and treatments that will have an everlasting effect on the subsequent life plan.[1]

The focus of this chapter is to highlight the differences between the diagnosis, treatment, and care of the child with cancer, as opposed to the adult with cancer, and in particular to examine how children's and adolescents' understanding of a cancer diagnosis and treatment is influenced by their level of cognitive development. It is not the intention here to discuss in detail specific medical treatment programmes or supportive medical care aimed to reduce side-effects of treatment. Such are to be found in a number of relevant texts (for a concise review see 'Recommended reading'). Throughout the chapter, reference will be made to the child and the family. In most cases this implies child or adolescent. However, there are issues specific to either the child or adolescent; as

these arise they will be discussed under separate headings.

Childhood cancer

Although the incidence of cancer in children and adolescents is extremely low, it remains the second most common cause of mortality following accidents in children over the age of 1 year. In the UK alone, nearly a quarter of all deaths in England and Wales in 2000–2002, in the age group 5 to 14 years, were recorded as being caused by cancer,[2] and although childhood cancer is rare, about 1 in 600 children develop cancer before the age of 15 years. However, universally two-thirds of children with access to optimal medical treatment and resources are cured, but the different types of cancer have highly variable cure rates and in fact the incidence of cancer diagnosis in young patients (15–24 years) is quite rare.

In Western populations, around 0.5% of all cancers occur in children aged under 15 years. The incidence rate is typically in the range of 110–130 per million children per year. Childhood cancers exhibit a diversity of histological type and anatomical site and are very different from those observed in adults: the carcinomas of the lung, female breast, stomach, and bowel are all extremely rare among children. Consequently, it is more appropriate for childhood tumours to be classified according to their histology, as opposed to adult cancers that are predominantly grouped by their site of origin. Children's cancers are generally described as belonging to those primarily affecting the haematopoietic system – the leukaemias – while others such as neuroblastoma and bone tumours are referred to as solid tumours.[3]

Paediatric tumours can also be divided into three broad groups. Embryonal cancers are due to faulty development of embryonal cells, where there is a proliferation of cells that closely resemble fetal tissue, for example neuroblastoma, rhabdomyosarcoma, and nephroblastoma (Wilms' tumour). Juvenile cancers arise due to malignant transformation in mature tissue, but are generally unique to the younger age group, such as osteosarcoma, Ewing's sarcoma, and Hodgkin's disease. Adult-type cancers rarely seen in children, but histologically identical to adult tumours, include renal cell carcinoma and nasopharyngeal carcinomas.

About one-third of all childhood cancers are leukaemias, and of these three-quarters are of the acute lymphoblastic type (ALL). Between one-quarter and one-fifth are brain and spinal tumours, of which astrocytoma is the most common histological type. The distinctive embryonal tumours (Wilms' tumour, neuroblastoma, retinoblastoma, and hepatoblastoma) account for 15% of registrations. Lymphomas account for a further 11%, with non-Hodgkin's lymphoma (NHL) somewhat more common than Hodgkin's disease.[4]

Different diagnostic groups have distinctive age distributions. The incidence of ALL is highest among children aged 2–4 years. Early age peaks in incidence are also found for the embryonal tumours; indeed for neuroblastoma, retinoblastoma, and hepatoblastoma the highest incidence is found in the first year of life. By contrast, Hodgkin's disease, osteosarcoma, and Ewing's sarcoma show a marked incidence with age that continues into early adulthood. The highest incidence of these cancers is seen in the adolescent population. Overall, childhood cancer is about one-third more common among boys than among girls. The male predominance is greatest in the lymphomas and less marked in leukaemia, brain tumours, and sarcomas of the bone and soft tissue.[4]

The patterns of incidence described are typically those of white populations throughout Europe, North America, and Australasia. There is, however, considerable systematic variation in many types of childhood cancer between different regions of the world and between ethnic groups in the same country.[5] In the US, black populations have a lower incidence of ALL, and the early childhood peak is much attenuated. By contrast, there is little evidence of ethnic variations in the incidence of childhood leukaemia in the UK; in particular, the pattern of occurrence of ALL among black people and children of South Asian ethnic origin is similar to that among white people, with a marked peak in early childhood.[6]

Little is known about the aetiology of most childhood cancers, but significantly the increase in the incidence of childhood and adolescent cancers has been demonstrated for a wide range of diagnoses. A study examining trends in childhood malignancy in the north west of England (1954–1958) identifed significant linear increases in ALL and Hodgkin's disease.[7] Although families of an affected child often link the disease to an environmental factor, such as exposure to smoking, insecticides, or ionising radiation, such a linkage can rarely be confirmed. For some diagnostic groups the high incidence at an early age and the cell type of origin strongly suggest that the causative factors occur before birth or even before conception. As a result, many aetiological studies of childhood cancer have been concerned with exposures occurring during the mother's pregnancy. The relationship between antenatal obstetric irradiation and subsequent cancer in the child was first established over 30 years ago by the work of Stewart *et al.*[8] At that time exposure to diagnostic X-rays in pregnancy was thought to have caused as many as 5% of all childhood cancers. Ultrasound has now superseded X-ray examination in pregnancy, and subsequent studies have concluded that there is no increased risk associated with antenatal ultrasound.[8,9]

The role of other environmental exposures in the aetiology of childhood cancer remains far from clear. The only well-established environmental causes in Western populations other than X-ray are intra-uterine exposure to diethylstilbestrol during pregnancy, which was linked with vaginal carcinomas.[10] Viruses are also known to play a role in the aetiology of some types of childhood cancer. It is established that the Epstein–Barr virus (EBV) is associated with Burkitt's lymphoma, and nasopharyngeal carcinoma and the hepatocellular carcinoma usually occur in patients who have had prenatal or early childhood exposure to the hepatitis B virus (HBV).[6] The analysis of childhood cancer offers a unique opportunity to study not only the cancer phenotype but also the genes that are important in normal embryonic development. Of particular importance was the discovery of a retinoblastoma predisposition gene. Approximately 25–30% of all cases of children diagnosed with retinoblastoma have a family history. In the familial form the retinoblastoma phenotype segregates in an autosomal dominant fashion. That is, it appears as though inheritance of the mutant gene is sufficient for tumorogenesis; thus the offspring of individuals carrying the mutant gene have a 50:50 chance of inheriting it. Another predisposition gene has been isolated for Wilms' tumour, and others are beginning to emerge.

The availability of these genes means that mutations in individual patients can be characterised in the tumours. As patterns emerge it is considered possible that particular mutations will be associated with a particular course of the disease, thereby allowing predictions about invasiveness, prognosis, and susceptibility to other tumours.[11]

The increasing complexity of treatments and the necessity for many disciplines to be involved has led to the centralisation of care for children with cancer into specialist units. In caring for children with cancer the primary aim is to cure the child with minimal physical and psychosocial cost to both the child and the family. Thus the approach to care requires the expertise of a multidisciplinary approach. In addition to the time trends in survival rates that are attributed to the development of more effective treatment, survival rates were noted to be substantially higher in paediatric oncology centres. The development of specialist units also gave clinicians the opportunity to specialise and to participate in clinical trials. As a result, large numbers of children with cancer are now entered into national and international trials.[12]

Childhood cancer treatments represent one of the great success stories of oncology. Thirty years ago, with the advent of chemotherapy, the first cures of leukaemia in children, previously unheard of, were being recorded.[13] Since that time multimodality therapy, especially chemotherapy combined with surgery and radiotherapy, has enabled the majority of children with cancer to survive. Children are reported as surviving into adulthood with normal or near-normal life expectancy and productive lives.[13] Thus, it is appropriate that those involved with their care make every effort to maximise survival and minimise the potential physical and psychosocial long-term complications. This goal can only be achieved when there is an exhaustive understanding of the unique differences between the diagnosis, treatment protocols, and approach to care of the child with cancer, as opposed to the adult with cancer.

Box 30.1 Cancer in childhood

- Childhood cancer is rare, affecting 1 in 600 children before the age of 15 years.
- Childhood cancers are classified according to their histology.
- Different diagnostic groups have distinctive age distributions.
- Systematic variation in some childhood cancers occurs in differing regions of the world.
- Childhood cancer is about one-third more common in boys.
- Childhood cancers respond more favourably to treatment than adult cancers.
- Centralisation of care, and advances in combination chemotherapy, surgical and radiotherapy techniques have significantly improved survival rates.
- Established environmental exposures in the aetiology of childhood cancers in Western populations are X-rays, exposure to diethylstilbestrol during pregnancy, and infection with hepatitis B and HIV.
- Predisposition genes in a small number of childhood cancers have been identified.
- There are unique differences between the diagnosis, treatment protocols, and approach to care of the child with cancer as opposed to that of the adult with cancer.

Setting care in context

Knowledge of two specialties is required by those caring for the child and adolescent – paediatrics and paediatric oncology. The complex care required of the child and adolescent with cancer has long dictated a team approach to treatment, and psychological care has become an increasingly necessary component. During the earlier years of successful treatment little attention was paid to the impact on the child, the family, and the immediate community. Success was uncommon and in most cases parents were warned of the high risk of death, although the emotional impact of waiting for this to happen was rarely addressed in an open manner.

The special needs of sick adolescents have received greater attention in the last 10–15 years and in the main are attributed to the Western world. The health care needs of this group are slowly being addressed, and adolescent medicine as a specialty is emerging. The period of adolescence is now understood to provide a critical example of psychosocial development that is highly subject to severe disruption by the symptoms of and treatment for cancer.

From the moment of diagnosis the child and the family have to face a myriad of practical and psychosocial problems associated with cancer treatments, altered lifestyle, and often a change in ambition. While some of these problems are inevitable, they can be minimised. Knowledgeable professional support is essential to help the child and family retain as much normality as possible.[14]

Essential to facilitating the best possible physical care and psychosocial adjustment of the child with cancer and their family is an in-depth knowledge of child and adolescent development. Factors related to a favourable adaptation to the diagnosis of cancer and treatment include the child's or adolescent's understanding of what is happening to them. The ability of the multidisciplinary team to address the complex questions of how the consequences of diagnosis and treatment interact with any given child's or adolescent's level of intellectual, emotional, and social development is important. A young person's understanding of what is happening and why it is happening will exert a major influence on his or her emotional response

to treatment. Similarly, when treatment interferes with normal developmental tasks, this needs to be anticipated and remedied.

The importance of those caring for the child and adolescent with cancer having a theoretical and working knowledge of developmental issues cannot be over-emphasised. Without such knowledge, decisions about the impact of a cancer diagnosis and subsequent treatment and care for the child and family will be less well informed.

Childhood and child development

To care for the child with cancer there is a need for those involved to understand the ways in which children's needs are understood in relation to their actual abilities, and the ways that these are perceived and interpreted through concepts of childhood. What does childhood mean? Public opinion, reinforced by philosophical and psychological theories, tends to perceive children as dependent, vulnerable, and lacking maturity to know how they will react to certain situations. A further commonly held view is that children are irrational. Even when it is accepted that children can understand, recall, and recount information, their ability to reason, to evaluate, and to assess information is questioned.[15]

Developmental psychologists, perhaps most influentially Piaget, whose research began in the 1920s, have taught that children understand fragments of knowledge slowly and it is unhelpful to teach children before the prescribed age of readiness. Piaget theorised that cognitive development (which, put simply, is the ability to reason and think) proceeded through age-related stages, which take place between birth and adulthood. Piaget's interest was not in the uniqueness of individual children but rather in the similarities between children of roughly equivalent age. Through interviewing children and studying his own children he found that at different times during development children appeared to be capable of different kinds of understanding. Piaget subsequently worked out the theory that logical thinking in children developed in age-related stages.

Piaget's theories have been refuted and criticised.[15] One of the main failings of the age stage approach is the failure to recognise the impact of experience upon development. It is claimed that Piaget looked at what children were unable to do rather than what they could achieve if helped by prompts and questions that make sense to them and engage their interest.[16] Nevertheless, Piaget helped to increase public understanding and respect for children, even though his work is reputed to have overlooked each child's experiences and views. It is therefore suggested that Piaget's stages of cognitive development to symbolic thought should be used as benchmarks, rather than formal expectations (see Box 30.2).

Other influential work related to child development includes that of Freud, Kohlberg, and Erikson, each of whom suggest that wisdom does not develop until at least adolescence.[17] However, more recent research and everyday evidence shows that young children are capable of cognitive complexity. The example in Personal account 30.1, the account of a 5-year-old boy who was being cared for at home in the terminal phase of his illness, illustrates this well.

Bluebond-Langner's research with seriously ill young children,[18] which has been concurred with more recently,[19] shows that they can have a mature understanding and can cope with and discuss complex and painful knowledge. This writer concludes that experience is more salient than age in determining children's understanding. There is a widely accepted view that it is wise not to assume a child is fine just because there is no obvious sign of anxiety or distress. Encouragement to talk and giving a reassuring cuddle may be needed but not requested.

Perhaps developmental theories that refer to age have remained influential because the concept of the ignorant child gradually moving through life towards adult understanding is more comfortable for adults to accept. The child's physical growth is so visible and in most cases obvious that it is easy to use this as a baseline on which to measure children's emotional and mental abilities. In reality, children mature at uneven rates and like adults they can be confident in one respect and not in another. Ability develops unevenly and depends on the experience of the child to a greater extent than the child's age. Another important issue is the widely varying

Personal account 30.1

A 5-year-old boy diagnosed with leukaemia had relapsed several times following unsuccessful treatment for his disease and was being cared for at home in the terminal phase of his illness.

He was the only child of elderly parents who believed that he was unaware of his impending death. It was a subject that neither the parents or those professionals involved with his care discussed with him. The child appeared to be 'comfortable' both physically and emotionally and did not ask questions about his situation.

Visiting the home on the day before his death, I noticed that his toys were positioned on the bed in two groups. When I inquired as to how he was feeling he replied, 'Fine thank you'. After a pause he pointed to one group of the toys on his bed and said, 'Those toys you can take back to the hospital, the other toys are going with me when I die'. Giving him a cuddle I thanked him and asked if there was anything else he wanted to talk about.

'Yes', he said, and after a long pause he continued to tell me who was best at giving his medicines through his 'wiggly' (central venous catheter) at the hospital and at home, and which medicines helped most with his 'hurts'. He clearly understood aseptic techniques and was critical of those he felt did not use the correct procedure. He also had a reasonable understanding of the drugs being used to control his pain.

views about childhood between cultures. The level of responsibility accepted by children in developing countries, such as the care of parents and other family members, is generally speaking at odds with the view of children's responsibilities in the Western world.

However, whatever boundaries of childhood are drawn, there remains a broad consensus that children are comparatively more vulnerable than adults, requiring special measures to protect and promote their needs. Certainly young children are vulnerable and their survival depends on the quality of care and commitment provided for them by the adults who have responsibility for them. Nevertheless, as Lansdown[20] argues, the vulnerability that we perceive in children is not an objective definition of their capacity. It is only partially drawn from the biological facts of

Box 30.2 Summary of Piaget's stages of children's cognitive development

The sensor–motor stage, age 0–2 years
Children begin to develop an understanding of themselves as separate and distinct from the environment, causality, time, and space. Learning is mainly through the senses and physical activity. Objects in general only appear to exist in terms of what babies can do with them; during the first year objects are simply things to act upon ('Can I suck it?', 'Can I hit it?'). Towards the end of the first year objects appear to become an interesting problem. The baby will spend time looking at, feeling, and exploring an object as if there is an attempt to understand what it is; they appear to ask themselves 'What is this object?', and will search for hidden objects, demonstrating that they know of their existence even if they are out of sight.

The pre-operational (or pre-logical) stage, age 2–7 years
Children at this stage learn much about the physical and social world. Some of this learning is spontaneous, while more is deliberately taught by parents and teachers. This is a time when children are capable of using language and symbolic thinking. This is apparent in their imaginative play. It is a time of egocentric thinking in which children are unable to take the views of others. Pre-operational children start from where they are, and to a greater or lesser extent distort reality in an attempt to make sense of it using ways of understanding they have already developed ('I'm sick and in hospital because I was naughty'). This is also a period when children can only attend to one aspect of a situation at a time.

The concrete operational stage, age 7–12 years
Thinking now becomes logical and children can attend to several aspects of an event at a time. They are now able to look at a situation from the point of view of someone else, and so overcome the earlier egocentrism. Whereas a pre-operational child thinks in absolutes – things are either black or white, good or bad, hurt or will not hurt – children in the concrete operational stage can see things relatively, things can be good or bad, hurt a little, or hurt a lot. Understanding at this stage generally remains in relation to absolute objects, not to events or relationships they have not yet experienced.

The formal operational stage, age 12 years and over
Thinking is now beyond the concrete stage and children can think abstractly and imagine or hypothesise about alternatives. Reasoning about objects, situations or people can be done symbolically without the need for the objects or events to be present or experienced. This is a time when thinking becomes more flexible and concrete, and children are able to combine information from a number of different sources.

childhood, and owes much to the social attitudes and perceptions that we impose. Children's vulnerabilities, according to Lansdown[20] and Franklin,[21] derive from historical attitudes and presumptions about the nature of childhood and are a social and political construct, not an inherent or inevitable consequence of childhood.

There may be many theoretical arguments offered as to when, where, how and at what age children should be encouraged to contribute to decisions affecting their lives. Respect for the visibility of childhood and for the value of what children say is not to deny the experience of childhood and the right to be a child. If children are to be encouraged to believe that their views are worth hearing and they can become active participants in society, we should respect their involvement and views from the earliest possible age and assist them to develop the necessary skills to achieve these goals, whether they are sick or well.

Adolescence and adolescent development

Ask a number of adults 'What is adolescence and who are adolescents?' and you will get a number of answers. However, it is likely that most will refer to the teenage years and the irritation of teenage behaviour, remarking that they have periods of acting childishly after seemingly achieving acceptable standards of maturity. The terms 'teenagers', 'adolescents', 'youth', and 'young people' are also likely to be used interchangeably.

Box 30.3 Childhood and child development

- Early developmental psychologists have taught that children understand knowledge at a prescribed chronological age.
- Traditional theories of childhood and children's considered inabilities are now challenged by current research findings and everyday evidence of competent children.
- Children are known to mature at different rates, and ability depends on the experience of the child more than on the child's age.
- Piaget's descriptions of age-related thinking stages in children should be used as benchmarks rather than formal expectations.
- Differences exist between cultures as to the concept of childhood and children's abilities.
- Research with seriously ill young children demonstrates that their understanding is not about abstract concepts but rather about intensely experienced illness and treatment.

Adolescence is defined as the process of growing up; that is, the transition of an individual from childhood to adulthood.[21,22] A broadly accepted definition of adolescence is that it represents the period between childhood and maturity, encompassing not only the physical changes of puberty and emerging sexuality but also the emotional, psychological, and social differences between adults and children. Perhaps the most influential approach to adolescence is Erikson's theoretical work on psychosocial development.[23] The period of adolescence has become associated with the process of acquiring identity and is described as a 'task' of adolescence, something that everyone does during this period of their life.

While the onset of adolescence is usually associated with the onset of puberty, the end of adolescence is less clearly defined. It also varies from culture to culture as far as the attainment of independence is concerned. Adolescence is also viewed as a relatively recent concept, one mainly confined to Western societies. In many different cultures there are rites of passage in which the child is initiated into the social roles of adulthood. For males in such cultures, psychological and social maturity

may only rarely converge. For females, ceremonial transitions such as marriage may be closely linked to physical events such as the first menstruation. Kuykendall refers to this as the social status acquisition approach whereby at various chronological ages individuals gain additional social privileges and status that can be used to define the stage of life they have reached.[24]

This approach is also reflected in modern ideas about the period of adolescence in Western societies that has been influenced by the introduction and extension of compulsory education, by legislation prohibiting the employment of young people under a certain age, and the development of services differentiating the adolescent from adults or children.

In 1980, the World Health Organisation considered 10–19 years as the period of adolescence, noting that this age range, which generally encompassed the time from onset of puberty to the legal age of majority, coincided with some population statistics. For the purposes of the International Youth Year, the United Nations defined youth as encompassing the age range 15–24 years. In 1986, the World Health Organisation study group, addressing the issue of young people's health and 'Health for all by the year 2000',[25] adopted a pragmatic approach to the issue of an appropriate age range by merging the two age ranges in the all-encompassing range of 10–24 years. Within this age range, three 5-year subdivisions of 10–14, 15–19, and 20–24 years were considered to be useful, noting that such a grouping facilitates cross-national comparisons of data and experience. For those of us working with adolescents, reference is usually made to periods of early adolescence (12–15 years, when increased awareness of body image, importance of peer relationships, and rebellious behaviour are commonplace); middle adolescence (15–18 years, when physical maturity is almost complete, and there is a realistic self-/body image and strong peer relationships are developed); and late adolescence (18–22 years, when concerns for the future and planning for the future become important). However, as with the limitations of using age as a sole indicator of child development, the above age grouping does not acknowledge the discrepancies between age and the biological and psychosocial stages of development or the variations due to personal and environmental factors.

Adolescence is also viewed as a time when young people become alienated from their parents and become influenced by their peers. While it is true that adolescents do have intense emotional interactions with their peers and a need for their approval, this does not mean that they turn away from their parents. However, there is probably no other developmental age that causes as much chaos and muddle within any family unit. This is a time when young people will question the fundamental values of their parents and other individuals, including caregivers. Rapoport and Rapoport, referring to the period of adolescence, support this view, stating that it is a time for experimenting and testing family and community norms and values.[26] Therefore, it is generally agreed that during adolescence there is a psychological shift in the individual's identity from being bound up with that of the parent to becoming an 'I'. An interesting point about this ego identity shift and the struggle to become independent is that the process is too threatening for the adolescent to go it alone, especially in the early days of adolescent development. Thus, generally they go through the process with their peers, they dress alike, eat the same foods, drink the same things, and have similar hairstyles.[26]

Uncertainties about their own identity and what the future may bring will come to the fore. Their need to compete with their peers and, at the same time to win social approval, is very strong and can place individuals in a situation of painful conflict. Such powerful feelings, which may be experienced for the first time, can lead to bewilderment and stress. It is at a time like this that the adolescent may revert to adopting a more comfortable and tested coping strategy used in earlier childhood years.

It is recognised that the above scenario offers many issues for reflection. However, the purpose of the account is to offer an example of an adolescent's reaction to a potentially bewildering and stressful event by adopting a known coping strategy, which is exhibited in more childlike behaviour. Frustration is one of the most common triggers of normal attention-seeking behaviour in both children and adolescents, and the reaction in both is usually similar. They make demands on themselves or others in an attempt to overcome a problem, and if the response is perceived as negative, the child or adolescent is likely to continue with attention-seeking behavioural responses in an attempt to achieve a quick and acceptable resolution.

Personal account 30.2

A 14-year-old boy diagnosed with non-Hodgkin's lymphoma had received his treatment either as an inpatient or an outpatient in a paediatric oncology unit. He had been involved with decisions about the management of his care and appeared to trust and be comfortable with the staff on the unit.

Attending for a routine outpatient appointment, he was found to have low haemoglobin and a blood transfusion was prescribed. As the paediatric unit was unable to accommodate him for this procedure he agreed to have the transfusion carried out in the adult day-care area.

During the procedure, a nurse from the paediatric unit visited the adolescent. On reaching the adult area the nurse was confronted by a member of the staff, who stated that she was not happy with the behaviour of the patient from the children's unit and offered the following account:

> He has been adjusting the rate of flow of his blood transfusion, I told him not to do it as it was dangerous and I readjusted the flow rate. Later when I returned to see how he was he had changed the rate again. The doctor also explained to the patient that this was unacceptable. Now look at him, we gave him some paints to do some painting as he said that he liked to paint and he has painted his face not the paper. You would think that at his age he would know how to behave, he's not exactly a child.

When invited to give his account of the issues raised, the adolescent offered the following:

> Why can't I adjust my transfusion here? I do it on the children's ward, I know it can be dangerous to let it go in too fast. Nobody asked me if I knew what I was doing they just assumed that I didn't. I didn't know what to do, they were treating me like a child.

Personal account 30.2 does, however, raise another issue worth discussing, that is the debate surrounding the provision of separate adolescent units in hospitals. Adolescent medicine in the main tends to fall between the expertise of paediatricians and that of adult medicine, and adolescents are frequently asked to choose between the company of adults or children. Many writers suggest that providing separate adolescent units is the answer to maintaining the process of adolescence in hospital. Indeed this view is supported by the recent publication of national guidelines.[27] Stiller states that young people of 15 years and older should have unhindered access to age-appropriate facilities and support when needed.[4] Muller *et al.* offer an alternative view, stating that well-prepared staff with appropriate knowledge and skills about adolescence could provide care whatever the architectural arrangements.[28] These writers do acknowledge that it may be advantageous to offer specialised units and staff, but at the same time they note that it should not be regarded as impossible to maintain optimal support for adolescents where special provision is not an option. They suggest that what is needed is a degree of motivation among staff to develop an understanding of the process of adolescence and to bring this to their patients, whatever the setting. Taking this a step further, the National Institute for Health and Clinical Excellence recommends that, more importantly, all health care professionals caring for children and young people with cancer should have training in age-appropriate communication skills.[27] They should be trained to communicate sensitively and effectively, and allowed sufficient time to do so. Facilities for imparting information, especially at the time of diagnosis, should be private and comfortable. Patients and parents/carers should be involved in treatment decisions at all stages of their treatment and care.

Cancer and the family

Quality-of-life issues have assumed increasing importance in discussions about care for the child with cancer and have brought with them the need to consider the whole life constellation around the illness. Leavitt stressed that in order to provide optimal patient care the family needs to be viewed as 'the unit facing illness', rather than simply a refuge or advocate for the patient.[29] One area that

Box 30.4   Adolescence and adolescent development

- Adolescence is generally defined as the period of transition from childhood to adulthood.
- Early, middle, and late periods of adolescence have their own developmental concerns.
- The onset of adolescence is usually associated with the commencement of puberty and the appearance of secondary sex characteristics.
- The end of adolescence is less clearly defined and varies from culture to culture as far as the attainment of adult independence is concerned.
- The period of adolescence is considered to be a process in which the child is confronted by a number of developmental tasks such as:
  - adjusting to a changing physique and sexual development
  - achieving a sense of independence from parents
  - acquiring the social skills of a young adult
  - achieving a sense of oneself as a worthwhile person
  - achieving a personal set of guiding norms and values.

has traditionally been considered somewhat more advanced in its understanding and provision of family-centred care is that of the sick child, notably the care of the child in hospital. Much of the impetus to consider the role of the family in illness care evolved from studies carried out in the 1950s and 1960s,[30,31] which began to demonstrate that the isolation of children from their families while in hospital had serious effects on the child's health and well-being. There is now substantial evidence in the literature that the health and well-being of the child's family is also affected when a child is sick, with most of the literature concentrating on families with a life-threatening or chronic illness.[32] Some of the aspects of childhood cancer that make psychological adjustment particularly difficult for family members include the life-threatening nature of the disease, the prospect of uncertain prognosis, and changes in family lifestyles (see, for example, the study by Dermatis and Lesko described in detail in research study 30.1).[33]

When caring for the child with cancer, part of the care will involve promoting health. Care therefore is concerned not only with the impact of the young person's health on the family but also

Research study 30.1

Dermatis H. and Lesko L.M. (1990). Psychological distress in parents consenting to child's bone marrow transplantation. *Bone Marrow Transplantation* **6**, 411–417.[33]

Aim of the study

To determine the nature and prevalence of psychological symptomatology in parents of children undergoing bone marrow transplantation and to investigate the manner in which certain psychosocial factors are related to parental distress associated with the informed consent process.

Method

Forty-six mothers and 15 fathers were assessed with respect to psychological distress, coping styles, quality of doctor–patient communication, and recall of bone marrow transplantation information after giving consent for the child to undergo the procedure. Research participants were given the Brief Symptom Inventory (BSI), a self-report measure of psychological distress, and the Ways of Coping (WOC) Checklist. Participants were also asked to complete a researcher-constructed scale concerning the quality of the communication between the doctor and parent during the consent discussion.

Results

Forty per cent of fathers and 60% of mothers exhibited significant psychological distress of a generalised nature. Mothers exhibited a broader range of specific psychological symptomatology, i.e. disturbed thinking and higher levels of depression and phobic anxiety, than did fathers. Consenting parents who were married exhibited significantly lower levels of global psychological distress than did mothers or fathers who were widowed, separated, or divorced. The quality of the doctor–parent communication was found to be the strongest negative correlate of global psychological distress.

Conclusions

The results indicate that mothers and fathers who gave consent for their children to have bone marrow transplantation exhibited statistically and clinically significant levels of psychological symptomatology. The strongest predictor of parental level of distress was the quality of the communication between the doctor and the parent. This finding suggests that where this was obtained from parents in an unhurried, empathetic and non-threatening manner, lower symptomatology resulted.

Limitations

This was a relatively small sample of parents, especially as the methodology applied to collect and analyse the data was orientated towards a quantitative research approach. There was failure to acknowledge that the finding that mothers' psychological distress was higher than the fathers' fits with clinical observations. Mothers frequently spend more time than fathers with the sick child in hospital, learning to deal with a foreign environment, caring for the child, and permitting the staff to perform frightening and invasive procedures. They also serve as the source of information about medical information to family and friends.

with the impact of the family on the health of the child. Interestingly, while the implications for the family of a child with cancer are frequently addressed in studies from the 1980s, to date the concept of the family for the most part is not defined. This is perhaps understandable, as in Western societies there have been numerous changes over the years in the nature of family life. Many children can now expect to live through periods of marriage, divorce, single parenthood,

and remarriage. Substantial numbers of children are likely to live in several configurations of the family; as a result, their experience of family is neither static nor constant.

Terkleson, addressing theories of family life, suggests that families are social organisations or units that have specific functions in relation to the developmental and situational needs of their own members, to their own maintenance as a family, and to the maintenance of society.[34] Caregiving, communication, problem solving, and decision making are cited as important aspects of family life, no matter what the particular family structure may be. Further, each family needs to be defined by its unique history, culture, and set of values.[35]

Whatever cultural or socio-economic family structure exists, when a child develops an acute or chronic illness various factors change for the family. The balance of daily life shifts as schedules alter to meet the new needs of the child. Parental roles and responsibilities alter in response to the child's changed and changing needs. Extended family members or friends may be called on for emotional support and advice. Other factors, such as sibling needs and financial concerns, may challenge families at the same time. Thomas reminds us that despite a child's medical problems families want to function to the greatest extent possible as normal families.[36] Bishop *et al.*, discussing family/professional collaboration for children with special health needs, state that in contrast to the family, professionals see a child in their care in circumscribed, problem-focused circumstances.[37] Therefore, these writers conclude that it is the family that is the constant in the child's life, while health care services and the personnel within these services fluctuate. They advocate that to keep a focus on the family's central role in the care of the child with special health care needs, it is necessary for health care professionals to recognise and understand the racial, ethnic, cultural, and socio-economic diversities of families.

Box 30.5 Issues for families affected by cancer

- Each family needs to be defined by its own unique history and set of values.
- The life-threatening nature of the child's disease, uncertain prognosis, and changes in family lifestyle contribute to making psychological adjustment difficult for the family.
- Coping and adjustment are influenced by ethnic, racial, cultural, and socio-economic family circumstances.
- The health and well-being of a family are affected when a child or adolescent is diagnosed with cancer.
- The health and well-being of the sick child are affected by the health and well-being of the family.

Approaches to treatment – an overview

Diagnosis

Childhood cancer is usually diagnosed in response to symptoms. This can be problematic as prognosis is primarily related to tumour burden, and clinical symptoms may not become evident until the tumour burden is considerable. Pallor, fatigue, and thrombocytopenic haemorrhage are characteristic symptoms of haematopoietic cancers, whereas palpable swelling, pain, and loss of function are usual symptoms of solid tumours. Techniques used in the diagnosis of childhood cancer include laboratory testing of blood, urine, bone marrow aspirates, and other specimens. X-ray examination, ultrasound, computerised tomography (CT) and magnetic resonance imaging (MRI) and other imaging techniques are used to describe the primary tumour and to detect its local and systemic spread.

Treatment

Most childhood cancers, and especially acute leukaemias and lymphomas, respond to various combinations of chemotherapeutic agents. In treating solid tumours, systemic chemotherapy is usually complemented by local therapy with surgery and radiotherapy. In the past, brain tumours have usually been treated with surgery and radiotherapy, irrespective of histology. With attempts to refine radiotherapy techniques and the development of new chemotherapy strategies, it is now considered important that histology is obtained in children if possible. In small children with deep inaccessible tumours, for example in the mid-brain or brainstem, this is often difficult, but stereotactic techniques may be useful. Under general anaesthesia and using a predetermined site based on CT or MRI imaging, the majority of children can now be biopsied with low morbidity.[38]

Because most childhood cancers proliferate and disseminate rapidly, 5-year survival rates before the use of systemic treatment were below 10%. Optimising and standardising systemic combination chemotherapy regimes in the last two decades has led to improvements in the prognosis of most childhood cancers, resulting in a rise in survival rates.[2]

Improved survival rates in some childhood cancers are due to the administration of very high doses of chemotherapy and radiation. This is only possible by infusing harvested bone marrow, either from the child or from a matched donor, following treatment. This procedure is now accepted as standard curative treatment in children with some historically poor prognosis leukaemias and solid tumours. Children undergoing high-dose therapy will face a potentially life-threatening situation, which in terms of management and support provides a challenging and often rewarding aspect of patient care.[38] Bone marrow transplantation (BMT) is the grafting of bone marrow from:

- a matched donor (usually a sibling) or another (allogeneic BMT)
- an identical twin (syngeneic BMT)
- oneself (autologous BMT).

Although the bone marrow is the main source of the haemopoietic stem cells, it is now known that a number of stem cells is present in circulating blood. Children who have received chemotherapy and experience myelosuppression show a marked rise in the peripheral stem cell population as the white cell count recovers.

Consequently, if stem cells are collected around this time and stored they can be used to assist in the restoration of haematopoiesis after a child has received megatherapy. The use of stem cells has impressively reduced the duration of neutropenia, which in turn has reduced the number of febrile episodes and promoted earlier healing of the gut mucosa. However, a bone marrow harvest is usually frozen in case the stem cells fail to engraft, thus providing a back-up. This aggressive multidisciplinary approach to care and the inclusion of children in state-of-the-art clinical trials has led to control of this rare disease, which would be difficult to investigate without the efforts of co-operative groups conducting similar protocols.[2]

Addressing needs – from diagnosis through treatment

When cancer is first suspected, the child or adolescent and family will in most cases be referred to a specialist oncology centre. Throughout all aspects of the child's management and care, nurses and members of the multidisciplinary team need to refer continually to knowledge based on the issues discussed in the first half of this chapter.

The needs of parents

The confirmation of a cancer diagnosis to the family of a child is an unenviable but necessary task.[38] The manner in which the information about the illness is given and the tone set by medical staff and members of the multidisciplinary team, both in the hospital and in the community, are of major importance throughout the family's cancer experience. A number of studies investigating the impact of a life-threatening illness, including a cancer diagnosis, conclude that the manner in which procedures were carried out and the way in which news was communicated to the family seemed to be far more important than the specifics

Box 30.6 Medical management of childhood cancer

- Childhood cancers are usually diagnosed in response to symptoms, which may not become apparent until the tumour burden is considerable.
- Various techniques are used to confirm the diagnosis; these include laboratory tests of blood, urine, etc, and imaging techniques such as CT and MRI scanning.
- Systemic combination chemotherapy regimes are used to treat paediatric cancers, as most childhood cancers proliferate and disseminate rapidly.
- Solid tumours are treated with systemic chemotherapy and complemented by localised therapy with surgery and/or radiotherapy.
- Brain tumours are routinely treated with surgery and radiotherapy but the addition of chemotherapy is now possible.
- BMT plays a significant role in the treatment of some haematological and solid childhood cancers.
- Aggressive multidisciplinary treatment and co-ordination of care has resulted in cure for two out of three children.
- Inclusion of children into national and international state-of-the-art clinical trials has led to improved survival.

Care strategy 30.1 Facilitating coping and understanding

To assist the child or adolescent and family to understand and cope with a cancer diagnosis a working knowledge is required of:

- the nature of cancer in children and adolescents
- the differences between adult and childhood cancers
- approaches to medical treatment
- side-effects associated with treatment programmes
- the importance of a team approach to the physical and psychosocial care of the family unit
- concepts of childhood and theories of child development
- concepts of adolescence and theories of adolescent development
- concepts of family and family structures
- cross-cultural variations in childhood and adolescence
- the potential impact that the diagnosis and treatment may have on the child or adolescent's developmental process
- the potential impact that the diagnosis and treatment may have on the family and individual family members
- long-term sequelae of cancer and its treatments.

of actual treatment.[33,38] Initial reactions of parents on hearing the diagnosis for the first time have been universally described in terms such as fear, shock, disbelief, numbness, and feeling guilty. Parents react in this way even when they have strongly suspected the nature of the illness before diagnosis.[39]

Many parents experience feelings of anger for many years after the treatment ends, and they have feelings of being robbed of a 'normal' life when they experience reminders of the costs of the cancer treatment. This can be perhaps allayed if there is open communication between professionals and parents, and this is seen as a prerequisite for success.

In response to the question, 'Can you remember your immediate reaction or feelings after being told of [child's name] diagnosis?', one mother replied:

It was like having a terrible nightmare that you woke up from and found was true. Our physical reaction was one of shock, feeling weak at the knees and shaky, and of disbelief, we also felt guilty and angry.

Ruccione *et al.*[40] discuss the contents of a letter that a mother of a young boy diagnosed with a spinal tumour wrote to the mother of a girl recently diagnosed with leukaemia:

The memories of our first days in hospital have been flooding back as I see all you are going through. I look at your faces and see a mirror image of what I looked like. The exhaustion, the fear, the disbelief, the pain and the grief – I was numb . . .

Such statements, often heard by paediatric oncology nurses and the paediatric team, reflect parents' emotional states after learning that their child has cancer. The illness has come seemingly without warning and for no comprehensible reason. Parents express concern as to the cause of the illness and may question themselves: 'Are we to blame?', 'Is it something we could have prevented?', 'Is it because I smoked during pregnancy?'. Even if they do not verbally express feelings of guilt, parents need to be reassured that they are not to blame.

As feelings of disbelief subside, anger is frequently the next reaction. Anger may be directed at the hospital staff. Nurses must be prepared to accept parental reactions and defences of anger, hostility, and rejection without taking such reactions as a personal assault and without withdrawing themselves from the situation. Reactions to the diagnosis may be further intensified as there may be the necessity to commence treatment immediately, which entails consenting and subjecting the child to intensive and frightening treatment programmes. Another dilemma parents have to face is what or how to tell the child or adolescent about their illness and what to tell brothers and sisters. The effects of the diagnosis will be far-reaching, affecting not only the immediate and extended family but also family friends and friends of the child or adolescent.

What, when, and how to tell the child, adolescent, or siblings about the illness is an issue that generates much debate. Following careful assessment of their level of development and family situation, it is now accepted that children and adolescents have a right to know about aspects of the disease and treatments.

It is clear that the diagnosis and treatment for childhood cancer involve major emotional stresses for parents. To cope with the child's illness parents must simultaneously maintain hope, care actively for the child, and delegate responsibility to medical specialists, develop trust with members of the multidisciplinary team, and attend to the immediate needs of the sick child and other family members, notably brothers or sisters, and plan for the future.

The watchwords for best patient care are stability, and knowledgeable, co-operative teamwork. Family members need to gain a feeling of stability and consistency of care, especially through the early days of treatment. They need to feel that staff are available to provide them with both information and the time to formulate questions. Much time is often needed for parents and families from all socio-economic backgrounds, asking the same questions several times before 'hearing' the answer. Koocher and O'Malley, investigating the psychological consequences of surviving childhood cancer, reported that it was important to families that carers gave a measure of realistic encouragement and hope along with the sense that they were cared about, and that the best possible care would be provided or found for their child.[41] Ruccione *et al.* found that among the most highly rated sources of information were physician, nurse, and social worker.[40] Of these, the most consistently highly rated, i.e. with the narrowest range of responses, were the physician and the nurse.

Research study 30.2

Calderwood M. and Koenen L. (1988). Parents' perspectives of paediatric oncology nursing services. *Nursing Management* **19**, 54–57.[42]

Aim of study
To discover which specific services or behaviours from nurses are important to parents.

Method
A sample of 184 parents was drawn from a list of parents whose children were seen in an oncology clinic. The sample included children with various types of cancer. A one-time-only mailed questionnaire was chosen to elicit views. The questionnaire was developed through discussions with clinic nurses, physicians, and administrative staff. Identifying that mail surveys generally have a lower return rate, the questionnaire was designed to make it short, understandable, and easy to complete. The Likert-type questionnaire dealt with two issues: the current clinic situation and the 'ideal' situation.

Results
Sixty-eight questionnaires were returned (37%). As only 64 were complete, data analysis included a 34% response rate. Frequency data were recorded for: mean, median, mode, standard deviation, coefficient of variation (%), standard error, and confidence indices of the 0.05 level of probability.

The most striking point was the high rating of items valuing nurses' technical skills and the time spent with nurses. The other highly rated items dealt with the importance of the nurse providing parents with initial survival skills. These included who to call and what to do if they were at all worried about the child. The items rated the lowest dealt with long-term rather than daily survival concerns; this included counselling on behaviour, and growth and developmental issues.

Limitations
There was no reference to the length of time since the child's diagnosis. It is known that issues of importance at the time of diagnosis may not be the same as therapy progresses.

The age of the children was not identified. Therefore, it is possible that the sample responses may have been skewed towards care issues relating to a particular age group.

Although the results are significant, the low response rate is puzzling.

Research study 30.2 demonstrates that parents value nurses' technical skills, especially when parents have gained an understanding of the knowledge and skills required to administer complicated and intense chemotherapy regimens.

A phenomenological study using a focused interviewing technique sought to gain knowledge and understanding of parents' experiences and perceptions of caring for their child's central venous catheter at home.[43] Interpretation of parents' accounts revealed three major themes: how parents experienced and dealt with learning to care for the central venous catheter, how parents experienced and dealt with the catheter at home, and how parents dealt with sharing the care of their child's catheter with others. During discussions with parents about the care of their child's central venous catheter, all six parents in the study raised concerns about the differences in knowledge and skills of nurses involved in the care outside the specialist hospital, i.e. in the community or at non-specialist hospitals:[43]

> Well the nurses are much better here [the specialist centre] than at other places, they know what they are doing.

> She [sic] the community nurse never knows much about the Hickman line. I could go to [hospital name] but the care for the Hickman line is nowhere near the standards they have got here [specialist centre]. If I was worried about the line I would ring here because other places you know . . .

The study was carried out in one geographical location, and generalisation of the results could be questioned. However, with the now accepted practice of involving parents in aspects of technical care, over time and through experience parents in any care setting may attain the status of 'expert parent'. As a result, parents become aware of limitations of professionals and enter a stage of 'guarded alliance'.[43]

In the Calderwood and Koenen study (Research study 30.2),[42] the parent's low rating of counselling on child behaviour and growth is interesting, as in clinical practice developmental concerns are seen to be important, although it is noted that these do not generally surface with parents until later in the therapy. This may not seem to be a crucial issue for the parents, but it is well documented and recognised in clinical practice that assisting the child's continuing growth and development physically and psychologically throughout the cancer experience is paramount.

It is essential that parents are helped to find the ability to cope, to provide a supportive environment for the entire family, and to meet the new demands created by the illness. Information about family members, how they interact with each other, their individual family roles, and previous illness experiences and stressful situations enables nurses and other team members to help families to recognise problems and assist them to find means of dealing with them.

Families need to develop a new system that will enable them to find guidelines to help them to cope. These may take many forms and differ as circumstances change, but they usually come in some sequence: before anything else there is a need for hard information about the child's condition, parents need to be restored to parenthood, and the team caring for the child should do so by sharing care as human beings.

It is acknowledged that the diagnosis of cancer in a child or young person often throws a family into crisis.[44] The patient faces the challenges of the disease, its symptoms, and side-effects of treatment. Many children and young people experience significant problems with body image and relationships with peers and potential partners, difficulties with schooling and other education or with employment, and in parallel the family experiences the shock and grief of a child faced with a life-threatening illness, and the family too will have significant psychosocial needs.

There are also many practical issues for families to face during treatment, such as increased costs of travel, work issues, living away from home, increased family stress plus caring for siblings. Psychosocial care comprises the psychological and social supportive care for a family during the stages of the illness; however these support needs are highly individual and will change as families and individuals move through the different stages of the care pathway.

Care strategy 30.2 Assisting parents to find the ability to cope and restructure their own lives and those of other family members

- Confirming the cancer diagnosis should be a planned event as parents vividly remember how, when, where, and the manner in which the diagnosis was given. The approach of the hospital and community team is known to affect the parents' initial and long-term ability to cope.
- Discuss and exchange information about members of the family, their individual roles, and how they interact with each other. Such information enables staff to assess with the parents the possible impact of the disease, and to assist with plans to deal with actual or potential problems.
- Enable parents to gain control of their emotions, giving them time and space.
- Assist parents to regain control over the situation by giving information about the disease, treatment, and side-effects. Information needs to be given and repeated as frequently as parents or other family members require.
- Support parenting roles by acknowledging the skills and knowledge that parents have about the sick child, and encourage and negotiate with them to participate in care to whatever level they choose.

The needs of the child

The nature of a child's reaction to his condition is not simply a reflection of how brave or cowardly he happens to be. Proper understanding and management of children with serious illness requires an appreciation of how the illness looks from the patient's point of view.[45]

Information needs of children

What to tell a child who has a life-threatening illness about the diagnosis and approaches to treatment tends to generate much discussion in an attempt to get it right. Certainly if children are to co-operate with frightening, painful, or uncomfortable procedures they must have an understanding of why. The impact of open communication patterns between the family, the child, and carers is clearly important. A known inverse relationship between a child's open discussion of illness and level of depression has been demon-

strated: greater openness assists adjustment. There is also clearly a relationship between sharing information on the diagnosis and late psychological adjustment among survivors.[41,45] Children may also have unknown fears and fantasies, which can be more frightening than the realities of the diagnosis and treatment. Such fears and fantasies cannot be adequately expressed in a climate of secrecy.

One study investigating information needs for children with cancer who were between 8 and 17 years of age, found that children want to be fully informed about their disease and its treatment and they do not want information withheld from them.[46] Individually, children and parents considered that they should be given information about prognosis, treatment, and all conceivable side-effects, not just those that are likely to occur. Parents, in contrast, wanted to shield their children about prognosis and treatment side-effects. This situation is not uncommon; in meetings with the parents and physician it is preferable that a nurse joins the parents to help them to express their fears and concerns about disclosure. The parents can be informed of the importance of communicating openly and honestly with the child and of the dangers of trying to shield the child from the facts. Bearison states that there are hardly any experiences that can be more frightening for a child than to have cancer.[47] Listening to children talk about their fears is difficult for adults. Thinking that we can protect children is a means of unconsciously trying to protect ourselves, thereby sometimes unwittingly denying children the opportunity to talk about their fears.

There are important differences between the way children understand what they experience and the way adults understand the same experience. These differences are not haphazard but can be predicted by reference to the child's stage of development, remembering that these stages are approximate. It is suggested that information gathering when dealing with children should be put before information giving. Another consideration is that when talking to young children the words used should be chosen carefully, avoiding potentially frightening words like 'cut', which may imply pain.[30]

The use of analogies must also be carefully thought out. Beales, cited in Muller *et al.*,[28] gives an example of a young boy with a chest complaint who had not previously given thought to what might be going on inside him. He was far from reassured when the doctor explained that his lungs were like balloons; all the balloons that he had known had extremely short lives, always bursting suddenly and unexpectedly and with a loud bang.

The most constructive approach for any explanation is listening to the child's own explanation. A question such as 'What do you think we can do to make you feel better?' or 'Why do you think you are in hospital?' is an approach that gives an opportunity to confirm to an anxious or uncertain child that certain practices and procedures will help to make things better, even if some of the procedures may make them uncomfortable at times.

Interestingly, the issues raised by the children in this study are similar to those expressed by children generally. Concerns about the cause of the disease were mostly expressed in relation to punishment as a result of wrong-doing or catching it from someone or something. Siblings also expressed concern about catching the illness and that they may have caused the illness because of a previous disagreement and having thought or verbalised an unkind outcome directed at the brother or sister. For example, children may wish one another dead if they cannot resolve differences. These concerns are also documented in the literature.[24,28,38]

Developmental needs

Play and education are considered to be the work of children. Both represent the basis of human development and creativity, not just a way of using up children's time while they grow into adults. The children in the study reported in Research study 30.3 indicated that distraction was important to assist them in coping with their

Research study 30.3

Hockenberry-Eaton M. and Minick P. (1994). Living with childhood cancer: children with extraordinary courage. *Oncology Nursing Forum* **21**, 1025–1030.[48]

Aim of study
To gain an understanding of the personal experience of school-age children with cancer.

Method
A sample of 21 children (11 males and 10 females) with cancer aged between 7 and 13 years was admitted to the study. A purposive sampling technique was used and a phenomenological research method was used to guide the study design and analysis. The interviewer obtained consent from parents and children. Children were asked to participate in a 30-minute audio-taped interview and were interviewed without the parents present.

Results
The children's perceptions of the cancer experience revealed four major themes: knowing, caring, feeling special, and getting used to it. Knowing about the type of cancer and treatment provided a sense of control that was extremely important for the children. However, despite the information given many did not understand why they got cancer and expressed numerous false ideas of disease transmission. One child thought she had got it from her cat or dog. The importance of human caring was emphasised throughout the interviews. Children felt a sense of security and support through human touch. In addition, it was important for the children to have a nurturing environment and to feel special; they also indicated that distraction was an effective intervention.

Limitations
The researchers felt that the small sample and the fact that the sample came from one geographical location may have limited the study's findings. Some may suggest that the cognitive development of school-age children limits their ability to articulate clearly what they perceive and distinguish as being helpful.

illness. One such distraction, which is important in the process of development, is the continuation with school and playgroup activities during hospitalisation and at home. Nurses can play a major role in helping children through difficult situations by implementing distraction methods through play and education.

There are many different types of play, each stimulating the development of a different aspect of a child's life. However, as with the sick child's understanding of what is happening, the particular form of play that engages a child will depend on the level of the child's maturity and individual interest. The potential for play to act as a vehicle for a child to express feelings has long been recognised by psychologists as having value in helping troubled children, and has led to the development of play therapy. Play therapy is based on the fact that play is the natural medium of self-expression. It is an opportunity that is given to the child to 'play out' feelings and problems, just as in certain types of adult therapy an individual 'talks out difficulties'.[49] Play therapy is usually defined as directive where the play is guided and interpreted, or non-directive where the direction is left to the child.

Play therapists are now considered to be necessary members of the paediatric team. Effective play therapy must give the child complete freedom to play out feelings of frustration, anxiety, insecurity, fear, and bewilderment. The beneficial use of play as a means of helping a child to understand medical procedures and what is happening needs to be considered and incorporated into all aspects of the child's care. Through play with toys and hospital equipment, children can, for example, be introduced to the reasoning for the placement of central venous catheters. Over time, through play and information giving, the child can be helped to gain an understanding of the need for the line. Many also become expert at knowing how the line should be used.

Education is said to be the single most important developmental factor affecting the child's adjustment. The information must, however, be pitched at a level commensurate with the patients' abilities to absorb and comprehend. This may require the use of special educational facilities, frequent repetition of information, or helping

parents to learn how to talk openly with their child about the illness.[41]

Considerable progress has been made in assessing and reducing children's distress during repetitive, painful, and unpleasant side-effects of medical procedures, such as bone marrow aspiration, lumbar puncture, or nausea and vomiting, and changes in physical appearance. Much of this progress is attributed to the recognition and understanding of the meaning the diagnosis and treatment have for the child. Knowledgeable staff are able to work with the child and family to determine the most appropriate approach, to reduce anxiety and to provide a heightened sense of self-control. For example, before subjecting a young child to a course of radiotherapy there is a need to have an understanding of child development, to know the child, to have discussions with the child, parents, play therapist, and other members of the paediatric team and the radiotherapy team, before deciding the best approach to getting the child through the procedure with minimal distress. This may be achieved through education and play, by watching another child undergoing the procedure, by giving sedation, or a general anaesthetic, or by a combination of any of the above.

Children's involvement in decision making
The growing debate about the status of children, and the broader debate around the rights of individuals have influenced the need to ensure that children are given the opportunity to articulate their concerns and to be involved in decision making about their affairs. This situation has been recognised and does not pose too many problems in the day-to-day care of the child with cancer. For example, a child is able to be involved in decision making about activities of daily living, about the most acceptable way of taking medication, about undergoing some diagnostic and medical procedures, and about which play and educational facilities engage their interest. However, there are other decision-making and consent issues that are faltering and uneven. Of particular importance in health care is the right or not of children to consent to medical interventions and participation in research. Arguably the most significant contribution to supporting the child's involve-

ment was the adoption by the United Nations General Assembly in 1998 of the UN Convention of the Rights of the Child.[50]

Care strategy 30.3 Development of appropriate intervention strategies for the child with cancer

- Knowledge of child development
- Knowledge of treatment programmes
- Knowledge of the unique structure of individual families
- Knowledge of individual family dynamics
- Co-operative team work, acknowledging skills and knowledge of colleagues
- Knowledge of supportive and relevant literature
- Understanding the importance of play and education
- Using appropriate communication skills that consider the child's developmental level and life experiences
- Flexibility and creativity when communicating with the child, e.g. use of diversional therapy
- Thinking carefully of the words used to communicate with children
- Considering when it is appropriate to use analogies
- Listening to the child and starting where the child is when entering into a conversation
- Involving the child in decision making.

The needs of the adolescent

Ettinger and Heiney write that the storm of adolescence may be particularly acute when overlaid with a diagnosis of cancer.[51] As with the child with cancer, the diagnosis in adolescence is a crisis,[52] and the impact of the disease on the adolescent threatens developmental milestones, to add to the psychological concerns raised by the illness itself. Understanding normal adolescent development provides a framework for identifying psychological concerns, predicting problems, and developing appropriate interventional strategies for adolescents with cancer.

Information needs
At the time of diagnosis the adolescent should be informed of the diagnosis and about treatment plans. Such communication helps to establish the trustworthiness of the professional, reduces the possibility of later serious emotional problems, and facilitates future discussions. Concealing the diagnosis is of little value; the adolescent may already be aware of the diagnosis or learn about it elsewhere.[18] Disclosure also prevents isolation, confusion, and stigmatisation. Generally the adolescent, like the adult, should have some control over the information received. Regardless of the potentially beneficial effects of disclosure in most cases, forcing unwanted information on an adolescent is disrespectful and may cause harm.[53] As with children, it is best to be led by adolescents themselves, and they should be asked if they want to know what is wrong with them.

Generally complicated explanations of the illness and how the treatment works are usually meaningless and not well understood.[54] However, adolescents will want to know and can understand what is to be done to them and what effect those interventions will have on their future.

Decision making
The debate about the rights of individuals and adolescents' involvement in consent to treatment and research is much to the fore; this will be discussed later (p. 597).

Developmental needs
The coping strategy identified in Research study 30.4 demonstrated that not thinking about the disease is interesting, as many researchers found denial critically important to the adolescent's adaptation to chronic illness.[55,56] Denial is thought to be part of normal adaptive processes and manifests itself in many different ways. Overcompensation in school activities, and intellectualisation of the disease and treatment is reported as being the adolescent's need to be 'normal'. The need for group identity, the common perception of adolescents that 'nothing will happen to me', and the strong need for autonomy appear to provide the rationale for this coping mechanism. Denial as a coping mechanism may appear irrational or inexplicable on its own, but when viewed in the context of known developmental principles it may be found to be meaningful and provide insight into the psychological functioning of the adolescent. However, denial may prove inadequate, and pathological behavioural and responses to

stressors are likely to be exhibited. These include hostility, projection of guilt and anger onto others, and withdrawal.[57]

As adolescence begins with the onset of puberty, concerns of the adolescent patient with cancer

Research study 30.4

Weekes D.P. and Kagan S.H. (1994). Adolescents completing cancer therapy: meaning, perception and coping. *Oncology Nursing Forum* **21**, 663–670.[58]

Aim of the study
To explore and describe adolescents' experiences and associated changes in coping strategies during the time period from 3 to 6 months before cancer therapy completion to 6 months after completion.

Method
A convenience sample of 13 adolescents (nine males and four females) with cancer, aged between 11 and 18 years, was included in the study. The study employed an exploratory, descriptive, longitudinal design. Parental consent and adolescent assent was obtained. A semi-structured interview eliciting information regarding the meaning and perceptions of therapy, changes at home, and coping strategies was used. The interviews were taped and lasted for about 1 hour.

Results
Three themes emerged from the data: meaning and perception of completing the cancer therapy (task accomplishment, movement towards a normal life); coping strategies before completion of therapy (positive thinking, not thinking about the treatments and 'busyness'); and coping strategies after completion of therapy (negotiation and selective forgetting).

Before completion, therapy was described by 77% of adolescents as invading every aspect of their lives.

Not thinking about the treatments was described by 92% of the adolescents; 'busyness' appeared to be a strategy used to dispel the notion of reduced capability. After therapy completion, adolescents reported that they could focus on getting back to a normal life. They also made reference to their parents being overvigilant of activities and time spent with friends.

Limitations
The adolescents included in the study came from one geographical area, which may limit the possibility of general application.

arise from the specific developmental tasks of that age. Concerns may be separated and relate to family relationships, body image and self-concept, loss of control, peer relationships and social isolation, sexuality, and the future. Considering the normal adolescent task of emotional separation from parents, most sick adolescents are often frustrated by the overprotectiveness of parents. Yet they remain ambivalent and want parental comfort when feeling ill, but not when feeling well. They are also concerned about worrying their parents and feel that they need to be strong for their parent.[59]

Cancer treatments result in undesirable changes, and concerns about appearance and altered self-perception are expressed by adolescents, especially as they relate to body image. They also worry intensely about looking different from their peers.[60] Sexuality issues are intertwined with peer relations and body image. There is a dearth of literature on sexuality and the adolescent cancer patient, with most information deriving from anecdotal reports. A situation is recalled when a 14-year-old male was devastated when he learnt that he was likely to be sterile as a consequence of his proposed treatment. Later when asked what he feared most about being sterile he replied, 'Not being able to have an erection'. It became evident that he was not sufficiently knowledgeable about reproduction and did not separate fertility and impotence. It is therefore important, when discussing information of this nature, to establish the adolescent patient's current knowledge. However, adolescents may not always be certain of their own values, and efforts to discuss intimate issues such as sexuality may meet with hostility. Anger should be accepted as a healthy reaction. Since all individuals have to come to terms with what may or may not be possible for them to achieve, it is better for adults to share problems with the adolescent, rather than trying to solve the unsolvable.

The physical and personal self are perhaps the most important areas of concern for the adolescent, and are linked with the major task of identity formation. Adolescents with cancer can be helped with their change in appearance, using a practical approach. Stressing the temporary nature of side-effects and linking these problems to the drugs that are responsible will help the adolescent to separate who they are as a person and how they look and feel as a result of their treatment.[61] This information is also valuable for their peers, who may have difficulty acknowledging changes in appearance and 'stay away' from confronting the issue.

Continuation of schoolwork and success in the student role will have a positive impact on self-esteem, and implications for future career options. The expectation should be that the adolescent patients will return to school as soon as possible and continue with schooling throughout treatment.

The social needs of the adolescent need to be accommodated and considered both in hospital and at home. Groups of peers visiting in hospital may be viewed by some as being disruptive, and it is possible that this may be so. Adolescent peers require courtesy and a positive approach. Confrontational attitudes by adults are not well received. Brook considers that adolescents' claims that they are misunderstood may be true, since many of the problems of adolescents are actually the problems of the adults who are having to deal with them (see Personal account 30.3).[22]

Personal account 30.3

> I was 16 years old and on the national championship hockey cheerleading team when I was diagnosed with an osteosarcoma. I never went back to school, and I'll never cheerlead again. I had a graft and a total knee replacement. I can't kneel, sit cross legged, or bend my knee all the way.

Care strategy 30.4 Development of appropriate intervention strategies for the adolescent with cancer

- Knowledge of adolescent development
- Knowledge of the adolescent's friends, social activities, goals, and achievements
- Knowledge of family structure and dynamics
- Use of appropriate communication skills
- Listening to the adolescent, respecting and acknowledging their views and opinions
- Being flexible and accommodating towards the need to continue with education, social activities, and peer interaction
- Involving the adolescent in decision making.

The needs of siblings

It is known that having a brother or sister with cancer can have a profound and sustained impact on a sibling. Emotional concerns of being left out, jealousy and resentment of the attention given to the sick brother or sister, and fears for their own health are relatively common. Closed communication systems in families may contribute to the development of behavioural and emotional problems.[41]

The effect on siblings will be similar to those effects of a child diagnosed with cancer. It will be dependent on the level of development, their age in relation to the sick child, and the family's reactions. It is usually frightening for a sibling to witness changes in the brother's or sister's appearance such as hair loss, weight loss or gain, or limb amputation. As a result of the fears and concerns they are experiencing, siblings may be reluctant to talk to parents as they may become unsure and feel insecure of their position in the family.[62] Siblings should not be neglected by members of the medical team, by other family members, or indeed by parents, at a time when the focus and attention is on the child with the diagnosis. They should be offered direct factual information at the time of diagnosis and throughout the course of treatment, be seen as an integral part of the family-centred approach to care, and acknowledged as important participants in the family's life throughout the illness. Enquiring how a brother or sister is and involving them in activities both in hospital and at home will give them a sense of importance and well-being. Involving siblings to whatever degree they want to be involved will also help to provide a real explanation of what is happening and help to address any fantasies that may be more frightening than the real thing.

Consent, decisions, and choices

Debates over the rights of children have had a high profile in recent years, with growing acceptance in national and international law that children are people, entitled to basic human rights. The most significant contribution to this profile was the adoption by the United Nations General Assembly in 1989 of the UN Convention on the

Rights of the Child. The Convention has been ratified by 177 countries as of September 1995, a level of support unprecedented in the history of the UN.[50] Article 12 of the convention stresses that all children who are able to express their views must be given the opportunity to participate in decisions that affect them. The right includes decisions made in the private domain of the family and in the public arena of health and education.

A commitment to respect the voice of the child does, however, represent a shift from the traditional understanding of the status of the child in the family and in society. A number of well-worn arguments can be made against involving children in decisions about their care, ranging from developmental theories through to concerns about their lack of ability to comprehend the gravity of important decisions.[63] In the UK, during a consultation exercise undertaken by the Children's Right Development Unit in 1993, 45 children between the ages of 5 and 18 years were approached to discuss their perceptions of how their rights were respected.[64] The children reflected a wide variety of life experiences, but common to the group was a deep sense of frustration that their views and experiences were not taken seriously at home, at school, or by policy makers.

An increased role for minor patients (i.e. those under the legal age of consent, in most cases under the age of 16 years) in medical decision making has been advocated in recent years. Underlying the concept of child assent (refers to acquiescence) are the child's basic right to be informed, and the physician's ethical duty to provide the child with relevant information about their illness and treatment. It is also noted that the child's dissent may be ethically binding in cases of non-therapeutic research or medical procedures that are not considered essential.[46]

Extensive debate about autonomy and the reasons for its importance are not always clear in discussions about children's autonomy. Children may mistakenly be assessed as not having the capacity for autonomy or other personal qualities, when they have not been given the opportunity to demonstrate their autonomy. Some practitioners are also sceptical about the rights of children. Claims that 'it has all gone too far' are not uncommon. A popular view seems to be that the rights of children can only be achieved by denying the rights of others, whether that is parents or those who work with children.[21] It has to be remembered, however, that not all children want to be involved in decisions about their treatment.[46,65] A general lack of research and experience in this area is likely to compound the views of some health care staff, who believe children are incapable of making decisions and consenting to treatment. There is also a lack of clarity about how to decide whether children are competent and have the capacity to understand the nature of the treatment. Each case needs to be examined in context. Respect for children requires recognition that they may wish to control, share in, or refer decision making. If adults believe that a decision is misguided then they can discuss it with the child in more detail. As with the adult patient, most children, if asked, do agree to treatment, most commonly because they trust the doctor and their parents, and believe that the cancer will get worse without the treatment and the treatment will fight the cancer. Involving children in decision making and in the process of consent can be disingenuous if one does not intend to respect a refusal.[53] It can also be argued that a young person, especially one who is ill and under stress, may be more willing to leave decisional authority to their parents. However, if a child or adolescent independently refuses treatment, that refusal should be carefully scrutinised and not hastily overridden.

Every effort should be made to understand the reason for refusal. Leikin advocates that if the refusal has been clarified and addressed and the minor continues to refuse therapy, their level of decision-making competence needs to be examined.[53] There is, however, a considerable lack of clarity about how to decide whether a child is competent. Alderson suggests that competence tests remain subjective and often ask children to show greater levels of competence than the average adult.[65] Such a position and the reluctance of some practitioners to involve young people because of their perceptions of the legal requirements indicate a need for a satisfactory framework for making decisions for children's health. Uncertainty and anxiety lead to some professionals being overcautious about involving children in decision making, even when they agree with the concept.

Another contentious issue is that if a child or adolescent under the age of legal consent refuses treatment for cancer, this may not be considered to be in the 'best interests of the child', as the majority of paediatric cancers responds to therapy. Overriding the child's decision in such cases is usually justified. However complex the issue of consent and decision making, the principle of respect for children's autonomy encourages us to accept that the best people to judge their interests are the children themselves. However, they are compromised if adults withhold information. Children will also often know far more than the adults realise. For example, one child was overheard talking to another in the playroom, saying:

> I heard them using words like 'tumour' and 'malignant' so I looked at these words on the internet, I then knew that I had cancer. I know what cancer is my auntie got cancer.

Death and the dying child

Sadly, today around 30% of children with cancer will die. Most will die from progression of their disease but a small number will die from side-effects of treatment.[66] At this time in the disease process, as at the time of diagnosis, the manner in which information is imparted to families and the emotions that information elicits are likely to remain vivid lifetime memories.[39] Families, notably parents, need to know that although the child is not going to be cured they are not being abandoned. They need to understand that palliative treatment and care will be available and how this can be organised. Survival may no longer be possible for the child, but rehabilitative potential is possible, if only for a short while.[41] When planning palliative care it is important to have knowledge of the family, individual family members, cultural and religious views and beliefs, and to be flexible so that families have as much choice and control as possible. The death of a child is one of

Care strategy 30.5   Facilitating understanding and competence

Respecting children's rights requires that they have adequate information appropriate to their level of development, experience, and abilities.

How informed is the child or adolescent about:

- the illness to be treated
- the purpose of the proposed treatment
- the benefits, such as relief of symptoms, i.e. less pain, feeling better
- side-effects, options available, and the implications of not having treatment
- the possible discomforts, such as pain, medications, and scarring
- the time needed for inpatient or outpatient care, disruptions to social activities and school?

Does the child or adolescent show an understanding of the information given:

- by asking questions about its meaning and/or accurately explaining its meaning
- by seeking reassurance about procedures and their benefits
- by answering questions about the information that clearly express an understanding
- by talking about the impact that the treatment might have now and in the future?

Does the child or adolescent need explanations:

- by repeating and rephrasing the information
- by giving more time for discussion
- with drawings, diagrams, books, photographs, play, or medical equipment
- with help from parents, family, peers, other patients, or other professionals?

the most traumatic events that can happen to any family, leaving a permanent mark on their lives.[66]

Children's understanding of death

The issue of how children learn to understand their world and the influence of developmental theories in relation to understanding and illness has previously been examined. A similar approach has been adopted in studying children's concepts of death, with a number of studies indicating that children's understanding is linked to age.[67]

Most of these studies agree that it is difficult for a child under 2 years of age to comprehend fully the meaning of death, the common view being that very young children's response to death is similar to their response to separation. Children over 2 and under 6 years of age are considered to have little knowledge and experience of death, and tend to view it as a reversible state, usually associated with separation and a loss of movement. This age group is also viewed as being unable to separate fact from fantasy: 'Bang, bang you're dead, now get up'. Children over the age of 7 years are said to have a complete or almost complete understanding of death. Adolescents will have a full understanding of death, but this is also a time when young people tend to believe that 'it will never happen to me', take risks in life, and are known to defy death. Therefore, adolescents in the terminal phase of cancer may move from periods of choosing to deny what is happening and getting on with life, to making choices and decisions to forego additional therapy with knowledge and maturity.

A more precise way of categorising children's concept of death is that based upon stages of their cognitive development rather than age alone. Reilly *et al.* studied children's understanding of death in relation to cognitive development.[68] As expected, children at more advanced levels gave more informed answers to questions, and all children between the ages of 5 and 10 years believed in personal mortality. This study and others suggest that many children with a serious illness can comprehend death and understand the ideas of their own death.[18,69] An early study by Spinetta of the dying child's awareness of death found that terminally ill children as young as 5 years were aware that their illness had serious implications, even when they had not been informed by others.[70] This was in striking contrast to their parents' beliefs about what their children knew. Children tend to appreciate more than adults expect, and their level of understanding will influence their concerns and the ways in which to work with them in order to help.[71]

Even when it is considered by professionals that a child is aware of the possibility of dying, there continues to be a need to listen to the child and to be led by the child in conversations. For example, a 7-year-old child with advanced disease stated that 'I'm really frightened of it'. This statement could easily have been interpreted as being frightened of death or dying. When children tell parents and carers how afraid they are it is not uncommon for adults to respond with statements such as, 'there's nothing to worry about, everything will be alright'. These kinds of messages are likely to convey to children that adults do not want to hear about their fears, and may lead to an eventual loss of trust. When the child was asked what was meant by 'it', the child replied, 'having more medicines'. Gently enquiring as to what the child meant indicated to the child that the adult was interested in the child's fears, and enabled further discussion. Reluctance to question children's ambiguous expressions and not being alert to their sometimes indirect approaches, such as playing dead with their toys, will only serve to distance the child from the adult. Children recognise the reluctance of adults to talk explicitly with them about their cancer and what is happening, and will use ambiguous expressions to maintain a kind of mutual pretence. Both children and adults need help to overcome their defences.[47] The guiding principle is to avoid lying and to let the child tell you how much to say; children will often end up answering their own questions in their own way. It is important to appreciate the child's perspective and to respond to their questions seriously and sensitively without being too probing or overpowering. Essential to this approach is that it is supported by professionals and parents involved with the child's care. Parents can be helped to communicate with their children in ways other than conversation, as some children will express themselves more readily through play or drawings. Giving parents the opportunity to anticipate awkward situations and to rehearse their response can be helpful. There are times, however, when it appears better to avoid confronting children or adolescents with stark realities and better not to challenge their use of adaptive denial or other psychological means of coping. This is not a statement in support of deception, but simply a statement that the physical and emotional climate of care can be more important than the factual knowledge that the child or adolescent has, or believes. That is to say, the child or adolescent and family members must feel cared about and know that all of their questions will be answered directly and honestly.[41] Whatever strategy is adopted, even the most open, the idea of facing a child's own death with the child is immensely difficult.[66]

Symptom management

Many of the symptoms experienced by children in the terminal phase of their illness give rise to both physical and psychological responses. It is therefore necessary to build up a clear picture of the child's actual and potential problems.

It is important to set realistic goals with parents and the child when symptom management and care is planned. It is possible to provide effective symptom relief for the majority of children, but there are some children who will have severe and resistant problems.[66] One of the worst fears for parents of a child with progressive cancer is that they will suffer pain; such fears are a realistic concern. A study carried out in a paediatric oncology centre in the UK found that of 76 children who died of progressive disease, 87% needed opioid analgesia.[72] This finding is likely to be repeated in other specialist centres where the physiological and psychological benefits of using opioids for severe pain control in children are understood and supported. The use of strong analgesics for pain control in children with progressive disease is known to cause unease with parents and also with professionals who are unfamiliar with their use. As pain control and the use of analgesia play a major role in the management of children with progressive disease, it will be examined here in some detail. A more comprehensive review of pain and other symptom management can be found in the recommended reading list at the end of the chapter.

Care strategy 30.6   Issues to be considered when assessing and planning symptom management for children and adolescents with advanced disease

- Nature of the cancer and usual metastatic pattern
- Previous cancer therapies used
- Potential benefits of palliative therapy, e.g. chemotherapy, radiotherapy, blood and platelet transfusion, nerve block, massage, relaxation techniques
- Nature of actual or potential physical symptoms, e.g. pain, nausea, vomiting, constipation, infection, bleeding, or lethargy
- Nature of actual or potential psychological symptoms, e.g. fears about pain, other physical symptoms, change in body image, lack of mobility, loss of control, reduced peer contact, threat to planned goals, and fear of death itself (depends on level of cognitive development)
- Child and adolescent development and concepts of death
- Family structure
- Previously demonstrated child, adolescent, and family coping strategies
- Where care is to take place, i.e. home, specialist centre, local hospital, or hospice
- Appropriate involvement of the multidisciplinary team in the specialist centre, the child's local hospital, local community, or hospice.

Pain assessment and measurement

There are many problems associated with assessment and measurement of pain in children and young people, such as their range of cognitive development and their limited means of expression. Varni *et al.* advocate a model of paediatric pain assessment that incorporates biomedical/disease variables, appreciation of cognitive developmental level, measurement of child psychological and social adjustment, and measurement of family environment.[73] Assessment and measurement of children's pain need to consider both the direct and indirect ways in which children may express their discomfort. Direct expression may include the type of cry, how much the child can describe the pain, facial expression, body movement, and how much the child's activities are restricted by the pain. Indirect expression may include hunger, thirst, demanding constant company, or becoming withdrawn, unusually quiet or disinterested in favourite activities.

Research into children's pain and its assessment has led to the development of a number of reliable assessment tools.[74,75] For babies, recording systems have been developed that depend on observations of body movement, type of cry and facial expressions. For older children, linear analogue scales, pain ladders, and photographs or drawings of ranked facial scales have been used. However, such data on their own will have little clinical relevance without an evaluation of the framework in which children perceive pain, the nature and diversity of their experiences, and their coping abilities.[76]

Generally, experienced nursing and medical staff working with terminally ill children and adolescents tend not to use pain measurement scales, and depend on multidimensional clinical observations and the parent's understanding of their own child's reaction to pain. Interestingly, a study that looked at this supposedly unscientific approach to pain measurement found that estimates of a child's physical and psychological pain by several experienced independent observers using a visual analogue scale and behavioural observations correlated well with each other.[77] It is suggested that this approach should not be dismissed, but should serve to promote further research.

In summary, there is a number of principles underlying clinical understanding of paediatric pain:

- children do suffer pain
- children with pain suffer, often silently
- assessment of child or adolescent pain requires a multidimensional approach
- the choice of pain-relief options needs to be based on advanced learning, research, and teaching
- the relief of pain should not be physically or psychologically painful.

Pain management

Following pain assessment, a plan of management can be made. This may include a number of approaches, such as palliative radiotherapy, palliative chemotherapy, use of mild to strong analgesia, steroids, antidepressants, anticonvulsants, and psychological approaches. The choice will also depend on what is acceptable to the child and parents; for example, palliative radiotherapy for a very young child may require the use of general anaesthesia. The reason for a period of fasting before the procedure and spending time in hospital during the recovery period will not be understood by a young child. Both situations are likely to cause distress for the child, and inevitably the family. Therefore, an alternative, less-distressing option for effective palliation would need to be considered.

Analgesia

Most children with progressive disease will develop pain gradually, so can be helped initially with mild analgesia, progressing to moderate or strong analgesia as the pain increases. Important to the prescribing of analgesics is the general principle of regular administration, depending on the length of action of the chosen drug. For mild pain paracetamol is usually the drug of choice. When pain is no longer relieved by regular paracetamol, a mild opioid such as dihydrocodeine can be prescribed. For severe pain, strong opioid analgesics are essential.[67] In the UK, the strong opioids recommended and used most widely are morphine preparations. Many myths and fears continue to prevail concerning pain and the use of strong analgesics, especially in children. Health care professionals who are unfamiliar with the use of strong opioids worry about addiction and side-effects such as respiratory depression. Respiratory depression is uncommon in patients receiving opioids for pain associated with cancer, and appears to be no more common in children than in adults receiving comparable plasma opioid levels.[78] Fears surrounding the issue of addiction are usually due to the confusion about physiological and psychological addiction to opioids. Physiological dependence will develop following regular administration, but this rarely presents a clinical problem. If a child's pain, for example, is decreased by the use of palliative chemotherapy then symptoms of withdrawal can be avoided by gradually decreasing the dose of opioids over a number of days. It is reported that there is no evidence that appropriate use of opioids for pain produces psychological addiction.[67] Parents and the child may also have inappropriate fears of side-effects and addiction; it is therefore important to give them time and opportunity to express their concerns, so that explanations can be given.

Where the child is to die

Unlike the adult with progressive cancer, comparatively few children with cancer die in hospital or in a hospice. To be cared for at home in familiar surroundings is almost always the choice of the child and the child's parents and family. The possibility of home care is now a reality owing to the development of community liaison or home care teams in a number of countries; these are usually attached to specialist centres. The expertise of specialist nurses is available to assist and support the child and family, and community-based health care professionals. This support is essential if a child is to die at home, as demands upon parents and the community-based team could be overwhelming, since both are unlikely to encounter dying children very often. Specialist nurses working alongside community colleagues are able to assess the child and family for physical and psychological discomfort, and to offer advice on measures to overcome problems. It is important if home care is the preferred choice of the child and family that they do not feel abandoned by the specialist centre. Families need to know that hos-

pital staff are still available to them, and should they decide to return to the hospital for the child to die, that this can be arranged. In practice this rarely happens; if it does, it is likely to be as a result of a medical emergency such as uncontrollable fitting. In most cases, children die at home with pain and symptoms well controlled. It is worth remembering that what is said, and how carers behave are important factors for parents and family members at this time, as at other significant times in the disease trajectory. There is evidence demonstrating that the time taken by parents and siblings to adapt is reduced in families where the child has died at home as opposed to hospital.[79] If hospital or hospice care is the preferred choice, this should be supported by the team at the specialist centre. As with home care the child and family should know that the plan of management has been carefully considered, is jointly agreed, and is in the best interests of the child and family.

Long-term issues and effects of surviving childhood cancer

The increasing numbers of survivors of childhood cancer provide evidence of the remarkable advances that have been made in paediatric oncology. In the late 1970s the percentage of children who would have been long-term survivors of cancer was around 30%,[80] but commensurate with the rapid advancement of treatment, current figures suggest that by the year 2010 at least one in every 9000 young adults will have been cured of childhood cancer.[81]

With increasing survival, the physical, emotional and social sequelae, which may impair the quality of life in the long term, become more important. Although many of those cured during childhood cancer or young adulthood will return to good health, others will experience significant sequelae. These can occur any time following completion of therapy. They include problems such as impairment of endocrine function (for some including infertility, and abnormal growth and development), cardiac and neurological impairment, cognitive decline and psychological effects, plus the increased risk of developing a second cancer. On average 4% of childhood cancer survivors develop a second primary malignancy within 25 years of diagnosis,[82] although for certain diagnoses this figure is higher.

Koocher and O'Malley report on a 4-year investigation carried out in the 1970s into the psychological, medical, and practical life problems of people who were successfully treated for cancer during childhood.[41] Although this is an early study, it is considered to be one of the most comprehensive investigations undertaken. Overall, this study reported that most survivors lead healthy adult lives, marry and have children, and maintain a quality of life consistent with others in the general population. As increasing numbers of children survive malignancies there are many implications for long-term survivors, which include the physical, psychological and social consequences of surviving childhood cancer.[83] A healthy adult psychological adjustment, however, is not assured. Virtually all the 117 survivors interviewed used some degree of denial as a coping mechanism, although the population varied widely with respect to adaptive and maladaptive applications of denial. Some of the findings that contributed to psychological concern for survivors were:

- the meaning of residual impairments resulting from cancer therapies
- the prospect for social acceptance and future relationships
- the ease of entry into the workplace
- the ability to obtain health and life insurance
- family communication, and the long-range impact the patterns of openness or secrecy may have on the survivors.

Many survivors and their parents recognise that they may have to deal with late effects from treatment as well as struggling to find a new 'normal life'.[83] A range of strong emotions are experienced as adjustments are made to the after-cancer life, and these can include fear of recurrence, anxiety, guilt and grief, as well as gratitude and joy. Survivors and their parents experience the whole spectrum of feelings about possible relapse, some never think about it and others state that it will be dealt with when it happens.[83] Many feel anxious when an anniversary or check-up is due, and often

parents are surprised when the feelings of recurrence vacillate over time. They go through a period of fearfulness followed by a long time when cancer is not thought about, and it is perfectly normal to be at different places of the spectrum at different times.

> I was just thinking that this state of vigilance and worry never seems to go away. I know parents of kids who are years out of treatment seem to do better with this, but it's not easy. Even when things are going well and you are sure it's just a cold, that worry is there. The thought at the back of your head thinks 'what if it's not just a cold?' I look forward to the day when that thought in the back of my head is not my first thought when my son is sick. In the last week my teenage son who is three months off treatment, has had a decreased appetite and been very tired. I know he's worried about the 'what if' question, but hasn't voiced it. He's just extra quiet, so we've mentioned that he just has a cold or something that's going around and he needs more sleep. But we all know that somewhere in the back of our heads, there are bells ringing. I know in my head that this is just a cold. But my heart whispers, 'what if'.

Some survivors and their parents find that they continue to have deep fears over an extended period of time.[83] The need for psychological support is paramount at this time.

Apajasalo et al.[84] noted that sophisticated data on specific problems are available, but very little is known about the quality of life of long-term survivors of childhood cancer. Based on previous reports and from their own observations, the researchers hypothesised that the health-related quality of life of adults surviving childhood cancer would be inferior to that of the normal population (see Research study 30.5 for a detailed summary).

In the Koocher and O'Malley study, denial and suppression are noted to be a major coping strategy adopted by survivors.[41] Denial is described as a primitive defence, which might be used in a major way by a child, someone with a mental illness, or someone in a crisis. The mature equivalent, which develops over time from denial, is suppression, the conscious choosing to put aside, not to consider certain disturbing or painful events. Interestingly, although survivors used this coping strategy, most remembered clearly what happened to them.

Research study 30.5

Apajasalo M., Sintonen H., Simes M.A. *et al.* (1996). Health-related quality of life of adults surviving malignancies in childhood. *European Journal of Cancer* **32A**, 1354–1358.[84]

Aim of the study
To establish whether the health-related quality of life of adults who had survived childhood cancer was inferior to that of the normal population, and further to attempt to establish whether the health-related valuations of survivors would differ from the valuations of the controls.

Method
A previously validated 15-dimensional questionnaire (15-D), which was considered to cover physical, social, and mental well-being aspects of health-related quality of life, was mailed to 220 survivors. One-hundred and twenty-nine adults who had previously completed the 15-D were chosen randomly as controls. There were no significant differences in the age, level of education, or employment status of the patients and control. The 15-D measure consisted of multiple choice questions, each representing one health-related dimension, e.g. mobility, vision, hearing, sleeping, eating, depression, distress, vitality, and sexual activity. Analysis of variance, the Mann–Whitney *U* test, multiple regression, and correlation coefficients were used to analyse results.

Results
There were no significant differences in the health-related valuations between the survivors and the controls. In statistical terms, the quality of life scores of the survivors were significantly better than those of the controls.

Conclusions
The observed excellent perceived health-related quality of life could be explained in many ways. One explanation may lie in the changes in personality and view of life brought about by the experience of surviving a life-threatening illness. Survivors may find their present life more satisfying and possible defects in their present health status less significant. This is supported by the finding that the most significant differences between survivors and controls were found in the most subjective dimensions, such as vitality and distress.

Limitations
Issues that are recognised by some survivors, such as perceived isolation, abnormal peer or family relationships, self-esteem, and body image, may not be sufficiently identified through a generic measure. In addition, fear of recurrence, employment and insurance problems, and potential social discrimination may lead to a situation in which survivors may ignore objective symptoms and findings. Denial mechanisms may compensate or overcompensate for the objectively measurable late effects.

It's been four years since my sarcoma was diagnosed and I don't even think about a relapse. Relapses happen most often in the first year, so the farther out I get the less likely it is to occur. But, honestly, I never worry about it.

Grief, loss and stress

As these survivors progress they often suffer some losses in the process.[83] A universal loss is the sense that the world is a safe place and that childhood cancer has robbed the entire family of that blissful belief in the natural order of things, that children will have a happy and carefree childhood and that children will never die before their parents. Grief and loss extends to other areas of life, such as the loss of abilities, life prospects or body parts. Grief over the loss of friends is universal. Not only must the survivors cope with the physical changes, but they must also deal with the alteration of self-image. Symbolically, the person one hoped to become dies or undergoes great change.

The feelings most often associated with the normal grieving process are denial, anxiety, fear and guilt, depression and anger. These are perfectly normal feelings and are often perceived by others as a problem when they are a natural response to a life-changing event. It is necessary and important to acknowledge these feelings in order to deal with what cannot be changed. These have to be separated from what is lost, in order to move on. Part of resolving grief is in sharing this with others, but expressing these feelings is often socially unacceptable. Survivors and parents struggle to balance gratitude for life with sadness over loss. These survivors and parents may not view these in the same way, and conflicts may arise, creating an inability to use each other for support.

During treatment children and adolescents are engaged in an arduous battle against their cancer. All of the time, energy and strength are directed toward dealing with immediate survival.[83] Many find it difficult to cope with what it means when treatments come to an end, and being cancer free does not mean that feelings are cancer free. Unresolved emotions may grow stronger and erupt unexpectedly.

Personal account 30.4

I had Hodgkin's when I was 15. I tried hard in university to put it behind me and to get on with my life. It just didn't work. Next to treatment that was the worst year of my life. It showed me that if I didn't deal with it consciously I was going to deal with it subconsciously. I had nightmares every night. I would wake up feeling like I had needles in my arms. Once I started dealing with it things improved. I had a wonderful teacher and really spilled my heart out to him that year.

According to the *Diagnostic and Statistical Manual of Mental Health Disorders*, post-traumatic stress disorders may be diagnosed if the person experienced one or more events that involved threatened death or physical injury, or a threat to their own or others' integrity. These parameters specifically include learning that one (or one's child) has a life-threatening disease. The provision of psychosocial support is paramount. The needs of individuals will change as the child moves through the journey. Psychological services have an important role to play at all stages along the journey, including after completion of treatment and into adult life.

Long-term follow-up

Long-term follow-up is now part of the overall management for children surviving cancer. This requires careful handling if patients are to attend, especially during the adolescent years, when the importance of adaptive denial is known to assist psychological coping. Attending for what appears to be an unnecessary appointment may threaten this coping mechanism. One way to overcome the problem is to stress to the individual the seriousness of the illness for which they were successfully treated and to encourage appropriate follow-up and routine health precautions. Health care professionals working with long-term survivors also need to be aware of both subtle and obvious consequences of cancer treatments. The survivor whose puberty is delayed, for example, may experience significant self-esteem problems, which could go unnoticed at a routine medical follow-up.

Recognising that such a symptom can be an issue, a sensitive practitioner can enquire and make referrals as indicated.[41] Therefore, the purpose of follow-up should be to consider the wellbeing of children with cancer, to ensure that they achieve normal or maximal growth, maturation, and psychosocial adaptation. Optimum management requires a multidisciplinary follow-up service in which a paediatric oncologist, paediatric endocrinologist, and paediatric clinical psychologist contribute. Long-term effects of treatment for childhood cancer are many and varied. Effects due to the toxicity of cancer therapies are currently known and understood; however, new problems may arise due to as-yet undescribed toxicity and evolution of tissue damage. Minimisation of these effects can be achieved by vigilant observation and a willingness on the part of clinicians to accept necessary modification of treatment, by early intervention and prevention, and with the co-operation of the multidisciplinary team. It is suggested that what is needed is that every new protocol should have a section built into it that makes provision for baseline assessment of organ function and psychological status. Well-designed prospective evaluation of treatment effects is also considered to be mandatory.[85] Rather than working to restore lost function, those caring for the child or adolescent with cancer and their family need to work collectively towards preventing or minimising early or late physical or psychological effects. It is not enough to 'mean well' when caring for the child or adolescent with cancer; it is essential to 'know well':[41]

A child's life is like a piece of paper on which every passerby leaves a mark.

Ancient Chinese proverb

References

1. Eiser C. (2004). *Children with Cancer – Quality of Life.* Mahwah, NJ: Lawrence Erlbaum Associates.
2. UK Childhood Cancer Research Group. (2004). *National Registry of Childhood Tumours.* www.ccrg.ox.ac.uk/datasets/nrct.htm (accessed 3 September 2007).
3. Pavlisis N. (2005). Improving care for children and adolescents within the frame of medical oncology. *Annals of Oncology* **16**, 181–188.
4. Stiller C.A. (1992). Aetiology and epidemiology. In Plowman P.N. and Pinkerton C.R. (eds.) *Paediatric Oncology: Clinical Practice and Controversies.* London: Chapman and Hall, pp. 17–45.
5. Bleyer W.A. (2002). Cancer epiemiology, diagnosis, treatment and survival in paediatrics. *Medical Paediatric Oncology* **38**, 1–10.
6. Voute P.A., Kalifa C. and Barrett A. (1998). *Cancer in Children: Clinical Management.* Oxford: Oxford University Press.
7. Blair V. and Birch J.M. (1994). Patterns and temporal trends in the incidence of malignant disease. *European Journal of Cancer* **30A**, 1490–1498.
8. Stewart A., Webb D. and Hewitt D. (1958). A survey of childhood malignancies. *British Medical Journal* **i**, 1495–1508.
9. Cartwright R.A., McKinney P.A. and Hopton P.A. (1984). Ultrasound examinations in pregnancy and childhood cancer. *Lancet* **ii**, 999–1000.
10. Kinnier-Wilson L.M. and Waterhouse J.A. (1984). Obstetric ultrasound and childhood malignancies. *Lancet* **ii**, 997–999.
11. Voute P.A., Barrett A., Bloom H.J., Lemerle J. and Neidhardt M.K. (1986). *Cancer in Children Clinical Management,* 2nd edition. Berlin: Springer.
12. Bleyer W., Tejada H. and Murphy S. (1997). National clinical cancer trials. *Journal of Adolescent Health* **21**, 366–373.
13. Nicholson A. (1990). Childhood cancer – an overview. In Thompson J. (ed.) *The Child with Cancer, Nursing Care.* London: Scutari Press.
14. Hammond G.D. (1986). Keynote address; the cure of childhood cancers. *Cancer* **58(suppl.)**, 407–413.
15. Siegal M. (1991). *Knowing Children.* Hove: Lawrence Erlbaum Associates.
16. Nicholson R. (1986). *Medical Research with Children, Ethics, Law and Practice.* Oxford: Oxford University Press.
17. Koocher G. and Saks M. (1993). *Children's Competence to Consent.* New York: Plenum Press.
18. Bluebond-Langner M. (1978). *The Private Words of Dying Children.* Princetown, NJ: Princetown University Press.
19. Nessim S. and Ellis J. (2001). *Cancervive.* Cambridge, MA: Houghton Mifflin Press.
20. Lansdown G. (1995). *Taking Part: Children's Participation in Decision Making.* London: Institute for Public Policy Research.
21. Franklin B. (1995). The case for children's rights: a progress report. In Franklin B. (ed.) *The Handbook of Children's Rights.* London: Routledge, pp. 85–96.
22. Brook C.G. (1985). *All About Adolescence.* Chichester: John Wiley.
23. Erikson E.H. (1968). *Identity, Youth and Crisis.* London: Faber and Faber.
24. Kuykendall J. (1989). Teenage trauma. *Nursing Times* **83**, 26–28.
25. World Health Organisation. (1986). *Young People's Health – A Challenge for Society.* Technical Report Series 731. Geneva: World Health Organisation.
26. Rapoport R. and Rapoport R. (1980). *Growing Through Life.* London: Harper and Row.
27. National Institute for Health and Clinical Excellence. (2005). *Improving Outcomes in Children and Young People with Cancer.* London: National Institute for Health and Clinical Excellence.
28. Muller D.J., Harris P.J. and Wattley L. (1986). *Nursing Children: Psychology, Research and Practice.* Lippincott Nursing Series. London: Harper and Row.
29. Leavitt M.B. (1989). Transition to illness; the family in hospital. In Gillis C.L., Highly B.L., Roberts B.M. and Martinson I.M. (eds.) *Towards a Science of Family Nursing.* Menlo Park, CA: Addison-Wesley, pp. 262–283.
30. Prugh D.G., Staub E.M., Sands H.H., Kirschbaum R.M. and Lenihan E.A. (1953). A study of the emotional reactions of children and families to hospitalisation and illness. *American Journal of Orthopsychiatry* **23**, 70–106.
31. Bowlby J. (1969). *Attachment and Loss,* Vol. 1. New York: Basic Books.
32. Koot H.M. and Wallender J.L. (2003). *Quality of Life in Child and Adolescent Illness: Concepts and Findings.* Oxford: Psychology Press.
33. Dermatis H. and Lesko L.M. (1990). Psychological distress in parents consenting to child's bone marrow transplantation. *Bone Marrow Transplantation* **6**, 411–417.

34. Terkleson K.G. (1980). Toward a theory of the family life cycle. In Carter E.A. and Goldrock M. (eds.) *The Family Life Cycle: A Framework for Family Therapy*. New York: Gardner.

35. Combrick-Graham M.D. and Thomas R.B. (eds.) (1985). A developmental model for family systems. *Family Process* **24**, 139.

36. Thomas R.B. (1987). Family adaptation to a child with a chronic condition. In Rose M.H. and Thomas R.B. (eds.) *Children with Chronic Conditions; Nursing in a Family and Community Context*. Orlando, FL: Grune and Stratton, pp. 112–118.

37. Bishop K.K., Woll J. and Arango P. (1994). Cited in Ahamann E. Family centred care: shifting orientation. *Paediatric Nursing* **March–April**, 20.

38. Pinkerton C.R., Cushing P. and Sepion B. (1994). *Childhood Cancer Management*. London: Chapman and Hall.

39. Woolley H., Stein A. and Forrest G.C. (1989). Imparting the diagnosis of a life-threatening illness in children. *British Medical Journal* **298**, 1623–1626.

40. Ruccione K., Kramer R.F., Moore I. and Perin G. (1991). Informed consent for treatment of childhood cancer: factors affecting parents' decision making. *Journal of Pediatric Oncology Nursing* **8**, 112–121.

41. Koocher G.P. and O'Malley J.E. (1981). *The Damocles Syndrome*. New York: McGraw-Hill.

42. Calderwood M. and Koenen L. (1988). Parents' perspectives of pediatric oncology nursing services. *Nursing Management* **19**, 54–57.

43. Thompson J. (1995). *Parents' Perceptions of Caring for their Child's Central Venous Catheter at Home*. MSc dissertation, Open University, North East Surrey College of Technology.

44. Beales G. (1983). The child's view of chronic illness. *Nursing Times* **79**, 50–51.

45. Slavin L., O'Malley J.E., Koocher G.P. and Foster D.J. (1981). Communication of the cancer diagnosis to paediatric patients: impact on long-term adjustment. *American Journal of Psychiatry* **139**, 179–183.

46. Ellis R. and Leventhal B. (1993). Information needs and decision-making preferences of children with cancer. *Psycho-oncology* **2**, 227–284.

47. Bearison D.J. (1991). *They Never Want to Tell You, Children Talk About Cancer*. Cambridge, MA: Harvard University Press.

48. Hockenberry-Eaton M. and Minick P. (1994). Living with childhood cancer: children with extraordinary courage. *Oncology Nursing Forum* **21**, 1025–1030.

49. Cheshcheir M.W. and Schulz K.M. (1981). The development of a capacity for concern in antisocial children: Winnicotts concept of human relatedness. *Clinical Social Work Journal* **17**, 24–39.

50. United Nations (1992). *The Convention on the Rights of the Child*. London: HMSO.

51. Ettinger R.S. and Heiney S. (1993). Cancer in adolescents and young adults. Psychological concerns, coping strategies and interventions. *Cancer* **71(suppl. 10)**, 3276–3280.

52. Eilerstein M. (2004). Value of professional collaboration in the care of children with cancer and their families. *European Journal of Cancer Care* **13**, 349–355.

53. Leikin S. (1993). The role of adolescents in decisions concerning their cancer therapy. *Cancer* **71(suppl. 10)**, 3342–3346.

54. Sussman E., Hersh S., Nannis E., Strope B. and Woodruff P. (1982). Conceptions of cancer; the perspectives of child and adolescent patients and their families. *Journal of Paediatric Psychology* **7**, 253–261.

55. Kagen L.B. (1976). Use of denial in adolescents with cancer. *Health and Social Work* **4**, 70–87.

56. Zelter L., Kellerman J. and Ellenburg L. (1980). Psychological interventions with adolescents. *Cancer Bulletin* **36**, 279–284.

57. Richie M.A. (1992). Psychological functioning of adolescents with cancer: a development perspective. *Oncology Nursing Forum* **19**, 1497–1501

58. Weekes D.P. and Kagan S.H. (1994). Adolescents completing cancer therapy: meaning, perception and coping. *Oncology Nursing Forum* **21**, 663–670.

59. Rudin M., Martinson I. and Gillis C. (1988). Measurement of psychological concerns of adolescents with cancer. *Cancer Nursing* **11**, 144–149.

60. Ohanian N. (1989). Informational needs of children and adolescents with cancer. *Journal of Paediatric Oncology Nursing* **6**, 94–97.

61. Ellis J. (1991). Coping with adolescent cancer: it's a matter of adaptation. *Journal of Paediatric Oncology Nursing* **8**, 10–17.

62. Eiser C. (1998). Practitioner view: long term consequences of childhood cancer. *Journal of Child Psychiatry and Psychology* **39**, 621–633.

63. Purssell E. (1995). Listening to children; medical treatment and consent. Guest editorial. *Journal of Advanced Nursing* **21**, 623–624.

64. Children's Rights Development Unit. (1994). *UK Agenda for Children*. London: Children's Rights Development Unit.

65. Alderson P. (1993). *Children's Consent to Surgery*. Milton Keynes: Open University Press.

66. Gonda T.A. and Ruark J.E. (1984). *Dying Dignified, The Health Professional's Guide to Care*. Menlo Park, CA: Addison-Wesley.

67. Goldman A. (1992). Care of the dying child. In Plowman P.N. and Pinkerton C.R. (eds.) *Paediatric Oncology:*

Clinical Practice and Controversies. London: Chapman and Hall.

68. Reilly T.P., Hasazi J.E. and Bond L.A. (1983). Children's conceptions of death and personal mortality. *Journal of Paediatric Psychology* **8**, 21–31.

69. Wass H. and Corr C.A. (1984). *Childhood and Death* Washington, DC. Hemisphere Publishing.

70. Spinetta J.J. (1974). The dying child's awareness of death. A review. *Psychological Bulletin* **81**, 256–260.

71. Lansdown R. and Benjamin G. (1985). The development of the concept of death in children aged 5–9 years. *Child Care Health and Development* **11**, 13–20.

72. Goldman A. and Bowman A. (1990). The role of oral controlled release morphine for pain relief in children with cancer. *Palliative Medicine* **4**, 279–285.

73. Varni J.W., Walco G.A. and Katz E.R. (1989). A cognitive–behavioural approach to pain associated with paediatric chronic pain. *Journal of Pain and Symptom Management* **4**, 238–241.

74. Bayer J. and Wells N. (1989). The assessment of pain in children. *Paediatric Clinics of North America* **36**, 837–854.

75. McGrath P.A. (1990). *Pain in Children: Nature, Assessment and Treatment*. New York: Guildford University Press.

76. McGrath P.A. (1989). Evaluating children's pain. *Journal of Pain and Symptom Management* **4**, 198–214.

77. McGrath P.A., DeVeber L.L. and Hearn M.T. (1985). Multidimensional pain assessment in children. In Fields H.L., Dubner R. and Cervero F. (eds.) *Advances in Pain Research and Therapy*. New York: Raven Press, pp. 387–393.

78. Armstrong D. (2005). *Cognitive and Late Effects Related to Childhood Cancer*. New York: Leukemia and Lymphoma Society, USA.

79. Mulhern R.K., Lauer M.E. and Hoffman R.G. (1983). Death of a child at home or in the hospital: subsequent psychological adjustment of the family. *Paediatrics* **71**, 743–747.

80. Mulhern G. (2003). *Reconfiguration in Paediatric Medicine*. London: British Association of Paediatric Surgeons.

81. Waterworth S. (1992). Long term effects of cancer. *British Journal of Nursing* **12**, 373–374, 376–377.

82. Wallace W.H. and Shalet S.M. (1992). Growth and endocrine function following treatment of childhood malignant disease. In Plowman P.N. and Pinkerton C.R. (eds.) *Paediatric Oncology: Clinical Practice and Controversies*. London: Chapman and Hall, pp. 186–216.

83. Keene W., Hobbie W. and Ruccione K. (2000). *Childhood Cancer Survivors: A Practical Guide to Your Future*. Cambridge: O'Reilly Associates.

84. Apajasalo M., Sintonen H., Simes M.A. *et al.* (1996). Health-related quality of life of adults surviving malignancies in childhood. *European Journal of Cancer* **32A**, 1354–1358.

85. Morris Jones P. (1992). Non-endocrine late effects of treatment. In Plowman P. and Pinkerton C.R. (eds.) *Paediatric Oncology: Practice and Controversies*. London: Chapman and Hall, pp. 189–216.

Recommended reading

1. Bearison D.J. (1991). *They Never Want to Tell You, Children Talk About Cancer*. Cambridge, MA: Harvard University Press.

2. Bluebond-Langner M. (1978). *The Private Words of Dying Children*. Princetown, NJ: Princetown University Press.

3. Keene W., Hobbie W. and Ruccione K. (2000). *Childhood Cancer Survivors: A Practical Guide to Your Future*. Cambridge: O'Reilly Associates.

4. National Institue for Health and Clinical Excellence. (2005). *Improving Outcomes in Children and Young People with Cancer*. London: National Institute for Health and Clinical Excellence.

5. Pinkerton C.R., Cushing P. and Sepion B. (1994). *Childhood Cancer Management*. London: Chapman and Hall.

6. Plowman P.N. and Pinkerton C.R. (1992). *Paediatric Oncology: Clinical Practice and Controversies*. London: Chapman and Hall.

7. Voute P.A., Kalifa C. and Barrett A. (1998). *Cancer in Children: Clinical Management*. Oxford: Oxford University Press.

This chapter is based on the original text from the first edition written by Jenny Thompson and updated for this new edition by Fay Scullion.

CHAPTER THIRTY-ONE

The needs of older people

Christopher Bailey

Introduction: a personal view

Some years ago my colleagues and I worked on a study of people over the age of 60 years who had cancer of the colon and rectum.[1-3] The main purpose of the study was to investigate the type of treatment and care older people were receiving, record the effects on functional status, and discover whether chronological age made a difference to the kind of treatment and care provided. Our study showed that for people with colorectal cancer, the likelihood of receiving adjuvant chemotherapy decreased significantly with age.[1] This finding was consistent with research from the US, which showed that rates of treatment with adjuvant chemotherapy decline markedly with age,[4] and with research in the Netherlands, where researchers found that older patients were more likely to receive single modality treatment.[5] Increased severity of co-morbidity in older people is sometimes given as a possible explanation for why older people receive less-aggressive treatment. In our study, however, the differences in the treatment people received were not explained by differences in morbidity, or in economic, mental or physical function, self-care capacity, physical or psychological symptom distress, activity level, or overall quality of life. Together with chronological age, one other factor did seem important in explaining why some over-60s received more extensive treatment than others: people with greater access to supportive relationships at home appeared to be more likely to be offered adjuvant chemotherapy.

For around 2 years, my colleagues and I had visited older people with colorectal cancer, both at home and in hospital. This was a valuable opportunity to talk in depth to older people and hear from them about the impact of illness and health care in later life.

The youngest person we spoke to was 60 and the oldest 95. While people of 60 years and upwards are often described as 'old' or 'older', categorising or labelling people in this way never captures the truth of their lives. We spoke to people of 90 whose lives were full and varied, and people of 90 whose lives were very restricted. It has become a cliché to say it, but there is no point trying to second guess the quality of a particular person's experiences on the basis of their age alone.

People's material circumstances differ widely, from luxurious to squalid, from homes with magnificent grounds to cluttered apartments with no room to move, where a commode, bed, and TV are squashed into one room. People can become isolated and despairing in luxury as well as in poverty, whether they are at home or in residential care, and whether they are alone or have a partner. Of course, older people with cancer lead fulfilled lives, whether or not they are alone. But my impression is that many of the people we visited were or had been frightened by what was happening to them and would have welcomed a means of addressing this. This may be as true for those spouses and partners who do not have cancer as for those who do.

Often in later life people's personal circumstances are complicated and demanding in most unexpected ways. One person, while materially and financially well cared for in specially built rooms in the family home, rarely spoke or interacted with other family members, even at meal times, and did not feel able to share the bath so used the sink in his room. Another, while cared for devotedly, was unable to respond or reciprocate because he had become so emotionally isolated. One man, who was in his 70s, was the oldest member of the household as well as the main carer for two or three younger but dependent family members with profound physical and mental problems. Another was the main source of family support for a partner who was in residential care. An elderly woman with cancer cried for the loss of her husband who had died 2 years before, and another recounted the loss of a grandchild 4 years previously, before telling me about her surgery.

Cancer can occur in the context of different or difficult lives, which older people often manage with little or no professional support. People who are experiencing fear, loneliness, grief, or the weight of responsibility have the added trauma of cancer and its treatment.

The most supportive, positive partners and families can experience painful confusion about the nature of a cancer diagnosis, the medical management of the illness, and the likely consequences. Many of the people I spoke to expressed powerful fears about the prospect of a colostomy or ileostomy; some found the practical aspects of stoma care unmanageable. Many experienced distressing and unexpected stoma 'accidents' or malfunctions, and got into the habit of avoiding supermarkets, hotels, restaurants, group holidays and activities, and long journeys because they felt unable to rely on their stoma in these circumstances.

My strong impression was that older people with colorectal cancer have an urgent need to reflect upon their illness, treatment, and care before and after their visits to hospital as a means of preparing for it emotionally and practically.

Reflecting on cancer, however, may mean accommodating a new kind of life story within what may already be a complicated or difficult life.

Older people and cancer

Facts and figures

It is no longer surprising to read or hear of statistics demonstrating how the proportion of older people in the populations of Western countries is changing. Often these figures are quoted in the context of a debate about health care, and in particular to illustrate the implications of demographic change for cancer and its care and treatment.

The percentage of people in the UK population aged 65 years and over has doubled since 1931 to 18% in 2001, but it is important to consider actual numbers as well as percentage increases.[6] To illustrate this point, Victor shows that from 1951–1971 the number of people aged 85 years and over rose by nearly 300%: in absolute terms, however, this represents an increase from 224 000 to 601 000.[6] This is especially important because, as Victor points out, ageing populations are associated with the same negative stereotypes attributed to individual older persons, and increased numbers of older people are seen as having negative consequences for health and social services.[6]

Victor draws attention to the importance of the relationship between social engagement and participation and quality of life in older age, emphasising that engagement with life (maintaining social relationships and productive activity, for example) is a key part of 'successful ageing':[7]

> . . . the promotion of and enhancement of social participation in later life could have benefits for the quality of life experienced by older people and be one approach to adding 'life to years' . . . [p.28].

In the UK women over the age of 65 years are more likely to be widowed, live alone, and have contact with friends and relatives than men:[7] in research showing that significantly more women than men reported that they were sometimes lonely (45% versus 28%), widowhood was shown to greatly increase vulnerability to loneliness.[7] But when the effect of this and other factors (e.g. living alone) is excluded, there is little difference between the prevalence of severe loneliness in older age between the sexes. Loneliness, Victor writes,[7] does not just impact upon quality of life. It is associated with a range of other negative health outcomes, including mortality, morbidity, depression, suicide, and health service use and there is, consequently, a clear case for developing interventions to promote social engagement in later life.

Writing about the experience of older people with cancer in the US, McCaffrey Boyle *et al.* emphasise the potential consequences of the 'gradual loss of supportive resources' that accompanies the co-morbidity and increasing incidence associated with cancer in older people:[8]

> Nearly one third of elderly people 65 years of age and over live alone. Most are women who have outlived their spouses and, in some cases have outlived their children and other relatives as well. The difficulties inherent to living alone may be intensified . . . by inadequate external social support networks, possibly resulting in unmet needs for long-term assistance with activities of daily living. These problems may be further exacerbated by loneliness, depression, and limited satisfaction with life [p.917].

In their 2004 position statement on cancer care in the older adult the Oncology Nursing Society and Geriatric Oncology Consortium (USA) point out that there has been failure to develop a body of knowledge to support care and treatment:[9]

> Empirical evidence that illuminates the unique needs of older adults with cancer is strikingly limited in proportion to the demographics of cancer in our ageing society. For example, patients older than 65 historically were excluded from clinical trials, resulting in a paucity of data relevant to this age group. Similarly, behavioural and social research has focused largely on younger adults, leading to a void in understanding the complex psychosocial needs of older adults with cancer [p.435].

A review of future trends and challenges for cancer services in England by the King's Fund pointed out that more than 220 000 people are diagnosed with cancer each year and that cancer causes over 128 000 deaths annually.[10] Cancer incidence increased by nearly one-third between 1971 and 2000, and is still increasing by 1.4% a year, due in part to an ageing population – more than 50% of cancers are diagnosed in people aged 70 years or over (rising to 75% in those aged 60 years or over), compared with 0.5% in children aged 14 years and under.[10] Ageing of the population is considered to be a major determinant of the future cancer burden.[11] The King's Fund review estimates that in the UK the proportion of people aged over 65 years will increase from 16% in 2004 to 23% by 2031, with clear consequences for health services:[10]

> If we assume that the risk of an individual getting cancer remains the same, there will be a substantial increase in demand for services as a result of the impact of demography alone [p.20].

In the European Union as a whole, it is estimated that there will be around 1.25 million cancer deaths in 2015. This, however, is some 155 000 less than the number projected for 2015 on the basis of demographic changes alone,[12] and it has been calculated that cancer mortality in older people is no longer rising systematically, and has in fact been declining in men since the 1980s.[13]

Treatment issues

It is not surprising given these statistics that cancer has been described as 'largely a disease of older persons',[14] and age as 'the greatest risk factor for developing cancer'.[15] There is a clear case to be made for cancer in older people to be treated as a priority both by policy makers and by health care professionals. Yet questions persist about how evenly the attention of policy makers, health care professionals, and researchers is divided between the age groups.

The question of whether the nature of malignant tumours changes with age is a vexed one, and the overall picture is mixed:[16]

> Some physicians believe that older people are more likely to have slow-growing cancers than the middle aged or young. Other physicians believe just the opposite . . . It seems that those who believe that slow-growing tumours are associated with old age are

correct as are those who believe that rapidly growing tumours are associated with old age. Both are correct, and site and stage are two important determinants . . . groups of old tumours are just as diverse as groups of old people [p.34].

Stage at diagnosis may increase with age, especially in cancer of the breast, cervix, ovary, and bladder, and melanoma. The inverse relationship between increasing age and stage at diagnosis in lung cancer and gastrointestinal cancer may be explained by incomplete staging: Hahn *et al.* point out that the extensive procedures necessary for staging these diseases may not be undertaken consistently in the elderly.[17]

The tendency for older people to have more advanced disease at diagnosis, the increased likelihood that they will be found to have metastatic disease,[18] and the implications that this may have for the effectiveness of any treatment that may be offered, have been cited as evidence for the need to prioritise early detection and screening in the elderly.[19] Faithfull points out that:[20]

The late presentation and diagnosis of cancers in the older person are frequently cited when considering the possible reasons for the increased mortality of older individuals with cancer. Cancers identified at an early stage are often limited in size and are less likely to have spread to other areas of the body. The advanced stage of disease at initial diagnosis in elderly people decreases the likelihood that optimal treatment will be used and . . . reduces opportunities for cure [p.62].

McCaffrey Boyle and Engelking suggest that older people may not seek advice promptly because of their great fear of cancer, and because they may believe that treatment is as bad or worse than the disease and that death is inevitable.[19] They argue that health care professionals may have a negative attitude towards cancer treatment in the elderly, and that the focus of health services is on sickness, not prevention and early detection. Faithfull concludes that because perceptions of health and illness are such an important influence on people's willingness to come forward for screening or early diagnosis, health services must be prepared to work for a different attitude to cancer in society in order to increase the effectiveness of their early-detection practices.[20]

One strongly stated point of view is that cancer in the elderly is 'surprisingly poorly treated' and the behaviour of cancer in older patients 'often poorly understood'.[21] This is, it is suggested, due to a lack of equity in the way that older people with cancer are approached:[21]

In current practice the elderly, disenfranchised as they are from entry into clinical trials, receive either untested treatments, inadequate treatment, or even none at all, at the whim of their clinician [p.1020].

There is, it is claimed:

. . . a myth that women over 70 will not live long because they are too frail . . . There is a deeply entrenched age bias. We still make decisions on age alone. The first thing a doctor asks a patient is how old they are.[22]

The European School of Oncology's report on cancer treatment in the elderly emphatically states that chronological age is not a reliable indicator of frailty and therefore cannot be used for selecting cancer treatment.[23] Instead, we should ask 'Which patients would benefit from which treatments?'.[24]

For some time now, researchers have been investigating the role of chronological age in treatment for cancer. In 1983 Begg and Carbone analysed 19 studies of chemotherapy for advanced cancer (lung, colon and rectum, stomach, sarcoma, head and neck, melanoma, and ovary) to compare elderly patients (aged 70 years and over) with other patients in terms of toxicity, response rate, and survival.[25] They suggest that, overall, toxic reactions in the elderly are similar to those in the non-elderly, although differences were observed in haematological reactions with some cancers. They concluded that response rates and survival curves were also similar in both groups. It has been suggested elsewhere that the importance of these findings for clinical practice is limited by the fact that the older patients involved may be generally healthier than elderly patients at large.[26]

Begg and Carbone point out that older patients in their study were comparable with the younger ones in terms of performance status and other measures.[25] They did find that with methotrexate and methyl-CCNU the older group of patients experienced significantly more haematological toxicity, but point out that as methotrexate is excreted by the kidneys and renal function in older people is known to be less effective, this finding is unsurprising. Their view overall is that elderly patients should be approached in the same way as younger ones in terms of clinical trials and chemotherapy, unless they have unusual medical problems. Exceptions to this principle include treatment with chemotherapeutic agents that are known to produce greater toxic effects in older patients, and cancers that are known to affect older people differently. Older patients with leukaemia, for example, appear to be more likely to die if they experience sepsis during remission-induction therapy.[27] They also point out that the physiological changes occurring with age may affect the metabolism or excretion of a drug following administration.

In 1989 Walsh *et al.* reviewed the literature in which older patients treated with chemotherapy are compared with younger ones.[27] They point out that some studies have shown that the elderly are less likely than younger patients to receive effective treatment, and that in particular there are indications that the elderly are less likely to receive chemotherapy as part of a course of treatment, even if differences in disease stage and co-morbidity are taken into account. They add, however, that their own work suggests that older patients are at a significantly higher risk of haematological side-effects with actinomycin-D, doxorubicin, methotrexate, methyl-CCNU, vinblastine, and etoposide. They conclude that 'a number of drugs have been implicated in causing more frequent episodes of toxicity in older patients' and that there is a 'well documented difference in response rates between younger and older leukaemia patients':

> However, these appear to be the exceptions. In general, chronological age is only a weak predictor of the likelihood of toxicity or non-response among chemotherapy recipients. Furthermore, what little predictive capacity chronological age does possess is attributable not to the impact of increased age alone, but to the effects of other patient characteristics that often, but not always, accompany longevity [p.73].

A recent study of lung cancer care in the UK pointed out that in this disease age at diagnosis is increasing and that reports of under-treatment of older patients are therefore a matter for concern.[28] In this study, older patients with lung cancer were less likely to receive active treatment 'of any sort':

> As would be expected, patients with good performance scores were much more likely to receive active therapy. However, a much lower level of chemotherapy use in older patients with confirmed SCLC [small-cell lung cancer] was observed in the subgroup with good performance scores and no chronic obstructive pulmonary disease (COPD). Similarly, the age related reduction in the surgical resection rate was observed even in those patients with good performance status, no significant COPD and graded as 'potentially operable' [p.174].

The researchers conclude that given the strength of evidence that factors other than age are more important in determining prognosis in lung cancer (e.g. performance status, stage, and some biochemical markers), 'patients should not be denied optimal treatment on the basis of chronological age alone' (p.175). They argue that research is available to show that:

- survival after surgery is independent of age: despite this, older people are less likely to receive surgery (e.g. for non-small-cell lung cancer)
- radiotherapy has been found to be effective and well tolerated in people aged over 80 years
- response rates in older patients receiving chemotherapy are comparable to those of younger patients.

Newcombe and Carbone interviewed 628 women recently diagnosed with breast or colorectal cancer.[29] Their analysis compared women aged less than 65 years with women aged 65 and over. Their findings include:

- no apparent difference in the percentage of women with breast cancer receiving surgery as primary therapy
- women aged 65 years and over received radiotherapy and adjuvant chemotherapy for breast cancer less often than the younger age group
- similar proportions of women in both age groups received surgery and radiotherapy for colorectal cancer

- chemotherapy for colorectal cancer was less common in the older age group
- older women were less likely to be referred to an oncologist.

Mor et al.,[18] who analysed data from a sample of over 1000 patients with breast, lung and colorectal cancer, argue that:

> . . . age-related differences in the receipt of post-diagnostic treatment suggest a deep and pervasive social 'ageism' influencing who receives aggressive treatment [p.387].

From the other side of the argument, however, it has been suggested that age-related differences in the treatment of breast cancer could be due not to age bias, but to differences in what constitutes the most appropriate therapy at a given age. Supporters of this view argue, for example, that there is little evidence that chemotherapy actually benefits older women with breast cancer,[30] so we should not be surprised if fewer older women receive this treatment. Conversely, if a treatment is known to benefit patients across the age groups, we would expect it to be provided equally if no age bias exists.

Guadagnoli et al. tested a number of hypotheses of this kind in a study of the treatment of early-stage breast cancer in nearly 750 newly diagnosed post-menopausal women, and concluded that use of adjuvant systemic therapy reflects our knowledge of treatment efficacy.[30] In women with node-negative disease, for example, no association between age and the use of hormonal therapy (tamoxifen) was found, but there was a negative association between age and likelihood of receiving chemotherapy. They add, however, that:

> . . . although the state of the art suggests that older patients are less likely than younger patients to benefit from chemotherapy, we may not yet have used the best designs to test the efficacy of this therapy in older patients [p.2342].

In recent work Rai and Stotter have argued that most women with breast cancer are likely to benefit from local treatment (i.e. radiotherapy/ surgery) in addition to systemic treatment, as they are 'fit enough to survive the local treatment and will live long enough to benefit' (p.863).[31] They point out that while elderly women with breast cancer are more likely to have significant medical problems, and the very elderly have a shorter life expectancy if judged on age alone, it is in reality very difficult to assess 'biological' (as opposed to chronological) age or life expectancy accurately. For historical reasons, they claim, there is an arbitrary 'cut-off point' of 70 years, after which women with breast cancer are considered for 'tamoxifen-only' (i.e. no surgery) treatment, but women can now be expected to live considerably longer after 70 years than they might have been in the past. Data from their own research show that there is a rapid rise in numbers of women with breast cancer who do not receive early surgery after the age of 70 years, and they suggest that this may be influenced by the availability of an alternative non-surgical treatment (tamoxifen), that the risks of surgery and anaesthesia may have been over-estimated (although older people do cope less well with complications), and that the life expectancy of elderly women may have been under-estimated. They conclude that:

> Age may have been used too rigidly to decide local treatment for elderly patients with breast cancer. Comprehensive multidisciplinary assessment is needed to make informed decisions and to optimize management of elderly patients. Breast cancer therapy should be defined by a woman's physiological age rather than chronological age. Increasing patient fitness with age requires more facilities for treatment of the older patient [p.865].

Care issues

While there are arguments for and against the presence of an age bias or 'ageism' in the treatment of older people with cancer, there is little doubt that the elderly are the focus of prejudice in our society. The negative view of ageing, it is suggested,[32] springs from the view that growing old involves a series of decrements or losses, so that ageing becomes a process of decay that affects us emotionally, intellectually, and socially.[32] Gross suggests that older people experience discrimination socially, in the family, and in employment because they are treated as dull, sickly, and inflexible.[32] In a culture that idealises youth, older adults tend to be viewed uniformly as deteriorating physically and mentally, as being socially isolated, and as being decreasingly productive members of society.[8] In response, perhaps, to the historical position of older people in society, Standard One of the Department of Health's *National Service Framework for Older People* now recognises the importance of 'rooting out' age discrimination, and stipulates that:

> NHS services will be provided, regardless of age, on the basis of clinical need alone. Social care services will not use age in their eligibility criteria or policies, to restrict access to available services.[33]

It would be comforting to believe that we have eliminated age bias or ageism in our care of older people, but unfortunately it probably still exists. Sharp argues that elderly patients, particularly those with mental health problems, do not match our idea of the 'ideal' patient: the traditional sick role involves being motivated to get better and co-operating with medical and nursing staff, and patients who do not meet our expectations in this respect are more likely to be disliked, and perhaps represent a threat to our sense of professional authority and therapeutic competence.[34]

In 1991 Reed and Bond wrote that:[35]

> ... the nursing care of long-stay elderly patients in hospital remains a routinised work system within a cure-dominated health care ethos. When cure is not possible it is patients who have 'failed the system'; it is they who are 'hopeless' cases and who 'block beds' [p.56].

Nursing, they imply, is partly responsible for perpetuating this system because instead of becoming 'dynamic and self-governing', it still takes its lead from the dominant medical ethos, is dominated by the idea of 'getting through the work', and treats patients as 'work objects'.

In their study of nurses' assessments of elderly patients in hospital, Reed and Bond observed nursing activities in a long-term care ward.[35] They comment that assessments:

> ... did not result in proposals for change in the way the patient was nursed. Changes proposed concerned how the existing routine of care could be implemented more effectively [p.58].

They refer to incidents in nurses' careers in which they are discouraged from 'wasting' themselves caring for older people, by colleagues and others who regard work in this area as low-status and unstimulating. They conclude that it is 'futile' to introduce practices like the nursing process which 'are at odds with nurses' value systems and levels of functioning':

> ... such activities become routinised into another administrative task to be completed ... It reinforces the inappropriateness of the medical model of care, emphasising cure or rehabilitation, for continuing care and chronically ill patients [p.63].

In 2000, Courtney *et al.* reviewed the research literature on attitudes of acute-care nurses towards older people.[36] They found that nurses 'generally hold slightly to moderately positive attitudes towards older people' (p.63), but that there are also many negative attitudes:

> Nurses felt ill at ease in the presence of older people and found them cantankerous and complaining, set in their ways and incapable of adjusting to new situations [p.66].

This may be due to 'emotional rejection' and 'stereotyping', which have:

> ... significant repercussions on the quality of care older patients may receive in the acute-care setting, particularly from nurses who do not prefer to work with patients 65 years and older [p.66].

The authors conclude that in the acute setting:

> ... older patients experience reduced independence, limited decision-making opportunities, increased probability of developing complications, little consideration of their ageing-related needs, limited health education and social isolation [p.62].

Latimer argues that 'older people' as a category is both absurd *and* inescapable: all of us, she says, are part of the process of creating this distinction, in part because of our fear of ageing, which we see as a series of physical losses rather than spiritual gains.[37] She uses an example from her research to illustrate how we may use the idea that ill-health in old age is biologically inevitable to ease our sense of responsibility for someone: in the light of biological inevitability we see not 'an acutely ill person' but 'an old person' 'whose illness is outside the domain of the medical ward' (p.144).

Latimer tells us that Jessie, who is 91 and has had a massive stroke, is 'refigured' by the ward sister:

Jessie is . . . put 'outside' one division, a class of patient (the person who is acutely ill), and into another class (that of old person whose difficulties are chronic and the consequence of a natural order of things, a progressive deterioration and decline) . . . there is no possibility of a heroic story of recovery . . . Jessie is a 'blocked bed' [p.144].

Koch and Webb interviewed 14 patients in their study of nursing care of the elderly in a large NHS hospital.[38] They identified two common themes in their accounts: 'routine geriatric style' and 'segregation'. Routine geriatric style, a term first coined in the 1970s,[39] is used by Koch and Webb to describe the conveyor belt approach to care that they see in the accounts they collected from patients. Patients, they say, were deprived of care, 'left unwashed, unsafe, and unfed', and felt that they could not draw attention to these issues for fear of making the situation worse:

. . . needs became reduced to nursing practices based on hygiene, pressure area care, medications and food, but even these needs were scarcely met [p.955].

People, write Koch and Webb, were treated as objects. One patient with metastatic cancer is quoted as saying:

I am sitting out of bed but I don't want to be here. They just sit everyone out of bed. I have to sit here until they put me back and I don't know when . . . I just sit here until they put me back to bed. I insisted to be put back yesterday, I was so ill. I was told off, they said 'don't dictate to me!'. I said I want to be put to bed, I feel very, very ill. Then sister came [p.955].

Koch and Webb also feel that patients resented being stereotyped as old (by having the letter 'G' for 'geriatric' on their case notes, for example). 'Old', they say, represented a state of decline and infirmity; patients rejected the idea of incapacity

or senility that 'old' evoked. There was unhappiness about being segregated into age-defined groups which, Koch says, reinforces the standardisation and depersonalisation of care. In fact, she argues, segregation and routine geriatric style go together, one reinforcing the other.

Koch and Webb believe that an important reason for the development of a distinctive way of caring for old people is the tendency (that they trace back to the French philosopher Descartes) to view individuals as a combination of mind-in-body, the mind contained within but distinct from the machine-like body:

. . . the machine or body can be entered, studied, and tampered with in order to be repaired. The body is the object of inquiry. The patient as subject fades into the background and becomes a biomedical object susceptible to medical intervention [p.957].

The machine-like body is seen as wearing out over time: Koch and Webb's implication seems to be that our age bias or ageism is connected to this, the idea that the older you are the more likely you are to be broken down, no longer productive, and therefore inconsequential. They recommend that geriatric medicine, with its focus on the health of the older person, and gerontology, with its focus on the nature of ageing, should be brought closer together to help to dispel stereotypical and ageist notions. Nurses, they say, should examine ageing, dispel its negative images, and 'promote the individual's health status rather than chronological age' (p.958).[38]

Harper believes that only acceptance of the mental and physical changes associated with later life as a 'normal and respectable component of the human condition' will enable us to resolve 'the current tension between spirit and body'.[40] As a feminist, she argues that the stigma attached to loss of control over the body is related to the dominance of male notions and expectations of control. In adulthood, she says, women are not accustomed to direct control of bodily functions such as menstruation, lactation, and childbirth. 'It can thus be argued', she says:

. . . that if absolute control of the body, defined by male experience, was not the overarching notion of adulthood, then the natural lack of control associated with extreme late life would not be so stigmatised [p.166].

Feminism, she concludes, may help us to develop a new concept of later life:

> . . . which fully accepts loss of bodily control, rejects the stigmatisation of the declining body . . . thus allowing the frailty of extreme later life to be fully integrated into mainstream social experience [p.170].

In the same way that chronological age *per se* is a poor basis for decisions about treatment, the assumption that there is a simple relationship between increasing age and frailty is a poor starting point for planning nursing care. Wenger believes that we expect a high level of dependency in people aged 80 years and over and that those who survive into their 80s are seen as a problem.[41] While acknowledging that there are more people in their 80s who are ill and impaired, she argues that only a small proportion are acutely dependent at any one time, and that most of the over-80s are relatively independent.

As areas for specialisation, the care and treatment of older people with cancer and the relationship between cancer and ageing are still in their infancy. A settled position has yet to be achieved on the criteria for medical decisions which:

> involve a delicate balance between limited life expectancy, risk of treatment complications, and the overall effects of cancer and cancer treatment on the patient's quality of life [p.33].[42]

At the same time, we must recognise that our perceptions of ageing may lead us to act as if those we categorise as old are less-legitimate recipients of a full range of health care resources simply because of their chronological age. As the Oncology Nursing Society and Geriatric Oncology Consortium position statement on cancer care in the older adult puts it:[9]

> Recognition of distinctions among chronologic age and biologic and functional age along with unique features of ageing in our society such as experience of comorbid illness, achievement of age appropriate social roles and thinning social support can foster a new paradigm for research and practice. Clinicians, researchers, educators, legislators and policy makers

must address themselves to this societal challenge and seek a new perspective on ageing and cancer, improved resources for research and education, more sophisticated investigation, targeted professional and public education and redesigned systems of care [p.435].

References

1. Bailey C., Corner J., Addington-Hall J., Kumar D., Nelson M. and Haviland J. (2003). Treatment decisions in older patients with colorectal cancer: the role of age and multidimensional function. *European Journal of Cancer Care* 12, 257–262.
2. Bailey C., Corner J., Addington-Hall J., Kumar D., Nelson M. and Haviland J. (2004). Older patients' experiences of treatment for colorectal cancer: an analysis of functional status and service use. *European Journal of Cancer Care* 13, 483–493.
3. Bailey C. (2001). Older patients' experiences of pre-treatment discussions: An analysis of qualitative data from a study of colorectal cancer. *Journal of Research in Nursing* 6, 736–746.
4. Schrag D., Cramer L.D., Bach P.B. and Begg C.B. (2001). Age and adjuvant chemotherapy use after surgery for stage III colon cancer. *Journal of the National Cancer Institute* 93, 850–857.
5. de Rijke J., Schouten L., Schouten H., Jager J., Koppejan A. and van den Brandt P. (1996). Age-specific differences in the diagnostics and treatment of cancer patients aged 50 years and older in the province of Limburg, The Netherlands. *Annals of Oncology* 7, 677–685.
6. Victor C.R. (2005). *The Social Context of Ageing: A Textbook of Gerontology.* London: Routledge.
7. Victor C.R., Scambler S.J., Marston L., Bond J. and Bowling A. (2006). Older people's experience of loneliness in the UK: does gender matter. *Social Policy and Society* 5, 27–38.
8. McCaffrey Boyle D., Engelking C., Blesch K.S., Dodge J., Sarna L. and Weinrich S. (1992). Oncology Nursing Society position paper on cancer and ageing: the mandate for oncology nursing. *Oncology Nursing Forum* 19, 913–933.
9. Oncology Nursing Society and Geriatric Oncology Consortium (2004). Joint position on cancer care in the older adult. *European Journal of Cancer Care* 13, 434–435.
10. Rosen R., Smith A. and Harrison A. (2006). *Future Trends and Challenges for Cancer Services in England: A Review of Literature and Policy.* London: King's Fund.
11. Edwards B.K., Howe H.L., Ries L.A. *et al.* (2002). Annual report to the nation on the status of cancer, 1973–1999, featuring implications of age and aging on U.S. cancer burden. *Cancer* 94, 2766–2792.

12. Quinn M.J., d'Onofrio A., Møller B. *et al.* (2003). Cancer mortality trends in the EU and acceding countries up to 2015. *Annals of Oncology* **14**, 971.

13. Levi F., Lucchini E., Negri E., Boyle P. and La Vecchia C. (2001) Changed trends in cancer mortality in the elderly. *Annals of Oncology* **12**, 1467–1477.

14. Dodd G.D. (1991). Cancer control and the older person. *Cancer* **68**, 2493–2495.

15. European School of Oncology Scientific Updates (1997). In Redmond K. and Aapro M.S. (eds.) *Cancer in the Elderly.* Amsterdam: Elsevier.

16. Holmes F.F. (1989). Clinical evidence for a change in tumour aggressiveness with age. *Seminars in Oncology* **16**, 34–40.

17. Hahn D.E.E., Bergman L., van Dam F.S.A.M. and Aaronson N.K. (1994). In Fentiman I.S. and Monfardini S. (eds.) *Cancer in the Elderly.* Oxford: Oxford University Press.

18. Mor V., Masterson-Allen S., Goldberg R.J. *et al.* (1985). Relationship between age at diagnosis and treatments received by cancer patients. *Journal of the American Geriatric Society* **33**, 585–589.

19. McCaffrey Boyle D. and Engelking C. (1993). Cancer in the elderly: the forgotten priority. *European Journal of Cancer Care* **2**, 101–107.

20. Faithfull S. (1994). Negative perceptions. *Nursing Times* **90**, 62–64.

21. Fentiman I., Tirelli U., Monfardini S. *et al.* (1990). Cancer in the elderly: why so badly treated? *Lancet* **335**, 1020–1022.

22. Elderly 'denied cancer surgery'. http://news.bbc.co.uk/1/hi/health/3223333.stm (accessed 13 August 2007).

23. Monfardini S., Aapro M., Ferrucci V., Scalliet P. and Fentiman I. (1993). Commission of the European Communities 'Europe Against Cancer' Programme European School of Oncology Advisory Report: Cancer Treatment in the Elderly. *European Journal of Cancer* **29A**, 2325–2330.

24. Yancik R. and Ries M.S. (1994). Cancer in older persons. *Cancer* **74**, 1995–2003.

25. Begg C.B. and Carbone P.P. (1983). Clinical trials and drug toxicity in the elderly: the experience of the Eastern Cooperative Oncology Group. *Cancer* **52**, 1986–1992.

26. Blesch K.S. (1988). The normal physiological changes of ageing and their impact on the response to cancer treatment. *Seminars in Oncology Nursing* **4**, 178–188.

27. Walsh S.J., Begg C.B. and Carbone P.P. (1989). Cancer chemotherapy in the elderly. *Seminars in Oncology* **16**, 66–75.

28. Peake D., Thompson S., Lowe D. and Pearson M.G. (2003). Ageism in the management of lung cancer. *Age and Ageing* **32**, 171–177.

29. Newcombe P.A. and Carbone P.P. (1993). Cancer treatment and age: patient perspectives. *Journal of the National Cancer Institute* **85**, 1580–1584.

30. Guadagnoli E., Shapiro C., Gurwitz J.H. *et al.* (1997). Age-related patterns of care: evidence against ageism in the treatment of early-stage breast cancer. *Journal of Clinical Oncology* **15**, 2338–2344.

31. Rai S. and Stotter A. (2005) Management of elderly patients with breast cancer: the time for surgery. *ANZ Journal of Surgery* **75**, 863–865.

32. Gross R.D. (1992). *Psychology: The Science of Mind and Behaviour.* London: Hodder and Stoughton.

33. National Service Framework for Older People. Standard One – Rooting Out Age Discrimination. www.dh.gov.uk/en/Policyandguidance/Healthandsocialcaretopics/Olderpeoplesservices/DH_4071271 (accessed 13 August 2007).

34. Sharp T. (1990). Old and in the way. *Nursing Standard* **14**, 54–55.

35. Reed J. and Bond S. (1991). Nurses' assessment of elderly patients in hospital. *International Journal of Nursing Studies* **28**, 55–64.

36. Courtney M., Tong S. and Walsh A. (2000). Acute-care nurses' attitudes towards older people: a literature review. *International Journal of Nursing Practice* **6**, 62–69.

37. Latimer J. (1997). Figuring identities: older people, medicine and time. In Jamieson A., Harper S. and Victor C. (eds.) *Critical Approaches to Ageing and Later Life.* Milton Keynes: Open University Press.

38. Koch T. and Webb C. (1996). The biomedical construction of ageing: implications for nursing care of older people. *Journal of Advanced Nursing* **23**, 954–959.

39. Baker D. (1983). 'Care' in the geriatric ward: an account of two styles of nursing. In Wilson-Barrett J. (ed.) *Nursing Research: Ten Studies in Patient Care.* Chichester: Wiley.

40. Harper S. (1997). Constructing later life/constructing the body: some thoughts from feminist theory. In Jamieson A., Harper S. and Victor C. (eds.) *Critical Approaches to Ageing and Later Life.* Milton Keynes: Open University Press.

41. Wenger G.C. (1986). What do dependency measures measure? Challenging assumptions. In Phillipson C., Bernard M. and Strang P. (eds.) *Dependency and Interdependency in Old Age: Theoretical Perspectives and Policy Alternatives.* London: Croom Helm.

42. Bennahum D.A., Forman W.B., Vellas B. and Albarede J.L. (1997). Life expectancy, comorbidity, and quality of life: a framework of reference for medical decisions. *Clinics in Geriatric Medicine* **13**, 33–53.

CHAPTER THIRTY-TWO

Ethnicity, difference, and care

Yasmin Gunaratnam

Introduction

The number of cancer deaths in the ethnic minority population will increase, both as a result of deprivation/social status and because ethnic minorities present to the health services with an already untreatable advanced disease . . . Do we meet the needs of patients from ethnic minority groups or do we provide culturally insensitive care? Is health care provision a friendly service for ethnic minorities or not? Is it the culture we should be concerned with or inequality and discrimination arising from social differences?[1]

The NHS and Department of Health must give even greater prominence to race equality as part of our drive to improve health. We must: . . . pay greater attention to meeting the service needs of people from ethnic minorities. This will help us to meet the standards both for improved services and health outcomes in the long term and to hit our short term targets.[2]

When people affected by cancer are unable to communicate effectively with their healthcare team, difficulties often arise in identifying symptoms and understanding advice or guidance. This is the case across all ethnic groups. However, language barriers and cultural misunderstanding often prevent well-intentioned healthcare staff and managers from communicating information in a culturally sensitive way, which will further exacerbate any existing difficulties.[3]

Inside every patient there is a poet trying to get out.[4]

The quotations above provide some indication of the ambivalent tensions and different facets of

thinking that frame this discussion on ethnicity, cancer, and nursing care. First, there is the epidemiological evidence of an increase in cancer and of disparities in health status amongst 'minority ethnic' groups and the connections between these and equity in service provision. Second, at the level of care, language 'barriers' and cultural insensitivity are key concerns. And third, in the autobiographical writing of Anatole Broyard, who had prostate cancer: 'Inside every patient there is a poet trying to get out',[4] we can hear something of the aesthetics of the communicative struggle for recognition in the patient experience. Rather than suppressing or glossing over these tensions, I want to use them to look at how we might develop more complex and ethical approaches in responding to the needs of patients from a diversity of backgrounds.

Challenges and contexts

The challenges for such approaches are considerable, not only in relation to meeting patients' needs, but also in addressing the varying levels and contexts in which nurses work. There are times, such as when we are interpreting epidemiological or ethnic monitoring data, when it is difficult to avoid using broad and sweeping ethnic categorisations. The third of the national surveys of NHS patients uses the broad categories of 'Black', 'South Asian' and 'White'.[5] Nevertheless, the finding that amongst cancer patients, 32% of South Asian patients did not completely understand their diagnosis, compared to 25% of black patients and 19% of all patients can be a valuable starting point in exploring differential experiences of care within services. What is important when we work with such categorisations of ethnicity is that we are aware of what is gained and what is lost in the process of categorisation, abstraction and generalisation.

In the everyday, face-to-face interactions of nursing, the meanings of categorisations such as 'Bengali grandmother', 'Bosnian teenager' or 'Mixed-race child' need more radical questioning. At times, knowledge about the cultural and religious beliefs of particular groups can be useful in examining and contextualising patient need and experience. Yet, when the meanings of differences in patient choice or behaviour are interpreted primarily in relation to cultural difference – what Pearson has termed 'culturalist' interpretations[6] – the holistic exploration of need, in all of its complexity, can be restricted and we can lose sight of the full human experience of cancer.

There are several different ways of thinking about holistic care in nursing; for me, the quotation from Anatole Broyard comes closest to capturing what I have come to appreciate as the artistry of meaningful holistic care in practice. In my interpretation, what Broyard is talking about when he says 'Inside every patient there is a poet trying to get out' is something of the delicate, chaotic, mysterious and unpredictable dimensions of lived experiences of identity and illness.[4] These are the dimensions that are not easily recognised or captured by large-scale survey research, by technical and bureaucratic approaches to equity, such as target setting, or by many 'cultural awareness' approaches to nurse education and training. What I take from Broyard is that in order to provide holistic care, health care professionals have to learn to read and respond to the 'poetry' inside every patient – and within themselves. They must learn to engage with the complicated, hidden, and often non-rational ways in which a person's body, unique life experiences, emotions and social positioning are a part of their experiences of illness and of care giving.

Drawing upon existing research sources, my own qualitative research conducted in a hospice,[7] and an ongoing project for The Policy Research Institute on Ageing and Ethnicity (PRIAE), this chapter will use a psychosocial approach to the relationships between ethnicity, cancer and nursing care. The first sections of the chapter are scene-setting sections, outlining in brief the concepts of 'race', ethnicity, and culture, and providing an overview of the epidemiological data on ethnicity and cancer. The subsequent sections move on to address the conceptual, practical, and ethical challenges and threats to providing holistic care that is responsive to difference.

'Race', ethnicity, and culture

It is not possible to discuss the needs of 'minority ethnic' cancer patients without examining what we mean by the interrelated terms 'race', 'ethnicity', and 'culture'. This is far from an academic exercise. Ideas and knowledge about 'race', ethnicity, and culture have played a pivotal part in systems of socio-economic power and exploitation.[8] At the level of cancer nursing, how we think about, and what we count as being 'ethnic' or 'cultural', has consequence for all of our interactions and care practices. It can have effects upon judgements about how we perceive someone is handling a diagnosis of cancer; whether we comply with or challenge a family's requests to withhold information about a diagnosis from a patient; how we negotiate bodies, touch and space in everyday, hands-on, nursing care;[9] and the skills and knowledge that we think we need in order to provide 'culturally competent' care.

In broad terms, 'race', ethnicity, and culture are now recognised as being entangled social and political constructs, rather than categories that reflect reliable and stable scientific 'facts'.[8,10] Nevertheless, distinctions have been drawn:

• 'race' has been theorised as a concept that has a political history in being used to categorise and to pass off social and cultural differences as biological and genetic difference. However, genetic evidence does not support the existence of distinct 'race's. There is more genetic variation at the individual, rather than the group level.[11] Many writers therefore use the term 'race' in inverted commas to mark their unease with using a concept that has no reality as a fact, but which still influences thinking about the nature of differences such as skin colour or emotionality

- ethnicity is used most commonly to refer to shared, cultural, religious and /or geographical origins[8]
- culture, has been seen as more fluid, a shared 'way of life', or as 'comprised of shared rules, values, beliefs and meanings that act as guidelines for decisions about a population's lifestyle activities'.[12]

Epidemiological research on cancer centres upon the concepts of ethnicity and culture, as do many of the discussions about intercultural nursing care. However, there are conceptual, technical, and political difficulties in operationalising the concepts in research, and in working with them in practice. Most significantly, ideas about 'race', although outdated, continue to inflect and infect ideas about ethnicity and culture (for an example, see Research study 32.1).

I will address some of the difficulties of working with the concepts in the next sections where I examine research on ethnicity and cancer and discuss my own conceptual framework.

Ethnicity and cancer

It has been acknowledged by several researchers that knowledge about ethnicity and cancer in the UK is currently unreliable. Data on risk factors for cancers, cancer incidence and mortality have been compromised by the poor recording of ethnicity in cancer registration datasets,[14] and the use of 'country of birth' as a proxy for ethnicity in death registration records, where ethnicity *per se*, is not recorded.

In a meta-analysis of research on ethnicity, health and health care conducted for the Department of Health, Aspinall and Jacobson highlight four main limitations of current research on ethnicity and cancer:[13]

- the poor recording of information on ethnic group in cancer registration data
- the lack of recording of ethnicity in death registration records and the use of 'country of

Research study 32.1

Aspinall P. and Jacobson B. (2004). *Ethnic Disparities in Health and Health Care: A Focused Review of the Evidence and Selected Examples of Good Practice*. London: London Health Observatory.[13]

This meta-analysis of research on ethnicity and cancer has found that:

- 'Few studies are available of cancer incidence by ethnic group. There is evidence that South Asian incidence rates (for all sites combined) are significantly lower than for non-South Asians.
- However, rates for childhood and early adult cancer were similar or higher than non-South Asian rates.'
- 'South Asian rates were significantly higher than non-South Asian rates for Hodgkin's disease in males, cancer of the tongue, mouth, oesophagus, thyroid gland, and myeloid leukaemia in females, and cancer of the hypopharynx, liver and gall bladder in both sexes.'
- 'Other studies report a low incidence of colorectal cancer amongst South Asians but significantly higher rates of oral cancer amongst South Asians and nasopharyngeal cancer amongst the Chinese.'
- 'Mortality ratios for lung cancer are elevated for men and women born in Scotland and Ireland but low in both genders in other migrant groups; generally low mortality ratios for breast cancer found in all the migrant groups.'
- 'While no studies of variations in prostate cancer rates between ethnic groups have been conducted in the UK, there is some indicative evidence relating to mortality and considerable evidence from other countries that suggest that rates are substantially higher in the black groups . . . There have been no comprehensive studies of equity of access to cancer services for minority ethnic groups, but the third of the national surveys of NHS patients suggests many areas of disadvantage.'

birth' has meant that much of the knowledge that has been gained about mortality is based upon the experience of migrants to the UK

- findings on cancer incidence rates and ethnicity are largely based on particular ethnic groups (notably those categorised as 'South-Asian') and localised research
- the reporting of cancer frequency/burdens and the broad categories of ethnicity that have been used 'frequently conceal variations in risk between distinct ethnic sub-groups'.

Despite these limitations, broad patterns of cancer incidence in different ethnic groups have been identified (see Commentary 32.1). In comparison to the 'native' populations of England and Wales, cancer incidence for Scottish, Irish, 'West Indian', and 'South Asian' migrants in England and Wales is lower, as is cancer mortality, calculated through Standardised Mortality Ratios (SMRs).[15] However, mortality ratios for lung cancer are higher for male, Irish and Scottish migrants, and are also relatively high for migrant women from Scotland and Ireland.[16] While the incidence of cancer is relatively low in groups categorised as being 'minority ethnic' (independent of age), researchers have predicted that there will be an increase in cancer within these groups as the different populations age.

In a summary of the data, Gill *et al.* (quoted in Aspinall and Jacobson[13]) state:

> Overall, cancers tend to be less common in ethnic minority groups than in the 'white' comparison population (but a dominant problem, nonetheless). Some cancers are strikingly less common, e.g. lung cancer – relating to lower smoking prevalence. For some cancers, the SMRs are strikingly different from the population as a whole. Oropharyngeal cancers are commonest in South Asian groups and prostate cancer in African groups.[17]

In making sense of the findings of the research on ethnicity and cancer, two main considerations – relating to ethnic categorisation and the complexity of experience – need to be borne in mind, particularly with regard to the poetry of lived experience.

Broad categories

While all research on ethnicity has to rely on some form of categorisation of ethnic identity, it is vital to recognise that the categories used in research are both flawed and objectifying.[10] They do not tell us about the meanings and effects of ethnicity in individual lives and they do not reflect within group differences such as differences of gender, age, religion, and socio-economic status, all of which can affect the incidence and the experience of cancer. As Firth has commented using the category of 'Indian':

Commentary 32.1 The impact of ideas about 'race' in nursing care

It can be difficult to recognise the ways in which what many of us see as outdated ideas about 'race' can affect contemporary nursing care. In my research with health professionals I have found that 'race'-based notions of difference, most often interrelated with culturalist thinking, can still play an active role in intercultural care. The following extract from a group discussion with hospice nurses provides a vivid example of the prevalence of ideas about 'race' in how judgements and interpretations are made about patients. In the extract a hospice team leader 'Tina' (a pseudonym) talks about a Nigerian patient who wanted to go to 'home' (to her country of origin) to die:

> *Tina*: Um, we had a lady . . . I think she was Nigerian . . . and we actually got her home on the plane . . .
>
> *Yasmin*: And what, and what do you think it was, um, about her motivations to go home? What was that about?
>
> *Tina*: Well I suppose that she had some sort of calling to go home. I mean by all appearances she looked sort of very modern, but I think she had some very, sort of traditional values which were quite important to her and maybe she had some sort of homing instinct or something.

In Tina's deliberations about why her patient wanted to go 'home' it is possible to see how 'race' in the notion of the biological drive of a 'homing instinct' overshadows any of the social or emotional dynamics that may have been involved in the patient's decision to return 'home'. In their eclipsing of subjectivity and other social relations, biological notions of 'race' can serve to dehumanise 'minority ethnic' patients and carers and can halt the exploration of the unique meanings of the choices that patients make. We can see this more clearly when we contrast Tina's account with the response of 'Nasreen' a Ugandan hospice patient, who when I asked why she wanted to go to Uganda to die, said simply: 'I'd love to die in my Mum's, or in my Dad's hands'.

Broad categories such as 'Indian' are not helpful, since an Indian can come from any part of the subcontinent, speak a wide range of languages, and be a member of a number of religious faiths and castes [social strata] . . . British South Asians also have very different migration patterns which could affect health and socio-economic status . . .[18]

In addition to the diversity of experience that can be obscured by ethnic categories, what is also apparent from Firth's observations is the existence of multiple and simultaneous identities and forms of social disadvantage. In their meta-analysis of the data on ethnic disparities in health, Aspinall and Jacobson have suggested that differences in health status that have been ascribed to ethnicity, reflect key social conditions, namely poverty and racism, in the lives of 'minority ethnic' populations.[13] They contend that:

In some areas of medical research and practice ethnic disparities in health continue to be attributed to genetic and non-specific 'cultural' explanations. However, the emerging evidence base suggests that socioeconomic factors and the experience of racism may be amongst the most important causes of these disparities.

What is important about this finding from Aspinall and Jacobson is that it suggests that the focus upon ethnicity as a single variable in research can obscure the influence of wider social and material influences on health inequalities. As Smaje[19] has argued:

. . . it is vital to recognise that the neat ethnic categories demanded by research (and typically assumed in everyday life) are partly fictional. Thus, insights derived from . . . research are best used to help formulate further questions about the social contexts within which both ethnicity and health experience are framed.[19]

Ethnicity, lifestyle and cancer

The second, related, consideration in interpreting the research on cancer incidence and ethnicity relates to the dynamic and moving nature of ethnic and cultural identities and their connections to health. Changes in diet, lifestyle, and economic status as a result of migration, settlement, and cultural mixing are known to have an impact upon the incidence of cancer. Several studies have shown that cancer incidence rates amongst migrants are rising to rates similar to that of the 'host' population within one or two generations.[15,20] Yet, despite the identification of these

changes, researchers still find it difficult to make reliable predictions about the relationships between changing cultural practices, lifestyles and cancer. This observation in the National Council for Palliative Care's report *20:20 Vision*[21] points to the influence of wider social and political processes in affecting future variations in the links between ethnicity, lifestyle, and disease incidence:

It should be noted that the extent to which migrants do adopt Western lifestyles or conversely retain their cultural and ethnic identity, may vary. For example, one trend amongst young Muslims is to emphasise and embrace traditional Muslim culture rather than gradually integrate into a Western lifestyle . . .

The relationship between epidemiology, ethnicity, migration, and ageing is already complex. Diversity of cultural attitudes makes that more so.

These complicated relationships can be further affected by the experience of illness itself. In my ethnographic study of a hospice, that involved 33 interviews with 23 migrant hospice service users from a range of African, South Asian and Caribbean backgrounds,[7] I found that the negotiation of cultural practices during illness is highly variable and idiosyncratic.[22] Patient choices about diet and food, for example, were not simply related to cultural and religious identifications, they also involved the negotiation of curiosity, sensual pleasure and evolving embodied experiences of disease and treatment. Some service users combined aspects of their 'traditional' diet with Western food, to take the 'hard work' out of food preparation, when fluctuations in appetite and nausea made eating unpredictable. Others chose English food from the hospice menu because they enjoyed the opportunity to try something different, and yet others made changes to their diet as a part of an awareness of 'healthy eating', often provoked by their illness. The varying nature of these choices has implications for how we interpret the findings of research on ethnicity and cancer incidence in the context of cancer care, and they also suggest that practitioners need to be aware of movements in the salience, vulnerability, and renegotiation of cultural and religious practices by patients throughout the illness trajectory.

A broad understanding of the research evidence on the relationships between ethnicity and cancer is clearly important for nurses in contextualising the current and future dynamics that can influence the experience of cancer and cancer service provision and care. The value of such an understanding lies in recognising both what the data mask and what they reveal. As Sheldon and Parker have argued: 'There is nothing so powerful as a large and available data set for encouraging the suspension of disbelief'.[23]

For the purposes of this discussion, and despite the recognised limitations of the data, it is important to point out that although broad epidemiological trends and ethnic categories can obscure the human experience of cancer, they can sometimes make visible patterns in the social structuring of experience, bringing questions of social context, equity and racism more explicitly to the forefront of cancer service provision and care.

Given the difficulties with using the concepts 'race', ethnicity, and culture, I want to make explicit my own analytic approach and the implications of this for nursing practice.

Working with and against categories of 'race', ethnicity, and culture

As in any field of study, there is a broad spectrum of theoretical approaches to the concepts of 'race', ethnicity, and culture. My approach has been influenced by ideas from post-structuralist, postcolonial and feminist theory.[10] Mulholland and Dyson have suggested that feminist and post-structuralist approaches to the concepts of 'race' and ethnicity have particular relevance to nursing because of their recognition of power relations and a questioning of categories of identity as based upon true and fixed essential differences.[24] That is, 'race', ethnicity and culture are not seen as unchanging 'essences' that define the very being and experiences of different individuals and groups, implying an 'internal sameness and external difference or otherness'.[25]

Such anti-essentialist approaches to 'race' and ethnicity can be valuable for nurses, Mullholland and Dyson argue, because:

> A full appreciation of the discredited nature of biological theories of 'race' . . . would enable nurses to evaluate the role played by ideas of 'race' in the delivery and experience of nursing care, and better address the dynamics of racism.
>
> . . . new approaches emphasize the interactive, complex and fluid nature of ethnic identifications . . . they . . . offer the potential for appreciating an ethnic dimension to patient need and nursing care, but in a manner that incorporates an understanding of the ethnicity of the patients as an identity constantly on the move.[24]

The recognition of identities as being 'on the move' is important in helping nurses to avoid the dangers of stereotyping and/or making assumptions about a patient's needs and experiences based upon their ethnicity or their religious dress, for example. Yet, the recognition that identities are dynamic and moving does not go far enough in addressing the tensions and contradictions of lived experience of ethnicity, culture and religion. For instance, while we might recognise the fluidity of identities at a conceptual level, individuals often talk about and experience themselves in ways that appear to fix their identities and erase the contradictions and tensions that they live with. In other words, while we might favour anti-essentialist approaches to ethnicity at a conceptual level, in real life people can experience or portray their ethnic, cultural, or religious identities in very uncompromising and essentialist terms.

James, a Kenyan patient with AIDS who I interviewed in my hospice research, talked about the particular tribe that he came from as being a 'proud people', telling me that: '. . . the ethnicity has got some proudness. They're a proud people . . . I still carry that pride within . . . you really have pride'. However, when I asked James whether he had any contact with the Kenyan community where he lived, he told me: 'No. No, and I don't want to have anything to do with the Kenyan community . . . with this disease, they tend to actually prey on you . . . they spread out rumours to the rest of the community, which is quite damaging'. In James' account it is possible to hear the painful tensions between being a 'proud Kenyan' and 'living with AIDS'.

Although James's experience relates to AIDS, cancer can also be a disease that carries social, moral, and religious meanings in different socio-economic, generational and cultural groups.[26,27] These meanings can threaten or fracture the belongingness and 'we-ness' of ethnic, cultural and religious identifications, but not always in ways that can be diminishing to patients. For example, particular attention has been given to cultural taboos about cancer in South Asian populations:

> Social and religious taboos within the Asian community are often barriers to the uptake of cancer screening . . . the imparting of cancer information needs to take place in an environment sympathetic to the social and cultural sensitivities of the community.[27]

Despite such taboos, the experience of cancer can enable some patients to challenge negative attitudes within their own communities. Nusrat, a Pakistani, Muslim woman with cancer, interviewed in Punjabi and Urdu, for the PRIAE research, was adamant that people with cancer:

> . . . should discuss their illness and thoughts with others. They shouldn't think about what others will think of them, or that within the family they will tell other people and create barriers for their children's weddings. This is very common within Asian society. They think that if people come to know about their illness, they won't be able to marry their children off, or people may think if the mother had cancer, then the children will also have it. You shouldn't think about this, you should tell others. So they can share your sorrow, they can share your sorrow. This is my principle and I will give this advice.

Nusrat's account displays a complex negotiation of psychosocial distance and closeness with a wider 'Asian society' in which the threat of social marginalisation in challenging cultural beliefs about cancer is recognised, but held against the possibility of a generous opening out of relationships in emotional support and empathy. By recognising tensions between individual struggles for authenticity and broader cultural identifica-

tions, nurses can begin to gain more in-depth insights into the varied and poetic meanings of identifications in the lives of 'minority ethnic' patients.

A significant challenge for nursing practice in working with the complexities of real-life experiences of ethnicity and cancer is how nurses might work both with and against ideas about 'race', ethnicity, and culture. What I mean by this is how nurses can be open to the ways in which the experiences of patients and carers might be affected by 'race', ethnicity, and culture, without making rigid assumptions about what these experiences are. This 'with' and 'against' approach is much more of an art than a science based upon the securities of typification and prescription. It implies a cognitive and emotional flexibility,[28] but also a 'doubleness'. By 'doubleness' I am referring to the need for nurses to work both with and against essentialist ideas about 'race', ethnicity, and culture, generating awareness that:

- a focus on ethnicity and culture in addressing the needs of 'minority ethnic' patients can obstruct a holistic appreciation of individual experience and need
- ethnic and cultural identifications can have real meaning and consequences in people's lives and these meanings need to be recognised and explored
- while ethnic and cultural identities can be given primacy in how some patients talk about themselves, these identities are always intimately and variously connected to other identities such as those of gender, class and sexuality
- some patients may resist or naturalise ethnic and cultural identifications, so that ethnicity-related need is not manifested
- the concepts of 'race', ethnicity, and culture, although flawed and politically 'dangerous', are important in addressing and challenging practices and processes of racism and discrimination.

In order to examine the relevance of these issues for cancer nursing care, I want to look at some of the close up detail of holistic care for patients from different ethnic and cultural backgrounds. I begin with a personal account (32.1) from a district nurse.

Personal account 32.1   The poetics of holistic care

The following extract is taken from a PRIAE interview between 'Rachel', a white, British district nurse and me, a British-Sri Lankan researcher. I use it as a starting point in discussing what the artistry and poetics of holistic care across difference might look like. In this story Rachel talks about a married couple from a Jamaican background:

Rachel: 'I've got a gentleman . . . he's dying of prostate cancer. He knows he's dying and she knows he's dying, but they can't actually verbalise it together and he's keeping himself awake at night coughing, coughing and coughing . . . and he keeps denying he's got pain, but you can see from his expressions that he's got physical as well as an awful lot of emotional pain and he'd actually ended up with retention of urine for 48 hours until he actually saw somebody in desperation and they weren't able to put a catheter in because the tumour was so large, they had to put it in through the abdomen. So it shows how much discomfort and pain he can tolerate. So if you think of the pain levels and the amount of pain he's in, dramatically under-expressed, so we talked to him about maybe giving him something to help him sleep at night, 'If there's a fire, I won't wake up', and his biggest fear is that if you give him something to help him sleep he won't wake up again and he'll die. So I think the cough is his way of trying to keep himself awake because he's afraid he'll die in his sleep.

. . . and they have a very strong faith which I think is what's helping them through the whole time and the priest comes and I think he's Roman Catholic and he seems to be the one that's pulling them together and forging that bond.

Yasmin: I was just wondering . . . you mentioned the physical pain, the symptoms, but it also seemed to me, emotional . . .

Rachel: Oh yes, incredible emotional pain, the fear of death and I think leaving his wife behind . . . my staff nurse had seen him first and she'd ordered . . . a very highfalutin pressure mattress . . . so I went to see them and said 'my colleague has ordered this for you, where do you normally sleep?' And the wife said 'Well, we've slept in the same bed for 43 years'. And I said 'Well how will you manage if we put your husband in a single bed?' 'Oh I'll sleep in a camp bed next to him'. I said 'Well at the moment things seem to be OK . . . if I get a double mattress . . . would that be more preferable?' And that was what she wanted . . . and that's what we've done.

I think we will probably need to get a hospital bed and a super-duper mattress another two weeks down the line, but we've given them another 3 or 4 weeks of sleeping next to each other in bed, which I think is much more important for the moment while they build up their trust of us and cope with the loss of each other.

Walking the tight-rope: the poetics of holistic care

In this rich account (Personal account 32.1) we can see and hear the poetry of holistic care in the ways Rachel's narrative moves between and weaves together varying aspects of the patient and carer experience. The couple's ethnicity, while relevant to the account, is not seen as determining and enveloping the breadth and layers of their experiences. Instead, Rachel evokes a much more complex intermingling of identities in which questions of age, gender, faith and sexuality also circulate, and we are able to appreciate something of the complicated and highly personal con-

nections between expressed and unexpressed pain, fear, and loss in the couple's lives. Through talk about the new bed and the changes it would entail to the couple's relationship, Rachel is able to explore some of the physical and emotional meanings of the advancing cancer. In this sense, the double mattress that Rachel provides for the couple enables a literal and symbolic 'containment' and 'holding' of their emotional and embodied experiences of illness,[29] while it also serves therapeutically to build up depth and trust in the nurse–patient relationship over time.[30]

I have used this account here because of the multiple levels of patient need and nursing skill that are highlighted and also because it is not based upon an emphasising of obvious ethnic and cultural differences such as language or cultural traditions. In disturbing the conventional exoticisation and categorisation of ethnic 'others', Rachel's account shows how the relevance of ethnicity to a 'minority ethnic' patient's needs and experiences cannot be pre-known or assumed. In some instances, patients' needs that are related to their ethnic and cultural identities may be prominent and articulated, while at other times they can be less manifest or can be evaded and/or resisted by patients. A clinical nurse specialist in a PRIAE interview described the oppositional tensions in his practice in intercultural care as 'walking a fine line' between cultural knowledge and openness, and responding to unpredictable (and unverifiable) emotional connections with patients:

> . . . you don't want to offend, but you don't want to appear ignorant either. So it's a fine line you walk actually and sometimes it's just a gut instinct that you're in there and sometimes you get a window opening of something and you just go with it . . .

The dangerous and precarious nature of this balancing act between knowledge and emotions in intercultural nursing care is given greater depth when we recognise that the negotiation and expression of ethnic, cultural, and/or religious identities by patients in health care relationships is far from benign. The non-manifestation of ethnic identity in relation to patient need can sometimes reflect a defensive and protective manoeuvring, a way of managing experiences of fear, powerlessness, or racism. At other times, it can involve a radical questioning and resistance of definition by ethnicity that challenges the dehumanising impulses of racism. Deciphering whether the non-manifestation of ethnicity-related need in a patient's care is either diminishing or empowering, evidence of holistic, or oppressive nursing care, places nurses in a highly ambivalent and political position.

A central argument that I want to pursue throughout this discussion is that interpreting the meanings of varied ethnic and cultural identifications in patients' lives is much more complicated, emotional, ethical, and political than current approaches to cultural sensitivity and competence suggest. Indeed, I am unhappy with using such terms as cultural competence as unproblematic

descriptions of practice, because they suggest that attention to identities and experiences of ethnic, cultural and/or religious difference is somehow outside the 'normal' parameters of holistic care. In its refusal to emphasise ethnicity, I believe Rachel's account allows us to explore a more open-ended, ambiguous and ambivalent version of what could be seen as cultural competence in nursing practice.

I would like you to keep Rachel's account in mind as we move through the following discussion where I will examine how holistic care for patients from different ethnic and cultural groups can be jeopardised and threatened in cancer nursing through:

- the emphasis upon culture and cultural knowledge for nurses
- notions of commonality and difference between patients and practitioners
- the lack of recognition of the emotional content of cancer nursing across difference.

Care strategy 32.1 outlines four fundamental requirements of holistic care that is responsive to difference.

Care strategy 32.1 The requirements of a responsive holistic practice (adapted from Gunaratnam[10])

I have identified four main requirements of a responsive holistic practice for nurses, in which care:

- must be able to take account of the connections and the distinctions between individual and collective experiences of ethnicity and culture and other social difference, how these dynamics are related, but also how they cannot be 'read off' each other
- must give attention to subjective, emotional experiences to bring questions of feeling and of experience into consideration, but always within a context of wider social relations
- must be able to generate complex and reflective practice even in those cases where rigid ethnic and cultural identifications appear to 'fit', are endorsed and are held onto by patients and carers
- must be able to commit itself to engage with and respect felt experiences of racial, ethnic and cultural difference, while working towards the dismantling of categorical thinking and racism.

The emphasis upon culture and cultural knowledge

A significant threat to the holistic care of 'minority ethnic' patients concerns culturalist approaches to intercultural care that predominate within contemporary nurse education and training programmes. Within the culturalist paradigm, the needs of 'minority ethnic' patients are seen primarily in relation to cultural and religious difference, arising from ethnicity.[31] 'Culturally competent' nurses can meet these needs through cultural knowledge, awareness and respect for different cultures.[32]

Kim-Godwin *et al.* describe cultural knowledge in the following terms:[17]

> Cultural knowledge refers to knowledge of integrated systems of learned behaviour that are characteristic of members of groups (for example, what a specific group of people think, say, do, make etc) as well as their system of attitudes, feelings, and values (Sawyer *et al.*, 1995)[33] ... When discussing knowledge or understanding of culturally different health values, beliefs, and practices, stereotyping is possible; however, generalization that acknowledges cultural differences is necessary (Galanti, 1997).[34] For example, it is important to acknowledge the importance of native healers in many cultures while still evaluating the appropriateness of a medical referral (Galanti, 1997).[34]

This quotation from Kim-Godwin *et al.* acknowledges the dangers for nurses of the 'doubleness' of working with and against the generalisations that are an unavoidable part of cultural knowledge. However, in the context of cancer care, I believe that the emotional anxieties, ethical dilemmas, and political questions that are raised for nurses in the process of using cultural knowledge in practice are underestimated. For instance, examination of ethical dilemmas that are related to disclosure of a diagnosis and truth telling in intercultural care suggests that cultural knowledge is much less important than the ability to negotiate the relationships between patient autonomy, constructions of cultural tradition, and the ability of patients and carers to discuss matters openly.[35] It is also the case that while cultural knowledge can provide a context to patient need, what is seen as 'cultural' can be a site of conflict within families and can also be a part of oppressive interpersonal

power relations that need to be recognised and explored by nurses.

From my experience of research, teaching, and training I have found that there are significant areas of contradiction in the relationships between having cultural knowledge and providing holistic nursing care to 'minority ethnic' patients. Although nurses often identify their lack of cultural knowledge as impeding intercultural care, when they tell stories about real-life care situations, they often do not remember the specific details of the ethnicity or cultural/religious identity of the patients in their accounts. The following extracts are from PRIAE interviews with nurses:

> I remember once, I can't remember where the patient was from, but we were told that when he died, the tradition was, I think he must have been from a Chinese background, I can't actually remember, but when he died the tradition was that they would try and bring him back to life . . .

> At the hospital, I can't remember what group of Muslims, but they were all bashing their heads against the walls . . .

> . . . there's another gentleman that . . . springs to mind who had travelled to America, whose family had paid for him to go to Mexico to have experimental chemotherapy . . . I can't remember where he was from . . .

The ambiguity of the identities of patients and carers in these nurse accounts suggest that the detail of cultural knowledge that nurses are seen as needing in intercultural care is overwhelmed in real-life practice by a more general attention to difference. This attention to difference can be indicative of ways of working that are responsive and holistic, addressing multiple experiences and needs. However, they can also involve processes of 'othering' in which ethnicity, although unnamed, comes to stand for – and obscure – a myriad of individual and social differences, creating false distances between an 'us' and 'them'. Indeed, I have found that professionals can be more willing to ascribe a wide range of behaviours, care choices, and preferences to cultural and religious difference when patients and carers come from 'minority ethnic' groups. In the following interview extract from my hospice study, a hospice social worker talks about how the labelling of what is 'cultural' functions in her multidisciplinary home care team:

> Oh in Home Care, the most quoted phrase which drives me up the wall, and I haven't quite worked out what to do about it is, 'it's cultural'. Anything that anybody does who's not white, that is at all different in some way, 'it's cultural' and what 'it's cultural' I think means is 'we therefore do not do anything with it', because that means 'it's cultural – therefore we leave it well alone'. So that can cover anything from 'no we don't like morphine', to denying that we are dying, to the family denying that.

What we can hear in the frustration evoked in this observation is how the label 'it's cultural' matters deeply in practice. It matters because what is thought of and categorised as being 'cultural' can work to restrict professional exploration with patients and carers who are 'not white', marking and legitimising particular no-go areas for professional intervention and support. What is of further relevance in this extract is how the behaviours and practices of white patients are positioned outside of the 'cultural'. In this way, whiteness is not primarily culturalised but is seen as being able to contain, integrate, and bend around the fullness and indeed 'normality' of human diversity. As Kirkham and Anderson have observed:

> In most health care theorising, White-dominant culture remains transparent and unspoken for the most part, positioned as 'normal' . . . 'being normal' is colonised by the idea of 'being white'.[36]

By pointing to the ways in which an emphasis upon culture and cultural knowledge can be problematic for nurses, I do not wish to suggest that awareness of cultural and religious patterns, beliefs, and traditions is unimportant. My intention is to encourage a critical and 'double' reflection on the modes through which constructions of ethnic and cultural difference can function to limit or enhance holistic care for 'minority ethnic' patients.

Closeness/distance – commonality and difference

The argument that culture can be overemphasised when nurses address the experiences of 'minority ethnic' patients and can also function to position the dominant white culture as 'normal', becomes more complicated when we address the increasingly multicultural nature of the NHS workforce in the UK. Although much of the nursing literature on intercultural care assumes that nurses are from a dominant white culture, issues of commonality and difference shadow concerns about the ability of health care professionals to meet the needs of 'minority ethnic' patients.[37,38] I will examine how notions of commonality and difference can compromise holistic cancer care for 'minority ethnic' patients, through discussions of cross-cultural communication.

Communicating across cultures

Language differences and problems of communication between cancer patients and health care practitioners are key areas of concern in the literature on cancer services and ethnicity. Fear, anxiety, and the stigma associated with cancer have been identified as making it more difficult for some patients to seek medical advice.[27] Furthermore, social differences and power relations between health care professionals and patients are recognised as inhibiting communication and patient participation in decision making, even when language is shared.[39] A report on cancer information for patients at the Christie Hospital in Manchester found that:

> Language, religion and cultural factors can affect Black and Ethnic Minorities [sic] ability to effectively use health services. Patients who speak little or no English are generally given less information and offered fewer choices. They cannot ask questions, voice worries, discuss important issues, ask for what they need or receive support. They cannot give genuinely informed consent.[40]

Although more services are now using trained interpreters and bilingual advocates, the identification of the need for professionals who can provide both linguistic and cultural interpretation for patients who do not speak English is a recurring theme in the literature on cancer, palliative care, and ethnicity.[41] Using the findings of qualitative interviews with 12 patients with advanced cancer from five Muslim and Hindu South Asian families in Bedfordshire, Randhawa et al. have concluded that:

... there was a feeling among many of those inter- viewed that not enough people were recruited from 'their community' who spoke their languages and understood their cultural and religious beliefs. It is clear that, to some interviewees, effective communica- tion does not simply entail the ability for patients and carers to speak the same language. It also involves a mutual understanding of religion and culture; the ability of a professional to appreciate and 'read' a whole way of life.[42]

As I have argued elsewhere, such approaches to cross-cultural communication that suggest that ethnic and cultural matching between a profes- sional and a patient can enable a professional to '"read" a whole way of life' need careful and criti- cal consideration.[43] This consideration needs to take account of how the interpreting role of bilin- gual staff can compromise their other areas of work,[44] and can lead to ethnicity-based divisions of care, particularly with regard to the emotional labour of cancer care. At the level of communica- tion, there is also a need to distinguish between the technical and the emotional: between linguis- tic and cultural interpretation and subjective mutuality and closeness.

There can be little doubt that language differ- ences can have a detrimental impact upon holistic care for patients who do not speak English. How- ever, ideas about 'mutual understanding' can be based upon essentialist ideas about ethnicity, culture, and religion that fail to recognise how the experience of illness, in addition to other social differences, can affect communication and identi- fications. The following extract from a PRIAE interview with a bilingual woman advocate working in a community palliative care team, illustrates how the advantages of shared ethnicity can turn into disadvantages with some patients:

I wouldn't even dream of asking a question about sexual intimacy . . . that would be one of the disad- vantages [of shared ethnicity] . . . going to see an elderly Asian patient with prostate cancer. If you had a particular list of questions you're supposed to ask, I couldn't ask the question about his sex life.

The assumption of what Shields has called 'communication as communion' that underlies suggestions that ethnic and cultural commonali-

ties between the patient and health care practi- tioner can lead to better understanding and communication,[45] presumes that a patient can be more open and 'readable' in care situations where language and culture are shared. This assumption does not recognise the resistance of some patients to subjective explorations by nurses,[46] and it does not recognise how the experience of cancer can disrupt feelings about ethnic and cultural com- monalities. As a white, British hospital clinical nurse specialist commented in a PRIAE interview:

I've . . . had Afro-Caribbean patients say to me that they don't want to be looked after by a nurse who may come from the same background as them, who may know people that know them and they're worried the details of their illness will get out and get amongst the community if they want to keep it to themselves.

From the interviews I have facilitated with 'minority ethnic' nurses, it is apparent that their 'insider' cultural and/or linguistic knowledge, in care situations where they come from a similar ethnic and cultural background as a patient, is not always enough to enable mutual understanding. Nurses have identified differences of gender and age and the site of cancer as factors that produce points of difference in the nurse–patient relation- ship. Indeed, some of the most interesting work on intercultural nursing is emerging from research- ers who are exploring the experiences of nurses from socially marginalised ethnic groups.

Qualitative research by Canales and Bowers on Latina nurses' educators in North America, has found a displacement of assumptions of ethnicity- based commonality and difference in favour of a recognition of processes of 'othering' and an active working towards connections with patients and the wider community settings in which nurses work.[47] In addressing these approaches that use the nurses' personal experiences of social margin- alisation as a starting point for practice, Canales and Bowers have identified processes of working with difference that are highly relevant to the development of approaches to holistic care in cancer nursing:

Their assumption that difference is not solely about specific cultural groups expands the boundaries for who is defined as 'cultural' and implies that in clinical practice, 'cultural' difference is encountered on a regular basis.

From the perspectives of these nurse educators, caring for Othered individuals and populations was not substantively different from caring for familiar groups . . . Their teaching practices reinforce that the Other is different for all of us. Who we are as self and whom we see as Other, varies for each person. This shift in thinking provides nurses with many possibilities for connecting with the Other and integrating this concept into all areas of nursing practice.[47]

Emotions, difference and organisational contexts

The emphasis upon cultural knowledge and a concern with relationships of commonality and difference in meeting the needs of 'minority ethnic' patients has been accompanied by attention to the emotional dynamics of intercultural nursing. Gerrrish *et al.*, in their examination of cultural competence, have drawn attention to nurses' emotions of fear and anxiety about 'things going wrong' in situations of intercultural care as blocking their openness to patients (see Box 32.1).[48] I will build upon this recognition of the emotional content of intercultural nursing, by examining how holistic care can be threatened by the heightened and convoluted emotions that can be provoked for nurses and patients in cancer care settings.

It has long been recognised that the structures and culture of cancer and palliative care settings can be organised and managed so that professionals can avoid engaging with difficult and painful emotions.[49,50] Isobel Menzies Lyth's pioneering study of nursing in a London general teaching hospital in the 1950s found that the objectification of patients through the structuring of nursing practices, decision making and delegation was a part of the organisational culture of the hospital: a 'social defence system' that functioned to help nurses avoid feelings of anxiety, guilt, doubt and uncertainty in working with illness and death.[51] For Menzies Lyth:

A social defence system develops over time as the result of collusive interaction and agreement, often

Box 32.1 Gerrish *et al.*'s 'Cultural competence' from Gerrish K., Husband C. and Mackenzie J. (1996). *Nursing for a Multi-Ethnic Society*. Buckingham: Open University Press[48]

Gerrish *et al.* conceptualise cultural competence as involving specific skills of 'cultural communicative competence' and more generic skills of 'inter-cultural communicative competence'.

By 'cultural communicative competence', the authors are referring to the more task-oriented requirement for practitioners to 'learn to understand the cultural values, behavioural patterns and rules for interaction in specific cultures'. The more process-oriented need for practitioners to be open and adaptable in their care practices is reflected in the notion of 'inter-cultural communicative competence'. Gerrish *et al.* suggest that there are three dimensions of intercultural communicative competence through which rigidity can be avoided and openness to difference can be pursued. These dimensions are:

- *the cognitive* – 'The cognitive dimension . . . is a creative flexibility in one's thought processes. It is a refusal to be dogmatic, or to insist on reducing new experiences to familiar or safe categories of understanding' (p.28)
- *the affective* – is seen as relating to emotions and can be either positive: 'an emotional openness to others', and/ or negative, marked by threat and an 'inner-directed, protective setting of boundaries' (p.28)
- *the behavioural* – is conceptualised as the ability to express the insights that are generated in the cognitive and the affective in action, 'the behavioural dimension is all about our ability to adapt and be flexible in new situations' (p.28).

unconscious, between members of the organisation as to what form it shall take.[51]

What is less well recognised in Menzies Lyth's work is that the nature of specific organisational 'defence systems' in health care settings are also entangled with wider social and political processes.[51] My argument is that there are specific interrelationships between the anxieties – and the organisational and personal defences that can accompany them – that are generated in working with serious illnesses, death, and dying and the anxieties and defences that are provoked in working with social and cultural differences in a health service with a stated commitment to race equality.

Solomon et al.,[52] in experiments on 'terror management' and self esteem in the field of social psychology, have suggested that the anxiety-buffering effects of shared 'cultural worldviews' developed in all societies to protect individuals from the existential angst of an awareness of death, can be threatened fundamentally by those with alternative worldviews (such as those arising from differences in ethnicity, religion, sexuality, or lifestyle). The value of terror management theory in addressing the demands of cancer nursing in multicultural contexts is the recognition that working with difference in an environment characterised by serious illness can be particularly threatening. It can be threatening because encountering different ways of life, values, and beliefs can agitate and uncover layers of anxiety, serving to question the most basic foundations of our personal and professional cultural worldviews such as those relating to knowledge, imagery, language, and disciplinary philosophies.

The following extracts taken from interviews with different professionals in my hospice study provide examples of how some dimensions of intercultural care can be affected by fear and anxiety:

> . . . when you are dealing with people from another culture . . . You don't know if you are using the right words, and even if you do speak the same language the depth of understanding of the other person's culture is very shallow on one side. In death we are so much dependent upon images and feelings that language is thrown into doubt . . . in the context of dying, we often have to reach out to people and take risks and I think I might be more reluctant to do that with people from a different culture.
>
> (chaplain)

> I think my concerns are about sticking my foot in it and that kind of thing inhibits me . . . I try to find the right way of trying not to offend anybody by calling them sort of, something that's not now PC [politically correct], it's really difficult and that makes me quite inhibited.
>
> (staff nurse)

> I don't actually think it is just a literal fear of being accused of being racist, I actually think it is a fear of triggering the rage and fury, maybe I should speak for myself, about white people's history of treatment of black people. That it is not just a 'You're a racist'. I mean . . . I know . . . it is devastating to be criticised. But . . . for me, it's like, it's not just that is it? It's like the whole history behind the kind of, I don't know, how much . . . does that immobilise us? Does that stop . . . me taking risks with families?
>
> (social worker)

What is striking in these extracts is how personal fears and anxieties can restrict and inhibit professional practice with racialised 'others', producing contorted and often imperceptible inequalities in care. At the level of patterns of racism and discrimination in cancer care settings, my argument is that it is not only that 'minority ethnic' patients and carers can receive suboptimal care, it is also that they do not receive the most creative, experimental and ground-breaking forms of practice that can come from risk taking and from practitioners who are enabled to recognise the full emotional content of working across difference.

Through the interviews that I have conducted with health care professionals, I have found that high-quality and innovative forms of practice frequently involve risk taking: trying something new and different, challenging service users, oneself, and colleagues, exploring intuitive hunches, and working outside established comfort zones.[53] The irony of the constriction of professional risk taking with 'minority ethnic' patients is that such constriction can also feed into and off some of the diminishing and entangled emotional dynamics between identities of difference and the illness experience in patient's lives.

Ahmad has addressed aspects of these dynamics in the connections he has made between forms of domination and subordination based upon colonialism and those that can be found in biomedicine and the professional–patient relationship. He argues that:

> Common to both is to some extent the complicity of the colonized. The legitimacy of colonial rule was rarely effectively challenged by the colonized . . . Likewise patients rarely challenge the hegemony of medicine or the expert status of the doctor . . . Notions of

appropriate and inappropriate behaviour in illness are dictated by medicine and relate directly to labels of 'good' and 'bad' patients.[54]

Ahmad's astute engagement with 'the complicity of the colonised' draws attention to the challenging and uncomfortable issue of whether patients from socially marginalised ethnic groups, through the emotional and interactional dynamics of the 'sick role'[55] can sometimes be complicit with oppressive relations of power within the health services. While I have found numerous examples in my research of patients who have been able to challenge what they have perceived as bad care practices, I have also found that the need to be a 'good patient' together with wider experiences of social exclusion can lead to low expectations of care and to the suppression of dissatisfaction. As Nussbaum has cautioned:[56]

> The poor and deprived frequently adjust their expectations and aspirations to the low level of life they have known. Thus, they may not demand . . . better health care.[56]

The poem in Personal account 32.2 has been produced from the transcript of a PRIAE interview with Ricardo, a non-English-speaking Portuguese man with cancer. Ricardo was a recent migrant to England and had been working as an office cleaner when his cancer was diagnosed. The poem uses only Ricardo's words, that I have reproduced using poetic techniques and structuring. In Ricardo's account, constructions of the 'good patient' and his linguistic and emotional inability to say 'I don't like cheese' provide a more complicated view of service inequalities and intercultural care, in which nurses need to recognise how experiences of social exclusion together with conscious and unconscious emotions of vulnerability and anxiety can affect patient accounts and experiences of care.

It is important to recognise that there is a particular lack of understanding in cancer care about the emotional and embodied pain of social exclusion: how experiences of racism might be 'remembered' by bodies, affecting physical care[9] and/or how the powerlessness and vulnerability of the illness experience might resonate with experiences of social exclusion. Although I have found

Personal account 32.2 'I don't like cheese'

You have to have the will
to survive.
I did not like the food.
There was no salt.
Sometimes I had cheese.
But I don't like cheese.
With the language barrier
I did not know how to say
'I don't like cheese'.
You have to have the will
and be stronger.
When you are in hospital
eat your meal.
Do the right thing.
Accept advice. Do everything right.
But I don't like cheese.

no recognition of these experiences in the nursing literature, my research with health care professionals and my personal experiences of in-depth interviews with patients has suggested that holding the emotional pain of social exclusion can be particularly difficult.[57]

The difficulty of engaging with emotional pain – and how we can avoid or deny it – has been recognised by the psychoanalyst Waddell in the distinction between 'servicing' (implying action) and 'serving' (which may constitute not 'doing' anything):

> 'Servicing' urges itself as a substitute for 'serving' because the not-acting of serving brings us in contact with feelings: feelings which are very hard to bear – the conscious phenomena of unconscious psychic pain . . . It may be more comfortable to be doing something, whether it is writing a prescription, making an interpretation, arranging a visit, than not doing so – although *not doing anything* does not constitute *doing nothing* [emphasis in original].[58]

In the context of cancer care, where emotions can be heightened, it is possible to see how the emphasis upon the rationalist acquisition of cultural knowledge for nurses discussed earlier can be a part of the 'servicing' role of nurses. In this role, the categorisation of patient need in relation to ethnicity, culture and/or religion can impede holistic care *and* function as a part of a professional and organisational 'defence system' that can serve to protect nurses from the emotional intensity of the anxieties that can be generated in working with illness and difference. In addition, the kaleidoscope of social and emotional dynamics that frame 'minority ethnic' patient experiences suggest that there can be tensions in a doubled nursing practice between the attention given to the social and cultural contexts of patient experience and the attention given to the emotional content of the nurse–patient relationship.

Conclusion

The psychosocial approach to the provision of holistic cancer care to 'minority ethnic' patients taken in this chapter provides new insights into how nurses might respond to the poetry of lived experiences of illness and difference. It has also identified inadequacies in culturalist approaches to intercultural nursing care that inform current thinking about cultural sensitivity and competence. In questioning the rationalist foundations of such approaches, I have sought to uncover some of the complex ethical, emotional, and political dimensions of nursing across difference, which can be marked by ambiguity and ambivalence. For me, the ambivalent, uneven, and evolving nature of such nursing practice is more adequately captured by the hesitant and softer notion of 'capability' rather than competence, the latter of which denotes the (unrealistic) rational mastery of a stable body of knowledge. In this softer approach to ethnicity, difference, and patient need, the false securities of cultural knowledge or the positioning of 'minority ethnic' professionals as 'cultural experts' become untenable, as nurses are enabled to recognise and be open to the slippery and poetic psychosocial dynamics of ethnicity as 'an absent presence, a present absence'[59] in lived experiences for both patients and themselves. At the same time, the ethical and inescapable political dimensions of care that is fully holistic, push practitioners to address how we are located, socially and emotionally, in wider systems of racism and discrimination in the organisational and social contexts in which we work.

References

1. Molassiotis A. (2004). Supportive and palliative care for patients from ethnic minorities in Europe: do we suffer from institutional racism? *European Journal of Oncology Nursing* **8**, 290–292.
2. Department of Health. (2004). *Race Equality Action Plan: Leadership and Race Equality in the NHS.* www.dh.gov.uk/PublicationsAndStatistics/Bulletins/BulletinArticle/fs/en?CONTENT_ID=4072494&chk=1e/oI7 (accessed 13 August 2007).
3. Macmillan Cancer Relief. (2002). *Macmillan Black and Ethnic Minority Toolkit, Effective Communication with South Asian People Affected by Cancer.* London: Macmillan Cancer Relief.
4. Broyard A. (1993). *Intoxicated by my Illness: and Other Writings on Life and Death.* New York: Fawcett Books.
5. Airey C., Becher H., Erens B. and Fuller E. (2002). *National Surveys of NHS Patients. Cancer: National Overview 1999/2000.* London: Department of Health.
6. Pearson M. (1986). The politics of ethnic minority health studies. In Rathewell T. and Phillips D. (eds.) *Health, Race and Ethnicity.* London: Croom Helm, pp. 100–116.
7. Gunaratnam Y. (1999). *Researching and Representing Ethnicity: a qualitative study of hospice staff and service users.* PhD thesis, University of London.
8. Hall S. (2000). Conclusion: the multi-cultural question. In Hesse B. (ed.) *Un/settled Multiculturalisms: Diasporas, Entanglements, Transruptions.* London: Zed Books, pp. 209–241.
9. Gunaratnam Y. (2004). 'Bucking and kicking': 'race', gender and embodied resistance in health care. In Apitzsch U., Bornat J. and Chamberlayne P. (eds.) *Biographical Methods and Professional Practice: An International Perspective.* Bristol: Policy Press, pp. 205–219.
10. Gunaratnam Y. (2003). *Researching 'Race' and Ethnicity: Methods, Knowledge and Power.* London: Sage.
11. Jones J. (1981). How different are human races? *Nature* **293**, 188–190.
12. Kim-Godwin Y., Clarke P. and Barton L. (2001). A model for the delivery of culturally competent community care. *Journal of Advanced Nursing* **35**, 918–925.
13. Aspinall P. and Jacobson B. (2004). *Ethnic Disparities in Health and Health Care: A Focused Review of the Evidence and Selected Examples of Good Practice.* London: London Health Observatory.
14. Harding S. and Allen E.J. (1996). Sources and uses of data on cancer among ethnic subgroups. *British Journal of Cancer* **74(suppl. 29)**, S17–S21.
15. Harding S. and Rosato M. (1999). Cancer incidence among first generation Scottish, Irish, West Indian and South Asian migrants living in England and Wales. *Ethnicity and Health* **4**, 83–92.

16. Wild S. and McKeigue P. (1997). Cross sectional analysis of mortality by country of birth in England and Wales 1970–92. *British Medical Journal* **314**, 705–710.

17. Gill P.S., Kai J., Bhopal R. and Wild S. *Black and Minority Ethnic Groups*. http://hcna.radcliffe-oxford.com/bemg-frame.htm (accessed 14 August 2007).

18. Firth S. (2001). *Wider Horizons: Care of the Dying in a Multicultural Society*. London: National Council for Hospice and Specialist Palliative Care Services.

19. Smaje C. (1996). The ethnic patterning of health: new directions for theory and research. *Sociology of Health and Illness* **18**, 139–171.

20. Ziegler R., Hoover R., Pike M. *et al.* (1993). Migration patterns and breast cancer risk in Asian-American women. *Journal of the National Cancer Institute* **85**, 1819–1827.

21. National Council for Palliative Care. (2005). *20:20 Vision*. London: National Council for Palliative Care.

22. Gunaratnam Y. (2001). Eating into multi-culturalism: hospice staff and service users talk food, 'race', ethnicity and identities. *Critical Social Policy* **21**, 287–310.

23. Sheldon T. and Parker H. (1992). The use of 'ethnicity' and 'race' in health research: a cautionary note. In Ahmad W.I.U (ed.) *The Politics of 'Race' and Health*. Bradford: Race Relations Unit, University of Bradford and Ilkley Community College, pp. 53–78.

24. Mulholland J. and Dyson S. (2001). Sociological theories of 'race' and ethnicity. In Culle L. and Dyson S. (eds.) *Ethnicity and Nursing Practice*. London: Palgrave, pp. 17–38.

25. Werbner P. (1997). Essentialising essentialism, essentialising silence: ambivalence and multiplicity in the constructions of racism and ethnicity. In Werbner P. and Modood T. (eds.) *Debating Cultural Hybridity: Multi-Cultural Identities and the Politics of Anti-Racism*. London: Zed Books, pp. 226–254.

26. Sontag S. (1977). *Illness as Metaphor*. New York: Farrar, Strauss and Giroux.

27. Cancerbackup. (2004). *Beyond the Barriers – Providing Cancer Information and Support for Black and Minority Ethnic Communities*. London: Cancerbackup.

28. Thomas V. (2001). The needs of people from minority ethnic groups. In Corner J. and Bailey C. (eds.) *Cancer Nursing: Care in Context*. Oxford: Blackwell Science, pp. 508–516.

29. Bion W. (1984). *Learning from Experience*, 2nd edition. London: Maresfield.

30. Cox M. (1988). *Structuring the Therapeutic Process: Compromise with Chaos*. London: Jessica Kingsley.

31. Culley L. (1996). A critique of multi-culturalism in health care: the challenge for nurse education. *Journal of Advanced Nursing* **23**, 564–570.

32. Papadopoulos I., Tilki M. and Taylor G. (1998). *Transcultural Care: a Guide for Health Care Professionals*. London: Quay Books.

33. Sawyer L., Regev H., Proctor S. *et al.* (1995). Matching versus cultural competence in research: methodological considerations. *Research in Nursing and Health* **18**, 556–567.

34. Galanti G. (1997). Caring *for Patients from Different Cultures: Case Studies from American Hospitals*, 2nd edition. Philadelphia, PA: University of Pennsylvania Press.

35. Werth J., Blevins D., Toussaint K. and Durham M. (2002). The influence of cultural diversity on end-of-life care and decisions. *American Behavioural Scientist* **46**, 204–219.

36. Kirkham S. and Anderson J. (2002). Postcolonial nursing scholarship: from epistemology to method. *Advances in Nursing Science* **25**, 1–17.

37. Department of Health. (2000). *The Vital Connection: An Equalities Framework for the NHS*. London: The Stationery Office.

38. Johns N. (2004). Ethnic diversity policy: perceptions within the NHS. *Social Policy and Administration* **38**, 73–88.

39. Social Action for Health. (2003). *Annual Report*. London: Social Action for Health.

40. Christie Hospital NHS Trust. (2002). *A Report on Cancer Information for Black and Ethnic Minority Patients at the Christie Hospital NHS Trust 2002*. Manchester: Christie Hospital NHS Trust.

41. Somerville J. (2001). The experience of informal carers within the Bangladeshi community. *International Journal of Palliative Nursing* **7**, 240–247.

42. Randhawa G., Owens A., Fitches R. and Khan Z. (2003). Communication in the development of culturally competent palliative care services in the UK: a case study. *International Journal of Palliative Nursing* **9**, 24–31.

43. Gunaratnam Y. (2004). Skin matters: 'race' and care in the health services. In Fink J. (ed.) *Care: Personal Lives, Social Policy*. Bristol: Polity Press, pp. 112–144.

44. Firth S. (1997). *Death, Dying and Bereavement in a British Hindu Community*. London: Peeters Leuven.

45. Shields R. (1996). Meeting or mis-meeting? The Dialogical challenge to Verstehen. *British Journal of Sociology* **47**, 275–294.

46. Porter S. (1996). Contra-Foucault: soldiers, nurses and power. *Sociology* **30**, 59–78.

47. Canales M. and Bowers B. (2001). Expanding conceptualizations of culturally competent care. *Journal of Advanced Nursing* **36**, 102–111.

48. Gerrish K., Husband C. and Mackenzie J. (1996). *Nursing for a Multi-Ethnic Society*. Buckingham: Open University Press.

49. Glaser B. and Strauss A. (1965). *Awareness of Dying.* Chicago: Aldine.

50. James N. (1992). Care = organisation + physical labour + emotional labour. *Sociology of Health and Illness* **14**, 487–509.

51. Menzies Lyth I. (1988). *Containing Anxiety in Institutions, Selected Essays.* London: Free Association Books.

52. Solomon S., Greenberg J. and Pyszczynski T. (1991). Terror management theory of self-esteem. In Synder C. and Forsyth D. (eds.) *Handbook of Social and Clinical Psychology: The Health Perspective.* New York: Pergamon, pp. 21–40.

53. Gunaratnam Y., Bremner I., Pollock L. and Weir C. (1998). Anti-discrimination, emotions and professional practice. *European Journal of Palliative Care* **5**, 122–124.

54. Ahmad W.I.U. (1993). *'Race' and Health in Contemporary Britain.* Milton Keynes: Open University Press.

55. Parson T. (1951). *The Social System.* Glencoe, IL: The Free Press.

56. Nussbaum M. (1995). Human capabilities, female human beings. In Nussbaum M. and Glover J. (eds.) *Women, Culture and Development.* Oxford: Oxford University Press, pp. 202–246.

57. Gunaratnam Y. (2003). More than words: dialogue across difference. In Sidell M., Jones J., Katz J., Peberdy A. and Douglas J. (eds.) *Debates and Dilemmas in Promoting Health: A Reader.* Basingstoke: Palgrave, pp. 112–121.

58. Waddell M. (1989). Living in two worlds: psychodynamic theory and social work practice. *Free Associations* **15**, 11–35.

59. Winant H. (1994). Racial formation and hegemony: global and local developments. In Rattansi A. and Westwood S. (eds.) *Racism, Modernity and Identity: On the Western Front.* Cambridge: Polity Press, pp. 266–289.

Further reading

Gunaratnam Y. (1997). Culture is not enough: a critique of multi-culturalism in palliative care. In Field D., Hockey J. and Small N. (eds.) *Death, Gender and Ethnicity.* London: Routledge, pp. 166–186.

Koffman J. and Higginson I. (2001). Accounts of carers' satisfaction with health care at the end of life: a comparison of first generation black Caribbeans and white patients with advanced disease. *Palliative Medicine* **15**, 337–345.

National Institute for Clinical Excellence. (2004). *Guidance on Cancer Services, Improving Supportive and Palliative Care for Adults with Cancer.* London: National Institute for Clinical Excellence.

CHAPTER THIRTY-THREE

Living with cancer long term: the implications of survival

David Wright

Long-term survival: introduction

There has been a dramatic increase in the survival rates from cancer in the Western world over recent decades. This has been as a result of a wide range of factors that include: improvements in early detection and treatment of cancer, significant advances in genetic research, the rapid translation of basic science into clinical practice, the modification of dose-limiting toxicities, an increase in cancer screening, enhanced rehabilitation and support interventions, and changes in socio-cultural factors, such as lifestyle, diet and exercise.[1,2] While increases in the rates of cancer survival are clearly something to be celebrated, they have as a consequence generated significant long-term physical and psychosocial difficulties for people affected by the disease.[3-5] This chapter explores these difficulties with particular reference to the experiences of adults with cancer, and will be divided into three sections. First, data on cancer survival and definitions are presented to reveal the complexity of conceptualising 'survivorship'. Second, specific attention is given to different problems faced by long-term cancer survivors. Each problem will include patient accounts from research to illustrate the significance of these problems in the lives of survivors. Finally, possible ways of managing the problems generated by long-term cancer survival will be considered with particular reference to nursing practice.

Long-term survival: facts, figures and definitions

The importance of supporting people living long term with cancer has become increasingly recognised in recent years. Supportive care is defined by the UK National Institute for Clinical Excellence as care that is:

> ... helping the patient and their family to cope with cancer and treatment of it – from pre-diagnosis, through the process of diagnosis and treatment, to cure, continuing illness or death and into bereavement. It helps the patient to maximise the benefits of treatment and to live as well as possible with the effects of the disease. It is given equal priority along with diagnosis and treatment.[5]

Evidence suggests that survival from cancer has increased dramatically in the Western world over recent decades.[1] In the US in the 1930s, it was estimated that only one in five patients survived cancer for 5 years or more, compared to one in two in the 1990s.[4] In 2002, there were 8.9 million cancer survivors in the US, with a survival rate of 60% amongst adults and 75% amongst children 5 years following a cancer diagnosis.[6] However, there are clear variations in rates between population backgrounds and different cancer types. For example, the 5-year survival rate for people diagnosed with Hodgkin's disease in the US has increased from 5% in the 1960s to 80% in the 1990s, while survival rates for US Caucasian lung cancer patients has remained around 14% for 20 years and is only 7% in the UK.[4,7] In the UK, testicular cancer patients have the highest 5-year relative survival rate at 95%, and that for pancreatic cancer is the lowest at 2%.

At present most cancers occur in people over 65 years, and with an ageing population, the incidence of cancer is rising. People affected by cancer in this age group are likely to have other illnesses in addition to their cancer that may make diagnosis and treatment more problematic. They are also more likely to have older carers, thus needing formal support services.[3] Considering the predicted increase in cancer burden related both to an ageing and a diversifying population, the impact of living long term following a cancer diagnosis is expected to increase in significance.[3]

Despite these evident trends in long-term survival, there is as yet no single definition of 'long-term survival' of cancer. Common definitions have related to specific aspects of survival. For example, issues relating to the after-effects of specific treatments have often been couched in terms of 'late' or 'delayed effects'.[2,8] The term 'survivorship' has often been used, particularly in the US, as an umbrella term to encompass all physiological and psychosocial aspects of living beyond diagnosis and treatment.[3] The US National Cancer Institute defines survivorship as 'physical, psychosocial and economic sequelae of cancer diagnosis and its treatment among both paediatric and adult survivors of cancer'.[3]

There is greater agreement over the definition of survivorship in terms of the number of years from diagnosis or treatment. Many define long-term survivorship as being at least 5 years on from diagnosis, given that cancer survival rates are traditionally expressed in these terms and because most recurrences occur within 5 years of diagnosis.[4] However, not everyone agrees with this definition, particularly as the incidents and intervals of recurrence do differ across different cancer groups.

The concept of 'survivorship' has often been associated with images of survivors of war and holocausts, raising the question, 'precisely what is it that is being survived?'.[9] The concept has been conceived of differently over time, often in relation to changing treatment regimens and survival rates. Early attempts to discuss cancer survival often focused on functional status, with psychological implications considered only in terms of the ability to perform tasks.[10] Since then, there has been a shift in the conceptualisation of survivorship to reflect a change in treatment away from radical surgery towards a greater use of chemotherapy and radiotherapy, and a greater recognition of the experiences of patients.[11] For example, Herold and Roetzheim suggested that patients diagnosed with cancer go through 'seasons of survival'.[12] The first phase, 'acute survival', relates to the period of diagnosis and treatment where, they suggest, the overarching concern is one of mortality. The second phase, 'extended survival', relates to the period of remission and a time of 'watchful waiting'. The third and final phase refers to a period of 'permanent survival', which equates to 'cure' and is represented by a period of reflection and re-entering society.[12] Others, however, have suggested that cancer survivorship exists as a 'continuum' whereby the needs and experiences of patients change continually as they live their lives beyond the point of diagnosis and treatment.[6]

However long-term survival is conceived, it is evident that such survival brings with it particular challenges. Each of these will now be considered and will be supported by examples taken from a project I recently completed for Macmillan Cancer Support, the Macmillan Listening Study.[13] The study involved a series of focus (consultation) groups conducted with a cross-section of cancer patients recruited across the UK.

The impact of long-term survivorship on adult patients

The impact of long-term survivorship on children and adolescents is well documented.[14] It is, for example, known that many survivors of cancer diagnosed in childhood experience both physical problems, such as late effects of chemotherapy and radiotherapy, and an increased risk of additional cancers, and psychosocial problems, such as adjustment difficulties and low self-esteem. However, the implications of long-term survival of adults diagnosed with cancer are somewhat less understood,[15] and thus, this will be a focus for this chapter.

Physiological consequences

Great emphasis has been placed on the various toxicities associated with radiotherapy and different drug treatments. These include, for example, the use of methotrexate in the treatment of gastrointestinal cancers causing abnormal liver function tests, hepatic fibrosis, and cirrhosis, and the use of steroids in bone cancers causing avascular necrosis. Surgical interventions may also cause physiological consequences. For example, women who have had a mastectomy have a 47% chance of developing lymphoedema within a year of surgery,[6] and fatigue and shoulder dysfunction may also occur.[11] It has also been shown that splenectomies can result in a high risk of bacterial infections.[2]

These varied physiological consequences of long-term cancer survival can significantly affect the quality of life of people following treatment for cancer. The following excerpts from transcripts from the Listening Study reveal how such difficulties can affect day-to-day functioning:[13]

> I have something that causes me a great deal of stress. I was given Taxol and Carboplatin and it said in the leaflets that I might experience a tingling in the toes and the fingers and it has left me with peripheral neuropathy, which has really affected by life. I can walk, which is fortunate, by my feet are permanently painful and I have trouble with earrings and doing buttons up and things like that . . . I've accepted it and I think I am well, I can walk, but a little bit more information would have helped.
>
> (Tracy)

> I had cancer of the rectum and since then I've had very bad diarrhoea. I can't go for a coach trip or I can't go very far in a car. When I stand in a queue in a supermarket, it comes over me and I've got to leave my stuff and dash to find a loo . . . My consultant said I had it because he had to cut down so low when he operated. So I asked my GP the other day, 'Will I always have this?'. 'Yes', he said, 'It won't get any better', and so I'm stuck. Wherever I go, I think 'Is there a toilet there?'.
>
> (Rose)

Long-term survivors are also often at greater risk of developing further cancers (a second primary cancer or recurrence).[1] This is due to a range of factors including genetics, lifestyle and habit (for example smoking), and treatment. The average risk for developing further cancers has been estimated to be 10 to 20 times greater in people who have had cancer than the general population, although this varies between different cancer types. For example, the likelihood of developing another cancer among lung cancer patients is 3.2% compared with 1.5–6% in testicular cancer patients.[12] People who have had Hodgkin's disease are at increased risk of developing leukaemia up to 10 years after diagnosis, after which the risk declines. In patients who have had cervical cancer treated with radiotherapy, however, second cancers can occur between 10 and 30 years after diagnosis.[12]

The fear of recurrence in itself generates a significant impact on the lives of cancer survivors with the concern that any new pain could be a sign of a secondary cancer:

> They operated on me and said 'It is fine now. Because we have found everything, it is fine now'. And at the same time I was threatened so much that the doctors told me 'This was the first attack, now if you get a second attack, we can't do anything'. And all the time, that fear is in my mind. Even if I sleep and I have got a little pain, I say, 'I am dying now'.
>
> (Komal)

There is therefore a need for nursing practitioners and other health professionals to recognise the potential long-term impact of cancer and its treatment on the people with cancer, to support their concerns and to provide appropriate information and advice where possible. Furthermore, as treatment regimens are constantly changing and are more often a combination of treatments involving radiotherapy, chemotherapy, and/or surgery, there is a need to continue to monitor the short- and long-term effects of treatment and their impact on a patients' quality of life.

Impact on quality of life

Quality-of-life measures have been developed and used to assess the overall long-term impact having cancer has on cancer survivors. These measures have incorporated various concerns, including the potential impact on physical, psychological, social, and spiritual functioning.[15] It has been suggested from these assessments that most long-term cancer survivors cope well and have a good quality of life following their cancer diagnosis.[16] For example, it has been documented that the majority of men and women surviving bone marrow transplant have reported 'good' to 'excellent' quality of life.[17] Similarly, it has been found that most women surviving ovarian cancer have reported little or no problem with physical well-being.[18] Furthermore, studies with long-term survivors of colorectal, breast and testicular cancer have revealed similar levels of quality of life to those of the general population.[19–21]

However, a problem with assessments of quality of life is that they tend to present an 'overall' picture and thus fail to address specific areas of concern for particular patients.[17,18] Long-term physical problems associated with cancer and its treatment can substantially affect quality of life. For example, the long-term quality of life of cancer survivors who had bone marrow transplant can be affected by a range of difficulties including eye problems, general pain, skin problems, constipation, pulmonary difficulties, nausea/vomiting, sleep disturbance, cognitive dysfunction, and dissatisfaction with sex and intimacy.[17] Similarly, ovarian cancer survivors can experience long-term physical side-effects including abdominal symptoms, difficulty in controlling bowels, gynaecological issues such as menopause, and sexual problems (such as decreased libido).[18] Oesophageal cancer survivors who have undergone oesophageal resection have reported severe long-term problems in swallowing food.[22] Survivors of Hodgkin's disease have also reported significant restrictions in physical functioning and a lower perceived overall health, which has undermined their quality of life.[23]

The experience of diarrhoea amongst survivors of colorectal cancers has been shown to affect their long-term quality of life. One survivor of colorectal cancer in the Listening Study[13] shared his experiences with this problem:

> I've got a problem with my bowel it's when I eat, if I eat something, within ten to fifteen minutes I must go to the toilet and you know there's no ifs or buts about it I've got to go. That's the effect it has on me. My tumour was low down and my consultant said to me it's because they cut so much.
>
> (Alex)

Similarly, Ingrid shared her experience of the long-term effects of her treatment for ovarian cancer:

> I had a surgical menopause, which is quite radical. I suffered quite a lot for that and I suppose still am, but in order to keep off the vaginal dryness in the skin, the hot flushes, [I was offered to] take HRT [hormone replacement therapy]
>
> (Ingrid)

Long-term physiological effects of cancer and its treatment can have an impact on the psychological and social well-being of survivors. For example, fatigue has been identified as a significant factor in affecting the emotional and cognitive functioning of survivors of oesophageal cancer, and dry mouth has been shown to be an important factor influencing poorer social functioning.[22]

The impact of long-term cancer survival on quality of life does not affect people uniformly but has been shown to be related to a range of factors including type of cancer, stage and age at diagnosis, nature of treatment, and socio-economic status.[24]

Psychological consequences

The long-term psychological implications following the onset of cancer have often been neglected by health professionals. This is due in part to patients tending to raise only physical problems with health care professionals and only discussing other matters when asked directly.[11] A range of psychological responses to survival have been identified, including denial, anger, hostility, and emotional repression, although there has been disagreement regarding how these responses should be interpreted. While many view these responses negatively, some commentators have suggested that they are important aspects of coping that should not be discouraged.[3] Commonly cited psychological consequences of long-term survivorship include a sense of vulnerability and insecurity,[2] a fear of recurrence,[2] depression or other psychiatric disorders,[12,25] and a poor body image.[7]

In the Listening Study,[13] the fear of recurrence was evident in numerous participants. As Alan describes:

It's always in the back of your mind. You know, you say to yourself, right, I'm going to get on with my life, to hell with it, but at the end of the day, I find that I get up in the morning, you wonder. I took a bad pain in my back and shoulder this last two months and every day I get up, whatever way I turn, it goes again and I just think to myself, 'Has this moved?' It's always in the back of your mind, it just doesn't go away.

(Alan)

One further psychological consequence of having had cancer identified by participants in the study was a certain 'blame mentality', and a sense of guilt in having cancer:

Linda: I do worry that we take on a huge amount when we get cancer. We take on a huge amount of responsibility for our own ailments . . . You know, have I been too porky? Was it that cake I ate?

Neil: Was it that coffee, my 24th I've had today!?

Linda: Absolutely. Did I not go on to decaffeinated soon enough and I do think that we need to be quite careful as well about taking it on ourselves.

The impact of these psychosocial consequences of survivorship is influenced by a range of factors including marital status, gender, level of education, nature of treatment, cancer type, co-morbidity, health status, and attitudes prior to diagnosis.[7,8,12] For example, Dobkin and Morrow suggest that long-term male survivors often experience a decrease in assertiveness and a poorer self-image, while female long-term survivors often experience little change.[8]

Evidence also suggests that there are positive psychological consequences of surviving cancer. Long-term survivors can experience greater appreciation of life, greater emotional intimacy, and a discovery of emotional strength and resilience.[4,8] As Liz put it:

I was diagnosed with colon cancer, I had an irreversible colonoscopy done. I had radiotherapy and I had chemotherapy. I finished that and I returned to full time work. And I'm having a ball, I really am, I learnt a lesson that there's more to life than just sitting watching paint peel . . . I know it sounds a terrible thing to say, but do you know there's a good side to cancer as well, it gives you a wake-up call, it really does.

(Liz)

Research has also sought to examine whether psychological status can directly influence cancer survival. The issue of whether 'positive thinking' can increase survival is highly contested. Many participants in the Listening Study held a firm belief that a positive attitude was an important factor both in terms of fighting cancer and in preventing recurrence:

I think one of the things that research has shown is that those who are positive are more likely to come out the other side than if you're negative, so fighting that depression is really important.

(Liz).

However, one recently published systematic review found little evidence to support the view that psychological coping (for example a fighting spirit, stoic acceptance or problem-focused coping) had any influence on the length of survival.[26] In contrast, Walker and colleagues have suggested that there is evidence that relaxation and imagery can generate a better immune response, and draw on findings from research into the psychoneuroimmunological effects of stress to suggest that psychological factors can potentially prolong survival.[27]

Evidence does suggest that levels of psychological distress among long-term survivors are generally similar to those of the general population.[28] However, it does appear that for a minority of survivors, there are higher levels of psychological distress. Fear of follow-up diagnostic tests, recurrence, or secondary cancers are common sources of ongoing psychological distress for some survivors.[18] The following exchange from one of the discussion groups in the Listening Study illustrates common concerns of secondary cancers:

Linda: If I have a headache, it's gone to my brain.

Audrey: You don't have headaches, you have brain tumours, don't you!

Linda: I cough, therefore it is in my lungs!

Research has found that survivors of colorectal and testicular cancer report significantly more psychological problems including depression and anxiety than the general population.[19,29] Again, fear of recurrence may persist for breast cancer survivors, impacting on their levels of anxiety and depression.[24] Breast cancer, Hodgkin's lymphoma, and leukaemia survivors have also been found to suffer post-traumatic stress disorders; some can experience such disorders more than 20 years after diagnosis.[30]

Survivors of lung, head, and neck cancers appear to be particularly vulnerable to psychological distress. Maliski *et al.*, for example, found that nearly one-third of the long-term lung cancer survivors involved in their study were clinically depressed, resulting in inadequate self-care.[31] Similarly, another study of head and neck cancer survivors treated with radiotherapy revealed that nearly one-third of participants reported high levels of distress 7–11 years after treatment when they were no longer receiving support.[32]

The experience of psychological difficulties is often related to a range of factors. The number of years of survivorship following diagnosis, for example, is an important factor in the level of psychological distress.[33] The experience of depressive symptoms is also related to the extent to which there is a long-term impact on quality of life, particularly with disruption to 'life-roles' (such as work, looking after a family, etc).[34] The risk of psychological problems has also been associated with low socio-economic status for survivors of colorectal and head and neck cancers.[19,32] Long-term survivors of head and neck cancers may be more susceptible to psychological problems due to the association of head and neck cancers with alcohol abuse and low social class.[32]

The experience of psychological distress by cancer patients typically decreases over time.[33] Numerous coping strategies have been used by cancer survivors, including positive thinking (using positive affirmations, relaxation), helping others, confronting reality, and spirituality.[35] In addition, evidence suggests that cancer survivors would also like a counselling programme to discuss long-term side-effects, and a support programme to be offered during their initial treatment.[18] It is evident, therefore, that nursing professionals can have role to play in supporting and alleviating the psychological consequences of long-term cancer survival.

The family and personal relationships

Cancer survival can have a significant impact on the family or personal relationships. Children, partners, and other relatives have been referred to as 'secondary survivors' of cancer. Consequently they can have physical and psychological responses to their relative's cancer, including depression, a sense of isolation, difficulties with sleep, financial concerns, and a sense of 'caregiver burden'.[3] Children of adults with cancer can be similarly affected, experiencing a fear of death and concerns about how they would manage in the future.[3] These experiences have been shown to vary in terms of gender amongst adults (with women reporting more distress than men), and developmental levels of children.[3]

The evidence is contradictory on the long-term impact cancer has on personal relationships. While some long-term survivors experience difficulty in establishing and maintaining intimate relationships, others have reported a sense of being closer to their partner following their diagnosis.[2] For example, female breast cancer survivors have expressed satisfaction with marital relationships,[20] as have survivors of chronic myeloid leukaemia.[36]

Similarly, evidence for the impact of cancer survivorship on friendships and social networks is also confused. It has been suggested, for example, that survivors of testicular cancer are more likely to retain friendships than the general population.[21] However, evidence also suggests that survivors of various cancers do report significant concerns about social and emotional support. Patients can, for example, experience a lack of support in their own lives where there are no new relationships and/or improvements in their existing relationships. Survivors of breast cancer have reported that while relatives may become closer, friends often avoided them.[37] Furthermore, Bush *et al.* found that in their study of bone marrow transplant recipients, nearly all participants reported that people became less supportive over time. This was found to be a particularly distressing aspect of long-term survival.[17]

Findings from the Listening Study revealed additional considerations for families of cancer survivors.[13] Many participants commented on what they perceived to be a lack of awareness of the support needs of families and friends:

> It's very important for your family to see you functioning normally, because I don't know about you, I mean I feel I can deal with breast cancer because it's happening to me, but the rest of my family can't deal with it, because they feel so totally incapable of helping me and anything that I can do to be as normal as possible is so important also for them and I think they get lost in this, because we tend to be the centre of attention and they get very lost in the whole thing and they're not supported in the way that we're supported.
>
> (Anita)

Anita went on to provide examples of the potential impact having cancer can have on the family:

> My cousin by marriage had prostate cancer, which he battled with for eleven years and his wife's parents have been very stressed by this and they've had illnesses over the period themselves, which I'm sure is down to how much they were worrying about the situation and being run down as a result of it as people do.
>
> (Anita)

Hence the concern of the impact of long-term survivorship of cancer goes beyond changes in the relationship between the person with the disease and his or her family to the impact cancer has on family members directly.

Sexual problems

Sexual problems are a relatively common occurrence in the general population of healthy individuals, but specific problems may result from cancer and its treatment. Sexual problems have been found amongst survivors of breast, gynaecological, and testicular cancer, as well as with leukaemia and lymphoma.[17,18,21,23,38] Ashing-Giwa *et al.* found in their study of Caucasian and African-American breast survivors that sexual function was the only area of concern.[39]

Long-term cancer survivors can experience difficulties with sexual relationships, often resulting from fatigue as a consequence of treatment, altered body image, or damage to or removal of sexual organs.[11] Among young breast cancer sur-

vivors, for example, vaginal dryness associated with hormones is commonly experienced, as is a lack of sexual desire, difficulty with arousal, a lack of sexual enjoyment, and a sense of embarrassment about their bodies.[38] The severity of vaginal dryness is clearly a significant factor impacting on the sexual function of long-term survivors. Survivors of breast cancer treated with adjuvant chemotherapy have reported greater sexual difficulties than the general population, with a lack of sexual interest, a lack of sexual enjoyment, and a lack of arousal being notable problems.[40]

Sexual difficulties are also prevalent in female survivors of clear cell adenocarcinoma of the vagina or cervix, with a reduced sexual interest/drive, inorgasmia, and painful intercourse being commonly cited problems.[34] These ongoing sexual problems have been so significant that they have been linked to depressive symptoms.

Survivors of testicular cancer have also reported impaired sexual life as a pronounced problem. Infertility, a decrease in sexual enjoyment, and a decrease in desire have been cited as being particularly prevalent amongst testicular long-term cancer survivors.[21] As a consequence of toxicity related to chemotherapy and radiotherapy, sperm banking has been used as a solution to infertility.[11]

Changes in body image since diagnosis also had an impact on reported sexual problems. One study of bone marrow transplant survivors revealed that over one-quarter of participants were dissatisfied with their appearance, which had an impact on their sexual functioning. They were also dissatisfied with their sexual appeal, ability to share warmth and intimacy, or interest in sexual thoughts or feelings.[17] Survivors of Hodgkin's disease have similarly reported significantly less satisfaction with their sexual lives compared with the general population.[23]

In the Listening Study, participants drew attention to the impact of cancer on sex and sexuality:

> That's another side to the after effects of cancer. Most of us here would have had intimate problems after our treatment. As a woman, if you've had breast cancer, that's bound to have interfered with your intimate life.

As a man, if you've had testicular cancer, that's bound to have interfered with your intimate life. In my case, I have a bag, it's bound to have interfered with my intimate life. I was more afraid than my partner was, but I didn't realise that until maybe, actually until July this year, my husband and I went on a cruise and I went to all sorts of trouble to try and make it as discreet as I possibly could and he said, 'I don't care, he said, I love you, it's not the bag'. And I was very lucky in that respect. It's not just having the chemotherapy and the radiotherapy, your life is different afterwards.

(Liz)

Hence, it is clear that there are significant problems with sexuality experienced by long-term cancer survivors that can potentially have a considerable impact on quality of life.

Employment, finances and insurance

Cancer and its treatment may impact on an individual's ability to work. Individuals may be discriminated against due to their cancer diagnosis or may be unable to work in the same capacity following their diagnosis and subsequent treatment.[7]

Barbara, a participant in the Listening Study, shared her experiences of discrimination in the police force:

My employers actually were very good they kept me on full pay because I think they thought I was going to die! But then when I went back to work to see the force doctor, because I'm a police officer, he threatened to sack me because he said, 'Because you've got a high risk of getting cancer again, I don't think you'll be effective as a police officer'. So on one hand they were very good financially 'til I got back to work, then the doctor said, 'Oh well, because you can get cancer again he said you're not going to be effective as an officer in the future'.

(Barbara)

The ability to work will, inevitably, have implications for the level of income and financial support. Relatives and friends may need to take time off work to support the person with cancer, which can add to the financial burden. Treatment may also be demanding financially where regular trips to hospital can be costly. Linda, for example, complained about the cost of treatment:

About state benefits and prescription charges and the wackiness in that some of us are getting DLA, Disability Living Allowance, and some of us aren't. Some of us, the GPs would sign the piece of paper that said you are not likely to live longer than six months and some of us they wouldn't. Some of the ailments that you can have where you get free prescriptions are less serious than the ailments we have. So why do we have to pay for prescriptions?

(Linda)

Little is known about employment or economic issues faced by long-term cancer survivors. The experiences of breast cancer survivors have been compared with those of the general population, where it was found that survivors did experience a reduction in total market earnings while the general population had a rise of annual earnings.[41] This was due, however, largely to a reduction in the number of hours worked rather than changes in pay level, and no significant differences were found between survivors and the healthy comparison group in changes in total income or assets.

It does appear that the majority of long-term survivors do not experience a change in their socio-economic position, although differences have been noted between cancer types.[42] Survivors of head and neck cancers, for example, have been found to be less likely to return to work than patients with reproductive, lymphatic, breast, or skin cancers, although this may be attributable to the fact that patients of this cancer type are typically older.

Problems obtaining insurance have also been commonly reported. van der Wouden *et al.*, for example, have found that of survivors who had tried to take out insurance or modify an existing insurance policy, nearly 90% had experienced difficulties.[42] Similarly, survivors of Hodgkin's disease have reported greater difficulty in obtaining life insurance in comparison with the general population.[23] This was commented on in the Listening Study:

Travel, that was a big part of my life, travelling, I loved to travel and I can't get travel insurance. I can, but it costs more than the holiday, you know and this is something else that I don't want to have to give up, but I'm having to accept it and I can't drive, either, because my eyesight's affected. So, I feel very much cut off, I can't work, I can't drive, I can't travel. Life has had to take a completely different turn.

(Fred)

Difficulties in obtaining financial loans have been noted by survivors of Hodgkin's disease, women with breast cancer, and men with testicular cancer.[21,23,41] van Tulder *et al.* have also found that survivors of Hodgkin's disease have had particular problems, for medical reasons, in obtaining a mortgage.[23] It is evident therefore from the little research undertaken in this area that some long-term cancer patients do face particular financial and employment difficulties.

Assessing the long-term impact of cancer on survivors

Formulating any overall assessment on the impact of long-term survivorship is difficult for, as Gotay and Muraoka comment, research undertaken in this area is typically too diverse in terms of study approaches and definitions to allow any conclusive or general comments to be generated.[4] There is still no standard definition of 'long-term survival'. While the definition of 5 or more years from the point of diagnosis appears to be the most commonly used criterion in long-term survivorship studies, it is apparent that certain cancer types may be excluded when using this definition, due to decreased numbers surviving beyond 5 years. The definition of a 'long-term' survivor therefore needs to be altered according to different cancers. Even within the area of quality of life, definitions and assessment tools are varied, making conclusive comments difficult to generate.

A recent review of the literature conducted by Foster *et al.*[15] has also highlighted further limitations with the cancer survivorship literature. First, much of the research conducted to date has drawn upon self-report postal questionnaires based on a variety of quality-of-life measurements. However, the use of qualitative methods may be more appropriate given the need to explore issues of survivorship in greater detail and in terms derived from the survivors' perspective.

Second, much of the evidence on survivorship is from the perspective of female breast cancer survivors and therefore does not represent the experiences of a wide range of different cancer types. As Bloom *et al.* comment, focusing on women with breast cancer may result in accessing mainly well-educated and employed participants.[38] Third, it is significant that research on long-term survivorship has predominantly been undertaken in the US and with Caucasian participants, again limiting the representativeness of available findings. This is compounded by the fact that most research in this area to date has been based on small population samples that, while being helpful for exploratory purposes, undermine their generalisation to wider populations.

Nevertheless, despite these limitations, several summary comments can be made. It is apparent that the majority of people living long term after cancer diagnoses have a good quality of life with few or no psychosocial consequences. Indeed for some a cancer diagnosis can yield a positive outcome whereby survivors can feel strengthened by the experience, have a greater appreciation of life, and refrain from taking life for granted.

However, a substantial minority of individuals do report long-term problems, and hence issues of survivorship do warrant attention. These include physical problems (limited movement, secondary cancers), psychological consequences (anxiety, depression, post-traumatic stress disorder), impacts on family and personal relationships (caregiver burden, declining social support), sexual problems (physical and psychological factors), and socio-economic problems (employment, insurance, and credit). Collectively these issues have been shown to affect the quality of life of many cancer survivors, although this does appear to vary between different cancer types, with long-term survivors of lung, head, and neck cancers seeming to be particularly vulnerable to difficulties. As a result of these difficulties, consideration must be given to the most effective and appropriate ways in which issues pertaining to long-term cancer survival can be managed. What this management may mean will now be discussed with particular attention to nursing practice.

Nursing practice and the management of long-term cancer survival problems

It is evident that there is a great need to recognise, manage and support long-term cancer survival difficulties in practice. How these are managed by health professionals has not been extensively considered. In one review of the literature conducted, no studies were found that involved interventions designed to prevent or alleviate psychosocial problems for people living long term with cancer.[43] Only one study was identified which compared the psychosocial well-being and quality of life of women with breast cancer who engaged in a randomised clinical trial that involved an 8-week support group intervention.[43] This intervention involved peer group discussion and education in different combinations. The study found no significant differences in psychosocial well-being or quality of life between breast cancer survivors in different intervention arms or with the general population.

However, research does suggest that there are areas where the difficulties experienced by long-term cancer survivors need to be addressed and supported. For example, cancer survivors have expressed a wish for the creation of counselling programmes to discuss long-term side-effects, and have felt that a support programme should be offered during their initial treatment.[18]

It is evident that psychological consequences of long-term survival are significant and warrant careful management. Thomas *et al.* have examined whether a carefully planned discharge from follow-up services could assist in the reduction of levels of anxiety in long-term cancer survivors.[44] They found that despite the provision of continued support, nearly one-third of those participating in their study refused to be discharged, largely due to the fear of a recurrence going undetected. Similar rates of anxiety were found with those who were discharged from the service after 4–5 months, thus suggesting that anxiety was not related to clinic attendance.[44]

Irrespective of the limited evidence available for the most effective means of managing long-term survival difficulties, the recognition of potential implications of long-term survival, the provision of appropriate information, and effective management and monitoring of problems is recommended for nursing practice. These recommendations have been made by cancer patients themselves. For example, participants in the Listening Study had clear ideas about how they would like long-term issues to be managed.

First, participants felt that health professionals should be sensitive and aware of the problems and issues faced by cancer survivors. There was a sense that such professionals failed to recognise the individual and unique needs or circumstances of patients:

> Well, I was offered HRT, I can't believe I was offered it, you know, with my disease [ovarian cancer], because of my problems, after surgical menopause . . . I refused it. I just feel doctors have, don't look into your individual needs.
>
> (Ingrid)

There was a strong sense from participants that nurses should provide an information-giving role, advising long-term survivors of potential difficulties, and acting as a source of advice for patients. In this regard, it was suggested that nurses should be a 'point of contact' for the ongoing concerns of long-term cancer survivors:

> *Audrey*: I get pain in my tummy or something like that, then it starts coming back and my mind goes into overdrive and what do I do then?
>
> *Linda*: Who do you ask?
>
> *Audrey*: You feel, I really can't ring the hospital, the oncology department, and say 'I have got a funny pain in my tummy, what do I do?'. So, you are left floundering. You need somebody. That was the time I actually rang the nurses really. I suppose they are there to help you in that way. And went and had a talk with them.
>
> (CG17)

In addition, the importance of information sharing was not related solely to concerns of alleviating or generating awareness of long-term problems, but was also needed to let cancer patients know what support services were available locally.

Nurses also have a role in the ongoing monitoring of long-term cancer survivors, as already described. However, patients have recommended that health professionals generally should provide better long-term health management:

> Planned maintenance. If you think we were an industrial country, we started with an amazing amount of factories and machines. If one breaks down, then that machine would be put under a specific plan of maintenance. If you are broken down then they should be looking to stop you breaking down again. And rather than go into emergency mode when you break down, they are very good in emergency mode, I think, the NHS. When you kick into that, they are second to none. But it's the in-between bit, where most of us live, most of our time.
>
> (Kevin)

Finally participants in the Listening Study also made recommendations for the management of long-term survival problems. In addition to the information, monitoring and management already outlined, the benefits of peer support were also recommended. As Stephanie stated:

> We all feel a little better after just talking, you know, so I think it does help a lot. It's someone to talk to other than the family. I mean we've all got over that stage where we were poorly and alone and we've pushed ourselves on but it's still at the back of your mind, you know. Do you do that kind of thing, do you think that kind of thing, it's hard to cope with being alone sometimes.
>
> (Stephanie)

These facets of support for long-term cancer survivors and their families – information, education, and peer support – have formed the basis of many management strategies of patient advocacy groups. These groups have been particularly active in the US, providing committed support for long-term survivors, and training programmes for health professionals.

The American Cancer Society, for example, has formed the Cancer Survivors Network, aiming to provide an online resource for cancer survivors, family, and friends. The Network allows members to browse discussion forums and correspond with others as well as providing information about support programmes and services that provide support for cancer survivors. Areas of support are diverse and include help for survivors of prostate cancer and assistance for female cancer patients concerning beauty techniques to help them restore their appearance and self-image.

Similarly, the National Coalition for Cancer Survivors (NCCS) was established in the US in 1986 and involved experts on employment and disability issues, health care and psychosocial and behavioural research.[45] A core concern of the NCCS is education, centring on the belief that cancer patients should better understand the impact of the disease 'on a physical, emotional, social and economic level'.[45] In an effort to provide such an education resource, the NCCS launched its 'Cancer Survival Toolbox' in 1998, in association with organisations such as the Oncology Nursing Society. Although the toolbox was aimed primarily at patients recently diagnosed with cancer, it is also of relevance to all those who have been affected by the disease. The Cancer Survival Toolbox has also been designed for use by health professionals who wish to support cancer survivors. Again, the need for understanding and awareness of survival issues, the necessity for information sharing, and the need to provide effective peer support is called for.

Consequently, while the literature on the most effective means of managing problems associated with long-term survival is sparse, it is possible to make recommendations on the basis of patients' views and the work of advocacy groups:

- nurses should remain aware of the varied physical and psychosocial implications of long-term survival on cancer patients
- nurses should remain sensitive to the concerns and difficulties of long-term cancer survivors and ensure that the care they provide is attuned to the specific needs of the survivor
- appropriate and effective sources of information should be provided to patients and their families at the point of diagnosis so that they can expect what may happen in the future
- where feasible, nurses should utilise the fact that they are seen as a potential 'point of contact' and be prepared to respond to queries or concerns associated with long-term cancer survival
- long-term cancer survivors and their families should be provided with information of counselling and support services, including peer support groups

- long-term survival problems should be monitored and managed, and follow-up programmes should be established where appropriate.

Conclusions

With improvements in treatment, it is inevitable that the numbers of long-term cancer survivors will continue to rise. It is necessary therefore that the difficulties long-term cancer survivors experience are identified and effectively managed. It is apparent from this chapter that while many long-term survivors appear to be living well, significant problems exist for a substantial number of survivors. Survivors of head, neck, or lung cancer appear to be the most vulnerable, although survivors of other cancers also report persistent problems. Consequently, a substantial proportion of individuals do experience challenges in the long term and thus may require appropriate additional formal and informal support.

The definition of long-term survival and quality of life needs further examination, and more research is needed to explore the long-term impact of survival on people and how this is managed. Nursing practitioners can support long-term cancer survivors by being aware and sympathetic of their problems, offer information and advice, and be part of ongoing monitoring programmes. The identification and management of problems faced by long-term cancer survivors is imperative for, as Western populations continue to age and diversify, the importance of survivorship issues is only set to increase in the near future.

References

1. Denmark-Wahnefried W., Aziz N.M., Rowland J.H. and Pinto B.M. (2005). Riding the crest of the teachable moment: promoting long-term health after the diagnosis of cancer. *Journal of Clinical Oncology* **23**, 5814–5830.
2. Ganz P.A. (2001). Late effects of cancer and its treatment. *Seminars in Oncology Nursing* **17**, 241–248.
3. Dow K.H. (2003). Seventh National Conference on Cancer Nursing Research keynote address: challenges and opportunities in cancer survivorship research. *Oncology Nursing Forum* **30**, 455–469.
4. Gotay C.C. and Muraoka M.Y. (1998). Quality of life in long-term survivors of adult-onset cancers. *Journal of the National Cancer Institute* **90**, 656–667.
5. National Council for Hospice and Specialist Palliative Care Services. (2002). *Definitions of Supportive and Palliative Care.* Briefing paper. London: National Council for Hospice and Specialist Palliative Care Services.
6. Tesauro G.M., Rowland J.H. and Lustig C. (2002). Survivorship resources for post-treatment cancer survivors. *Cancer Practice* **10**, 277–283.
7. Kornblith A.B., Herndon J.E., Zuckerman E. *et al.* (1998). Comparison of psychosocial adaptation of advanced stage Hodgkin's disease and acute leukemia survivors. Cancer and Leukemia Group B. *Annals of Oncology* **9**, 297–306.
8. Dobkin P.L. and Morrow G.R. (1987). Long-term side effects in patients who have been treated successfully for cancer. *Journal of Psychosocial Oncology* **3**, 23–51.
9. Little M. and Sayers E.J. (2004). The skull beneath the skin: cancer survival and awareness of death. *Psycho-oncology* **13**, 190–198.
10. Quigley K.M. (1989). The adult cancer survivor: psychosocial consequences of cure. *Seminars in Oncology Nursing* **5**, 63–69.
11. Ganz P.A. (1990). Current issues in cancer rehabilitation. *Cancer* **65(suppl. 51)**, 742–751.
12. Herold A.H. and Roetzheim R.G. (1992). Cancer survivors. *Primary Care: Clinics in Office Practice* **19**, 779–791.
13. Corner J., Wright D., Foster C. *et al.* (2006). *The Macmillan Listening Study: Listening to the Views of People Affected by Cancer about Cancer Research.* London: Macmillan Cancer Support.
14. Eiser C. and Havermans T. (1994). Long term social adjustment after treatment for childhood cancer. *Archives of Disease in Childhood* **70**, 66–70.
15. Foster C., Wright D., Hill H. and Hopkinson J. (2005). *What are the Implications of Long Term Survival for Cancer Patients?: A Review of the Evidence.* London and Southampton: Macmillan Cancer Relief and University of Southampton.
16. Pedro L.W. (2001). Quality of life for long-term survivors of cancer: influencing variables. *Cancer Nursing* **24**, 1–11.
17. Bush N.E., Haberman M., Donaldson G. and Sullivan K.M. (1995). Quality of life of 125 adults surviving 6–18 years after bone marrow transplantation. *Social Science and Medicine* **40**, 479–490.
18. Wenzel L.B., Donnelly J.P., Fowler J.M. *et al.* (2002). Resilience, reflection, and residual stress in ovarian cancer survivorship: a gynecologic oncology group study. *Psycho-oncology* **11**, 142–153.

19. Ramsey S.D., Berry K., Moinpour C., Giedzinska A. and Andersen M.R. (2002). Quality of life in long term survivors of colorectal cancer. *American Journal of Gastroenterology* **97**, 1228–1234.

20. Dorval M., Maunsell E., Deschenes L., Brisson J. and Masse B. (1998). Long-term quality of life after breast cancer: comparison of 8-year survivors with population controls. *Journal of Clinical Oncology* **16**, 487–494.

21. Joly F., Heron J.F., Kalusinski L. *et al.* (2002). Quality of life in long-term survivors of testicular cancer: a population-based case-control study. *Journal of Clinical Oncology* **20**, 73–80.

22. Hallas C.N., Patel N., Oo A. *et al.* (2001). Five-year survival following oesophageal cancer resection: psychosocial functioning and quality of life. *Psychology Health and Medicine* **6**, 85–94.

23. van Tulder M.W., Aaronson N.K. and Bruning P.F. (1994). The quality of life of long-term survivors of Hodgkin's disease. *Annals of Oncology* **5**, 153–158.

24. Weitzner M.A., Meyers C.A., Stuebing K.K. and Saleeba A.K. (1997). Relationship between quality of life and mood in long-term survivors of breast cancer treated with mastectomy. *Supportive Care in Cancer* **5**, 241–248.

25. Gotay C.C., Blaine D., Haynes S.N., Holup J. and Pagano I.S. (2002). Assessment of quality of life in a multicultural cancer patient population. *Psychological Assessment* **14**, 439–450.

26. Petticrew M., Bell R. and Hunter D. (2002). Influence of psychological coping on survival and recurrence in people with cancer: systematic review. *British Medical Journal* **325**, 1066.

27. Walker L.G., Heys S.D. and Eremin O. (1999). Surviving cancer: do psychosocial factors count? *Journal of Psychosomatic Research* **47**, 497–503.

28. Kurtz M.E., Wyatt G. and Kurtz J.C. (1995). Psychological and sexual well-being, philosophical/spiritual views, and health habits of long-term cancer survivors. *Health Care for Women International* **16**, 253–262.

29. Douchez J., Droz J.P., Desclaux B. *et al.* (1993). Quality of life in long-term survivors of nonseminomatous germ cell testicular tumors. *Journal of Urology* **149**, 498–501.

30. Amir M. and Ramati A. (2002). Post-traumatic symptoms, emotional distress and quality of life in long-term survivors of breast cancer: a preliminary research. *Journal of Anxiety Disorders* **16**, 195–206.

31. Maliski S.L., Sarna L., Evangelista L. and Padilla G. (2003). The aftermath of lung cancer – balancing the good and bad. *Cancer Nursing* **26**, 237–244.

32. Bjordal K. and Kaasa S. (1995). Psychological distress in head and neck cancer patients 7–11 years after curative treatment. *British Journal of Cancer* **71**, 592–597.

33. Grassi L. and Rosti G. (1996). Psychosocial morbidity and adjustment to illness among long-term cancer survivors. A six-year follow-up study. *Psychosomatics* **37**, 523–532.

34. Matthews A.K., Aikens J.E., Helmrich S.P. *et al.* (1999). Sexual functioning and mood among long-term survivors of clear-cell adenocarcinoma of the vagina or cervix. *Journal of Psychosocial Oncology* **17**, 27–45.

35. Halstead M.T. and Fernsler J.I. (1994). Coping strategies of long-term cancer survivors. *Cancer Nursing* **17**, 94–100.

36. Kiss T.L., Abdolell M., Jamal N. *et al.* (2002). Long-term medical outcomes and quality-of-life assessment of patients with chronic myeloid leukemia followed at least 10 years after allogeneic bone marrow transplantation. *Journal of Clinical Oncology* **20**, 2334–2343.

37. Wyatt G., Kurtz M.E. and Liken M. (1993). Breast cancer survivors: an exploration of quality of life issues. *Cancer Nursing* **16**, 440–448.

38. Bloom J.R., Stewart S.L., Chang S. and Banks P.J. (2004). Then and now: quality of life of young breast cancer survivors. *Psycho-oncology* **13**, 147–160.

39. Ashing-Giwa K., Ganz P.A. and Petersen L. (1999). Quality of life of African-American and white long term breast carcinoma survivors. *Cancer* **85**, 418–426.

40. Broeckel J.A., Thors C.L., Jacobsen P.B., Small M. and Cox C.E. (2002). Sexual functioning in long-term breast cancer survivors treated with adjuvant chemotherapy. *Breast Cancer Research and Treatment* **75**, 241–248.

41. Chirikos T.N., Russell-Jacobs A. and Cantor A.B. (2002). Indirect economic effects of long-term breast cancer survival. *Cancer Practice* **10**, 248–255.

42. van der Wouden J.C., Greaves-Otte J.G., Greaves J. *et al.* (1992). Occupational reintegration of long-term cancer survivors. *Journal of Occupational Medicine* **34**, 1084–1089.

43. Tomich P.L. and Helgeson V.S. (2002). Five years later: a cross-sectional comparison of breast cancer survivors with healthy women. *Psycho-oncology* **11**, 154–169.

44. Thomas S.F., Glynne-Jones R., Chait I. and Marks D.F. (1997). Anxiety in long-term cancer survivors influences the acceptability of planned discharge from follow-up. *Psycho-oncology* **6**, 190–196.

45. National Coalition for Cancer Survivors. (2004). *We Speak: 2004 Annual Report*. Silver Spring, MD: National Coalition for Cancer Survivors.

CHAPTER THIRTY-FOUR

Self-management and self-help

Claire Foster

Advances in the diagnosis and treatment of cancer mean that more people are living with cancer and problems associated with the disease process and treatment.[1] People living with such problems are generally managing these as part of their daily lives. Many people want to have an active role in tackling problems associated with their cancer, and find ways to manage problems themselves. This chapter explores what the research evidence tells us about what people do to help themselves when living with problems associated with their cancer and its treatment; the knowledge base to enable nurses and others to help support people affected by cancer to help themselves is currently limited. The terms self-management and self-help are used to describe activities that individuals engage in to help themselves manage particular problems they are facing associated with their cancer and its treatment.

Self-management

Self-management is not a well-defined concept for people living with cancer (unpublished observations Foster C., Hopkinson J., Hill H. and Wright D. (2005). Macmillan Cancer Support and University of Southampton) but it is relatively well defined within the literature relating to people living with long-term, chronic conditions such as arthritis and diabetes. In this context self-management:

. . . involves [the person with the chronic disease] engaging in activities that protect and promote health, monitoring and managing the symptoms and signs of illness, managing the impact of illness on functioning, emotions and interpersonal relationships and adhering to treatment [p.1].[2]

Self-management is also about enabling the person with the condition:

. . . to make informed choices, to adapt new perspectives and generic skills that can be applied to new problems as they arise, to practise new health behaviours, and to maintain or regain emotional stability [p.11].[3]

Having an active role in managing long-term health conditions is viewed as important, as it can empower patients to act for themselves, increase confidence in their ability to manage problems associated with the disease and its treatment, and enhance quality of life.[4,5] Self-management is:

. . . aimed at helping the participant become an active, not adversarial, partner with health care providers. Chronic disease is best treated by a balance of traditional medical care and the day-to-day practice of self management skills [p. 11].[3]

Self-management and medical care are likely to be enhanced by a collaborative approach.[6]

Patients and clinicians are both considered experts on the patients' problems; the consultation is, therefore, a meeting between experts in which the experiential expert (the patient) meets with the clarification expert (the physician). In this view, the object of the consultation is not to convert the patient to the physician's point of view, but to enlist the patient as a therapeutic ally and to negotiate mutually acceptable plans for enhancing the patient's well-being [p.1358].[7]

Key self-management tasks for chronic illness include:

- medical management (e.g. taking medication, adhering to dietary recommendations, using inhaler)
- lifestyle change (e.g. exercise, diet)
- managing emotional consequences of the chronic condition (e.g. fear, anger, frustration, depression)
- maintaining/changing and creating new and meaningful behaviours or life roles (e.g. moderating activity)
- communicating effectively with health care professionals.[8,9]

This approach acknowledges medical and psychosocial components, and is aimed at empowering individuals though proactive and adaptive strategies.

Self-management programmes have been established in the US, Canada, Australia, and more recently the UK.[10] These programmes are designed to enhance self-efficacy (confidence in one's ability to achieve a particular outcome) through skill mastery, role modelling, persuasion, reinterpretation of symptoms, problem solving, decision making, and action planning,[9] to help patients with the above tasks. The theory is that individuals learn by doing and this enhances self-efficacy and confidence to manage illness-related problems themselves. The programmes also prepare patients to collaborate with their health care professionals and the health care system.

Self-management programmes have been effective for people with arthritis, who have reported increased perceptions of control, improved quality of life, reduced pain (despite greater disability), less depressed mood, and fewer visits to their physician in the 4 years following the programme.[3,11] Similar benefits have been reported by those attending courses for people with various chronic

conditions.[12] People with cancer have not been included in published research relating to self-management programmes to date.

There is clear interest in and emphasis on patient self-management in the UK. Recent policy from the Department of Health is encouraging a move towards partnership between health professionals and patients. A clear example is the piloting of the Expert Patient Programme for patients living with chronic conditions.[13] The central message of this programme is that having an active role in managing one's own chronic condition enhances quality of life.

Changes in health care provision

Our health care system was initially set up to tackle acute conditions, and as such the role of the health care provider was to diagnose and treat.[8] With acute conditions the patient is generally inexperienced and relies on the expertise of the health care professional. In recent times, chronic conditions have become the focus of the health care system. With long-term conditions, the role of the health care provider is different as people affected by the condition develop expertise about the condition, manage it, and live with the consequences on a daily basis.

> When you leave the clinic, you still have a long term condition. When the visiting nurse leaves your home, you still have a long term condition. In the middle of the night, you fight the pain alone. At the weekend, you manage without your home help. Living with a long term condition is a great deal more than medical or professional assistance.[14]

Coulter emphasises the need for patients to be encouraged to see themselves as active participants in their health and illness (including shaping health policy), and that health care professionals have to change their behaviour to accommodate this new role by becoming facilitators.[15] Active partnerships between patients and health care professionals would call for a 'culture change' in the NHS. Self-management programmes prepare patients to collaborate with health care professionals and navigate the health care system. If such a culture change is to take place it would seem sensible that this is a collaborative effort between health care professionals and patients.

To enable true partnership between health care professionals and people affected by cancer, and to help support individuals to enhance their physical and psychosocial well-being, we need to build a better understanding of what people do to help themselves. Failure to address the social nature of illness (the context in which individuals live e.g. socio-economic, cultural elements and how people manage to support themselves) may affect the ability to provide services that are acceptable to service users.[16] In order to explore the social nature of cancer and what people do to help themselves it is necessary to conduct carefully designed research which would enable consideration of these issues.

Living with cancer

There is undoubtedly a need to explore what people do to help themselves when living with cancer, both within and beyond self-management programmes – in particular, to know whether this enhances a sense of control or confidence in one's ability to manage symptoms and other problems associated with cancer and its treatment. A recent literature review has explored self-management and self-help by people living with cancer (unpublished observations Foster C., Hopkinson J., Hill H. and Wright D. (2005). Macmillan Cancer Support and University of Southampton). The evidence identified in this review is summarised in this section.

Three terms are frequently used to describe actions that people engage in to help them live with their cancer and associated problems: self-care, self-management, and self-help. Self-care and self-management are frequently used interchangeably. For the purposes of this chapter the term self-management by people living with cancer will be used to describe the following:

- usual, *everyday self-care* such as eating, exercise, washing and dressing. These behaviours may be modified according to symptoms experienced or efforts to prevent future difficulties and can therefore be proactive or reactive

- *medical management* of the cancer, symptoms or disease process by the patient. Examples would be self-medication for pain, vomiting, or other symptoms. These actions could be initiated to avoid or control disease symptoms and treatment side-effects, and may be proactive (to prevent) or reactive (to control or treat).

This definition of self-management is clearly narrower than that used in the chronic illness literature, but reflects the research evidence to date.

Self-help is a term used to refer to a vast array of activities. They are activities that people may engage in which are non-medical, to enhance physical and/or psychosocial well-being. Examples include attending support groups, use of complementary and alternative therapies (hereafter referred to as CAM), and information seeking. Self-help can be proactive (to prevent problems or maintain current state) or reactive (in response to particular need or difficulty) (unpublished observations Foster C., Hopkinson J., Hill H. and Wright D. (2005). Macmillan Cancer Support and University of Southampton).

Symptoms and other consequences following a cancer diagnosis

Cancer is often referred to as a chronic or long-term condition, however this is contested.[17] Although the nature of cancer is changing and more people are surviving and living with the disease, it does not sit easily alongside chronic conditions such as diabetes, arthritis, or depression. The term *cancer* describes a set of diseases with different causes, symptoms, treatment options, and prognoses. Many people diagnosed with cancer may have been symptom free. A cancer diagnosis brings great uncertainty, and is often followed by immediate, aggressive, physically, and emotionally demanding treatment which can have visible effects (e.g. scarring, hair loss, weight loss/gain) and/or impair functions of the body (e.g. digestive problems, erectile dysfunction). Treatment can cause symptoms and side-effects that are often immediate and may remain following treatment. These side-effects can be debilitating. Where an individual may effectively have been cured of their cancer, some people continue to experience long-term effects (such as physical and psychosocial problems) many years following treatment.[18] Problems are often complex, and some patients may need long-term support that is frequently provided by informal carers in the home or community. In addition, with an ageing population the number of people living with cancer is set to rise, and many will have multiple conditions. Although mortality associated with cancer remains high in many instances, there has been a necessary shift in emphasis towards 'living with cancer' and how people affected by cancer can be supported to do this. While we can draw on the literature relating to chronic conditions, to inform our understanding of self-management (i.e. what it is, what it means, how it may be effective in helping people to live with cancer), it is important to have in mind that a diagnosis of cancer is different in many respects from living with long-term conditions where the function of treatment is often to alleviate or prevent symptoms.

How do people with cancer manage symptoms and other consequences of cancer and treatment themselves?

Self-management
There is very little research evidence to indicate what people do to help themselves live with symptoms or the progression of cancer. A handful of studies have focused on self-management to:

- alleviate side-effects associated with treatment (chemotherapy and radiotherapy)
- make dietary modification to promote health.

There is almost no evidence to suggest how people self-manage particular symptoms beyond treatment.

Common side-effects associated with chemotherapy (adjuvant and palliative) include: fatigue, sleep difficulty, nausea and vomiting, reduced appetite, changes in taste/smell, mouth sores, and weakness. Patients have reported managing side-effects by sleeping, distraction, reading, watching TV, changing eating patterns, and cleaning their mouth more often.[19] Delay of more than 24 hours in initiating self-management strategies for particular symptoms is unusual. However, delay may occur when symptoms are severe or debilitating,[20] and when patients are experiencing fatigue.[21] Self-management strategies used to tackle specific symptoms have been reported to give some degree of relief,[21] or rated as 'moderately effective'.[20]

A prospective study has explored self-management by women with breast cancer (stage I or II) during and post radiotherapy.[22] Self-management strategies included managing feelings (e.g. distraction, verbally expressing feelings), managing stress (e.g. writing in a diary, cognitive restructuring, reading, taking a holiday, visiting friends, shopping), living life to the fullest/having more appreciation of life, resting, taking exercise, changing diet, and communicating effectively with health care professionals. Reasons for initiating self-management strategies included the view that this was a more natural and sensible course of action.[21]

No research appears to specifically explore self-management by people in terms of medical treatment and related activities. Some researchers mention (unspecified) medication and anti-emetic medication taken by patients in response to nausea and vomiting which was rated as moderately effective.[21] There is no evidence to indicate what enables people to medically self-manage problems associated with cancer and treatment.

In terms of health promotion, self-management strategies to reduce the risk of recurrence or detect early signs of cancer include dietary change (reducing meat/dessert intake and increasing fruit/vegetable consumption) following diagnosis of localised breast cancer treated with surgery,[23] and having symptoms checked for early diagnosis.[24]

Self-help
Studies investigating aspects of self-help indicate that people engage in a number of self-help activities for their perceived psychological, social and physical benefits when living with cancer. Examples include attending support groups, establishing support networks (both formal and informal), use of complementary and alternative medicine

(CAM), and seeking information. Patients may engage in self-help activities in response to a particular problem or to prevent or ward off problems.

Accessibility of groups and the belief that the group will provide a safe environment to express feelings, meet others in a similar situation, make new friends, learn more about cancer and treatment, and share problems has been related to support group attendance.[25] People with strong emotional support from their family or friends may be less likely to attend a support group than those that do not have such support.[26] Women attending a self-help group have reported enjoying helping others in the group, receiving a high degree of support from the group in return, and feeling empowered by offering support to others.[26] Men have reported being more assertive and taking responsibility for their health following support group attendance.[27]

Many studies refer to *complementary* therapies: things people do to enhance physical and psychological well-being alongside conventional treatment (although the term 'alternative' is at times used to describe what appear to be complementary actions). Essentially, studies report anything and everything that people do in an attempt to enhance physical and/or psychological well-being when living with cancer, and this is generally complementary to conventional health care. Few studies report use of alternative therapies – that is those chosen instead of conventional health care.

Boon *et al.* have described factors that influence decision making in relation to CAM use: fixed factors (e.g. gender, age, cancer type, stage) which are not amenable to change, and flexible factors (e.g. knowledge, attitudes, beliefs, availability) which are.[28] Younger patients and those educated to a higher level appear more likely to use CAM.[29] Availability and accessibility of CAM are clearly important for use.[30] Literature about CAM has been described as more readily available and appealing than biomedical literature.[31] The relationship with a CAM practitioner has also been described as appealing. Family and friends are often sources of knowledge and information about CAM,[32,33] and physicians are less likely to be informed of use.[34]

Attitudes and beliefs are key to CAM use. Use has been associated with holistic views about health rather than dissatisfaction with conventional medicine,[35] although previous negative experiences with conventional medicine have been associated with more CAM use.[30] Some patients may see conventional treatment as incompatible with active patient involvement in disease management.[36] Where CAM is viewed to have some influence over cancer it is more likely to be used.[28,30] Where CAM is viewed as important for psychological well-being, motivations for use include: a need to gain/increase/maintain sense/illusion of control, improve quality of life, maintain hope, reduce stress, and enhance coping.[29,37,38]

Sources of information about cancer include the internet, leaflets, books, community education, friends with cancer, and friends who are health care professionals.[39] People have reported seeking information to gain a sense of control, increase their confidence and security, and enable active participation in decision making.[40] Information may be avoided to bypass subsequent feelings of worry, through fear or because information is perceived as negative and/or depressing. Women with metastatic breast cancer have reported seeking information and perceived that it helped them with their own situation and personal future planning.[41] They have also reported seeking information regarding their medical situation, symptoms and how to act on them, treatment options, how to obtain counselling, homecare services, how to access CAM, and how to talk to relatives about cancer.[41]

The internet is a popular source of information. Internet use to access cancer-related information has been described as potentially empowering among breast cancer patients on chemotherapy.[42] Accessibility, familiarity, and trust were key factors influencing internet use. Information found on the internet is often used in discussions with health care professionals.

Limitations of the research evidence

Research into self-management by people living with cancer is scarce, although more is known about self-help. There are numerous limitations of the evidence. For example, there is little or no consideration of age, gender, or ethnicity in relation to self-management or self-help by people living with cancer. Nor are cancer sites or stage of the disease considered. This matters, because in order to support people in ways most appropriate to their needs or circumstances it is necessary to know if people have different needs at different times in their life, if there are gender differences, and differences according to ethnicity, socioeconomic status and so on. Cross-sectional studies (assessment at one time point) do not allow for exploration of change over time. Various recruitment strategies have been used, including individuals responding to advertisements, attending support groups, patients receiving CAM, and clinical populations. In order to have a broad picture of what people do to help themselves when living with cancer it is important to go beyond those who are already engaged in self-help groups or related activities, and include individuals who are engaging in self-management of symptoms and other problems in their own homes, and those who would like to engage in self-management but need support to do so. There is evidence to suggest that some people may be more motivated to engage in self-management or self-help than others,[43] and careful consideration of recruitment strategies is needed.

Very little work has explored the benefits to individuals affected by cancer in helping themselves in relation to their health, although benefits are assumed or inferred. In order to support people we need to know what they are doing to help themselves and how this may change over time. At present it is difficult to ascertain this from the evidence, as this is an undeveloped area. The research generally has not set out to explore what people do to help themselves; rather it describes particular activities that individuals engage in when faced with cancer.

Why might supporting self-management and self-help be beneficial to patients?

There is a need to develop an appropriate theoretical framework to explore self-management by people affected by cancer. Self-management programmes have been informed by behaviour change models, and social learning theory in particular.[44] Becoming more skilled at managing problems associated with a chronic condition has been shown to enhance quality of life.[5] Self-management models consider a person's 'readiness to change' in relation to a health issue, and focus on enhancing self-efficacy (confidence in one's ability to achieve a particular outcome). With enhanced self-efficacy comes a sense of empowerment.

Cancer is a life-threatening condition which is often greatly feared and accompanied by a sense of powerlessness and lack of control. Enhancing one's sense of control may be highly important for people living with uncertainty.[45] People living with cancer have described the need to do something to maintain an illusion of control or a sense of security in acting for oneself.[28,37] There may be a particularly powerful impetus for some patients to do something when little can be offered by conventional treatment (for example, watchful waiting in prostate cancer), conventional treatment has adverse effects, or people wish to continue to do something after their treatment has ended and they are living long term after a cancer diagnosis. Self-management programmes may not be appropriate for all people, and certainly many find ways to manage problems associated with their health themselves. A better understanding of what people do to help themselves when living with cancer and how this may be of benefit is required. This may enable sharing of self-management strategies with other people living with cancer.

Summary

In order to help improve the lives of people living with cancer and the health care they experience, we need to know what people are doing to help themselves at all stages of their cancer journey and how this can best be supported. People living with cancer have described the importance of regaining and maintaining a sense of control in doing something for themselves.[28,30] Having an active role in managing long-term health conditions has been demonstrated to empower people to act for themselves, increase confidence in their ability to manage problems associated with the disease and its treatment, and enhance quality of life.[4,5] This has yet to be demonstrated for people living with cancer. The self-management literature for chronic conditions is likely to inform the development of new research, keeping in mind that cancer is different in many respects.

To enable partnership between health care professionals and people living with cancer, and to help support individuals to enhance their physical and psychosocial well-being, there is a need to build a better understanding of what people do to help themselves. Failure to address the social nature of illness (for example socio-economic, cultural elements, and how people manage to support themselves) may affect the ability to provide services that are acceptable to service users. Clearly there is an urgent need to establish a strong evidence base to inform how best to support people affected by cancer to help themselves in living with cancer. It will be necessary to conduct carefully designed research to enable consideration of these issues.

References

1. Cancer Research UK. (2004). *Cancer Incidence, Survival and Mortality in the UK and EU.* CancerStats Monograph. London: Cancer Research UK.
2. Gruman J. and Von Korff M. (1996). *Indexed Bibliography on Self Management for People with Chronic Disease.* Washington DC: Center for Advancement in Health.
3. Lorig K.R., Mazonson P. and Holman H.R. (1993). Evidence suggesting that health education for self-management in patients with chronic arthritis has sustained health benefits while reducing health care costs. *Arthritis and Rheumatism* **36**, 439–446.
4. Barlow J.H., Bancroft G.V. and Turner A.P. (2005). Self-management training for people with chronic disease: a shared learning experience. *Journal of Health Psychology* **10**, 863–872.
5. Lorig K.R., Sobel D.S., Ritter P.L., Laurent D. and Hobbs M. (2001). Effect of a self-management program on patients with chronic disease. *Effective Clinical Practice* **4**, 256–262.
6. Von Korff M., Gruman J., Schaefer J., Curry S.J. and Wagner E.H. (1997). Collaborative management of chronic illness. *Annals of Internal Medicine* **127**, 1097–1102.
7. Butler C., Rollnick S. and Stott N. (1996). The practitioner, the patient and resistance to change: recent ideas on compliance. *Canadian Medical Association Journal* **154**, 1357–1362.
8. Lorig K.R. and Holman H.R. (2003). Self-management education: history, definition, outcomes and mechanisms. *Annals of Behavioural Medicine* **26**, 1–7.
9. Barlow J.H., Bancroft G.V. and Turner A.P. (2005). Self-management training for people with chronic disease: a shared learning experience. *Journal of Health Psychology* **10**, 863–872.
10. Holman H.R. and Lorig K.R. (2004). Patient self-management: a key to effectiveness and efficiency in care of chronic disease. *Public Health Reports* **119**, 239–243.
11. Barlow J.H., Williams B. and Wright C.C. (1999). 'Instilling the strength to fight the pain and get on with life': learning to become an arthritis self manager through an adult education programme. *Health Education Research* **14**, 915–919.
12. Wright C.C., Barlow J.H., Turner A.P. and Bancroft G.V. (2003). Self management training for people with chronic disease: an exploratory study. *British Journal of Health Psychology* **8**, 465–476.
13. Department of Health. (2001). *The Expert Patient: A New Approach to Chronic Disease Management for the 21st Century.* London: Stationery Office.
14. Department of Health. (2005). *Supporting People with Long Term Conditions: An NHS and Social Care Model to Support Local Innovation and Integration.* London: Department of Health.
15. Coulter A. (2002). *The Autonomous Patient: Ending Paternalism in Medical Care.* London: Nuffield Trust.
16. Miewald C.A. (1997). Is awareness enough? The contradictions of self-care in a chronic disease clinic. *Human Organisation* **56**, 353–363.
17. Tritter J.Q. and Calnan M. (2002). Cancer as a chronic illness? Reconsidering categorization and exploring experience. *European Journal of Cancer Care* **11**, 161–165.
18. Foster C., Wright D., Hill H. and Hopkinson J. (2005). *Psychosocial Implications of Living Long-term with Cancer.* London: Macmillan Cancer Support.
19. Nail L.M., Jones L.S., Greene D., Schipper D.L. and Jensen R. (1991). Use and perceived efficacy of self-care activities in patients receiving chemotherapy. *Oncology Nursing Forum* **18**, 883–887.
20. Musci E.M. and Dodd M.J. (1990). Predicting self-care with patients and family members' affective states and family functioning. (Study of self-care activities by patients and their families during chemotherapy). *Oncology Nursing Forum* **17**, 394–400.
21. Richardson A. and Ream E.K. (1997). Self-care behaviours initiated by chemotherapy patients in response to

fatigue. *International Journal of Nursing Studies* **34**, 35–43.

22. Seegers C., Walker B.L., Nail L.M. *et al.* (1998). Self-care and breast cancer recovery. *Cancer Practice* **6**, 339–345.

23. Maunsell E., Drolet M., Brisson J., Robert J. and Deschenes L. (2002). Dietary change after breast cancer: extent, predictors, and relation with psychological distress. *Journal of Clinical Oncology* **20**, 1017–1025.

24. Braun K.L., Mokuau N., Hunt G.H., Kaanoi M. and Gotay C.C. (2002). Supports and obstacles to cancer survival for Hawaii's native people. [see comment]. *Cancer Practice* **10**, 192–200.

25. Deans G., Bennett-Emslie G.B., Weir J., Smith D.C. and Kaye S.B. (1988). Cancer support groups – who joins and why? *British Journal of Cancer* **58**, 670–674.

26. Pilisuk M., Wentzel P., Barry O. and Tennant J. (1997). Participant assessment of a nonmedical breast cancer support group. *Alternative Therapies in Health and Medicine* **3**, 72–80.

27. Gray R.E., Fitch M., Davis C. and Phillips C. (1997). Interviews with men with prostate cancer about their self-help group experience. *Journal of Palliative Care* **13**, 15–21.

28. Boon H., Brown J.B., Gavin A. and Westlake K. (2003). Men with prostate cancer: making decisions about complementary/alternative medicine. *Medical Decision Making* **23**, 471–479.

29. Henderson J.W. and Donatelle R.J. (2004). Complementary and alternative medicine use by women after completion of allopathic treatment for breast cancer. *Alternative Therapies in Health and Medicine* **10**, 52–57.

30. Boon H., Brown J.B., Gavin A., Kennard M.A. and Stewart M. (1999). Breast cancer survivors' perceptions of complementary/alternative medicine (CAM): making the decision to use or not to use. *Qualitative Health Research* **9**, 639–653.

31. Montbriand M.J. (1993). Freedom of choice: an issue concerning alternate therapies chosen by patients with cancer. *Oncology Nursing Forum* **20**, 1195–1201.

32. Edgar L., Remmer J., Rosberger Z. and Fournier M.A. (2000). Resource use in women completing treatment for breast cancer. *Psycho-oncology* **9**, 428–438.

33. Eng J., Ramsum D., Verhoef M. *et al.* (2003). A population-based survey of complementary and alternative medicine use in men recently diagnosed with prostate cancer. *Integrative Cancer Therapies* **2**, 212–216.

34. Lengacher C.A., Bennett M.P., Kip K.E. *et al.* (2002). Frequency of use of complementary and alternative medicine in women with breast cancer. *Oncology Nursing Forum* **29**, 1445–1452.

35. Steginga S., Occhipinti S. and Dunn J. (2001). The supportive care needs of men with prostate cancer. *Psycho-oncology* **10**, 66–75.

36. Verhoef M.J. and White M.A. (2002). Factors in making the decision to forgo conventional cancer treatment. *Cancer Practice* **10**, 201–207.

37. Truant T. and Bottorff J.L. (1999). Decision making related to complementary therapies: a process of regaining control. *Patient Education and Counseling* **38**, 131–142.

38. Kao G.D. and Devine P. (2000). Use of complementary health practices by prostate carcinoma patients undergoing radiation therapy. *Cancer* **88**, 615–619.

39. Braun K.L., Mokuau N., Hunt G.H., Kaanoi M. and Gotay C.C. (2002). Supports and obstacles to cancer survival for Hawaii's native people.[see comment]. *Cancer Practice* **10**, 192–200.

40. Rees C.E. and Bath P.A. (2001). Information-seeking behaviors of women with breast cancer. *Oncology Nursing Forum* **28**, 899–907.

41. Gray R.E., Greenberg M., Fitch M. *et al.* (1998). Information needs of women with metastatic breast cancer. *Cancer Prevention and Control* **2**, 57–62.

42. Pereira J.L., Koski S., Hanson J., Bruera E.D. and Mackey J.R. (2000). Internet usage among women with breast cancer: an exploratory study. *Clinical Breast Cancer* **1**, 148–153.

43. van der Weg F. and Streuli R.A. (2003). Use of alternative medicine by patients with cancer in a rural area of Switzerland. *Swiss Medical Weekly* **133**, 233–240.

44. Bandura A. (1982). Self-efficacy mechanism in human agency. *The American Psychologist* **37**, 122–147.

45. Brennan J. (2004). *Cancer in Context: A Practical Guide to Supportive Care.* Oxford: Oxford University Press.

CHAPTER THIRTY-FIVE

User involvement in cancer services

David Wright and Jenny Walton

Introduction

There has been growing interest in the involvement of service users in the development and organisation of health services in recent decades. In the US, patient advocacy groups presently enjoy significant influence over the co-ordination and provision of health and social care services. In the UK, recent white papers from the Department of Health, such as *Choosing Health* and *Our Health, our Care, our Say*, have involved extensive public consultations and recommend that service users should be supported in the management of their own conditions, thus illustrating a shift towards a more collaborative approach to health care.[1,2]

The development and organisation of cancer services have also been affected by these trends. In the UK, for example, influential publications such as the 1995 Calman–Hine report and the *NHS Cancer Plan* published in 2000, have both acknowledged the importance of a patient-centred approach to the planning and delivering of cancer services.[3,4] However, while there has been much discussion of the importance of user involvement, details of precise mechanisms through which users of cancer services can be consulted have typically remained vague.

Consequently, this chapter will assess the various strategies used to involve service users in the development and organisation of cancer services. This chapter is divided into three sections: first, a background to user involvement will be presented with reference to policy and historical context; second, the relative benefits and challenges to user involvement will be discussed; third, different strategies for user involvement will be presented with reference to examples. Jenny Walton, one of the co-authors of this chapter, has extensive experience as a patient representative for cancer services. She has provided a personal account that will be used to illustrate issues raised in this chapter.

User involvement in developing and monitoring cancer services: a historical and policy context

Conceptualising and defining 'users'

The concept of health service 'user' has evolved considerably over recent decades. Traditionally, the patient has been seen as a consumer of health services, literally using their economic resources (or lack of resources) to purchase health care. The medical profession, by contrast, has typically held a more central role in the formation and co-ordination of health services. The health care system was therefore viewed to be patriarchal, whereby patients were seen as 'passive recipients' of health care in relation to that of the 'expert' health professional.[5] This model of patients as passive users of health care services has remained dominant where patients have used the services provided rather than having an input into their shape or delivery. In this regard, perceiving patients in this manner has perpetuated a 'provider-led' system where control and decision making has rested with the health professional.[5]

Commentators have criticised the perception of patients as users of health care as disempowering, and the assumption that patients represent some undifferentiated community of service users. Hence, there is an underlying assumption that all patients share equal access to health care services, which thus fails to appreciate differences in use and experiences between certain groups or individuals.[6-8] Similarly, there is an assumption of a 'hierarchy of deservedness', whereby 'normal' or 'average' patients are privileged above minority concerns (e.g. the elderly and ethnic minorities).[9,10]

In response, greater emphasis has been placed in viewing patients as active 'citizens' in health care, thus according them a greater role in commenting on and developing health care services. This shift towards perceiving patients as citizens subverts the traditional 'provider-led' model of service development and delivery, and holds health practitioners accountable to the needs of the patient.[11] This 'democratic' model of patient involvement redistributes power between health professionals and patients to generate a more equivalent relationship.[5,11]

A purely 'citizen-based' approach, however, has also been criticised for providing only a collective view of patients' priorities and needs without appreciating individual perspectives.[5] Hence, patient-based consultation groups or lobbying organisations may fail to represent the views of all potential patients (for example, where disability groups may exclude mental illness as a form of disability).[9] Furthermore, it has been suggested that the greater emphasis on patient choice associated with citizenship status is 'neo-paternalistic' in that patients may be forced to make choices when they may not wish to do so.[5] It has been suggested, therefore, that patients should be seen to exist somewhere between the 'consumer'/'citizen' extremes, thus placing them in a co-operative and collaborative partnership with health care professionals.[6,12]

The concept of 'user' is further complicated by the fact that it is multifaceted. It has been dem-onstrated for example that the term 'user' does not solely include patients and their carers but may also include members of the general public, potential patients, and public, community and voluntary organisations. Health professionals may also define themselves as 'users', and evidence suggests that professionals working in hospices are more likely to see themselves in this manner than other professional groups.[13] Despite these complexities, the phrase 'user' is still commonly used and will be adopted in this chapter.

A historical context of user involvement

User involvement in health services is not a recent phenomenon, but has been recognised over recent decades. Inequalities in the dynamic between patients and health professionals resulting from the 'power' associated with specialist knowledge were recognised in the 1950s.[14] In the 1960s and 1970s, the importance of patient autonomy and the right for service users to be involved in planning and delivering health services was acknowledged in the *Declaration of Helsinki* and by the World Health Organisation.[15,16]

Since then, there has been growing recognition of the importance of increased participation of service users in health care. This has particularly been the case in the US and Canada.[17,18] From the UK perspective, an overview of influential reports and legislation since the 1990s illustrates the burgeoning importance of user involvement. In 1990, for example, the *Community Care Act*[19] required local authorities to consult with patients and carers, and in 1992, *Local Voices*[20] recommended user involvement to help establish priorities and develop and monitor services. *The New NHS: Modern Dependable*, published in 1997, sought to 'rebuild confidence in the NHS as a public service, accountable to patients, open to the public and shaped by their views'.[21]

In 2000, *the NHS Plan* discussed a range of initiatives aimed at improving service-user involvement, including the formation of patient advocacy and liaison services, and patient forums in all NHS trusts to provide user input into local services.[22] As a result of these publications, various organisations were established in the UK, several of which are still in existence:

- *Patient Advice and Liaison Services* (PALS) – an organisation employed by and responsible to health care trusts providing assistance and information for patients, and monitoring problems arising
- *Independent Complaints Advocacy Services* (ICAS) – a service commissioned by the now defunct Commission for Patient and Public Involvement in Health
- *Overview and Scrutiny Committees* (OSCs) – an organisation that reviews local NHS provisions for health improvement and inequalities
- *patient forums* – independent statutory bodies located in every NHS trust and primary care trust to monitor and review services from a patient perspective and to represent the views of local communities.[23]

The development and organisation of cancer services has also been influenced by the trend towards greater user involvement. For example, in 1995, the Calman–Hine report was published in the UK.[3] This report detailed an agenda for reforming the organisation and delivery of cancer services in England and Wales, and established a general principle of patient engagement in cancer services. The report stated that:

> The development of cancer services should be patient centred and should take account of patients', families' and carers' views and preferences as well as those of professionals involved in cancer care. Individuals' perceptions of their needs may differ from those of the professional [p. 6].

However, despite these clear recommendations, there was little detail about how services should be patient centred. Hence, 'the Calman–Hine report creates the potential for considerable user involvement but operationally it requires much development'.[24] The recommendations of the Calman–Hine report were developed further in the *NHS Cancer Plan*, published in 2000, which stated that 'Users and their carers should have choice, voice and control over what happens to them at each step in their care' (p. 66).[4] They went on to suggest that at a local level 'Cancer networks should take account of the views of patients and carers when planning services' (p. 69).[4] However, again, there are few recommendations given about

precisely how services users should be involved in planning services.[13]

Various strategies have been adopted however in the UK to support user involvement. For example, in 1982, Cancerlink was founded by health professionals and people affected by cancer, to help people seeking support, provide a format through which views could be expressed, and to direct interested people to cancer self-help and support groups.[24] In addition, as a result of the Calman–Hine report and the *NHS Cancer Plan*, Cancer Networks have been established throughout England and in parallel developments in Wales, Scotland and Northern Ireland to assist with the co-ordination of cancer services. Many of the networks have patient forums to ensure patient representation in the planning of local services.

Despite recent advances in user involvement both within cancer and more generally, and the UK governments' emphasis on the relevance of user involvement, evidence suggests that overall, there has been relatively little involvement of the public in the development of health care services in recent years. For example, Milewa *et al.* and Pickard *et al.* have reported little involvement of patients in primary care trusts,[25,26] while Elston and Fulop found minimal involvement of patients in the development of health improvement programmes.[27] Furthermore, while there is increasing emphasis of the benefits that can accrue from involving patients in determining the shape of health services, the effectiveness of user involvement has been undermined by tokenism and a tendency for health care agencies to play the 'user card' in an attempt to outbid competitors.[7,28]

User-involvement strategies in cancer services have also developed considerably on the European, US and global arena. In Western Europe, for example, organisations such as Europa Donna and the European Breast Cancer Coalition have been established to represent the interests of women with breast cancer in relation to local, national and European organisations and institutions. Europa Donna aims to increase the awareness of breast cancer, improve the level of understanding about treatments and other cancer-related issues, and ensure that services and professionals are responsive to the needs of women with breast cancer.

In the US, there has been a notable history of service user activism and involvement through organisations such as The National Breast Cancer Coalition, founded in 1991, and the Lance Armstrong, founded in 1997. The National Breast Cancer Coalition has been particularly effective in educating and empowering people affected by breast cancer and representing their interests. The organisation has a particularly strong lobbying capacity and has influenced public policy, science, and industry in the US. The coalition also provides information, training and support to those affected by breast cancer, and actively attempts to increase public awareness of breast cancer.

At an international level, the International Union Against Cancer (UICC) has formed patient forums to promote timely access to cancer services and greater patient involvement in health care decision making. The forums allow people affected by cancer to share experiences and issues relating to their quality of life and the quality of care. In addition the forums provide an opportunity for greater advocacy, as well as raising the awareness of cancer and disseminating and obtaining information.

Contrasting the user-involvement activities within the UK with those in the US and elsewhere does reveal certain notable differences. In the UK, the NHS has enabled the development of a system-wide structure for greater service-user involvement. However, in the US and internationally, user-involvement organisations are often centred on the political mobilisation of patient groups, often aiming for greater patient advocacy and lobbying power.

Benefits and barriers to user involvement

The benefits of involving service users

It has been suggested that the evidence for the impact of user involvement on the quality and structure of health care services is limited.[29] In part, this is no doubt due to the fact that it is only in recent years that user involvement has been given serious consideration. There is now accumulating evidence that user involvement can benefit both the patient and the organisation and delivery of health services.

From the patients' perspective, it has been suggested that involvement in health services can result in improved health outcomes.[13] Evidence from research conducted outside cancer has suggested that user involvement in health care can improve physical symptoms and reduce anxiety and depression.[15] It has also been suggested that user involvement in consultations and health services can increase patient satisfaction.[13,30] Specific benefits to the patient can include a sense of personal growth, increased confidence and self-perception, greater sense of control, a greater understanding and knowledge of their conditions, health care needs and services, an increased trust in health professionals, more appropriate use of health services, and a greater ability to discuss issues with health care professionals.[30]

However, it has also been suggested that the level of patient satisfaction that is derived from their involvement in services is dependent on their preferred level of participation.[15] Not all users may want to get involved, and thus it is inappropriate to impose choice and decision making on patients.[15,16] As Gattellari et al. state:[15]

> One may argue that imposing choice on patients is as detrimental as imposing advice, and neither approach reflects the tenets of shared decision making [p. 1867].

Patients and carers may choose to get involved for altruistic reasons, while others become involved as a means of coping or making sense of their own illness. Users may become involved as a result of a bad experience, such as delayed detection, lack of continuity of care, or poor communication skills associated with breaking bad news. For example, in Personal account 35.1, Jenny shares her experiences of cancer and provides reasons for getting involved in cancer services: a sense of anger at the disease, dissatisfaction with the service she had received, and a need to promote rare cancers.

In addition to the benefits for patients, user involvement can aid health care professionals

Personal account 35.1

I have had cancer of the vulva. For a time, as I stumbled along that rocky, uncertain and scary journey, I felt so alone. No one within the medical teams who looked after me asked if either I or my husband (my carer) was in need of help. We were not offered written information or psychological support. But then, we knew no different and thought it was up to us to cope, alone.

After I'd gone through the being scared stage, then the resignation that there was nothing I could do except stay positive whenever possible (not as easy as it sounds) and try to keep my body as active as it would allow, anger crept into my whole being. I'd contracted a sneaky disease and, through no fault of my own, turned from being a physically and mentally very fit and able person to feeling like a worn out wreck.

Because of circumstances – no one's fault – I didn't have the reassurance of continuity. Circumstances necessitated my attendance at four different hospitals. After stamping the proverbial foot, I now see the same person, my consultant, each time I go into hospital, whether it is for a clinic appointment or to have surgery. It used to feel degrading, being asked to strip off from the waist down for a different man each time I went along, someone who did not know me or my case. Excluding nurses, I've been attended by one woman and 10 men! Not a comfortable situation to be in. I also wish I'd been given more information about exactly what was going to be done during the procedure – I was given some, but not all details.

Having the kind of cancer I did was, to say the least, embarrassing at first. It took me about 12 months to be able to say openly that I had had vulval cancer and to describe especially, the misleading symptoms I had experienced. Eventually, I decided to promote vulval cancer awareness. The media, however, was reluctant to help. This was not a subject fit for an audience, I was told, even though it might contain important life-saving information.

It is a deep need to aid in the fight against cancer that keeps me involved. Approximately a third of my daytime hours is accounted for in this respect. I have been asked on a number of occasions if I would perhaps be better off keeping away 'from all that cancer', especially on days when I may feel extra tired and perhaps even low in spirits. But the truth is, being amongst fellow cancer patients and carers actually strengthens my ability to cope with the uncertainty of the future.

and the organisation of the health services. User involvement can help to identify health needs and thus provide a mechanism through which services can be matched to those needs.[31] This can promote efficient and effective service provision for local populations.[13] Furthermore, a patient-centred and responsive approach to providing cancer services can result in improved quality of care.[29]

Involving users can also be helpful in providing effective information to patients and carers about cancer, treatment and health care services, resulting in improved compliance and patient satisfaction.[13,30] Users can also become involved in the management and decision making of their own treatment, which again can have implications for levels of compliance.[15,30] It has also been suggested that patients can be valuable in the monitoring and evaluation of cancer services, although evidence suggests this is undertaken less frequently and is less recognised by health professionals.[13]

Patients can also serve as educators for health professionals, sharing their experiences of cancer and advising on good practice, such as breaking bad news.[15] For example, in Personal account 35.2, Jenny shares her experiences of informing cancer nurses about her rare cancer:

Personal account 35.2

Nurses didn't know what my cancer was all about. I'd be asked questions, such as, 'What are the symptoms?', and 'Will you be able to have sex again?'. Their understanding of this rare cancer was abysmal. It is amazing how, after the two vulvectomies, these good ladies would expect me to get out of bed and sit on a chair within a couple of days of surgery. Fortunately for today's vulvectomy patients, ongoing education of gynae cancer nurses – certainly within my own cancer network – now includes a talk from a patient. When I go along to a training day to talk to trainees, it is amusing to watch their faces grimacing as they 'see' my story unfolding. I often am asked to speak at medical conferences, too, in order to illustrate the other side of a cancer case history. I am amazed, and gratified, that this always results in professionals from all spheres of the medical world coming to me afterwards and expressing their thanks, especially because 'We didn't realise . . .'.

The barriers to involving service users

Having recognised the potential benefits of involving users in cancer services, it is necessary to consider the various challenges and barriers that may inhibit such involvement.

One of the chief barriers to user involvement is a resistance on the part of health professionals towards an alternative, patient-derived perspective.[13] This resistance can be attributed to numerous factors, including a belief that input to cancer services requires specialist knowledge and skills that service users do not have, and a paternalistic, professional protectionism that perceives cancer patients as typically vulnerable people.[15,16,32,33] Consequently, it has been suggested that effective user involvement is more than adopting suitable structures and policies, but requires a significant culture shift within the health service.[15,25,33]

Resistance to user involvement may also be attributed to a fundamental challenge to the belief of how health services should be provided. This is felt acutely by nursing professionals who perceive their role as 'patient advocates' and thus have particularly protective attitudes towards patients. As Daykin et al. state:[33]

> A key element of the occupational strategy that nurses have adopted in seeking autonomy as a professional group has been to lay claim to a professional knowledge base that is seen as distinct from that of biomedicine.[34] Central to this is knowledge about care as opposed to cure, and related skills such as advocacy that, it is claimed, arise from the close position in relation to patients that nurses occupy in their day-to-day work.[35] Ironically, the prospect of users speaking for themselves through processes of user involvement can be potentially threatening to such an agenda [p. 280].

A further barrier to user involvement is the challenge of identifying patient and carer representatives. This is particularly problematic when seeking to involve typically under-represented sections of society.[13] It has been suggested, for example, that breast cancer patients are often well represented, while other groups, such as men, or those with rarer cancers are left out.[15,24] Particular difficulties have also been found with involving black and minority ethnic groups.[13]

Techniques for identifying user representatives have often involved approaching patients and carers from pre-existing user-support groups.[36] However, these groups often involve atypical representatives, and typically do not reflect the views or experiences of rarer cancers, diverse ethnicities, rural communities or people in the advanced stage of disease.[36] Consequently an 'inverse care law' can exist where those most in need of representation are least likely to have an opportunity of getting involved and thus having their voices heard. Furthermore, as Gattellari et al. suggest, only those who are relatively well usually get involved, thus limiting the representativeness of the outcomes of such involvement.[15] Hence, 'prescribing increased patient involvement for all may well be a form of paternalism in which the well community dictates what is best for patients' (p. 1867).[15] In addition, it has been suggested that the representativeness of users can be undermined as they become 'institutionalised' or 'professionalised' as a result of their involvement.[13] However, it has also been discussed that gaining experience through involvement does not negate the experiences or the perspective that a service user can bring.[37]

A further barrier to user involvement is the resource intensiveness of such activity in terms of finance and time. Fostering effective involvement requires considerable time in establishing groups, building up trust and confidence (particularly with black and minority ethnic groups), and developing the requisite skills and knowledge.[13] Similarly, from the health care professionals' perspective, there is a lack of understanding about user involvement, and hence time is also required for providing training and developing skills.[31,33] Health care professionals may find it difficult to find the time to commit to user-involvement training events, or consultation exercises, or to include patient-involvement strategies within their clinical practice.[16,29] Inevitably, supporting such activities requires significant levels of financial investment, resources that are not usually available to community or voluntary organisations.[29]

Further challenges have been identified that can potentially undermine the effectiveness of user-involvement activity.[13] Users are typically consulted in exercises led by health professionals, and are thus often not in a position of control over the consultation process. This can result in users' views being collected with no formal requirement to respond to them in any way.[29] Also, users involved in consultation exercises often do not receive any feedback on the outcomes of their involvement, resulting in feelings of being unappreciated or their views being sidelined. Where users' views and priorities differ from those of health professionals, these differences need to be managed effectively to ensure that there is adequate and unbiased input from all parties over service issues.

There can be problems of confidentiality, with many consultation exercises effectively being little more than complaints procedures, resulting in reports in which health professionals are 'named and shamed'.[13] This can result in those health professionals losing confidence, losing faith in user involvement activities, adopting a more defensive medical practice, and generating a greater wariness of patients.

It is evident, therefore, that user-involvement activities can generate numerous benefits and challenges. To minimise the difficulties, user-involvement activities have to be undertaken sensitively, with considerable planning, and with the consultation of the multidisciplinary team. The various strategies that can be adopted for involving users will be discussed in the final section of this chapter.

How to involve users in cancer services

Conducting baseline assessments and approaching users

Before approaching users or identifying which strategies to use to engage patients or carers, it is necessary to establish a 'vision and set of core principles' for user involvement.[38] The aims of user involvement must be clearly formulated with a clear account of how the service or organisation will respond to the consultation exercise. Failure to specify aims and objectives will result in patients and carers being paid 'lip service', identifying issues without indicating how they will be put into practice.

Having set out these core principles, it is necessary to assess current performance, examining strengths and weaknesses of current user-involvement practice, and learning from such activity, should it exist.[38] It then may be helpful to conduct a baseline assessment to identify the local demographics, potential areas through which users can be identified, and community needs. After this, service users can be identified and approached.

There are several mechanisms through which users can be involved. One approach is to identify users through existing community organisations and institutions. The National Centre for the Coordination of Health Technology Assessment, for example, has recruited patients through self-help groups, patients' representative groups, campaign groups and charities.[39] There are concerns, however, that identifying users in this manner can exclude those who do not have equal access to these groups, such as ethnic minorities, those with rarer cancers, and those living in rural areas.[28,36] Consequently, user-involvement exercises have been undertaken using either a total sample of patients or a random sample within a particular organisation or geographical region. Brown and Doran, for example, randomly sampled 214 women in five postcode areas in Australia to participate in a study determining local health care priorities.[40] Mixed strategies have also been used. In the Macmillan Listening Study, for example, a UK-wide project exploring the research views and priorities of people affected by cancer, user representatives were identified through the patient forums of all cancer networks. In order to involve often under-represented groups, however, such as those from diverse ethnic backgrounds and those at the end of life, other users were identified purposively through other sites.[37]

Differences of opinion exist over whether users from the same background (i.e. all patients) or from different backgrounds (i.e. patients, researchers, practitioners, and other stakeholders) be consulted. A significant challenge in involving a mixed group is the effective management of the power differentials between health service practitioners and health service users.[36] There is a tendency, for example, for health professionals to feel defensive when presented with the views and experiences of patients.[41] Conversely, patients can feel 'helpless' or that they are 'troublemakers' when raising their experiences in the presence of professionals.[42] As Johnson *et al.* note, it is wrong to assume that all participants have an equal input into consultation exercises, due to certain individuals and organisations having a stronger and more coherent voice than others.[43] Barnes presents a contrary view and suggests that patients may be so reactive against the 'official agenda' that this inhibits effective collaboration.[9] Further difficulties have also been reported where practitioners, community members, and researchers have such disparate attitudes and beliefs that attempting to achieve a consensus view is difficult.[44]

Strategies for involving users

Nursing professionals can potentially play a key role in involving users in cancer services. The *Manual of National Cancer Services Standards*, for example, stated that cancer networks in the UK must identify lead nurses whose responsibilities included ensuring a network-wide user perspective to inform the development of cancer services.[45] It is important, therefore, that nursing staff are aware of the different strategies than can be used for involving users in the delivery and organisation of cancer services. Patients and carers differ in the level of involvement they seek, although Gattellari *et al.* suggest that most cancer patients fail to achieve their desired level of involvement in cancer services.[15] It is thus important that nurses tailor user-involvement strategies to the preferences of patients and carers.

Strategies for involving users exist on a continuum from low level, often viewed as tokenistic, forms of involvement to more developed forms of engaging with services users (see Figure 35.1). Minimum forms of involvement are concerned with providing or collecting information from patients and carers, and are often seen as 'passive' forms of involvement.[13,31] The provision of information often centres on giving patients or carers details of the cancer, prognosis, and treatment. The paternalism traditionally associated with health care services has meant that information has often been filtered, such that patients are only given information that is deemed appropriate. The nursing profession, however, is well placed to support information giving, given that patient education is a core component of nursing care.[46] Furthermore, nurses are a popular source of information for patients.[47] In one study, for example,

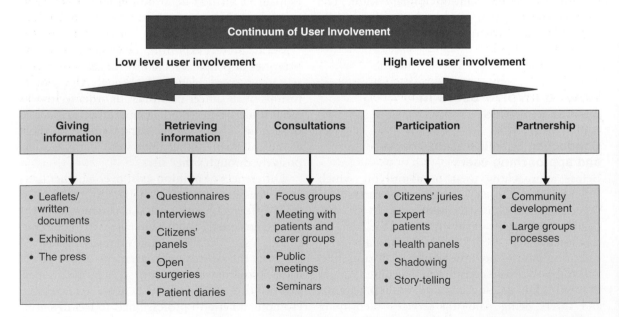

Figure 35.1   Continuum of user involvement. Reproduced with permission from the East of England Strategic Health Authority.

breast care nurses were considered to be a more effective source of information than the general staff.[48]

Providing information to patients about their progress and treatment has been identified as an effective means for reducing anxiety, developing coping skills, and enhancing recovery.[46] Different means of providing information include setting up exhibitions (such as in schools, shopping centres, and community centres), providing written documents such as information leaflets, involving the press, using videos, and providing information verbally.[38,46]

Evidence suggests, however, that information needs differ by patient type (where, for example, younger patients are more likely to require information), by sex (where men appear less likely to seek information), and by time since diagnosis.[14,46,49] In one survey of breast cancer patients, it was found that at the point of diagnosis, information needs are most likely to be concerned with the likelihood of cure, the extent of the disease, and treatment types.[48] After 21 months, however, patients required information on the risk of cancer for other family members, although information on the likelihood of cure remained important. It has been suggested, therefore that nurses should provide information that is appropriate to the stage of cancer.[50]

In terms of retrieving information from patients or carers, common techniques include the use of questionnaires, citizens' panels, and complaints procedures.[13,23] Other methods that can be used include open surgeries (where members of the public can discuss health care issues with a representative of health care organisations), patient diaries (where users can keep a personal written record of their treatment or care), or structured or semi-structured one-to-one interviews.[23]

Other, more developed approaches to user involvement have been used less frequently. Hence, patients and carers have typically not been involved in planning or evaluating cancer services.[13] However, more developed forms of user involvement include meetings with patients and carer groups, public meetings, or seminars through which patients and carers can contribute to local health care service issues.[23] As discussed earlier, should these techniques be adopted, attempts

have to be made to ensure that the views of those often under-represented in voluntary groups are included, such as those in receipt of palliative care services, those in rural locations, those with rarer cancers, and representatives from diverse ethnic minority groups.[36]

More-developed strategies for involving users include the development of cancer partnership groups within the UK and 'expert patients'.[29,51] The latter refers to people who have experiences of a particular condition and are prepared to share with others their knowledge about living with it, often in the context of self-management programmes such as the Expert Patient Programme in the UK. Other developed means of supporting user involvement are shadowing (where staff accompany users as they use services in order to obtain a different perspective of the patients' experience), and story telling (a patient-centred approach where a patient tells their story to a staff member from a different clinical area). Community development initiatives are another approach that involves community members identifying their own needs and the means by which they can be addressed.[23]

As most examples of user-involvement activities in cancer services have typically been passive information-giving or -collecting strategies, evaluations of how users have influenced the development and organisation of cancer services has remained under-developed. However, there are examples of cancer services being changed or provided in light of service-user input. For example, in Personal account 35.3, Jenny provides a detailed example of how cancer services in her region have been improved through the involvement of a 'patient involvement group'.

Jenny therefore provides an example from her own personal experience of influencing cancer services at various levels, from being involved in information giving to influencing the structure of local services and acting in a lobbying capacity for cancer-related issues.

Supporting service users

Involving services users in cancer services can raise many issues over how they can be supported. For example, 'consultation overload' may occur where the same patient or carer representative

Personal account 35.3

With a couple of clinical nurse specialists and other gynaecological patients, I was involved at the start of a gynae cancer support group within our region. Although no one else had had the same cancer as me, I could empathise with the other ladies and their problems. I learned a lot, too, about how different treatments for the same types of cancer might be necessary. That inevitably opened my eyes to the fact there were other groups of people who actually worked at improving cancer services on a local and national level, rather than supporting each other. I joined our local Patient Involvement Group, one of three spread across the Cancer Network. Each of the groups is made up of patients, carers and health professionals, all working together to improve the cancer services within our area.

I am pleased to have been involved with the production of information booklets for patients with my type of cancer, for my own network and for Cancerbackup.

The Patient Involvement Group, which is neither a complaints committee nor a support group, has been responsible for many changes as well as additions to how the cancer service is delivered. For example, we have produced, and keep updated, a directory of cancer self-help and support groups; our members have had input into the design brief of a major capital build – the network's new oncology/haematology centre. Some have worked with the Cancer Services Collaborative and the Cancer Service Improvement Programme to influence future patient care, and we have had input into the Breaking Bad News guidance policy, nurse training, patient consultation leaflets, patient surveys, and have held 'Cancer Awareness' events. Our influence has brought hospital pharmacy hours in line with last outpatient clinic closure, and we have patient/carer representatives on all the management and locality boards, and site-specific groups within our network.

Various ongoing Patient Involvement Group projects include the production of a general information booklet specifically aimed at those affected by cancer within our region, encouraging and assisting the local hospitals trust to investigate the feasibility of opening a couple of oncology drop-in centres, and exploring ways of assisting patients with the cost of wigs. However, the most prominent work currently being undertaken is that of the groups' campaign against the bridge tolls in our area. Hundreds of patients and carers have to travel weekly in order to receive life-saving treatment. As most people realise, once contracting a disease that suddenly prevents someone from working, there is not just the frightening aspect of 'will I or won't I die?', but the unexpected drop in income while, at the same time, having to find heavy travelling costs for treatment, prescription payments for necessary drugs, a change of wardrobe because of weight loss, and payment for special equipment to help the patient manage in the home. So, here, where crossing the bridge is the way to possible extension of life, it was decided that if concessions could be made, it would, in one small way, help ease financial problems.

participates in more than one project. This is a particular concern where patients are unwell and the responsibilities of being involved in consultation exercises may affect their health. There may be confidentiality issues where, for example, a patient or carer may be privy to information concerning particular services.

There are also issues of remuneration. Questions arise over whether patients or carers should be paid for their services. These are often couched in ethical terms: would the users be involved were it not for the offer of payment, in which case, is such involvement coercive? However, there are other considerations. For example, there may be tax implications in offering payment to users, and this may have an impact on benefits.[37]

Finally, involvement in cancer services as a user representative may be emotionally demanding.

For example, patients or carers may be presented with certain patient experiences that they could find distressing.

In response to these challenges, certain guiding principles should be in place at the start of any user-involvement exercise. Service users should be fully informed of what is expected of them before agreeing to take part, and they should be able to stop their involvement at any time of their choosing without having to give an explanation why. Service users should, where appropriate, sign a terms of agreement form that sets out the responsibilities and the need for confidentiality. The strategy for user involvement should be established in advance, and financial issues should be resolved before patients and carers commit to being involved. Finally, appropriate support should be provided for patients or carers involved in any consultation exercise if this is deemed appropriate, and may include peer support, clinical supervision or counselling.

Conclusion

User involvement in the organisation and delivery of health care services in general, and cancer services in particular have developed considerably over recent decades. The traditional paternalistic model of health service users being placed in a passive relationship to the powerful role of the 'expert' health professional has been subverted by the concept of patients and carers as active citizens in their health care. However, to date, user-involvement strategies have usually been low key, often centring on providing or obtaining information from patients or carers rather than involving them in any meaningful way in shaping or evaluating cancer services.

The potential for user involvement is considerable, and numerous strategies have been identified, from providing information leaflets to Expert Patient Programmes, and community-development initiatives. Nursing professionals play a key role in supporting user involvement in cancer services. In the UK, government policy has highlighted the importance of nurses in supporting a patient-centred approach to the organisation of local cancer services. Research has also indicated that nurses are a preferred source for information about cancer and treatment. It has also been suggested that, as 'patient education' is a core component of nursing practice, nursing professionals should be supportive of user-involvement initiatives. However, it also appears that the recommendations for giving patients and carers greater influence over cancer services can profoundly challenge fundamental beliefs of nursing practice.

Emerging evidence from research and personal experience illustrate that patients and carers can make a valuable contribution to the organisation and delivery of cancer services. Through careful planning of user-involvement activities and a commitment from health care professionals to collaborate with service users, cancer services can become more attuned and responsive to the very people they seek to serve.

References

1. Department of Health. (2004). *Choosing Health: Making Healthy Choices Easier.* London: Department of Health.
2. Department of Health. (2006). *Our Health, our Care, our Say.* London: Department of Health.
3. Department of Health and the Welsh Office. (1995). *A Policy Framework for Commissioning Cancer Services. A Report by the Expert Advisory Group on Cancer to the Chief Medical Officers of England and Wales.* London and Cardiff: Department of Health and the Welsh Office.
4. Department of Health. (2000). *The NHS Cancer Plan: A Plan for Investment, a Plan for Reform.* London: Department of Health.
5. Anderson W. and Gillam S. (2001). The elusive NHS consumer: 1948 to the NHS Plan. *Economic Affairs* **21**, 14–18.
6. Hickey G. and Kipping C. (1998). Exploring the concept of user involvement in mental health through a participation continuum. *Journal of Clinical Nursing* **7**, 83–88.
7. Mort M. and Wiston G. (1996). The user card: picking through the organisational undergrowth in health and social care. *Contemporary Political Studies* **2**, 1133–1140.
8. Dolan P., Cookson R. and Ferguson B. (1999). Effect of discussion and deliberation on the public's views of priority setting in health care: focus group study. *British Medical Journal* **318**, 916–919.
9. Barnes M. (1999). Users as citizens: collective action and the local governance of welfare. *Social Policy and Administration* **33**, 73–90.
10. Atkinson J.M. and Elliott J. (1994). Evaluation and consumers. In Titterton M.I. (ed.) *Caring for People in the Community: New Agenda for Welfare.* London: Jessica Kingsley Publishers, pp. 153–167.
11. Beresford P. (2003). User involvement in research: exploring the challenges. *NT Research* **8**, 36–46.
12. Tovey P. and Adams J. (2001). Primary care as intersecting social worlds. *Social Science and Medicine* **52**, 695–706.
13. Tritter J., Barley V., Daykin N. *et al.* (2003). Divided care and the Third Way: user involvement in statutory and voluntary sector cancer services. *Sociology of Health and Illness* **25**, 429–456.
14. Gamble K. (1998). Communication and information: the experience of radiotherapy patients. *European Journal of Cancer Care* **7**, 153–161.
15. Gattellari M., Butow P. and Tattersal M. (2001). Sharing decisions in cancer care. *Social Science and Medicine* **52**, 1865–1878.
16. Evans S., Tritter J., Barley V. *et al.* (2003). User involvement in UK cancer services: bridging the policy gap. *European Journal of Cancer Care* **12**, 331–338.

17. Williams D. (1991). Policy at the grassroots: community-based participation in health care policy. *Journal of Professional Nursing* **7**, 271–276.

18. Gray R., Fitch M., Greenberg M. and Shapiro S. (1995). Consumer participation in cancer system planning. *Journal of Palliative Care* **11**, 27–33.

19. Department of Health. (1990). *The Community Care Act.* London: Department of Health.

20. Department of Health. (1992). *Local Voices.* London: Department of Health.

21. Department of Health. (1997). *The New NHS: Modern Dependable.* London: Department of Health.

22. Department of Health. (2001). *Health and Social Care Act.* London: Department of Health.

23. Department of Health. (2001). *Involving Patients and the Public in Healthcare.* London: Department of Health.

24. Gott M., Stevens T., Small N. and Ahmedzai S. (2002). Involving users, improving services: the example of cancer. *British Journal of Clinical Governance* **7**, 81–85.

25. Milewa T., Harrison S., Ahmad W. and Tovey P. (2002). Citizens' participation in primary healthcare planning: innovative citizenship practice in empirical perspective. *Critical Public Health* **12**, 39–53.

26. Pickard S., Marshall M., Rogers A. *et al.* (2002). User involvement in clinical governance. *Health Expectations* **5**, 187–198.

27. Elston J. and Fulop N. (2002). Perceptions of partnership: a documentary analysis of Health Improvement Programmes. *Public Health* **116**, 207–213.

28. Barnes M. and Wistow G. (1994). Learning to hear voices: listening to users of mental health services. *Journal of Mental Health* **3**, 525–540.

29. Richardson A., Sitzia J. and Cotterell P. (2005). Working the system. Achieving change through partnership working: an evaluation of cancer partnership groups. *Health Expectations* **8**, 210–220.

30. Department of Health. (2004). *Patient and Public Involvement in Health: The Evidence for Policy Implementation.* London: Department of Health.

31. Poulton B. (1999). User involvement in identifying health needs and shaping and evaluating services: is it being realised? *Journal of Advanced Learning* **30**, 1289–1296.

32. Daykin N., Rimmer J., Turton P. *et al.* (2002). Enhancing user involvement through interprofessional education in healthcare: the case of cancer services. *Learning in Health and Social Care* **1**, 122–131.

33. Daykin N., Sanidas M., Tritter J. *et al.* (2004). Developing user involvement in a UK cancer network: professionals' and users' perspectives. *Critical Public Health* **14**, 277–294.

34. Witz A. (1992). *Professions and Patriarchy.* London: Routledge.

35. Daykin N. and Clarke C. (2001). They'll still get the bodily care. Discourses of care and relationships between nurses and health care assistants in the NHS. *Sociology of Health and Illness* **22**, 249–363.

36. Stevens T., Wilde D., Hunt J. and Ahmedzai S. (2003). Overcoming the challenges to consumer involvement in cancer research. *Health Expectations* **6**, 1–8.

37. Wright D., Corner J., Hopkinson J. and Foster C. (2005). Participatory research as a strategy for patient involvement in health research: learning from the Macmillan Listening Study. *Health Expectations* **8**, 1–10.

38. Department of Health. (2003). *Strengthening Accountability: Involving Patients and the Public. Practice Guidance. Section 11 of the Health and Social Care Act 2001.* London: Department of Health.

39. Oliver S., Milne R., Bradburn J. *et al.* (2001). Involving consumers in a needs-led research programme: a pilot project. *Health Expectations* **4**, 18–28.

40. Brown W. and Doran F. (1996). Women's health: consumers views for planning local health promotion and health care priorities. *Australian and New Zealand Journal of Public Health* **20**, 149–154.

41. Winter R. and Munn-Giddings C. (2001). *A Handbook for Action Research in Health and Social Care.* London: Routledge.

42. Park P. (1999). People, knowledge, and change in participatory research. *Management Learning* **30**, 141–157.

43. Johnson N., Ravnborg H.M., Westermann O. and Probst K. (2001). User participation in watershed management and research. *Water Policy* **3**, 507–520.

44. Boutilier M., Mason R. and Rootman I. (1997). Community action and reflective practice in health promotion research. *Health Promotion International* **21**, 69–78.

45. Department of Health. (2000). *Manual of National Cancer Services Standards.* London: Department of Health.

46. Mills M. and Sullivan K. (1999). The importance of information giving for patients newly diagnosed with cancer: a review of the literature. *Journal of Clinical Nursing* **8**, 631–642.

47. Bilodeau B. and Degner L. (1996). Informational needs, sources of information and decisional roles in women with breast cancer. *Oncology Nursing Forum* **23**, 691–696.

48. Luker K., Beaver K., Leinster S. and Glynn Owens R. (1996). Informational needs and sources of information for women with breast cancer: a follow up study. *Journal of Advanced Nursing* **23**, 487–495.

49. Leydon G., Boulton M., Moynihan C. *et al.* (2006). Cancer patients' information needs and information

seeking behaviour: in depth interview study. *British Medical Journal* **320**, 909–913.

50. Rees C. and Bath P. (2000). The information needs and source preferences of women with breast cancer and their family members: a review of the literature published between 1988 and 1998. *Journal of Advanced Nursing* **31**, 833–841.

51. Department of Health. (2000). *Saving Lives, Our Healthier Nation*. London: Department of Health.

CHAPTER THIRTY-SIX

Palliative care and cancer

Sheila Payne

Introduction

The rationale for including a chapter on palliative care tucked away in the final part of a book predominantly concerned with treating cancer may seem obvious, because sadly, not all cancer patients survive. Palliative care is often equated with death and dying. In this chapter, I will endeavour to present a more proactive vision of palliative care, in which supportive and palliative care are conceptualised as concurrent programmes of management with other anti-cancer therapeutic regimes. Nurses have been crucially important in introducing and developing hospice and palliative care services throughout the world.[1–3] Nursing work has always included the palliation of distressing symptoms, the care of patients approaching death, the laying out of the body, and the care of newly bereaved relatives. In the latter part of the 20th century, the emergence of the modern hospice movement has provided an impetus to reconceptualising the delivery of some aspects of this care.[4] Nursing has been central to these developments, both in specialist contexts such as in hospices, hospital teams and community teams, and more broadly in delivering care to terminally ill people in a range of settings. Palliative care in the UK is now regarded as integral to cancer care services, and recent policy initiatives have sought to recommend standards of service provision.[5]

While death is a universal given, the process of dying is largely determined by social, economic, and health care factors.[6] In this chapter, the terminology associated with palliative care will be explored and problematised. It will be argued that changes in terminology go beyond mere semantics and have a profound influence upon how services are conceptualised and the extent of their remit. A description of the environments in which palliative care is delivered is provided. Readers will be introduced to some of the origins of palliative care. It has been suggested that palliative care represents a remarkable success story, as by the turn of the century it had emerged from a small specialist service for those dying from certain types of cancer to being now recognised as a global public health issue applicable to all types of anticipated dying.[7] Fifty-six million people die in the world each year,[8] and it is estimated that 60% of dying people could benefit from palliative care.[9] While there are approximately 8000 hospice or palliative care services in over 100 countries, many people with advanced disease are not able to access this type of care.[10] The majority of this chapter will therefore consider whether palliative care can be regarded as a success story and what factors may limit its future development. The emerging critique of palliative care will be addressed mainly in relation to the concerns of nurses working with adult cancer patients and their families.

This chapter is written from a predominantly Western perspective, drawing largely upon the British health care context and research evidence. It is acknowledged that nurses working in resource-poor countries may face different challenges in delivering palliative care to people with cancer. There are multiple 'voices' in the experience of advanced cancer, but some remain hidden or unrepresented in texts such as this, despite attempts to elicit and value 'service user' views (for example the Macmillan Cancer Voices project). I am mindful that there is little evidence about the needs and views of advanced cancer patients from different ethnic minority backgrounds, those with serious mental health problems or learning disabilities, and socially excluded or institutionalised people.[11] Likewise much less is known about the preferences and experiences of older people nearing the end of life.[12]

What is palliative care? Definitions and terminology

Evidence indicates that terms like 'palliative care' and 'supportive care' are poorly understood and lack consensus.[13,14] Until recently the lack of a universally agreed definition of specialist palliative care services has bedevilled progress. A number of terms including: end of life care, palliative care, hospice care, terminal care, and supportive care have been used to describe the health and social care delivered to those with advanced cancer and those near death. The lack of clarity is potentially problematic because of differences in expectations and concerns about appropriate access and referral to services.[14] Terminology is influenced by the historical development and the nature of end-of-life health care services in different countries and changes over time (see Box 36.1). In the UK, terminology relating to end-of-life care has undergone a number of transitions from hospice care and terminal care in the 1960s and 1970s, to palliative care towards the turn of the century. In the new century two new terms have become more widely used. Supportive care has emerged as an accepted term for services that are provided in addition to curative treatments for cancer patients.[5,15] While the term end-of-life care was first applied to care of dying patients in Canada, it is now widely used in North America, and in the UK tends to refer to more than the terminal phase. Clark and Seymour provide

an insightful account of these transitions in terminology in relation to the UK context.[4] They have noted how terminology has changed as tensions in the boundaries between generalist and specialist skills, activities and services have become more contentious. For the purposes of this chapter, the term 'palliative care' will be used forthwith.

The World Health Organisation has defined palliative care as encompassing physical, psychological, social, and spiritual aspects of care (see Box 36.2).[16] In the UK, specialist palliative care services are predominately accessed by patients with cancer, but there is a growing recognition that this type of care should be available to all patients regardless of their medical diagnosis (see Box 36.3).[17] Foley has argued, from a North American perspective, that access to high-quality end-of-life care for all is an international public health issue because dying with dignity is universally valued.[7]

Box 36.1 Terminology associated with health care services for dying people and their families in the UK

- Hospice care
- Terminal care
- Continuing care
- Care of the dying
- Palliative care
- End-of-life care
- Supportive care

Box 36.2 World Health Organisation (WHO) Definition of Palliative Care[16]

Palliative care is an approach that improves the quality of life of patients and their families facing the problems associated with life-threatening illness, through the prevention and relief of suffering by means of early identification and impeccable assessment and treatment of pain and other problems, physical, psychosocial and spiritual.

Box 36.3 The features of palliative care

Palliative care:

- provides relief from pain and other distressing symptoms
- affirms life and regards dying as a normal process
- intends neither to hasten nor postpone death
- integrates the psychological and spiritual aspects of patient care
- offers a support system to help patients live as actively as possible until death
- offers a support system to help the family cope during the patient's illness and in their own bereavement
- uses a team approach to address the needs of patients and their families, including bereavement counselling, if indicated
- will enhance quality of life, and may also positively influence the course of illness
- is applicable early in the course of illness, in conjunction with other therapies that are intended to prolong life, such as chemotherapy or radiation therapy, and include those investigations needed to better understand and manage distressing clinical complications.

The National Council for Hospices and Specialist Palliative Care Services[18] differentiates between:

- *general palliative care* which 'is provided by the usual professional carers of the patient and family with low to moderate complexity of palliative care need', and
- *specialist palliative care services* which 'are provided for patients and their families with moderate to high complexity of palliative care need. They are defined in terms of their core service components, their functions and the composition of the multi-professional teams that are required to deliver them.'

Nurses are key workers in providing direct physical care and in managing and co-ordinating physical care provided by others to patients near the end of life, and supporting their family caregivers.

Where is palliative care delivered?

The delivery of palliative care is not restricted to a clinical environment and can be accomplished anywhere the patient and family feel comfortable. Cancer nurses need to take account of the religious and cultural beliefs of the person and family receiving care. No single model of care is right for all patients at all times; instead service providers should aim to provide a range of options so choices can be made. The professional ethical and legal framework in which cancer nurses work will differ by country, but nurses should be guided by the principles of palliative care stated above. The following examples indicate common environments for delivering palliative care.

Home

Most people remain at home during the majority of their terminal illness and their families or friends deliver care.[19] Where general palliative care is available, it is most commonly provided by community nurses visiting people in their homes. In Britain in 2001, the government invested in an extensive 3-year programme of education for community nurses in the principles of palliative care aimed at improving care delivered at home. Evaluation studies show that those community nurses who attended the educational courses appeared to have increased their knowledge and confidence in their skills.[20] There are different models of nursing in the community, but the following may be available.

- teams of community care nurses (district nurses) who may be directly or indirectly linked to general practitioners and other primary medical care services. These nurses deliver direct hands-on nursing care at home and may consult with specialist palliative care nurses
- specialist palliative care nurses who are independent of generalist primary care services, but sometimes work with multidisciplinary palliative care teams and are linked to hospices. They provide support and consultancy to community nurses and general practitioners about palliative care at home
- specialist palliative care nurses who are linked to a hospice or similar service and provide

direct hands-on nursing care to patients at home.

Hospitals

In many Western countries, the majority of people die in hospitals, but there are concerns about the poor quality of care and high use of invasive treatments right up to the end of life.[21,22] Hospital-based specialist palliative care support teams were developed initially to provide consultancy services within hospitals, to promote better pain and symptom control, and increase skills and knowledge in general nurses. It has proved to be difficult to demonstrate their value and efficacy.[23] Some hospital-based teams also have their own ward areas with inpatient beds. Hospital-based specialist palliative care teams usually involve nurses, medical staff, and other professionals in providing advice to other health professionals. Working in an advisory capacity may bring with it particular tensions within the hospital, and Box 36.4 summarises some of these challenges.

Box 36.4   The challenges of delivering specialist palliative care in hospitals[2]

- Non-acceptance of palliative care as a specialty with specialist knowledge
- Divergent opinions between nurses and doctors about who has palliative care needs
- Power sharing between professional disciplines
- Poor communication
- Acceptance of advice and this being acted upon, especially for nurses
- Access to free/cheap medication
- Difficulties with opioid prescribing
- Role ambiguity for nurses
- Lack of resources (both human and financial).

Day care and drop-in clinics

Palliative care is also provided by day care services which enable patients to have social and rehabilitative activities, nursing care, and medical surveillance one or more days per week. They also offer opportunities for families to have respite from their caring duties. Palliative day care services have developed predominantly in the UK and the nature and aims of the activities offered

vary widely. Evidence from a number of research studies indicates that they are popular with certain types of patients but it is difficult to demonstrate their efficacy using robust outcome measures.[24]

Hospices

Hospices in the UK are generally thought of as specialist buildings in which inpatient or day care is provided to patients with advanced disease. In the UK, hospice care is overwhelmingly provided to people with cancer, although attempts are increasingly being made to enable those with non-malignant diseases to access services.[25,26] Hospices vary in a number of ways including their design, organisation, sources of funding, and bed capacity. Most UK hospices provide a range of services in addition to inpatient beds, including bereavement support services, respite care, social care teams, rehabilitative and complementary therapies, chaplaincy and spiritual support, counselling, and psychological therapies. Nursing in hospices is usually undertaken within a multidisciplinary team, working alongside doctors, social workers, chaplains, therapists, and voluntary staff to support patients and family members.

Origins of palliative care

Historically it has largely been women, both family members and others, who have been centrally concerned with the physical care of the dying. According to Clark, a number of influential pioneers were women who sought to improve the care of the dying, such as Jeanne Garnier in France, Mary Aikenhead in Ireland and Rose Hawthorne in the US.[27] In the UK, Dame Cicely Saunders, who founded St Christopher's Hospice, London, in 1967, originally qualified as a nurse before studying social work and later medicine.[28] Most of these women were motivated by personal experience, tragedies, religious calling and philanthropy.

A number of social and technological transitions during the latter part of the 20th century in many industrialised countries led to increasing hospitalisation for the dying. The following factors have been attributed to the development of the modern hospice movement:

- medicine becoming more technical and cure orientated, leading to the marginalisation of those who were dying
- the imperative to treat leading to a tendency to continue treatment even with little evidence of benefit
- emphasis on those with curable conditions led to the neglect of those with chronic illness and the dying
- concerns about morphine use and addiction
- medical paternalism and communication practises such as non-disclosure of diagnosis and prognosis, which was motivated out of a concern to 'protect' patients from the painful truth of their dying status
- health care was organised hierarchically with nurses positioned as 'medical handmaidens'.

So despite nurses having an important role in caring for those near the end of life, many were not in a position to influence changes in care or challenge medical practices. Few nurses had the motivation or power to influence policy developments.

The modern hospice movement developed from new conceptual understandings and a desire to address perceived inadequacies in the care of dying patients.[27] Research in the latter part of the 20th century in a number of industrialised countries indicated the extent of the impact of cancer and other chronic conditions on the psychological and social welfare of patients. In the UK, a number of cancer charities (such as Macmillan Cancer Support and Marie Curie Cancer Care) in conjunction with statutory health care services, responded to these and other concerns, by developing posts for specialist nurses leading to the recognition of clinical nurse specialist (CNS) roles.

Most palliative care nursing is delivered by *general qualified nurses* in hospitals, care homes, and patients' homes. These nurses need to be aware of the principles of palliative care; including attention to the physical, psychological, social and spiritual care of patients and their families, and to know how and when to access additional support in dealing with complex problems.

Nurses with additional qualifications and expertise in palliative care are described as *special-ist palliative care nurses*. These nurses may work in hospitals, hospices, or the community both to provide direct care to patients and families and also provide advice to other health professionals. Many of these nurses work independently but some are part of multidisciplinary teams. The role of specialist palliative care nursing is varied and complex, and includes symptom control and supportive care for patients and families, co-ordination and communication between other services, empathy, and respect for the dignity and preferences of those in their care.[29–32]

The role of specialist palliative care nurses has been developed in the UK largely through the funding made available from a cancer charity now called Macmillan Cancer Support. These specialist nurses tend to use the title 'Macmillan' nurse. Research evidence demonstrates that a large proportion (89%) of their role involves direct face-to-face contact with patients, and that the commonest reason for referral is for emotional support.[29,30] Most of these nurses do not provide 'hands-on' direct nursing care but offer support and information to patients. They also work behind the scenes in co-ordinating care and offering specialist advice to generalists including general practitioners and community nurses. Their work serves to promote better standards of palliative care by disseminating good practice and current evidence. They are therefore an important resource in trying to improve palliative care provision. However, they have predominantly focused their work on people with cancer, which results in few services for those with other conditions.

Palliative care – a success story?

Dying and death, like pregnancy and birth, are life transitions that touch all those involved. It is therefore not surprising that providing good end-of-life care should be regarded as more than good physical care of the body and the control of difficult symptoms. For example, improvement in the management of pain, especially of pain that is associated with terminal cancer, is arguably one of the major achievements of specialist palliative care.[33] The development of the WHO pain ladder, based on early research by Saunders, Twycross and others,[34] has transformed clinical practice. This, combined with other technologies associated with analgesia delivery (the syringe driver) and pharmaceutical developments, especially oral morphine preparations, means that the majority of cancer patients with advanced disease can anticipate adequate pain management.[35] In many resource-poor countries a key challenge to effective palliative care is access to medication, especially adequate supplies of opioids. These drugs need to be legally acceptable, affordable, and available when needed, including at night and at weekends. In some countries there remain major barriers to the ready availability of opioids, or specific preparations such as oral morphine, because of concerns about morphine addiction or trafficking. Per capita consumption of morphine between countries remains very variable and is of concern to the WHO.[36] It indicates that pain control remains less than optimal in many areas of the world.

The concept of 'total pain', which developed from the work of Cicely Saunders,[33] neatly draws our attention to the interdependency of physical, psychological, social, or spiritual elements in the experience and alleviation of pain. There are two ways of interpreting the concept of 'total pain': it may be viewed as enabling and empowering for cancer nurses who use it to attend to more than just the physical aspects of care; alternatively it can be seen as coercive and potentially invasive for patients, as all aspects of their functioning, both physical and psychosocial, come under scrutiny. Clark has argued, from a Foucauldian perspective, that this, unintentionally, is potentially more invasive in patients' lives than a concern only with the physical aspects of pain management because it legitimates the exploration of not only patients' physical bodies by nurses but also their minds, their social relationships, and even their existential concerns.[33] The concept of 'total pain' mapped out new territories for nurses. No longer was it sufficient for nurses to tend the physical bodies of dying patients, but their psychological, social and spiritual state fell within the remit of nursing work. For a critical account of how nurses conceptualise and deal with symptom control in palliative care see Corner.[37]

Psychological care

One area in which palliative care nursing work has carved out its territory is in psychological support. Specialist palliative care nurses in the UK, US, and other Western countries are increasingly involved in providing psychological care.[1,30] It has long been recognised that a diagnosis of cancer and the experience of cancer treatment has an emotional, cognitive and social impact on patients and families. Evidence suggests that a sizeable proportion of patients will experience psychological morbidity, with by far the most common disorders being depression and anxiety.[38] Reviews of the research literature indicate that between 3% and 69% of people with advanced cancer experience depression.[39,40] Much of this variability can be accounted for by differences in how and when patients are assessed and the criteria used to classify depression. Sadly, there is also evidence that much of this morbidity goes unrecognised and untreated.[41] For example, Lloyd Williams and Payne found that many people, including nurses, regard depression as an inevitable part of end-stage disease and thus are not sensitised to recognising this as treatable pathology.[42]

The symptoms of depression include three components (behaviours, cognitions and emotions) as shown in Box 36.5. The criteria for diagnosis of clinical depression are that symptoms should be persistent rather than transitory, and should have lasted for at least 2 weeks. Clinical depression is a severely disabling condition which is potentially life threatening because of the risk of suicide, and seriously reduces the quality of life of the patient and family. There are gender (women are more likely to express depressed feelings than men), age-related and cultural differences in the expression of emotions, which should be taken into account when assessing patients for psychological distress. Consideration of the list of symptoms of depression in Box 36.5 shows that for patients with advanced cancer there are a number of problems in discriminating between clinical depression, 'normal' sadness, and symptoms of their illness. To complicate the recognition of depression in palliative care patients, there are two further confounding factors; namely symptoms resulting from the disease process and treatment side-effects. For example, weakness, anorexia, and fatigue are all common features of advanced cancer. Many patients, especially older people with advanced cancer may suffer from a number of co-morbidities that may also

Box 36.5 Behavioural, cognitive, and emotional indictors of depression

- *Behaviours* – such as agitated restlessness or sluggishness (slow movements), loss of energy (feeling tired all the time), anorexia, weight changes (increases or decreases), sleep disturbance (more or less, especially early morning wakening), loss of interest in activities.
- *Cognitions* – such as apathy, feelings of worthlessness, self-reproach, guilt, sense of failure, self-punishment, indecisiveness, thoughts of death or suicide.
- *Emotions* – such as a lack of pleasure in everyday events, sadness, crying.

cloud the picture. Depression may be associated with other psychological disorders including dementia and, perhaps most commonly, anxiety.

In the UK, the National Institute for Clinical Excellence (NICE) (2004) guidance recommends a four-tiered model of psychological assessment, support and intervention based upon the complexity of the needs of patients and the expertise of professionals involved (shown in Figure 36.1).[5] It proposes that all cancer nurses have an important role in the recognition of psychological support needs and should be able to provide compassionate and effective communication. Those with additional skills such as CNSs have a role in screening for depression, anxiety, and other psychological problems using standardised measures such as the Hospital Anxiety and Depression Scale,[43] or other tools. They may also have the skills to deliver well-defined simple interventions to support patients and help with stress manage-

Level	Group	Assessments	Interventions
1	All health and social care professionals	Recognition of psychological needs	Effective information-giving, compassionate communication and general psychological support
2	Health and social care professionals with additional expertise	Screening for psychological distress	Psychological interventions (such as anxiety management and problem solving)
3	Trained and accredited professionals	Assessed for psychological distress and diagnosis of some psychopathology	Counselling and specific psychological therapies, such as cognitive behavioural therapy (CBT) and solution-focused therapy, delivered according to an explicit theoretical framework
4	Mental health specialists – clinical psychologists and psychiatrists	Diagnosis of psychopathology	Specialist psychological and psychiatric interventions

(Left vertical axis arrow label: Self-help and informal support)

Figure 36.1 Recommended model of professional, psychological assessment and support. National Institute for Clinical Excellence (2004). *Guidance on Cancer Services: Improving Supportive and Palliative Care for Adults with Cancer – the Manual.* London: NICE. Available from www.nice.org.uk. Reproduced with permission.

ment, for example. At the third level, properly trained and accredited practitioners may deliver specific interventions such as counselling or cognitive-behavioural therapy. Finally, some cancer patients may experience such complex or long-standing types of psychopathology that assessment and intervention by experienced mental health specialists such as liaison psychiatrists or clinical psychologists are required. Cancer nurses need to be aware of the limits of their expertise and be prepared to make appropriate referrals.

Much psychological morbidity goes unrecognised and therefore untreated because nurses are reluctant to question people directly about their feelings, and patients fail to report their concerns because they fear wasting professional's time, are afraid that they may be construed as ungrateful or 'weak willed', or do not believe that nurses are interested in their psychological state.[44] Some patients fail to disclose feelings of depression because they fear that more medication may be prescribed. While nurses are comfortable and generally feel skilled in assessing pain and other physical symptoms, many are reluctant to assess for depression, and lack confidence in psychological assessment.[45] Research has shown that even if clinical nurse specialists in palliative care did recognise depression or other psychological problems, they delayed referring the patient for further assessment and treatment, or reported that medical colleagues were reluctant to respond to their suggestions.[46] Yet the evidence indicates that even in late-stage cancer, depression may be treatable by pharmacological and non-pharmacological interventions.[47]

Resilience and hardiness

One of the main problems in the way psychological care is often construed is to emphasise the abnormal or pathological ways to respond. Relatively little attention is focused on the way that the majority of people affected by cancer manage to contain their distress, carry on with their everyday lives and maintain good relationships with those around them. These are remarkable achievements but we tend not to celebrate or study them. Little is known about the individual differences that predict who will manage these difficult challenges and who will be overwhelmed by the experience of cancer. In my view, most people with cancer are very resilient and cope well with the challenges facing them. They are forgiving and understanding of the inadequacies of health care systems and of the ineptitude of novice cancer nurses and junior doctors.[48,49]

Psychological research shows that some people have personalities that are better able to deal with difficult and challenging situations. Kobasa introduced the notion of 'hardiness' as a personality trait.[50] There were three key characteristics: commitment (active involvement in life), control (a belief in the ability to influence life events), and challenge (a stance that regards change as normal and not threatening). People with these attributes are more likely to be optimistic, deal better with stressful situations, and engage in healthy behaviours. Cancer nurses may like to support their patients in ways that reduce passivity and help them to engage in these psychologically healthy ways of responding to cancer. We also need to recognise that people have intrinsic (e.g. their personality, life experiences) and extrinsic (e.g. family, community, religion, money) resources. It is important not to create dependency upon health care services.

Recognition of families and carers

From the outset, palliative care philosophy has incorporated families and carers as well as patients within the remit of service provision. There has been recognition that cancer affects families and that carers are crucially important throughout the experience of cancer, but evidence suggests that many cancer nurses do not realise the nature or demands of care provided by family members.[51] Typically family carers strive to maintain 'normal' family functioning, provide emotional support to patients, and mediate between service providers to obtain resources. In the UK the NICE guidance offered a broad and inclusive definition of families and carers (see Box 36.6) that made no assumptions of kinship or sexual orientation.[5]

According to the British General Household Survey conducted in 2000, there are approximately seven million carers.[52] Most provide care

Box 36.6 Definitions of family and carers (p.126)[5]

. . . those related through committed heterosexual or same sex partnerships, birth and adoption, and others who have strong emotional and social bonds with a patient. Carers, who may or may not be family members, are lay people in a close supportive role who share in the illness experience of the patient and who undertake vital care work and emotion management.

for those with chronic illness, or disabilities, and for frail older people. It is difficult to estimate the numbers of those providing care for a person nearing the end of life, as much will depend upon the definition of palliative care used and whether the remit extends to those with chronic life-limiting diseases such as dementia, heart failure, and end-stage renal disease. Evidence suggests that greater numbers of people provide care at some point in their lives than 10 years ago. More women (3.9 million) than men (2.9 million) provide care; and the majority are middle-aged (between 45 and 64 years), but increasingly older people over 65 years are involved in caring.[52] In palliative care, there is more likely to be within-generational than intergenerational caregiving. Carers are usually family members, but changing social patterns such as divorce, geographical mobility, increased longevity, and declining birth rates, may mean that for some people, friends, neighbours, or employed care workers (for example, for older people living in care homes) may provide more meaningful relationships than distant kin. Increasing numbers of older people are living in single-person households, especially older women, and for these people no readily identifiable carer may be available. These people may have few viable choices except institutional care when they face the end of life.

Much of the early research on carers emphasised the domestic and personal care tasks that were performed; this lead to a picture of carers being physically burdened by the labour of caring, which has been critiqued by Nolan.[53] In addition to providing care for the ill person, carers often take on additional responsibilities in managing the home, family finances, childcare, and care of other dependents such as older relatives. In a study of carers of those with cancer, 21% of carers were already carers before the cancer diagnosis.[54] It is only recently that patients and carers have been invited to contribute directly to national debates on health and social care or become involved in the planning and delivery of services and contribute to the design and conduct of research in health care.[55–57] Even with these new 'user-involvement' policies, carers in palliative care tend to be regarded as proxies for patients who are too ill or otherwise unable to articulate their own views, rather than as having a mandate to speak about their own concerns.

In the broad context of health and social care in the UK, family carers lie at the heart of community care policy, and over the last decade services to support family carers have moved from the margins of social policy to occupy 'centre stage',[58] representing one of the most striking developments in the policy arena.[59]

Notwithstanding such advances, a major review of the recent literature has identified several unresolved issues in relation to carer support, including:

- *when* is support best provided?
- *how* is support best provided?
- *what* are the intended aims of support?
- *who* is the perceived beneficiary?[60]

Consequently, despite an explosion of research into family care over the last two decades, predominantly in the context of care for older people,[61] there remains little evidence for the effectiveness of services.[62] In the context of palliative care, a systematic review of the research literature indicates that carers have many challenges and demands but there is little evidence about how best to help them.[63] For example, a review of the literature on palliative care respite failed to demonstrate strong evidence of its efficacy.[64] A probable cause of the problem lies in the fact that services are often inflexible and fail to provide care and support that carers see as being of sufficient quality and readily available when they are required.[65,66] All too often the outcomes of services are not those that carers see as important,[66] and there is a general failure to engage fully with carers as co-experts in care delivery.[67] Consequently, services are often viewed as obstructing or inhibiting carers' goals, rather than facilitating them.[67]

Family carers are increasingly being relied upon to provide the majority of daily care, including the management of the physical, emotional, and psychological consequences of advanced disease, but professional service providers often are unaware of the complexity and nature of the caring role assumed by families. The impact of family carers' policy changes in the UK and those that promote greater choice of place of care and death, which have resulted in an emphasis on community care and the movement away from care delivered in hospices, remains unclear. The NICE guidance recommends that a separate key worker is appointed specifically to assess the needs of carers, provide them with information when it is required, and co-ordinate available services and help them to access resources.[5] These suggestions have largely yet to be implemented in practice and it is too soon to determine their impact on carers.

Bereavement support

As part of the continuing care of families which extends after the death of patients, many palliative care services regard the provision of bereavement support as an integral part of their remit.[68] Until recently the UK NHS has contributed little to bereavement support, with the exception of spiritual support to families from hospital chaplains at the time of death and, in a minority of cases, psychiatric treatment for those with complicated grief reactions.[69] In the community, bereavement support has largely been delivered through faith groups and other self-help networks, and by voluntary organisations such as Cruse. Most bereavement services are based on the assumption that loss through death challenges coping abilities, and that supportive interventions may facilitate post-death adaptation, reduce complicated grief reactions, and promote well-being. Palliative care services can be regarded as pioneers in developing these types of services. The nature and quality of interactions with nurses in the period before a person with cancer dies may also help families

accept this life transition. For example, helping a person to die with dignity, with optimal symptom control, and with attention to their spiritual and cultural needs, may in retrospect be seen as comforting to bereaved families.

Evidence from a survey conducted in the UK of all bereavement support services provided by hospices and specialist palliative care services demonstrated that there was considerable diversity in the nature, organisation, and extent of services.[70] The most commonly provided support activities were individual support, telephone support, written information, memorialisation events, and group support. Most services were led by paid staff who had qualifications in either nursing, counselling, or social work, and over two-thirds involved volunteers in the delivery of bereavement support. The researchers found that 80% of the adult bereavement services were implementing or planning changes to their service either in response to perceived difficulties and/or to expand existing services. Over one-fifth of services reported they had insufficient paid or voluntary staff. This survey suggested that bereavement support services were an under-resourced element of palliative care provision with many services dependent upon relatively few staff. The situation for childhood bereavement services was reported to be similar,[71] with an even greater diversity of organisational structure and provision.

In the UK the NICE guidance[5] suggested that a three-tier model of bereavement support be implemented for all families and carers of cancer patients, in which all health care providers should provide information about local services to bereaved people (level 1).[5] Those in need of more comprehensive support should be offered support from professionals and/or volunteers (level 2), and a minority of people at high risk of complicated bereavement reactions should be referred to specialist services (level 3). Evidence from organisational case study research conducted in five bereavement services in England indicated that while levels 1 and 2 appeared to be provided, services had yet to develop robust referral mechanisms to suitable specialist providers at level 3.[72] Box 36.7 offers some practical suggestions for cancer nurses.

Box 36.7 Practical suggestions for supporting cancer patients and their families near the end of life

- As people approach the end of life, they and their families experience numerous losses and anticipate even more losses.
- Experiencing loss is a normal part of everyone's life and most people are resilient and have sufficient resources, in terms of their personal experiences of coping, existential understandings, family and friends to draw upon.
- People cope with loss in different ways at different times. One way is to assert control and maintain autonomy but this may not be right or culturally appropriate for all people.
- Family members are not all the same, they may respond in different ways to the experiences they face, for example some may require a lot of information and others less. Nurses should not assume that communication is good between family members. Communicating just with a 'main' carer risks excluding others.
- Patients and families often fear the process of dying and nurses can help by explaining what support and symptom control is available at each step.
- Once the patient dies, bereaved people draw upon their cultural, social and spiritual understandings to provide a meaning for their loss and to determine their behaviour and expression of their grief.
- Bereaved people may display their grief in many ways in different environments and these displays are largely socially proscribed. A failure to appear distressed when they are with you does not mean that they can not or will not display their distress elsewhere.
- Grief hurts both physically and psychologically, and because of the loss of the dead person, the bereaved person may no longer have their normal sources of support.
- Bereaved people experience changes in their identity and social roles, for example a wife becomes a widow, a mother may become childless, which changes how they are perceived by others and eventually how they perceive themselves.
- Providing an opportunity for a bereaved person to talk about the dead person, the process of dying, and the death may be helpful, especially when they have concerns about the adequacy of care or feel there may have been some omissions such as a failure to recognise cancer recurrence early enough. In talking through their experiences, bereaved people may be helped to construct a story about the dead person and their final illness; this may be comforting.
- Not all bereaved people need additional support but a minority may have complex bereavement reactions which mean that referral to support organisations such as Cruse or other agencies might be welcomed. This should be considered when the nature of the death is very traumatic or unexpected, or the person has concurrent losses or other stresses.

Communication and information

There has been a remarkable transformation in health-related communication practices in most Westernised countries over the last 30 years. In cancer care the disclosure of diagnosis is now almost universal and to a lesser extent so is information about prognosis.[73] While these changes have paralleled the growth of the modern hospice movement, it is less clear that they can be solely attributed to palliative care. The early research of Glaser and Strauss conducted in the US in the 1950s described patterns of communication (called awareness contexts) between dying patients, relatives, and hospital staff which sought to conceal the truth.[74] They challenged the value of these practices and demonstrated that rather than protecting people from worrying and confronting the

reality of dying, they served to isolate and disempower patients, and prevented supportive communication with their families and health care providers. From the outset, hospice philosophy espoused 'open' awareness communication practices in which patients and families were encouraged to freely and honestly talk with staff about their predicament and their concerns. Field and Copp have argued that actual communication practices in palliative care are better described as 'conditional' awareness, where information is tempered to the desires and tolerance of individuals on a daily basis.[75]

Concurrently there have been social changes in Western countries where increasingly cultures place high value and emphasis on individual autonomy and personal rights. This is reflected in cancer care practice by an increasing emphasis on patient involvement in making treatment decisions and other choices. To achieve this more participatory style of health professional–patient interaction requires patterns of communication that go beyond merely issuing 'medical orders', and for nurses, ensuring that these 'orders' are complied with. Thus arose, from about the 1980s onwards, a growing body of research and education in communication skills in cancer care contexts. There is now robust evidence that communication skills can be taught and that, following training, improvements in skills are retained over time and can be demonstrated to be used in clinical situations.[76] The opening up of full and honest communication with patients has transformed cancer nursing practice. No longer do nurses need to be skilled in techniques of evasion and the use of euphemisms. It is now common for patients to be encouraged to participate in making 'care plans' in relation to their cancer treatment. However, concerns remain about the quality of cancer nurses' communication skills and their ability to elicit all the concerns of patients,[77] and their ability to recognise the minority of patients who do not wish to engage in open communication. Based on a doctoral research study, Jarrett and Payne argued that cancer patients work with cancer nurses to maintain normal social conversational conventions and what are described as 'comfortable' conversations.[78] They found that patients go out of their way to make sure they do not threaten the status of nurses by questioning their knowledge or asking difficult questions.

In palliative care, patients are being encouraged to express preferences about place of care and indicate choices about the extent of treatment offered near the end of life. These are described as advance directives or 'living wills'. While they have been widely adopted in North America, there is less evidence about their acceptability and efficacy in Britain.[79] Finlay has advocated that 'death plans' be introduced into specialist palliative care, to allow patients and their families to express their wishes about important aspects of end-of-life care such as terminal sedation and resuscitation.[80] This requires nurses and doctors to have the confidence and ability to address very difficult topics. To really engage patients in preparing their own plans will require considerable communication skills and an openness to empower patients to make choices, some of which may not fit with what the nurse considers to be 'right or proper'. This much more radical approach requires a shift in the balance of power and is likely to prove to be a new challenge for cancer nurses.

Multidisciplinary working

One of the key features of early hospice management structure was an engagement in multidisciplinary working. Typically, organisational structures were 'flat' rather than hierarchical. Doctors, nurses, social workers, and volunteers collaborated together to provide integrated care. There were fewer professional boundaries than was the norm in other health care contexts. James and Field, in their reflections on transitions in organisational systems of hospice services during their first 20 years, argued that professional boundaries were blurred in the early days but re-emerged with the formal recognition of palliative medicine as a specialty (in 1987 in the UK).[81]

Nurses are a core component of the multidisciplinary team in palliative care. They may have a leadership or collaborative role. Teams vary in size and in professional composition, but it is common for nurses to work with other nurses and medical staff. In addition, multidisciplinary teams in palliative care may include social workers, physiotherapists, occupational therapists, pharmacists, psychologists, and counsellors. It may be necessary to refer patients to other professionals with specialist expertise such as speech and language therapists or nutritionists. Nurses will also work with non-professional staff such as care assistants and domestic workers, and in some services volunteer workers (who may or may not hold professional qualifications).

The rhetoric of 'multidisciplinary' or 'interdisciplinary' teams emerged in the 1990s within cancer and palliative care. Little critical scrutiny of the composition or effectiveness of teams in palliative care appears in the literature, instead they are generally assumed to be a 'good thing'. Cox and James offer a more challenging analysis of team working, drawing upon three paradoxes.[82,83] The first highlights the inward orientation of many teams, yet the necessity for palliative care teams to work with other organisations and agencies. The second emphasises that working in teams may be mutually supportive in the face of institutional demands but managers often regard teams as strategies to deliver institutional imperatives. Third, team working means engaging with the 'inward' complexity of interactions with colleagues but current health care policy emphasises 'outward' responsiveness to the service users' agenda. Therefore working in teams offers both benefits such as being supported in decision making and shared responsibility, but also challenges such as dealing with interpersonal conflict and constraints.

The hospice as a social movement

The hospice emerged in response to perceived inadequacy in the care of dying cancer patients in the UK. However, in a remarkably short timespan the vision of palliative care has engaged the public imagination and spread in different versions to many parts of the world. In the UK and some other countries, the early hospices were supported by charitable giving, and the imperative for service development has largely been driven outside of central health care planning. What was it about these services that appealed to individual and community generosity? Were the types of care offered – holistic, person-centred, family orientated, and nurturing – a radical alternative to those offered within mainstream health care services? In the UK, charitably funded (independent) hospices typically emphasised their 'homely' non-clinical environment, the individual nature of care, and the 'warmth' and supportiveness of their staff and volunteers.[84] This was at a time when dying in acute care hospitals was characterised as being in a coldly clinical busy 'cure-orientated' environment, isolating, lacking in individualised care, with the perils of either under- or over-treatment.[21] Not surprisingly, alternatives to this awful reality were eagerly sought and hospices offered one solution. More cynically, Lawton proposed that hospices also functioned to sequestrate those who were dying in difficult and complex ways ('dirty dying'), away from the public gaze and

served to protect society from the threat to social order that they posed.[85] While there are some merits to her argument, it fails to account for the large numbers of people who choose to volunteer to work within hospices.

Hospices that derive the majority of their funding from charitable sources are under tremendous pressure to contain their costs. Volunteers represent one way to achieve this. Moreover, their contribution in terms of free labour and fund-raising effort has been, and in many places continues to be, vital to the survival of hospices. In New Zealand volunteers donated 322 672 hours of labour to hospices in 1999.[86] In Britain, research has demonstrated that employing voluntary staff is cost-effective and contributes to the quality of services.[87] Hospices can be seen as a social movement because of the large number of people who readily engage with them by volunteering their labour.

For example, in Kerala, India, public participation in delivering palliative care support in people's homes has been described by Graham and Clark.[88] Their observations illustrate how Neighbourhood Network Groups in Palliative Care (NNPC) have been established by medical staff and social activists to co-ordinate care provided by local volunteers to dying people in their homes. This resource-poor and rural area of the world has achieved a sustainable community-directed service which offered coverage of 70% of people in 2 years. According to Graham and Clark, 'volunteers undertook practical tasks, such as helping families wash and change patients and spent time asking about symptoms and other problems' (p.38).[88] They were supported by professionals in dealing with more complex symptom-control issues. This example shows how supporting patients with advanced disease may draw upon community strengths and not merely be regarded as the work of health professionals.

An emerging critique of palliative care

Palliative care has been predominantly developed in the context of adults with cancer, but it is also appropriate for those with other chronic diseases.

It cannot be assumed that the skills learned within the context of predominantly middle-aged people dying of cancer can be readily transferred to other groups.[17] Even for those with cancer, some groups of people appear to be under-served by current palliative care services such as those who are:

- economically deprived
- living in inner-city or rural areas
- in older age, especially late old age
- living in certain institutions (e.g. prisons and care homes)
- have learning difficulties and/or mental health problems
- are from minority groups.

Addressing the inequalities within palliative care provision should be high on the agenda.[89] A review of the evidence from the US indicates that poverty largely determines the type and quality of services that an individual can access when they have palliative care needs.[90] Living on a low income is likely to have multiple effects such as less access to choice of medical treatment and health care providers, limited capacity to pay for treatment-related costs such as medications, equipment and supplementary items, and less access to rehabilitative and supportive interventions. Even in countries with statutory provision of health care such as the UK, there is evidence that poor people are more likely to be burdened by disease, die earlier than their richer countrymen, and have more limited access to poorer-quality health care. An unpublished public health audit conducted in Sheffield (a post-industrial city in the North of England) indicated that people living in the more economically deprived areas of the north and east of the city were less likely to access specialist palliative care services than those in the south and west where the hospice was sited.[91]

Geographical inequality relates to the challenges of delivering specialist palliative care services in rural areas where the low density of population, difficulties relating to terrain, and limited road network, or in island communities, add to the complexity. Telemedicine and other technologies offer imaginative solutions. Ingleton *et al.* reported on a primary care-based supportive intervention to improve palliative care in an area of rural Wales (Powys).[92] They highlighted how improving the knowledge, skills, and confidence of general practitioners and community nurses served to enable more patients to remain at home for palliative care.[93]

Cancer is predominantly a disease of older people, but specialist palliative care services have not adequately addressed the needs of older people.[94,95] Within a US public health context,[96] a model was developed which described older patients' dying trajectories, in order to seek a better understanding of access to and use of health and social care services in the last year of life. The authors proposed a typology of four dying trajectories:

- sudden death such as road traffic accidents or myocardial infarctions
- diseases with anticipated and predictable terminal trajectories such as cancer
- disease with episodic crises and unpredictable trajectories such as heart failure and chronic obstructive pulmonary disease
- slow and progressive decline and frailty associated with multiple co-morbidities and dementia.

Lunney *et al.* suggest that this model can capture the nature of clinical courses which can enhance the evaluation of health care patterns at the end of life, and indicate where palliative care interventions are required.[96] Most current palliative care services are provided to those with the second typology of dying. It is not clear how current service configurations are best able to deal with the latter types of dying. Seymour *et al.* have conducted a comprehensive review of the issues for services to older people near the end of life and made recommendations for improving care.[79] An increasing proportion of older people die within institutions such as care homes. Froggatt has highlighted concerns about the quality of services provided to older people resident in care homes.[97] She suggests that merely applying models from specialist palliative care are inadequate because care homes tend to have fewer and less-well-qualified staff. She also highlights a tension for care home staff that, while at any one time one or two residents may be dying, the rest of the residents are living, and activities in the home should be directed towards the needs of both groups.

Evidence from the US, Canada and Britain indicates that attempts have been made to improve the conditions of those inmates dying in prisons.[98] Penal policies differ by country and by state in the US, with much larger numbers being imprisoned without possibility of parole in North America than in Britain. In the US, initiatives have been developed within penal institutions to use volunteer prisoners to offer companionships and support for other dying prisoners during their palliative phase.[99] British prison health service policy has been to facilitate early release of dying prisoners on parole, whenever possible. Prison health care services have to face the challenges of offering care in the context of predominantly custodial systems. They increasingly draw upon the expertise of local palliative care specialists.[100]

Some cancer patients' lives are challenged by other conditions such as learning disabilities, mental health problems, and sensory deficits. Services do not always take into account those with differing needs, and cancer nurses may not know how best to help. Little attention has been directed towards the needs of cancer patients who have learning disabilities.[101] For example, they are likely to have special needs for information and communication.[102] Cancer nurses may not feel skilled in helping people with pre-existing psychiatric problems, and their mental health needs may be neglected through ignorance. As more people are treated for cancer in late old age, the risk of concurrent cognitive deficit and dementia becomes more likely. Palliative care services are not usually designed to accommodate the needs of those with dementia.[46,103] People with sensory deficits may find that communication is poor, because specially designed information is unavailable. Liaison working between experts in learning disability, mental health, and elderly care and cancer nurses are likely to benefits all these groups.

Evidence suggests that minority ethnic groups make less use of cancer and specialist palliative care services than anticipated; the reasons for this are unclear.[104] There are many explanations to account for differences in ethnic patterns of health, including artefactual, material, cultural, social selection, the consequences of migration, the effects of racism, and genetic factors,[98] There is an emerging literature that has started to recognise end-of-life issues for different cultural groups and problematise the construction of 'ethnicity' and the responses of services. A number of innovative solutions have been tested to help services respond to cultural diversity.

Conclusions

This chapter has reviewed the progress of palliative care and highlighted the achievements made in the last four decades. It has of necessity been selective, which leaves much unsaid, for example about ethical issues, spiritual care, professional nursing roles, education, and research. These have not been neglected because they are unworthy of debate. I end by considering the challenges facing nurses. Performance by nurses in developing and delivering palliative care has been impressive, they have been central to many of the innovations. However, they will need to sharpen their practice and be prepared to set more ambitious targets to address the inequalities of service provision identified above. The National Council for Palliative Care published a document indicating the anticipated challenges facing services in the next 20 years.[105] They suggest that palliative care will need to take account of an ageing population where co-morbidities complicate the experience of cancer, greater consumer 'voice' and rising expectations, social changes in communities with more people living alone, greater cultural and ethnic diversity, and all this within the context of reduction in availability of the workforce to provide care, especially to deliver health and social care at home. It is important not to feel overwhelmed by the magnitude of these challenges. There are already innovations in service delivery that offer potential improvement in care such as the introduction of integrated care pathways,[106,107] although it is important that they do not reduce nursing care to formulaic responses. Cancer nurses have an important role to play in combining with others in the multidisciplinary team and at the policy level in setting targets, developing their performance, and initiating organisational changes to services.

References

1. Ferrell B.R. and Coyle N. (eds.) (2001). *Textbook of Palliative Nursing*. Oxford: Oxford University Press.
2. Payne S., Seymour J. and Ingleton C. (eds.) (2004). *Palliative Care Nursing: Principles and Evidence for Practice*. Maidenhead: Open University Press.
3. Payne S., Seymour J. and Ingleton C. *Palliative Care Nursing: Principles and Evidence for Practice*, 2nd edition. Maidenhead: Open University Press (In preparation).
4. Clark D. and Seymour J. (1999). *Reflection on Palliative Care*. Buckingham: Open University Press.
5. National Institute for Clinical Excellence. (2004). *Supportive and Palliative Care Guidance for Adults with Cancer*. London: National Institute for Clinical Excellence.
6. Field D., Hockey J. and Small N. (eds.) (1997). *Death, Gender and Ethnicity*. London: Routledge.
7. Foley K.M. (2003). How much palliative care do we need? *European Journal of Palliative Care* **10**, 5–7.
8. World Health Organization. (2002). Report: *Preventing Risks, Promoting Healthy Life*. www.who.int/mediacentre/releases/pr84/en/ (accessed 14 August 2007).
9. Davies E. and Higginson I.J. (2004). *The Solid Facts: Palliative Care*. Copenhagen: World Health Organization.
10. Wright M. (2003). *Models of Hospice and Palliative Care in Resource Poor Countries: Issues and Opportunities*. London: Hospice Information.
11. Oliviere D. and Monroe B. (eds.) (2004). *Death, Dying and Social Differences*. Oxford: Oxford University Press.
12. Seymour J., Witherspoon R., Gott M., Ross H. and Payne S., Help the Aged. (2004). *Thinking about the Future: Promoting Comfort, Choice and Well Being for Older People at the End of their Lives*. Bristol: Policy Press.
13. Praill D. (2000). Who are we here for? (editoral). *Palliative Medicine* **14**, 91–92.
14. Payne S., Sheldon F., Jarrett N. *et al.* (2002). Differences in understandings of specialist palliative care amongst service providers and commissioners in South London. *Palliative Medicine* **16**, 395–402.
15. Department of Health. (2000). *The NHS Cancer Plan: A Plan for Investment, a Plan for Reform*. London: HMSO.
16. Sepulveda C., Marlin A., Yoshida T. and Ullrich A. (2002). Palliative care: The World Health Organization's global perspective. *Journal of Pain and Symptom Management* **24**, 91–96.
17. Addington-Hall J.M. and Higginson I.J. (eds.) (2001). *Palliative Care for Non-cancer Patients*. Oxford: Oxford University Press.
18. National Council for Hospice and Specialist Palliative Care Services. (2002). *Definitions of Supportive and Palliative Care*. London: National Council for Hospice and Specialist Palliative Care Services.
19. Addington-Hall J.M. (2004). Referral patterns and access to specialist palliative care. In Payne S., Seymour J. and Ingleton C. (eds.) *Palliative Care Nursing: Principles and Evidence for Practice*. Maidenhead: Open University Press, pp. 90–107.
20. Hughes P., Noble B., Payne S., Ingleton I. and Parker C. (2006). Evaluating an education programme in general palliative care for community nurses: how long do the effects last? *International Journal of Palliative Nursing* **12**, 123–131.
21. Mills M., Davies, T.O. and Macrae W.A. (1994). Care of dying patients in hospital. *British Medical Journal* **309**, 583–586.
22. Edmonds P. and Rogers A. (2003). 'If only someone had told me . . .' A review of the care of patients dying in hospital. *Clinical Medicine* **3**, 149–152.
23. Higginson I.J., Finlay I., Goodwin G.M. *et al.* (2002). Do hospital-based palliative teams improve care for patients or families at the end of life? *Journal of Pain and Symptom Management* **23**, 96–106.
24. Hearn J. and Myers K. (2001). *Palliative Day Care in Practice*. Oxford: Oxford University Press.
25. Eve A. and Higginson I. (2000). Minimum dataset activity for hospice and palliative care services in the UK 1997/8. *Palliative Medicine* **14**, 395–404.
26. National Council for Palliative Care. (2005). *Minimum Data Sets Project Update*. London: National Council for Palliative Care.
27. Clark D. (2004). History, gender and culture in the rise of palliative care. In Payne S., Seymour J. and Ingleton C. (eds.) *Palliative Care Nursing: Principles and Evidence for Practice*. Maidenhead: Open University Press, pp. 39–54.
28. Clark D. (2000). Palliative care history: ritual process. *European Journal of Palliative Care* **7**, 50–55.
29. Corner J., Clark D. and Normand C. (2002). Evaluating the work of clinical nurse specialists in palliative care. *Palliative Medicine* **16**, 275–277.
30. Skilbeck J., Corner J., Bath P. *et al.* (2002). Characterising the Macmillan nurse caseload. *Palliative Medicine* **16**, 285–296.
31. Clark D., Seymour J., Douglas H.-R. *et al.* (2002). Explaining diversity in the organisation and costs of Macmillan nursing. *Palliative Medicine* **16**, 375–385.
32. Corner J., Halliday D., Haviland J. *et al.* (2003). Exploring nursing outcomes for patients with advanced cancer following intervention by Macmillan specialist palliative care nurses. *Journal of Advanced Nursing* **41**, 561–574.

33. Clark D. (1999). 'Total pain', disciplinary power and the body in the work of Cicely Saunders, 1958–1967. *Social Science and Medicine* **49**, 727–736.

34. Twycross R.G. and Wilcock A. (2001). *Symptom Management in Advanced Cancer*, 3rd edition. Oxford: Radcliffe Medical Press.

35. Winslow M., Clark D., Seymour J. *et al.* (2004). Changing technologies of cancer pain relief: case studies of innovation. *Progress in Palliative Care* **12**, 123–134.

36. Clark D. and Wright M. (2003). *Transition in End of Life Care: Hospice and Related Developments in Eastern Europe and Central Asia*. Buckingham: Open University Press.

37. Corner J. (2004). Working with difficult symptoms. In Payne S., Seymour J. and Ingleton C. (eds.) *Palliative Care Nursing: Principles and Evidence for Practice*. Maidenhead: Open University Press, pp. 241–259.

38. Lloyd Williams M. (2003). Screening for depression in palliative care. In Lloyd Williams M. (ed.) *Psychosocial Issues in Palliative Care*. Oxford: Oxford University Press, pp. 105–118.

39. Payne S. (1998). Depression in palliative care patients: a literature review. *International Journal of Palliative Nursing* **4**, 184–191.

40. Pessin H., Potash M., and Breitbart W. (2003). Diagnosis, assessment, and treatment of depression in palliative care. In Lloyd Williams M (ed.) *Psychosocial Issues in Palliative Care*. Oxford: Oxford University Press, pp. 81–104.

41. Maguire G.P. (1995). Psychosocial interventions to reduce affective disorders in cancer patients: research priorities. *Psycho-oncology* **4**, 113–119.

42. Lloyd Williams M. and Payne S. (2003). A qualitative study of nurses' views on depression in palliative care patients. *Palliative Medicine* **17**, 334–338.

43. Zigmond A.S. and Snaith R.P. (1983). The Hospital Anxiety and Depression Scale. *Acta Psychiatrica Scandinavica* **67**, 361–370.

44. Lloyd Williams M. (2001). Screening for depression in palliative care patients: a review. *European Journal of Cancer Care* **10**, 31–35.

45. Skilbeck J. and Payne S. (2003). Emotional support and the role of Clinical Nurse Specialists in palliative care. *Journal of Advanced Nursing* **43**, 521–530.

46. Lloyd-Williams M. and Payne S. (2002). Can multi-disciplinary guidelines improve the palliation of symptoms in the terminal phase of dementia. *International Journal of Palliative Nursing* **8**, 370, 372–375.

47. Lloyd Williams M. (2004). Are antidepressants effective in cancer patients? *Progress in Palliative Care* **12**, 217–219.

48. Costain Schou K. and Hewison J. (1999). *Experiencing Cancer: Quality of Life in Treatment*. Buckingham: Open University Press.

49. The A.-M. (2002). *Palliative Care and Communication: Experiences in the Clinic*. Buckingham: Open University Press.

50. Kobasa S.C. (1979). Stressful life events, personality and health: an inquiry into hardiness. *Journal of Personality and Social Psychology* **37**, 1–11.

51. Payne S. (2004). Carers and caregivers. In Oliviere D. and Monroe B. (eds.) *Death, Dying and Social Differences*. Oxford: Oxford University Press, pp. 181–198.

52. Maher J. and Green H. (2002). *Carers 2000. Office of National Statistics*. London: The Stationery Office.

53. Nolan M. (2001). Positive aspects of caring. In Payne S. and Ellis-Hill C. (eds.) *Chronic and Terminal Illness: New Perspectives in Caring and Carers*. Oxford: Oxford University Press, pp. 22–43.

54. Thomas C., Morris S.M. and Harman J.C. (2002). Companions through cancer: the care given by informal carers in cancer contexts. *Social Science and Medicine* **54**, 529–544.

55. The National Cancer Alliance. (1996). *'Patient-Centred Cancer Services?' What Patients Say*. Oxford: The National Cancer Alliance.

56. Department of Health (1999/2000). *National Surveys of NHS Patients Cancer National Overview 1999/2000*. London: HMSO.

57. Crawford M., Rutter D., Manley C. *et al.* (2002). Systematic review of involving patients in the planning and development of health care. *British Medical Journal* **325**, 1263–1269.

58. Johnson J. (1998). The emergence of care as policy. In Brechin A., Walmsley J., Katz J. and Peace S. (eds.) *Care Matters: Concepts, Practice and Research in Health and Social Care*. London: Sage, pp. 139–153.

59. Moriarty J. and Webb S. (2000). *Part of Their Lives: Community Care for Older People with Dementia*. Bristol: Policy Press.

60. Nolan M.R., Ryan T., Enderby P. and Reid D. (2002). Towards a more inclusive vision of dementia care practice and research. *Dementia: The International Journal of Social Research and Practice* **1**, 193–211.

61. Fortinsky R.H. (2001). Health care triads and dementia care: integrative framework and future directions. *Aging and Mental Health* **5(suppl. 1)**, S35–S48.

62. Zarit S.H. and Leitsch S.A. (2001). Developing and evaluating community based intervention programmes for Alzheimer's patients and their caregivers. *Aging and Mental Health* **5(suppl. 1)**, S84–S98.

63. Harding R. and Higginson I.J. (2003). What is the best way to help caregivers in cancer and palliative care? A

systematic literature review of interventions and their effectiveness. *Palliative Medicine* **17**, 63–74.

64. Ingleton C., Payne S., Nolan M. and Carey I. (2003) Respite in palliative care: a review and discussion of the literature. *Palliative Medicine* **17**, 567–575.

65. Braithwaite V. (2000). Contextual or generic stress outcomes: making choices through care giving appraisals. *The Gerontologist* **40**, 706–717.

66. Qureshi H., Bamford C., Nicholas E., Patmore C. and Harris J.C. (2000). *Outcomes in Social Care Practice: Developing an Outcome Focus in Care Management and Use Surveys*. York: Social Policy Research Unit, University of York.

67. Nolan M.R., Lundh U., Grant G. and Keady J. (eds.) (2003). *Partnerships in Family Care: Understanding the Caregiving Career*. Maidenhead: Open University Press.

68. Payne S. and Lloyd-Williams M. (2003). Bereavement care. In Lloyd-Williams M. (ed.) *Psychosocial Issues in Palliative Care*. Oxford: Oxford University Press, pp. 149–164.

69. Payne S. (2004). Depression in palliative care. *Cancer Nursing Practice* **3**, 12–15.

70. Field D., Reid D., Payne S. and Relf M. (2004). A national postal survey of adult bereavement support in hospice and specialist palliative care services in the UK. *International Journal of Palliative Nursing* **10**, 569–579.

71. Rolls L. and Payne S. (2003). Childhood bereavement services: a survey of UK provision. *Palliative Medicine* **17**, 423–432.

72. Payne S., Field D., Relf M. and Reid D. (2004). *Evaluating Bereavement Support Provided to Older People by Hospices, 2nd Annual Report to The Health Foundation*. Sheffield: Palliative and End-of-life Care Research Group, University of Sheffield.

73. Christakis C.A. (1999). *Death Foretold: Prophecy and Prognosis in Medical Care*. Chicago: The University of Chicago Press.

74. Glaser B.G. and Strauss A.L. (1965). *Awareness of Dying*. Chicago: Aldine Publishing Company.

75. Field D. and Copp G. (1999). Communication and awareness about dying in the 1990s. *Palliative Medicine* **13**, 459–468.

76. Heaven C. and Maguire P.M. (1996). Training hospice nurses to elicit patient concerns. *Journal of Advanced Nursing* **23**, 280–286.

77. Booth K., Maguire P.M., Butterworth T. and Hillier V.F. (1996). Perceived professional support and the use of blocking behaviours by hospice nurses. *Journal of Advanced Nursing* **24**, 522–527.

78. Jarrett N.J. and Payne S.A. (2000). Creating and maintaining 'optimism' in cancer care communication. *International Journal of Nursing Studies* **37**, 81–90.

79. Seymour J.E., Gott M., Bellamy G., Clark D., Sam H. and Ahmedzai S. (2004). Planning for the end of life: the views of older people about advance statements. *Social Science and Medicine* **59**, 57–68.

80. Finlay I. (2001). Death plans (editorial). *Palliative Medicine* **15**, 179–180.

81. James N. and Field D. (1992). The routinisation of hospice. *Social Science and Medicine* **34**, 1363–1375.

82. Cox K. and James V. (2004). Professional boundaries in palliative care. In Payne S., Seymour J. and Ingleton C. (eds.) *Palliative Care Nursing: Principles and Evidence for Practice*. Maidenhead: Open University Press, pp. 605–619.

83. Payne M. (2000). *Teamwork in Multi-professional Care*. London: Macmillan.

84. Seymour J., Ingleton C., Payne S. and Beddow V. (2003). Specialist palliative care: patients' experiences. *Journal of Advanced Nursing* **44**, 24–33.

85. Lawton J. (2000). *The Dying Process. Patients' Experiences of Palliative Care*. London: Routledge.

86. The New Zealand Palliative Care Strategy. (2001). www.moh.govt.nz/ (accessed 14 August 2007).

87. Field D., Ingleton C. and Clark D. (1997). The costs of unpaid labour: the use of voluntary staff in the King's Mill Hospice. *Health and Social Care in the Community* **5**, 198–208.

88. Graham F. and Clark D. (2005). Addressing the basics of palliative care. *International Journal of Palliative Nursing* **11**, 36–39.

89. Ahmed N., Bestall J., Ahmedzai S. *et al.* (2004). Systematic review of the problems and issues of accessing specialist palliative care by patients, carers and health and social care professionals. *Palliative Medicine* **18**, 525–542.

90. Hughes A. (2005). Poverty and palliative care in the US: issues facing the urban poor. *International Journal of Palliative Nursing* **11**, 6–13.

91. Carlisle R. (2002). *Sheffield Palliative and Supportive Care Corporate Health Needs Assessment*. Sheffield: North Sheffield PCT.

92. Ingleton C., Morgan J., Hughes P. *et al.* (2003). Carer satisfaction with end-of-life care in Powys, Wales. *Health and Social Care in the Community* **12**, 43–52.

93. Ingleton C., Clark D., Hughes P., Yap T. and Noble B. (2004). Evaluation of a scheme to enhance palliative care in rural Wales. *Supportive Care in Cancer* **12**, 683–691.

94. Seymour J., Clark D. and Philp I. (2001). Palliative care and geriatric medicine: shared concerns, shared challenges. *Palliative Medicine* **15**, 269–270.

95. Davies E. and Higginson I. (eds.) (2004). *Better Palliative Care for Older People*. Copenhagen: World Health Organization Europe.

96. Lunney J.R., Lynn J. and Hogan C. (2002). Profiles of older medicare decedents. *Journal of the American Geriatrics Society* **50**, 1108–1112.

97. Froggatt K.A. (2001). Palliative care and nursing homes: where next? *Palliative Medicine* **15**, 42–48.

98. Koffman J. and Camps M. (2004). No way in: including the excluded at the end of life. In Payne S., Seymour J. and Ingleton C. (eds.) *Palliative Care Nursing: Principles and Evidence for Practice.* Maidenhead: Open University Press, pp. 364–384.

99. Ratcliff M. (2002). Hospice care for prisoners – the US experience. *Hospice Information Bulletin* **1**, 1–2.

100. Bolger M. (2004). Offenders. In Oliviere D. and Monroe B. (eds.) *Death, Dying and Social Differences.* Oxford: Oxford University Press, pp. 133–148.

101. Cardy P. (2005). Learning disability and palliative care. *International Journal of Palliative Nursing* **11**, 14.

102. Read S. (2005). Learning disability and palliative care: recognizing pitfalls and exploring potential. *International Journal of Palliative Nursing* **11**, 15–20.

103. McCarthy M., Addington-Hall J.M. and Altmann D. (1997). The experience of dying with dementia: a retrospective study. *International Journal of Geriatric Psychiatry* **12**, 404–409.

104. Firth S. (2001). *Wider Horizons.* London: National Council for Hospices and Specialist Palliative Care Services.

105. National Council for Palliative Care. (2005). *20:20 Vision.* London: National Council for Palliative Care.

106. Ellershaw J. and Ward C. (2003). Care of the dying patient: the last hours or days of life. *British Medical Journal* **326**, 30–34.

107. Thomas K. (2003). The Gold Standards Framework in community palliative care. *European Journal of Palliative Care* **10**, 113–115.

CHAPTER THIRTY-SEVEN

Research and cancer care

Jessica Corner

Research is a dynamic process, through which knowledge is generated. It can also be seen as an important force for change, given that the goal of research is constant improvement and discovery. The need for research into cancer, its treatment and care is unquestionable. It is a moral and ethical duty to ensure that people with cancer are receiving optimal treatment, and that their needs are established, understood, and catered for, also that the various forces and conditions that create the construction of cancer treatment and care are more clearly understood, so that these can be redefined and taken forward as appropriate. This may be by conducting studies into the biological and genetic causes of the disease, developing and evaluating new treatments, or researching new and better ways of caring. In nursing, there is increasing interest in how research can be used as a means of developing practice in a way that is more immediate than relying on practitioners to read the results of published studies.

Research has always played a prominent part in the management of cancer. Since there remains uncertainty over who will be cured of cancer and cancer treatment often has a major impact on quality of life, those working in the specialty of oncology have constantly sought to identify more effective cancer treatments. The success of cancer research is beginning to deliver longer survival of people with cancer, and this is also opening up important new avenues for research into the needs of people living with cancer and issues around coping with the disease after initial treatment is completed. Researchers from other disciplines such as psychology and sociology have studied the emotional and social consequences of cancer to both the sufferer and family or friends. Nurses too are increasingly using and undertaking research; in particular, they are studying the needs of people affected by cancer and nursing effectiveness in relieving problems related to cancer or its treatment. More generally, changes in health care internationally are driving changes in the management of research and its funding. This in turn affects research into cancer treatment and care. There is a recognition that in health care, research needs more planning and a strategic direction.

Following the publication of the Cancer Plan for England in 2000,[1] major developments in the organisation and management of cancer research in the UK have been initiated. The National Cancer Research Institute (NCRI) was established in 2001 with the aim of accelerating progress in cancer research in the UK for the benefit of people with cancer. This is an umbrella body which brings together the major research funding bodies for UK cancer research into a partnership organisation. The role of the NCRI is to take a strategic oversight of cancer research in the UK, identify gaps and opportunities in current research, facilitate collaboration between funding bodies, and monitor progress in areas deemed to be of strategic importance. The NCRI's work began with an analysis of the £335 million spent each year on cancer research in the UK funded by the NCRI partner bodies. A Cancer Research Database for the NCRI was established, which records information on all research supported through the partner organisations. Every research project was coded using an internationally recognised coding system – the Common Scientific Outline (CSO). Analysis of these data by the NCRI, published in 2002,[2] revealed a huge volume of research activity;

the proportion of spend by type of research through the NCRI funding bodies is shown in Figure 37.1. However, the analysis also reveals a relative lack of investment in research in key areas – notably prevention, which made up only 2% of funded research, and cancer control and outcomes research which made up only 6% of funded research. The latter encompasses research that would broadly cover much of the research relevant

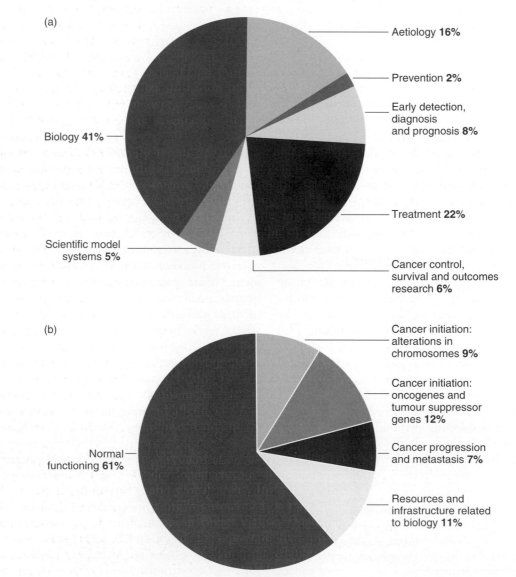

Figure 37.1 (a) Proportion of total NCRI partners spend by Common Scientific Outline category and (b) subdivision of Common Scientific Outline biology category. Reprinted with permission from National Cancer Research Institute (2002). *Strategic Analysis: an Overview of Cancer Research in the UK Directly Funded by the NCRI Partner Organisations*. London: National Cancer Research Institute.[2]

to nursing practice (patient care, pain and symptom management, surveillance behaviour and education, supportive and palliative care, and cost-effective health care delivery). Similarly, when different cancer types were reviewed there was a mismatch between cancer mortality and research investment so that some cancer types, most notably lung cancer, received relatively little investment compared with burden of disease, if mortality is taken as a crude indicator of this (see Figure 37.2). These findings have stimulated further strategic reviews into the areas of cancer control and early detection, supportive, and palliative care, and into lung cancer with a view to increase capacity to undertake research in these areas and to stimulate increased research activity through strategic investment.

The publication of guidance, based on a systematic review of research literature by the National Institute for Clinical Excellence (NICE) into supportive and palliative care revealed strengths and weaknesses in the evidence base

related to supportive and palliative care.[3] In reviewing the evidence collated for the review, the NCRI concluded that while research into patients' needs has been undertaken there is a paucity of evidence relating to how best to meet these needs. Research into psychological support, information giving, specialist palliative care, and face-to-face communication has been undertaken. In contrast, little research has been conducted in relation to complementary therapies, user involvement, spiritual support, support for families and carers, bereavement support, co-ordination and integration of care, social care, rehabilitation, cultural differences, underserved groups care settings, or symptoms other than pain.[4] The review of supportive and palliative care research has led to an initiative to establish collaborative networks of researchers across the UK. Two networks, one co-ordinated from the University of Southampton and a second co-ordinated from King's College, University of London have been awarded infrastructure to support the development of

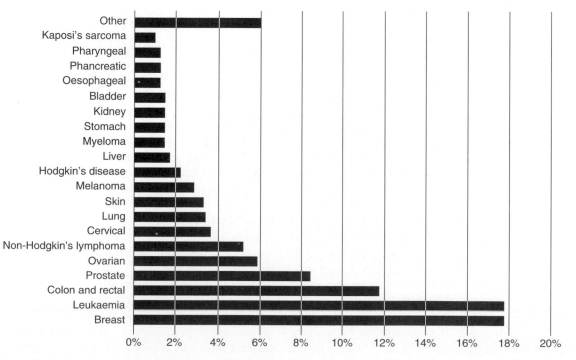

Figure 37.2   Percentage of total NCRI partners' spend by disease site. Reprinted with permission from National Cancer Research Institute (2002). *Strategic Analysis: an Overview of Cancer Research in the UK Directly Funded by the NCRI Partner Organisations.* London: National Cancer Research Institute.[2]

supportive and palliative care research over a 5-year period. These initiatives are demonstrating the effectiveness of the NCRI in stimulating research into areas of importance to nurses.

Research and cancer treatment

Clinical trials and cancer

Clinical trials of new treatments have been the mainstay of research in cancer care and are a dominant part of the environment of cancer centres. Cancer treatment is largely experimental, and research is a driving force behind much of service development. Unfortunately, little attention has been paid to the impact this has on care, or the treatment packages on offer to patients. Because of the experimental nature of much cancer treatment, many people will have their treatment while involved in a clinical trial, particularly if they are being treated in a specialist cancer-treatment centre. Cancer nurses are therefore frequently involved in administering experimental cancer treatments, or talking through issues surrounding clinical trials and experimental treatments with people with cancer and their families. Cancer nurses can find themselves having ambivalent attitudes to such experimental treatments and the ethics of user involvement in clinical trials. Nurses working in cancer therefore need to have an understanding of the issues surrounding clinical trials and cancer, and of an individual's rights regarding participation in these.

Clinical trials are the means by which the efficacy of a new treatment is established. Since new treatments for cancer are continually being developed, it is necessary to determine whether existing established treatments should be replaced by these new developments. The ultimate goal is to improve the rates of disease remission, survival, and quality of life. Increasingly, cost and economic evaluation is also becoming an important feature of clinical trials, since cancer treatment is costly and governments are requiring tangible, measurable benefits of treatment to be assessed against the costs.

Clinical trials for new treatments are conducted in three phases (see Box 37.1). The principles on which each is based are somewhat different, as are the dilemmas. The principles that justify such studies are a careful assessment of the likelihood of achieving a medical advance versus any risks to the person undergoing treatment. This is most difficult in phase I and II trials where the likelihood of benefit to those participating, who already have advanced disease and where standard treatments have already failed, is minimal, whereas the likelihood of adverse effects could be significant. There is a need for participating subjects to have given informed consent to all aspects of the study, including potential adverse effects, and without pressure, or the fear that their care might be adversely affected if they refuse to participate.[5] In addition, studies must be governed by the 'uncertainty principle', that is there must be genuine uncertainty as to the therapeutic effectiveness of the treatment, and a likelihood that this can be determined through the trial.[6]

Phase III trials are larger studies usually involving a comparison of a new drug or treatment with an existing treatment. People who are identified as eligible to take part are considered to be representative of the wider population of those with the same condition and are known as a sample. Those agreeing to take part are then usually allocated at random to receive one or other of the treatments. Participants are then studied over time to examine how they fare according to certain identified outcome criteria. Common outcome indicators are: tumour response (reduction in size of the tumour, classified either as non-response, partial response, or complete response, i.e. no evidence of tumour following treatment); length of survival; toxicity or side-effects experienced.

Quality of life

Quality of life is an important component to outcome assessment in clinical trials of cancer treatments. In the past, studies were criticised because they did not sufficiently take into account the individual's experience of treatment.[8] Researchers conducting early clinical trials of new treatments were preoccupied with increasing the survival rates of invariably fatal cancers. Progress in the treatment of such cancers (for example, leukaemia in childhood, and testicular cancers) led to other factors such as the physical and

Box 37.1   Clinical trials

A clinical trial is a planned experiment designed to elucidate the most appropriate treatment for future patients with a given medical condition. Results based on a limited sample of patients are used to make inferences about how treatment should be conducted in the general population of patients who will require treatment in the future.[7] Clinical trials involving a new drug, chemotherapy, or radiotherapy treatment for cancer are classified into three phases.

Phase I trials
These are conducted to determine drug safety, bio-availability, and drug metabolism, usually through dose-escalation studies in which patient volunteers are subjected to increasing doses of the drug. There is little or no likelihood of benefit to the patient and therefore patients consenting to take part are really doing so for the benefit of future patients.

Phase II trials
These are small-scale studies of the effectiveness and safety of a drug. Different doses of the drug are given to different groups of patients to help to identify the therapeutic dose and activity of the drug. Again, patients are usually invited to take part in a phase II trial when other more conventional treatments have failed, therefore there may be only a small likelihood of the patient benefiting.

Phase III trials
New drugs with known effectiveness are compared with standard treatment regimes in a trial of a large number of patients. Patients are usually randomly allocated to the different treatments under comparison. Efficacy of different treatments is evaluated using outcomes such as disease response, survival, and changes in performance status, which is a crude measure of an individual's functional state on a scale from 0 (representing fully mobile and functional) to 4 (completely dependent, or moribund), as well as quality of life, and economic effects or costs.

long-term cost of treatment to the individual becoming a greater priority. In addition, the requirement to seek the person's viewpoint has increasingly been recognised and there is criticism of a failure to respond to this in cancer trials. A wide variety of quality-of-life measures has been developed for use in clinical trials. Quality-of-life tools address one or all of a number of domains

of the potential impact cancer and its treatment may have on an individual. These are as follows:

- *physical well-being* – perceived and observed bodily function or disruption (for example, pain, nausea, and fatigue). It encompasses the degree to which the individual is experiencing disease symptoms, treatment side-effects and general physical problems
- *functional well-being* – the ability to perform activities of daily living such as walking, feeding, bathing, and dressing oneself; taking part in social activities and ability to work
- *emotional well-being* – usually assessments are made of the extent of psychological morbidity from anxiety and depression
- *social well-being* – the extent of social support needed and available, disruptions to family functioning, intimacy, and sexual functioning.[9]

Established quality-of-life measures are available for use in studies; these may be generic (developed for measuring health status regardless of the nature of illness) or cancer specific (developed to take account of the particular needs and issues facing people with cancer and developed and tested with populations of people with cancer). The advantage of the latter is that they are designed for use in studies with people who have cancer and results can be readily compared with those from other studies. Generic measures may be useful if data from a population of patients with cancer are to be compared with those of the general population. Box 37.2 shows measures most commonly used in cancer quality-of-life studies.

Quality-of-life measures can be used as outcomes measures to investigate the quality of survival following treatment for cancer, or assess the late physical or psychological consequences of treatment. They can be used to predict mortality or likely duration of survival from cancer, since good or poor quality of life can predict outcomes from the disease. Quality-of-life measures have more recently been used as part of clinical practice to assist in the identification of ongoing problems that people may have during or following treatment for cancer. Quality-of-life studies have shown a wide variety of disruptions caused by cancer treatment; some of these have been helpful

Box 37.2 Commonly used quality-of-life measures

Source: Sprangers M.A.G. (2002). Quality of life assessment in oncology. *Acta Oncologica* **41**, 229–237.[10]

Generic instruments
- Sickness Impact Profile
- Nottingham Health Profile
- EQ 5D.

Cancer-specific instruments
- Rotterdam Symptom Checklist
- Functional Living Index
- Cancer Rehabilitation Evaluation System Short Form (CARES-SF)
- Functional Assessment of Cancer Therapy – General (FACT-G), with additional cancer site-specific modules
- EORTC Core Quality of Life Questionnaire (EORTC QLQ-C30), with additional cancer site-specific modules.

Domain-specific instruments
- Multidimensional Fatigue Inventory (MFI)
- McGill Pain Questionnaire
- Hospital Anxiety and Depression Scale (HADS).

in determining the relative value of different treatments. An example of this is the collective evidence of studies on the differences for women having mastectomy as opposed to conservative surgery for breast cancer, such as lumpectomy. Fallowfield has collated a number of studies, which seem to show that conservative treatment may not yield the lower rates of psychological morbidity anticipated from the less-physically mutilating treatment.[11] Rather, Fallowfield suggests that this is a more complicated issue; in studies where they were given a choice over their treatment, women fared better regardless of the type of surgery they received. Fallowfield's conclusions are supported by a recent economic evaluation of the two treatments: although breast-conserving treatment is more costly than mastectomy, when the benefits to quality of life are taken into account and economic outcomes are considered, the differences between the two treatments are much smaller.[12] Another example is a systematic review by Langeveld *et al.* of studies of quality

of life in young adult survivors of cancer in childhood.[13] Thirty studies were included in the review, and although not all the studies show consistent results the authors conclude that most participants were in good health physically and psychologically, with the exception of those with bone tumours. Children treated for central nervous system and acute lymphoblastic leukaemia were at risk educationally. While survivors of childhood cancer were relatively well, many reported facing job discrimination and difficulty in obtaining health and life insurance as a result of their cancer diagnosis, and were worried about their reproductive and future health. The review reveals a need for further detailed research of the long-term consequences for children successfully treated for cancer. It is the cumulated evidence from studies using quality-of-life measures that allows insights into such aspects of treatment to be explored.

The difficulty in making the assessment of quality of life part of all clinical trials, and a meaningful and practical tool for clinical practice, are well recognised and may raise ethical dilemmas. For example, measuring quality of life in clinical trials may identify problems that are not then acted upon; there are difficulties in obtaining complete data on all patients since in longitudinal studies attrition of participants who are less well can bias results, as can the tendency of participants to change their responses over time. Interpretation of the results of studies, and understanding when a change in quality of life is clinically meaningful, and the validity and reliability of instruments are problematic.[14] There is evidence to suggest that scores indicated using a standard quality-of-life instrument may not accord with what individuals report during face-to-face interviews,[15] and completing these measures can be emotionally distressing and can prompt an emotional reaction.[16] Recently, work has been undertaken to test the value of quality-of-life measurement in clinical settings using touch screen technology, and has proved useful in enhancing doctor–patient communication about ongoing problems during and after cancer treatment.[17]

Some criticism of the measurement approach to quality of life has been expressed in the nursing literature.[15] Established measures of quality of life have predetermined the aspects to be measured for the patient; these are usually in the form of a series of items to be rated by the patient. The problem with this is that it does not allow the unique and individual experience of cancer and its related problems to be expressed. It is impossible to know whether the items selected for inclusion in the tool, or the scores yielded for that individual, truly represent their quality of life, and this is an issue of validity in measurement. Benner argues for studies using a phenomenological approach to the study of quality of life.[18] Such studies attempt to access the individual experience, through the person's own eyes, using in-depth, open-ended interviews, from which detailed accounts of experiences can be derived. According to Benner, it is only by undertaking such studies that real insight into patient needs and agendas can be gained.[18] In phenomenologically orientated studies, the domains of inquiry would be somewhat different from those identified by Cella,[9] and would encompass:

- the changing experience of the body
- changing social relationships as a result of illness
- changing tasks and demands of different stages of the disease process and disease trajectory
- predictable responses and effective coping strategies for treatment side-effects and sequelae
- the particular – what the illness interrupts, threatens, and means to the individual.[18]

Faithfull has combined both a phenomenological perspective and a well-established quality-of-life tool (the EORTC QLQ-30) in order to gain deeper understanding of the symptoms patients experience when undergoing pelvic radiotherapy for cancers of the bladder and prostate.[19,20] This allowed both data on symptom severity using the EORTC QLQ-30 scale, and detailed information about the meaning of symptoms and their impact on patients' lives to be gathered. The use of a standard measure such as the EORTC QLQ-30 was useful in that it made comparisons with other patient groups possible, and was useful as a measure of change within this group of patients over time. However, open-ended interviews allowed the researcher to develop much deeper

understanding of the needs and difficulties that patients were facing. Combined-method approaches such as this have a lot of potential for nursing research.

Economic evaluation

With the growing pressure on health services internationally to contain escalating health care costs, economic evaluations of all new cancer treatments are increasingly being demanded by health planners. These evaluations are designed to give information on the cost-effectiveness of such treatments, and to enable comparisons with existing best methods of management. The introduction of new treatments therefore increasingly will have to be justified in relation to their costs, in terms of both quality of life for individuals receiving them, and the economic costs.[21] Techniques for the economic evaluation of treatments vary. These may take the form of:

- *cost-effectiveness studies* – undertaken to compare different health care interventions with different consequences, and comparing the different levels of effectiveness of these with their costs
- *cost-utility studies* – for example, calculating quality-of-life-adjusted years or QALYs. Here the analysis takes into account a trade-off between length and quality of life as a result of different treatments
- *cost–benefit studies* – where all the consequences of interventions, the changes in length and quality of life, and their expense are expressed in financial terms.

From these it is possible to assess whether the total value of the extra benefits from one intervention exceeds the extra costs involved if it is also more expensive. In reality, economic evaluation is complex, and many factors influence the validity of costs and benefits in relation to new and existing cancer treatments; they are, however, going to become an increasingly common factor in health care research, and nurses need to become familiar with considering economic issues when scrutinising research into cancer treatments and in undertaking their own research. Moore *et al.*, for example, incorporated an economic evaluation into a randomised controlled trial of nurse-led follow-up for people with lung cancer; this included collecting data on patterns of service use in the months after completing cancer treatment and estimating the costs of care for nurse-led care and for conventional medical follow-up.[22] Those cared for by nurses had fewer medical consultations, and chest X-rays, were more likely to die at home, made no greater call on other professionals or services, and were no more likely to be re-admitted to hospital. There were no significant differences in costs between the two service models. The conclusion drawn was that nurse-led care was not more costly, but there were indications that a larger study might reveal that nurse-led care was less costly and led to a more appropriate mixture and location of care than conventional medical follow-up.

Ethical issues in cancer research

All research raises ethical issues about the manner in which a study is conducted, and the checks and safeguards for individuals involved, or who may be affected by the research itself or its findings. This is particularly the case when the research involves vulnerable individuals such as people with cancer or their families and carers, and where the research may involve the experimental use of new treatments. The principles on which research involving human subjects should be based were first laid down in the *Declaration of Helsinki* in 1964.[23] These reinforce the necessity for the justification of all research in terms of the balance of the potential benefits to the person involved as a research subject against inherent risks, and identify the importance of informed consent. Worldwide agreement on research ethics and European legislation such as the *European Convention on Human Rights*,[24] and the *European Clinical Trials Directive*,[25] set down stringent regulations for conducting research and principles for protecting human subjects in research. Potential subjects must be adequately informed of the aims, anticipated benefits and hazards of the study. Consent must be given voluntarily, without pressure or incentive to take part; subjects should also understand that they can withdraw from the study at any time, and that non-participation will not prejudice their treatment or care in any way. In most instances, consent would be required to be given in writing and witnessed by an independent observer. Participants in research also have rights that need to be protected by the researcher, such as the right to anonymity and confidentiality of any data about them used in the study. Participants in studies involving experimental cancer treatments known to be toxic, as well as in apparently less-hazardous studies, such as interviews with individuals about their disease and needs for care, need to be protected. Studies using qualitative research methods, such as tape recording of in-depth interviews with participants, are increasingly being recognised as having ethical implications, and are potentially exploitative of vulnerable individuals.[26]

Studies involving patients or patient data are required to be scrutinised by an ethics committee, and in the UK also to be approved through research governance processes.[27] Researchers are required to submit detailed proposals or protocols of the research study to the research governance body and local research ethics committee. These should include sufficient detail for the following to be made clear to the committee:

- the scientific merit of a study (since inadequate research is also unethical)
- the potential hazards and risks to the paticipant
- the means by which informed consent will be obtained
- copies of written information for participants regarding the study
- assurances over the protection of anonymity, confidentiality, and other rights of any individual taking part in a study.

In addition, the committee requires that researchers declare any potential conflict of interest they may have in conducting a study, such as receiving payment by a pharmaceutical company for undertaking the work, if this could encourage bias in interpreting the results of a study. Clinicians undertaking studies involving the evaluation of a new drug or other treatments are also subject to stringent monitoring and registration requirements, depending on the country in which the research is taking place, for example the European Clinical Trials Directive sets out requirements for the management of clinical trials involving new pharmaceutical products. There are also international systems in place for the notification of adverse effects of experimental drugs and treatments. The Royal College of Nursing has published useful guidance for nurses undertaking or involved in the management of medical research.[28]

While there is increasing scrutiny of research into new cancer treatments through local ethics and multicentre research ethics committees, the nature of cancer treatment is such that much treatment offered, particularly in specialist centres, is experimental. Nurses working in cancer care will frequently find themselves caring for people who are participating in clinical trials, and they may be asked to administer experimental treatments. The ethical issues surrounding clinical trials have been the subject of much discussion and debate. Hazel Thornton, a woman diagnosed with breast cancer, was asked to take part in a trial of different treatments for ductal carcinoma of her breast. As a result of her experience she has actively campaigned for greater involvement of patients in the design of such trials.[29] Personal account 37.1 contains an excerpt of Hazel Thornton's writing on this, which gives insight into the dilemmas people with cancer may face in giving consent. The work of Beaver *et al.* suggests that more than half of women diagnosed with breast cancer would adopt a very passive role in decision making about their treatment if given a choice.[30] This makes it difficult for nurses to understand their own role in working with people undergoing experimental treatment. Professional bodies for nursing give useful guidance here; for example, the Royal College of Nursing advises that in acting as a witness to a patient giving informed consent, nurses should 'satisfy themselves' that this has been freely given and that the person understands what they are giving consent to and any risks involved.[28] In the event of the research being seen to have an adverse effect on the subject, the nurse has an obligation to intervene by informing the researcher and appropriate person in authority.

Increasingly, some of these issues are being addressed through the involvement of people with cancer in the design and monitoring of clinical trials. This trend towards the 'user as commissioner' allows co-operation and shared responsibility in planning and designing clinical trials and in particular in the preparation of information for participants so that it is clear and assists decision making. As Hazel Thornton says:

> . . . this approach demonstrates a new attitude to research that is not imposed on the patients, but which has been devised and executed as an expression of the appreciation of the ideal that, as this research is for the patient, the patients have been allowed to exercise their responsibility by participating in designing and planning trials which might more clearly express their desired outcomes, thereby providing trials in which they might be pleased to participate.[29]

The experience of people participating in clinical trials has until recently received little attention. Cox interviewed 55 people participating in phase I clinical trials about their experiences.[31] While participants were very positive about their decision to participate and wanted to contribute – this was in the context of being recently told they had untreatable disease. It offered hope, but also felt like 'the only option'; as their doctor had offered them the treatment, most felt it was the 'right' thing to accept. Understanding of the purpose of the trial was limited; more than half could not state the purpose of the trial. The study reveals that there are powerful reasons for accepting participation, which call into question the extent to which 'true' informed consent is achieved in all situations. The burden of trial participation later led participants to question their decision, and as they received information about their response to treatment, which was inevitably limited, trial participants developed a feeling that the harm was too great or disillusionment took over, though many wanted to persevere. The end of participation/ withdrawal from the experimental treatment was distressing and led to feelings of abandonment. Participants wanted information about the outcome of the trial but had not received this. Despite the difficulties, the majority at follow-up said they would make the same decision about

Personal account 37.1

Extract from Thornton H. (1992). Breast cancer trials: a patient's viewpoint. *Lancet* **339**, 44–45, reproduced with permission.[29]

The practice of 'informed consent' before inclusion in randomised controlled trials is well known. My invitation to participate in such a trial is well known. My invitation came 2 weeks after an operation to remove an abnormal piece of breast tissue. I was handed a leaflet that explained the need for the DCIS [ductal carcinoma in situ] trial and which listed the treatment options. The booklet *Living with Breast Cancer*, published by the UK Health Education Authority, was given to me and I was advised to telephone Cancerbackup to obtain information on radiotherapy and tamoxifen. I was asked to come back in 2 weeks with my decision and was assured that, if I declined, my aftercare would not be affected.

A lay person's dilemma is clear. A woman is given a diagnosis that she has never heard of before and a leaflet indicating four widely differing treatment options: no further treatment, a 4–5-week course of X-ray therapy to the breast, one tamoxifen tablet daily for 5 years, or both radiotherapy and tamoxifen. This scenario begs the question: What is informed consent?

I sought every means to inform myself during the next 2 weeks about DCIS and its treatments, and about randomised controlled trials. I quickly became aware that without the facts of my case, e.g. size of DCIS, volume of tissue removed, state of marked excision margins, histological sub-type, and oestrogen receptor status, it would be impossible to speculate on the likely effects of the four treatments on offer. I was fortunate to have excellent sources of information.

My instinctive reaction against radiotherapy for this noninvasive condition was reinforced by several experienced and well-informed doctors and radiotherapists . . . radiotherapy is included in two out of the four treatment options in the trial; my feeling was that, because I was unwilling to undergo radiotherapy, I could not take part in this study . . . Without the supplementary information that I was able to obtain myself, I cannot understand how a woman can properly judge the proposal that has been put to her. Even with such information it is a haphazard assessment for the lay person. I was astonished that . . . women were asked to co-operate in a study where the range of treatments was so wide. To suggest that randomised controlled trials are necessary and to ask your average woman-in-the-street to have to decide whether or not to take part at the moment she has just been told she has a carcinoma would seem to be asking just too much.

participation. The findings of this study point to a need for much greater care and attention to the experience of trial participants, whose needs are too readily overlooked in the interests of successful completion of important clinical research.

User involvement in research

In response to a recognition of the important perspective of service users in research there has been increasing commitment to involving people with cancer in the design and conduct of research. The value of user involvement has been acknowledged by funding bodies and governmental organisations internationally, in order to ensure that studies are relevant to the general public, that research questions and methods are appropriate and accessible and in assisting in the dissemination of research findings.[32] In England the Department of Health has strongly advocated the involvement of patients and the public in the organisation and delivery of health care and established patient involvement forums in both service delivery and research contexts.[33] Evidence of involving service users in the design and conduct of studies is now a prerequisite for funding from many public bodies in the UK, and the National Cancer Research Institute has an active consumer liaison forum, and patient forums within national cancer research networks have been established. Likewise in the US and Australia, bodies such as the National Cancer Institute involve advocacy groups in advising on national research agendas and act as representatives on research advisory groups.

Nursing research and cancer care

The enormous potential for nurses to undertake research in cancer care is obvious. The number of nurses working in cancer settings, and the move of basic and post-basic nurse education into the higher education setting has meant that nurses are increasingly becoming equipped to conduct studies into areas of their practice. The growth of advanced practice and nurse specialist roles, where systematic evaluation of practice and service inno vation are inherent, will increasingly require nurses to undertake research as part of their roles. The number of nurses undertaking PhD study continues to grow, and therefore internationally there is a network of nurses in key positions who can play a pivotal role in instigating programmes of research and facilitating others to initiate studies. The need for research into aspects of cancer care is ever more apparent. Nursing needs an evidence base for its practice, not just to provide information on how best to provide effective care, but also to offer evidence for the need for specialist nursing intervention at a time when the value of all health care settings and interventions is being called into question.

Over the last 25 years, a number of attempts have been made to identify priorities for the focus of nursing research in cancer care. Oberst's priority-setting study using the Delphi technique was the first to attempt to do this systematically.[34] A panel of 575 nurses was surveyed and asked to identify priorities for cancer nursing research. A list of problem statements was generated from the responses, which was then returned to the panel members to rate in terms of the value these may have for nursing research and patient welfare. In two further rounds of the survey, consensus was reached over the items and their ranked order. For areas with the greatest potential for improving patient welfare, items relating to problems surrounding physiological responses to cancer treatment, especially chemotherapy, and relief of patients' physical discomfort, including pain, were given highest priority. Items judged to have the highest value to practising nurses surrounded the need for organisational support systems for the practitioner, and educational and communication needs. Recently Browne *et al.*[35] have surveyed members of the European Oncology Nursing Society using the Delphi approach.[35] The top priorities for research from the perspective of European nurses are shown in Box 37.3.

Box 37.3   Priority areas for cancer nursing research[35]

1. Needs of patients related to communication, information and education
2. Symptom management, particularly pain, nausea and vomiting, and fatigue
3. Experiences of disease and its treatment with particular reference to psychological experiences
4. Cancer nursing research issues such as research facilitation and utilisation
5. Cancer nursing education issues such as nurses' educational needs.

The most recent research priority setting survey has been that of the USA Oncology Nursing Society's membership conducted in 2004.[36] This was conducted online. One-hundred and seventeen topics under seven categories were listed: symptom management, behavioural and psychosocial aspects of cancer, communication and decision making, health services, health-promotion/disease-prevention behaviours, cancer continuum of care, and special cancer populations. The top five priorities identified through the survey were: quality of life, patient and family education, and participation in decision making about treatment and pain. The survey reflects the fact that increasingly nurses are relying on the results of research to guide their practice and to develop and improve their nursing interventions. Nursing research in cancer care has been defined as:

> . . . the impact of the disease and its treatment on the individual and his or her family, and the efficacy of nursing care in alleviating/ameliorating disease or treatment induced problems and needs.[37]

As such, it has a distinct and complementary orientation to medical research, which largely concerns itself with the assessment of disease outcome in response to treatment using end-points such as duration of survival, tumour response, treatment toxicity, and cost versus quality-of-life estimates. In contrast, nursing research has focused on the consequences to the individual of their cancer and its treatment at any stage of the disease process, and on investigating the most effective methods of providing supportive care.

Two broad areas of research encapsulate nursing practice in cancer care:

1. patients, problems, systematic methods of assessment, and studies related to the management of these
2. the experiences and needs of patients, survivors, close relatives, and significant others, and methods of facilitating coping and adjusting to cancer.

It has been recommended that research into cancer care should be promoted by the development of ongoing coherent programmes of research by groups of nurses according to agreed priorities. Centres conducting such research programmes should also be in a position to offer research training. Programmes of research could be built using a framework similar to that of clinical trials for anti-cancer agents, using multiphase studies, which incorporate theory-generating and exploratory/descriptive phases, before moving onto more traditional intervention studies, for example:

- *phase 1* – exploration of a problem (e.g. descriptive studies of the level and nature of fatigue following chemotherapy or the symptom of breathlessness in lung cancer)
- *phase 2* – development and piloting of an intervention/problem-management strategy
- *phase 3* – formal evaluation of the intervention, using clinical trials, evaluation research, and multicentre studies.[37]

It has, however, been recognised that there exist a number of barriers to nurses developing a strong research base in cancer care; Payne identifies a lack of research training in basic and post-basic nursing education as contributing to the difficulty of establishing research.[38] Neither bachelor's nor master's programmes in nursing could really be described as offering anything more than an introduction to research. Real research training in other disciplines is not considered to start until higher degree level, such as in PhD programmes. The lack of funding available for nursing research, the difficulty of access to skilled research supervision, and the lack of time in busy clinical posts for research are significant constraints. Payne also

argues that there is no money or status to be gained for the majority of nurses who might contemplate undertaking research, and a powerful anti-intellectual ethos apparent in some parts of nursing may militate against its development. Since this critique was published, considerable developments have been made in nursing research and the number of nurses internationally sustaining research careers in cancer care is growing, although securing funding and recognition for nursing research remains a considerable challenge. Despite these difficulties for nursing in establishing its research base, a range of work has been conducted that continues to be highly influential for practice, and suggests an important future for nursing research in cancer care.

Ross *et al.*, commissioned by the National Coordinating Centre for Service Delivery and Organisation Research and Development in England to identify priorities for nursing and midwifery research, used a three-stranded approach through – the views of service users, the views of stakeholders (professionals, leaders, organisations), and a literature analysis.[39] Priorities identified were appropriate, timely and effective interventions, individualised services, continuity of care, staff capacity, and quality and user involvement (see Figure 37.3). As found by Payne, a key issue for developing a strong evidence base of nursing and midwifery research was reported to be building capacity. The need for continuity and coherence in building substantial research investigations rather than multiple small studies, methodological development for intervention studies, and encouraging innovation and creativity through investigator-led as well as policy-driven research, was felt to be highly important.

Recently, a groundbreaking study has been undertaken to identify the research priorities of people with cancer.[40] A team of researchers used a participatory approach and worked with a group of 13 patients and carers who were trained to take on the roles of co-researchers and jointly led the research. Priorities were identified in a series of focus groups with over 100 people who were either undergoing cancer treatment or had completed it. There were also focus groups held with individuals usually excluded from studies, such as people with advanced disease, older people and

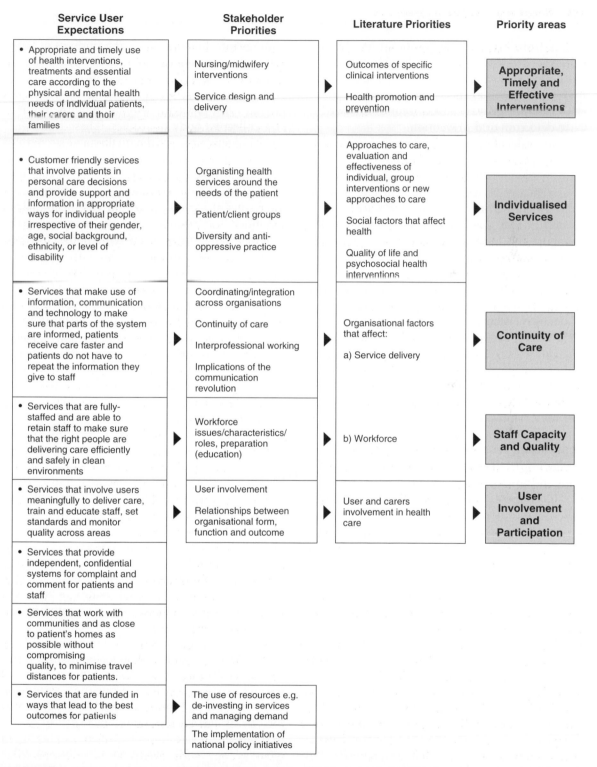

Figure 37.3 Framework for identifying research priorities for nursing and midwifery research in service organisation and delivery. Reprinted with permission from Ross F., Smith E., Mackenzie A. and Masterson A. (2004). Identifying research priorities in nursing and midwifery service delivery and organization: a scoping study. *International Journal of Nursing Studies* **41**, 547–558.[39]

people from South Asian communities. The priorities accord with those identified by Ross *et al.*,[39] with impact of cancer on life being the top priority for people with cancer, while research into the causes of cancer was ranked second, followed by early detection and prevention.

Core tasks of research for cancer nursing practice can be listed under five headings:

1. systematic reviews of the current state of knowledge/evidence in any given area
2. studies that develop and test research instruments and measures, or research approaches
3. development of detailed understanding of cancer-related problems or client needs
4. evaluation of existing or new practices aimed at enhancing care or alleviating problems
5. detailed evaluation of existing and new services in cancer care.

A range of research methods and techniques has been used in studies; these vary according to the particular question the study aims to answer and the orientation of the researcher.

Systematic research reviews

Reviewing the literature to ascertain the current state of knowledge and level and type of research that has previously been undertaken in any given field is a traditional precursor to undertaking any study. Over recent years, there has been growing interest in the use of more systematic techniques of research synthesis. Traditional reviews, conducted by a single researcher describing and giving a critical overview of previously conducted research, have a number of problems. They are inherently open to bias since the reviewer can be highly selective in both the studies chosen for the review and the level of detail and critical evaluation presented. In addition, one of the most problematic areas of reviewing the literature lies in the area of determining what actions should be taken as a result of a collective body of evidence from the totality of studies conducted. This is particularly the case when decisions are being made about the effectiveness of treatments or new interventions. For this reason, methods of systematic review have been developed. Systematic reviews are also heralded as a means of getting research

findings into practice, since the findings of larger volumes of studies can be examined and recommendations made for practitioners.

Integrative review and meta-analysis techniques use statistical procedures to combine the findings of a collective body of studies. These techniques allow judgements over the quality and strength of the findings of individual studies to be weighted, and then these weightings can be taken into account for the statistical analysis.[41] Theoretically the results of a carefully conducted meta-analysis are much less open to bias on the part of the reviewer than more traditional methods. However, these techniques are not without their critics.[42] The quality of any systematic review lies in the coverage of the review. What is important is the confidence one has in the retrieval of all studies in a given area. This may mean accessing unpublished studies, since it is known that a large response bias exists towards the publication of studies that show a positive effect of treatment or intervention, rather than a negative one. The latter are much more likely to be rejected or never submitted for publication.

Searching the literature is a difficult and complex process. Online computer searching using databases such as Medline and CINAHL is known to yield very low retrieval rates (some estimates suggest between 30% and 50% of published studies).[43] Retrieval is much improved by supplementing searching with hand-searching journals and retrieving studies referenced by other authors. The second area of difficulty lies in the judgements made about studies during analysis. Determining effect, size, and quality of studies is difficult, and often inadequately reported by the original authors.

These techniques yield the most useful data when a large volume of studies focused on intervention and/or outcomes exists. Since a dearth of research exists in cancer nursing, systematic reviewing can be problematic. However, it was used by Smith *et al.* to examine American oncology nursing research.[44] Of 428 research studies retrieved over a 10-year publication period, 90% were purely descriptive and therefore not amenable to meta-analysis techniques. Forty-two intervention studies were, however, of sufficient quality to examine this way. Using the meta-analytic technique, cancer nursing interventions were found overall to be significantly effective, with membership of the intervention group improving success by 22%.

Richardson *et al.* reviewed the evidence base to support cancer nursing between 1980 and 2000, using systematic review techniques, and identified 446 research papers – an enormous and growing body of research.[45] Noted is the lack of clear focus and utility of much of the work to the kinds of decisions needed to guide practice in cancer nursing. Little research activity has been focused on the development and testing of interventions to assist with the problems and needs of people affected by cancer.

Studies that develop and test research instruments and measures, or research approaches

In order for cancer nursing research to develop, further methodological work is essential to develop measures for use in studies focused on patients and/or carer outcomes, and detailed work needs to be undertaken on research approaches and designs most suited to answering the kinds of questions nurses are asking. Traditionally, nursing has looked to the methods employed by related disciplines such as biomedicine, psychology, and sociology. In some instances nurses have developed research instruments specifically for use in nursing studies; in others, research designs and instruments have been taken from other established health disciplines and applied to nursing situations.

Quality of life is one area in which cancer nurses have been active, and a number of quality-of-life measures have been developed by nurses; for example, Mast has reviewed quality-of-life research in cancer nursing and has found work using unidimensional scales where quality of life is measured as a single dimension, studies that treat it as a multidimensional entity in which these are measured within a single instrument, and studies that have used multiple separate scales.[46] More recent studies show a trend towards the development and use of scales specific to different cancers, and towards evaluating the outcomes of nursing interventions.

Quality-of-life research in cancer is a large and growing field; in the main, nursing research has had little impact to date on this field more generally, and measures developed by nurses have in most instances not been used more widely by researchers from other disciplines. This raises the question of whether there is a need for measures developed specifically for nursing research, since it will not be possible directly to compare results obtained from these with studies conducted by other health professionals who use standard measures. One frustration for nursing is, however, the lack of research instruments available to assess outcomes in areas of nursing interest, since these frequently combine physical, functional, and psychological aspects of any given problem. This has led nurses to seek alternative approaches to acquire information and insight into the lives of people who are ill, through the use of qualitative research methods.[47]

Development of detailed understanding of cancer-related problems or client needs

Since one of the most important areas of focus for nursing research is the problems and needs of people with cancer, imposed either by the disease itself or as a result of treatment, nursing research in cancer care has concentrated on a whole variety of different problems. Pain management and fatigue are two prominent examples. There is now a growing body of research into the problem of fatigue in cancer, which is led by nurses. Studies have been undertaken to develop measures and assessment tools for the problem,[48] as has work to define and understand the term in the context of cancer. Other studies, such as those by Richardson and Ream,[48] Glaus,[49] and Krishnasamy[50] have used different approaches to gather data to give insight into the symptom and its pattern during chemotherapy or in advanced disease, and have compared fatigue in patients with cancer with reports of fatigue amongst healthy individuals, as well as comparing the reports of people with cancer with the assessments of professionals. Furthermore, ongoing work is under way to explore and evaluate possible interventions to alleviate the problem, and there also exist international collaborations for dissemination of information discovered from fatigue studies and from multicentre studies.[51]

Evaluation of new or existing practices aimed at enhancing care or alleviating problems

Cancer nursing research is increasingly being used to evaluate nursing interventions, so that there is an emerging evidence base for the specialty, although in reality this is new and emergent. Much of the research into cancer nursing to date has been descriptive and focused on delineating patient problems and/or describing nursing approaches and inadequacies in relation to these. There are, however, a growing number of examples where knowledge is being generated about practice.

An example of this is our work on breathlessness in lung cancer.[52,53] We set out to develop and evaluate a nursing approach to the management of breathlessness in lung cancer using the research process as a vehicle for this. We reviewed the literature to examine the problem of breathlessness, and to identify strategies used in other fields, such as chronic pulmonary disease rehabilitation, to identify possible intervention approaches. We then conducted a pilot study, which recorded the experiences of patients with breathlessness and randomly allocated a small group of consenting patients either to attend a nursing clinic where a therapeutic approach to breathlessness was offered, or to be followed up as a control group. This pilot study allowed the intervention strategy to be developed and articulated, as well as producing some useful evaluation data indicating that this approach was promising. The approach has now been evaluated more formally in a multicentre randomised controlled trial in six centres around the UK.[53] The research process offers a useful framework for the development and evaluation of cancer nursing as a therapeutic endeavour.

Detailed evaluation of existing and new services in cancer care

This area of research encompasses a wide range of studies; for example, work evaluating nursing roles and practices. Wilkinson's work on factors that influence how nurses communicate with cancer patients reflects a body of earlier work on the quality of care delivered to patients revealed through a number of studies of nurses' communication skills.[54]

An area that is currently very important is studies evaluating new, extended roles for nursing in the cancer arena. McCorkle et al. used a randomised clinical trial of home nursing for lung cancer patients, in which 166 patients were assigned to either a specialist cancer home care nurse, care from regular home care nurses, or an office-based care group.[55] Patients receiving home care were shown to have less symptom distress and greater independence than the office care group. More recently Moore et al. demonstrated the value of nurse-led follow-up for people with lung cancer compared with conventional medically led care.[22] People who experienced nurse-led care were highly satisfied and had equivalent health outcomes compared with individuals who had experienced conventional, medically led care. They were also more likely to die at home rather than in a hospice. A range of studies have been completed into the effectiveness of nurse-managed care in a variety of situations, such as monitoring patients undergoing radiotherapy, and follow-up for patients with lung and breast cancer. In these studies, nurse-managed care has been compared with conventional medical care for outcomes such as quality of life, symptom management, and cost. Overall, nurse-led care in cancer compares well with other models of care on a range of indicators such as patient satisfaction, quality of life, and service costs.[56]

Methodological issues for nursing research in cancer care

In the process of developing research into cancer care, as with many other areas of health care, nurses have found themselves questioning the methodological traditions on which prevailing research has been based. Traditional research methods, exemplified by the randomised controlled trial employed in much of health care research, have been felt to be too narrow and limiting to answer the kinds of questions nurses have wanted to pose about the nature of the experience of having cancer, or the needs of patients, or for evaluating nursing interventions. As in the wider field of social sciences, this has led to a schism and the emergence of opposing methodological camps, according to the research methods felt to be most valid. This is seen at its most extreme in the 'quantitative versus qualitative methods debate'. Unfortunately, the model of measurement, prediction, and causal inference upon which quantitative and experimental research relies does not easily fit a world where health, illness, recovery, and participation in care are frequently the variables one is attempting to measure. Methods are most commonly represented by experimental research, where causal relationships between variables are examined and controlled, and observations are quantified and analysed to determine statistical probabilities and the certainty of a particular outcome.

Over the past 20 years, important contributions to cancer care have been made by nurses using methods derived from both schools. Bryman is critical of the 'quantitative versus qualitative methods debate', since the literature has until recently concentrated on the distinct and incompatible nature of these two methodologies, rather than on the value of particular research techniques in answering specific questions.[57] According to Bryman, the discussions also confuse the epistemological (issues relating to the philosophical principles on which research methods are based) and technical aspects of data collection and analysis. The epistemological arguments have tended to exaggerate the differences between the method types, rather than suggest where each may be relevant.

These issues have been played out in cancer research, with quantitative methods being predominant in medical research with clinical trials, and in psychological research using standardised measures of anxiety, depression, and quality of life. The distinction between the 'hard' science pursued by medical clinicians and the 'soft' science pursued by nurses has exaggerated further the idea of methodological encampments occupied by distinct professional groups, and frequently issues of power, status, and funding are played out in the debate.

Many researchers are now trying to move beyond such polarised views of research by encouraging greater eclecticism in methods, and greater fluidity and flexibility in methods adopted for a given study, which should be determined by the specific question being pursued and the methods most suited to answering it.[58] It is also increasingly

recognised that qualitative methods encompass a wide range of particular research methods, each with its own tradition and philosophical origins. So studies derived from ethnographic, phenomenological, or ethnomethodological schools will be quite different in approach, even though they may all use qualitative methods. This means that researchers need to be quite clear about the particular approach they are using in any given study.

Qualitative methods have been championed to a large extent by nurses, who have been attracted to the use of material gained through the use of in-depth, semi-structured interview techniques to gain deeper insight into the experiences and needs of cancer sufferers. These methods provide insightful and moving accounts of what it is like to receive a diagnosis of cancer and to undergo cancer treatment. However, the notion that such methods offer a superior means by which to access the 'true' meaning of experience of cancer, and that researchers can access this in some way through post hoc analysis of interview data, is an unlikely one. Bailey *et al.* have systematically reviewed the contribution of qualitative nursing research to palliative care, offering a critique of the quality of published studies by nurses in this field.[59] The review reveals a substantial body of work undertaken, but work that is of variable quality and value in terms of the extent to which it contributes to new thinking or to theoretical ideas about the practice of palliative care.

Critical for nursing research in cancer care is that rigorous methods are utilised to pursue questions relevant to the experience of patients with cancer and their carers, and to the practice of nursing.[60] Nurses need to be confident in conducting such studies, and in being members of, and taking on leadership roles in, multidisciplinary research teams. The research agendas in health care have in the past been heavily dominated by basic scientists and medical clinicians. Increasingly, these agendas are changing so that they are directed to questions surrounding effective health care and the needs of individuals and client groups. Nursing has an important and central role to play in determining the direction such research agendas take, and in conducting the research generated as a result. Cancer patients and their families and carers also have a vital role in this process; nurses could also play a significant role in making this possible for them because of their close and intimate role in their care.

Nursing research and practice development

Recently, practice development has been adopted as a goal for researchers,[61] to encourage researchers in nursing to act responsively towards the needs of practising nurses, so that they use research to develop their practice and effectiveness. The features of practice development research using this approach are:

- consensus with consumers of research over questions to be asked and the design of studies aiming to answer these
- collaborative inquiry (with both nurses as clinicians, and patients and carers as consumers as partners in all stages of the research process)
- radical deconstruction and reconstruction of health care situations and problems for consumers of services. During this process all the features of the problems and the context in which these arise and are treated and cared for, are taken apart. All elements are examined for their ability to help or hinder healing, adjustment or alleviation, alternative approaches to the problem developed, and the environments in which such problems are managed or adapted
- creative use of methods of dissemination, such as practice reviews, and practitioner as partner researcher in multicentre studies.

Cancer care research and the future

Throughout this book, there has developed an extended critique of current approaches to the management and care of people with cancer, and an examination of the contribution cancer nurses can make to the environment of care and the nature of care delivered. There are numerous opportunities for nurses to change the culture of care for cancer and to play a central role in any reformulated system that may emerge. Central to

such change and development is research, which can act as a powerful force to initiate change, and to offer evaluations of existing and new systems of care. For this to happen, however, nurses need to become much more effective users of research, and to become recognised as expert researchers themselves. For it is research that generates the knowledge on which all systems of care rest.

The prevailing knowledge base is derived from information generated from clinical trials and the biomedical tradition. Currently, there is a dearth of high-quality nursing research focused on intervention, or new and different models of care, and of research with a true consumer focus. While this situation is improving, cancer nurses need to be much more proactive. Important agenda-setting work has been undertaken in cancer nursing research. This has been to some extent overtaken by the multidisciplinary health services research agenda. Nurses cannot afford to remain outside this, but need to seek positions of power and leadership within it. Only then will there be a flow of funding to support programmes of nurse-led research. What is needed now is for the nursing research agenda in cancer to be placed centre stage, and for it to be seen as aimed at radical change, so that the potential for nursing research to change the agenda for cancer care in general can be realised.

References

1. Department of Health. (2000). *The NHS Cancer Plan: A Plan for Investment, a Plan for Reform*. London: Department of Health.
2. National Cancer Research Institute. (2002). *Strategic Analysis: An Overview of Cancer Research in the UK Directly Funded by the NCRI Partner Organsiations*. London: National Cancer Research Institute.
3. National Institute for Clinical Excellence. (2004). *Service Guidance on Improving Supportive and Palliative Care for Adults with Cancer*. London: National Institute for Clinical Excellence. http://guidance.nice.org.uk/csgsp (accessed 9 August 2007).
4. National Cancer Research Institute. (2004). *Supportive and Palliative Care Research in the UK: Report of the NCRI Strategic Planning Group on Supportive and Palliative Care*. London: National Cancer Research Institute.
5. Tattersall M.L. and Jones R.J. (1992). Issues in informed consent. In Williams C.J. (ed.) *Introducing New Treatments for Cancer*. Chichester: John Wiley.

6. Stenning S. (1992). 'The Uncertainty Principle': selection of patients for clinical trials. In Williams C.J. (ed.) *Introducing New Treatments for Cancer.* Chichester: John Wiley.

7. Pocock S.J. (1983). *Clinical Trials: A Practical Approach.* Chichester: John Wiley.

8. Clark A. and Fallowfield L. (1986). Quality of life measurement in patients with malignant disease: a review. *Journal of the Royal Society of Medicine* **79**, 165–169.

9. Cella D.F. (1994). Quality of life: concepts and definitions. *Journal of Pain and Symptom Management* **9**, 186–192.

10. Sprangers M.A.G. (2002). Quality of life assessment in oncology. *Acta Oncologica* **41**, 229–237.

11. Fallowfield L. (1990). *Quality of Life: The Rising Measurement in Health Care.* London: Souvenir Press.

12. Polsky D., Mandlebatt J.S., Weeks J.C. *et al.* (2003). Economic evaluation of breast cancer treatment: considering the value of patient choice. *Journal of Clinical Oncology* **21**, 1139–1146.

13. Langeveld N., Stam H., Grootenhuis M. and Last B. (2002). Quality of life in young adult survivors of childhood cancers. *Supportive Care in Cancer* **10**, 579–600.

14. Hopwood P. (1992). Progress, problems and priorities in quality of life research. *European Journal of Cancer* **28A**, 1748–1752.

15. Cox K. (2003). Assessing quality of life of patients in phase I and II anti-cancer drug trials: interviews versus questionnaires. *Social Science and Medicine* **56**, 921–934.

16. Plant H., Bredin M., Krishnasamy M. and Corner J. (2000). Working with resistance, tension and objectivity: conducting a randomized controlled trial of a nursing intervention for breathlessness. *Journal of Research in Nursing* **5**, 426–434.

17. Wright P.A., Selby P.J., Gillibrand A. *et al.* (2003). Feasibility and compliance of automated measurement of quality of life in oncology practice. *Journal of Clinical Oncology* **21**, 374–382.

18. Benner P. (1985). Quality of life: a phenomenological perspective on explanation, prediction and understanding in nursing science. *Advances in Nursing Science* **8**, 1–14.

19. Faithfull S. (1995). 'Just grin and bear it and hope that it will go away': coping with urinary symptoms from pelvic radiotherapy. *European Journal of Cancer Care* **4**, 158–165.

20. Aaronson N.K., Ahmedzai S., Bergman B. *et al.* (1993). The EORTC QLQ-C30: a quality of life instrument for use in international clinical trials in oncology. *Journal of the National Cancer Institute* **85**, 365–376.

21. Van der Scheuren E., Kesteloot K. and Cleemput I. (2000). Federation of European Cancer Societies Full Report. Economic evaluation of cancer care: questions and answers on how to alleviate conflicts between rising needs and expectations and tightening budgets. *European Journal of Cancer* **35**, 13–36.

22. Moore S., Corner J., Haviland J. *et al.* (2002). Nurse led follow up and conventional medical follow up in management of patients with lung cancer: randomized trial. *British Medical Journal* **325**, 1145–1147.

23. World Medical Association. (1964). *Declaration of Helsinki: Recommendations Guiding Medical Doctors in Biomedical Research Involving Human Subjects.* Helsinki: World Medical Association.

24. Human Rights Act 1998. www.hmso.gov.uk/acts/acts 1998/ (accessed 9 August 2007).

25. Woods K. (2004). Editorial. Implementing the European Clinical Trials Directive. *Bitish Medical Journal* **328**, 240–241.

26. Smith L. (1992). Ethical issues in interviewing. *Journal of Advanced Nursing* **17**, 98–103.

27. Fontenela M. and Rycroft M.J. (2006). Research governance and ethics: a resource for novice researchers. *Nursing Standard* **20**, 41–46.

28. Royal College of Nursing. (2004). *Research Ethics: Guidance for Nurses Involved in Research or any Investigative Project Involving Human Subjects.* London: Royal College of Nursing.

29. Thornton H. (1992). Breast cancer trials: a patient's viewpoint. *Lancet* **339**, 44–45.

30. Beaver K., Luker K.A., Owens R.G., Leinster S.J. and Bejner L. (1996). Treatment decision making in women newly diagnosed with breast cancer. *Cancer Nursing* **19**, 8–19.

31. Cox K. (2000). Enhancing trial management: recommendations from a qualitative study of trial patients experiences. *Psych-oncology* **9**, 314–322.

32. Hanley J., Bradburn J., Barnes M. *et al.* (2003). *Involving the Public in NHS, Public Health and Social Care Research: Briefing Notes for Researchers,* 2nd edition. Eastleigh: INVOLVE.

33. Department of Health. (2006). *Our Health, Our Say.* London: Department of Health.

34. Oberst M.T. (1978). Priorities in cancer nursing research. *Cancer Nursing* **3**, 281–290.

35. Browne N., Robinson L. and Richardson A. (2002). A Delphi survey on the research priorities of Euopean oncology nurses. *European Journal of Oncology Nursing* **6**, 133–144.

36. Berger A.M., Berry D.L., Christopher K.A. *et al.* (2005). Oncology Nursing Society year 2004 research priorities survey. *Oncology Nursing Forum* **32**, 281–290.

37. Corner J. (1993). Building a framework for nursing research in cancer care. *European Journal of Cancer Care* **2**, 112–116.

38. Payne S. (1993). Constraints for nursing developing a framework for cancer care research. *European Journal of Cancer Care* **2**, 117–120.

39. Ross F., Smith E., Mackenzie A. and Masterson A. (2004). Idenitfying research priorities in nursing and midwifery service delivery and organization: a scoping study. *International Iorunal of Nursing Studies* **41** 547–558

40. Corner J., Wright D., Foster C. *et al.* (2006). *The Macmillan Listening Study: Listening to the Views of People Affected by Cancer about Cancer Research.* London: Macmillan Cancer Support.

41. Cooper H.M. (1984). *The Integrative Research Review.* Beverly Hills, CA: Sage.

42. Eysenck H.J. (1984). Meta-analysis: an abuse of research integration. *Journal of Special Education* **8**, 41–59.

43. Dickerson K., Scherer R. and Le Febvre C. (1995). Identifying relevant studies for systematic reviews. In Chalmers I. and Altman D.G. (eds.) *Systematic Reviews.* London: BMJ Publishing.

44. Smith M.C., Holcombe J.K. and Stullenberger E. (1994). A meta-analysis of intervention effectiveness for symptom management in oncology nursing. *Oncology Nursing Forum* **2**, 1201–1210.

45. Richardson A., Miller M. and Potter H. (2001). Developing, delivering and evaluating nursing services: building the evidence base. *Journal of Research in Nursing* **6**, 726–735.

46. Mast M.E. (1995). Definition and measurement of quality of life in oncology nursing research: review and theoretical implications. *Oncology Nursing Forum* **22**, 957–964.

47. Corner J., Halliday D., Haviland J. *et al.* (2003). Exploring nursing outcomes for patients with advanced cancer following intervention by Macmillan specialist palliative care nurses. *Journal of Advanced Nursing* **41**, 561–574.

48. Richardson A. and Ream E. (1996). The experience of fatigue and other symptoms in patients receiving chemotherapy. *European Journal of Cancer Care* **5(suppl.)**, 24–30.

49. Glaus A. (1996). A qualitative study to explore the concept of fatigue/tiredness in cancer patients and healthy individuals. *European Journal of Cancer Care* **5(suppl.)**, 8–23.

50. Krishnasamy M. (2000). Fatigue in advanced cancer – meaning before measurement. *International Journal of Nursing Studies* **37**, 401–414.

51. Given B., Given C.W., McCorkle R. *et al.* (2002). PIN nd fatigue management. results of a nursing randomized clinical trial. *Oncology Nursing Forum* **29**, 949–956.

52. Corner J., Plant H., Warner L., A'Hern R. and Bailey C. (1996). Non-pharmacological intervention for the management of breathlessness in lung cancer. *Palliative Medicine* **10**, 299–305.

53. Bredin M., Corner J., Krishnasamy M. *et al.* (1999). Multicentre randomized controlled trial of nursing intervention for breathlessness in patients with lung cancer. *British Journal of Medicine* **318**, 901–904.

54. Wilkinson S. (1991). Factors which influence how nurses communicate with cancer. *Journal of Advanced Nursing* **16**, 677–688.

55. McCorkle R., Benoliel J.Q., Donaldson G. *et al.* (1989). A randomised clinical trial of home nursing care for lung cancer patients. *Cancer* **64**, 1375–1382.

56. Corner J. (2003). The role of nurse-led care in cancer management. *The Lancet Oncology* **4**, 631–636.

57. Bryman A. (1988). *Quantity and Quality in Social Research.* London: Routledge.

58. Pope C. and Mays N. (1996). Qualitative methods in health and health services research. In Pope C. and Mays N. (eds) *Qualitative Research in Health Care.* London: BMJ Publishing.

59. Bailey C., Froggat K., Field D. and Krishnasamy M. (2002). The nursing contribution to qualitative research in palliative care 1990–1999: a critical evaluation. *Journal of Advanced Nursing* **40**, 48–60.

60. Krishnasamy M. and Plant H. (1998). Developing nursing research with people. *International Journal of Nursing Studies* **35**, 79–84.

61. Manley K. and McCormack B. (2003). Practice development: purpose, methodology, facilitation and evaluation. *Nursing in Critical Care* **8**, 22–29.

Index